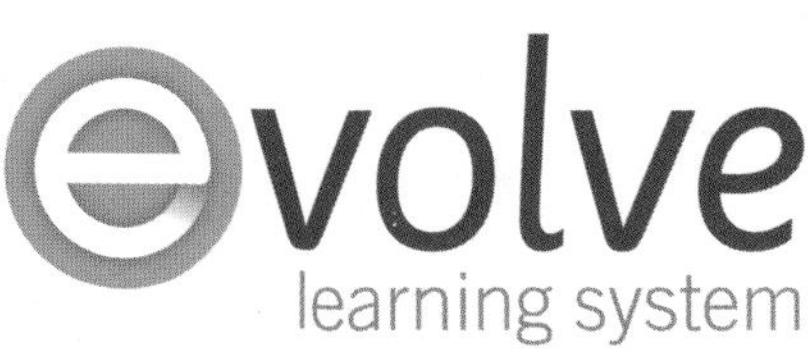

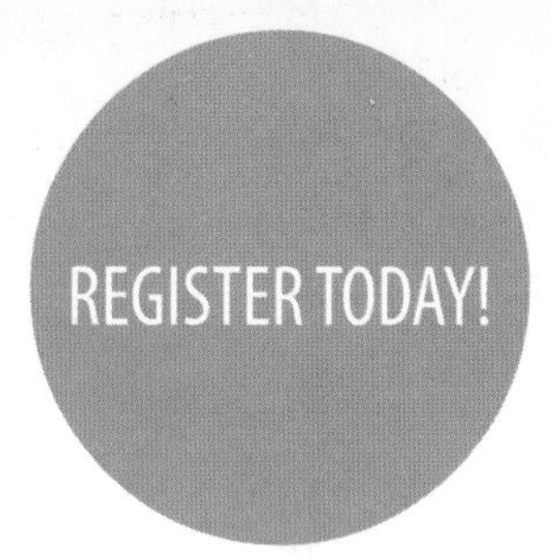

To access your Student Resources, visit:

http://evolve.elsevier.com/Lowdermilk/Maternity

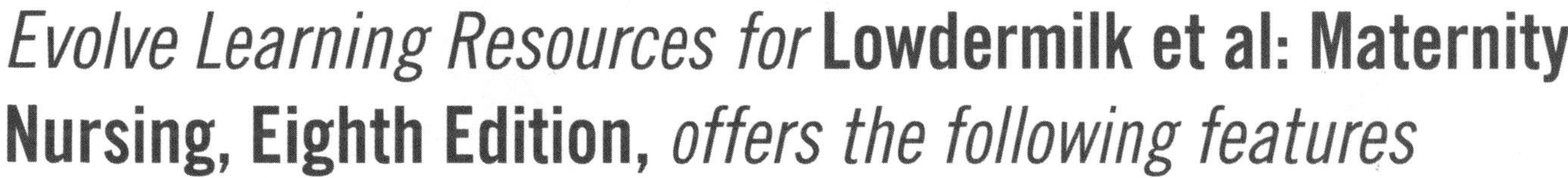

Evolve Learning Resources for **Lowdermilk et al: Maternity Nursing, Eighth Edition,** *offers the following features*

- **Anatomy Reviews**
- **Animations**
- **Answers to Critical Thinking Exercises**
- **Assessment Videos**
- **Audio Glossary**
- **Audio Summaries**
- **Care Plan Constructor**
- **Childbirth Videos**
- **Critical Thinking Exercises**
- **Nursing Skills**
- **Resources**
- **Review Questions**
- **Spanish Guidelines**

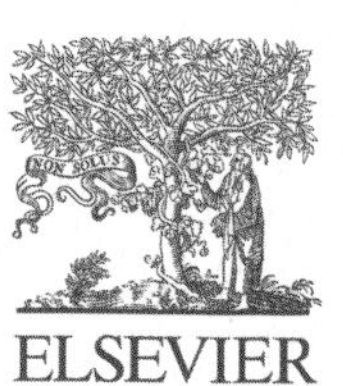

REVISED REPRINT

8th Edition

Maternity Nursing

Deitra Leonard Lowdermilk, RNC, PhD, FAAN
Clinical Professor Emerita, School of Nursing
University of North Carolina at Chapel Hill
Chapel Hill, North Carolina

Shannon E. Perry, RN, CNS, PhD, FAAN
Professor Emerita, School of Nursing
San Francisco State University
San Francisco, California

Kitty Cashion, RN, BC, MSN
Clinical Nurse Specialist
University of Tennessee Health Science Center
College of Medicine
Department of Obstetrics & Gynecology
Division of Maternal-Fetal Medicine
Memphis, Tennessee

MOSBY

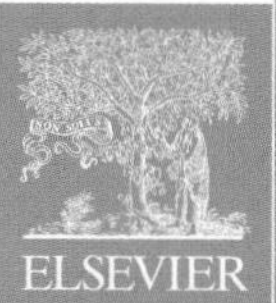

ELSEVIER

Associate Editor
Kathryn Rhodes Alden, EdD, MSN, RN, IBCLC
Clinical Associate Professor, School of Nursing
University of North Carolina at Chapel Hill
Chapel Hill, North Carolina

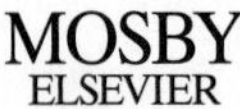

3251 Riverport Lane
Maryland Heights, MO 63043

MATERNITY NURSING, EIGHTH EDITION REVISED REPRINT ISBN: 978-0-323-24191-5
Copyright © 2014, by Mosby, an imprint of Elsevier Inc.
Copyright © 2010, by Mosby, an affiliate of Elsevier Inc.

All rights reserved. No part of this publication may be reproduced or transmitted in any form or by any means, electronic or mechanical, including photocopying, recording, or any information storage and retrieval system, without permission in writing from the publisher. Permissions may be sought directly from Elsevier's Rights Department: phone: (+1) 215-239-3804 (US) or (+44) 1865 843830 (UK); fax: (+44) 1865 853333; e-mail: healthpermissions@elsevier.com. You may also complete your request on-line via the Elsevier website at www.elsevier.com/permissions.

Notice

Knowledge and best practice in this field are constantly changing. As new research and experience broaden our knowledge, changes in practice, treatment, and drug therapy may become necessary or appropriate. Readers are advised to check the most current information provided (i) on procedures featured or (ii) by the manufacturer of each product to be administered, to verify the recommended dose or formula, the method and duration of administration, and contraindications. It is the responsibility of the practitioner, relying on his or her own experience and knowledge of the patient, to make diagnoses, to determine dosages and the best treatment for each individual patient, and to take all appropriate safety precautions. To the fullest extent of the law, neither the Publisher nor the Authors/Editor assume any liability for any injury and/or damage to persons or property arising out of or related to any use of the material contained in this book.

The Publisher

Previous editions copyrighted 2006, 2003, 1999, 1995, 1991, 1987, 1983.
Nursing Diagnoses–Definitions and Classifications 2009-2011 © 2009, 2007, 2005, 2003, 2001, 1998, 1996, 1994 NANDA International. Used by arrangement with Wiley–Blackwell Publishing, a company of John Wiley and Sons, Inc.

ISBN: 978-0-323-24191-5

Managing Editor: Laurie K. Gower
Publishing Services Manager: Deborah L. Vogel
Project manager: Pat Costigan
Design Direction: Maggie Reid

Working together to grow libraries in developing countries

www.elsevier.com | www.bookaid.org | www.sabre.org

ELSEVIER BOOK AID International Sabre Foundation

Printed in the United States of America

Last digit is the print number: 9 8 7 6 5 4 3 2 1

About the Authors

Deitra Leonard Lowdermilk is Clinical Professor Emerita, School of Nursing, University of North Carolina at Chapel Hill. She received her BSN from East Carolina University and her MEd and PhD in Education from UNC CH. She is certified in In-Patient Obstetrics by the National Certification Corporation. She is a Fellow in the American Academy of Nursing. In addition to being a nurse educator for more than 34 years, Dr. Lowdermilk has clinical experience as a public health nurse and as a staff nurse in labor and delivery, postpartum, and newborn units, and has worked in gynecologic surgery and cancer care units.

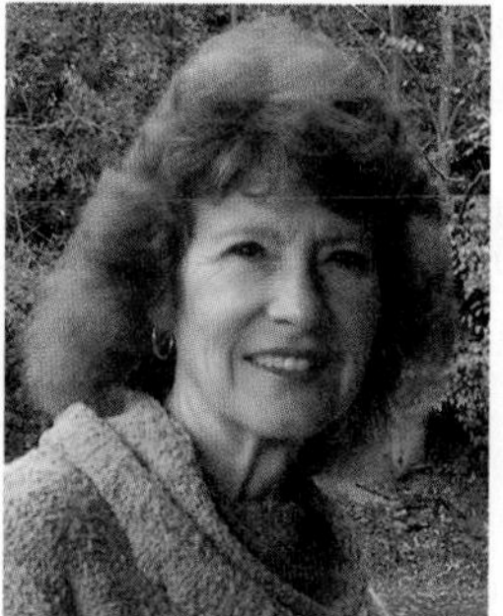

Dr. Lowdermilk has been recognized for her expertise in nursing education. She has repeatedly been selected as Classroom and Clinical Teacher of the Year by graduating seniors. She was a recipient of the Educator of the Year Award from both the District IV Association of Women's Health, Obstetric and Neonatal Nurses (AWHONN) and the North Carolina Nurses Association. She also received the 2005 AWHONN Excellence in Education Award.

She is active in AWHONN, having served as Chair of the North Carolina Section of AWHONN and as chair and member of various committees in AWHONN at the national, district, state, and local levels. She has acted as guest editor for the *Journal of Obstetric, Gynecologic, and Neonatal Nursing* and served on editorial boards for other publications.

Dr. Lowdermilk's most significant contribution to nursing has been to promote excellence in nursing practice and education in women's health through integration of knowledge into practice. In 2005 she received the first Distinguished Alumni Award from East Carolina University School of Nursing for her exemplary contributions to the nursing profession in the area of maternal-child care and the community. She was also Alumna of the Year for East Carolina University in 2005, and was selected as one of the 100 Incredible ECU Women in 2007 for Outstanding Leadership Among Women in the first 100 years of the university's founding.

Shannon E. Perry is Professor Emerita, School of Nursing, San Francisco State University. She received her diploma in nursing from St. Joseph Hospital School of Nursing, Bloomington, Illinois; a Baccalaureate in Nursing from Marquette University; an MSN from the University of Colorado Medical Center, Denver; and a PhD in Educational Psychology from Arizona State University. She completed a 2-year postdoctoral fellowship in perinatal nursing at the University of California, San Francisco, as a Robert Wood Johnson Clinical Nurse Scholar.

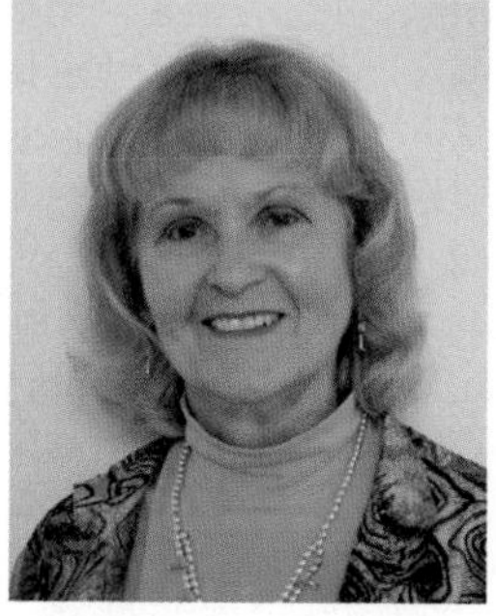

Dr. Perry has had clinical experience as a staff nurse, head nurse, and supervisor in surgical nursing, obstetrics, pediatrics, gynecology, and neonatal nursing. She has served as expert witness and legal consultant. She has taught in schools of nursing in several states and was Interim Director and Director of the School of Nursing and Director of a Child and Adolescent Development Baccalaureate Program at SFSU. She was Marquette University College of Nursing Alumna of the Year in 1999, the University of Colorado School of Nursing Distinguished Alumna of the Year in 2000, and received the San Francisco State University Alumni Association Emeritus Faculty Award in 2005.

She is a Fellow in the American Academy of Nursing, a nursing consultant to the International Education Research Foundation, and co-chair of INESA, the International Nursing, Education, Services, and Accreditation Task Force.

Dr. Perry's experience in international nursing includes teaching international nursing courses in the United Kingdom, Ireland, Italy, Thailand, Ghana, and China and participating in health missions in Ghana, Kenya, and Honduras. For her "exemplary contributions to nursing, public service, and selfless commitment and passion in shaping the future of international health," she received the President's Award from the Global Caring Nurses Foundation, Inc., in 2008.

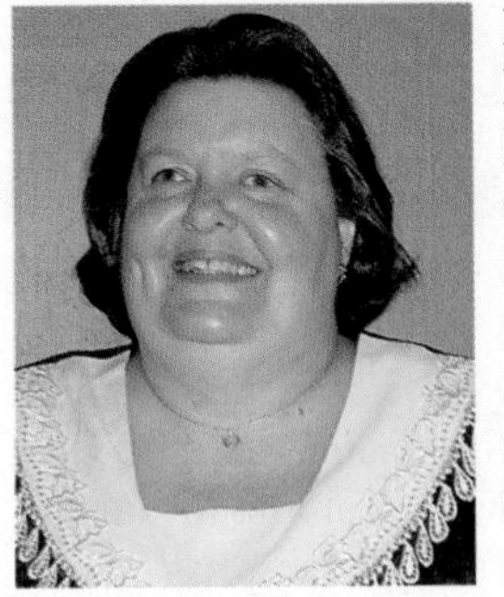

Kitty Cashion is a Clinical Nurse Specialist in the Maternal-Fetal Medicine Division at The University of Tennessee Health Science Center in Memphis, College of Medicine, Department of Obstetrics and Gynecology. She received her BSN from the University of Tennessee College of Nursing in Memphis and her MSN in Parent-Child Nursing from Vanderbilt University School of Nursing in Nashville, Tennessee. Ms. Cashion is certified as a High Risk Perinatal Nurse through the American Nurses Credentialing Center (ANCC).

Ms. Cashion's job responsibilities at the University of Tennessee include providing education regarding low and high risk obstetrics to staff nurses in West Tennessee community hospitals. In addition, she works part-time as a staff nurse in Labor and Delivery at The Regional Medical Center at Memphis (The MED). For more than 15 years, Ms. Cashion has taught Labor and Delivery clinical for students at Northwest Mississippi Community College in Senatobia, Mississippi, and Union University in Germantown, Tennessee.

Ms. Cashion has been an active AWHONN member, holding office at both the local and state levels. She has also served as an officer and board member of the Tennessee Perinatal Association and as an active volunteer for the Tennessee Chapter of the March of Dimes Birth Defects Foundation.

Ms. Cashion has contributed many chapters to maternity nursing textbooks over the years. She also co-authored a series of Virtual Clinical Excursions workbooks to accompany six obstetric nursing textbooks published by Elsevier. More recently, she served as an Associate Editor for *Maternity Nursing,* 7th edition and as one of the editors of *Clinical Companion for Maternity & Women's Health Care,* 9th edition.

ABOUT THE ASSOCIATE EDITOR

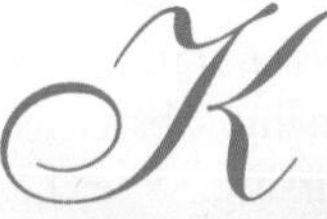

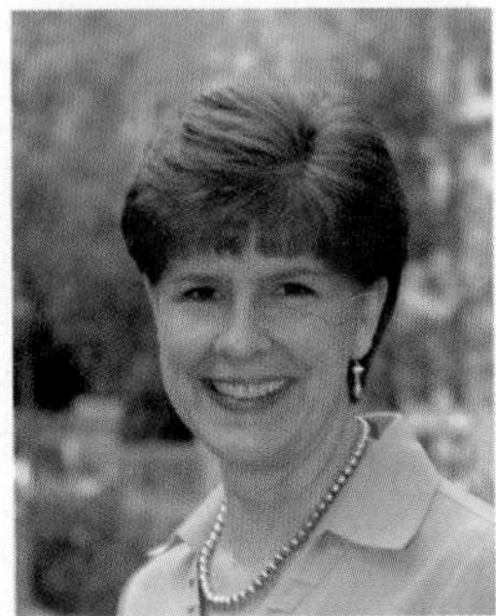

Kathryn Rhodes Alden is Clinical Associate Professor, University of North Carolina at Chapel Hill School of Nursing. She received a BSN from the University of North Carolina at Charlotte, an MSN from the University of North Carolina at Chapel Hill, and a doctorate in adult education from North Carolina State University.

Dr. Alden has had clinical experience as a staff nurse in pediatrics and neonatal intensive care. She has worked in administrative and quality improvement roles in nursing. She has taught in the baccalaureate nursing program at the University of North Carolina at Charlotte. For the past 21 years, Dr. Alden has served on the faculty at the University of North Carolina at Chapel Hill School of Nursing, where she coordinates the maternal-newborn nursing course in the undergraduate program and serves as lead academic counselor for the nursing school. She has been recognized and awarded for her clinical teaching expertise. Dr. Alden has been instrumental in the use of human patient simulation at UNC Chapel Hill; she has written numerous simulation scenarios and recently developed two obstetrical simulation cases for Elsevier. She co-authored a chapter on "Enhancing Patient Safety in Nursing Education through Patient Simulation" in *Patient Safety and Quality: An Evidence-Based Handbook for Nursing,* published by the Agency for Healthcare Research and Quality (AHRQ).

Dr. Alden is an international board certified lactation consultant and works part-time as a lactation consultant for Rex Healthcare in Raleigh, North Carolina. She teaches prenatal breastfeeding classes to expectant parents and has provided continuing education programs on breastfeeding throughout the state of North Carolina.

She has authored a variety of chapters in maternity texts for Elsevier on endocrine and metabolic disorders of pregnancy; newborn nutrition, assessment, and nursing care; and postpartum care. Her research interests focus on predictors of academic success and retention in baccalaureate nursing students.

Contributors

Pat Mahaffee Gingrich, RNC, MSN, WHNP
Clinical Assistant Professor, School of Nursing
University of North Carolina at Chapel Hill
Chapel Hill, North Carolina

Edward L. Lowdermilk, BS, RPh
Clinical Pharmacist
Piedmont Health Services
Siler City, North Carolina

Diana L. McCarty, RNC, MSN
Clinical Assistant Professor, School of Nursing
University of North Carolina at Chapel Hill
Chapel Hill, North Carolina

INSTRUCTOR AND STUDENT ANCILLARIES

Audience Response Questions, Curriculum Guides, PowerPoint Slides, Review Questions, Test Bank
Barbara Pascoe, RN, BA, MA
Director, The Family Place
Concord Hospital
Concord, New Hampshire

Instructor's Manual, Study Guide
Julie White, RN, MSN
Clinical Instructor, Graduate Entry Program
College of Nursing, Maternal/Child Department
University of Illinois at Chicago
Chicago, Illinois

Reviewers

Martha Barry, RN, MS, CNM
Adjunct Clinical Instructor
University of Illinois at Chicago
Chicago, Illinois

Beverly Bowers, PhD, RN, CNS
Assistant Professor, College of Nursing
University of Oklahoma Health Sciences Center
Oklahoma City, Oklahoma

Johnett Benson Soros, MSN, RN, NP
Assistant Professor, College of Nursing
Kent State University
Ashtabula, Ohio

Charlotte Stephenson, RN, DSN, CLNC
Clinical Professor, College of Nursing
Texas Woman's University
Houston, Texas

Deborah A. Terrell, PhD, RN, CFNP
Associate Professor
Harry S Truman College
Chicago, Illinois

Preface

This eighth edition of *Maternity Nursing* focuses on the care of women during their reproductive years. Childbearing issues and concerns, including neonatal care, are the primary focus; concerns of the family in the childbearing cycle and the promotion of wellness and the management of common health problems of women are also addressed. Contemporary issues and care arising in the 21st century are included.

The specialty of maternity and women's health nursing offers both challenges and opportunities. Nurses are challenged to assimilate knowledge and develop the technical and critical thinking skills needed to apply that knowledge to practice. Each woman and family present a new challenge because their individual needs must be identified and met. However, the opportunities are sufficiently extraordinary to make this one of the most fulfilling specialties of nursing practice.

The goal of nursing education is to prepare today's student to meet the challenges of tomorrow. This preparation must extend beyond the mastery of facts and skills. Nurses must be able to combine competence with caring, critical thinking, and clinical decision making. They must address both the physiologic and the psychosocial needs of patients. They must look beyond the condition and see the woman as an individual with distinctive needs but also in the context of her family, her culture, and her community. Above all, nurses must strive to improve nursing practice on the basis of evidence.

In a time of shrinking financial and personnel resources for health care, nurses can use evidence-based practice to produce measurable outcomes that validate their unique role in the health care delivery system.

Maternity Nursing was developed to provide students with guidance for acquiring the knowledge and skills they need to become competent, critically thinking, caring nurses able to make clinical decisions based on evidence. This edition has been revised and refined in response to comments and suggestions from educators, clinicians, and students. It includes the most accurate, current, and clinically relevant information available. Many exciting changes are noted throughout the book. However, we have retained the underlying philosophy that has been the strength of the previous editions: Pregnancy and childbirth and developmental changes in a woman's life are natural processes. We have also retained a strong integrated focus on the family and evidence-based practice.

Approach

Professional nursing practice continues to evolve and adapt to society's changing health priorities. The delivery system offers opportunities for nurses to alter the practice of maternity and women's health nursing and to improve the way care is given. Consumers of maternity and women's health care vary in age, ethnicity, culture, language, social status, marital status, and sexual preference. They seek care from obstetricians, gynecologists, family practice physicians, nurse-midwives, nurse practitioners, and other health care providers in a variety of health care settings, including the home. Increasingly, many are self-treating, using a variety of alternative and complementary therapies.

Nursing education must reflect these changes. Clinical education must be planned to offer students a variety of maternity and women's health care experiences in settings that include hospitals and birth centers, homes, clinics and private physicians' offices, shelters for the homeless or women in need of protection, and other community-based settings. The changing needs of nursing students also must be addressed. Today's nursing students are challenged to learn more than ever before and often in less time than their predecessors. Students are diverse. They may be high school graduates, college students, or older adults with families. They may be men or women. They may have college degrees in other fields and be interested in changing to a nursing career through a traditional or accelerated nursing curriculum, or they may pursue education online. They may represent various cultures; English may not be their primary language.

This eighth edition of *Maternity Nursing* is designed to meet the learning needs of women and their families during their childbearing years and students in all types of nursing programs. This edition presents tighter, focused content in a clearly written and easily readable manner while retaining the comprehensiveness of previous editions.

To ensure a logical and consistent presentation of material, *Care Management* has been used again as an organizing framework for discussion in the nursing care chapters. This approach incorporates the nursing process and collaborative care approach to demonstrate how nurses work with other health care providers to give the most comprehensive care to women, newborns, and their families. Assessment, nursing diagnoses, expected outcomes, nursing interventions, and evaluation of care are highlighted throughout the chapters for emphasis. Nursing Care Plans,

Nursing Process boxes, and Critical Thinking/Clinical Decision Making boxes reinforce the problem-solving approach to patient care. In chapters that focus on complications of childbearing and reproductive conditions, medical care is often the priority for patient care. Therefore in these discussions the specific condition is discussed first, followed by discussion of medical and nursing management, including home care.

Health care today emphasizes *wellness.* This focus is an integral part of our philosophy. Likewise, the developmental changes that a woman experiences throughout her life are considered natural and normal. In women's health care the goal is promotion of wellness for the woman through knowledge of her body and its normal functions throughout her reproductive years. Health care also helps her develop an awareness of conditions that require professional intervention. The unit on women's health care emphasizes the wellness aspect of care. This unit has been placed before the units on pregnancy because many of the aspects of assessment and care can be applied to later chapters. Pregnancy and childbirth are also part of a natural developmental process. We believe that students need to thoroughly understand and recognize the normal processes before they can identify complications and comprehend their implications for care. Therefore we present the entire normal childbearing cycle before discussing potential complications.

Patient instruction for self-management is an essential component of nursing care for women and newborns. In recognition of integrative health care models that provide both traditional and nontraditional health care and in seeking to provide options for women that encourage them to take more responsibility for their health, we have integrated and highlighted content on alternative and complementary therapies; an icon (🌿) is placed in the margin to call attention to these therapies. The chapter on women's health promotion and screening emphasizes teaching for self-care to promote wellness and encourage preventive care. The chapter on assessment and care of the newborn and family includes teaching for new parents and infants at home. Special boxed features highlight teaching guidelines and patient instructions for self-management throughout the text. Information in these boxes can be used in inpatient, outpatient, and home care settings. To implement *preventive care,* perinatal and women's health nurses must be able to recognize signs and symptoms of emergent problems. Throughout the discussion of assessment and care, we alert the nurse to signs of potential problems and provide boxed information highlighting warning signs and emergency situations. Safety alerts are included to prepare the nurse for unexpected occurrences.

Today's perinatal and women's health nurses will encounter women from diverse backgrounds. The first chapter includes a discussion of cultural implications and focuses on specific customs related to childbearing and women's health. This chapter also stresses the importance of assessing both the nurse's and the patient's cultural beliefs. *Cultural considerations* are integrated throughout the text to emphasize the wide range of ethnic diversity and its effects on maternity and women's health. Boxes throughout the text highlight cultural aspects of care. The chapter also includes a discussion of care in the community and home that prepares the student to provide maternity and women's health care in a variety of settings. *Community Activity boxes* are included in the nursing care chapters to emphasize that care can take place wherever the woman and her family are located.

To truly meet the specific needs of each woman, the nurse must include family members and significant others in the plan of care. The nurse is often the family's primary advocate. Consideration of the family is integrated throughout the chapters on pregnancy, labor and birth, postpartum, and newborn care. Issues concerning grandparents, siblings, and different family constellations are addressed.

Evidence-based practice is an integral part of nursing education and practice. Evidence-based practice is incorporated by including Evidence-Based Practice boxes in each chapter and placing an icon (❋) next to content for which there is research evidence of its effectiveness. Students and practicing nurses will be challenged to think critically as they seek to improve patient outcomes by questioning traditional nursing practices that have no scientific basis. Maternity and women's health nurses confront ethical and legal challenges daily and increasingly will face situations involving genetic issues. Nurses must develop a reflective stance that assesses the new reproductive and women's health technologies and policies in light of their potential to influence human well-being. Information on legal tips and ethical considerations is integrated throughout the text to emphasize these issues as they relate to maternal and women's health nursing. Content on genetics and the nurse's role has been updated and expanded.

Features

This eighth edition features a contemporary design and spacious presentation. Students will find that the logical, easy-to-follow headings and attractive full-color design highlight important content and increase visual appeal. Hundreds of color photographs, many of them new, and drawings throughout the text illustrate important concepts and techniques to further enhance comprehension.

Each chapter includes a list of *Key Terms and Definitions* that alerts students to new vocabulary; these terms are then boldfaced within the chapter. *Learning Objectives* focus students' attention on the important content to be mastered. *Web Resources* that can be found on the companion website are listed at the beginning of each chapter to provide the student with additional information. Each chapter ends with *Key Points,* which summarize important content. *References* have been updated significantly, with most citations being less than 5 years old and all chapters including citations within 1 year of publication. The following are more of the outstanding features:

- *Care Management* is the organizing framework used consistently to discuss nursing care. The five steps of the nursing process are incorporated into this framework.
- *Nursing Care Plans and Nursing Process boxes* are included to help students apply the nursing process in the clinical setting. The Nursing Care Plans and Nursing Process boxes use only NANDA-approved nursing diagnoses, describe expected outcomes for patient care, provide rationales for interventions, and include evaluation of care.
- *Procedure* boxes are included to provide students with examples of various approaches to the implementation of care.
- *Patient Instructions for Self-Management* boxes emphasize guidelines for the patient to practice self-management and provide information to help students transfer learning from the hospital to the home setting.
- *Emergency* boxes alert students to the signs and symptoms of various emergency situations and provide interventions for immediate implementation.
- *Nursing Alerts* highlight critical information for the student.
- *Evidence-Based Practice* is incorporated throughout in **NEW** boxes that integrate findings from studies on selected clinical practices and changing practice. In addition, research findings from various sources–as well as those summarized in the *Cochrane Pregnancy and Childbirth Database*–that confirm effective practices or identify practices that have unknown, ineffective, or harmful effects, are integrated throughout the text and identified by this icon in the margin. ( )
- *Signs of Potential Complications* are included in chapters that cover uncomplicated pregnancy and childbirth. Although childbearing is a normal process, nurses need to know that complications may occur.
- *Alternative and Complementary Therapies* are discussed for many women's health and pregnancy-related problems and are identified in the text by this icon in the margin. ( )
- *Cultural Considerations* boxes describe beliefs and practices about pregnancy, childbirth, parenting, and women's health concerns and the importance of understanding cultural variations when providing care.
- *Legal Tips* and *Ethical Considerations* are integrated throughout to provide students with relevant information to deal with these important areas in the context of maternity and women's health nursing.
- *Medication Guide* boxes include key information about medications used in maternity and women's health care, including their indications, adverse effects, and nursing considerations.
- *Critical Thinking/Clinical Decision Making Exercises* are integrated into the chapters to guide the students in applying their knowledge and in increasing their ability to think critically about maternity and women's health care issues. Answers to these exercises are provided on the Evolve site.
- *Community Activity* exercises are new to each chapter and focus on maternal and newborn activities that can be pursued in local community settings.
- *Historic Milestones in Maternity Care* in Chapter 1 provide a perspective on the advances in care of women and infants.
- *Teaching Guidelines* emphasize the information needed by the nurse to teach the patient about self-management, infant care, and health promotion.

Organization

This eighth edition of *Maternity Nursing* is composed of six units organized to enhance understanding and learning and to facilitate easy retrieval of information.

Introduction to Maternity Nursing begins with an overview of 21st century maternity and women's health nursing practice. It addresses the family as a unit of care, incorporating culture and community aspects of care. This chapter provides an understanding of these concepts in relation to maternity and women's health nursing.

Unit One, *Reproductive Years,* is a reorganized unit on women's health. Three chapters discuss health promotion, physical assessment of women, common reproductive concerns, and contraception, abortion, and infertility.

Unit Two, *Pregnancy,* describes nursing care of the woman and her family from conception through preparation for childbirth. Genetics content has been expanded. A chapter on maternal and fetal nutrition emphasizes the important aspects of care, highlights cultural variations on diet, and stresses the importance of early recognition and management of nutritional problems.

Unit Three, *Childbirth,* focuses on collaborative care among physicians, nurse-midwives, nurses, and women and their families during the processes of labor and birth. Separate chapters deal with the nurse's role in management of discomfort during labor and childbirth and fetal monitoring. These chapters familiarize students with current childbirth practices and focus on interventions to support and educate the woman and her family.

Unit Four, *Postpartum Period,* deals with a time of significant change for the entire family. The mother requires both physical and emotional support as she adjusts to her new role. Chapters on assessment and care during the fourth trimester focus on these needs. The chapter on transition to parenthood discusses family dynamics in response to the birth of a child and describes ways nurses can facilitate parent-infant adjustment.

Unit Five, *The Newborn,* addresses physiologic adaptations of the newborn and assessment and care of the newborn and family, including anticipatory guidance for the first few days at home and home follow-up care. Information on the nutritional needs of the newborn and nursing care associated with breastfeeding and formula feeding are highlighted in a separate chapter.

Unit Six, *Complications of Childbearing,* discusses the conditions that place the woman, fetus, infant, and family at risk. This unit includes a chapter on assessment of high risk pregnancies, two chapters on pregnancy at risk (preexisting and gestational conditions), a chapter on labor and birth complications, a chapter on postpartum complications, and a chapter on the high risk newborn which includes tables describing birth trauma and congenital anomalies. Care management focuses on achieving the best possible outcomes and supporting the woman and family when expectations are not met. Loss and grief issues of the family experiencing a fetal or neonatal loss are integrated throughout the chapters in this unit.

The text concludes with a detailed, cross-referenced Index and Glossary.

TEACHING/LEARNING PACKAGE

Several ancillaries to this text have been developed for instructors and students to use in classroom and clinical settings.

- ***Evolve.*** Evolve is an innovative website that provides a wealth of content, resources, and state-of-the-art information on maternity and pediatric nursing. Evolve's wide array of information includes course resources for instructors (Instructor's Manual, Test Bank, Image Collection, PowerPoint Slides, Audience Response Questions) and learning resources for students (Case Studies, NCLEX-style Review Questions, Nursing Skills, Assessment Videos, Animations, Nursing Care Plans, Spanish Guidelines, and more).
- ***Instructor's Electronic Resource.*** The innovative electronic resources for the instructor (available online) contains the following components:
  - *Instructor's Manual* contains learning objectives, chapter outlines and accompanying teaching strategies, learning activities, and curriculum guides for courses of varying lengths.
  - *Electronic Test Bank in ExamView format* contains more than 500 NCLEX-style test items, including new alternate format questions. An answer key with page references to the text, rationales, and NCLEX-style coding is included.
  - *Electronic Image Collection*, containing more than 500 full-color illustrations and photographs from the text, helps instructors develop presentations and explain key concepts. All images can be printed as acetates for overhead projection.
  - *PowerPoint Slides*, with lecture outlines for each chapter of the text, assist in presenting materials in the classroom.
  - *Audience Response Questions* for i-clicker and other systems provide additional review of content in the classroom.
  - A *Curriculum Guide* that includes a proposed class schedule and reading assignments for courses of varying lengths is provided. This gives educators suggestions for using the text in the most essential manner or in a more comprehensive way. Also, answers are provided for the Critical Thinking/Clinical Decision Making Exercises found in the text.
- ***Study Guide.*** This comprehensive and challenging study aid presents a variety of questions to enhance learning of key concepts and content from the text. Multiple-choice and matching questions are included, as well as Critical Thinking Case Studies. Answers for all questions are included at the back of the study guide.
- ***Virtual Clinical Excursions: CD and Workbook Companion.*** A CD-ROM and workbook have been developed as a virtual clinical experience to expand student opportunities for critical thinking. This package guides the student through a computer-generated virtual clinical environment and helps the user apply textbook content to virtual patients in that environment. Case studies are presented that allow students to use this textbook as a reference to assess, diagnose, plan, implement, and evaluate "real" patients using clinical scenarios. The state-of-the-art technologies reflected on this CD-ROM demonstrate cutting edge learning opportunities for students and facilitate knowledge retention of the information found in the textbook. The clinical simulations and workbook represent the next generation of research-based learning tools that promote critical thinking and meaningful learning.
- ***Simulation Learning System.*** The *Simulation Learning System* (SLS) is an online toolkit that effectively incorporates medium- to high-fidelity simulation into nursing curricula with scenarios that promote and enhance the clinical decision-making skills of students at all levels. The SLS offers a comprehensive package of resources including leveled patient scenarios, detailed instructions for preparation and implementation of the simulation experience, debriefing questions that encourage critical thinking, and learning resources to reinforce student comprehension.

ACKNOWLEDGMENTS

The eighth edition of *Maternity Nursing* would not have been possible without the contributions of many people. First we want to thank the many nurse educators, clinicians, and nursing students who made comments and suggestions about the manuscript that led to this collaborative effort. We wish to welcome Kitty Cashion as an author in this eighth edition and thank Kathy Alden who continues her role as an Associate Editor. Special thanks go to the contributors of the seventh edition. Their expertise and knowledge of current clinical practice and research added to the relevance and accuracy of the materials presented and provided a strong base for this revision. We especially thank Pat Gingrich for contributing to the Evidence-Based Practice boxes, Ed Lowdermilk for assisting with the Medication Guides, and Diana McCarty for her contributions to the Community Activity boxes.

We are also appreciative of the critiques given by the reviewers, especially in their attention to validating the accuracy of the content and their challenge to present content differently and include new ideas. These combined efforts have resulted in a revision that incorporates the most recent research and current information about the practice of maternity and women's health care. We offer thanks for shared expertise and photographs to the staff and patients of the University of North Carolina at Chapel Hill Women's Hospital; Leonard Nihan (Sea-Band International); Polly Perez (Cutting Edge Press); and Barbara Harper (Global Maternal/Child Health Association, Inc.).

We would also like to thank the following photographers: Cheryl Briggs, RN, Annapolis, MD; Kim Molloy, Knoxville, IA; Michael S. Clement, MD, Mesa, AZ; Ed Lowdermilk, Chapel Hill, NC; Amy and Ken Turner, Cary, NC; Judy Meyr, St. Louis, MO; Wendy Wetzel, Flagstaff, AZ; Patricia Hess, San Francisco, CA; Brian Sallee, Las Vegas, NV; Sara Kossuth, Los Angeles, CA; Julie Perry Nelson, Loveland, CO; Chris Rozales, San Francisco, CA; Eugene Doerr, Leitchfield, KY; Mahesh Kotwal, MD, Phoenix, AZ; Marjorie Pyle, RNC, Lifecircle, Costa Mesa, CA; H. Gil Rushton, MD, Washington, DC; Edward S. Tank, MD, Portland, OR; David A. Clarke, Philadelphia, PA; Paul Vincent Kuntz, Houston, TX; Leslie Altimier, Cincinnati, OH; Shari Sharp, Chapel Hill, NC; Sharon Johnson, Petaluma, CA; Dale Ikuta, San Jose, CA; Roni Wernik, Palo Alto, CA; Jodi Brackett, Phoenix, AZ; Bernadine Cunningham, Phoenix, AZ; Tricia Olson, North Ogden, UT: Jason Gardin, Marana, AZ; Nicole Larson, Eden Prairie, MN; Rebekah Vogel, Fort Collins, CO; Margaret Spann, New Johnsonville, TN; and Freida Belding, Munfordville, KY.

Special words of gratitude are extended to Robin Carter, Executive Editor; Laurie Gower, Managing Editor; Ann Rogers, Senior Project Manager; and Margaret Reid, Designer, for their encouragement, inspiration, and assistance in the preparation and production of this text. These talented and hardworking people helped change our manuscript into a beautiful book by editing the manuscript, designing an attractive format for our special features, and overseeing the production of the book from start to finish. We continue to be especially thankful to Laurie Gower, who always had time to answer our questions, kept track of innumerable details, found just the right photo or resource, obtained that elusive permission, and always reassured us that we were doing a great job and were going to finish on time.

Deitra Leonard Lowdermilk
Shannon E. Perry
Kitty Cashion

Contents

UNIT THREE
Childbirth

CHAPTER 1

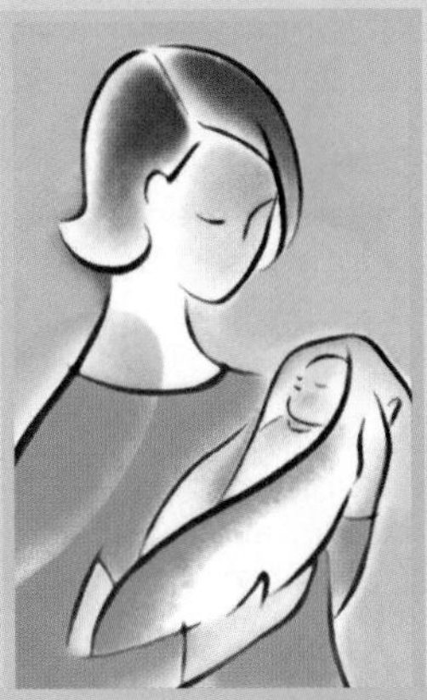

21st Century Maternity Nursing: Culturally Competent, Family and Community Focused

SHANNON E. PERRY

LEARNING OBJECTIVES

- *Evaluate contemporary issues and trends in maternity nursing.*
- *Compare selected biostatistical data among races and countries.*
- *Explain risk management and standards of practice in the delivery of nursing care.*
- *Discuss legal and ethical issues in perinatal nursing.*
- *Examine the* Healthy People 2010 *goals related to maternal and infant care.*
- *Describe the main characteristics of contemporary family forms.*
- *Identify key factors influencing family health.*
- *Relate the impact of culture on childbearing families.*
- *Compare community-based health care and community health (population- or aggregate-focused) care.*
- *List indicators of community health status and their relevance to perinatal health.*
- *Describe how home care fits into the maternity continuum of care.*
- *Discuss safety and infection control principles as they apply to the care of patients in their homes.*

KEY TERMS AND DEFINITIONS

binuclear family Family after divorce in which the child is a member of both the maternal and the paternal nuclear households

Cochrane Pregnancy and Childbirth Database Database of up-to-date systematic reviews and dissemination of reviews of randomized controlled trials of health care

continuum of care Range of clinical services provided for an individual or group that reflects care given during a single hospitalization or care for multiple conditions over a lifetime

cultural competence Awareness, acceptance, and knowledge of cultural differences and adaptation of services to acknowledge and support the culture of the patient

cultural context Setting in which one considers the individual's and the family's beliefs and practices (culture)

cultural knowledge Knowledge that includes beliefs and values about each facet of life and is passed from one generation to the next

cultural relativism Learning about and applying the standards of another person's culture to activities within a particular culture

ethnocentrism Belief in the rightness of one's culture's way of doing things

evidence-based practice Practice based on knowledge that has been gained through research and clinical trials

extended family Family that includes the nuclear family and other people related by blood

family dynamics Interaction and communication among family members

genogram Pictorial representation of family relationships and health history

home health care Care that is provided within the home

homosexual (lesbian or gay) family Family that consists of same-sex adults and children from previous heterosexual unions, conceived through therapeutic insemination, or adopted

KEY TERMS AND DEFINITIONS—cont'd

integrative health care Complementary and alternative therapies in combination with conventional Western modalities of treatment

low-birth-weight (LBW) infants Babies born weighing less than 2500 g (5½ lbs)

nuclear family Family that consists of parents and their dependent children

preterm infants Infants born before 37 weeks of gestation

reconstituted family Also called blended, combined, or remarried family; includes stepparents and stepchildren

single-parent family Family in which a child lives with one parent because of divorce, separation, desertion, or death of a parent; birth to a single parent; or adoption

standard of care Level of practice that a reasonable, prudent nurse would provide

telehealth Use of communication technologies and electronic information to provide or support health care when participants are separated by distance

vulnerable populations Groups who are at increased risk of developing physical, mental, or social health problems or who are more likely to have worse outcomes from these health problems than the population as a whole

walking survey Technique of using one's senses while traveling through a community to obtain information about sociocultural characteristics and the environment, housing, transportation, and local community agencies

WEB RESOURCES

Additional related content can be found on the companion website at evolve

http://evolve.elsevier.com/Lowdermilk/Maternity/

- NCLEX Review Questions
- Critical Thinking Exercise: Community Resources for Families
- Critical Thinking Exercise: Cultural Health and the Family
- Nursing Care Plan: Community and Home Health Care
- Nursing Care Plan: The Family Newly Immigrated from a Non-English-Speaking Country
- Nursing Care Plan: Incorporating the Infant into the Family

Maternity nursing encompasses care of childbearing women and their families through all stages of pregnancy and childbirth, as well as the first 4 weeks after birth. Throughout the prenatal period, nurses, nurse practitioners, and nurse-midwives provide care for women in clinics and physicians' offices and teach classes to help families prepare for childbirth. Nurses care for childbearing families during labor and birth in hospitals, in birthing centers, and in the home. Nurses with special training may provide intensive care for high risk neonates in special care units and for high risk mothers in antepartum units, in critical care obstetric units, or in the home. Maternity nurses teach about pregnancy; the process of labor, birth, and recovery; breastfeeding; and parenting skills. They provide continuity of care throughout the childbearing cycle. An excellent model for nurses who care for women and children is the International Confederation of Midwives' (www.internationalmidwives.org) Vision for Women and Their Health.

Although tremendous advances have taken place in the care of mothers and their infants during the past 150 years (Box 1-1), serious problems exist in the United States related to the health and health care of mothers and infants. Lack of access to prepregnancy and pregnancy-related care for all women and lack of reproductive health services for adolescents are major concerns. Sexually transmitted infections, including acquired immunodeficiency syndrome (AIDS), continue to affect reproduction adversely.

Racial and ethnic diversity is increasing within North America. The U.S. Census Bureau (2008) estimates that by the year 2050, 46% of the population will be European-American, 30% will be Hispanic, 15% will be African-American, and 9.2% will be Asian-American. Significant disparity exists in health outcomes among people of various racial and ethnic groups despite the great strides in public health that the United States has made.

CONTEMPORARY ISSUES AND TRENDS

Healthy People 2020 Goals

Healthy People 2020 is the U.S. agenda for improving health. The goals of *Healthy People 2020* are based on assessments of major risks to health and wellness, changes in public health priorities, and issues related to the health preparedness and prevention of the United States.

Every 10 years the U.S. Department of Health and Human Services (USDHHS) revises and updates this

BOX 1-1

Historic Milestones in the Care of Mothers and Infants

1847—James Young Simpson in Edinburgh, Scotland, used ether for an internal podalic version and birth; first reported use of obstetric anesthesia

1861—Ignaz Semmelwies wrote *The Cause, Concept, and Prophylaxis of Childbed Fever*

1906—First program for prenatal nursing care established

1908—Childbirth classes started by the American Red Cross

1909—First White House Conference on Children

1911—First milk bank in the United States established in Boston

1912—U.S. Children's Bureau established

1915—Radical mastectomy is effective treatment for breast cancer

1916—Margaret Sanger established first American birth control clinic in Brooklyn, NY

1918—Condoms became legal in the United States

1923—First U.S. hospital center for premature infant care established at Sarah Morris Hospital in Chicago

1928—Penicillin to treat bacterial infections discovered

1929—The modern tampon (with an applicator) invented and patented

1933—Sodium pentothal used as anesthesia for childbirth

1933—*Natural Childbirth* published by Grantly Dick-Read

1935—Sulfonamides introduced as cure for puerperal fever

1941—Penicillin used as treatment for infection

1941—Papanicolaou (Pap) tests introduced

1942—Premarin approved by the U.S. Food and Drug Administration (FDA) as treatment for menopausal symptoms

1950—Disposable diaper invented

1953—Virginia Apgar, an anesthesiologist, published Apgar scoring system of neonatal assessment

1956—Oxygen determined to cause retrolental fibroplasia (now known as retinopathy of prematurity)

1958—Edward Hon reported on the recording of the fetal electrocardiogram from the maternal abdomen (first commercial electronic fetal monitor produced in late 1960s)

1958—Ian Donald, a Glasgow physician, was first to report clinical use of ultrasound to examine the fetus

1959—*Thank You, Dr. Lamaze* published by Marjorie Karmel

1959—Cytologic studies demonstrate that Down syndrome is associated with a particular form of nondisjunction now known as trisomy 21

1960—American Society for Psychoprophylaxis in Obstetrics (ASPO/Lamaze) formed

1960—International Childbirth Education Association formed

1960—Birth control pill approved by the FDA

1962—Thalidomide found to cause birth defects

1963—Title V of the Social Security Act amended to include comprehensive maternity and infant care for women who were low income and high risk

1965—Supreme Court ruled married people have the right to use birth control

1967—Rh_o(D) immune globulin produced

1968—Rubella vaccine available

1969—Nurses Association of the American College of Obstetricians and Gynecologists (NAACOG) founded; renamed Association of Women's Health, Obstetric, and Neonatal Nurses (AWHONN) and incorporated as a 501(c)3 organization in 1993

1969—Mammogram became available

1972—Special Supplemental Food Program for Women, Infants, and Children (WIC) started

1973—Abortion legalized

1974—First standards for obstetric, gynecologic, and neonatal nursing published by NAACOG

1975—The Pregnant Patient's Bill of Rights published by the International Childbirth Education Association

1976—First home pregnancy kits approved by FDA

1976—Intrauterine device for birth control approved by the FDA

1978—Louise Brown, first test-tube baby, born

1987—Safe Motherhood Initiative launched by World Health Organization and other international agencies

1991—Society for Advancement of Women's Health Research founded

1992—Office of Research on Women's Health authorized by U.S. Congress

1992—Depo Provera approved by FDA

1993—Female condom approved by FDA

1993—Human embryos cloned at George Washington University

1993—Family and Medical Leave Act enacted

1994—DNA sequences of BRCA1 and BRCA2 identified

1994—Zidovudine guidelines published to reduce mother to fetus transmission of HIV

1996—FDA mandated folic acid fortification in all breads and grains sold in United States

1998—Newborns' and Mothers' Health Act put into effect

1998—First emergency contraception pill for pregnancy prevention in women who had unprotected sex approved by FDA

2000—Working draft of sequence and analysis of human genome completed

2006—Human papillomavirus vaccine available

2010—Patient Protection and Affordable Care Act (PPACA) signed into law

2010—U.S. Supreme Court upheld individual mandate but not Medicaid expansion provisions of PPACA

2012—Scientists reported findings of Encyclopedia of DNA Elements (ENCODE) Project showing 80% of human genome is active

BOX 1-2

United Nations Millennium Development Goals

Goal 1—Eradicate extreme poverty and hunger
Goal 2—Achieve universal primary education
Goal 3—Promote gender equality and empower women
Goal 4—Reduce child mortality
Goal 5—Improve maternal health
Goal 6—Combat HIV/AIDS, malaria, and other diseases
Goal 7—Ensure environmental sustainability
Goal 8—Develop a global partnership for development

Source: *UN millennium development goals.* Internet document available at www.un.org/millenniumgoals (accessed July 1, 2013).
AIDS, Acquired immunodeficiency syndrome; *HIV,* human immunodeficiency virus.

agenda. *Healthy People 2020,* has four recommended overarching goals: (1) attaining high-quality, longer lives free of preventable disease, disability, injury, and premature death; (2) achieving health equity, eliminating disparities, and improving the health of all groups; (3) creating social and physical environments that promote good health for all; and (4) promoting quality of life, healthy development, and healthy behaviors across all life stages (www.healthypeople.gov/2020/about/default.aspx). Of the objectives of *Healthy People 2020,* 33 are related to maternal, infant, and child health.

Millennium Development Goals

The Millennium Development Goals (MDGs) are eight goals to be achieved by 2015 that respond to the world's main development challenges. The MDGs are drawn from the actions and targets contained in the Millennium Declaration that was adopted by 189 nations and signed by 147 heads of state and governments during the United Nations Millennium Summit in September 2000 (www.un.org/millenniumgoals/goals.html). Goals 3 through 5 of the MDGs relate specifically to women and children (Box 1-2).

Integrative Health Care

Integrative health care encompasses complementary and alternative therapies in combination with conventional Western modalities of treatment. Many popular alternative healing modalities offer human-centered care based on philosophies that recognize the value of the patient's input and honor the individual's beliefs, values, and desires. The focus of these modalities is on the whole person, not just on a disease complex. Patients often find that alternative modalities are more consistent with their own belief systems and allow for more patient autonomy in health care decisions (Fig. 1-1). Complementary and alternative therapies are identified throughout the text with an icon:

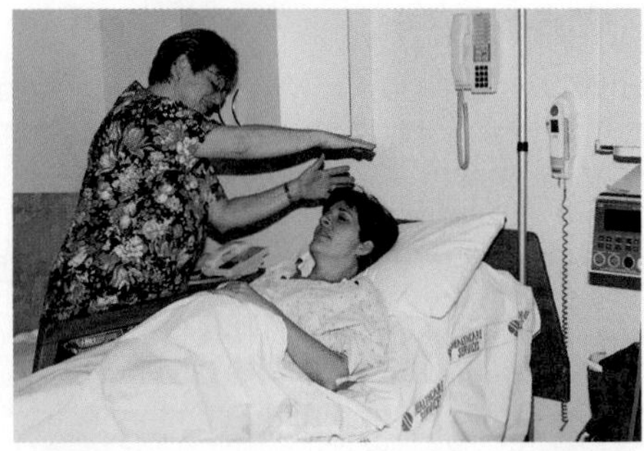

Fig. 1-1 Healing touch with pregnant patient. (Courtesy Wendy Wetzel, Flagstaff, AZ.)

Problems with the U.S. Health Care System

Structure of the health care delivery system

The changing health care delivery system offers opportunities for nurses to alter nursing practice and improve the way care is delivered through managed care, integrated delivery systems, and redefined roles. Consumer participation in health care decisions is increasing, information is available on the Internet, and care is provided in a technology-intensive environment (Tiedje, Price, & You, 2008).

Nurses have been critically important in developing strategies to improve the well-being of women and their infants and have led the efforts to implement clinical practice guidelines and to practice using an evidence-based approach. Through professional associations, nurses have a voice in setting standards and influencing health policy by actively participating in the education of the public and of state and federal legislators (e.g., www.nursingworld.org; www.cna-nurses.ca; www.awhonn.org). For example, in 2008 the American Nurses Association (ANA) published *ANA's Health System Reform Agenda,* and in 2009 a nurse was appointed the Administrator of the Health Resources and Services Administration, the agency that oversees approximately 7000 community clinics that serve low-income and uninsured people (Obama chooses UND's Mary Wakefield as Health Resources and Services Administration Leader, February 20, 2009).

Reducing medical errors

Medical errors are the leading cause of death in the United States and result in as many as 98,000 deaths per year (Gauthier & Serber, 2005). In Canada, adverse events are implicated in up to 23,750 deaths per year (French, 2006). Since the Institute of Medicine released its 1999 report, *To Err Is Human: Building a Safer Health System,* a concerted effort has been under way to analyze causes of errors and develop strategies to prevent them. Recognizing the multifaceted causes of medical errors, the Agency for Healthcare Research and Quality (2000) prepared a *Patient Fact Sheet* with *20 Tips to Help Prevent Medical Errors* for patients and the public. Patients are encouraged to be

BOX 1-3

National Quality Forum's Serious Reportable Events Pertaining to Maternal and Child Health

- Infant discharged to the wrong person
- Maternal death or serious injury associated with labor or birth in a low risk pregnancy while being cared for in a health care facility
- Death or serious injury of a neonate associated with labor or birth in a low risk pregnancy
- Artificial insemination with the wrong donor sperm or wrong egg

Source: The National Quality Forum: *National Quality Forum updates endorsement of serious reportable events in healthcare.* Internet document available at www.qualityforum.org (accessed July 1, 2013).

BOX 1-4

Selected Safe Practices for Better Health Care

- Ask each patient or legal surrogate to "teach back" in his or her own words key information about the proposed treatments or procedures for which he or she is being asked to provide informed consent.
- Ensure that care information is transmitted and appropriately documented in a timely manner and in a clearly understandable form to patients and to all of the patients' health care providers/professionals, within and between care settings, who need that information in order to provide continued care.
- Standardize a list of "Do Not Use" abbreviations, acronyms, symbols, and dose designations that cannot be used throughout the organization.
- Comply with current Centers for Disease Control and Prevention (CDC) hand hygiene guidelines.

Source: National Quality Forum. (2010). *Safe practices for better healthcare—2010 update.* Internet document available at www.qualityforum.org (accessed July 1, 2013).

knowledgeable consumers of health care and ask questions of providers, including physicians, midwives, nurses, and pharmacists.

In 2002 the National Quality Forum published a list of Serious Reportable Events in health care. The list was updated in 2006 and 2011 with a total of 29 events. Of these events, four pertain directly to maternity and newborn care (Box 1-3). The National Quality Forum also published *Safe Practices for Better Healthcare* (www.qualityforum.org). The 34 safe practices included should be used in all applicable health care settings to reduce the risk of harm that results from processes, systems, and environments of care. Box 1-4 contains a selection of practices from that document.

In August 2007, the Centers for Medicare & Medicaid Services issued a rule that denies payment for eight hospital-acquired conditions effective October 2008 (O'Reilly, 2008). Five of the conditions are also on the National Quality Forum list. Conditions that might pertain to maternity nursing include a foreign object retained after surgery, air embolism, blood incompatibility, falls and trauma, and catheter-associated urinary tract infection. Almost 1300 U.S. hospitals waive costs associated with serious reportable events (O'Reilly).

High cost of health care

Health care is one of the fastest-growing sectors of the U.S. economy. Currently, 17.4% of the gross domestic product is spent on health care (Squires, 2012). A shift in demographics, an increased emphasis on high-cost technology, higher incidence of obesity, and the liability costs of a litigious society contribute to the high cost of care. Most researchers agree that caring for the increased number of low-birth-weight (LBW) infants in neonatal intensive care units contributes significantly to the overall health care costs.

Midwifery care has helped contain some health care costs. However, not all insurance carriers reimburse nurse practitioners and clinical nurse specialists as direct care providers; nor do they reimburse for all services provided by nurse-midwives, a situation that continues to be a problem. Nurses must become involved in the politics of cost containment because they, as knowledgeable experts, can provide solutions to many health care problems at a relatively low cost.

Limited access to care

Barriers to access must be removed so pregnancy outcomes can be improved. The most significant barrier to access is the inability to pay. The number of uninsured people in the United States in 2010 was 49.9 million or 16.3% of the population (DeNavas-Walt, Proctor, & Smith, 2011). Lack of transportation and dependent child care are other barriers. In addition to a lack of insurance and high costs, a lack of providers for low-income women exists. Many physicians either refuse to take Medicaid patients or take only a few such patients. This circumstance presents a serious problem because a significant proportion of births are to mothers who receive Medicaid.

Efforts to reduce health disparities

Significant disparities in morbidity and mortality rates are experienced by African-Americans, Native Americans, Hispanics, Alaska Natives, and Asians/Pacific Islanders in comparison with Caucasians. Shorter life expectancy, higher infant and maternal mortality rates, more birth defects, and more sexually transmitted infections are found among these ethnic and racial minority groups by comparison. The disparities are thought to result from a complex interaction among biologic factors, environment, and health behaviors. Disparities in education and income are associated with differences in occurrence of morbidity and mortality.

The Health Resources and Services Administration (HRSA) Health Disparities Collaboratives are part of a national effort with the goal of eliminating disparities and improving delivery systems of health care for all people in the United States who are cared for in HRSA-supported health centers (Calvo, 2006). The National Institutes of Health has a commitment to improve the health of minorities and provides funding for research and training of minority researchers (www.nih.gov). The National Institute of Nursing Research (www.ninr.nih.gov) has included the goal of reducing disparities in its strategic plan and supports research for this purpose. A broad public health perspective is needed to reduce these disparities (Satcher & Higginbotham, 2008).

Trends in Fertility and Birthrate

Fertility trends and birthrates reflect women's needs for health care. Box 1-5 defines biostatistical terminology useful in analyzing maternity health care. In 2009 the *fertility rate,* the number of births per 1000 women from 15 to 44 years of age, was 66.7 (Kochanek et al., 2012). The highest *birthrates* (the number of births per 1000 women) were for women between ages 25 and 29 (110.5 per 1000). The teen birthrate was 39.1 per 1000. More than one third of all births in the United States in 2009 were to unmarried women, with much variation in proportion among racial groups (non-Hispanic black, 72.8%; Hispanic, 53.2%; non-Hispanic white, 29%) (Kochanek et al., 2012). Births to unmarried women are often related to less-favorable outcomes such as LBW or preterm birth. A large number of teenagers are typically found in the unmarried group. In 2009, the birthrate to women under 20 years of age was 39.1 per 1000 (Kochanek et al., 2012).

BOX 1-5

Maternal-Infant Biostatistical Terminology

Abortus—An embryo or fetus that is removed or expelled from the uterus at 20 weeks of gestation or less, weighs 500 g or less, or measures 25 cm or less

Birthrate—Number of live births in 1 year per 1000 population

Fertility rate—Number of births per 1000 women between the ages of 15 and 44 (inclusive), calculated on a yearly basis

Infant mortality rate—Number of deaths of infants under 1 year of age per 1000 live births

Maternal mortality rate—Number of maternal deaths from births and complications of pregnancy, childbirth, and puerperium (the first 42 days after termination of the pregnancy) per 100,000 live births

Neonatal mortality rate—Number of deaths of infants under 28 days of age per 1000 live births

Perinatal mortality rate—Number of stillbirths and number of neonatal deaths per 1000 live births

Stillbirth—An infant who at birth demonstrates no signs of life such as breathing, heartbeat, or voluntary muscle movements

Low Birth Weight and Preterm Birth

The risks of morbidity and mortality increase for newborns weighing less than 2500 g (5 lb, 8 oz)–LBW infants. Multiple births contribute to the incidence of LBW. In 2009 the incidence of LBW births was 8.1%, and the incidence of very low-birth-weight (VLBW; less than 1500 g [3.3 lb]) births was 1.4% (Kochanek et al., 2012). Racial disparity exists in the incidence of LBW. Non-Hispanic black babies are twice as likely as non-Hispanic white babies to be LBW and to die within the first year of life. By race the incidence of LBW for non-Hispanic black births was 13.6%; for non-Hispanic white births, 7.1%; and for Hispanic births, 6.9%. Cigarette smoking is associated with LBW, prematurity, and intrauterine growth restriction. In 2005, 10.7% of pregnant women smoked, a proportion that has declined slightly from 2004 (Kochanek et al., 2012).

The proportion of **preterm infants** (i.e., those born before 37 weeks of gestation) was 12.1% in 2009. Racial variation in rates has been found: 17.4% for non-Hispanic black births, 12.1% for Hispanic births, and 11.9% for non-Hispanic white births (Kochanek et al., 2012). Multiple births accounted for 3.4% of births in 2006, with most of the increase associated with increased use of fertility drugs and older age at childbearing (Kochanek et al.).

Infant Mortality in the United States

A common indicator of the adequacy of prenatal care and the health of a nation as a whole is the *infant mortality rate,* the number of deaths of infants younger than 1 year of age per 1000 live births. The neonatal mortality rate is the number of deaths of infants younger than 28 days of age per 1000 live births. The perinatal mortality rate is the number of stillbirths plus the number of neonatal deaths per 1000 live births. The preliminary infant mortality rate for 2009 was 6.4 (Kochanek et al., 2012). The infant mortality rate continues to be higher for non-Hispanic black babies (13.3 per 1000) than for non-Hispanic white babies (5.66 per 1000) and Hispanic babies (5.55 per 1000) (Kochanek et al.). Limited maternal education, young maternal age, unmarried status, poverty, and lack of prenatal care appear to be associated with higher infant mortality rates. Poor nutrition, smoking and alcohol use, and maternal conditions such as poor health or hypertension are also important contributors to infant mortality. To address the factors associated with infant mortality, a shift must occur from the current emphasis on high-technology medical interventions to a focus on improving access to preventive care for low-income families.

International Trends in Infant Mortality

The infant mortality rate of Canada (5.1 per 1000 in 2008 [data not available for 2009]) ranks twenty-fifth, and that of the United States ranks thirtieth (6.4 per 1000 in 2009) when compared with other industrialized nations (Kochanek et al., 2012). One reason for this statistic is the high rate of LBW infants born in the United States compared with other countries.

Maternal Mortality Trends

The fifth Millennium Development Goal is to improve maternal health and reduce the maternal mortality rate by 75% between 1990 and 2015. Worldwide, approximately 800 women die each day of problems related to pregnancy or childbirth, with hemorrhage being the leading cause of death. Great disparities exist in maternal mortality rate between developing and developed countries. For example, in the United States in 2007 the annual maternal mortality rate (number of maternal deaths per 100,000 live births) was 12.7 (USDHHS, HRSA, Maternal and Child Health Bureau, 2010), whereas the rate in Africa in 2010 was 500 (World Health Organization [WHO], 2012).

In the United States, significant racial differences exist in the rates: black or African-American women have a maternal mortality rate three times higher than that of non-Hispanic white women. The maternal mortality rate was 28.4 per 100,000 for black or African-American women, in contrast with 10.5 per 100,000 for non-Hispanic white women (USDHHS, HRSA, Maternal and Child Health Bureau, 2010). The *Healthy People 2020* goal of 11.4 maternal deaths per 100,000 poses a significant challenge.

Increase in High Risk Pregnancies

The number of high risk pregnancies has increased, which means that a greater number of women are at risk for poor pregnancy outcomes (www.nlm.nih.gov/medlineplus/highriskpregnancy.html). Escalating drug use (ranging from 11% to 27% of pregnant women, depending on geographic location) has contributed to higher incidences of prematurity, LBW, congenital defects, withdrawal symptoms in infants, and learning disabilities. Alcohol use in pregnancy has been associated with miscarriages, mental retardation, LBW, and fetal alcohol syndrome.

The twin birth rate was 33.2 per 1000 in 2009. The downward trend in the birthrate of higher-order multiples (triplet, quadruplet, and greater) continued in 2009, with a rate of 153.5 per 100,000 (Kochanek et al., 2012). More than one third of women in the United States are obese (body mass index of 30 or greater), with adults ages 40 to 59 having the highest prevalence. Obesity in women demonstrates significant racial disparities: 49.6% of non-Hispanic black women, 45.1% of Mexican-American women, and 33% of non-Hispanic white women ages 20 years and over are obese (Flegal, Carroll, Ogden, et al., 2010; Shields, Carroll, & Ogden, 2011). Almost 20% of women who give birth in the United States are obese. The two most frequently reported maternal medical risk factors are hypertension associated with pregnancy and diabetes, both of which are associated with obesity. Obesity in pregnancy is associated with the use of increased health care services and hospital stays that are longer (Chu et al., 2008).

High-Technology Care

Advances in scientific knowledge and the large number of high risk pregnancies have contributed to a health care system that emphasizes high-technology care. Maternity care has extended to preconception counseling, more and better scientific techniques to monitor the mother and fetus, more definitive tests for hypoxia and acidosis, and neonatal intensive care units. Virtually all labors in hospital settings are monitored electronically despite the lack of evidence of the efficacy of such monitoring. The numbers of assisted labors and births are increasing. Internet-based information is available to the public that enhances interactions among health care providers, families, and community providers. Point-of-care testing is available. Personal data assistants are used to enhance comprehensive care; the medical record is increasingly in electronic form. *Telehealth* is an umbrella term for the use of communication technologies and electronic information to provide or support health care when the participants are separated by distance. Telehealth permits specialists, including nurses, to provide health care and consultation when distance separates them from those needing care. This technology has the potential to save billions of dollars annually for health care, but these technologic advances have also contributed to higher health care costs.

Care during Pregnancy and Childbirth

Safe motherhood

The Centers for Disease Control and Prevention (CDC) began working with national and international groups in 2001 to develop and implement programs to promote safe motherhood (Jones, 2008). Maternal mortality and morbidity is a measure of a nation's commitment to the status of women and their health. The leading causes of pregnancy-related deaths in the United States are hemorrhage, blood clots, hypertension, infection, stroke, amniotic fluid embolism, and heart muscle disease. The CDC estimates that more than half of these deaths can be prevented with better access to care, better quality care, and positive changes in the health and lifestyle habits of women. The CDC continues to invest resources to improve positive outcomes and prevent negative outcomes of pregnancy (Jones).

Childbirth practices

Prenatal care may promote better pregnancy outcomes by providing early risk assessment and promoting healthy behaviors such as improved nutrition and smoking cessation. In 2006, 69.9% of all women received care in the first trimester. Disparity can be seen in the use of prenatal care by race and ethnicity; Native American, Hispanic, or non-Hispanic black women were more than twice as likely as non-Hispanic white women to receive late care (i.e., care beginning in the third trimester or no care at all) (Heron, Sutton, Xu, et al., 2010). In spite of this statistic, substantial gains have been made in the use of prenatal care since the early 1990s, which is attributed to the expansion in the 1980s of Medicaid coverage for pregnant women.

Women can choose physicians or nurse-midwives as primary care providers. In 2009, physicians attended 92% and nurse-midwives attended approximately 7.4% of all births (Martin, Hamilton, Ventura, et al., 2011). Hospital births accounted for 99% of births. Of the out-of-hospital births, 67% were in the home, 27% in free-standing birth centers, 0.9% in clinics or physician's offices, and 5% other or not specified (Martin et al., 2007). Cesarean births increased to 32.9% of live births in the United States in 2009, the highest rate ever in the United States, whereas the rate of vaginal births after cesarean declined (Martin, Hamilton, Ventura, et al., 2011). This cesarean rate is significantly higher than the *Healthy People 2020* goal of 23.9%.

Certified nurse-midwives are registered nurses with education in the two disciplines of nursing and midwifery. Certified midwives (direct-entry midwives) are educated only in the discipline of midwifery. In the United States, certification of midwives is through the American College of Nurse-Midwives, the professional association for midwives in the United States. The Royal College of Midwives is the professional association for midwives in the United Kingdom. In Canada the Association of Ontario Midwives is the professional association, and the College of Midwives of Ontario is the regulatory body for midwives in Ontario; the other provinces of Canada have similar regulatory bodies. Many national associations belong to the International Confederation of Midwives, which is composed of 83 member associations from 70 countries in the Americas and Europe, Africa, and the Asia-Pacific region.

With family-centered care, fathers, partners, grandparents, siblings, and friends may be present for labor and birth. Fathers or partners may be present for cesarean births. Fathers may participate by "catching the baby" or cutting the umbilical cord or both (Fig. 1-2). Doulas–trained and experienced female labor attendants–may be present to provide a continuous, one-on-one caring presence throughout the labor and birth. Newborn infants remain with the mother and mothers are encouraged to breastfeed immediately after birth. Parents participate in the care of their infants in nurseries and neonatal intensive care units.

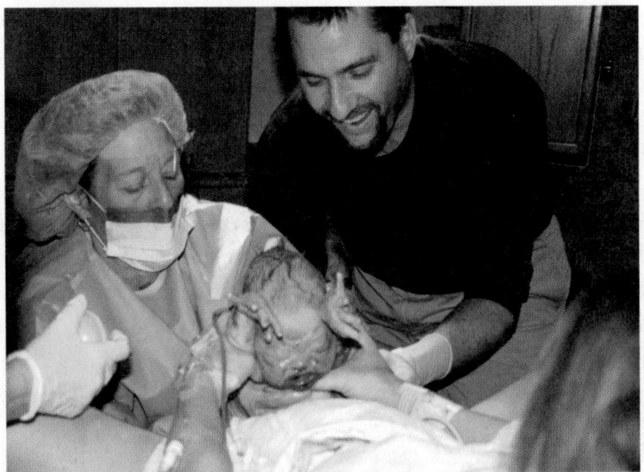

Fig. 1-2 Father "catching" newborn son. Mother is reaching down to help birth the baby. (Courtesy Darren and Julie Nelson, Loveland, CO.)

Neonatal security in the hospital setting is of concern. A significant number of cases of "baby-napping" and of sending parents home with the wrong baby have been reported. Security systems are being placed in nurseries, and nurses are required to wear photo identification or some other security badge.

Discharge of a mother and baby within 24 hours of birth has created a growing need for follow-up or home care. Legislation has been enacted to ensure that mothers and babies are permitted to stay in the hospital at least 48 hours after vaginal birth and 96 hours after cesarean birth, although they may choose to leave earlier. Focused and efficient teaching is necessary to enable the parents and infant to make a safe transition from hospital to home.

Involving Consumers and Promoting Self-Management

Self-management is appealing to both patients and the health care system because of its potential to reduce health care costs. Maternity care is especially suited to self-management because childbearing is essentially health focused, women are usually well when they enter the system, and visits to health care providers can present the opportunity for health and illness interventions. Measures to improve health and reduce risks associated with poor pregnancy outcomes and illness can be addressed. Topics such as nutrition education, stress management, smoking cessation, alcohol and drug treatment, prevention of violence, improvement of social supports, and parenting education are appropriate for such encounters.

International Concerns

Female genital mutilation is the removal of part or all of the female external genitalia for cultural or nontherapeutic reasons (WHO Study Group, 2006). Worldwide, many women undergo such procedures. With the growing number of immigrants from Africa and other countries where female genital mutilation is practiced, nurses in the U.S. and Canada will increasingly encounter women who have undergone the procedure. Women who have undergone the procedure are significantly more likely to have adverse obstetric outcomes resulting in one or two additional perinatal deaths per 100 births (WHO Study Group, 2006). The International Council of Nurses and other health professionals have spoken out against the procedures as harmful to women's health and a violation of human rights.

TRENDS IN NURSING PRACTICE

Evidence-Based Practice

Evidence-based practice–providing care based on evidence gained through research and clinical trials–is increasingly emphasized. Although not all practice can be evidence based, practitioners must use the best available information on which to base their interventions. The *Standards for Professional Nursing Practice in the Care of Women and Newborns* (AWHONN, 2009) and the *Standards for Professional Perinatal Nursing Practice and Certification in Canada* (AWHONN, 2002) include an evidence-based approach to practice. Discussion of nursing care and evidence-based nursing boxes throughout this text provide examples of evidence-based practice (see Evidence-Based Practice box).

Cochrane Pregnancy and Childbirth Database

The Cochrane Collaboration, which includes the Cochrane Pregnancy and Childbirth Database, oversees up-to-date, systematic reviews of randomized controlled trials of health care and disseminates these reviews. The premise of the project is that these types of studies provide the most reliable evidence about the effects of care.

The evidence from these studies should encourage practitioners to implement useful measures and abandon those that are useless or harmful. Studies are ranked in six categories:

1. Beneficial forms of care
2. Forms of care that are likely to be beneficial
3. Forms of care with a trade-off between beneficial and adverse effects
4. Forms of care with unknown effectiveness
5. Forms of care that are unlikely to be beneficial
6. Forms of care that are likely to be ineffective or harmful

Practices that have been reviewed by the Collaboration are identified with this symbol throughout this text: ❊ Other evidenced-based practices are indentified with the same icon.

Joanna Briggs Institute

Founded in 1995 as an initiative of the Royal Adelaide Hospital and the University of Adelaide in Australia, the Joanna Briggs Institute (JBI) uses a collaborative approach for evaluating evidence from a range of sources (www.joannabriggs.edu.au). The JBI has formed collaborations with a variety of universities and hospitals around the world, including in the United States and Canada. It provides another source for perinatal nurses to access information to support evidence-based practice.

EVIDENCE-BASED PRACTICE

Searching for and Evaluating the Evidence

Pat Gingrich

Throughout this text, you will see Evidence-Based Practice boxes. These boxes provide examples of how a nurse might conduct an inquiry into an identified practice question. Curiosity and access to a virtual or real library are all the nurse needs to be confident that his or her practice has a sound foundation of evidence.

A literature search may reveal up to three levels of evidence. The first level consists of primary studies. The strongest of these are randomized controlled trials. Well-designed studies, even small ones, each add another piece to the puzzle.

These primary studies may be combined into the second level of evidence. In systematic analyses such as those in the Cochrane Database, the researcher uses methods to identify all studies relevant to a particular question. If the data are similar enough, they can be pooled into a metaanalysis. If the evidence is strong, some analyses will form the basis for recommendations for practice and to guide further inquiry.

At the tertiary level, professional organizations such as the Agency for Healthcare Research and Quality (AHRQ) (www.ahrq.gov) or the Academy of Breastfeeding Medicine (ABM) (www.bfmed.org) may decide to address a broad practice question by sorting through all the available primary and secondary evidence in addition to consulting experienced clinicians. After thoughtful review the committee of experts in the organization then crafts its consensus statement. These recommendations for best practice stand on the shoulders of the systematic analysts, who stand on the many shoulders of the primary researchers.

Provided the professional organization is well respected and the process is rigorous, these guidelines in the consensus statement carry enormous authority. Individuals and institutions may choose to adopt these guidelines with confidence. An example of this process is the Association of Women's Health, Obstetric and Neonatal Nurses (AWHONN) (www.awhonn.org) Late Preterm Infant Initiative. This initiative began in 2005 in response to the confusion that surrounded the care of infants who do not qualify for neonatal intensive care admission yet require extra vigilance. Nurseries can adapt these recommendations to their specific institutions, enabling nurses to become more effective at caring for the unique problems of this population of neonates. As is the case with AWHONN, most professional organizations make their guidelines available free of charge on their websites.

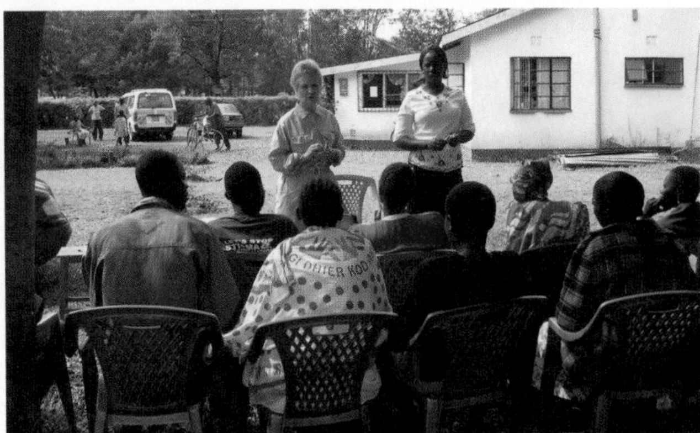

Fig. 1-3 Nurse teaching breast self-examination with the assistance of an interpreter to traditional birth attendants (TBAs) in a rural clinic in Kenya (both men and women serve as TBAs). Women may detect lumps but usually do not seek care unless pain is associated with the lump. (Courtesy Shannon Perry, Phoenix, AZ.)

A Global Perspective

As the world becomes smaller because of travel and communication technologies, nurses and other health care providers are gaining a global perspective and participating in activities to improve the health and health care of people worldwide. Nurses participate in medical outreach, providing obstetric, surgical, ophthalmologic, orthopedic, or other services; attend international meetings; conduct research; and provide international consultation (Fig. 1-3). International student and faculty exchanges occur. More articles about health and health care in various countries are appearing in nursing journals. Several schools of nursing in the United States are World Health Organization Collaborating Centers.

STANDARDS OF PRACTICE AND LEGAL ISSUES IN DELIVERY OF CARE

Nursing standards of practice in perinatal nursing have been described by several organizations, including the ANA (for maternal-child health nursing), AWHONN (for perinatal nurses) (Box 1-6), the American College of Nurse-Midwives (ACNM) (for midwives), and the National Association of Neonatal Nurses (NANN) (for neonatal nurses). These standards reflect current knowledge, represent levels of practice agreed on by leaders in the specialty, and can be used for clinical benchmarking.

In addition to these more formalized standards, agencies have their own policy and procedure books that outline standards to be followed in that setting. In legal terms, the standard of care is that level of practice that a reasonably prudent nurse would provide. In determining legal negligence, the care given is compared with the standard of care. If the standard was not met and harm resulted, negligence occurred. The number of legal suits in the perinatal area has typically been high. As a consequence, malpractice insurance costs are high for physicians, nurse-midwives, and nurses who work in labor and delivery.

BOX 1-6

Standards of Care for Women and Newborns

STANDARDS THAT DEFINE THE NURSE'S RESPONSIBILITY TO THE PATIENT

Assessment—Collection of health data of the woman or newborn

Diagnosis—Analysis of data to determine the nursing diagnosis

Outcome Identification—Identification of expected outcomes that are individualized

Planning—Development of a plan of care

Implementation—Performance of interventions for the plan of care, including coordination of care and health teaching and promotion

Evaluation—Evaluation of the effectiveness of interventions in relation to expected outcomes

STANDARDS OF PROFESSIONAL PERFORMANCE THAT DELINEATE ROLES AND BEHAVIORS FOR WHICH THE PROFESSIONAL NURSE IS ACCOUNTABLE

Quality of Practice—Systemic evaluation of nursing practice

Education—Participation in educational activities to maintain knowledge and competencies that reflect current evidence-based practice

Professional Practice Evaluation—Self-evaluation of own nursing practice in relation to professional standards and guidelines, legal responsibilities, and current evidence-based practices

Ethics—Use of ethical decision making guide such as the ANA Code of Ethics for nurses to guide practice

Collegiality—Contribution to the development of peers, students, and others

Collaboration and Communication—Involvement of women, families/significant others, health care providers, and the community in the provision of patient care

Research—Use of research findings in practice; participation in research activities that are appropriate to the education, position, and practice of the nurse

Resource and Technology—Consideration of factors related to safety, effectiveness, and costs in planning and delivering patient care

Leadership—Participation in a variety of leadership roles within the work setting including role model, consultant, and change agent; participation in professional organizations

Source: Association of Women's Health, Obstetric, and Neonatal Nurses (AWHONN) (2009). *Standards for professional nursing practice in the care of women and newborns* (7th ed.). Washington, DC: AWHONN.

LEGAL TIP **Standard of Care**

When you are uncertain about how to perform a procedure, consult the agency procedure book and follow the guidelines printed therein. These guidelines are the standard of care for that agency.

Quality and Safety Education for Nurses (QSEN) provides nurses with the competencies to improve the quality and safety of the health care systems in which they practice (Cronenwett, Sherwood, Barnsteiner, et al., 2007). The competencies identified by the Institute of Medicine (IOM, 2003) are patient-centered care, teamwork and collaboration, evidence-based practice, quality improvement, safety, and informatics. QSEN competencies for each chapter are listed in the Appendix.

Risk Management

Risk management is an evolving process that identifies risks, establishes preventive practices, develops reporting mechanisms, and delineates procedures for managing lawsuits. Nurses should be familiar with concepts of risk management and their implications for nursing practice. These concepts can be viewed as systems of checks and balances that ensure high-quality patient care from preconception until after birth. Effective risk management minimizes the risk of injury to patients and the number of lawsuits against nurses. Each facility or site develops site-specific risk management procedures based on accepted standards and guidelines. The procedures and guidelines must be reviewed periodically.

To decrease risk of errors in the administration of medications, The Joint Commission developed a list of abbreviations, acronyms, and symbols *not* to use (Table 1-1). In addition, each agency must develop its own list.

Sentinel Events

The Joint Commission describes a sentinel event as "an unexpected occurrence involving death or serious physical or psychological injury, or the risk thereof. Serious injury specifically includes loss of limb or function." These events are called *sentinel* because they signal a need for an immediate investigation and response (The Joint Commission, 2010). Reportable sentinel events in perinatal nursing include any maternal death related to the process of birth, any perinatal death not related to a congenital condition in an infant with a birth weight greater than 2500 g, severe neonatal hyperbilirubinemia (bilirubin greater than 30 mg/dL), and infant discharge to the wrong family (The Joint Commission, 2010).

ETHICAL ISSUES IN PERINATAL NURSING

Ethical concerns and debates have multiplied with the increased use of technology and with scientific advances. For example, with reproductive technology, pregnancy is now possible in women who thought they would never bear children, including some who are menopausal or postmenopausal. Should scarce resources be devoted to achieving pregnancies in older women? Is giving birth to a child at an older age worth the risks involved? Should older parents be encouraged to conceive a baby when they may not live to see the child reach adulthood? Should a woman who is HIV positive have access to assisted reproduction services? Should third-party payers assume the costs of reproductive technology such as the use of induced ovulation and in vitro fertilization? Questions about informed consent and allocation of resources must be addressed with innovations such as intrauterine fetal surgery, fetoscopy, therapeutic insemination, genetic engineering, stem cell research, surrogate childbearing, surgery for infertility, "test-tube" babies, fetal research, and treatment of VLBW babies. The introduction of long-acting contraceptives has created moral choices and policy dilemmas for health care providers and legislators (i.e., should some women [substance abusers, women with low incomes, or women who are HIV positive] be required to take the contraceptives?) With the potential for great good that can come from fetal tissue transplantation, what research is ethical? What are the rights of the embryo? Should cloning of humans be permitted? Discussion and debate about these issues will continue for many years. Nurses and patients, as well as scientists, physicians, attorneys, lawmakers, ethicists, and clergy, must be involved in the discussions.

TABLE 1-1

The Joint Commission "Do Not Use" List*

ABBREVIATION	POTENTIAL PROBLEM	PREFERRED TERM
U (for unit)	Mistaken as zero, four, or cc	Write "unit."
IU (for international unit)	Mistaken as IV (intravenous) or 10 (ten)	Write "international unit."
Q.D., QD, q.d., qd (daily)	Mistaken for each other; period after the Q mistaken for "I" and "O" mistaken for "I"	Write "daily."
Q.O.D., QOD, q.o.d., qod (every other day)		Write "every other day."
Trailing zero (X.0 mg)†	Decimal point is missed	Write X mg.
Lack of leading zero (.X mg)		Write 0.X mg.
MS	Can mean morphine sulfate or magnesium sulfate	Write "morphine sulfate."
MSO_4 and $MgSO_4$	Confused for one another	Write "magnesium sulfate."

*Applies to all orders and all medication-related documentation that is handwritten (including free-text computer entry) or on preprinted forms.
†Exception: A "trailing zero" may be used only where required to demonstrate the level of precision of the value being reported, such as for laboratory results, imaging studies that report size of lesions, or catheter or tube sizes. It may not be used in medication orders or other medication-related documentation.
Source: *Official "Do not use" list.* Internet document available at www.jointcommission.org/assets/1/18/Do_Not_Use_List.pdf (accessed July 1, 2013).

RESEARCH IN PERINATAL NURSING

Research plays a vital role in the establishment of a maternity nursing science. Research can validate that nursing care makes a difference. For example, although prenatal care is clearly associated with healthier infants, no one knows exactly which nursing interventions produce this outcome. Many possible areas of research exist in maternity and women's health care. The clinician can identify problems in the health and health care of women and infants. Nurses should promote research funding and conduct research on maternity and women's health, especially concerning the effectiveness of nursing strategies for these patients.

Ethical Guidelines for Nursing Research

Research with perinatal patients may create ethical dilemmas for the nurse. For example, participating in research may cause additional stress to a woman concerned about outcomes of genetic testing or one who is waiting for an invasive procedure. Obtaining amniotic fluid samples or performing cordocentesis poses risks to the fetus. Nurses must protect the rights of human subjects (i.e., patients) in all of their research. For example, nurses may collect data on or care for patients who are participating in clinical trials. The nurse ensures that the participants are fully informed and aware of their rights as subjects. The nurse may be involved in determining whether the benefits of research outweigh the risks to the mother and the fetus. Following the ANA ethical guidelines in the conduct, dissemination, and implementation of nursing research helps nurses ensure that research is conducted ethically.

THE FAMILY IN CULTURAL AND COMMUNITY CONTEXT

Nursing Care Plan: Incorporating the Infant into the Family

The family and its **cultural context** play an important role in defining the work of maternity nurses. Despite modern stresses and strains, the family forms a social network that acts as a potent support system for its members. Family care-seeking behavior and relationships with providers are all influenced by culturally related health beliefs and values. Ultimately, all of these factors have the power to affect maternal and child health outcomes. The current emphasis in working with families is on wellness and empowerment for families to achieve control over their lives.

The Family in Society

The social context for the family can be viewed in relation to social and demographic trends that define the population as a whole. Current U.S. census data indicate that the racial and ethnic diversity of the population has grown dramatically in the last three decades. This increased diversity–first manifested among children and soon to be evident in the older population–is projected to increase in the future.

Each family sets up boundaries between itself and society. People are conscious of the difference between "family members" and "outsiders," or people without kinship status. Some families isolate themselves from the outside community; others have a wide community network to whom they can turn for help in times of stress. Although boundaries exist for every family, family members set up channels through which they interact with society. These channels also ensure that the family receives its share of social resources.

Family Organization and Structure

The **nuclear family** has long represented the traditional American family in which male and female partners and their children live as an independent unit, sharing roles, responsibilities, and economic resources (Fig. 1-4). In contemporary society this idealized family structure actually represents only a relatively small number of families. The **binuclear family** is an alternate form of the traditional nuclear family arrangement that results from divorce. Children of remarried parents then become members of both the maternal and paternal nuclear households. In joint custody the court assigns divorcing parents equal rights to and responsibilities for the minor child or children.

Reconstituted families, or blended families (i.e., those formed as the result of divorce and remarriage), consist of unrelated family members (stepparents, stepchildren, and stepsiblings) who join together to create a new household. These family groups frequently involve a biologic or adoptive parent whose spouse has not adopted the child.

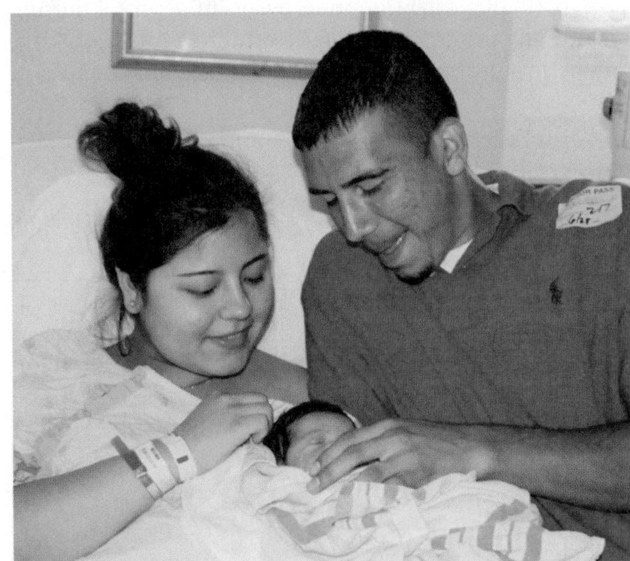

Fig. 1-4 Nuclear family. (Courtesy Cheryl Briggs, RN, Annapolis, MD.)

Many nuclear families have other relatives living in the same household. These **extended family** members may be grandparents, aunts or uncles, or other people related by blood (Fig. 1-5). For some groups, such as African-American and Latin-American women, the family network is an important resource in terms of preventive health behavior.

Single-parent families comprise an unmarried biologic or adoptive parent who may or may not be living with other adults. The single-parent family may result from the loss of a spouse by death, divorce, separation, or desertion; from either an unplanned or a planned pregnancy; or from the adoption of a child by an unmarried woman or man. This family structure has become a common and acceptable choice in society, with current estimates at one fifth of Caucasian families, one third of Hispanic families, and more than one half of African-American families in the United States. In many cases the single-parent family tends to be vulnerable economically and socially, creating an unstable and deprived environment for the growth potential of children. Single mothers are more likely to live in poverty and have poor perinatal outcomes.

Other family configurations, which are less well documented, include children in families whose parents are cohabiting and an increasing number of **homosexual (lesbian and gay) families,** who may live together with or without children. Children in homosexual families may be the offspring of previous heterosexual unions, conceived by one member of a lesbian couple through therapeutic insemination, or adopted.

FAMILY NURSING

Family plays a pivotal role in health care, representing the primary target of health care delivery for maternal and newborn nurses. The core concepts of patient- and family-centered care are dignity and respect, information sharing, participation, and collaboration (Johnson et al., 2008). When treating the patient and family with respect and dignity, health care providers listen to and honor perspectives and choices of the patient and family. They share information with families in ways that are positive, useful, timely, complete, and accurate. The family is supported in participating in the care and decision making at the level of their choice.

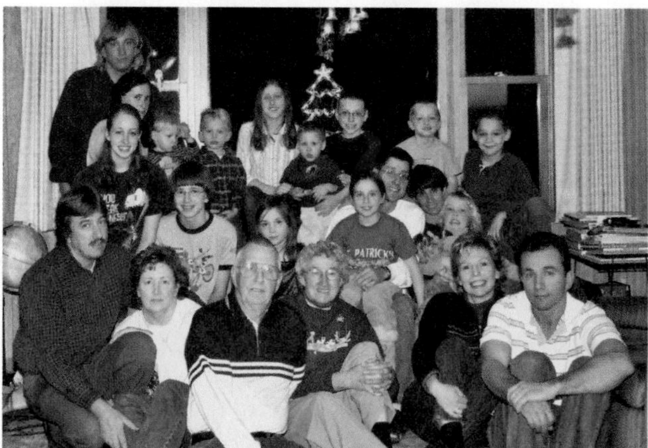

Fig. 1-5 Extended family. (Courtesy Rosemary Toohill, LeRoy, IL.)

Family Assessment

When selecting a family assessment framework, an appropriate model for a perinatal nurse is one that is a health-promoting rather than illness-care model. The low risk family can be assisted in promoting a healthy pregnancy, childbirth, and integration of the newborn into the family. The high risk perinatal family has illness-care needs, and the nurse may be able to meet those needs while also promoting the health of the childbearing family.

Family Theories

A family theory can be used to describe families and how the family unit responds to events both within and outside the family. Each family theory makes certain assumptions about the family and has inherent strengths and limitations. Most nurses use a combination of theories in their work with families. Application of theoretical concepts can guide assessment and interventions for the family.

Because so many variables affect ways of relating, the nurse must be aware that most family members will interact and communicate with each other in ways that are very different from those of the nurse's own family of origin. Most families will hold at least some beliefs about health that are very different from those of the nurse. In some instances, their beliefs will conflict with principles of health care management predominant in the Western health care system.

Graphic Representations of Families

A family **genogram** (family tree format depicting relationships of family members over at least three generations) (Fig. 1-6) provides valuable information about a family and can be placed in the nursing care plan for easy access by care providers. An ecomap, a graphic portrayal of social relationships of the patient and family, may also help the nurse understand the social environment of the family and identify support systems available to them (Fig. 1-7) (Rempel, Neufeld, & Kushner, 2007). Software is available to generate genograms and ecomaps (www.interpersonaluniverse.net).

CULTURAL FACTORS RELATED TO FAMILY HEALTH

Cultural Context of the Family

Culture of an individual is influenced by religion, environment, and historic events and plays a powerful role in the individual's behavior and patterns of human interaction.

Culture is not static; it is an ongoing process that influences people throughout their entire lives, from birth to death.

Cultural knowledge includes beliefs and values about each facet of life and is passed from one generation to the next. Cultural beliefs and traditions relate to food; language; religion; art, health, and healing practices; kinship relationships; and all other aspects of community, family, and individual life. Culture also has been shown to have a direct effect on health behaviors. Values, attitudes, and beliefs that are culturally acquired may influence perceptions of illness, as well as health care–seeking behavior and response to treatment. The impact of these influences must be assessed by health professionals in providing health care and developing effective intervention strategies. Cultural sensitivity, compassion, and a critical awareness of **family dynamics** and social stressors that affect health-related decision making are critical components in developing an effective plan of care.

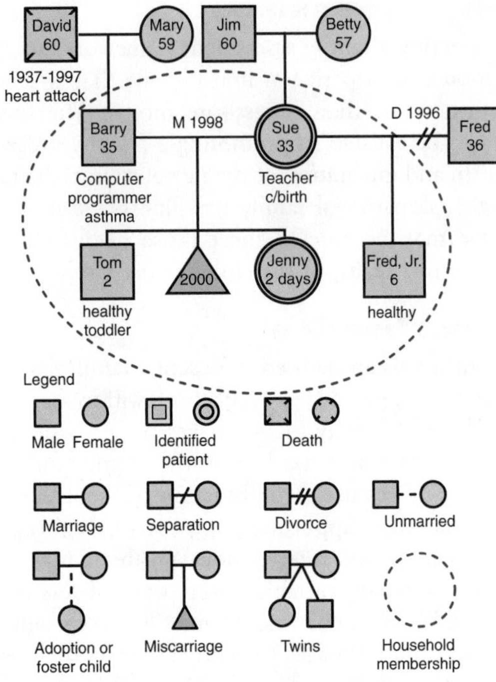

Fig. 1-6 Example of a family genogram.

Nurses must be aware that some factors may prevent some health care practitioners from providing optimal care, whereas others can enhance nursing practice. Understanding the concepts of ethnocentrism and cultural relativism may help nurses care for families in a multicultural society.

Ethnocentrism refers to the view that one's own culture's way of doing things is best. Although the United States and Canada are culturally diverse, the prevailing practice of health care is based on the beliefs and practices held by members of the dominant culture, primarily Caucasians of European descent. From this biomedical perspective, pregnancy and childbirth are viewed as processes with inherent risks that are most appropriately managed by using scientific knowledge and advanced technology.

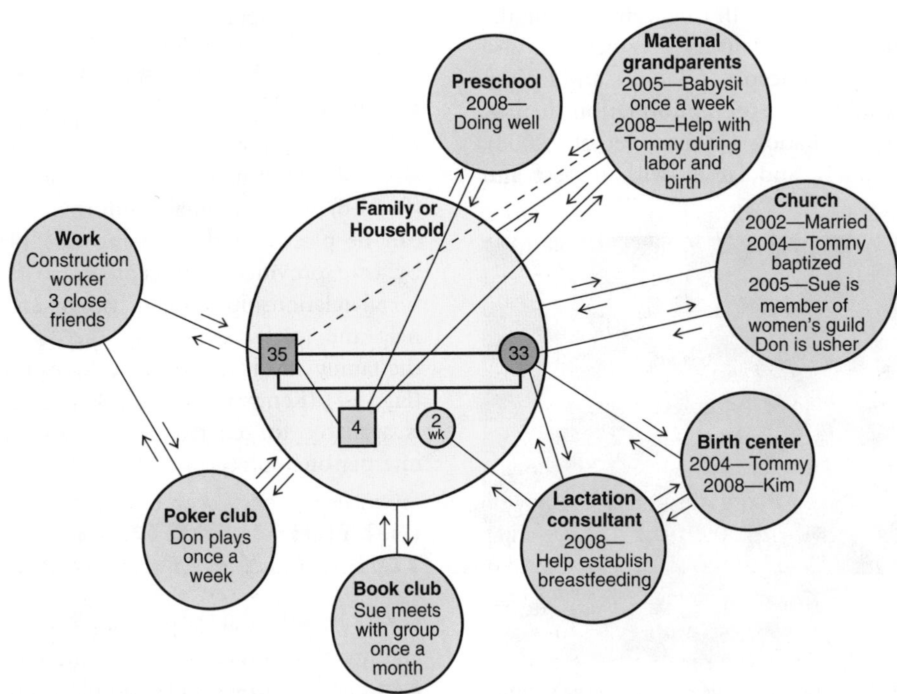

Fig. 1-7 Example of an ecomap. An ecomap describes social relationships and depicts available supports.

The medical perspective stands in direct contrast with the belief systems of many cultures. Among many women, birth is traditionally viewed as a completely normal process that can be managed with a minimum of involvement from health practitioners. When encountering behavior in women who are unfamiliar with the biomedical model, the nurse may become frustrated and impatient. The nurse may label the woman's behavior inappropriate and believe that it conflicts with *good* health practices. If the Western health care system provides the nurse's only standard for judgment, the behavior of the nurse is called ethnocentric.

Cultural relativism is the opposite of ethnocentrism. It refers to learning about and applying the standards of another's culture to activities within that culture. The nurse recognizes that people from different cultural backgrounds comprehend the same objects and situations differently. In other words, culture determines viewpoint.

Cultural relativism does not require nurses to accept the beliefs and values of another culture. Instead, nurses recognize that the behavior of others may be based on a system of logic different from their own. Cultural relativism affirms the uniqueness and value of every culture.

Childbearing Beliefs and Practices

Nurses working with childbearing families care for families from many different cultures and ethnic groups. To provide culturally competent care, the nurse must assess the beliefs and practices of patients. A nurse should consider all aspects of culture, including communication, space, time orientation, and family roles, when working with childbearing families.

Communication

Communication often creates the most challenging obstacle for nurses working with patients from diverse cultural groups. Communication is not merely the exchange of words. Instead, it involves (1) understanding the individual's language, including subtle variations in meaning and distinctive dialects; (2) appreciating individual differences in interpersonal style; and (3) accurately interpreting the volume of speech, as well as the meanings of touch and gestures. For example, members of some cultural groups tend to speak more loudly, with great emotion, and with vigorous and animated gestures when they are excited; this tendency is true whether their excitement is related to positive or negative events or emotions. Therefore the nurse should avoid rushing to judgment regarding a patient's intent when the patient is speaking, especially in a language not understood by the nurse. In these situations the nurse must avoid instantaneous responses that may well be based on an incorrect interpretation of the patient's gestures and meaning. Instead, the nurse should withhold an interpretation of what has been communicated until clarification of the patient's intent becomes possible. The nurse needs to enlist the assistance of a person who can help verify the patient's true intent and meaning of the communication (see Critical Thinking/Clinical Decision Making box).

Critical Thinking/Clinical Decision Making

Culturally Competent Care in the Emergency Department

Felicia, a 37-year-old woman, accompanied by her 16-year-old son, Jose, is admitted to the emergency department (ED) with profuse vaginal bleeding. Felicia's primary language is Spanish, and she speaks very little English; Jose is fluent in Spanish and English. No health care professionals present in the ED speak Spanish. The nurse assigned to care for Felicia must obtain a health history and perform an assessment. She wants to provide culturally competent care for Felicia.

1. Evidence—Does sufficient evidence exist to determine the extent to which culturally competent care exists?
2. Assumptions—What assumptions can be made about culturally competent care and the role language plays in providing that care?
   a. How the nurse, who speaks no Spanish, can effectively communicate with Felicia
   b. How the nurse can obtain a health history with questions about vaginal bleeding, sexual activity, and pregnancy if Jose is the only person available who speaks Spanish
   c. How the nurse can provide culturally competent teaching
   d. Appropriate teaching materials and resources; appropriate questions to gain information about sexual activity and possibility of pregnancy
3. What implications and priorities for nursing care can be drawn at this time?
4. Does the evidence objectively support your conclusion?
5. Are there alternative perspectives to your conclusion?

Use of interpreters

Inconsistencies between the language of patients and that of providers present a significant barrier to effective health care. Because of the diversity of cultures and languages within the United States and Canadian populations, health care agencies are increasingly seeking the services of interpreters (of oral communication from one language to another) or translators (of written words from one language to another) to bridge these gaps and fulfill their obligation for culturally and linguistically appropriate health care (Box 1-7). Finding the best possible interpreter in the circumstance is also critically important. A substantial number of personal attributes and qualifications contribute to an interpreter's potential to be effective. Ideally, interpreters should have the same native language and be

Critical Thinking Exercise: Cultural Health and the Family

Nursing Care Plan: The Family Newly Immigrated from a Non-English-Speaking Country

BOX 1-7

Working with an Interpreter

Step 1: Before the Interview
- Outline your statements and questions. List the key pieces of information you want or need to know.
- Learn something about the culture so that you can converse informally with the interpreter.

Step 2: Meeting with the Interpreter
- Introduce yourself to the interpreter and converse informally. This is the time to find out how well he or she speaks English. No matter how proficient or what age the interpreter is, be respectful. Some ways to show respect are to ask a cultural question to acknowledge that you can learn from the interpreter or learn one word or phrase from the interpreter.
- Emphasize that you want the patient to ask questions because some cultures consider this inappropriate behavior.
- Make sure that the interpreter is comfortable with the technical terms you need to use. If not, take some time to explain them.

Step 3: During the Interview
- Ask your questions and explain your statements (see Step 1).
- Make sure that the interpreter understands which parts of the interview are most important. You usually have limited time with the interpreter, and you want to have adequate time at the end for patient questions.
- Try to get a *feel* for how much is *getting through.* No matter what the language is, if in relating information to the patient the interpreter uses far fewer or far more words than you do, *something else* is going on.
- Stop every now and then and ask the interpreter, "How is it going?" You may not get a totally accurate answer, but you will have emphasized to the interpreter your strong desire to focus on the task at hand. If language problems exist: (1) speak *slowly,* (2) use gestures (e.g., fingers to count or point to body parts), and (3) use pictures.
- Ask the interpreter to elicit questions. This may be difficult, but it is worth the effort.
- Identify cultural issues that may conflict with your requests or instructions.
- Use the interpreter to help problem solve or at least give insight into possibilities for solutions.

Step 4: After the Interview
- Speak to the interpreter and try to get an idea of what went well and what could be improved. This will help you to be more effective with this or another interpreter.
- Make notes on what you learned for your future reference or to help a colleague.

Remember:
Your interview is a *collaboration* between you and the interpreter. *Listen* as well as speak.

Notes
- The interpreter may be a child, grandchild, or sibling of the patient. Be sensitive to the fact that the child is playing an adult role.
- Be sensitive to cultural and situational differences (e.g., an interview with someone from urban Germany will likely be different from an interview with someone from a transitional refugee camp).
- Younger females telling older males what to do may be a problem for both a female nurse and a female interpreter. This is not the time to pioneer new gender relations. Be aware that in some cultures it is difficult for a woman to talk about some topics with a husband or a father present.

Courtesy Elizabeth Whalley, PhD, San Francisco State University.

of the same religion or have the same country of origin as the patient. Interpreters should have specific health-related language skills and experience and help bridge the language and cultural barriers between the patient and the health care provider. The person interpreting should also be mature enough to be trusted with private information. However, because the nature of nursing care is not always predictable, and because nursing care that is provided in a home or community setting does not always allow expert, experienced, or mature adult interpreters, ideal interpretive services are sometimes impossible to find when they are needed. In crisis or emergency situations, or when family members are having extreme stress or emotional upset, using relatives, neighbors, or children as interpreters may be necessary. If this situation occurs, the nurse must ensure that the patient is in agreement and comfortable with using the available interpreter to assist. Language line (www.languageline.com) is an interpretation service available for telephone, video, and on-site interpretation by trained medical interpreters. The service provides both translation and interpretation services in 176 languages.

When using an interpreter, the nurse respects the family by creating an atmosphere of respect and privacy. Questions should be addressed to the woman and not to the interpreter. Even though an interpreter will of necessity be exposed to sensitive and privileged information about the family, the nurse should take care to ensure that confidentiality is maintained. A quiet location free from interruptions is the ideal place for interpretive services to take place. In addition, culturally and linguistically appropriate educational materials that are easy to read, with appropriate text and graphics, should be available to assist the woman and her family in understanding health care information.

Personal space

Cultural traditions define the appropriate personal space for various social interactions. Although the need for personal space varies from person to person and with the situation, the actual physical dimensions of comfort zones differ from culture to culture. Actions such as touching, placing the woman in proximity to others, taking away personal possessions, and making decisions for the woman can decrease personal security and heighten anxiety. Conversely, respecting the need for distance allows the woman to maintain control over personal space and support personal autonomy, thereby increasing her sense of security. For example, many Asian groups have reserved attitudes about physical contact, and touching a woman may at times create anxiety when health care is delivered. Nurses must touch patients. However, they frequently do so without any awareness of the emotional distress they may be causing.

Time orientation

Time orientation is a fundamental way in which culture affects health behaviors. People in cultural groups may be relatively more oriented to past, present, or future. Those who focus on the past strive to maintain tradition or the status quo and have little motivation for formulating future goals. In contrast, individuals who focus primarily on the present neither plan for the future nor consider the experiences of the past. These individuals do not necessarily adhere to strict schedules and are often described as "living for the moment" or "marching to the beat of their own drummer." Individuals oriented to the future maintain a focus on achieving long-term goals.

The time orientation of the childbearing family may affect nursing care. For example, talking to a family about bringing the infant to the clinic for follow-up examinations (events in the future) may be difficult for the family that is focused on the present concerns of day-to-day survival. Because a family with a future-oriented sense of time plans far in advance and thinks about the long-term consequences of present actions, they may be more likely to return as scheduled for follow-up visits. Despite the differences in time orientation, each family may be equally concerned for the well-being of its newborn.

Family roles

Family roles involve the expectations and behaviors associated with a member's position in the family (e.g., mother, father, grandparent). Social class and cultural norms also affect these roles, with distinct expectations for men and women clearly determined by social norms. For example, culture may influence whether a man actively participates in pregnancy and childbirth, yet maternity care practitioners working in the Western health care system expect fathers to be involved. This circumstance can create a significant conflict between the nurse and the role expectations of very traditional Mexican or Arab families, who usually view the birthing experience as a female affair. The way that health care practitioners manage such a family's care molds its experience and perception of the Western health care system.

In maternity nursing the nurse supports and nurtures the beliefs that promote physical or emotional adaptation to childbearing. However, if certain beliefs might be harmful, the nurse should carefully explore them with the woman and use them in the reeducation and modification process. Nurses should exercise sensitivity in working with every family, being careful to assess the ways in which they apply their own mixture of cultural traditions.

Developing Cultural Competence

Cultural competence has many names and definitions, all of which have subtle shades of difference but which are essentially the same: multiculturalism, cultural sensitivity, and intercultural effectiveness. Cultural competence involves acknowledging, respecting, and appreciating ethnic, cultural, and linguistic diversity. Culturally competent professionals act in ways that meet the needs of the patient and are respectful of ways and traditions that may be very different from their own. In today's society, nurses must develop more than technical skill. At every level of preparation and throughout their professional lives, nurses must engage in a continual process of developing and refining attitudes and behaviors that will promote culturally competent care.

Cultural Considerations

Questions to Ask to Determine Cultural Expectations about Childbearing

1. What do you and your family believe you should do to remain healthy during pregnancy?
2. What are the things you can or cannot do to improve your health and the health of your baby?
3. Do you have any special dietary needs or foods that you cannot eat?
4. Do you or your family have concerns or fears about hospitalization for childbirth?
5. Whom do you want with you during your labor?
6. What actions are important for you and your family to take after the baby's birth?
7. What do you and your family expect from the nurse or nurses caring for you?
8. How will family members participate in your pregnancy, childbirth, and parenting?

In addition to issues of preserving and promoting human dignity, the development of cultural competence is of equal importance in terms of health outcomes. Nurses who relate effectively with patients are able to motivate them in the direction of health-promoting behaviors. Rust and colleagues (2006) developed a CRASH Course in Cultural Competency for health care personnel. This course includes the essential components of culturally competent health care (Box 1-8).

One strategy to teach cultural competence in nursing education is to have international clinical placements or experiences (Perry & Mander, 2005; Sloand, Bower, & Groves, 2008). In such placements, students may experi-

BOX 1-8

CRASH Course in Cultural Competence

- **C**ulture
- Show **R**espect
- **A**ssess or **A**ffirm differences
- Show **S**ensitivity and **S**elf-awareness
- Do it all with **H**umility

Source: Rust, G., Kondwani, K., Martinez, R., Dansie, R., Wong, W., Fry-Johnson, Y., et al. (2006). A CRASH-course in cultural competence. *Ethnicity and Diseases, 16* (2 Suppl 3), 29-36.

ence being in the minority, not knowing the language, eating unfamiliar foods, not having a ready source of safe drinking water, using primitive bathroom facilities, and having a shortage of equipment and supplies. Students come away with an appreciation for the problems of non-native speakers having limited access to care and being dependent on health care workers who may not appreciate the stress and fears of being cared for in an unfamiliar environment.

Integrating Cultural Competence with the Nursing Care Plan

Critical Thinking Exercise: Community Resources for Families

In many cultures, family members make most of the decisions for the patient; therefore the central relationship between the nurse and the patient is mediated directly by the family. The nurse must recognize the cultural importance of family in supporting the patient, guiding decision making, and preserving cultural integrity in the health care interaction.

Nursing care is delivered in multiple cultural contexts. These contexts include the cultures of the patient, the nurse, and the health care system, as well as the larger culture of the society in which health care is delivered. If any of these cultural groups is excluded from the nurse's assessment and consideration, nursing care may fail to achieve its goals and may be culturally insensitive.

COMMUNITY AND HOME CARE

Nursing Care Plan: Community and Home Care

A major shift in health care delivery is an increased emphasis on brief hospital stays that serve to reduce the financial burden for individuals, agencies, and insurance carriers. By minimizing inpatient length of stay, much of acute care nursing has been transferred to home-based nursing services in local communities demonstrating the need for comprehensive, community-based care that is culturally relevant for mothers, infants, and families.

In the community, health care ranges from individual care to group and community services and from primary prevention to tertiary care experiences and home visiting. Depending on the needs of the individual family unit, independent self-management, ambulatory care, home care, low risk hospitalization, or specialized intensive care may be appropriate at different points along this continuum (see Fig. 1-9).

In community-based health care, both the aggregate (a group of people who have shared characteristics) and the population become the focus of intervention. Health professionals are required not only to determine health priorities, but also to develop successful plans of care to be delivered in the health clinic, the community health center, or the patient's home. This home- and community-based delivery system presents unique challenges for perinatal and maternity nurses.

COMMUNITY HEALTH PROMOTION

Best practices in community-based health initiatives involve both understanding of community relationships and resources and participation of community leaders. The emphasis on community-based health promotion has grown in recent years, with recognition that many health issues require the collaborative efforts of a diverse community network to achieve public health goals (Cottrell, Girvan, & McKenzie, 2006). These efforts are particularly relevant in relation to maternal-newborn health, which is affected by multiple public health issues: lack of health insurance, teen pregnancy, substance abuse, and the consequences of inadequate prenatal care.

Assessing the Community

Community assessment is a complex but well-defined process through which the unique characteristics of the populations and their special needs are identified to plan and evaluate health services for the community as a whole. The purpose of this process is to identify direct service and advocacy needs of the targeted aggregate or group and to improve health for the community.

In community health assessment, data are collected, analyzed, and used to educate and mobilize communities, develop priorities, garner resources, and plan actions to improve public health. Many models and frameworks of community assessment are available, but the actual process often depends on the extent and nature of the assessment to be performed, the time and resources available, and the way the information is to be used (www.assessnow.info/resources/models-of-community-health-assessment).

Data Collection and Sources of Community Health Data

Measures of community health include access to care, level of provider services available, and other social and economic factors. Consideration of individual, interpersonal, community, organizational, and policy-level data and the interaction of these factors are important in providing a comprehensive framework for community health promotion. A community assessment model (Fig. 1-8) is

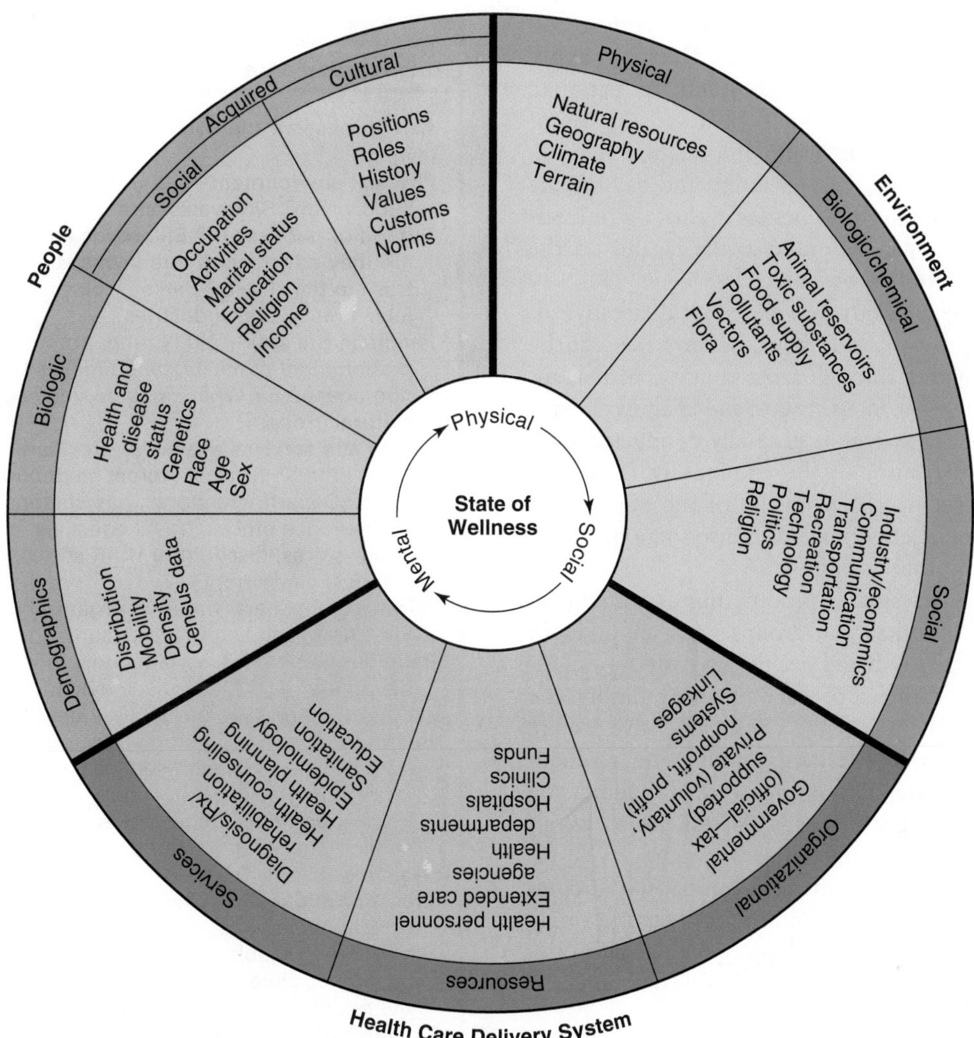

Fig. 1-8 Community health assessment wheel. (From Clemen-Stone, S. [2002]. Community assessment and diagnosis. In S. Clemen-Stone, S. McGuire, & D. Eigsti [Eds.], *Comprehensive community health nursing: Family, aggregate, and community practice,* [6th ed.] St. Louis: Mosby.)

often used to provide a comprehensive guide to data collection.

The most critical community indicators of perinatal health relate to access to care, maternal mortality, infant mortality, LBW, first trimester prenatal care, and rates for mammography, Papanicolaou tests, and other similar screening tests.

Access to health care relates not only to the *availability* of health department services, hospitals, public clinics, or other sources of care, but also to *accessibility* of care. In many areas where facilities and providers are available, geographic and transportation barriers render the care inaccessible for certain populations. This circumstance is particularly true in rural areas or other remote locations. The trend is growing in the United States to have walk-in clinics in grocery and drug stores, which are easily accessible locations.

Health departments at the city, county, and state level are a valuable resource for annual reports of births and deaths. Maternal and infant death rates are particularly important because they reflect health outcomes that may be preventable. Local health departments also compile extensive statistics about birth complications, causes of death, and leading causes of morbidity and mortality for each age group.

Information from individual census tracts within a community helps to identify subpopulations or aggregates whose needs may differ from those of the larger community. For example, women at high risk for inadequate prenatal care according to age, race, and ethnic or cultural group may be readily identified, and outreach activities may be targeted appropriately.

Other sources of useful information are hospitals and voluntary health agencies. The perinatal health nurse also may explore existing community health program reports, records of preventive health screenings, and other informal data. Established programs often provide reliable indicators of the health-promotion and disease-prevention characteristics of the population.

Professional publications are a rich and readily accessible source of information for all nurses. The Internet has increased the availability and accessibility of national, state, and local health data as well. However, the use of Internet-based resources for health information requires some caution, given that data reliability and validity are difficult to verify. (Some guidelines for evaluation of Internet health resources can be found at the Health on the Net Foundation website www.hon.ch.)

Data collection methods may be either qualitative or quantitative and may include visual surveys that can be completed by walking through a community, participant observation, interviews, focus groups, and analysis of existing data. A **walking survey** is generally conducted by a walk-through observation of the community (Box 1-9), taking note of specific characteristics of the population, economic and social environment, transportation, health care services, and other resources.

As part of the assessment process, nurses working in multiethnic and multicultural groups need an in-depth assessment of culturally based health behaviors.

Analysis and synthesis of data obtained during the assessment process help generate a comprehensive picture of the community's health status, needs, and problem areas, as well as its strengths and resources for addressing these concerns. The goals of this process are to assign priorities to community health needs and to develop a plan of action for correcting them. A comparison of community health data with state and national statistics may be useful in the identification of appropriate target populations and interventions to improve health outcomes.

BOX 1-9

Community Walk Through

As you observe the community, take note of the following:

Physical environment—Older neighborhood or newer subdivision? Sidewalks, streets, and buildings in good or poor repair? Billboards and signs? What are they advertising? Are lawns kept up? Is there trash in the streets? Parks or playgrounds? Parking lots? Empty lots? Industries?

People in the area—Old, young, homeless, children, predominant ethnicity, language? Is the population homogeneous? What signs do you see of different cultural groups?

Stores and services available—Restaurants: chain, local, ethnic? Grocery stores: neighborhood or chain? Department stores, gas stations, real estate or insurance offices, travel agencies, pawn shops, liquor stores, discount or thrift stores, newspaper stands?

Social—Clubs, bars, fraternal organizations (e.g., Elks, American Legion), museums?

Religious—Churches, synagogues, mosques? What denominations? Do you see evidence of their use other than on religious or holy days?

Health services—Drug stores, doctors' offices, clinics, dentists, mental health services, veterinarians, urgent care facilities, hospitals, shelters, nursing homes, home health agencies, public health services, traditional healers (e.g., herbalists, palmists)?

Transportation—Cars, bus, taxi, light rail, sidewalks, bicycle paths, access for disabled persons?

Education—Schools, before- and after-school programs, child care, libraries, bookstores? What is the reputation of the schools?

Government—What is the governance structure? Does the town or city have a mayor? City council? Are meetings open to the public? Do you see signs of political activity (e.g., posters, campaign signs)?

Safety—How safe is the community? What is the crime rate? What types of crimes are committed? Are police visible? Is a fire station nearby?

Evaluation of the community based on your observations—What is your impression of the community? Is the environment pleasing? Are services and transportation adequate? How difficult is it for residents to obtain needed services (i.e., how far do they have to travel)? Would you want to live in this community? Why or why not?

VULNERABLE POPULATIONS IN THE COMMUNITY

Assessment of population health includes indicators related to diverse groups and cultures, particularly disenfranchised or "vulnerable" community members (www.crosshealth.com). Health disparities are conditions that disproportionately affect certain racial, ethnic, or other groups. African-Americans, Hispanics or Latinos, Native Americans, Pacific Islanders, and Asian-Americans are all considered **vulnerable populations** because they are more likely to have poor health and die prematurely.

Women

Women comprise 51% of the U.S. population, representing a very diverse and largely "at-risk" group in relation to health (USDHHS, 2007). One of the primary factors compromising women's health is lack of access to acceptable-quality health care, which may take many forms: lack of health insurance, living in a medically underserved area, or an inability to obtain needed services, particularly basic services such as prenatal care. For example, some rural areas have few obstetricians, pediatricians, and nurse-midwives; women may have to travel hundreds of miles for this kind of care. Women often have lower incomes and less education and are therefore considered at high risk. Infant mortality is nearly two times higher for mothers without a high school education when compared with women who have this level of education.

Women with underlying health conditions are at especially high risk for poor obstetric outcomes for both themselves and their infants. (See previous discussion of Increase in High Risk Pregnancies, p. 7.) These are the patients for whom the community-based perinatal nurse will be providing care, and their needs are complex, demanding high levels of expertise and skill.

Within the larger group of vulnerable women, a considerable number of subgroups present challenges to the community-based perinatal nurse.

Adolescent girls

The adolescent population in the United States generally is considered healthy. Yet this group of women is often vulnerable because of high risk behaviors. Adolescent girls, especially those from minorities and low-income or disrupted families, are more likely to engage in early sexual activity and other high risk behaviors, with both immediate and long-term health consequences. Female adolescents in the United States also experience a high rate of teen pregnancy, with 4 out of 10 becoming pregnant before the age of 20 years. Sexually transmitted infection (STI) rates, primarily chlamydia and gonorrhea, are highest among adolescent and young adult women (USDHHS, 2007).

Although adolescents are concerned about becoming pregnant, they still engage in unprotected sex. Adolescents also use a variety of sources for health information (i.e., the media, friends, and sex education); yet they are often misinformed, particularly about STIs and HIV transmission. These factors have significant implications for perinatal outcomes and emphasize the importance of aggressive prevention programs and community outreach related to sexuality, teen pregnancy, and substance abuse.

Older women

In 2005 the U.S. population consisted of 20.4 million women over the age of 65 years. This figure represents over 57% of the population ages 65 and older. Although women have a longer life expectancy than men, they are more likely to have chronic illnesses, less likely to use preventive services, and ultimately spend more on health care by comparison (USDHHS, 2007).

However, a great deal of emphasis has been placed on preventive interventions that are effective in delaying or controlling age-related changes. Improving self-management activities such as diet and exercise are important health-promotion elements for this population.

Incarcerated women

The number of incarcerated women in the United States has continued to climb in recent years, increasing at a significantly greater rate than for men. In 2010, nearly 113,000 women were in prison, with the highest number of these prisoners being non-Hispanic black women (Sipes, 2012). Many of these women report a history of sexual and physical abuse.

The lifestyle choices of this group, including risky sexual relationships, illicit drug use, and smoking, place them at high risk for STIs, HIV, and AIDS; other chronic and communicable diseases; and complicated pregnancies (USDHHS, 2007).

Women and the migrant work force

An estimated three million migrant and seasonal farm workers reside in the United States, 21% of whom are women. Diverse ethnic and cultural groups are represented among migrant workers; however, 75% of these workers were born in Mexico (U.S. Department of Labor, 2005).

Numerous reproductive health issues exist for migrant women, including less consistent use of contraception and increased rates of STIs. Migrants are less likely to receive early prenatal care and have a greater incidence of inadequate weight gain during pregnancy than do other poor women.

Primary health care services are largely provided by a sizable number of migrant health centers, of which more than 400 are scattered throughout the United States. Routine prenatal care and screening and treatment for hypertension and diabetes are provided. Community health nurses frequently encounter the challenges of providing culturally and linguistically appropriate care while facing numerous health issues.

Homeless women

Homelessness among women is an increasing social and health issue in the United States. Although exact numbers are unknown, estimates suggest that women make up one third of America's two to three million homeless people. As women are increasingly affected by poverty, homelessness is becoming more prevalent for families and children, particularly among rural populations.

Health issues among the homeless are numerous and result primarily from a lack of preventive care and resources in general. Homeless women face many health issues, related both to lifestyle factors and to the vulnerability resulting from being homeless. In addition to extreme poverty, women are at increased risk for illness and injury; many have been victims of domestic abuse, assault, and rape.

Although little is known about pregnancy in this population, approximately 20% of women do become pregnant while homeless. Conversely, pregnancy and recent birth are highly correlated with becoming homeless (American College of Obstetricians and Gynecologists [ACOG], 2005). In addition to risk factors related to inadequate nutrition, inadequate weight gain, anemia, bleeding problems, and preterm birth, homeless women face multiple barriers to prenatal care: transportation, distance, and wait times. Most women also underuse available prenatal services. The unsafe environment and high risk lifestyles often result in adverse perinatal outcomes.

Refugees and immigrants

Along with their profound resilience and determination, refugees and immigrants have brought rich diversity to the United States in several important dimensions, including cultural heritage and customs, economic productivity, and enhanced national vitality. At the same time, multiple challenges accompany the dramatic influx of individuals and families from other countries.

Although 73% of immigrants are legal citizens, this population is disproportionately affected by health disparities related to cultural and language barriers, no usual source of care, and lack of insurance. Women without U.S. citizenship are less likely to have a usual source of care (26.1%) and are more likely to be without health insurance coverage (45.5%). Nearly 25% of these women have not seen a health care provider in the past year (USDHHS, 2007).

Refugee status imposes a particular type of vulnerability on affected individuals and groups. In general, refugees are more likely to live in poverty than are immigrants. Over time, health disparities that adversely affect health and well-being actually decline for the immigrant population as they become part of American society.

Individuals with low literacy

Individuals and groups who have less than a high school education or for whom English is a second language often lack the skills necessary to seek medical care and function adequately in the health care setting. Communication barriers may affect access to care, particularly in such areas as making appointments, applying for services, and obtaining transportation.

Health literacy involves a spectrum of abilities, ranging from reading an appointment slip to interpreting medication instructions (www.hsph.harvard.edu/healthliteracy). Disparities in preventive care, early screening for cancer, and use of health care services, particularly among minority women, have also been linked to language barriers (Ferguson, 2008).

Health literacy must be viewed as a component of culturally and linguistically competent care. These skills must be assessed routinely to recognize a problem and accommodate patients with limited literacy skills.

HOME CARE IN THE COMMUNITY

Home health care is an important component of health care delivery along the perinatal **continuum of care** (Fig. 1-9). The growing demand for home health care is based on several factors:

- Interest in family birthing alternatives
- Shortened hospital stays
- New technologies that facilitate home-based assessments and treatments
- Reimbursement by third-party payers

As health care costs continue to rise, and because millions of American families lack health insurance, the demand for innovative, cost-effective methods of health care delivery in the community becomes greater. The integration of clinical services changes the focus of care to a continuum of services that is increasingly community based.

COMMUNITY ACTIVITY

Make an appointment with the clinic staff to visit a community health clinic that serves pregnant women. What are the qualifications of the clinic's staff (i.e., does the clinic have registered nurses, licensed practical or vocational nurses, nutritionists, social workers, childbirth educators, lactation consultants)? Is a laboratory available? What clientele does the clinic serve (i.e., what racial and ethnic groups are served)? Is the staff representative of those racial and ethnic groups? Is the staff bilingual? Are educational materials available in languages of the women served by the clinic? Is the clinic located near public transportation for ease of access? Is the setting "friendly" (i.e., available reading materials, a play area for children, a restroom, a drinking fountain, a public telephone)? What could improve the setting? Would you be willing to seek care in the clinic?

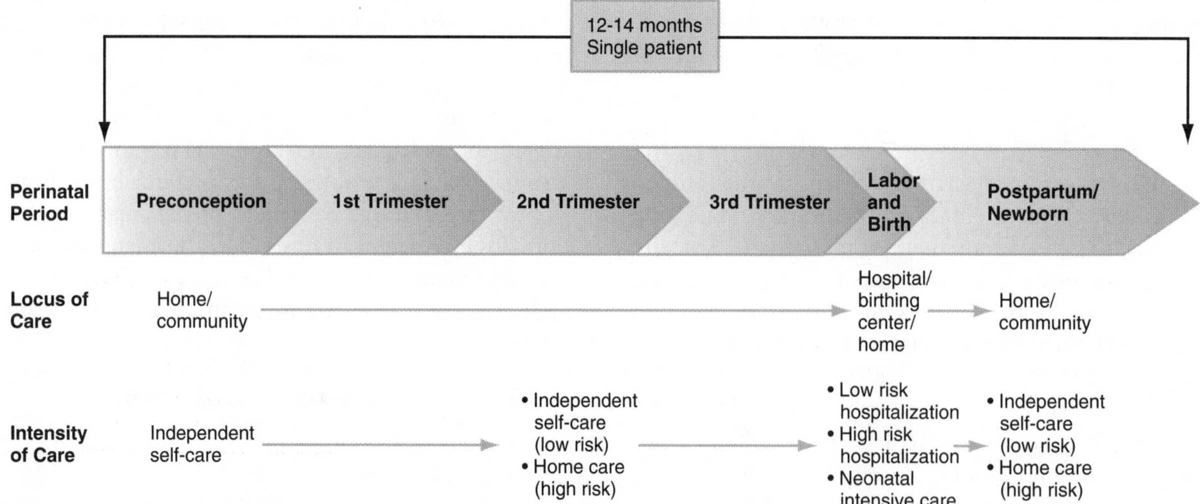

Fig. 1-9 Perinatal continuum of care.

Telephonic nursing care through services such as *warm lines,* nurse advice lines, and telephonic nursing assessments is a valuable means of managing health care problems and bridging the gaps among acute, outpatient, and home care services. Some providers are using the Internet to communicate with patients who have an Internet service provider.

Nursing care that occurs by telephone is interactive and responsive to immediate health care questions about particular health care needs. Warm lines are telephone lines that are offered as a community service to provide new parents with support, encouragement, and basic parenting education. Nurse advice lines, or toll-free nurse consultation services, are often supported by third-party payers or by health maintenance organization or managed care organization nurse case managers and are designed to provide answers to medical questions. Because of liability concerns, some agencies require that nurses staffing answer lines use a scripted answer to questions so that it is known exactly what advice was given; documentation supports the content of advice given.

KEY POINTS

- Maternity nursing encompasses care of women and their infants and families during the childbearing cycle.
- Nurses caring for women can play an active role in shaping health care systems to be responsive to the needs of contemporary women.
- Childbirth practices have changed to become more family focused and to allow alternatives in care.
- Canada ranks twenty-fourth and the United States ranks twenty-sixth among industrialized nations in infant mortality.
- Integrative medicine combines modern technology with ancient healing practices and encompasses the whole body, mind, and spirit.
- Perinatal practice is increasingly evidence based.
- *Healthy People 2010* provides goals for maternal and infant health; *Healthy People 2020* is currently in preparation.
- Ethical concerns have multiplied with increasing use of technology and scientific advances.
- Contemporary American society recognizes and accepts a variety of family forms.
- The family is a social network that acts as an important support system for its members.
- Family theories provide nurses with useful guidelines for understanding family function.
- Family socioeconomics, response to stress, and culture are key factors influencing family health.
- The reproductive beliefs and practices of a culture are embedded in its economic, religious, kinship, and political structures.
- To provide quality care to women in their childbearing years and beyond, nurses should be aware of the cultural beliefs and practices important to individual families.
- A community is defined as a locality-based entity composed of systems of societal institutions, informal groups, and aggregates that are interdependent, the function of which is to meet a wide variety of collective needs.
- Of necessity, most changes aimed at improving community health involve partnerships among community residents and health workers.
- Methods of collecting data useful to the nurse working in the community include walking surveys, analysis of existing data, informant interviews, and participant observation.
- Vulnerable populations are groups of people who are at increased risk for developing physical, mental, or social health problems.
- Telephonic nurse advice lines, telephonic nursing assessments, and warm lines are low-cost health care services that facilitate continuous patient education, support, and health care decision making, even though health care is delivered in multiple sites.

Audio Chapter Summaries Access an audio summary of these Key Points on evolve

References

Agency for Healthcare Research and Quality. (2000). *20 Tips to help prevent medical errors: Patient Fact Sheet*: AHRQ Publication No. 00-PO38. (2000). Rockville, MD: Agency for Healthcare Research and Quality. Available at www.ahrq.gov/consumer/20tips.htm (accessed February 25, 2009).

American College of Obstetricians and Gynecologists. (2005). ACOG committee opinion, number 312, August 2005: Healthcare for homeless women. *Obstetrics & Gynecology*, *106*, 429-434.

American Nurses Association. (2008). *ANA's Health System Reform Agenda.* Silver Spring, MD. Internet document available at http://www.nursingworld.org/MainMenuCategories/HealthcareandPolicyIssues/HealthSystemReform/Agenda/ANAsHealthSystemReformAgenda.aspx (accessed June 7, 2009).

Association of Women's Health, Obstetric, and Neonatal Nurses (AWHONN). (2009). *Standards for professional nursing practice in the care of women and newborns* (7th ed). Washington, DC: AWHONN.

Association of Women's Health, Obstetric, and Neonatal Nurses (AWHONN). (2002). *Standards for professional perinatal nursing practice and certification in Canada.* Washington, DC: AWHONN.

Banks, E., Meirik, O., Farley, T., Akande, O., Bathija, H., Ali, M. (2006). Female genital mutilation and obstetric outcome: WHO collaborative prospective study in six African countries. *Lancet*, *367*(9525), 1835-1841.

Calvo, A. (2006). *HRSA Health disparities collaborative: Executive Summary–Septem-*

ber, 2006. Internet document available at www.healthdisparities.net/hdc/html/home.aspx (accessed February 25, 2009).

Chu, S. Y., Bachman, D. J., Callaghan, W. M., Whitlock, E. P., Dietz, P. M., Berg, C. J., et al. (2008). Association between obesity during pregnancy and increased use of health care. *New England Journal of Medicine*, *358*(14), 1444-1453.

Cottrell, R., Girvan, J., & McKenzie, J. (2006). *Health promotion and education* (3rd ed.). San Francisco: Pearson Benjamin Cummings.

Cronenwett, L., Sherwood, G., Barnsteiner, J., et al. (2007). Quality and safety education for nurses. *Nursing Outlook*, *55*(3), 122-131.

DeNavas-Walt, C., Proctor, B. D., & Smith, J. (2007). *US Census Bureau, Current Population Reports, P60-233, Income poverty, and health insurance coverage in the United States: 2006*. Washington, DC: US Government Printing Office.

DeNavas-Walt, C., Proctor, B., & Smith, J. (2011). *U.S. Census Bureau, Current Population Reports, P60-239, Income poverty, and health insurance coverage in the United States: 2010*. Washington, DC: U.S. Government Printing Office.

Ferguson, B. (2008). Health literacy and health disparities. The role they play in maternal and child health. *Nursing for Women's Health*, *12* (4), 286-298.

Flegal, K. M., Carroll, M. D., Ogden, C. L., et al. (2010). Prevalence and trends in obesity among US adults, 1999-2008. *Journal of the American Medical Association*, *303*(3), 235-241.

French, J. (2006). Medical errors and patient safety in health care. *Canadian Journal of Medical Radiation Technology*, *37*(4), 9-13.

Gauthier, A., & Serber, M. (2005). *A need to transform the US health care system: Improving access, quality, and efficiency*, The Commonwealth Fund, October 3, 2005. Internet document available at www.commonwealthfund.org/publications/publications_show.htm?doc_id=302833 (accessed February 25, 2009).

Harrison, P., & Karlberg, J. (2004). *Prison and jail inmates at midyear 2003*. Bureau of Justice Statistics Bulletin. Washington, DC: US Department of Justice.

Heron, M., Sutton P., Xu, J., et al. (2010). Annual summary of vital statistics 2007. *Pediatrics*, *125*(1), 4-15.

Institute of Medicine. (2003). *Health professions education: A bridge to quality*. Washington, DC: National Academies Press.

The Joint Commission. (2011). *Sentinal events, 2010*. www.jointcommission.org/assets/1/6/2011_CAMAC_SE.pdf.

Johnson, B., Abraham, M., Conway, J., Simmons, L., Edgman-Levitan, S., Sodomka, P., et al. (2008). *Partnering with patients and families to design a patient- and family-centered health care system*, Bethesda, MD: Institute for Family-Centered Care.

Jones, W. K. (2008). *Safe motherhood at a glance: Promoting health for women before, during, and after pregnancy*. Atlanta, GA: USDHHS, CDC. Internet document available at www.cdc.gov/nccdphp/publications/aag/pdf/drh.pdf (accessed February 25, 2009).

Kochanek, K. D., Kirmeyer, S. E., Martin, J. A., et al. (2012). Annual summary of vital statistics 2009. *Pediatrics*, *129*, 338-348.

Martin, J. A., Hamilton, B. E., Sutton, P. D., Ventura, S. J., Menacker, F., Kirmeyer, S., et al. Centers for Disease Control and Prevention National Center for Health Statistics National Vital Statistics System. (2007). Births: Final data for 2005. *National Vital Statistics Reports*, *56*(6), 1-104.

Martin, J. A., Hamilton, B. E., Ventura, M. A., et al. (2011). *Births: Final data for 2009, National Vital Statistics Reports*, *60*(1). Hyattsville, MD: National Center for Health Statistics.

National Quality Forum (NQF). (2010). *Safe practices for better healthcare–2010 update: A consensus report*. Washington, DC: NQF.

Obama chooses UND'S Mary Wakefield as Health Resources and Services Administration Leader. (February 20, 2009). Internet document available at www.GrandForksHerald.com/event/article/id/107444 (accessed February 26, 2009).

O'Reilly, K. B. (2008). *No pay for "never event" errors becoming standard*. Internet document available at www.ama-assn.orog/amednews/2008/01/07/prsc0107.htm (accessed June 5, 2009).

Rempel, G., Neufeld, A., & Kushner, K. (2007). Interactive use of genograms and ecomaps in family caregiving research. *Family Nursing*, *13*(4), 403-419.

Roehr, B. (2008). Pressure mounts to cut US spending on health care. *BMJ*, *336*(7638), 236-237.

Rust, G., Kondwani, K., Martinez, R., Dansie, R., Wong, W., Fry-Johnson, Y., et al. (2006). A crash-course in cultural competence. *Ethnicity and Disease*, *16*(2 Suppl 3), 29-36.

Satcher, D., & Higginbotham, E.J. (2008). The public health approach to eliminating disparities in health. *American Journal of Public Health*, *98*(3), S8-S11.

Shalo, S. (2007). In the news. The price of committing error. *American Journal of Nursing*, *107*(8), 20.

Sipes, L. A. (2012). *Statistics on women offenders*. www.corrections.com/news/article/30166-statistics-on-women-offenders.

Sloand, E., Bower, K., & Groves, S. (2008). Challenges and benefits of international clinical placements in public health nursing. *Nurse Educator*, *33*(1), 35-38.

Squires, D. A. (2012). Explaining high health care spending in the United States: An international comparison of supply, utilization, prices, and quality. *The Commonwealth Fund*, 10.

Tiedje, L. B., Price, E., & You, M. (2008). Childbirth is changing. What now? *MCN American Journal of Maternal/Child Nursing*, *33*(3), 144-150.

U.S. Census Bureau. (2008). Press release: *An older and more diverse nation by midcentury*. www.census.gov/newsroom/releases/archives/population/cb08-123.html.

U.S. Department of Health and Human Services (USDHHS) (2007). Health Resources and Services Administration: *Women's health USA 2007*. Internet document available at www.mchb.hrsa.gov/whusa_07/ (accessed February 26, 2009).

U.S. Department of Health and Human Services (USDHHS). (2010). Health Resources and Services Administraiton (HRSA), Maternal and Child Health Bureau: *Women's health USA 2010*. Rockville, MD: USDHHS.

U.S. Department of Labor. (2005). *The national agricultural workers survey, 2005*. Internet document available at www.doleta.gov/agworker/naws.cfm (accessed February 26, 2009).

World Health Organization. (2012). *Trends in maternal mortality: 1990-2010*. Internet document available at www.unfpa.org/public/home/publications/pid/10728 (accessed July 27, 2013).

World Health Organization study group on female genital mutilation and obstetric outcome, Banks, E., Meirik, O., Farley, T., Akande, O., Bathija, H., & Ali, M. (2006). Female genital mutilation and obstetric outcome: WHO collaborative prospective study in six African countries. *Lancet*, *367*(9525), 1835-1841.

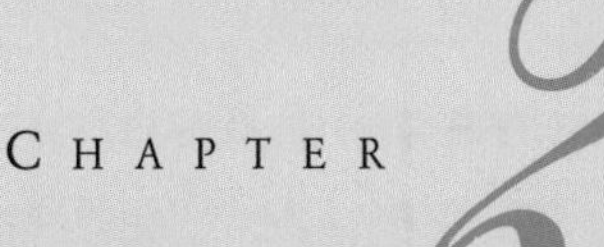

CHAPTER 2

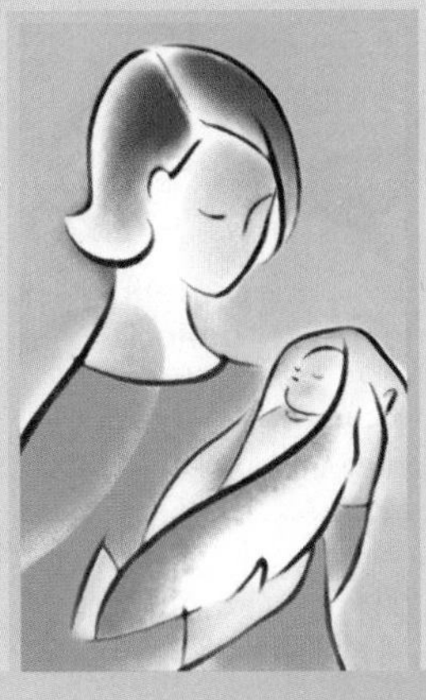

Assessment and Health Promotion

DEITRA LEONARD LOWDERMILK

LEARNING OBJECTIVES

- *Identify the structures and functions of the female reproductive system.*
- *Compare the hypothalamic-pituitary, ovarian, and endometrial cycles of menstruation.*
- *Identify the four phases of the sexual response cycle.*
- *Identify the reasons why women enter the health care delivery system, including preconception care.*
- *Discuss the financial, cultural, and gender barriers to seeking health care.*
- *Explain the conditions and characteristics that increase health risks, specifically age, substance abuse, nutritional and physical status, medical conditions, and intimate partner violence.*
- *Outline the components of taking a woman's history and performing a physical examination.*
- *Discuss how the assessment and physical examination can be adapted for women with special needs.*
- *Identify the correct procedure for assisting with and collecting specimens for Papanicolaou testing.*
- *Review health promotion and prevention suggestions for common health risks.*

KEY TERMS AND DEFINITIONS

breast self-examination (BSE) Systematic examination of her breasts by the woman

climacteric The period of a woman's life when she is passing from a reproductive to a nonreproductive state, with regression of ovarian function; the cycle of endocrine, physical, and psychosocial changes that occurs during the termination of the reproductive years; also called climacterium

cycle of violence Violence against a woman that (usually) occurs in a pattern consisting of three phases: period of increasing tension, the abusive episode, and a period of contrition and kindness

Kegel exercises Pelvic floor muscle exercises to strengthen the pubococcygeal muscles

menarche Onset, or beginning, of menstrual function

menopause From the Greek words mensis (month) and pausis (cessation), the actual permanent cessation of menstrual cycles; so diagnosed after 1 year without menses

menstrual cycle A complex interplay of events that occur simultaneously in the endometrium, the hypothalamus and pituitary glands, and the ovaries that results in ovarian and uterine preparation for pregnancy

menstruation Periodic vaginal discharge of bloody fluid from the nonpregnant uterus that occurs from the age of puberty to menopause

ovulation Periodic ripening and discharge of the ovum from the ovary, usually 14 days before the onset of menstrual flow

Papanicolaou (Pap) test (or smear) Microscopic examination using scrapings from the cervix, endocervix, or other mucous membranes that will reveal, with a high degree of accuracy, the presence of premalignant or malignant cells

perimenopause Period of transition of changing ovarian activity before menopause and through the first few years of amenorrhea

KEY TERMS AND DEFINITIONS—cont'd

preconception care Care designed for health maintenance and health promotion for the general and reproductive health of all women of childbearing potential

prostaglandins (PGs) Substances present in many body tissues, having roles in many reproductive tract functions and used to induce abortions and for cervical ripening for labor induction

sexual response cycle Phases of physical changes that occur in response to sexual stimulation and sexual tension release

squamocolumnar junction Site in the endocervical canal where columnar epithelium and squamous epithelium meet; also called transformation zone

vulvar self-examination (VSE) Systematic examination of the vulva by the woman

WEB RESOURCES

Additional related content can be found on the companion website at evolve

http://evolve.elsevier.com/Lowdermilk/Maternity/

- NCLEX Review Questions
- Anatomy Review: Adult Female Pelvis
- Anatomy Review: External Female Genitalia
- Anatomy Review: Female Breast
- Anatomy Review: Female Pelvic Organs
- Animation: Breasts
- Animation: Female Accessory Sex Glands
- Animation: Female External Genitalia
- Animation: Female Reproductive Ducts
- Animation: Menstrual Cycle: Uterine
- Animation: Ovaries
- Animation: Ovarian Cycle
- Animation: Ovulation
- Case Study: Health Assessment
- Critical Thinking Exercise: Women's Health and Safety
- Nursing Care Plan: The Battered Woman
- Skill: Breast Self-Examination
- Spanish Guidelines: Menstruation
- Spanish Guidelines: Physical Examination
- Spanish Guidelines: Recognizing Violence in a Relationship

Anatomy Review: External Female Genitalia

Animation: Female External Genitalia

Animation: Female Accessory Sex Glands

Many women initially enter the health care system because of some reproductive system–related situation, such as pregnancy; irregular menses; desire for contraception; or episodic illness, such as vaginal infection. Once women are in the system, however, one of the health care provider's responsibilities is to recognize the need for health promotion and preventive health maintenance and to provide these services as part of lifelong care for women. This chapter reviews female anatomy and physiology, including the menstrual cycle. It also covers physical assessment and screening for disease prevention for women in their reproductive years. In addition, the chapter discusses barriers to seeking health care and gives an overview of conditions and circumstances that increase health risks in the childbearing years. Anticipatory guidance suggestions for health promotion and prevention are also included.

FEMALE REPRODUCTIVE SYSTEM

External Structures

The external genital organs, or *vulva,* include all structures visible externally from the pubis to the perineum (Fig. 2-1). The *mons pubis* is a fatty pad that lies over the anterior surface of the symphysis pubis. In the postpubertal woman, the mons is covered with coarse curly hair. The *labia majora* are two rounded folds of fatty tissue covered with skin that extend downward and backward from the mons pubis. These folds are highly vascular structures that develop hair on the outer surfaces after puberty and protect the inner vulvar structures. The *labia minora* are two flat, reddish folds of tissue visible when the labia majora are separated. Anteriorly, they fuse to form the *prepuce* (a hoodlike covering of the clitoris) and the *frenulum* (a fold of tissue under the clitoris). The labia minora join to form a thin flat tissue called the *fourchette* underneath the vaginal opening at the midline. The *clitoris* is a small structure composed of erectile tissue with numerous sensory nerve endings located underneath the prepuce.

The vaginal *vestibule* is an almond-shaped area enclosed by the labia minora that contains openings to the urethra, Skene glands, vagina, and Bartholin glands. The urethra is not a reproductive organ but is considered here because of its location. Usually this structure is approximately 2.5 cm below the clitoris. The Skene glands are located on each side of the urethra and produce mucus, which aids in lubrication of the vagina. The vaginal opening is in the lower portion of the vestibule and varies in shape and size. The hymen, a connective tissue membrane, surrounds the vaginal opening. Bartholin glands (see Fig. 2-1) lie under the constrictor muscles of the vagina and are located posteriorly on

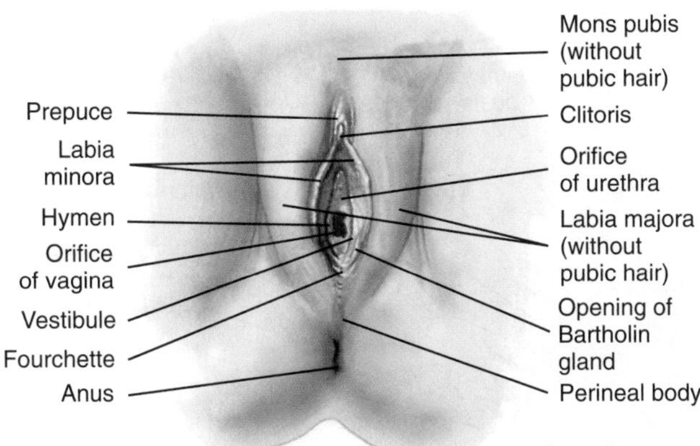

Fig. 2-1 External female genitalia.

the sides of the vaginal opening, although the ductal openings are not usually visible. During sexual arousal the glands secrete clear mucus to lubricate the vaginal introitus.

The area between the fourchette and the anus is the *perineum,* a skin-covered muscular area that covers the pelvic structures. The perineum forms the base of the perineal body, a wedged-shaped mass that serves as an anchor for the muscles, fascia, and ligaments of the pelvis. The pelvic organs are supported by muscles and ligaments that form a sling.

Internal Structures

The internal structures include the vagina, uterus, uterine tubes, and ovaries. The *vagina* is a fibromuscular, collapsible tubular structure that extends from the vulva to the uterus and lies between the bladder and rectum. During the reproductive years the mucosal lining is arranged in transverse folds called *rugae.* These rugae allow the vagina to expand during childbirth. Estrogen deprivation that occurs after childbirth, during lactation, and at menopause causes dryness and thinness of the vaginal walls and smoothing of the rugae. Vaginal secretions are acidic (pH 4 to 5), which reduces the vagina's susceptibility to infections. The vagina serves as a passageway for menstrual flow, as a female organ of copulation, and as a part of the birth canal for vaginal childbirth. The uterine cervix projects into a blind vault at the upper end of the vagina. Anterior, posterior, and lateral pockets called *fornices* surround the cervix. The internal pelvic organs can be palpated through the thin walls of these fornices.

The *uterus* is a muscular organ shaped like an upside-down pear that sits midline in the pelvic cavity between the bladder and the rectum above the vagina. Four pairs of ligaments support the uterus: the cardinal, uterosacral, round, and broad. Single anterior and posterior ligaments also support the uterus. The *cul-de-sac of Douglas* is a deep pouch, or recess, posterior to the cervix and formed by the posterior ligament.

The uterus is divided into two major parts: an upper triangular portion called the *corpus* and a lower cylindric portion called the *cervix* (Fig. 2-2). The *fundus* is the dome-shaped top of the uterus and is the site where the uterine tubes enter the uterus. The isthmus (lower uterine segment) is a short, constricted portion that separates the corpus from the cervix.

Animation: Female Reproductive Ducts

The uterus serves many purposes. It receives and implants the fertilized ovum and nourishes it throughout the pregnancy. During childbirth, the uterus is responsible for the expulsion of the fetus. It also is the organ for cyclic menstruation.

The uterine wall consists of three layers: the endometrium, the myometrium, and part of the peritoneum. The endometrium is a highly vascular lining made up of three layers, the outer two of which are shed during menstruation. The myometrium is made up of layers of smooth muscles that extend in three different directions (longitudinal, transverse, and oblique) (Fig. 2-3). Longitudinal fibers of the outer myometrial layer are mostly in the fundus, and this arrangement assists in expelling the fetus during the birth process. The middle layer contains fibers from all three directions, which form a figure-eight pattern encircling large blood vessels. This arrangement assists in constricting blood vessels after childbirth and controls blood loss. Most of the circular fibers of the inner myometrial layer are around the site where the uterine tubes enter the uterus and around the internal cervical os (opening). These fibers help keep the cervix closed during pregnancy and prevent menstrual blood from flowing back into the uterine tubes during menstruation.

The cervix is made up of mostly fibrous connective tissues and elastic tissue, enabling it to stretch during vaginal childbirth. The opening between the uterine cavity and the canal that connects the uterine cavity to the vagina (endocervical canal) is the internal os. The narrowed opening between the endocervix and the vagina is the external os, a small circular opening in women who have never been pregnant. The cervix feels firm (similar to the end of a nose) with a dimple in the center, which marks the external os.

The outer cervix is covered with a layer of squamous epithelium. The mucosa of the cervical canal is covered with columnar epithelium and contains numerous glands that secrete mucus in response to ovarian hormones. The **squamocolumnar junction**, where the two types of cells meet, is usually just inside the cervical os. This junction is also called the *transformation zone* and is the most common site for neoplastic changes. Cells from this site are scraped for the Papanicolaou (Pap) test (or smear) (see p. 51).

The *uterine (fallopian) tubes* attach to the uterine fundus. Broad ligaments support these tubes that range from 8 to 14 cm in length. The uterine tubes provide a passage between the ovaries and the uterus for the passage of the ovum.

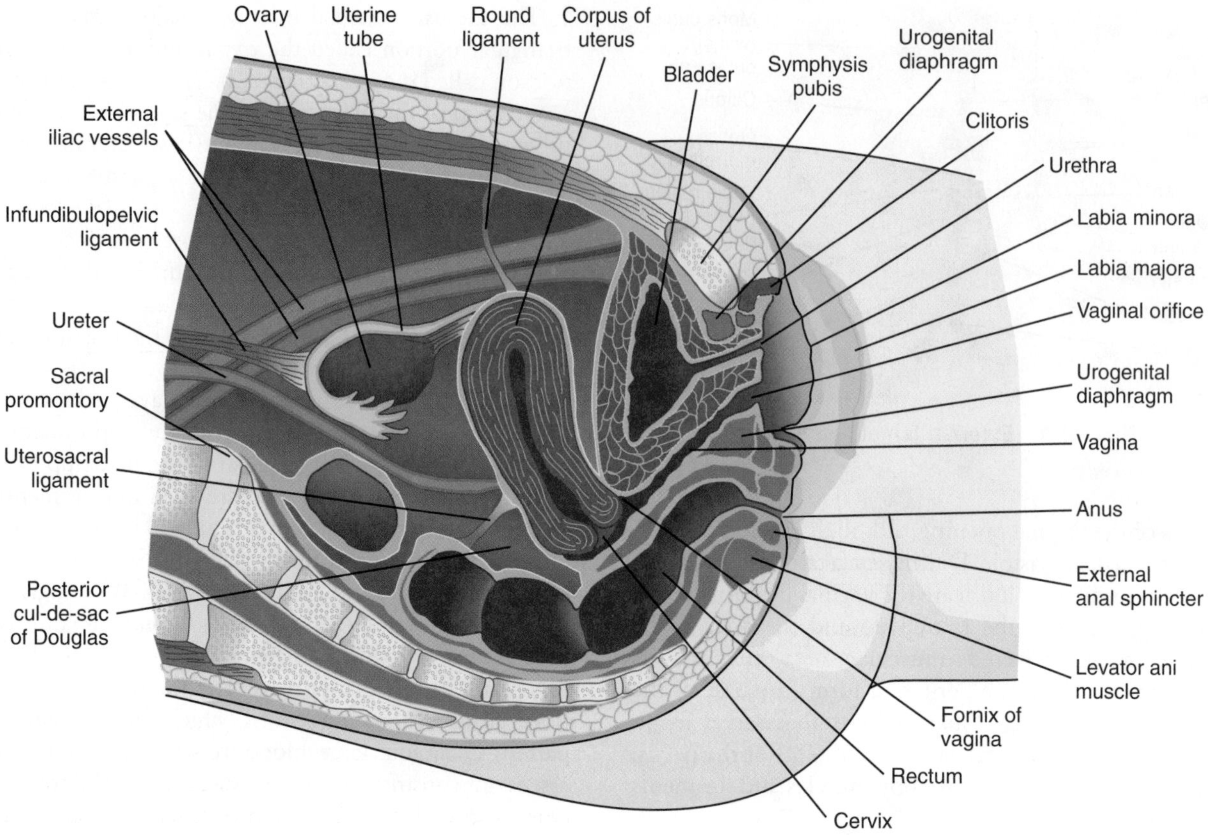

Fig. 2-2 Midsagittal view of female pelvic organs, with woman lying supine.

Anatomy Review: Female Pelvic Organs

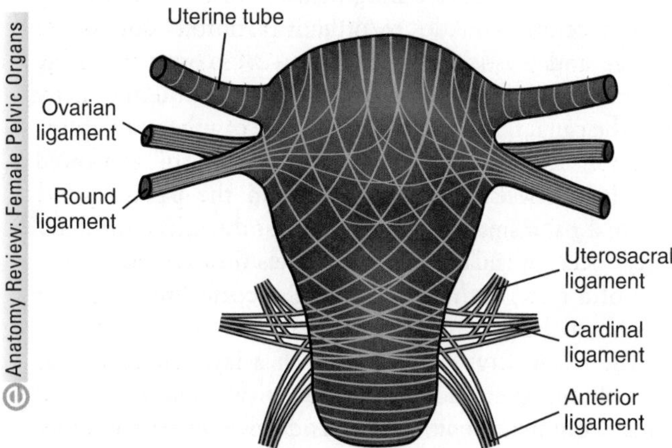

Fig. 2-3 Schematic arrangement of directions of muscle fibers. Note that uterine muscle fibers are continuous with supportive ligaments of uterus.

Anatomy Review: Adult Female Pelvis

The *ovaries* are almond-shaped organs located on each side of the uterus below and behind the uterine tubes. During the reproductive years, they are approximately 3 cm long, 2 cm wide, and 1 cm thick. They diminish in size after menopause. The two functions of the ovaries are ovulation and production of estrogen, progesterone, and androgen.

Bony Pelvis

The bony pelvis serves three primary purposes: protection of the pelvic structures, accommodation of the growing fetus during pregnancy, and anchorage of the pelvic support structures. Two innominate (hip) bones (consisting of the ilium, ischium, and pubis), the sacrum, and the coccyx make up the four bones of the pelvis (Fig. 2-4). Cartilage and ligaments form the symphysis pubis, sacrococcygeal, and two sacroiliac joints that separate the pelvic bones. The pelvis is divided into two parts: the false pelvis and the true pelvis (Fig. 2-5). The false pelvis is the upper portion above the pelvic brim or inlet. The true pelvis is the lower curved bony canal, which includes the inlet, the cavity, and the outlet through which the fetus passes during vaginal birth. Variations that occur in the size and shape of the pelvis are usually a result of age, race, and injury. Pelvic ossification is complete by approximately 20 years of age.

Breasts

The breasts are paired mammary glands located between the second and sixth ribs (Fig. 2-6). Approximately two thirds of the breast overlies the pectoralis major muscle, between the sternum and midaxillary line, with an extension to the axilla referred to as the *tail of Spence.* The lowest

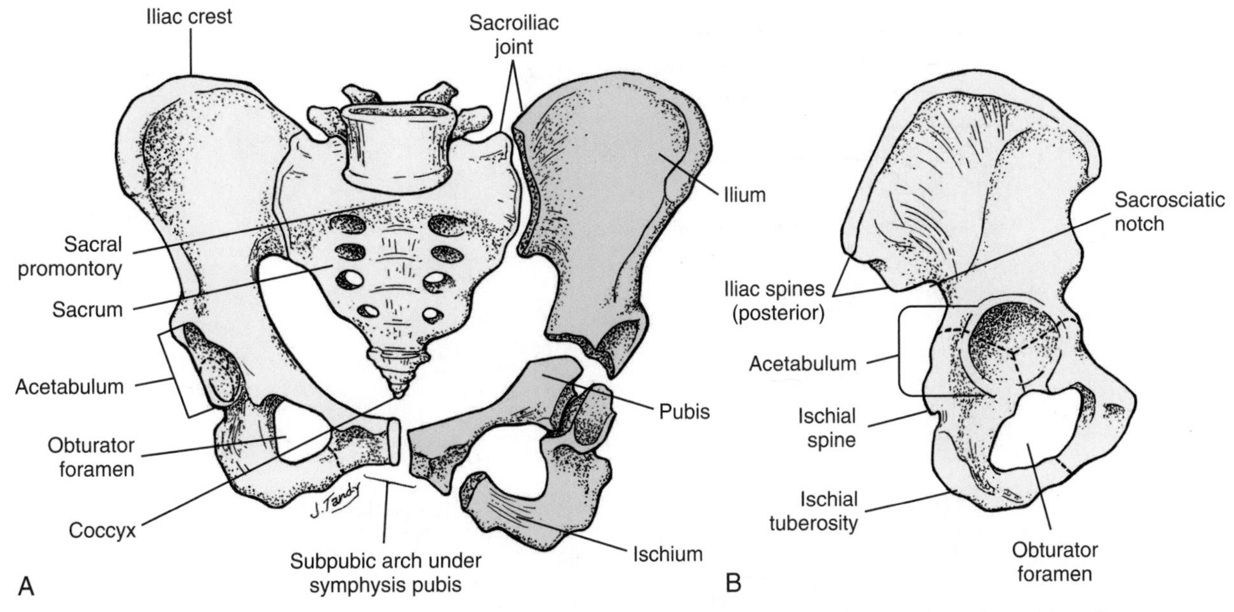

Fig. 2-4 Adult female pelvis. **A,** Anterior view. **B,** External view of innominate bone (fused).

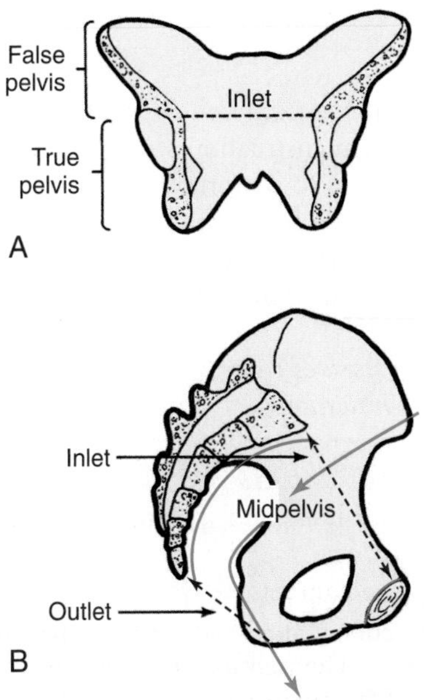

Fig. 2-5 Female pelvis. **A,** Cavity of false pelvis is shallow. **B,** Cavity of true pelvis is an irregularly curved canal *(arrows).*

third of the breast lies over the serratus anterior muscle. Connective tissue called fascia attach the breast to the muscles.

The breasts of healthy mature women are approximately equal in size and shape but are often not absolutely symmetric. The size and shape vary depending on the woman's age, heredity, and nutrition. However, the contour should be smooth with no retractions, dimpling, or masses. Estrogen stimulates growth of the breast by inducing fat deposition in the breasts, development of stromal tissue (i.e., an increase in its amount and elasticity), and growth of the extensive ductile system. Estrogen also increases the vascularity of breast tissue. The increase in progesterone at puberty causes maturation of mammary gland tissue, specifically the lobules and acinar structures. During adolescence, fat deposition and growth of fibrous tissue contribute to the increase in the gland's size.

Findings from several studies using ultrasound imaging to investigate the anatomy of the breast found differences from previous descriptions (Geddes, 2007; Love & Barsky, 2004; Ramsay, Kent, Hartmann, & Hartmann, 2005). Each mammary gland is made of a number of lobes, which are divided into lobules. Lobules are clusters of acini. An acinus is a saclike terminal part of a compound gland emptying through a narrow lumen or duct. The acini are lined with epithelial cells that secrete colostrum and milk. Just below the epithelium is the myoepithelium (*myo,* or muscle), which contracts to expel milk from the acini.

The ducts from the clusters of acini that form the lobules merge to form larger ducts draining the lobes. Ducts from the lobes converge in a single nipple (mammary papilla) surrounded by an areola. The anatomy of the ducts is similar for each breast but varies among women. Protective fatty tissue surrounds the glandular structures and ducts. *Cooper's ligaments,* or fibrous suspensory, separate and support the glandular structures and ducts. Cooper's ligaments provide support to the mammary glands while permitting their mobility on the chest wall (see Fig. 2-6). The round nipple is usually slightly elevated above the breast. On each breast the nipple projects slightly upward and laterally. It contains 4 to 20 openings from the milk ducts. The nipple is surrounded by fibromuscular tissue and covered by wrinkled skin (the areola).

Anatomy Review: Female Breast
Animation: Breasts

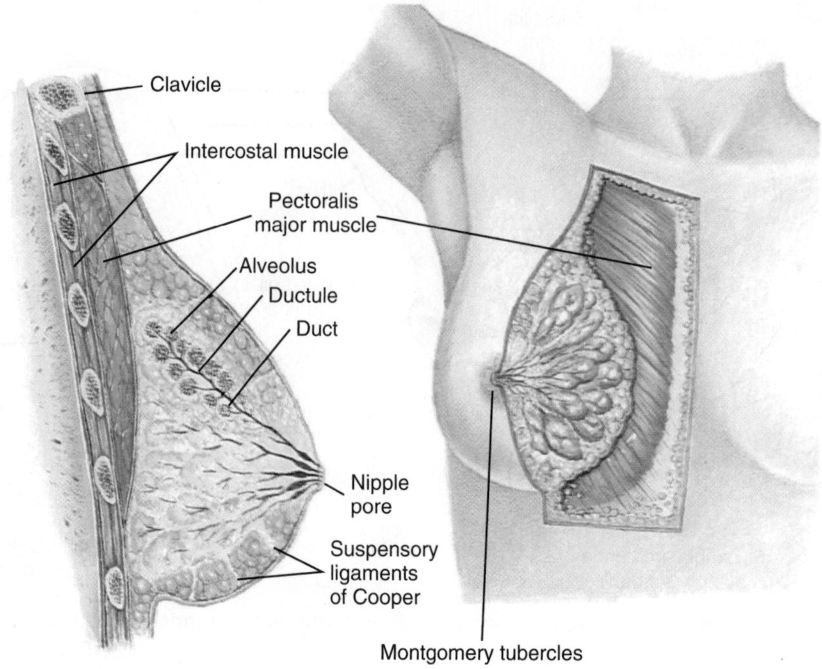

Fig. 2-6 Anatomy of the breast, showing position and major structures. (From Seidel, H., Ball, J., Dains, J., & Benedict, G. [2006]. *Mosby's guide to physical examination* [6th ed.]. St. Louis: Mosby.)

Except during pregnancy and lactation, there is usually no discharge from the nipple.

The nipple and surrounding areola are usually more deeply pigmented than the skin of the breast. Sebaceous glands called *Montgomery tubercles* directly beneath the skin (see Fig. 2-6) give the areola its rough appearance. These glands secrete a fatty substance thought to lubricate the nipple.

The vascular supply to the mammary gland is abundant. The skin covering the breasts contains an extensive superficial lymphatic network that serves the entire chest wall and is continuous with the superficial lymphatics of the neck and abdomen. In the deeper portions of the breasts, the lymphatics form a rich network as well. The primary deep lymphatic pathway drains laterally toward the axillae.

The breasts change in size and nodularity in response to cyclic ovarian changes throughout reproductive life. Increasing levels of both estrogen and progesterone in the 3 to 4 days before menstruation increase vascularity of the breasts, induce growth of the ducts and acini, and promote water retention. As a result, breast swelling, tenderness, and discomfort are common symptoms just before the onset of menstruation. After menstruation, cellular proliferation begins to regress, acini begin to decrease in size, and retained water is lost. In time, after repeated hormonal stimulation, small persistent areas of nodulations may develop just before and during menstruation, when the breast is most active. The physiologic alterations in breast size and activity reach their minimal level approximately 5 to 7 days after menstruation stops. The best time for a woman who wishes to perform a **breast self-examination (BSE)** is during this phase of the menstrual cycle or whenever the breasts are not tender or swollen (see Patient Instructions for Self-Management box).

Skill: Breast Self-Examination

Critical Thinking/Clinical Decision Making

Breast Self-Examination

Jessie is a 21-year-old college student who has come to the student health clinic for contraception advice. During her consultation with the nurse, Jessie asks about doing a breast self-examination (BSE). Her roommate told her she really needs to do them every month. What advice or counseling would you give Jessie?

1. Evidence—Is there sufficient evidence to draw conclusions about what intervention is needed?
2. Assumptions—Describe the underlying assumptions about the following issues:
   a. Risk factor assessment for breast cancer
   b. Screening for breast cancer
   c. Research on BSE
   d. BSE practices
3. What implications and priorities for nursing care can be drawn at this time?
4. Does the evidence objectively support your conclusion?
5. Are there alternative perspectives to your conclusion?

PATIENT INSTRUCTIONS FOR SELF-MANAGEMENT

Breast Self-Examination

If you choose to perform a breast self-examination, the best time is when breasts are not tender or swollen.

How to examine your breasts:

1. Lie down and put a pillow under your right shoulder. Place your right arm behind your head (Fig. 1).

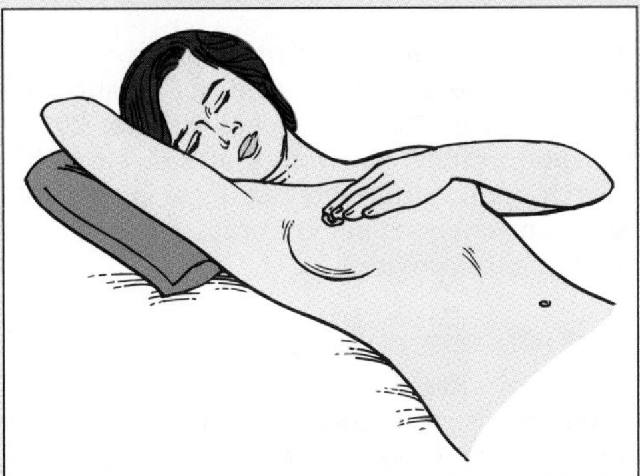

Fig. 1

2. Use the finger pads of your three middle fingers on your left hand to feel for lumps or thickening. Your finger pads are the top third of each finger. Use circular motions of the finger pads to feel the breast tissue.
3. Press firmly enough to know how your breast feels. Use light pressure to feel the tissue just under the skin, medium pressure for a little deeper, and firm pressure to feel the breast tissue close to the chest and ribs. A firm ridge in the lower curve of the breast is normal.
4. Move around the breast in a set way, such as using an up and down or vertical line pattern (Fig. 2). Go up to the collar bone and down to the ribs and from your underarm on the side to the middle of your chest. Use the same technique every time. It will help you to make sure that you have gone over the entire breast area and to remember how your breast feels.

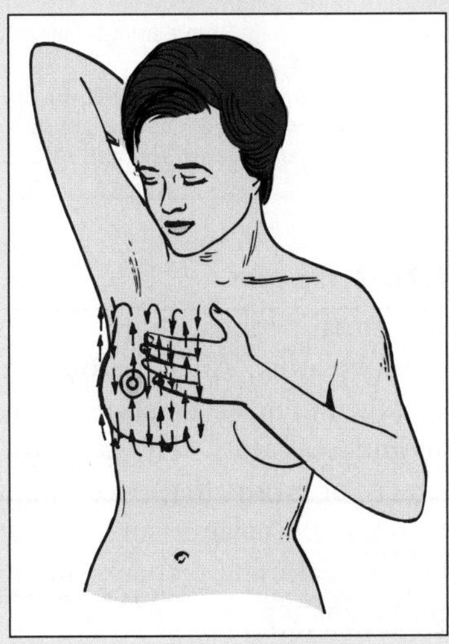

Fig. 2

5. Now examine your left breast using the finger pads of your right hand.
6. You may want to check your breasts while standing in front of a mirror. See if there are any changes in the way your breasts look: dimpling of the skin, changes in the nipple, or redness or swelling.
7. You may also want to perform an extra breast self-examination while you are in the shower (Fig. 3). Your soapy hands will glide over the wet skin, making it easy to check how your breasts feel.

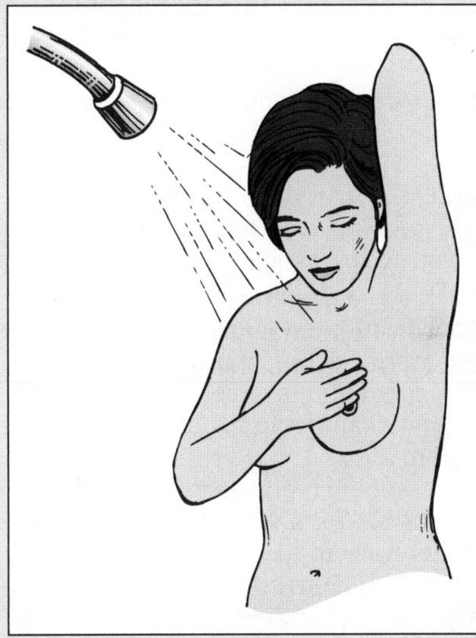

Fig. 3

8. Checking the area between the breast and the underarm and the underarm itself is important. Examine the area above the breast to the collarbone and to the shoulder while you are standing or sitting up with your arms lightly raised.
9. If you find any changes, see your health care provider right away.

Source: American Cancer Society. (2008). *How to perform a breast self-exam.* Internet document available at www.cancer.org (accessed June 4, 2009).

EVIDENCE-BASED PRACTICE

Teaching Women Breast Self-Examination: Is It Worthwhile?

Pat Gingrich

ASK THE QUESTION

Does teaching women breast self-examination (BSE) actually result in fewer deaths from breast cancer?

SEARCH FOR EVIDENCE

Search strategies: Professional organization guidelines, metaanalyses, systematic reviews, randomized controlled trials, nonrandomized prospective studies, and retrospective studies since 2006

Search databases: Cumulative Index to Nursing and Allied Health Literature, Cochrane, Medline, National Guideline Clearinghouse, and websites for the Association of Women's Health, Obstetric and Neonatal Nurses, American College of Obstetricians and Gynecologists, American Cancer Society, and National Cancer Institute

CRITICALLY ANALYZE THE DATA

The ideal screening test for breast cancer would have a high sensitivity for breast cancer in an early, curable stage, thus decreasing mortality. Moreover, it would have a high specificity, meaning few false positives and thus few unnecessary diagnostic tests. Screening for breast cancer has conventionally consisted of a BSE monthly, a clinical breast examination (CBE) yearly, and a screening mammogram every 1 to 2 years after 40 years of age. Of these, the screening mammogram has been the gold standard, responsible for a 15% to 20% decrease in mortality in a metaanalysis of seven trials, representing one half million women (Gotzsche & Nielsen, 2006). Mammograms are limited by their cost, discomfort, geographic availability, skilled interpretation, exposure to radiation, and high false-positive rates.

Mammograms are usually accompanied by a CBE given by a trained examiner. Since the 1970s, women were also routinely taught to perform a BSE. The assumption was that BSE was a low-tech screening tool for women to detect tumors in the early, more treatable stages. This theory was challenged by a classic metaanalysis of two randomized controlled trials involving 388,535 women in Russia and Shanghai, which found no difference in cancer mortality between groups taught BSE and control groups without the BSE education (Kosters & Gotzche, 2003, updated 2007). In fact, the BSE group was twice as likely to undergo unnecessary biopsy with benign results as the control group. The authors noted poor compliance with breast examinations but commented about the possibility that BSE may have decreased mortality in some countries.

Breast cancer screening recommendations from the National Cancer Institute (NCI) include a CBE and a screening mammogram (National Cancer Institute, 2007). The NCI organization guidelines note that BSE alone has not been shown to reduce mortality but do encourage women to be alert to any changes in their breasts and report them to their health care provider.

IMPLICATIONS FOR PRACTICE

BSE is a low-tech, low-cost technique that can empower some women to discover breast changes earlier. Whether this technique will decrease mortality is unclear. BSE and CBE may also result in unnecessary testing. A Breast Health Global Initiative panel recommends "breast health awareness," a combination of education and SBE that may provide the greatest value by promoting breast awareness in low-resource areas (Smith et al., 2006). Nurses should offer to teach the technique to women who wish to learn. However, some women are not comfortable examining their breasts or find it frightening. All women should be taught to follow the recommended guidelines for CBE yearly and mammograms based on age and personal history.

References:

Gotzsche, P. C. & Nielsen, M. (2006). Screening for breast cancer with mammography. In *The Cochrane Database of Systematic Reviews 2006,* Issue 4, CD0001877.

Kosters, J. P. & Gotzsche, P. C. (2003). Regular self-examination or clinical examination for early detection of breast cancer. In *The Cochrane Database of Systematic Reviews 2003,* Issue 2, CD003373.

National Cancer Institute. (2007). *What you need to know about breast cancer.* Internet document available at www.cancer.gov/cancertopics/wyntk/breast/page5#screening3 (accessed January 8, 2009).

Smith, R., Caleffi, M., Albert, U., Chen, T., Duffy, S., Franceschi, D., et al. (2006). Breast care in limited-resource countries: Early detection and access to care. *Breast Journal,* 12(Supp 1): S16-S20.

ⓔ Spanish Guidelines: Menstruation

Menstruation

Menarche and puberty

Puberty is a broad term that denotes the entire transitional stage between childhood and sexual maturity. Although young girls secrete small, rather constant amounts of estrogen, a marked increase occurs between 8 and 11 years of age. The term **menarche** denotes first menstruation. In North America, menarche occurs in most girls at approximately 13 years of age.

Although pregnancy can occur in exceptional cases of true precocious puberty, most pregnancies in young girls occur after the normally timed menarche. All girls would benefit from knowing that pregnancy can occur at any time after the onset of menses.

Menstrual cycle

Initially, menstrual periods are irregular, unpredictable, painless, and anovulatory. After the ovary produces adequate cyclic estrogen to make a mature ovum, periods tend to be regular and ovulatory. The **menstrual cycle** is a complex interplay of events that occur simultaneously in the endometrium, hypothalamus and pituitary glands, and ovaries. The menstrual cycle prepares the uterus for pregnancy. When pregnancy does not occur, menstruation follows. **Menstruation** is the periodic uterine bleeding that begins approximately 14 days after ovulation. The average length of a menstrual cycle is 28 days, but variations are common. The first day of bleeding is designated as day 1 of the menstrual cycle, or menses (Fig. 2-7). The average

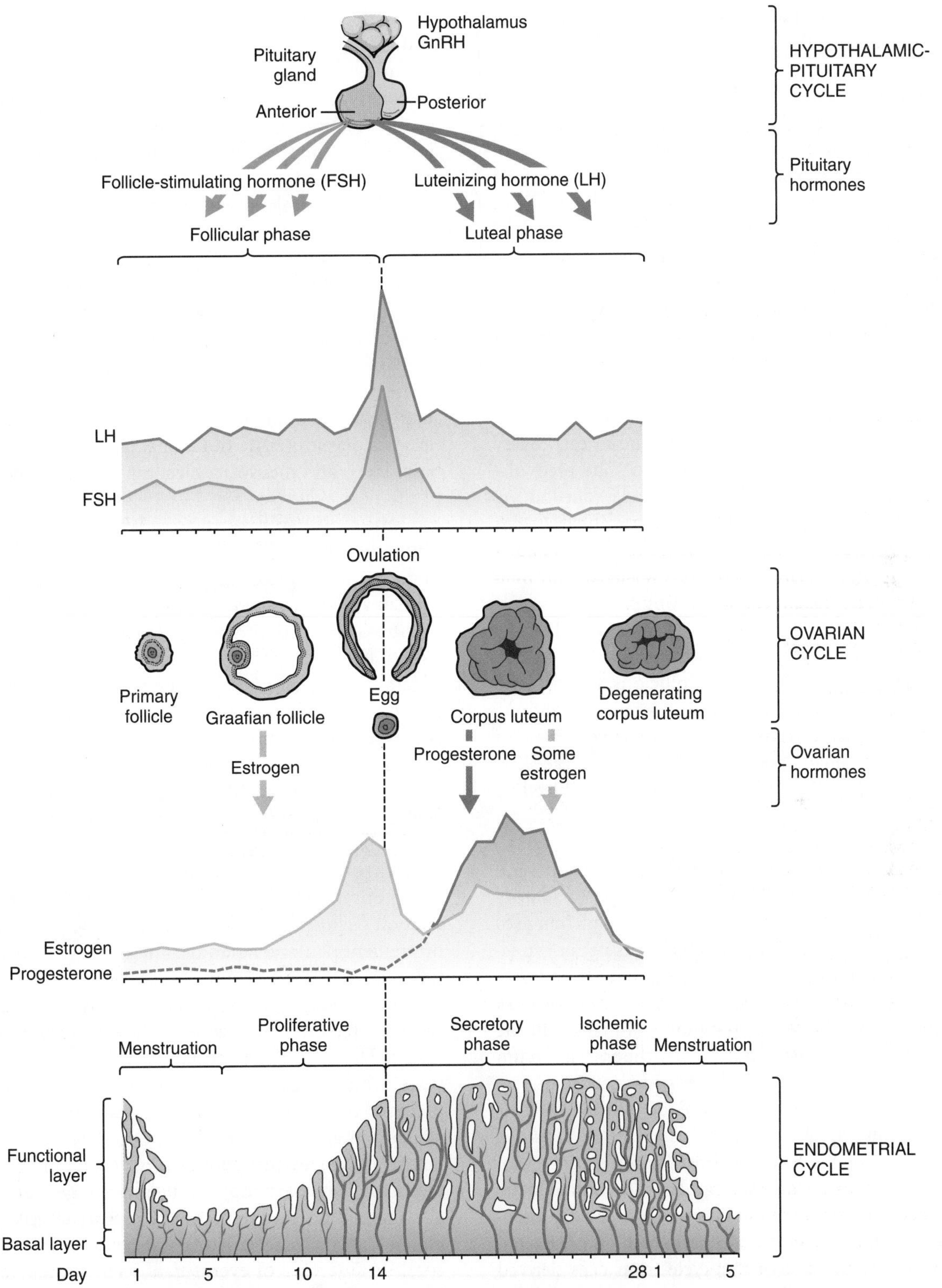

Fig. 2-7 Menstrual cycle: hypothalamic-pituitary, ovarian, and endometrial.

duration of menstrual flow is 5 days (range of 1 to 8 days), and the average blood loss is 50 ml (range of 20 to 80 ml), but these vary greatly (Fehring, Schneider, & Raviele, 2006). The woman's age, physical and emotional status, and environment also influence the regularity of her menstrual cycles.

Hypothalamic-pituitary cycle. Toward the end of the normal menstrual cycle, blood levels of estrogen and progesterone fall. Low blood levels of these ovarian hormones stimulate the hypothalamus to secrete gonadotropin-releasing hormone (GnRH). In turn, GnRH stimulates anterior pituitary secretion of follicle-

Animation: Menstrual Cycle: Uterine

Animation: Ovaries

stimulating hormone (FSH) that stimulates development of ovarian graafian follicles and their production of estrogen. Estrogen levels begin to fall, and hypothalamic GnRH triggers the anterior pituitary release of luteinizing hormone (LH). A marked surge of LH and a smaller peak of estrogen (day 12; see Fig. 2-7) precede the expulsion of the ovum **(ovulation)** from the graafian follicle by approximately 24 to 36 hours. LH peaks at approximately the thirteenth or fourteenth day of a 28-day cycle. If fertilization and implantation of the ovum do not occur by this time, the corpus luteum regresses. Levels of progesterone and estrogen decline, menstruation occurs, and the hypothalamus is once again stimulated to secrete GnRH. This process is the *hypothalamic-pituitary cycle.*

Animation: Ovarian Cycle

Ovarian cycle. The primitive graafian follicles contain immature oocytes (primordial ova). Before ovulation, from 1 to 30 follicles begin to mature in each ovary under the influence of FSH and estrogen. The preovulatory surge of LH affects a selected follicle. The oocyte matures, ovulation occurs, and the empty follicle begins its transformation into the corpus luteum. This follicular phase (preovulatory phase) (see Fig. 2-7) of the ovarian cycle varies in length from woman to woman and accounts for almost all variations in ovarian cycle length (Fehring et al., 2006). On rare occasions (approximately 1 in 100 menstrual cycles), more than one follicle is selected and more than one oocyte matures and undergoes ovulation.

Animation: Ovulation

After ovulation, estrogen levels drop. For 90% of women, only a small amount of withdrawal bleeding occurs, so it goes unnoticed. In 10% of women bleeding is sufficient for it to be visible, resulting in what is known as *midcycle bleeding.*

The luteal phase begins immediately after ovulation and ends with the start of menstruation. This postovulatory phase of the ovarian cycle usually requires 14 days (range of 13 to 15 days). The corpus luteum reaches its peak of functional activity 8 days after ovulation, secreting both estrogen and progesterone. Coincident with this time of peak luteal functioning, the fertilized ovum is implanted in the endometrium. If no implantation occurs, the corpus luteum regresses, steroid levels drop, and menstruation occurs.

Endometrial cycle. The endometrial cycle is divided into four phases (see Fig. 2-7). During the *menstrual phase,* shedding of the functional two thirds of the endometrium (the compact and spongy layers) is initiated by periodic vasoconstriction in the upper layers of the endometrium. The basal layer is always retained, and regeneration begins near the end of the cycle from cells derived from the remaining glandular remnants or stromal cells in the basalis.

The *proliferative phase* is a period of rapid growth lasting from approximately the fifth day to the time of ovulation. The endometrial surface is completely restored in approximately 4 days, or slightly before bleeding ceases. From this point on, an eightfold to tenfold thickening occurs, with a leveling off of growth at ovulation. The proliferative phase depends on estrogen stimulation derived from ovarian follicles.

The *secretory phase* extends from the day of ovulation to approximately 3 days before the next menstrual period. After ovulation, larger amounts of progesterone are produced. The fully matured secretory endometrium reaches the thickness of heavy, soft velvet. It becomes luxuriant with blood and glandular secretions, a suitable protective and nutritive bed for a fertilized ovum.

Implantation of the fertilized ovum generally occurs approximately 7 to 10 days after ovulation. If fertilization and implantation do not occur, the corpus luteum, which secretes estrogen and progesterone, regresses. With the rapid fall in progesterone and estrogen levels, the spiral arteries go into spasm. During the *ischemic phase,* the blood supply to the functional endometrium is blocked, and necrosis develops. The functional layer separates from the basal layer, and menstrual bleeding begins, marking day 1 of the next cycle (see Fig. 2-7).

Other cyclic changes. When the hypothalamic-pituitary-ovarian axis functions properly, other tissues undergo predictable responses. Before ovulation the woman's basal body temperature (BBT) is often below 37° C; after ovulation, with rising progesterone levels, her BBT rises. Changes in the cervix and cervical mucus follow a generally predictable pattern. Preovulatory and postovulatory mucus is viscous (thick), so sperm penetration is discouraged. At the time of ovulation, cervical mucus is thin and clear. It appears, feels, and stretches like egg white. This stretchable quality is termed *spinnbarkeit.* Some women experience localized lower abdominal pain, termed *mittelschmerz,* that coincides with ovulation.

Climacteric. The **climacteric** is a transitional phase during which ovarian function and hormone production decline. This phase spans the years from the onset of premenopausal ovarian decline to the postmenopausal time when symptoms stop. **Menopause** refers to the last menstrual period. Unlike menarche, however, menopause can be dated only with certainty 1 year after menstruation ceases. The average age at natural menopause is 51 to 52 years, with an age range of 35 to 60 years. Menopause is preceded by a period known as the **perimenopause,** during which ovarian function declines. Ova slowly diminish, and menstrual cycles are anovulatory, resulting in irregular bleeding; the ovary stops producing estrogen, and eventually menses no longer occurs. This period lasts approximately 5 years (range 2-8 years) (Speroff & Fritz, 2005).

Prostaglandins

Prostaglandins (PGs) are oxygenated fatty acids classified as hormones. The different kinds of PGs are distinguished by letters (PGE, PGF), numbers (PGE_2), and letters of the Greek alphabet ($PGF_{2\alpha}$). PGs are produced in most organs of the body, most notably by the endometrium. Menstrual blood is a potent PG source. PGs affect smooth-muscle contractility and modulation of hormonal activity. Indirect evidence supports the effects of PGs on ovulation, fertility, and changes in the cervix and cervical mucus that affect receptivity to sperm, tubal and uterine motility, sloughing of endometrium (menstruation), onset of abortion (spontaneous and induced), and onset of labor (term and preterm).

Sexual Response

The hypothalamus and anterior pituitary gland in females regulate the production of FSH and LH. The target tissue for these hormones is the ovary, which produces ova and secretes estrogen and progesterone. A feedback mechanism involving hormone secretion from the ovaries, hypothalamus, and anterior pituitary aids in the control of the production of sex cells and steroid sex hormone secretion.

Sexual stimulation results in vasocongestion (congestion of blood vessels, usually venous) that causes vaginal lubrication and engorgement and distention of the genitals. This venous congestion occurs to a lesser degree in the breasts and other parts of the body. Arousal is characterized by myotonia (increased muscular tension), resulting in voluntary and involuntary rhythmic contractions. Examples of sexually stimulated myotonia are pelvic thrusting, facial grimacing, and spasms of the hands and feet (carpopedal spasms).

The **sexual response cycle** is divided into four phases: excitement phase, plateau phase, orgasmic phase, and resolution phase. The four phases occur progressively, with no sharp dividing line between any two phases. Specific body changes take place in sequence. The time, intensity, and duration for cyclic completion also vary for individuals and situations. Table 2-1 compares male and female body changes during each of the four phases of the sexual response cycle.

TABLE 2-1

Four Phases of Sexual Response

REACTIONS COMMON TO BOTH SEXES	REACTIONS IN WOMEN	REACTIONS IN MEN
EXCITEMENT PHASE		
Heart rate and blood pressure increase. Nipples become erect. Myotonia begins.	Clitoris increases in diameter and swells. External genitals become congested and darken. Vaginal lubrication occurs; upper two thirds of vagina lengthen and extend. Cervix and uterus pull upward. Breast size increases.	Erection of the penis begins; penis increases in length and diameter. Scrotal skin becomes congested and thickens. Testes begin to increase in size and elevate toward the body.
PLATEAU PHASE		
Heart rate and blood pressure continue to increase. Respirations increase. Myotonia becomes pronounced; grimacing occurs.	Clitoral head retracts under the clitoral hood. Lowest third of vagina becomes engorged. Skin color changes occur—red flush may be observed across breasts, abdomen, or other surfaces.	Head of penis may enlarge slightly. Scrotum continues to grow tense and thicken. Testes continue to elevate and enlarge. Preorgasmic emission of two or three drops of fluid appears on the head of the penis.
ORGASMIC PHASE		
Heart rate, blood pressure, and respirations increase to maximal levels. Involuntary muscle spasms occur. External rectal sphincter contracts.	Strong rhythmic contractions are felt in the clitoris, vagina, and uterus. Sensations of warmth spread through the pelvic area.	Testes elevate to maximal level. Point of "inevitability" occurs just before ejaculation and an awareness of fluid in the urethra. Rhythmic contractions occur in the penis. Ejaculation of semen occurs.
RESOLUTION PHASE		
Heart rate, blood pressure, and respirations return to normal. Nipple erection subsides. Myotonia subsides.	Engorgement in external genitalia and vagina resolves. Uterus descends to normal position. Cervix dips into seminal pool. Breast size decreases. Skin flush disappears.	Fifty percent of erection is lost immediately with ejaculation; penis gradually returns to normal size. Testes and scrotum return to normal size. Refractory period (time needed for erection to occur again) varies according to age and general physical condition.

REASONS FOR ENTERING THE HEALTH CARE SYSTEM

Women's health assessment and screening focus on a systems evaluation beginning with a thorough history and physical examination. During the assessment and evaluation, the responsibility for self-management, health promotion, and enhancement of wellness are emphasized. Nursing care includes assessment, planning, education, counseling, and referral as needed, as well as commendations for good self-management that the woman has practiced. This process enables women to make informed decisions about their own health care.

Preconception Counseling

Preconception health promotion provides women and their partners with information that is needed to make decisions about their reproductive future. Preconception counseling guides couples on how to prevent unintended pregnancies, stresses risk management, and identifies healthy behaviors that promote the well-being of the woman and her potential fetus (Moos, 2006).

All providers who treat women for well-woman care or other routine care should incorporate preconception health screening as part of the routine care for women of reproductive age (Johnson et al., 2006). The initiation of activities that promote healthy mothers and babies must occur before the period of critical fetal organ development, which is between 17 and 56 days after fertilization. By the end of the eighth week after conception and certainly by the end of the first trimester, any major structural anomalies in the fetus are already present. Because many women do not realize that they are pregnant and do not seek prenatal care until well into the first trimester, the rapidly growing fetus may be exposed to many types of intrauterine environmental hazards during this most vulnerable developmental phase.

Preconception care is important for women who have had a problem with a previous pregnancy (e.g., miscarriage, preterm birth). Although causes are not always identifiable, in many cases, problems can be identified and treated and may not recur in subsequent pregnancies. Preconception care is also important to minimize fetal malformations. For example, the woman may be exposed to teratogenic agents such as drugs, viruses, and chemicals, or she may have a genetically inherited disease. Preconception counseling can educate the woman about the effects of these agents and diseases, which can help prevent harm to the fetus or allow the woman to make an informed decision about her willingness to accept potential hazards should a pregnancy occur (Atrash, Johnson, Adams, Cordero, & Howse, 2006).

A model for preconception care of women of reproductive age targets all women from menarche to menopause at every encounter, not just in maternity and women's health. Providing optimal health care for women whether or not they desire to conceive can result in a high level of preconception wellness (Moos, 2006). Suggested components of preconception care, such as health promotion, risk assessment, and interventions, are outlined in Box 2-1.

Pregnancy

A woman's entry into health care is often associated with pregnancy, either for diagnosis or for actual care. Suspicion of pregnancy occurs most commonly when a woman is late with her menses. A woman should enter prenatal care within the first 12 weeks of pregnancy; this allows for early pregnancy counseling, especially for the woman who has had no preconception care. Extensive discussion of pregnancy is found in Unit Two.

Well-Woman Care

Current trends in the health care of women have expanded beyond a reproductive focus. A holistic approach to women's health care includes a woman's health needs throughout her lifetime. This view is one that goes beyond simply her reproductive needs. Women's health assessment and screening focus on a multisystem evaluation emphasizing the maintenance and enhancement of wellness.

Fertility Control and Infertility

Almost half of the pregnancies in the United States each year are unintended even with birth control use (Trussell, 2007). Education is the key to encouraging women to make family planning choices based on preference and actual risk-to-benefit ratios. Women who enter the health care system seeking contraceptive counseling can be assisted to use a chosen method correctly (see Chapter 4 for further discussion).

Women also enter the health care system because of their desire to achieve a pregnancy. Approximately 15% of couples in the United States have some degree of infertility. Infertility can cause emotional pain for many couples, and the inability to produce an offspring sometimes results in feelings of failure and inordinate stress on the relationship. Steps toward prevention of infertility should be undertaken as part of ongoing routine health care, and such information is especially appropriate in preconception counseling. For additional information about infertility, see Chapter 4.

Menstrual Problems

Irregularities or problems with the menstrual period are among the most common concerns of women and often cause them to seek help within the health care system. Common menstrual disorders include amenorrhea, dysmenorrhea, premenstrual syndrome, endometriosis, and menorrhagia or metrorrhagia. These problems are discussed in Chapter 3.

Perimenopause

Although fertility is greatly reduced during the perimenopausal period, women are urged to maintain some method

BOX 2-1

Components of Preconception Care

HEALTH PROMOTION: GENERAL TEACHING
- Nutrition
  - Healthy diet, including folic acid
  - Optimal weight
- Exercise and rest
- Avoidance of substance abuse (tobacco, alcohol, "recreational" drugs)
- Use of risk-reducing sex practices
- Attending to family and social needs

RISK FACTOR ASSESSMENT
- Chronic diseases
  - Diabetes, heart disease, hypertension, asthma, thyroid disease, kidney disease, anemia, mental illness
- Infectious diseases
  - HIV/AIDS, other sexually transmitted infections, vaccine preventable diseases (e.g., rubella, hepatitis B)
- Reproductive history
  - Contraception
  - Pregnancies—unplanned pregnancy, pregnancy outcomes
  - Infertility
- Genetic or inherited conditions (e.g., sickle cell anemia, Down syndrome, cystic fibrosis)
- Medications and medical treatment
  - Prescription medications (especially those contraindicated in pregnancy), over-the-counter medication use, radiation exposure
- Personal behaviors and exposures
  - Smoking, alcohol consumption, illicit drug use
  - Overweight or underweight; eating disorders
  - Folic acid supplement use
  - Spouse or partner and family situation, including intimate partner violence
  - Availability of family or other support systems
  - Readiness for pregnancy (e.g., age, life goals, stress)
  - Environmental (home, workplace) conditions
  - Safety hazards
  - Toxic chemicals
  - Radiation

INTERVENTIONS
- Anticipatory guidance or teaching
  - Treatment of medical conditions and results
  - Medications
  - Cessation or reduction in substance use and abuse
  - Immunizations (e.g., rubella, tuberculosis, hepatitis)
- Nutrition, diet, weight management
- Exercise
- Referral for genetic counseling
- Referral to and use of:
  - Family planning services
  - Family and social needs management

AIDS, Acquired immunodeficiency syndrome; *HIV,* human immunodeficiency virus.

of birth control because pregnancies can still occur. Most women seeking health care at this time do so because of irregular bleeding that may accompany the perimenopause. Others are concerned about vasomotor symptoms (hot flashes and flushes). All women need to have factual information, the dispelling of myths, a thorough examination, and periodic health screenings.

BARRIERS TO SEEKING HEALTH CARE

Financial Issues

The United States spends more on health care than any other industrialized nation, yet major problems still exist. In the United States, disparity among races and socioeconomic classes affects many facets of life, including health. Limited money and awareness can lead to a lack of access to care, delay in seeking care, few prevention activities, and little accurate information about health and the health care system. Women use health services more often than do men but are more likely than men to have difficulty in financing the services. They are twice as often underinsured (i.e., they have limited coverage with high-cost copayments or deductibles). Eighteen percent of women have no health insurance (National Women's Law Center, 2007). Insurance coverage varies significantly by age, marital status, race, and ethnicity. Caucasians of all ages are more likely than African-Americans, Hispanics, and other racial or ethnic groups to have private insurance (Agency for Healthcare Research and Quality, 2005). Single, separated, or divorced individuals are less likely to have insurance. Often, unmarried teenagers, who are usually covered by their parents' medical insurance, do not have maternity coverage because policies have inclusion statements that cover only the employee or spouse. More than twice as many women as men are insured by Medicaid (Patchias & Waxman, 2007). In most states, Medicaid includes special benefits for pregnant women, but they are limited to treatment of pregnancy-related conditions and terminated 60 days after the birth. Midwifery care has helped contain some health care costs, but reimbursement issues still exist in some areas.

COMMUNITY ACTIVITY

Investigate the resources in your community for women with the following health care needs, taking into account different age, language, and cultural needs. Evaluate the services and information provided, especially related to ease and access, cost (insurance), confidentiality, and follow-up care.

A. A 16-year-old girl who is sexually active and wants birth control

B. A 35-year-old woman who wants prenatal care and speaks only Spanish

C. A 29-year-old woman who smokes and needs a Pap test

Cultural Issues

Although they are most significant, financial considerations are not the only barriers to obtaining quality health care. As our nation becomes more racially, ethnically, and culturally diverse, the health of minority groups becomes a major issue. Providers must consider culturally based differences that could affect the treatment of diverse groups of women, and the women themselves must discuss with their health care providers the practices and beliefs that could influence their management responses or willingness to comply (Callister, 2005). For example, women in some cultures value privacy to such an extent that they are reluctant to disrobe and, as a result, avoid physical examination unless absolutely necessary. Other women rely on their husbands to make major decisions, including those affecting the woman's health. Religious beliefs may dictate a plan of care, as with birth control measures or blood transfusions. Some cultural groups prefer folk medicine, homeopathy, or prayer to traditional Western medicine, and yet others attempt combinations of some or all practices.

Cultural Considerations

Female Genital Mutilation

Female circumcision occurs in women of many different ethnic, cultural, and religious backgrounds worldwide. Although circumcision is usually performed during childhood, some communities circumcise infants or older females. It is generally acknowledged as a violation of human rights of young girls and women, and the World Health Organization and other organizations have advocated for the practice to be abandoned.

The procedure involves the removal of a portion of the clitoris but may extend to the removal of the entire clitoris and labia minora. Additionally, the labia majora, which are often stitched together over the urethral and vaginal openings, may be affected. The procedure has no health benefits.

The extent of the circumcision site affects the seriousness of complications. Common complications include bleeding, pain, local scarring, keloid or cyst formation, and infection. Impaired drainage of urine and menstrual blood may lead to chronic pelvic infections, pelvic and back pain, and chronic urinary tract infections. Some women may require surgery before vaginal examination, intercourse, or childbirth if the vaginal opening is obstructed.

Nurses in the United States and Canada and other western countries are providing care to a growing number of women who have emigrated from the Middle East, Asia, and Africa, where female circumcision is more common than in other areas. Nurses must be sensitive to the unique needs of these women, especially if these women have concerns about maintaining or restoring the intactness of the circumcision after childbirth.

Sources: Kelly, E., & Hillard, P. (2005). Female genital mutilation. *Current Opinion in Obstetrics and Gynecology, 17*(5), 490-494; Turner, D. (2007). Female genital cutting: Implications for nurses. *Nursing for Women's Health, 11*(4), 366-372.

Gender Issues

Gender influences provider-patient communication and may influence access to health care in general. The most obvious gender consideration is that between men and women. Researchers have reported significant male-female differences in receipt of major diagnostic and therapeutic interventions, especially with cardiac and kidney problems. Women tend to use primary care services more often (and, some believe, more effectively) than men. The sex of the provider plays a role because studies have shown that female patients have tests such as the Pap test and mammogram more consistently if they are seen by female providers.

Sexual orientation may produce another barrier. Lesbian women have primary erotic attractions and relations with other women. Some lesbians may not disclose their orientation to health care providers because they may be at risk for hostility, inadequate health care, or breach of confidentiality (Goldberg, 2005-2006). To offset stereotypes, providers should develop an approach that does not assume that all patients are heterosexual. Revising forms to be inclusive of sexual diversity and providing an environment that promotes acceptance and inclusiveness are two strategies suggested by researchers (Goldberg, 2005-2006; Roberts, 2006).

HEALTH RISKS IN THE CHILDBEARING YEARS

Maintaining optimal health is a goal for all women. Essential components of health maintenance are the identification of unrecognized problems and potential risks and the education or promotion needed to reduce them. This concept is especially important for women in their childbearing years because conditions that increase a woman's health risks are not only of concern to her well-being but also are potentially associated with negative outcomes for both mother and baby in the event of a pregnancy. Prenatal care is the prime example of prevention that is practiced after conception. However, prevention and health maintenance are needed before pregnancy because many of the mother's risks can be identified and eliminated or at least modified. An overview of conditions and circumstances that increase health risks in the childbearing years follows.

Age

Adolescence

All teens undergo progressive growth of sexual characteristics and also undertake developmental tasks of adolescence, such as establishing identity, developing sexual preference, emancipating from family, and establishing career goals. Some of these situations can produce great stress for the adolescent, and the health care provider should treat her very carefully. Female teenagers who enter the health care system usually do so for screening (Pap tests start 3 years after sexual activity begins or by age 21) or because of a problem such as episodic illness or accident. Gynecologic problems are often associated with menses (either bleeding irregularities or dysmenorrhea), vaginitis or leukorrhea, sexually transmitted infections (STIs), contraception, or pregnancy. The adolescent is also at risk for depression (Huff, Abuzz, & Omar, 2007).

Teenage pregnancy. Pregnancy in the teenager who is 16 years of age or younger often introduces additional stress into an already stressful developmental period. The emotional level of such teens is commonly characterized by impulsiveness and self-centered behavior, and they often place primary importance on the beliefs and actions of their peers. In attempts to establish a personal and independent identity, many teens do not realize the consequences of their behavior, and planning for the future is not part of their thinking processes.

Teenagers usually lack the financial resources to support a pregnancy and may not have the maturity to avoid teratogens or to have prenatal care and instruction or follow-up care. Children of teen mothers may be at risk for abuse or neglect because of the teen's inadequate knowledge of growth, development, and parenting.

Young and middle adulthood

Because women ages 20 to 40 have a need for contraception, pelvic and breast screening, and pregnancy care, they may prefer to use their gynecologic or obstetric provider also as their primary care provider. During these years, the woman may be "juggling" family, home, and career responsibilities with resulting increases in stress-related conditions. Health maintenance includes not only pelvic and breast screening, but also promotion of a healthy lifestyle, that is, good nutrition, regular exercise, smoking cessation, moderate or no alcohol consumption, sufficient rest, stress reduction, and referral for medical conditions and other specific problems. Common conditions in well-woman care include vaginitis, urinary tract infections, menstrual variations, obesity, sexual and relationship issues, and pregnancy.

Parenthood after age 35 years. The woman older than 35 is at risk for age-related conditions that can affect pregnancy. For example, a woman with type 2 diabetes may not have had expression of her diabetes at age 22 but may have full-blown disease at age 38. Other chronic or debilitating diseases or conditions increase in severity with time, and these, in turn, may predispose the woman to increased risks during pregnancy (National Women's Health Resource Center, 2008). Of significance to women in this age group is the risk for having a baby with certain genetic anomalies (e.g., Down syndrome), and the opportunity for genetic counseling should be available to all (March of Dimes Foundation, 2006b) (see Chapter 5).

Late reproductive age

Women of later reproductive age are often experiencing change and reordering personal priorities. Generally, the goals of education, career, marriage, and family have been achieved, and now the woman has increased time and opportunity for new interests and activities. Conversely, divorce rates are high at this age, and children leaving home may produce an "empty nest syndrome," resulting in levels of depression. Chronic diseases also become more apparent. Most problems for the well woman are associated with perimenopause (e.g., bleeding irregularities, vasomotor symptoms). Health-maintenance screening continues to be of importance because some conditions such as breast disease or ovarian cancer occur increasingly often during this stage.

Social and Cultural Factors

Differences exist among people from different socioeconomic levels and ethnic groups with respect to risk for illness and distribution of disease and death. Some diseases are more common among people of selected ethnicity, for example, sickle cell anemia in African-Americans, Tay-Sachs disease in Ashkenazi Jews, adult lactase deficiency in Chinese, beta thalassemia in Mediterranean peoples, and cystic fibrosis in northern Europeans. Cultural and religious influences also increase health risks because the woman and her family may have life and societal values and a view of health and illness that dictate practices different from those expected in the Judeo-Christian Western model. These practices may include food taboos or frequencies, methods of hygiene, effects of climate, care-seeking behaviors, willingness to undergo screening and diagnostic procedures, and value conflicts.

Socioeconomic contrasts result in major health differences, as exemplified in birth outcomes. The rates of perinatal and maternal deaths, preterm births, and low-birth-weight babies are higher in disadvantaged populations (Martin et al., 2008). Social consequences for poor women as single parents are great because many mothers with few skills are caught in the bind of having insufficient income to afford child care. These families generate fewer and fewer resources and increase their risks for health problems. Multiple roles for women in general produce overload, conflict, and stress, resulting in higher risks for psychologic illnesses.

Substance Use and Abuse

Cigarettes, caffeine, and alcohol are legal substances that can be addicting or harmful, especially to pregnant woman and her fetus or newborn. The inappropriate use of prescription and illicit drugs continues to increase and is found in all ages, races, ethnic groups, and socioeconomic strata. Addiction to substances is seen as a biopsychosocial disease, with several factors leading to risk. These factors include biogenetic predisposition, lack of resilience to stressful life experiences, and poor social support. Women are less likely than men to abuse drugs, but the rate in women is increasing significantly. Substance-abusing pregnant women create severe problems for themselves and their offspring, including interference with optimal growth and development and addiction. In many instances the use of substances is identified through screening programs in prenatal clinics and obstetric units.

Smoking

Cigarette smoking is a major preventable cause of illness and death. Smoking is linked to cardiovascular heart disease, various types of cancers (especially lung and cervical), chronic lung disease, and negative pregnancy outcomes. Tobacco contains nicotine, which is an addictive substance that creates a physical and a psychologic dependence. Cigarette smoking impairs fertility in both women and men, may reduce the age for menopause, and increases the risk for osteoporosis after menopause. Passive, or secondhand, smoke contains similar hazards and presents additional problems for the smoker, as well as harm for the nonsmoker. Smoking during pregnancy is known to cause a decrease in placental perfusion and is a cause of low birth weight (Kliegman, 2006).

Caffeine

Caffeine is a stimulant that is found in society's most popular drinks: coffee, tea, and soft drinks. It is a stimulant that can affect mood and interrupt body functions by producing anxiety and sleep interruptions. Heart arrhythmias may be made worse by caffeine, and interactions with certain medications such as lithium can occur. Birth defects have not been related to caffeine consumption; however, high intake has been related to an increase in the risk of miscarriage (Weng, Odouli, & Li, 2008).

Alcohol

Women aged 35 to 49 years have the highest rates of chronic alcoholism, but women aged 21 to 34 have the highest rates of specific alcohol-related problems. Approximately one third of alcoholics are women, and many relate the onset of their drinking problem to stressful events. Women who are problem drinkers are often depressed, and they have more motor-vehicle injuries and a higher incidence of attempted suicide than women in the general population. Also, they are at particular risk for alcohol-related liver damage (Centers for Disease Control and Prevention, 2008).

Prescription drugs

Psychotherapeutic drugs. Stimulants, sleeping pills, tranquilizers, and pain relievers are used by a small percentage of American women. Such drugs can bring relief from undesirable conditions such as insomnia, anxiety, and pain, but because the drugs have a mind-altering capacity, misuse can produce psychologic and physical dependency in the same manner as illicit drugs. Risk-to-benefit ratios should be considered when such drugs are used for more than very short periods. All of these categories of drugs have some effect on the fetus when taken during pregnancy, and their use should be monitored very carefully.

Depression is the most common mental health problem in women. Many kinds of medications are used to treat depression (National Women's Health Resource Center, 2006a). All of these psychotherapeutic drugs can have some effect on the fetus when taken during pregnancy and must be carefully monitored.

Illicit drugs

Cocaine. Cocaine is a powerful central nervous system stimulant that is addictive because of the tremendous sense of pleasure or good feeling that it creates. It can be snorted, smoked, or injected. Cocaine affects all of the major body systems. Among other complications, it produces cardiovascular stress that can lead to heart attack or stroke, liver disease, central nervous system stimulation that can cause seizures, and even perforation of the nasal septum. Users are often poorly nourished and commonly have STIs. If the user is pregnant, incidences of miscarriage, preterm labor, small-for-dates babies, abruption of placenta, and stillbirth are increased. Anomalies have also been reported (March of Dimes Foundation, 2006a).

Heroin. Heroin is an opiate that is usually injected but can be smoked or snorted. It produces euphoria, relaxation, relief from pain, and "nodding out" (apathy, detachment from reality, impaired judgment, and drowsiness). Signs and symptoms are constricted pupils, nausea, constipation, slurred speech, and respiratory depression (Stuart & Laraia, 2005). Users are at increased risk for acquiring human immunodeficiency virus (HIV) and hepatitis B, C, and D viruses, primarily because of sharing needles that contain contaminated blood. Perinatal effects include interference with fetal growth, premature rupture of membranes, preterm labor, and prematurity.

Marijuana. Marijuana is a substance derived from the cannabis plant. It is usually rolled into cigarettes and smoked, but it may also be mixed into food and eaten. It produces an intoxicating and sensory-distorting "high." Marijuana smoke has the same characteristics as tobacco smoke: both readily cross the placenta and have the effect of increasing carbon monoxide levels in the mother's blood, which reduces the oxygen supply to the fetus. Fetal abnormalities are possible (Stuart & Laraia, 2005).

Other illicit drugs. A sizable number of other street drugs pose risk to users. Variations of stimulants, such as *speed,* methamphetamine *(meth),* and *ice,* produce signs and symptoms similar to cocaine. Sedatives such as *downers, yellow jackets,* or *red devils* are used to "come down" from a high. Hallucinogens alter perception and body function. Phencyclidine hydrochloride (PCP; *angel dust*) and lysergic acid diethylamide *(LSD)* produce vivid changes in sensation, often with agitation, euphoria, paranoia, and a tendency toward antisocial behavior. Their use may lead to flashbacks, chronic psychosis, and violent behavior (Stuart & Laraia, 2005).

Nutrition

Good nutrition is essential for optimal health. A well-balanced diet helps prevent illness and is also used to treat certain health problems. Conversely, poor eating habits, eating disorders, and obesity are linked to disease and debility.

Nutritional deficiencies

Overt disease caused by the lack of certain nutrients is rarely seen in the United States; however, insufficient amounts or imbalances of nutrients do pose problems for individuals and families. Overweight or underweight status, malabsorption, listlessness, fatigue, frequent colds and other minor infections, constipation, dull hair and thin nails, and dental caries are examples of problems that can be related to poor nutrition and indicate the need for further nutritional assessment. Poor nutrition, especially related to obesity and excessive fat and cholesterol intake, may lead to more serious conditions and is said to contribute to four of the six leading causes of death in the United States: diseases of the heart, malignant neoplasms, cerebrovascular diseases, and diabetes (Kung, Hoyert, Xu, & Murphy, 2008).

Obesity

During the last 20 years, obesity in the United States has increased dramatically. Estimates indicate that one third of women older than 20 years are obese (body mass index [BMI] 30 or higher), and two thirds of women older than 20 years are obese or overweight (BMI 25 to 25.9) (National Women's Health Resource Center, 2006b). In the United States the prevalence of obesity is highest among non-Hispanic black women, followed by Hispanic women and non-Hispanic white women (Ogden, Carroll, Curtin, McDowell, Tabak, & Flegal, 2006). The BMI is defined as a measure of an adult's weight in relation to his or her height, specifically the adult's weight in kilograms divided by the square of his or her height in meters (see Chapter 8).

Overweight and obesity are known risk factors for diabetes, heart disease, stroke, hypertension, gallbladder disease, osteoarthritis, sleep apnea, and some types of cancer (uterine, breast, colorectal, kidney, and gallbladder) (American Cancer Society, 2009). In addition, obesity is associated with high cholesterol, menstrual irregularities, hirsutism (excessive body and facial hair), stress incontinence, depression, complications of pregnancy, increased surgical risk, and shortened life span (U.S. Department of Health and Human Services & U.S. Department of Agriculture, 2005). Obesity-related pregnancy complications include macrosomia, gestational diabetes, hypertensive disorders, preterm birth, and cesarean birth. Pregnant women who are morbidly obese are at increased risk for intrauterine growth restriction and intrauterine fetal demise (Smith, Hulsey, & Goodnight, 2008).

Other considerations

Other dietary extremes also can produce risk. For example, insufficient amounts of calcium can lead to osteoporosis, too much sodium can aggravate hypertension, and megadoses of vitamins can cause adverse effects in several body systems. Fad weight-loss programs and "yo-yo dieting" (repeated weight gain and weight loss) result in nutritional imbalances and, in some instances, medical problems. Such diets and programs are not appropriate for weight maintenance. Adolescent pregnancy produces special nutritional requirements because the metabolic needs of pregnancy are superimposed on the teen's own needs for growth and maturation at a time when eating habits are less than ideal.

Anorexia nervosa

Some women have a distorted view of their bodies and, no matter what their weight, perceive themselves to be much too heavy. As a result, they undertake strict and severe diets and rigorous extreme exercise. This chronic and rarest of eating disorders is known as *anorexia nervosa.* A coexisting depression usually accompanies anorexia. Women can carry this condition to the point of starvation, with resulting endocrine and metabolic abnormalities. If nutritional status is not corrected, significant complications of arrhythmias, cardiomyopathy, and congestive heart failure occur and, in the extreme, can lead to death. The condition commonly begins during adolescence in young women who have some degree of personality disorder. They gradually lose weight over several months, have amenorrhea, and are abnormally concerned with body image. The condition requires both psychiatric and medical interventions (Wolfe, 2005).

Bulimia nervosa

Bulimia refers to secret, uncontrolled binge eating alternating with methods to prevent weight gain: self-induced vomiting, taking laxatives or diuretics, strict diets, fasting, and rigorous exercise. Bulimia usually begins in early adulthood (ages 18 to 25) and is found primarily in young women. Complications can include dehydration and electrolyte imbalance, gastrointestinal (GI) abnormalities, dental problems, and cardiac arrhythmias (Wolfe, 2005).

Physical Fitness and Exercise

Exercise contributes to good health by lowering risks for a variety of conditions that are influenced by obesity and a sedentary lifestyle. It is effective in the prevention of cardiovascular disease and in the management of chronic conditions such as hypertension, arthritis, diabetes, respiratory disorders, and osteoporosis. Exercise also contributes to stress reduction and weight maintenance. Women report that engaging in regular exercise improves their body image and self-esteem and acts as a mood enhancer. Aerobic exercise produces cardiovascular involvement because increasing amounts of oxygen are delivered to working muscles. Anaerobic exercise, such as weight training, improves individual muscle mass without stress on the cardiovascular system. Because women are concerned about both cardiovascular and bone health, weight-bearing aerobic exercises such as walking, running, racket sports, and dancing are preferred. Excessive or strenuous exercise can lead to hormonal imbalances, resulting in amenorrhea and its consequences. Physical injury is also a potential risk.

Stress

Stress in women often occurs because of multiple roles in which coping with job and financial responsibilities conflict with parenting and home. To add to this burden, women are socialized to be caretakers, which is emotionally draining in itself. Also, they may find themselves in positions of minimal power that do not allow them to have control over their everyday environments. Some stress is normal and, in fact, contributes to positive outcomes. Many women thrive in busy surroundings. However, excessive or high levels of ongoing stress trigger physical reactions in the body, such as rapid heart rate, elevated blood pressure, slowed digestion, release of additional neurotransmitters and hormones, muscle tenseness, and weakened immune system. Consequently, constant stress can contribute to clinical illnesses such as flare-ups of arthritis or asthma, frequent colds or infections, GI upsets, cardiovascular problems, and infertility. Psychologic signs such as anxiety, irritability, eating disorders, depression, insomnia, and substance abuse also have been associated with stress.

Sexual Practices

Potential risks related to sexual activity are undesired pregnancy and STIs. The risks are particularly high for adolescents and young adults, who engage in sexual intercourse at earlier and earlier ages. Adolescents report many reasons for wanting to be sexually active, among which are peer pressure, desire to love and be loved, experimentation, enhancement of self-esteem, and enjoyment. However, many teens do not have the decision-making or values-clarification skills needed to take this important step at a young age and also lack a good knowledge base regarding contraception and STIs. They also do not believe that becoming pregnant or getting an STI will happen to them.

Although some STIs can be cured with antibiotics, many can cause significant problems. Possible sequelae include infertility, ectopic pregnancy, neonatal morbidity and mortality, genital cancers, acquired immunodeficiency syndrome, and even death (Centers for Disease Control and Prevention, Workowski, & Berman, 2006) (see Chapter 3). No method of contraception offers complete protection.

Spanish Guidelines: Recognizing Violence in a Relationship

NURSING ALERT A comprehensive sexual assessment should be integrated into all health histories.

Medical Conditions

Most women of reproductive age are relatively healthy. However, certain medical conditions that occur during pregnancy can have deleterious effects on both mother and fetus. Of particular concern are risks from all forms of diabetes, urinary tract disorders, thyroid disease, hypertensive disorders of pregnancy, cardiac disease, and seizure disorders. Effects on the fetus vary and include intrauterine growth restriction, macrosomia, anemia, prematurity, immaturity, and stillbirth. Effects on the mother can also be severe. See Chapter 20 for information on specific conditions.

Gynecologic Conditions Affecting Pregnancy

Gynecologic conditions may contribute negatively to pregnancy by causing infertility, miscarriage, preterm labor, and fetal and neonatal problems. Most of these conditions are discussed in Chapter 3 and include pelvic inflammatory disease, endometriosis, STIs and other vaginal infections, uterine fibroids, and uterine deformities such as bicornuate uterus. Gynecologic and other cancers also affect women's health. Risk factors depend on the type of cancer (Table 2-2).

Environmental and Workplace Hazards

Environmental hazards in the home, workplace, and community can contribute to poor health at all ages. Environmental hazards can affect fertility, fetal development, live birth, and the child's future mental and physical development. Everyone is at risk from air pollutants such as tobacco smoke, carbon monoxide, smog, suspended particles (dust, ash, and asbestos), and cleaning solvents; noise pollution; pesticides; chemical additives; and poor preparation of food. Workers also face safety and health risks caused by ergonomically poor workstations and stress. Risk assessments should continue to be in effect to identify and understand environmental public health problems.

Violence against Women

Violence against women is a major health care problem worldwide. In the United States, almost one in four women each year are affected, resulting in millions of dollars in annual medical costs (Family Violence Prevention Fund, 2009) (http://endabuse.org). Women of all races and of all ethnic, educational, religious, and socioeconomic backgrounds are affected. The magnitude of the problem may be far greater than the statistics indicate because violent crimes against women are underreported as a result of fear, lack of understanding, and stigma surrounding violent situations.

Maternity and women's health nurses, by the very nature of their practice, are in a unique position to conduct case findings, provide sensitive care to women

TABLE 2-2

Gynecologic and Other Cancers

CANCER	RISK FACTORS	SIGNS AND SYMPTOMS	COMMENTS
Cervical	Human papillomavirus (HPV) infection is the most common cause. Other risk factors include early age of first sexual intercourse, cigarette smoking, human immunodeficiency virus infection, possible other sexually transmitted infections (e.g., chlamydia), and multiple sexual partners.	Abnormal spotting or vaginal bleeding is the primary sign.	Preinvasive cancer is more common than invasive cancer.
Endometrial	Estrogen-related exposures such as nulliparity, unopposed estrogen therapy, infertility, early menarche, and late menopause; obesity, hypertension, diabetes, and family history of breast or ovarian cancer.	Abnormal uterine bleeding is the cardinal sign.	Use of birth control pills and pregnancy appear to provide some protection against endometrial cancer. It occurs most frequently in Caucasian women and after menopause.
Ovarian	Risk factors include family history of ovarian or breast cancer and having no children or having them late in life. Risk increases with age.	Abdominal enlargement accompanied by persistent vague digestive symptoms is the most common sign.	Ovarian cancer is the most malignant of all gynecologic cancers, accounting for the most deaths from these cancers.
Vulvar, vaginal, uterine tube	Cancers of the vulva and vagina have been linked to HPV and herpes simplex virus; the cause of uterine tube cancer is unknown.	Lesions are often the first sign of vulvar cancer. Women with vaginal or uterine tube cancer may be asymptomatic or have vaginal bleeding.	Occurrence is uncommon.
Lung	Cigarette smoking is the most important risk factor. Other risks include exposure to certain industrial substances, organic chemicals (e.g., radon, asbestos), and radiation.	A persistent cough, blood-tinged sputum, chest pain, and recurring pneumonia or bronchitis	Lung cancer is the leading cause of cancer deaths in women.
Breast	Family history, inherited genetic mutations (BRCA1 and BRCA2), early menarche, late menopause, nulliparity or having children later in life, and possibly postmenopausal use of estrogen. Risk increases with age.	Earliest sign is having an abnormality that shows up on a mammogram before it can be detected by the woman or a clinician.	Breast cancer is the second leading cause of cancer deaths in women.
Colon	A personal or family history of colorectal cancer or polyps, inflammatory bowel disease, and a high-fat, low-fiber diet. Risk increases with age.	Signs include rectal bleeding, blood in the stool, and a change in bowel habits.	Colon cancer is the third most common cancer in women.

Sources: American Cancer Society (ACS). (2009). *Cancer facts and figures, 2009.* New York: ACS; DiSaia, P. & Creasman, W. (2007). *Clinical gynecologic oncology* (7th ed.). Philadelphia: Mosby.

experiencing abusive situations, engage in prevention activities, and influence health care and public policy toward decreasing the violence.

Intimate partner violence

Intimate partner violence (IPV), *wife battering, spouse abuse,* and *domestic violence* or *family violence* are all terms applied to a pattern of assaultive and coercive behaviors that includes physical, sexual, and psychologic attacks, as well as economic coercion usually inflicted by a male partner in a marriage or other heterosexual, significant, intimate relationship. IPV is the preferred term (Krieger, 2008).

Relationship violence rarely consists of a single episode, but rather is a pattern that may start with intimidation or threats and progress to more aggressive physical and sexual acts, resulting in injury to the woman. Common elements of battering are economic deprivation, sexual abuse, intimidation, isolation, and stalking and terrorizing victims and their children. Pregnancy is often a time when violence begins or escalates (Krieger, 2008) (see Chapter 7).

Characteristics of women in battering relationships. Every segment of society is represented among abused women; race, religion, social background, age, and educational level are not significant factors in differentiating women at risk. Battered women may believe they are to blame for the situation because they are "not good enough wives." Many women have low self-esteem and may have histories of IPV in their families of origin. Social isolation seems to be another characteristic of battered women, which may result from stigma, fear, or restrictions placed on them by their partners.

Cycle of violence: the dynamics of battering. According to the cycle of violence concept, battering is neither random nor constant; rather, it occurs in repeated cycles (Fig. 2-8). A three-phase cyclic pattern to the battering behavior has been described as a period of increasing tension leading to the battery, which is then followed by a period of calm and remorse in which the male partner displays kind, loving behavior and pleas for forgiveness. This "honeymoon" phase lasts until stress or other factors cause conflict and tension to mount again toward another episode of battering. Over time, the tension and battering phases last longer and the calm phase becomes shorter until no honeymoon phase exists (Walker, 1984).

ⓔ Nursing Care Plan: The Battered Woman
ⓔ Critical Thinking Exercise: Women's Health and Safety
ⓔ Case Study: Health Assessment

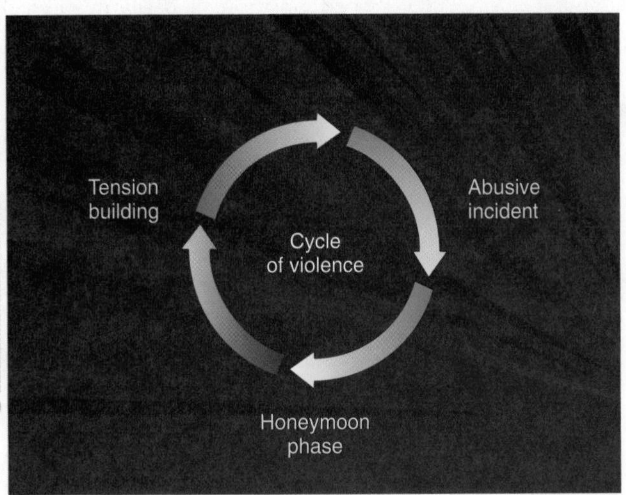

Fig. 2-8 Cycle of violence. (Courtesy Barbara Rynerson, Chapel Hill, NC.)

Sexual abuse and rape

The rate of sexual assault or rape in women age 12 or older was 1.8 per 1000 in 2007 (Family Violence Prevention Fund, 2009). Many female sexual abuse and assault victims experience posttraumatic stress disorder (PTSD). Common psychopathologic consequences are dissociative identity disorder, borderline personality disorder, and generalized anxiety disorder. Although pregnant or postpartum patients with these diagnoses may come to the attention of maternity nurses, women who experience symptoms of PTSD, sexual dysfunction, depression, anxiety, or substance abuse problems are more likely to be seen in gynecologic practice.

Rape is an act of violence rather than a sexual act. Rape is a legal and not a medical entity and, in its strictest sense, is the penile penetration of the female sex organ or labia without the woman's consent. *Sexual assault,* a term used interchangeably with *rape,* is also an act of force and has a much broader definition to include unwanted or uncomfortable touches, kisses, hugs, petting, intercourse, or other sexual acts. States may also use different legal definitions of rape.

Medical considerations for the rape victim include treatment of physical injuries, prophylactic treatment for STIs, and prophylaxis for pregnancy (emergency contraception) (see Chapter 4). Emergency departments and ambulatory care facilities usually follow protocols for examination, collection of evidence and photographing injuries, treatment, and providing information on community resources for victims of violence.

HEALTH ASSESSMENT

Interview

At a woman's first visit, she is often expected to fill out a form with biographic and historical data before meeting with the examiner. The nurse is usually responsible for ensuring that the woman's name, age, marital status, race, ethnicity, address, phone numbers, occupation, and date of visit are recorded. The interview should be conducted in a private, comfortable, and relaxed setting and in an unhurried manner (Fig. 2-9). The woman is addressed by her title and name (e.g., Mrs. Chang), and the nurse introduces herself or himself using name and title. Phrasing questions in a sensitive and nonjudgmental manner is

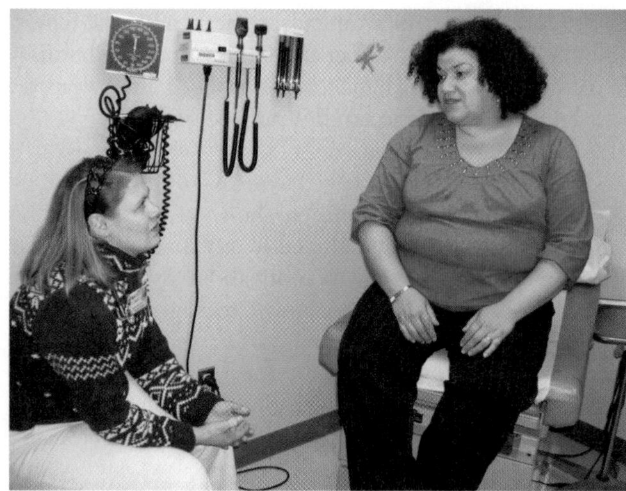

Fig. 2-9 Nurse interviews woman as part of annual physical examination. (Courtesy Ed Lowdermilk, Chapel Hill, NC.)

important. The woman's culture should be considered in case modifications in the examinations should be needed. For example, a female examiner may be preferred, or disrobing completely for an examination may be inappropriate for the woman. The nurse is cognizant of a woman's vulnerability and assures her of strict confidentiality. Many women are uninformed, misguided by myths, or afraid they will appear ignorant by asking questions about sexual or reproductive functioning. The woman is assured that no question is irrelevant. The history begins with an open-ended question such as, "What brings you in to the office/clinic/hospital today? Anything else? Tell me about it."

Communication may be hindered by different beliefs even when the nurse and patient speak the same language. Examples of communication variations are listed in the Cultural Considerations box.

Cultural Considerations

Communication Variations

- *Conversational style and pacing:* Silence may show respect or acknowledgment that the listener has heard. In cultures in which a direct "no" is considered rude, silence may mean *no*. Repetition or loudness may mean emphasis or anger.
- *Personal space:* Cultural conceptions of personal space differ based on one's culture. Someone may be perceived as distant for backing off when approached or aggressive for standing too close.
- *Eye contact:* Eye contact varies among cultures from intense to fleeting. In an effort to refrain from invading personal space, avoiding direct eye contact may be a sign of respect.
- *Touch:* The norms about how people should touch each other vary among cultures. In some cultures, physical contact with the same sex (embracing, walking hand in hand) is more appropriate than that with an unrelated person of the opposite sex.
- *Time orientation:* In some cultures, involvement with people is more valued than being *on time*. In other cultures, life is scheduled and paced according to clock time, which is valued over personal time.

Source: Mattson, S. (2000). Striving for cultural competence: Providing care for the changing face of the U.S. *AWHONN: Lifelines, 4*(3), 48-52.

Women with Special Needs

Women with emotional or physical disorders have special needs. Women who are visually, aurally, emotionally, or physically disabled should be respected and involved in the assessment and physical examination to the full extent of their abilities. The assessment and physical examination can be adapted to each woman's individual needs.

Communication with a woman who is hearing impaired can be accomplished without difficulty. Most of these women read lips, write, or both; therefore an interviewer who speaks and enunciates each word slowly and in full view may be easily understood. If a woman is not comfortable with lip reading, she may use an interpreter. The visually impaired woman needs to be oriented to the examination room and may have her guide dog with her. As with all patients, the visually impaired woman needs a full explanation of what the examination entails before proceeding. For example, before touching the woman, the nurse explains, "Now I am going to place a cuff on your right arm to take your blood pressure." Ask the woman if she would like to touch each of the items that will be used in the examination to reduce her anxiety.

Many physically disabled women cannot comfortably lie in the lithotomy position for the pelvic examination. Specially designed examination tables are available in some clinics. When this equipment is not available, several alternative positions may be used, including a lateral (side-lying) position, a V-shaped position, a diamond-shaped position, and an M-shaped position (Piotrowski & Snell, 2007) (Fig. 2-10). Ask the woman what has worked best for her previously. If she has not had a pelvic or a comfortable examination in the past, show her a picture of various positions and ask her which one she prefers. The nurse's support and reassurance can help the woman to relax, which will make the examination go more smoothly.

Abused women

Nurses should screen all women entering the health care system for potential abuse. It is important to keep in mind the possibility that violence against this woman may have occurred. Help for the woman may depend on the sensitivity with which the nurse screens for abuse, the discovery of abuse, and subsequent intervention. The nurse must be familiar with the laws governing abuse in the state in which she or he practices.

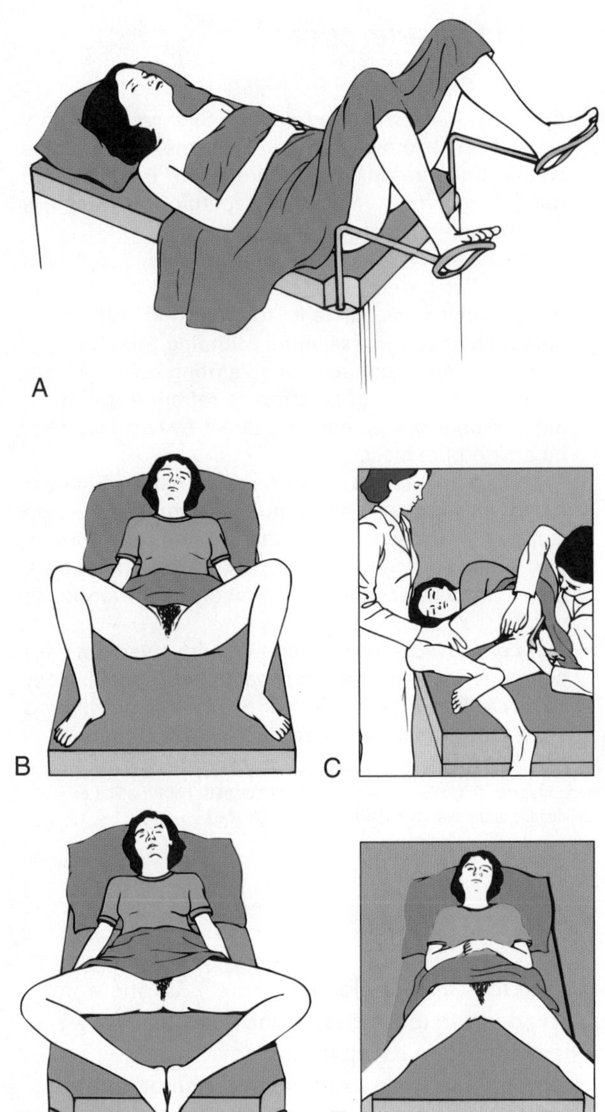

Fig. 2-10 Lithotomy and variable positions for women who have a disability. **A,** Lithotomy position. **B,** M-shaped position. **C,** Side-lying position. **D,** Diamond-shaped position. **E,** V-shaped position.

Spanish Guidelines: Physical Examination

Pocket cards listing emergency numbers (abuse counseling, legal protection, and emergency shelter) may be available by calling the local police department or women's shelter or going to an emergency department or 24-hour clinic. These emergency numbers should be on hand in the setting where screening is performed. An abuse assessment screen can be used as part of the interview or written history (Fig. 2-11). If a male partner is present, he should be asked to leave the room because the woman may not disclose experiences of abuse in his presence or he may try to answer questions for her to protect himself.

Fear, guilt, and embarrassment may keep many women from giving information about family violence. Clues in the history and evidence of injuries on physical examination should give a high index of suspicion. The areas most commonly injured in women are the head, neck, chest, abdomen, breasts, and upper extremities. Burns and bruises in patterns resembling hands, belts, cords, or other weapons and multiple traumatic injuries may be seen.

Adolescents

As a young woman matures, she should be asked the same questions that are included in any history. Particular attention should be paid to hints about risky behaviors, eating disorders, and depression. A teenager may or may not be sexually active. After rapport has been established, talking to a teen with the parent (or partner or friend) out of the room is best. Questions should be asked with sensitivity and in a gentle and nonjudgmental manner (Seidel, Ball, Dains, & Benedict, 2006).

History

As previously mentioned, at a woman's first visit, she is often expected to fill out a form with biographic and historical data before meeting with the examiner. This form aids the health care provider in completing the history during the interview. Most forms include information about the following categories:

- Biographic data
- Reason for seeking care
- Present health or history of present illness
- Past health
- Family history
- Review of systems
- Functional assessment (activities of daily living)

Box 2-2 describes a complete health history based on the above categories.

Physical Examination

In preparation for the physical examination, the woman is instructed on undressing and is given a gown to wear during the examination. She is usually given the opportunity to undress privately. Objective data are recorded by system or location. A general statement of overall health status is a good way to start. Findings are described in detail.

- *General appearance:* age, race, sex, state of health, posture, height, weight, development, dress, hygiene, affect, alertness, orientation, cooperativeness, communication skills
- *Vital signs:* temperature, pulse, respiration, blood pressure
- *Skin:* color; integrity; texture; hydration; temperature; edema; excessive perspiration; unusual odor; presence and description of lesions; hair texture and distribution; nail configuration, color, texture, condition, or presence of nail clubbing
- *Head:* size, shape, trauma, masses, scars, rashes, or scaling; facial symmetry; presence of edema or puffiness
- *Eyes:* pupil size, shape, reactivity, conjunctival injection, scleral icterus, fundal papilledema, hemorrhage, lids, extraocular movements, visual fields and acuity

ABUSE ASSESSMENT SCREEN

1. Have you ever been emotionally or physically abused by your partner or someone important to you?

YES ☐ NO ☐

2. Within the last year, have you been hit, slapped, kicked, or otherwise physically hurt by someone?

YES ☐ NO ☐

If YES, by whom ____________________

Number of times ____________________

Mark the area of injury on body map.

3. Within the last year, has anyone forced you to have sexual activities?

YES ☐ NO ☐

If YES, by whom ____________________

Number of times ____________________

4. Are you afraid of your partner or anyone you listed above?

YES ☐ NO ☐

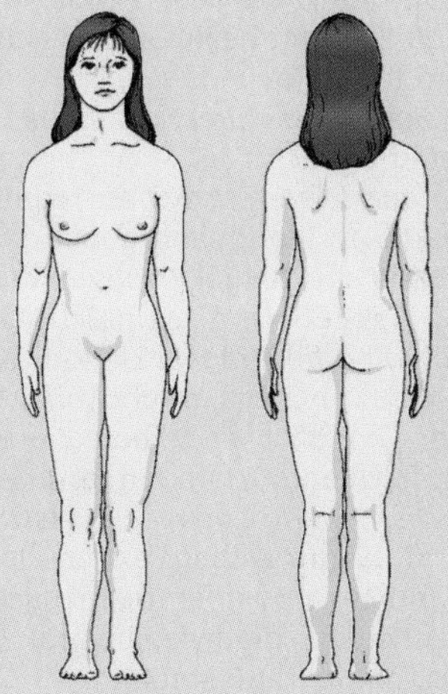

Fig. 2-11 Abuse assessment screen. (Modified from the Nursing Research Consortium on Violence and Abuse.)

- *Ears:* shape and symmetry, tenderness, discharge, external canal, and tympanic membranes; hearing–Weber should be midline (loudness of sound equal in both ears) and Rinne negative (no conductive or sensorineural hearing loss); should be able to hear whisper at 3 feet
- *Nose:* symmetry, tenderness, discharge, mucosa, turbinate inflammation, frontal or maxillary sinus tenderness; discrimination of odors
- *Mouth and throat:* hygiene, condition of teeth, dentures, appearance of lips, tongue, buccal and oral mucosa, erythema, edema, exudate, tonsillar enlargement, palate, uvula, gag reflex, ulcers
- *Neck:* mobility, masses, range of motion, trachea deviation, thyroid size, carotid bruits
- *Lymphatic:* cervical, intraclavicular, axillary, trochlear, or inguinal adenopathy; size, shape, tenderness, and consistency
- *Breasts:* skin changes, dimpling, symmetry, scars, tenderness, discharge or masses; characteristics of nipples and areolae
- *Heart:* rate, rhythm, murmurs, rubs, gallops, clicks, heaves, or precordial movements
- *Peripheral vascular:* jugular vein distention, bruits, edema, swelling, vein distention, Homans sign, or tenderness of extremities
- *Lungs:* chest symmetry with respirations, wheezes, crackles, rhonchi, vocal fremitus, whispered pectoriloquy, percussion, and diaphragmatic excursion; breath sounds equal and clear bilaterally
- *Abdomen:* shape, scars, bowel sounds, consistency, tenderness, rebound, masses, guarding, organomegaly, liver span, percussion (tympany, shifting, dullness), costovertebral angle tenderness
- *Extremities:* edema, ulceration, tenderness, varicosities, erythema, tremor, or deformity
- *Genitourinary:* external genitalia, perineum, vaginal mucosa, cervix, inflammation, tenderness, discharge, bleeding, ulcers, nodules, masses, internal vaginal support; bimanual and rectovaginal palpation of the cervix, uterus, and adnexae
- *Rectal:* sphincter tone, masses, hemorrhoids, rectal wall contour, tenderness, and stool for occult blood
- *Musculoskeletal:* posture, symmetry of muscle mass, muscle atrophy, weakness, appearance of joints, tenderness or crepitus, joint range of motion, instability, redness, swelling, or spine deviation
- *Neurologic:* mental status, orientation, memory, mood, speech clarity and comprehension, cranial nerves II to XII, sensation, strength, deep tendon and superficial reflexes, gait, balance, and coordination with rapid alternating motions

Pelvic Examination

Many women are intimidated by the gynecologic portion of the physical examination. The nurse in this instance can take an advocacy approach that supports a partnership relationship between the woman and the care provider. Preparing the adolescent for her first speculum

BOX 2-2

Health History and Review of Systems

Identifying data: Name, age, race, sex, marital status, occupation, religion, and ethnicity

Reason for seeking care: A response to the question, "What problem or symptom brought you here today?" If the woman lists more than one reason, focus on the one she thinks is most important.

Present health: Current health status is described with attention to the following:

- *Use of safety measures:* seatbelts, bicycle helmets, designated driver
- *Exercise and leisure activities:* regularity
- *Sleep patterns:* length and quality
- *Sexuality:* Is she sexually active? With men, women, or both? Risk-reducing sex practices?
- *Diet, including beverages:* 24-hour dietary recall; caffeine: coffee, tea, cola, or chocolate intake
- *Nicotine, alcohol, illicit or recreational drug use:* type, amount, frequency, duration, and reactions
- *Environmental and chemical hazards:* home, school, work, and leisure setting; exposure to extreme heat or cold, noise, industrial toxins such as asbestos or lead, pesticides, diethylstilbestrol (DES), radiation, cat feces, or cigarette smoke

History of present illness: A chronologic narrative that includes the onset of the problem, the setting in which it developed, its manifestations, and any treatments received are noted. The woman's state of health before the onset of the present problem is determined. If the problem is long standing the reason for seeking attention at this time is elicited. The principal symptoms should be described with respect to the following:

- *Location*
- *Quality or character*
- *Quantity or severity*
- *Timing (onset, duration, frequency)*
- *Setting*
- *Factors that aggravate or relieve*
- *Associated factors*
- Woman's perception of the meaning of the symptom

Past health:

- *Infectious diseases:* measles, mumps, rubella, whooping cough, chickenpox, rheumatic fever, scarlet fever, diphtheria, polio, tuberculosis (TB), hepatitis
- *Chronic disease and system disorders:* arthritis, cancer, diabetes, heart, lung, kidney, seizures, thyroid, stroke, ulcers, sickle cell anemia
- *Adult injuries, accidents*
- *Hospitalizations, operations, blood transfusions*
- *Obstetric history*
- *Allergies:* medications, previous transfusion reactions, environmental allergies
- *Immunizations:* diphtheria, pertussis, tetanus, polio, measles, mumps, rubella (MMR), hepatitis B, varicella, influenza, pneumococcal vaccine, last TB skin test
- *Last date of screening tests:* Pap test, mammogram, stool for occult blood, sigmoidoscopy or colonoscopy, hematocrit, hemoglobin, rubella titer, urinalysis, cholesterol test; electrocardiogram, last vision, dental, hearing examination
- *Current medications:* name, dose, frequency, duration, reason for taking, and compliance with prescription medications; home remedies, over-the-counter drugs, vitamin and mineral or herbal supplements used over a 24-hour period

Family history: Information about the ages and health of family members may be presented in narrative form or as a family tree or genogram: age, health or death of parents, siblings, spouse, children. Check for history of diabetes; heart disease; hypertension; stroke; respiratory, renal, or thyroid problems; cancer; bleeding disorders; hepatitis; allergies; asthma; arthritis; TB; epilepsy; mental illness; human immunodeficiency virus infection; or other disorders.

Screen for abuse: Has she ever been hit, kicked, slapped, or forced to have sex against her wishes? Has she been verbally or emotionally abused? Does she have a history of childhood sexual abuse? If yes, has she received counseling or does she need referral?

Review of systems: It is probable that all questions in each system will not be included every time a history is taken. Some questions regarding each system should be included in every history. The essential areas to be explored are listed in the following head-to-toe sequence. If a woman gives a positive response to a question about an essential area, more detailed questions should be asked.

- *General:* weight change, fatigue, weakness, fever, chills, or night sweats
- *Skin:* skin, hair, and nail changes; itching, bruising, bleeding, rashes, sores, lumps, or moles
- *Lymph nodes:* enlargement, inflammation, pain, suppuration (pus), or drainage
- *Head:* trauma, vertigo (dizziness), convulsive disorder, syncope (fainting); headache: location, frequency, pain type, nausea and vomiting, or visual symptoms present
- *Eyes:* glasses, contact lenses, blurriness, tearing, itching, photophobia, diplopia, inflammation, trauma, cataracts, glaucoma, or acute visual loss
- *Ears:* hearing loss, tinnitus (ringing), vertigo, discharge, pain, fullness, recurrent infections, or mastoiditis
- *Nose and sinuses:* trauma, rhinitis, nasal discharge, epistaxis, obstruction, sneezing, itching, allergy, or smelling impairment
- *Mouth, throat, and neck:* hoarseness, voice changes, soreness, ulcers, bleeding gums, goiter, swelling, or enlarged nodes
- *Breasts:* masses, pain, lumps, dimpling, nipple discharge, fibrocystic changes, or implants; breast self-examination practice
- *Respiratory:* shortness of breath, wheezing, cough, sputum, hemoptysis, pneumonia, pleurisy, asthma, bronchitis, emphysema, or TB; date of last chest x-ray
- *Cardiovascular:* hypertension, rheumatic fever, murmurs, angina, palpitations, dyspnea, tachycardia, orthopnea, edema, chest pain, cough, cyanosis, cold extremities, ascites, intermittent claudication (leg pain caused by poor circulation to the leg muscles), phlebitis, or skin-color changes

BOX 2-2

Health History and Review of Systems—cont'd

- *Gastrointestinal:* appetite, nausea, vomiting, indigestion, dysphagia, abdominal pain, ulcers, hematochezia (bleeding with stools), melena (black, tarry stools), bowel-habit changes, diarrhea, constipation, bowel-movement frequency, food intolerance, hemorrhoids, jaundice, or hepatitis; sigmoidoscopy, colonoscopy, barium enema, ultrasound
- *Genitourinary:* frequency, hesitancy, urgency, polyuria, dysuria, hematuria, nocturia, incontinence, stones, infection, or urethral discharge; menstrual history (e.g., age at menarche, length and flow of menses, last menstrual period [LMP], dysmenorrhea, intermenstrual bleeding, age at menopause or signs of menopause), dyspareunia, discharge, sores, itching
- *Sexual health and sexual activity:* with men, women, or both; contraceptive use; sexually transmitted infections
- *Peripheral vascular:* coldness, numbness and tingling, leg edema, claudication, varicose veins, thromboses, or emboli
- *Endocrine:* heat and cold intolerance, dry skin, excessive sweating, polyuria, polydipsia, polyphagia, thyroid problems, diabetes, or secondary sex characteristic changes
- *Hematologic:* anemia, easy bruising, bleeding, petechiae, purpura, or transfusions
- *Musculoskeletal:* muscle weakness, pain, joint stiffness, scoliosis, lordosis, kyphosis, range-of-motion instability, redness, swelling, arthritis, or gout
- *Neurologic:* loss of sensation, numbness, tingling, tremors, weakness, vertigo, paralysis, fainting, twitching, blackouts, seizures, convulsions, loss of consciousness or memory
- *Mental status:* moodiness, depression, anxiety, obsessions, delusions, illusions, or hallucinations
- *Functional assessment:* ability to care for self

examination is especially important because she will develop perceptions that will remain with her for future examinations. What the examination entails should be discussed with the teen while she is dressed. Models or illustrations can be used to show exactly what will happen. All of the necessary equipment should be assembled so that no interruptions occur. Pediatric specula that are 1 to 1.5 cm wide can be inserted with minimal discomfort. If the teen is sexually active, a small adult speculum may be used.

Have the woman empty her bladder before the procedure. This will make the examination less uncomfortable, and palpation of the pelvic organs will be easier. The woman is assisted into the lithotomy position (see Fig. 2-10, *A*) for the pelvic examination. When she is in the lithotomy position, the woman's hips and knees are flexed with the buttocks at the edge of the table, and her feet are supported by heel or knee stirrups.

Some women prefer to keep their shoes or socks on, especially if the stirrups are not padded. Many women express feelings of vulnerability and strangeness when in the lithotomy position. During the procedure the nurse assists the woman with relaxation techniques, such as taking slow deep breaths. Distraction is another technique that can be used effectively (e.g., placement of interesting pictures on the ceiling over the head of the table).

Many women find it distressing to attempt to converse in the lithotomy position. Most women appreciate an explanation of the procedure as it unfolds, as well as coaching for the type of sensations they may expect. Generally, however, women prefer not to have to respond to questions until they are again upright and at eye level with the examiner. Questioning during the procedure, especially if they cannot see their questioner's eyes, may make women tense.

External inspection

The examiner sits at the foot of the table for the inspection of the external genitals and for the speculum examination. To facilitate open communication and to help the woman relax, the woman's head is raised on a pillow, and the drape is arranged so that eye-to-eye contact can be maintained. In good lighting, external genitals are inspected for sexual maturity, including the clitoris, labia, and perineum. After childbirth or other trauma, healed scars may be seen.

External palpation

The examiner proceeds with the examination using palpation and inspection. The examiner wears gloves for this portion of the assessment. Before touching the woman, the examiner explains what is going to be done and what the woman should expect to feel (e.g., pressure). The examiner may touch the woman in a less sensitive area such as the inner thigh to alert her that the genital examination is beginning. This gesture may put the woman more at ease. The labia are spread apart to expose the structures in the vestibule: urinary meatus, Skene glands, vaginal orifice, and Bartholin glands (Fig. 2-12). To assess the Skene glands, the examiner inserts one finger into the vagina and "milks" the area of the urethra. Any exudate from the urethra or the Skene glands is cultured. Masses and erythema of either structure are assessed further. Ordinarily the openings to the Skene glands are not visible; prominent openings may be seen if the glands are infected (e.g., with gonorrhea). During the examination the examiner keeps in mind the data from the review of systems, such as history of burning on urination.

The vaginal orifice is examined. Hymenal tags are normal findings. With one finger still in the vagina, the

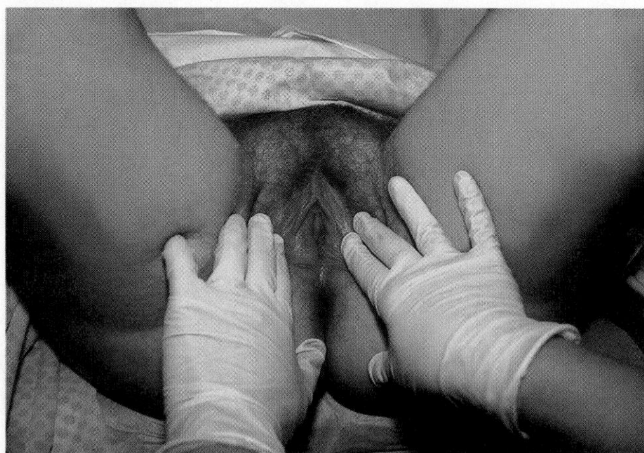

Fig. 2-12 External examination. Separation of the labia. (From Wilson, S.F., & Giddens, J.F. [2009]. *Health assessment for nursing practice* [4th ed]. St. Louis: Mosby.)

examiner repositions the index finger near the posterior part of the orifice. With the thumb outside the posterior part of the labia majora, the examiner compresses the area of Bartholin glands located at the 8 o'clock and 4 o'clock positions and looks for swelling, discharge, and pain.

The support of the anterior and posterior vaginal wall is assessed. The examiner spreads the labia with the index and middle finger and asks the woman to strain down. Any bulge from the anterior wall (urethrocele or cystocele) or posterior wall (rectocele) is noted and compared with the history, such as difficulty to start the stream of urine or constipation.

The perineum (area between the vagina and anus) is assessed for scars from old lacerations or episiotomies, thinning, fistulas, masses, lesions, and inflammation. The anus is assessed for hemorrhoids, hemorrhoidal tags, and integrity of the anal sphincter. The anal area is also assessed for lesions, masses, abscesses, and tumors. If the patient has a history of STI, the examiner may want to obtain a culture specimen from the anal canal at this time. Throughout the genital examination the examiner notes the odor. Odor may indicate infection or poor hygiene.

Vulvar self-examination. The pelvic examination provides a good opportunity for the practitioner to emphasize the need for regular **vulvar self-examination** (VSE) or *genital self-examination (GSE)* and to teach this procedure. A VSE should be performed as part of preventive health care by all women who are sexually active or 18 years of age or older to assess for signs of STIs or for signs of precancer or cancer. The examination can be performed by the practitioner and woman together using a mirror. A simple diagram of the anatomy of the vulva can be given to the woman along with instructions to perform the examination herself that evening to reinforce what she has learned. She performs the examination in a sitting position with adequate lighting, holding a mirror in one hand and using the other hand to expose the tissues surrounding the vaginal introitus. She then systematically examines the mons pubis, clitoris, urethra, labia majora, perineum, and perianal area and palpates the vulva, noting any changes in appearance of abnormalities, such as ulcers, lumps, warts, blisters, sores, and changes in pigmentation.

Internal examination

A vaginal speculum consists of two blades and a handle and comes in a variety of types and styles. A vaginal speculum is used to view the vaginal vault and cervix (see Procedure box: Assisting with Pelvic Examination). The closed speculum is gently placed into the vagina and inserted to the back of the vaginal vault. The blades are opened to reveal the cervix and are locked into the open position. The cervix is inspected for position and appearance of the os: color, lesions, bleeding, and discharge (Fig. 2-13). Cervical findings that are not within normal limits include ulcerations, masses, inflammation, and excessive protrusion into the vaginal vault. Anomalies, such as a cockscomb (a protrusion over the cervix that appears similar to a rooster's comb), a hooded or collared cervix (seen in *DES daughters*–women whose mothers ingested diethylstilbestrol [DES]), or polyps are noted.

Collection of specimens. The collection of specimens for cytologic examination is an important part of the gynecologic examination. Infection can be diagnosed through examination of specimens collected during the pelvic examination. Possible infections include *Candida albicans, Trichomonas vaginalis,* bacterial vaginosis, β-hemolytic streptococci, *Neisseria gonorrhoeae, Chlamydia trachomatis,* and herpes simplex virus (see Chapter 3). Once the diagnoses have been made, treatment can be instituted.

Papanicolaou (Pap) test. Carcinogenic conditions, potential or actual, can be determined by examination of cells from the cervix collected during the pelvic examination. This examination is termed a **Papanicolaou (Pap) test** (see Procedure box–Papanicolaou [Pap] Test).

Vaginal examination

After the specimens are obtained, the vagina is viewed when the speculum is rotated. The speculum blades are unlocked and partially closed. As the speculum is withdrawn, it is rotated and the vaginal walls are inspected for color, lesions, rugae, fistulas, and bulging.

Bimanual palpation

The examiner stands for this part of the examination. A small amount of lubricant is placed on the first and second fingers of the gloved hand for the internal examination. To prevent tissue trauma and contamination, the thumb is abducted and the ring and little fingers are flexed into the palm (Fig. 2-14).

The vagina is palpated for distensibility, lesions, and tenderness. The cervix is examined for position, shape, consistency, motility, and lesions. The fornix around the cervix is palpated.

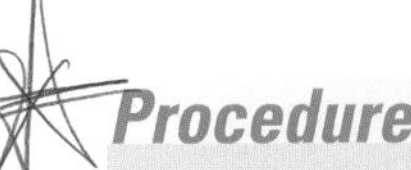

Procedure

Papanicolaou (Pap) Test

- In preparation, make sure the woman has not douched, used vaginal medications, or had sexual intercourse for 24 to 48 hours before the procedure. Reschedule the test if the woman is menstruating. Midcycle is the best time for the test.
- Explain to the woman the purpose of the test and what sensations she will feel as the specimen is obtained (e.g., pressure but not pain).
- The woman is assisted into a lithotomy position. A speculum is inserted into the vagina.
- The cytologic specimen is obtained before any digital examination of the vagina is made or endocervical bacteriologic specimens are taken. A cotton swab may be used to remove excess cervical discharge before the specimen is collected.
- The specimen is obtained by using an endocervical sampling device (Cytobrush, Cervex-brush, spatula, or broom) (see Figs. *A* and *B*). If the two-sample method of obtaining cells is used, the Cytobrush is inserted into the canal and rotated 90 to 180 degrees, followed by a gentle smear of the entire transformation zone by using a spatula. Broom devices are inserted and rotated 360 degrees five times. They obtain endocervical and ectocervical samples at the same time. If the patient has had a hysterectomy, the vaginal cuff is sampled. Areas that appear abnormal on visualization will require colposcopy and biopsy. If using a one-slide technique, the spatula sample is smeared first. This is followed by applying the Cytobrush sample (rolling the brush in the opposite direction from which it was obtained), which is less subject to drying artifact; then the slide is sprayed with preservative within 5 seconds.
- The ThinPrep or SurePath Pap Test is a liquid-based method of preserving cells that reduces blood, mucus, and inflammation. The Pap specimen is obtained in the manner described above except that the cervix is not swabbed before collection of the sample. The collection device (brush, spatula, or broom) is rinsed in a vial of preserving solution that is provided by the laboratory. The sealed vial with solution is sent off to the appropriate laboratory. A special processing device filters the contents, and a thin layer of cervical cells is deposited on a slide, which is then examined microscopically. The AutoPap and Papnet tests are similar to the ThinPrep test. If cytology is abnormal, liquid-based methods allow follow-up testing for human papillomavirus (HPV) DNA with the same sample.
- Label the slides or vial with the woman's name and site. Include on the form to accompany the specimens the woman's name, age, parity, and chief complaint or reason for taking the cytologic specimens.
- Send specimens to the pathology laboratory promptly for staining, evaluation, and a written report, with special reference to abnormal elements, including cancer cells.
- Advise the woman that repeated tests may be necessary if the specimen is not adequate.
- Instruct the woman concerning routine checkups for cervical and vaginal cancer. Women vaccinated against HPV should follow the same screening guidelines as unvaccinated women. Current recommendations of the U.S. Preventive Services Task Force (USPSTF) (2012) and the American Cancer Society (ACS) (2012) for Pap tests are that women ages 21 through 65 be screened every 3 years, or for women ages 30 through 65 every 5 years (if they had a pap test plus HPV test that were both negative). These guidelines recommend no screening in women younger than 21, although if a girl becomes sexually active, the guidelines recommend that she get a Pap test within 3 years of initiating sexual activity or at age 21—whichever comes first. Women with high risk factors such as exposure to diethylstilbestrol (DES) in utero, those treated for cervical intraepithelial neoplasia (CIN) 2, CIN 3, cervical cancer, or human immunodeficiency virus (HIV) may need more frequent screening.
- Young women who have been treated with excisional procedures for dysplasia have had an increase in premature births. A large majority of the cervical dysplasias in adolescents caused by HPV resolve on their own without treatment. It is important to avoid unnecessary instrumentation and procedures that negatively affect the cervix. Women who have had a complete hysterectomy for noncancerous reasons who have no history of high-grade CIN may have routine cervical cytology testing discontinued. Women who are older than 65 years who have not had serious cervical precancer or cancer in the past 20 years may discontinue cervical cancer screening (American Cancer Society, 2012).
- Record the examination date on the woman's record.
- Communicate findings to the woman per agency protocol.

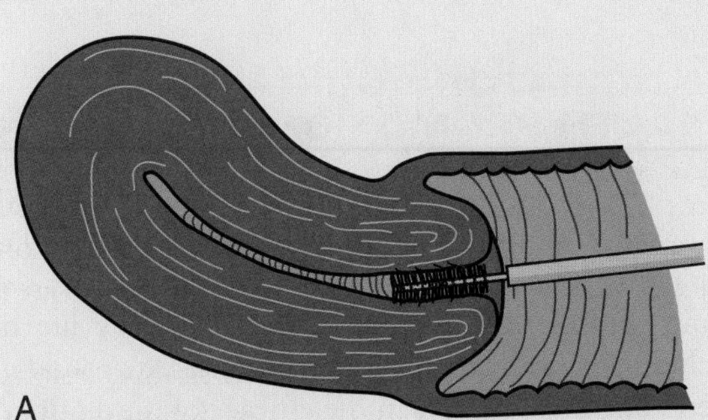

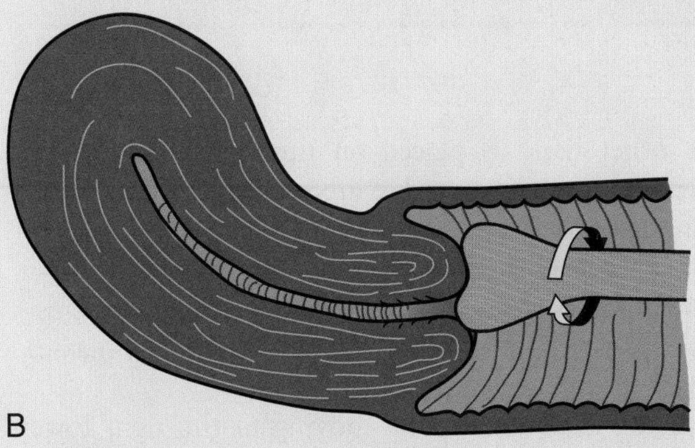

A, Collecting cells from endocervix using a Cytobrush. **B,** Obtaining cells from the transformation zone using a wooden spatula. (From Lentz, G.M., Lobo, R.A., Gershenson, D.M., et al. [2012]. *Comprehensive gynecology* [6th ed.]. St. Louis: Mosby.)

Procedure

Assisting with Pelvic Examination

- Wash hands. Assemble equipment (see figure below).
- Ask the woman to empty her bladder before the examination (obtain a clean-catch urine specimen as needed).
- Assist with relaxation techniques. Have the woman place her hands on her chest at approximately the level of the diaphragm, and ask her to breathe deeply and slowly.
- Encourage the woman to become involved with the examination if she shows interest. For example, a mirror can be placed so that she can see the area being examined.
- Assess for and treat signs of problems such as supine hypotension.
- Warm the speculum in warm water if a prewarmed one is not available.
- Instruct the woman to bear down when the speculum is being inserted.
- Apply gloves and assist the examiner with collection of specimens for cytologic examination, such as a Pap test. After handling specimens, remove the gloves and wash the hands.
- Lubricate the examiner's fingers with water or water-soluble lubricant before the bimanual examination.
- Assist the woman at the completion of the examination to a sitting position and then a standing position.
- Provide tissues to wipe the lubricant from the perineum.
- Provide privacy for the woman while she is dressing.

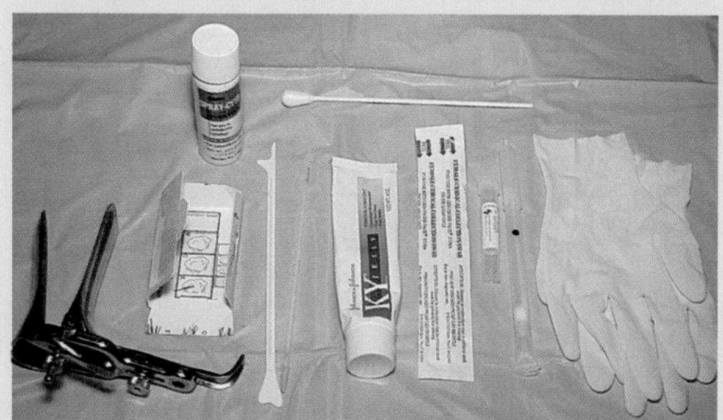

Equipment used for pelvic examination. (Courtesy Michael S. Clement, MD, Mesa, AZ.)

The other hand is placed on the abdomen halfway between the umbilicus and symphysis pubis and exerts pressure downward toward the pelvic hand. Upward pressure from the pelvic hand traps reproductive structures for assessment by palpation. The uterus is assessed for position, size, shape, consistency, regularity, motility, masses, and tenderness.

With the abdominal hand moving to the right lower quadrant and the fingers of the pelvic hand in the right lateral fornix, the adnexa is assessed for position, size, tenderness, and masses. The examination is repeated on the woman's left side.

Just before the intravaginal fingers are withdrawn, the woman is asked to tighten her vagina around the fingers as much as she can. If the muscle response is weak, the woman is assessed for her knowledge about Kegel exercises.

Rectovaginal palpation

To prevent contamination of the rectum from organisms in the vagina (e.g., *N. gonorrhoeae*) the examiner must change gloves, add fresh lubricant, and then reinsert the index finger into the vagina and the middle finger into the rectum (Fig. 2-15). Insertion is facilitated if the woman strains down. The maneuvers of the abdominovaginal examination are repeated. The rectovaginal examination permits assessment of the rectovaginal septum, the posterior surface of the uterus, and the region behind the cervix and the adnexa. The vaginal finger is removed and folded into the palm, leaving the middle finger free to rotate 360 degrees. The rectum is palpated for rectal tenderness and masses.

After the rectal examination, the woman is assisted into a sitting position, given tissues or wipes to cleanse herself, and given privacy to dress. The woman often returns to the examiner's office for a discussion of findings, prescriptions for therapy, and counseling.

Pelvic examination during pregnancy is discussed in Chapter 7.

Laboratory and Diagnostic Procedures

The following laboratory and diagnostic procedures are ordered at the discretion of the clinician: complete blood count or hemoglobin and hematocrit, total blood cholesterol, fasting plasma glucose, urinalysis for bacteria, syphilis serology (Venereal Disease Research Laboratory [VDRL] test or rapid plasma reagin test [RPR]) and other screening tests for STIs, mammogram, tuberculin skin test, hearing test, electrocardiogram, chest x-ray film, fecal occult blood, flexible sigmoidoscopy, and bone mineral density scan. Results of tests usually are reported by phone call or letter. HIV and drug screening may be offered or encouraged with informed consent, especially in high-risk populations; these results are usually reported in person.

ANTICIPATORY GUIDANCE FOR HEALTH PROMOTION AND PREVENTION

Knowledge alone is not enough to bring about healthy behaviors. The woman must be convinced that she has some control over her life and that healthy life habits, including periodic health examinations, are a sound investment. She must believe in the efficacy of prevention, early detection, and therapy and in her ability to perform self-management practices.

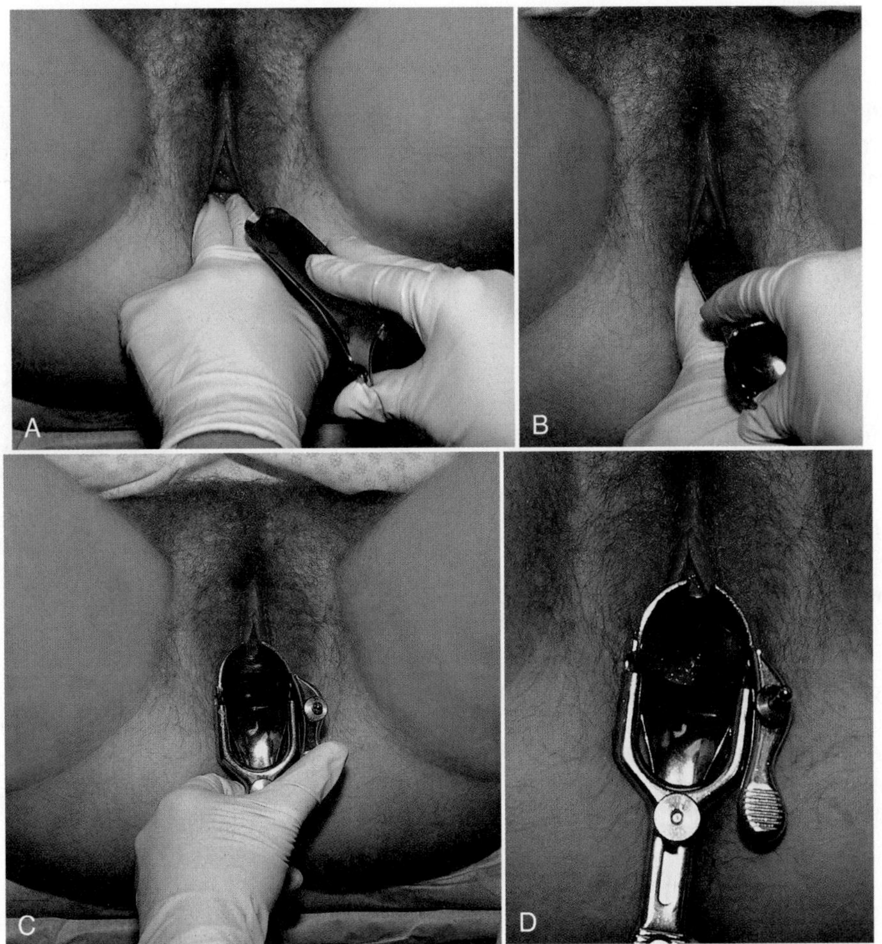

Fig. 2-13 Insertion of speculum for vaginal examination. **A,** Opening of the introitus. **B,** Oblique insertion of the speculum. **C,** Final insertion of the speculum. **D,** Opening of the speculum blades. (From Wilson, S.F., & Giddens, J.F. [2009]. *Health assessment for nursing practice* [4th ed]. St. Louis: Mosby.)

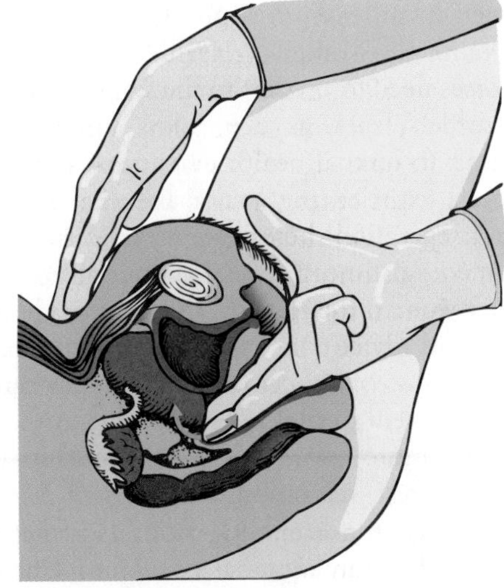

Fig. 2-14 Bimanual palpation of the uterus.

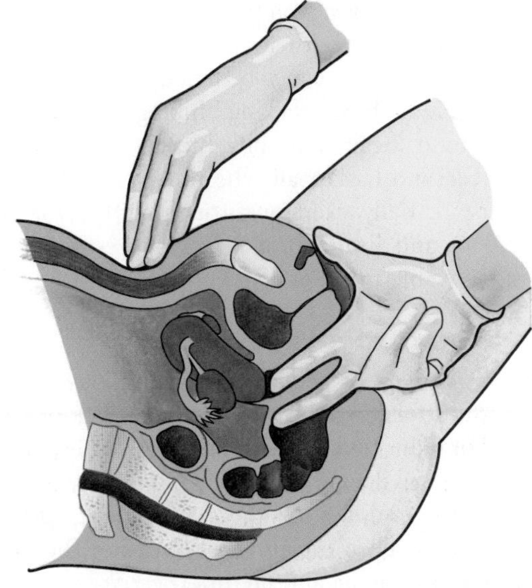

Fig. 2-15 Rectovaginal examination. (From Seidel, H., Ball, J., Dains, J., & Benedict, G. [2006]. *Mosby's guide to physical examination* [6th ed.]. St. Louis: Mosby.)

Nutrition

To maintain good nutrition, women should be counseled to eat a variety of foods. Foods low in saturated fat and cholesterol, moderate sodium and sugar intake, whole grain products, and a variety of fruits and vegetables should be selected (see www.MyPyramid.gov). At least four to six glasses of water in addition to other fluids such as juices should be included in the diet daily. Coffee, tea, soft drinks, and alcoholic beverages should be used in moderation (U.S. Department of Health and Human Services & Department of Agriculture, 2005). Red meats and processed meats, as well as refined grains, should be limited (American Cancer Society, 2009).

Most women do not recognize the importance of calcium to health, and their diets are insufficient in calcium. Women who are unlikely to get enough calcium in the diet may need calcium supplements in the form of calcium carbonate, which contains more elemental calcium than other preparations.

The diet can be assessed using a standard assessment form–a 24-hour recall is adequate and quick–and then food likes and dislikes, including cultural variations and typical food portions and dietary habits, should be discussed and incorporated into counseling. Referral to a weight-reduction program or support group may be beneficial.

Exercise

Physical activity and exercise counseling for women of all ages should be undertaken at schools, work sites, and primary care settings. American Heart Association (2009) recommendations include 30 to 60 minutes of moderate to vigorous activity on most days of the week at 50% to 75% of the maximum heart rate. Activities do not need to be strenuous to bring health benefits; including activities as part of a regular health routine is what is important. Activities that are especially beneficial when performed regularly include brisk walking, hiking, stair climbing, aerobic exercise, jogging, running, bicycling, rowing, swimming, soccer, and basketball. The nurse should stress the importance of daily exercise throughout life for weight management and health promotion, suggesting exercises that are enjoyable to the individual (Fig. 2-16).

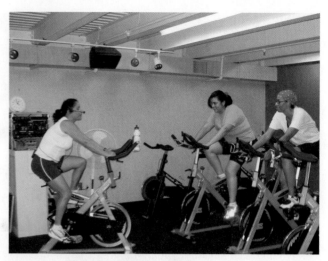

Fig. 2-16 Exercise should be a part of one's regular health routine. A cycle class is fun and provides moderate to vigorous exercise. (Courtesy Shari Rivera Sharp, Chapel Hill, NC.)

Kegel exercises

Kegel exercises, or pelvic floor muscle exercises, were developed to strengthen the supportive pelvic floor muscles to control or reduce incontinent urine loss. These exercises are also beneficial during pregnancy and postpartum. They strengthen the muscles of the pelvic floor, providing support for the pelvic organs and control of the muscles surrounding the vagina and urethra (Berzuk, 2007).

A research utilization project focused on continence for women was conducted by the Association of Women's Health, Obstetric and Neonatal Nurses (www.awhonn.org). Educational strategies for teaching women how to perform Kegel exercises were compiled by nurse researchers who were involved in the project are described in the Teaching Guidelines box.

Stress Management

Because it is neither possible nor desirable to avoid all stress, women need to learn how to manage stress. The nurse should assess each woman for signs of stress using therapeutic communication skills to determine risk factors and the woman's ability to function.

Some women must be referred for counseling or other mental health therapy. Women are two to three times as likely as men to suffer from depression, anxiety, or panic attacks (National Women's Health Resource Center, 2006a). Nurses need to be alert to the symptoms of serious mental disorders, such as depression and anxiety, and make referrals to mental health practitioners when necessary. Women experiencing major life changes, such as divorce and separation, bereavement, serious illness, and unemployment, also need special attention.

For many women the nurse is able to provide comfort, reassurance, and advice concerning helping resources, such as support groups. Many centers offer support groups to help women prevent or manage stress. The nurse can help them become more aware of the relationship between good nutrition, rest, relaxation, and exercise or diversion and their ability to deal with stress. In the case of role overload, determining what needs immediate attention and what can wait is important. Practical advice includes regular breaks, taking time for friends, developing interests outside of work or the home, setting realistic goals, and learning self-acceptance. Anticipatory guidance

TEACHING GUIDELINES

Kegel Exercises

DESCRIPTION AND RATIONALE

Kegel exercise, or pelvic floor muscle exercise, is a technique used to strengthen the muscles that support the pelvic floor. This exercise involves regularly tightening (contracting) and relaxing the muscles that support the bladder and urethra. By strengthening these pelvic muscles, a woman can prevent or reduce accidental urine loss.

TECHNIQUE

The woman needs to learn how to target the muscles for training and how to contract them correctly. One suggestion for teaching is to have the woman pretend she is trying to prevent the passage of intestinal gas. Have her use this tightening motion on the muscles around her vagina and the upper pelvis. She should feel these muscles drawing inward and upward. Other suggested techniques are to have the woman pretend she is trying to stop the flow of urine in midstream or to have her think about how her vagina is able to contract around and move up the length of the penis during intercourse.

The woman should avoid straining or bearing-down motions while performing the exercise. She should be taught how bearing down feels by having her take a breath, hold it, and push down with her abdominal muscles as though she were trying to have a bowel movement. Then the woman can be taught how to avoid straining down by exhaling gently and keeping her mouth open each time she contracts her pelvic muscles.

SPECIFIC INSTRUCTIONS

1. Each contraction should be as intense as possible without contracting the abdomen, thighs, or buttocks.
2. Contractions should be held for at least 10 seconds. The woman may have to start with as little as 2 seconds per contraction until her muscles get stronger.
3. The woman should rest for 10 seconds or more between contractions so that the muscles have time to recover and each contraction can be as strong as the woman can make it.
4. The woman should feel the pulling up over the three muscle layers so that the contraction reaches the highest level of her pelvis.

OTHER SUGGESTIONS FOR IMPLEMENTATION

1. At first the woman should set aside approximately 15 minutes a day to do the Kegel exercises.
2. The woman may want to put up reminders, such as notes on her bathroom mirror, her refrigerator, her television, or her calendar, to do the exercises.
3. Guidelines for practicing Kegel exercises suggest performing between 24 and 100 contractions a day; however, positive results can be achieved with only 24 to 45 a day.
4. The best position for learning how to do Kegel exercises is to lie supine with the knees bent. Another position to use is on the hands and knees. Once the woman learns the proper technique, she can perform the exercises in other positions such as standing or sitting.

Sources: Sampselle, C. (2000). Behavioral interventions for urinary incontinence in women: Evidence for practice. *Journal of Midwifery & Women's Health, 45*(2), 94-103; Sampselle, C. (2003). Behavior interventions in young and middle-aged women: Simple interventions to combat a complex problem. *American Journal of Nursing, 103*(suppl), 9-19; Sampselle, C. Wyman, J., Thomas, K., Newman, D., Gray, M., Dougherty, M., et al. (2000). Continence for women: A test of AWHONN's evidence-based protocol. *Journal of Obstetric, Gynecologic, and Neonatal Nursing, 29*(1), 312-317.

for developmental or expected situational crises can help women plan strategies for dealing with potentially stressful events.

Role playing, relaxation techniques, biofeedback, meditation, desensitization, imagery, assertiveness training, yoga, diet, exercise, and weight control are techniques nurses can include in their repertoire of helping skills. Insufficient time prevents one-on-one assistance in many situations, but the more nurses know about these resources, the better able they are to intervene, counsel, and direct women to appropriate resources. Careful follow-up of all women experiencing difficulty in dealing with stress is important.

Substance Use Cessation

All women at all ages will receive substantial and immediate benefits from smoking cessation. However, this task is not easy, and most people stop several times before they accomplish their goal (Box 2-3). Many are never able to do so. Those who wish to stop smoking can be referred to a smoking-cessation program where individualized methods can be implemented. At the very least, individuals should be guided to self-help materials available from the March of Dimes Birth Defects Foundation, American Lung Association, and American Cancer Society. During pregnancy, women seem to be highly motivated to stop or at least to limit smoking. Insult to the fetus can be reduced or even prevented if cessation is accomplished by the end of the first trimester (Bernstein, Mongeon, Badger, Solomon, Heil, & Higgins, 2005).

Counseling women who appear to be drinking excessively or using drugs may include strategies to increase self-esteem and teaching new coping skills to resist and maintain resistance to alcohol abuse and drug use. Appropriate referrals should be made, with the health care provider arranging the contact and then following up to be sure that appointments are kept. General referral to sources of support should also be provided. National groups that provide information and support for those who are chemically dependent are listed in the Web Resources (online). Many of these organizations have local branches or contacts that are listed in the telephone book.

BOX 2-3

Interventions for Smoking Cessation: The Five As

ASK

What was her age when she started smoking?
How many cigarettes does she smoke a day? When was her last cigarette?
Has she tried to quit?
Does she want to quit?

ASSESS

What were her reasons for not being able to quit before, or what made her start again?
Does she have anyone who can help her?
Does anyone else smoke at home?
Does she have friends or family who have quit successfully?

ADVISE

Give her information about the effects of smoking on pregnancy and her fetus, on her own future health, and on the members of her household.

ASSIST

Provide support; give self-help materials.
Encourage her to set a quit date.
Refer to a smoking-cessation program, or provide information about nicotine replacement products (not recommended during pregnancy) if she is interested.
Teach and encourage use of stress-reduction activities.
Provide for follow-up with a phone call, letter, or clinic visit.

ARRANGE FOLLOW-UP

Arrange to monitor the woman to find out about smoking-cessation status.
Make a phone call around the time of her quit date. Assess her status at every prenatal visit.
Congratulate her on her success, or provide support for her if she relapses.
Referral to intensive treatment may be necessary.

Source: American College of Obstetricians and Gynecologists, Committee on Health Care for Underserved Women, Committee on Obstetric Practice. (2005). ACOG Committee Opinion No. 316, October, 2005. Smoking cessation during pregnancy. *Obstetrics and Gynecology*, 106(4), 883-888.

Sexual Practices that Reduce Risk

Prevention of STIs is based on the reduction of high risk behaviors by educating toward a behavioral change. Behaviors of concern include multiple and casual sexual partners and unsafe sexual practices. The abuse of alcohol and drugs is also a high risk behavior resulting in impaired judgment and thoughtless acts. Specific self-management measures to reduce risk are described in Chapter 3.

In addition to information about the prevention of STIs, women of childbearing years need information regarding contraception and family planning (see Chapter 4).

Health Screening Schedule

Periodic health screening includes history, physical examination, education, counseling, and selected diagnostic and laboratory tests. This regimen provides the basis for overall health promotion, prevention of illness, early diagnosis of problems, and referral for appropriate management. Such screening should be customized according to a woman's age and risk factors. In most instances, it is completed in health care offices, clinics, or hospitals; however, portions of the screening are now being carried out at events such as community health fairs. An overview of health screening recommendations for women older than 18 years of age is found in Table 2-3.

Health Risk Prevention

Often, simple safety factors are forgotten or perceived not to be important; yet injuries continue to have a major impact on health status among all age groups. Being aware of hazards and implementing safety guidelines will reduce risks. The nurse should frequently reinforce commonsense concepts that will protect the individual, such as wearing seat belts at all times in a moving vehicle and protecting the skin from ultraviolet light with sunscreen and clothing.

Health Protection

Nurses can make a difference in stopping violence against women and preventing further injury. Educating women that abuse is a violation of their rights and facilitating their access to protective and legal services constitute a first step. Also, encouraging health care institutions to implement appropriate IPV assessment and intervention programs is needed. Other helpful measures for women to discourage their fall into abusive relationships are promoting assertiveness and self-defense courses; suggesting support and self-help groups that encourage positive self-regard, confidence, and empowerment; and recommending educational and skills development classes that will enhance independence or at least the ability to take care of oneself. Numerous national and local organizations provide information.

NURSING ALERT Nurses should be knowledgeable about reporting requirements and community services for women who have been sexually assaulted or abused.

TABLE 2-3

Health Screening Guidelines and Immunization Recommendations for Women Ages 18 Years and Older

INTERVENTION	RECOMMENDATION*
PHYSICAL EXAMINATION	
Blood pressure	Every visit, but at least every 2 years
Height and weight	Every visit, but at least every 2 years
Pelvic examination	Annually until age 70; recommended for any woman who has ever been sexually active
BREAST EXAMINATION	
Clinical examination	Every 3 years, ages 20 to 39; after age 40 with periodic examination, preferably annually
High risk	Annually after age 18 with history of premenopausal breast cancer in first-degree relative
Risk groups	
Skin examination	Family history of skin cancer or increased exposure to sunlight every 3 years between ages 20 and 40; annually after age 40; monthly mole self-examinations also recommended
Oral cavity examination	History of mouth lesions or exposure to tobacco or excessive alcohol at least annually
LABORATORY AND DIAGNOSTIC TESTS	
Blood cholesterol (fasting lipoprotein analysis)	Between ages 20 and 45 only if high risk; Beginning at age 45 if level is within normal limits, every 5 years; more often if abnormal levels or have risk factors for coronary artery disease
Papanicolaou (Pap) test	Between ages 21 and 65—every 3 years with only Pap test done Between ages 30 and 65—every 5 years if Pap test plus human papillomavirus (HPV) test done After age 65 and 3 negative tests and no risks and after total hysterectomy for benign disease—women may choose to stop screening
Mammography†	Every 1 to 2 years between ages 40 and 49 or earlier if at high risk Annually after age 40 Annually after age 50 Biennially, ages 50 to 74 After age 75, discuss with your health care provider
Colon cancer screening	Use 1 of these 3 methods: • Fecal occult blood test annually ages 50 to 74 • Flexible sigmoidoscopy every 5 years ages 50 to 74 • Colonoscopy every 10 years ages 50 to 74 Screen more often if family history of colon cancer or polyps After age 75, discuss with your health care provider
Hearing screen	Starting at age 18, then every 10 years until 49 Every 3 years after age 50 Annually with exposure to excessive noise or when loss is suspected
Vision screen	At least once between ages 20 and 29; at least twice between ages 30 and 39; Every 2 to 4 years between ages 40 and 64; every 1 to 2 years after age 65
Risk groups	
Fasting blood sugar	Annually with family history of diabetes or gestational diabetes or if significantly obese; every 3 to 5 years for all women older than 45 years
Thyroid-stimulating hormone (TSH) test	As determined by the health care provider
Sexually transmitted infection test (e.g., gonorrhea, syphilis, herpes)	As needed if sexually active with multiple partners and engaging in risky sexual behaviors
Chlamydia test	If sexually active, yearly until age 25; after age 25, test as needed when sexually active with new or multiple partners
Human immunodeficiency virus (HIV) test	At least once between ages 18 and 64 to determine HIV status; test if there is a high risk for HIV infection

Continued

TABLE 2-3

Health Screening Guidelines and Immunization Recommendations for Women Ages 18 Years and Older—cont'd

INTERVENTION	RECOMMENDATION*
Tuberculin skin test	Annually with exposure to persons with tuberculosis or in risk categories for close contact with the disease
Endometrial biopsy	At menopause for women at risk for endometrial cancer; repeat as needed
Bone mineral density testing	All women age 65 and older at least once; repeat testing as needed; younger women with risk for osteoporosis may need periodic screenings
IMMUNIZATIONS	
Tetanus-diphtheria-pertussis (Td/Tdap)	Tdap vaccine once; then booster is given every 10 years
Measles, mumps, rubella	Once if born after 1956 and no evidence of immunity
Hepatitis A	Primary series of two injections for all who are in risk categories
Hepatitis B	Primary series of three injections for all who are in risk categories
Influenza	Annually
Pneumococcal	1-2 doses between ages 19 and 64; 1 dose after age 65
Herpes zoster (shingles)	One dose at age 65
Human papillomavirus (HPV) vaccine	Primary series of three injections for girls ages 9 to women 26 years old; intended for those not previously exposed to HPV

Data from American Cancer Society (ACS). (2012). *Cancer prevention and early detection facts and figures.* Atlanta: Author; Centers for Disease Control and Prevention (CDC) Advisory Committee on Immunization Practices. (2012). *Recommended adult immunization schedule, United States.* www.cdc.gov/vaccines; Centers for Disease Control and Prevention (CDC). (2010). Sexually transmitted diseases treatment guidelines. *MMWR Recommendations and Reports* 59(RR12),1–109; National Women's Health Information Center. (2012). *Screenings tests for women.*, www.4woman.gov; U.S. Preventive Services Task Force. (2012). *Screening for cervical cancer.* www.preventiveservicestaskforce.org/uspstf/uspscerv.htm.

*The information in this table is only a guide; health care providers will individualize the timing of tests and immunizations for each woman.

†Note: No consensus has been reached regarding mammograms for women between 40 and 49 years of age; therefore various recommendations are listed. Women are urged to discuss circumstances with their health care providers.

KEY POINTS

- The female reproductive system consists of external and internal structures.
- Normal feedback regulation of the menstrual cycle depends on an intact hypothalamic-pituitary-gonadal mechanism.
- The female's reproductive tract structures and breasts respond predictably to changing levels of sex hormones across her life span.
- The myometrium of the uterus is uniquely designed to expel the fetus and promote hemostasis after birth.
- Prostaglandins play an important role in reproductive functions by their effect on smooth-muscle contractility and modulation of hormones.
- Culture, religion, socioeconomic status, personal circumstances, the uniqueness of the individual, and stage of development are among the factors that influence a person's recognition of need for care and response to the health care system and therapy.
- The changing status and roles of women affect their health needs and their ability to cope with problems.
- Assessment is more comprehensive and learning is best in a safe environment in which the atmosphere is nonjudgmental and sensitive and the interaction is strictly confidential.
- Preconception care allows identification and possible remediation of potentially harmful personal and social conditions, medical and psychologic conditions, and environmental conditions before conception.
- Conditions that increase a woman's health risks also increase risks for her offspring.
- Violence against women is a major social and health care problem in the United States.
- Periodic health screening, including history, physical examination, and diagnostic and laboratory tests, provides the basis for overall health promotion, prevention of illness, early diagnosis of problems, and referral for management.
- Health promotion and illness prevention assist women to actualize their health potential by increasing motivation, providing information, and suggesting how to access specific resources.

Audio Chapter Summaries Access an audio summary of these Key Points on evolve

References

Agency for Healthcare Research and Quality. (2005). *Women's health care in the United States. Selected findings from the 2004 national healthcare quality and disparities report.* Internet document available at www.ahrq.gov (accessed June 1, 2009).

American Cancer Society (ACS). (2009). *Cancer facts and figures 2009.* New York: ACS.

American Heart Association. (2009). *Physical activity and cardiovascular health: Questions and answers.* Internet document available at www.americanheart.org (accessed June 6, 2009).

Atrash, H., Johnson, K., Adams, M., Cordero, J., & Howse, J. (2006). Preconception care for improving perinatal outcomes: The time to act. *Maternal and Child Health Journal, 10*(5 Suppl), S3-S11.

Bernstein, I., Mongeon, J., Badger, G., Solomon, L., Heil, S., & Higgins, S. (2005). Maternal smoking and its association with birth weight. *Obstetrics and Gynecology, 106*(5 Part 1), 986-991.

Berzuk, K. (2007). A strong pelvic floor: How nurses can spread the word. *Nursing for Women's Health, 11*(1), 54-62.

Callister, L. (2005). What has the literature taught us about culturally competent care of women and children? *MCN The American Journal of Maternal/Child Nursing, 30*(6), 380-388.

Centers for Disease Control and Prevention. (2008). *Quick stats. General information on alcohol use and health.* Internet document available at www.cdc.gov/alcohol/quickstats/general_info.htm (accessed June 18, 2009).

Centers for Disease Control and Prevention (CDC), Workowski, K., & Berman, S. (2006). Sexually transmitted diseases treatment guidelines 2006. *Morbidity and Mortality Weekly Report. Recommendations and Reports, 55*(RR11), 1-94.

Family Violence Prevention Fund. (2009). *Get the facts: The facts on domestic, dating and sexual violence.* Internet document available at www.endabuse.org (accessed June 5, 2009).

Fehring, R., Schneider, M., & Raviele, K. (2006). Variability in the phases of the menstrual cycle. *Journal of Obstetric, Gynecologic, and Neonatal Nursing, 35*(3), 376-384.

Geddes, D. (2007). Inside the lactating breast: The latest anatomy research. *Journal of Midwifery & Women's Health, 52*(6), 556-563.

Goldberg, L. (2005-2006). Understanding the lesbian experience: What perinatal nurses should know to promote women's health. *AWHONN Lifelines, 9*(6), 463-467.

Huff, M., Abuzz, G., & Omar, H. (2007). Detecting and treating depression among adolescents presenting for reproductive care: Realizing opportunities. *Journal of Pediatric and Adolescent Gynecology, 20*(6), 371-376.

Johnson, K., Posner, S., Biermann, J., Cordero, J., Atrash, H., Parker, C. et al. (2006). Recommendations to improve preconception health and health care–United States. A report of the CDC/ATSDR preconception care work group and the select panel on preconception care. *Morbidity and Mortality Weekly Report. Recommendations and Reports, 55*(RR06), 1-23.

Kliegman, R. (2006). Intrauterine growth restriction. In R. Martin, A. Fanaroff, & M. Walsh (Eds.). *Fanaroff and Martins's neonatal–perinatal medicine: Diseases of the fetus and infant.* Philadelphia: Mosby.

Krieger, C. (2008). Intimate partner violence: A review for nurses. *Nursing for Women's Health, 12*(3), 224-233.

Kung, H., Hoyert, D., Xu J., & Murphy, S. (2008). Deaths: Final data for 2005. *National Vital Statistics Reports, 56*(10), 1-120.

Love, S., & Barsky, S. (2004). Anatomy of the nipple and breast ducts revisited. *Cancer, 101*(9), 1947-1957.

March of Dimes Foundation. (2006a). *Illicit drug use in pregnancy.* Internet document available at www.marchofdimes.com/professionals/14332_1169.asp (accessed June 4, 2009).

March of Dimes Foundation, (2006b). *Pregnancy after 35.* Internet document available at www.marchofdimes.com/printableArticles/14322_1155.asp (accessed June 4, 2009).

Martin, J., Kung, H., Mathews, T., Hoyert, D., Strobino, D., Guyer, B., & Sutton, S. (2008). Annual summary of vital statistics: 2006. *Pediatrics, 121*(4), 788-801.

Moos, M. (2006). Preconception care: Every woman, every time. *AWHONN Lifelines, 10*(4), 332-334.

National Women's Health Resource Center. (2008). Pregnancy & women age 35+. *National Women's Health Report, 30*(2), 1-4.

National Women's Health Resource Center. (2006a). *Depression.* Internet document available at www.healthywomen.org.healthtopics/depression (accessed June 5, 2009).

National Women's Health Resource Center. (2006b). Women and obesity. *National Women's Health Report, 28*(4), 1-7.

National Women's Law Center. (2007). *Making the grade on women's health: A national and state-by-state report card, 2007* Internet document available at www.nwlc.org (accessed June 2, 2009).

Ogden, C., Carroll, M., Curtin, L., McDowell, M., Tabak, C., & Flegal, M. (2006). Prevalence of overweight and obesity in the US–1999-2004. *Journal of the American Medical Association, 295*(13), 1549-1555.

Patchias, E., & Waxman, J. (2007). Women and health coverage: The affordability gap. *Issue Brief (Commonwealth Fund)* April, *25*, 1-12.

Piotrowski, K., & Snell, L. (2007). Health needs of women with disabilities across the life span. *Journal of Obstetric, Gynecologic, and Neonatal Nursing, 36*(1), 79-87.

Ramsay, D., Kent, J., Hartmann, R., & Hartmann, P. (2005). Anatomy of the lactating breast redefined with ultrasound imaging. *Journal of Anatomy, 206*(6), 525-534.

Roberts, S. (2006). Health care recommendations for lesbian women. *Journal of Obstetric, Gynecologic, and Neonatal Nursing, 35*(5), 583-591.

Seidel, H., Ball, J., Dains, J., & Benedict, G. (2006). *Mosby's guide to physical examination* (6th ed.). St. Louis: Mosby.

Smith, S., Hulsey, T., & Goodnight, W. (2008). Effects of obesity on pregnancy. *Journal of Obstetric, Gynecologic, and Neonatal Nursing, 37*(2), 176-184.

Speroff, L., & Fritz, M. (2005). *Clinical gynecologic endocrinology and infertility* (7th ed.). Philadelphia: Lippincott Williams & Wilkins.

Stuart, G., & Laraia, M. (2005). *Principles and practices of psychiatric nursing* (8th ed.). St. Louis: Mosby.

Trussell, J. (2007). The cost of unintended pregnancies in the United States. *Contraception, 75*(3), 168-170.

U.S. Department of Health and Human Services & U.S. Department of Agriculture. (2005). *Dietary guidelines for Americans 2005.* Hyattsville, MD: U.S. Department of Agriculture.

Walker, L. (1984). *The battered woman syndrome* (Vol. 6). New York: Springer.

Weng, X., Odouli, R., & Li, D. (2008). Maternal caffeine consumption during pregnancy and the risk of miscarriage: A prospective cohort study. *American Journal of Obstetrics and Gynecology, 198*(3), 279.e1-279.e8.

Wolfe, B. (2005). Reproductive health in women with eating disorders. *Journal of Obstetric, Gynecologic, and Neonatal Nursing, 34*(2), 255-263.

CHAPTER 3

Common Concerns

DEITRA LEONARD LOWDERMILK

LEARNING OBJECTIVES

- *Differentiate the signs and symptoms among common menstrual disorders.*
- *Develop a nursing care plan for the woman with primary dysmenorrhea.*
- *Outline patient teaching about premenstrual syndrome.*
- *Relate the pathophysiologic aspects of endometriosis to associated symptoms.*
- *Consider the use of alternative therapies for menstrual disorders.*
- *Describe the prevention of sexually transmitted infections in women.*
- *Differentiate the signs, symptoms, diagnoses, and management of women with bacterial and viral sexually transmitted infections.*
- *Differentiate the signs, symptoms, and management of selected vaginal infections.*
- *Explain the effects on and management of pregnant women who have human immunodeficiency virus (HIV) infection.*
- *Review the principles of infection control, including Standard Precautions and precautions for invasive procedures.*
- *Discuss the pathophysiologic features of selected benign breast conditions and malignant neoplasms of the breasts found in women.*
- *Discuss the emotional effects of benign and malignant neoplasms.*
- *Compare alternatives for treatment for the woman with a lump in her breast.*

KEY TERMS AND DEFINITIONS

amenorrhea Absence or cessation of menstruation

dysfunctional uterine bleeding (DUB) Excessive uterine bleeding with no demonstrable organic cause

dysmenorrhea Painful menstruation beginning 2 to 6 months after menarche, related to ovulation or to organic disease such as endometriosis, pelvic inflammatory disease, or uterine neoplasm

endometriosis Tissue closely resembling endometrial tissue located outside the uterus

fibroadenoma Firm, freely movable, solitary, solid, benign breast tumor

fibrocystic changes Benign changes in breast tissue

leiomyoma Benign smooth-muscle tumor

lumpectomy Removal of a wide margin of normal breast tissue surrounding a breast cancer

menorrhagia Abnormally profuse or excessive menstrual flow

metrorrhagia Abnormal bleeding from the uterus, particularly when it occurs at any time other than the menstrual period

modified radical mastectomy Surgery that includes the removal of the breast and fascia over the pectoralis major muscle

oligomenorrhea Abnormally light or infrequent menstruation

pelvic inflammatory disease (PID) Infection of internal reproductive structures and adjacent tissues usually secondary to sexually transmitted infections

premenstrual syndrome (PMS) Syndrome of nervous tension, irritability, weight gain, edema, headache, mastalgia, dysphoria, and lack of coordination occurring during the last few days of the menstrual cycle preceding the onset of menstruation

radical mastectomy Surgery that includes the total removal of the breast, as well as the underlying pectoralis major and pectoralis minor muscles

simple mastectomy Surgery that includes the removal of the breast without the underlying muscle or fascial tissue

WEB RESOURCES

Additional related content can be found on the companion website at evolve

http://evolve.elsevier.com/Lowdermilk/Maternity/

- NCLEX Review Questions
- Animation: Pelvic Inflammatory Disease
- Case Study: Breast Cancer
- Nursing Care Plan: Breast Cancer
- Nursing Care Plan: Endometriosis
- Nursing Care Plan: Premenstrual Syndrome
- Nursing Care Plan: Sexually Transmitted Infections

Throughout her life, the average woman is likely to have some concerns related to her menstrual and gynecologic health and will experience bleeding, pain, or discharge associated with her reproductive organs or functions. In addition, during a woman's life span, she may experience infections associated with her reproductive or sexual life. Many women will seek out nurses as advisors, counselors, and health care providers for these concerns. Nurses must have accurate, up-to-date information to meet these women's needs. This chapter provides information on common menstrual problems, sexually transmitted infections (STIs), and selected other infections that affect reproductive functions, and benign breast conditions. Breast cancer is also included because it is the most common reproductive system cancer occurring in women.

MENSTRUAL PROBLEMS

Women typically have menstrual cycles for approximately 40 years. Once the predictable pattern of monthly bleeding is established, women may worry about any deviation from that pattern or what they have been told is normal for all menstruating women. A sign such as amenorrhea or excessive menstrual bleeding is often a source of severe distress and concern for a woman as it causes her to wonder what is wrong.

Amenorrhea

Amenorrhea, the absence or cessation of menstrual flow, is a clinical sign of a variety of disorders. Although the criteria used to determine when amenorrhea is a clinical problem are not universal, you should evaluate the following circumstances: (1) the absence of both menarche and secondary sexual characteristics by age 14; (2) the absence of menses by age 16½, regardless of presence of normal growth and development (primary amenorrhea); or (3) a 6- to 12-month cessation of menses after a period of menstruation (secondary amenorrhea) (Speroff & Fritz, 2005).

Amenorrhea is most commonly a result of pregnancy, although it may occur from any defect or interruption in the hypothalamic-pituitary-ovarian-uterine axis (see Chapter 2). It may also result from anatomic abnormalities; other endocrine disorders, such as hypothyroidism or hyperthyroidism; chronic diseases, such as type 1 diabetes; medications, such as phenytoin (Dilantin); eating disorders; strenuous exercise; emotional stress; and oral contraceptive use.

Hypogonadotropic amenorrhea reflects a problem in the central hypothalamic-pituitary axis. In rare instances a pituitary lesion or genetic inability to produce FSH and LH is at fault. More commonly, it results from hypothalamic suppression as a result of two principal influences: stress (in the home, school, or workplace) or a body fat-to-lean ratio that is inappropriate for an individual woman, especially during a normal growth period (Lobo, 2007d). Research has demonstrated a biologic basis for the relationship of stress to physiologic processes. Exercise-associated amenorrhea can occur in women undergoing vigorous physical and athletic training and is associated with many factors, including body composition (height, weight, and percentage of body fat); type, intensity, and frequency of exercise; nutritional status; and the presence of emotional or physical stressors (Lobo). Amenorrhea is one of the classic signs of anorexia nervosa, and the interrelatedness of disordered eating, amenorrhea, and altered bone mineral density has been described as the female athlete triad (Lebrun, 2007). Calcium loss from bone, comparable to that seen in postmenopausal women, may occur with this type of amenorrhea.

Assessment of amenorrhea begins with a thorough history and physical examination. An important initial step is to confirm that the woman is not pregnant. Specific components of the assessment process depend on a woman's age–adolescent, young adult, or perimenopausal–and whether she has previously menstruated.

Management

When amenorrhea is caused by hypothalamic disturbances, the nurse is an ideal health professional to assist women because many of the causes are potentially reversible (e.g., stress, weight loss for nonorganic reasons). When a stressor known to predispose a woman to hypothalamic amenorrhea is identified, initial management involves addressing the stressor. Together the woman and nurse plan how to decrease or discontinue medications known to affect menstruation, correct weight loss, deal more effectively with psychologic stress, and eliminate substance abuse. Deep-breathing exercises and relaxation techniques are simple yet effective stress-reduction measures. Referral for biofeedback or massage therapy also may be useful. In some instances, referral for psychotherapy is indicated.

If a woman's exercise program is contributing to her amenorrhea, several options exist for management. She may decide to decrease the intensity or duration of her training, if possible, or to gain some weight, if appropriate. Accepting this alternative is often difficult for women who are committed to a strenuous exercise regimen. Some young women athletes do not understand the consequences of low bone density or osteoporosis; nurses can point out the connection between low bone density and stress fractures. If the woman continues to have low estrogen levels, instituting estrogen therapy, as well as calcium supplementation for osteoporosis prevention, is sometimes necessary (Lobo, 2007d).

Cyclic Perimenstrual Pain and Discomfort

Cyclic perimenstrual pain and discomfort (CPPD) is a concept developed by a nurse science team for a research project for the Association of Women's Health, Obstetric and Neonatal Nurses (AWHONN) (AWHONN, 2003; Collins Sharp, Taylor, Thomas, Killeen, & Dawood, 2002). This concept includes dysmenorrhea, premenstrual syndrome, and premenstrual dysphoric disorder, as well as symptom clusters that occur before and after the menstrual flow starts. CPPD is a health problem that can have a significant impact on the quality of life for a woman. The following discussion focuses on the three main conditions of CPPD.

Dysmenorrhea

Dysmenorrhea, pain during or shortly before menstruation, is one of the most common gynecologic problems in women of all ages. Many adolescents have dysmenorrhea in the first 3 years after menarche. Young adult women ages 17 to 24 years are most likely to report painful menses. Approximately 75% of women report some level of discomfort associated with menses, and approximately 15% report severe dysmenorrhea (Lentz, 2007b); however, the amount of disruption in women's lives is difficult to determine. Researchers have estimated that up to 10% of women with dysmenorrhea have severe enough pain to interfere with their functioning for 1 to 3 days a month. Menstrual problems, including dysmenorrhea, are relatively more common in women who smoke and who are obese. Severe dysmenorrhea is also associated with early menarche, nulliparity, and stress (Lentz). Traditionally dysmenorrhea is differentiated as primary or secondary. Symptoms usually begin with menstruation, although some women have discomfort several hours before onset of flow. The range and severity of symptoms are different from woman to woman and from cycle to cycle in the same woman. Symptoms of dysmenorrhea may last several hours or several days.

> ***Critical Thinking/Clinical Decision Making***
>
> **Management of Dysmenorrhea**
>
> Cheri, 16, has come to the Adolescent Health Clinic for a check up. She reports that she has "really bad cramps" for the first 2 days of her period. She has been taking Midol Menstrual Complete but says it does not help "a lot." She wants to know if anything else can be done to relieve her pain. How should the nurse respond?
>
> 1. Evidence—Is evidence sufficient to draw conclusions about what advice the nurse should give?
> 2. Assumptions—Describe underlying assumptions about the following issues:
>   a. Causes and symptoms of primary dysmenorrhea
>   b. Cyclic perimenstrual pain and discomfort
>   c. Self-help strategies (e.g., comfort measures, medications)
> 3. What implications and priorities for nursing care can be drawn at this time?
> 4. Does the evidence objectively support your conclusion?
> 5. Do alternative perspectives to your conclusion exist?

Pain is usually located in the suprapubic area or lower abdomen. Women describe the pain as sharp, cramping, or gripping or as a steady dull ache. For some women, pain radiates to the lower back or upper thighs.

Primary dysmenorrhea

Primary dysmenorrhea is a condition associated with ovulatory cycles. Research has shown that primary dysmenorrhea has a biochemical basis and arises from the release of prostaglandins with menses. During the luteal phase and subsequent menstrual flow, prostaglandin F_2-alpha (PGF_{2a}) is secreted. Excessive release of PGF_{2a} increases the amplitude and frequency of uterine contractions and causes vasospasm of the uterine arterioles, resulting in ischemia and cyclic lower abdominal cramps. Systemic responses to PGF_{2a} include backache, weakness, sweats, gastrointestinal symptoms (anorexia, nausea, vomiting, and diarrhea), and central nervous system symptoms (dizziness, syncope, headache, and poor concentration). Pain usually begins at the onset of menstruation and lasts 8 to 48 hours (Lentz, 2007b).

Primary dysmenorrhea usually appears 6 to 12 months after menarche when ovulation is established. Anovulatory bleeding, common in the few months or years after menarche, is painless. Because both estrogen and progesterone are necessary for primary dysmenorrhea to occur, it is experienced only with ovulatory cycles. This problem is more common among women in their late teens and early twenties than in women in older age groups; the incidence declines with age. Psychogenic factors may influence symptoms, but symptoms are definitely related to ovulation and do not occur when ovulation is suppressed.

Management. Management of primary dysmenorrhea depends on the severity of the problem and the individual woman's response to various treatments. Important components of nursing care are information and support. Because menstruation is so closely linked to reproduction and sexuality, menstrual problems such as dysmenorrhea can have a negative influence on sexuality and self-worth. Nurses can correct myths and misinformation about menstruation and dysmenorrhea by providing facts about what is normal. Nurses must support their patients' feelings of positive sexuality and self-worth.

Often, you can offer more than one alternative for alleviating menstrual discomfort and dysmenorrhea, which gives women options to try and decide which works best for them. Heat (heating pad or hot bath) minimizes cramping by increasing vasodilation and muscle relaxation and minimizing uterine ischemia. Massaging the lower back can reduce pain by relaxing paravertebral muscles and increasing the pelvic blood supply. Soft, rhythmic rubbing of the abdomen (effleurage) is useful because it provides a distraction and an alternative focal point. Biofeedback, transcutaneous electrical nerve stimulation (TENS), progressive relaxation, Hatha yoga, acupuncture, and meditation are also used to decrease menstrual discomfort, although evidence is insufficient to determine their effectiveness (Lentz, 2007b).

Exercise helps relieve menstrual discomfort through increased vasodilation and subsequent decreased ischemia. Exercise also releases endogenous opiates (specifically beta-endorphins), suppresses prostaglandins, and shunts blood flow away from the viscera, resulting in reduced pelvic congestion. One specific exercise that nurses can suggest is pelvic rocking.

In addition to maintaining good nutrition at all times, specific dietary changes are helpful in decreasing some of the systemic symptoms associated with dysmenorrhea. Decreased salt and refined sugar intake 7 to 10 days before expected menses may reduce fluid retention. Natural diuretics such as asparagus, cranberry juice, peaches, parsley, or watermelon may help reduce edema and related discomforts. Decreasing red meat intake may also help minimize dysmenorrheal symptoms.

Medications used to treat primary dysmenorrhea include prostaglandin synthesis inhibitors, primarily nonsteroidal antiinflammatory drugs (NSAIDs) (Lentz, 2007b) (Table 3-1). NSAIDs are most effective if started several days before menses or at least by the onset of bleeding. All NSAIDs have potential gastrointestinal side effects, including nausea, vomiting, and indigestion. Warn all women taking NSAIDs to report dark-colored stool because this may be an indication of gastrointestinal bleeding.

NURSING ALERT If one NSAID is ineffective, a different one may often be effective. If the second drug is unsuccessful after a 6-month trial, combined oral contraceptive pills (OCPs) may be used. Women with a history of aspirin sensitivity or allergy should avoid all NSAIDs.

OCPs prevent ovulation and can decrease the amount of menstrual flow, which can decrease the amount of prostaglandin, thus decreasing dysmenorrhea. There is evidence that combined OCPs can effectively treat dysmenorrhea (Lentz, 2007b). OCPs may be used in place of NSAIDs if the woman wants oral contraception and has primary dysmenorrhea. OCPs have side effects, and women who do not need or want them for contraception may not wish to use them for dysmenorrhea. OCPs also may be contraindicated for some women.

Over-the-counter (OTC) preparations that are formulated for primary dysmenorrhea include the same active ingredients (e.g., ibuprofen, naproxen sodium) as prescription preparations. However, the labeled recommended dose is often subtherapeutic. Preparations containing acetaminophen are even less effective because acetaminophen does not have the antiprostaglandin properties of NSAIDs.

Alternative and complementary therapies are increasingly popular and used in developed countries. Therapies such as acupuncture, acupressure, biofeedback, desensitization, hypnosis, massage, reiki, relaxation exercises, and therapeutic touch have been used to treat pelvic pain (Dehlin & Schuiling, 2006). Herbal preparations have long been used for the management of menstrual problems, including dysmenorrhea (Table 3-2). Herbal medicines can be valuable in treating dysmenorrhea; however, women must understand that these therapies are not without potential toxicity and may cause drug interactions. Women should use herbal preparations from well-established companies. It is also important to know that research is limited about the effectiveness of use (Dehlin & Schuiling, 2006).

Secondary dysmenorrhea

Secondary dysmenorrhea is menstrual pain that develops later in life than primary dysmenorrhea, typically after age 25. It is associated with pelvic abnormalities such as adenomyosis, endometriosis, pelvic inflammatory disease, endometrial polyps, submucous or interstitial myomas (uterine fibroids), or use of an intrauterine device (IUD). Pain often begins a few days before menses, but it can be present at ovulation and continue through the first days of menses or start after menstrual flow has begun. In contrast to primary dysmenorrhea, the pain of secondary dysmenorrhea is often characterized by dull, lower abdominal aching radiating to the back or thighs. Women often experience feelings of bloating or pelvic fullness. Treatment is directed toward removal of the underlying pathology. Many of the measures described for pain relief of primary dysmenorrhea are also helpful for women with secondary dysmenorrhea.

TABLE 3-1

Nonsteroidal Antiinflammatory Agents Used to Treat Dysmenorrhea

DRUG	BRAND NAME AND STATUS	RECOMMENDED DOSAGE (ORAL)	COMMON SIDE EFFECTS	COMMENTS	CONTRAINDICATIONS
Diclofenac	Cataflam Rx	50 mg tid or 100 mg initially, then 50 mg tid up to 150 mg/day	Nausea, diarrhea, constipation, abdominal distress, dyspepsia, heartburn, flatulence, dizziness, tinnitus, itching, rash	Enteric coated: immediate release	For all NSAIDs: Do not give if patient has hemophilia or bleeding ulcers, do not give if patient has had an allergic or anaphylactic reaction to aspirin or another NSAID, do not give if patient is taking anticoagulant medication.
Ibuprofen	Motrin Rx	400 mg q 6-8 hrs	See diclofenac	If GI upset occurs, take with food, milk, or antacids; avoid alcoholic beverages; do not take with aspirin; stop taking and call care provider if rash occurs	
	Advil OTC, Nuprin OTC, Motrin IB OTC	200 mg q 4-6 hrs up to 1200 mg/day			
Ketoprofen	Orudis Rx	25-50 mg q 6-8 hrs up to 300 mg/day	See diclofenac	See ibuprofen	
	Orudis KT OTC, Actron OTC	12.5 mg q 6-8 hrs up to 75 mg/day			
Meclofenamate	Meclofenamate	100 mg tid up to 300 mg	See diclofenac	See ibuprofen	
Mefenamic acid	Ponstel Rx	500 mg initially, then 250 mg q 6 hr	See diclofenac	Very potent and effective prostaglandin-synthesis inhibitor; antagonizes already formed prostaglandins; increased incidence of adverse GI side effects	
Naproxen	Naprosyn Rx	500 mg initially, then 250 mg q 6-8 hr up to 1250 mg/day	See diclofenac	See ibuprofen	
Naproxen sodium	Anaprox Rx	550 mg initially, then 275 mg q 6-8 hr or 550 mg q12 hr up to 1375 mg/day	See diclofenac	See ibuprofen	
	Aleve OTC	440 mg initially, then 220 mg q 6-8 hr up to 660 mg/day			
Celecoxib	Celebrex	400 mg initially, then 200 mg bid	See diclofenac	See ibuprofen	

Data from Facts and Comparisons. (2012). *Nonsteroidal antiinflammatory drugs.* www.factsandcomparisons.com; Lentz, G.M. (2012). Primary and secondary dysmenorrhea, premenstrual syndrome, and premenstrual dysphoric disorder: etiology, diagnosis, and management. In Lentz, G.M., Lobo, R.A., Gershenson, D.M., et al. (Eds.). *Comprehensive gynecology* (6th ed.). Philadelphia: Mosby; U.S. Department of Health and Human Services, U.S. Food and Drug Administration. (2008). *Medication guide for nonsteroidal antiinflammatory drugs (NSAIDs).* www.fda.gov/CDER/drug/infopage/COX2/NSAIDmedguide.htm.

GI, Gastrointestinal; *NSAID,* nonsteroidal antiinflammatory drug; *OTC,* over the counter.

TABLE 3-2
Herbal Therapies for Menstrual Disorders

SYMPTOMS OR INDICATIONS	HERBAL THERAPY	ACTION
Menstrual cramping	Black haw	Uterine antispasmodic
	Ginger	Antiinflammatory
	Valerian	Uterine antispasmodic
Premenstrual discomfort	Black cohosh root	Estrogen-like LH suppressant; binds to estrogen receptors
	Chaste tree fruit	Decreases prolactin levels
Tension, breast pain	Bugleweed	Antigonadotropic; decreases prolactin levels
Dysmenorrhea	Potentilla	Uterotonic
	Dong quai	Antiinflammatory; possibly analgesic activity
Menorrhea, metrorrhagia	Shepherd's purse	Uterotonic

Sources: Bascom, A. (2002). *Incorporating herbal medicine into clinical practice.* Philadelphia: FA Davis; Fugh-Berman, A., & Awang, D. (2001). Black cohosh. *Alternative Therapies in Women's Health, 39*(11), 81-85; Dog, L. (2001). Conventional and alternative treatments for endometriosis. *Alternative Therapies, 7*(6), 50-56; Stevinson, C., & Ernst, E. (2001). Complementary/alternative therapies for premenstrual syndrome: A systemic review of randomized controlled trials. *American Journal of Obstetrics and Gynecology, 185*(1), 227-235.
LH, Luteinizing hormone.

Premenstrual Syndrome and Premenstrual Dysphoric Disorder

Approximately 30% to 80% of women experience mood or somatic symptoms (or both) that occur with their menstrual cycles (Lentz, 2007b). Establishing a universal definition of **premenstrual syndrome (PMS)** is difficult, given that so many symptoms have been associated with the condition, and at least two different syndromes have been recognized: PMS and *premenstrual dysphoric disorder* (PMDD).

PMS is a complex, poorly understood condition that includes one or more of a large number (more than 100) of physical and psychologic symptoms beginning in the luteal phase of the menstrual cycle, occurring to such a degree that lifestyle or work is affected, and followed by a symptom-free period. Symptoms include fluid retention (abdominal bloating, pelvic fullness, edema of the lower extremities, breast tenderness, and weight gain); behavioral or emotional changes (depression, crying spells, irritability, panic attacks, and impaired ability to concentrate); premenstrual cravings (sweets, salt, increased appetite, and food binges); and headache, fatigue, and backache.

PMDD is a more severe variant of PMS in which 3% to 8% of women have marked irritability, dysphoria, mood lability, anxiety, fatigue, appetite changes, and a sense of feeling overwhelmed (Lentz, 2007b).

A diagnosis of PMS is made when the following criteria are met (American College of Obstetrics and Gynecology [ACOG], 2000; AWHONN, 2003):

- Symptoms consistent with PMS occur in the luteal phase and resolve within a few days of menses onset.
- Symptom-free period occurs in the follicular phase.
- Symptoms are recurrent.
- Symptoms have a negative impact on some aspect of a woman's life.
- Other diagnoses that better explain the symptoms have been excluded.

For a diagnosis of PMDD, the following criteria must be met (American Psychiatric Association [APA], 2000):

- Five or more affective and physical symptoms are present in the week before menses and are absent in the follicular phase of the menstrual cycle.
- At least one of the symptoms is irritability, depressed mood, anxiety, or emotional lability.
- Symptoms interfere markedly with work or interpersonal relationships.
- Symptoms are not caused by an exacerbation of another condition or disorder.
- These criteria must be confirmed by prospective daily ratings for at least two menstrual cycles (APA, 2000).

Nursing Care Plan: Premenstrual Syndrome

The causes of PMS and PMDD are unknown. Researchers have theorized that PMS has a significant psychologic component or may result from cultural beliefs that lead to the menstrual cycle being associated with a variety of negative reactions. In reality, PMS is most likely not a single disorder but is rather a collection of different problems (Lentz, 2007b). Much controversy exists regarding PMS. The existence, diagnosis, and causes of PMS are controversial. Explore current feminist, medical, and social science literature for more information on these topics.

Management

Little agreement exists on management. A careful, detailed history and daily log of symptoms and mood fluctuations spanning several cycles may give direction to a plan of management. Any changes that assist a woman with PMS to exert control over her life have a positive impact. For this reason, lifestyle changes are often effective in the treatment of PMS.

Education is an important component of the management of PMS. Nurses can advise women that self-help modalities often result in significant symptom improvement. Women have found a significant number of complementary and alternative therapies to be useful in managing the symptoms of PMS. Diet and exercise changes are a useful way to begin and provide symptom relief for some women. Suggest that women refrain from smoking and limit their consumption of refined sugar (less than 5 tbsp/day), salt (less than 3 g/day), red meat (up to 3 oz/day), alcohol (less than 1 oz/day), and caffeinated beverages. Also, encourage them to include whole grains, legumes, seeds, nuts, vegetables, fruits, and vegetable oils in their diet. Three small-to-moderate-sized meals and three small snacks a day that are rich in complex carbohydrates and fiber help reduce symptoms (Lentz, 2007b). Use of natural diuretics (see section on dysmenorrhea management) also helps reduce fluid retention as well. Nutritional supplements may assist in symptom relief. Calcium (1000-1200 mg daily), magnesium (300-400 mg daily), and vitamin B_6 (100-150 mg daily) have been reported to be moderately effective in relieving symptoms, have few side effects, and are safe. Daily supplements of evening primrose oil are also useful in relieving breast symptoms with minimal side effects. Other herbal therapies have long been used to treat PMS; Table 3-2 lists specific suggestions.

Regular exercise (aerobic exercise three to four times a week), especially in the luteal phase, is widely recommended for relief of PMS symptoms (Lentz, 2007b). A monthly program that varies in intensity and type of exercise according to PMS symptoms is best. Women who exercise regularly seem to have less premenstrual anxiety than do nonathletic women. Researchers believe aerobic exercise increases beta-endorphin levels to offset symptoms of depression and elevate mood. Yoga, acupuncture, hypnosis, chiropractic therapy, and massage therapy have all been reported to have a beneficial effect on PMS. Further research is needed for all of these suggested therapies.

Nurses can explain the relationship between cyclic estrogen fluctuation and changes in serotonin levels, that serotonin is one of the brain chemicals that assist in coping with normal life stresses, and how the different management strategies recommended help maintain serotonin levels. Counseling, in the form of support groups or individual or couple counseling, is helpful. Stress-reduction techniques also may assist with symptom management (Lentz, 2007b).

If these strategies do not provide significant symptom relief in 1 to 2 months, medication is often begun. Many medications have been used in treatment of PMS, but no single medication alleviates all PMS symptoms. Medications often used in the treatment of PMS include diuretics, prostaglandin inhibitors (NSAIDs), progesterone, and OCPs. Selective serotonin reuptake inhibitors such as Fluoxetine (Sarafem or Prozac) are U.S. Food and Drug Administration (FDA)-approved agents for PMS. Use of these medications results in a decrease in emotional symptoms, especially depression (Lentz, 2007b).

Endometriosis

Endometriosis is the presence and growth of endometrial tissue outside of the uterus. The tissue may be implanted on the ovaries, cul-de-sac, uterine ligaments, rectovaginal septum, sigmoid colon, pelvic peritoneum, cervix, or inguinal area (Fig. 3-1). Endometrial lesions have been found in the vagina and in surgical scars; on the vulva, perineum, and bladder; and in sites far from the pelvic area, such as the thoracic cavity, gallbladder, and heart. A chocolate cyst is a cystic area of endometriosis in the ovary. Old blood causes the dark coloring of the cyst's contents.

Endometrial tissue contains glands and stoma and responds to cyclic hormonal stimulation in the same way that the uterine endometrium does but is often out of phase with it. During the proliferative and secretory phases of the cycle the endometrial tissue grows. During or immediately after menstruation the tissue bleeds, resulting in an inflammatory response with subsequent fibrosis and adhesions to adjacent organs.

Endometriosis is a common gynecologic problem, affecting from 6% to 10% of women of reproductive age (Lobo, 2007b). Although the condition usually develops in the third or fourth decade of life, endometriosis occurs in approximately 10% of adolescents with disabling pelvic

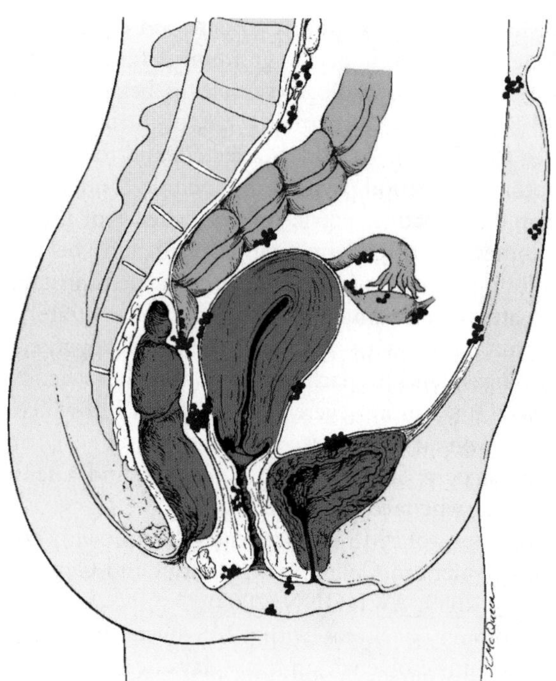

Fig. 3-1 Common sites of endometriosis. (From Lobo, R. [2007b]. Endometriosis. In V. Katz, G. Lentz, R. Lobo, & D. Gershenson [Eds.]. *Comprehensive gynecology* [5th ed.]. Philadelphia: Mosby.)

pain or abnormal vaginal bleeding (ACOG, 2005). The condition is found equally in Caucasian and African-American women, is slightly more prevalent in Asian women, and may have a familial tendency for development (Lobo, 2007b). Endometriosis may worsen with repeated cycles, or it may remain asymptomatic and undiagnosed, eventually disappearing after menopause.

Several theories have been offered to account for the cause of endometriosis, yet the causes and pathologic features of this condition are poorly understood. One of the most widely accepted, long-debated theories is transtubal migration or retrograde menstruation. According to this theory, endometrial tissue is regurgitated or mechanically transported from the uterus during menstruation to the uterine tubes and into the peritoneal cavity, where it implants on the ovaries and other organs.

Symptoms vary among women, from nonexistent to incapacitating. Severity of symptoms can change over time and may be disconnected from the extent of the disease. The major symptoms of endometriosis are dysmenorrhea, infertility, and deep pelvic dyspareunia (painful intercourse). Women also experience chronic noncyclic pelvic pain, pelvic heaviness, or pain radiating into the thighs. Many women report bowel symptoms such as diarrhea, pain with defecation, and constipation secondary to avoiding defecation because of the pain. Less common symptoms include abnormal bleeding (hypermenorrhea, menorrhagia, or premenstrual staining) and pain during exercise as a result of adhesions (Lobo, 2007b).

Management

Treatment is based on the severity of symptoms and the goals of the woman or couple. Women without pain who do not want to become pregnant need no treatment. Women with mild pain who may desire a future pregnancy may use NSAIDs for pain relief. Women who have severe pain and can postpone pregnancy may be treated with continuous OCPs that have a low estrogen-to-progestin ratio to shrink endometrial tissue. However, when this therapy stops, women often experience high rates of recurrence of pain and other symptoms.

Hormonal antagonists that suppress ovulation and reduce endogenous estrogen production and subsequent endometrial lesion growth are currently used to treat mild to severe endometriosis in women who wish to become pregnant at a future time. Gonadotropin-releasing hormone (GnRH) agonist therapy (leuprolide, nafarelin [Synarel], goserelin acetate [Zoladex]) acts by suppressing pituitary gonadotropin secretion. FSH and LH stimulation to the ovary declines noticeably, and ovarian function decreases significantly. The hypoestrogenism results in hot flashes in almost all women. In addition, minor bone loss sometimes occurs, most of which is reversible within 12 to 18 months after the medication is stopped. Leuprolide (3.75 mg intramuscular injection given once a month) or nafarelin (200 mcg administered twice daily by nasal spray) are both effective and well tolerated. Both medications reduce endometrial lesions and pelvic pain associated with endometriosis and have posttreatment pregnancy rates similar to that of danazol therapy (Lobo, 2007b). Common side effects of these drugs are similar to those of natural menopause–hot flashes and vaginal dryness. Some women report headaches and muscle aches. These medications are not given to adolescents as the hypoestogenic state that occurs can affect bone mineralization (ACOG, 2005).

Danazol (Danocrine), a mildly androgenic synthetic steroid, suppresses FSH and LH secretion, thus producing anovulation with resulting decreased secretion of estrogen and progesterone and regression of endometrial tissue. Bothersome side effects include masculinizing traits in the woman–weight gain, edema, decreased breast size, oily skin, hirsutism, and deepening of the voice–all of which often disappear when treatment is discontinued. Other side effects are amenorrhea, hot flashes, vaginal dryness, insomnia, and decreased libido. Some women report migraine headaches, dizziness, fatigue, and depression. In addition, some women experience decreases in bone density that are only partially reversible. Danazol should never be prescribed when pregnancy is suspected, and contraception should be used with it because ovulation may not be suppressed. Danazol can produce pseudohermaphroditism in female fetuses. The drug is contraindicated in women with liver disease and should be used with caution in women with cardiac and renal disease (Lobo, 2007b).

Surgical intervention is often needed for severe, acute, or incapacitating symptoms. A woman's age, desire for children, and location of the disease influence decisions regarding the extent and type of surgery. For women who do not want to preserve their ability to have children, the only definite cure is hysterectomy and bilateral salpingo-oophorectomy (BSO) (total abdominal hysterectomy [TAH] with BSO). In women who are in their childbearing years and who want children if the disease does not prevent pregnancy, surgery or laser therapy is used to carefully remove as much endometrial tissue as possible to maintain reproductive function (Lobo, 2007b).

Short of TAH with BSO, endometriosis recurs in approximately 40% to 50% of women, regardless of the form of treatment. Therefore, for many women, endometriosis is a chronic disease with conditions such as chronic pain or infertility. Counseling and education are critical components of nursing care of women with endometriosis. Women need an honest discussion of treatment options with potential risks and benefits of each option reviewed. Because pelvic pain is a subjective, personal experience that can be frightening, support is important. Sexual dysfunction resulting from dyspareunia may be present and may necessitate referral for counseling. Some locations have support groups for women with endometriosis. The nursing care measures discussed in the section on dysmenorrhea are appropriate for managing chronic pelvic pain associated with endometriosis (see Nursing Care Plan).

NURSING CARE PLAN *Endometriosis*

Nursing Care Plan: Endometriosis

NURSING DIAGNOSIS Acute pain related to menstruation secondary to endometriosis

Expected outcome *Woman will verbalize a decrease in intensity and frequency of pain during each menstrual cycle.*

Nursing Interventions/*Rationales*

- Assess location, type, and duration of pain and history of discomfort *to determine the severity of dysmenorrhea.*
- Administer analgesics *to assist with pain relief.*
- Administer hormone-altering medications if ordered *to suppress ovulation.*
- Provide nonpharmacologic methods such as heat *to increase blood flow to the pelvic region.*

NURSING DIAGNOSIS Deficient knowledge related to unfamiliarity with treatment, as evidenced by patient statements

Expected outcome *Woman will verbalize correct understanding of the use of self-management methods and prescribed therapies.*

Nursing Interventions/*Rationales*

- Assess the woman's current understanding of the disorder and related therapies *to validate the accuracy of the knowledge base.*
- Give information to the woman regarding the disorder and treatment regimen *to empower the woman to become a partner in her own care.*

NURSING DIAGNOSIS Situational low self-esteem related to infertility as evidenced by the patient's statements of decreased self-worth

Expected outcome *Woman will verbalize positive feelings of self-worth.*

Nursing Interventions/*Rationales*

- Provide therapeutic communication *to validate feelings and provide support.*
- Refer the woman to a support group *to enhance feelings of self-worth through group communication.*

NURSING DIAGNOSIS Anxiety related to possible invasive surgical procedure as evidenced by the patient's verbal report

Expected outcome *Woman will report a decreased number of anxious feelings.*

Nursing Interventions/*Rationales*

- Provide the opportunity to discuss feelings *to identify source of anxiety.*
- Reinforce information provided *to keep expectations realistic and dispel myths or inaccuracies.*
- Provide emotional support *to encourage verbalization of feelings.*

NURSING DIAGNOSIS Risk for injury related to disease progression

Expected outcome *Woman will report any changes in health status to the health care provider.*

Nursing Interventions/*Rationales*

- Teach the woman to report any changes in health status *to initiate prompt treatment.*
- Review side effects of medications *to recognize possible rationales for changes in health status.*
- Encourage ongoing communication with the health care provider *to promote trust and comfort.*

Alterations in Cyclic Bleeding

Women often experience changes in amount, duration, interval, or regularity of menstrual cycle bleeding. Commonly, women worry about menstruation that is infrequent or scanty (**oligomenorrhea**), is excessive (**menorrhagia**), or occurs between periods (**metrorrhagia**).

Treatment depends on the cause and may include education and reassurance. For example, tell women that OCPs can cause scanty menstrual flow and midcycle spotting. Progestin intramuscular injections and implants can also cause midcycle bleeding. A single episode of heavy bleeding may signal an early pregnancy loss such as a miscarriage or ectopic pregnancy. This type of bleeding is often thought to be a period that is heavier than usual, perhaps delayed, and is associated with abdominal pain or pelvic discomfort. When early pregnancy loss is suspected, hematocrit and pregnancy tests are indicated.

Uterine **leiomyomas** (fibroids or myomas) are a common cause of menorrhagia. Fibroids are benign tumors of the smooth muscle of the uterus with an unknown cause. Fibroids occur in approximately one fourth of women of reproductive age; the incidence of fibroids is higher in African-American women than in Caucasian, Asian, or in Hispanic women (Katz, 2007). Other uterine growths ranging from endometrial polyps to adenocarcinoma and endometrial cancer are common causes of heavy menstrual bleeding, as well as intermenstrual bleeding.

Treatment for menorrhagia depends on the cause of the bleeding. If the bleeding is related to contraceptive method (e.g., an IUD), provide factual information and reassurance and discuss other contraceptive options. If bleeding is related to the presence of fibroids, the degree of disability and discomfort associated with the fibroids and the woman's plans for childbearing will influence treatment decisions. Treatment options include medical and surgical management. Most fibroids can be monitored by frequent examinations to judge growth, if any, and correction of anemia, if present. Warn women with metrorrhagia to avoid using aspirin because of its tendency to increase bleeding. Medical treatment is directed toward temporarily reducing symptoms, shrinking the myoma, and reducing its blood supply (Katz, 2007). This reduction is often accomplished with the use of a GnRH agonist. If the woman wishes to retain childbearing potential, a myomectomy may be performed. Myomectomy, or removal of the tumors only, is particularly difficult if multiple myomas must be removed. If the woman does not want to preserve her childbearing function, or if she has severe symptoms (severe anemia, severe pain, considerable disruption of lifestyle), uterine artery embolization (procedure that blocks blood supply to fibroid), endometrial ablation (laser surgery or electrocoagulation), or hysterectomy (removal of uterus) may be performed.

Dysfunctional uterine bleeding

Abnormal uterine bleeding (AUB) is any form of uterine bleeding that is irregular in amount, duration, or timing and is not related to regular menstrual bleeding. Box 3-1 lists possible causes of AUB. Although often used interchangeably, the terms AUB and **dysfunctional uterine bleeding (DUB)** are not synonymous. DUB is a subset of AUB defined as "excessive uterine bleeding with no demonstrable organic cause (genital or extragenital)" (Lobo, 2007a, p. 915). DUB is most commonly caused by anovulation. When no surge of LH occurs, or if insufficient progesterone is produced by the corpus luteum to support the endometrium, it will begin to involute and shed. This process most often occurs at the extremes of a woman's reproductive years–when the menstrual cycle is just becoming established at menarche or when it draws to a close at menopause. DUB also occurs with any condition that gives rise to chronic anovulation associated with continuous estrogen production. Such conditions include obesity, hyperthyroidism and hypothyroidism, polycystic ovarian syndrome, and any of the endocrine conditions discussed in the sections on amenorrhea and oligomenorrhea. A diagnosis of DUB is made only after ruling out all other causes of abnormal menstrual bleeding (Lentz, 2007a).

The most effective medical treatment of acute bleeding episodes of DUB is administration of oral or intravenous estrogen. Dilation and curettage may be done if the bleeding has not stopped in 12 to 24 hours. An oral conjugated estrogen and progestin regimen is usually given for at least 3 months. If the woman wants contraception, she should continue to take OCPs. If she has no need for contraception, the treatment may be stopped to assess the woman's bleeding pattern. If her menses does not resume, a progestin regimen (e.g., medroxyprogesterone, 10 mg each day for 10 days before the expected date of her menstrual period) may be prescribed after ruling out pregnancy. This is done to prevent persistent anovulation with chronic unopposed endogenous estrogen hyperstimulation of the endometrium, which can result in eventual atypical tissue changes (Lobo, 2007a).

If hormonal therapy does not control the recurrent, heavy bleeding, ablation of the endometrium through laser treatment may be performed (Lobo, 2007a). Nursing roles include informing women of their options, counseling and providing education as indicated, and referring to the appropriate specialists and health care services.

BOX 3-1

Possible Causes of Abnormal Uterine Bleeding

ANOVULATION
- Hypothalamic dysfunction
- Polycystic ovary syndrome

PREGNANCY-RELATED CONDITIONS
- Threatened or spontaneous miscarriage
- Retained products of conception after elective abortion
- Ectopic pregnancy

LOWER REPRODUCTIVE TRACT INFECTIONS
- Chlamydial cervicitis
- Pelvic inflammatory disease

NEOPLASMS
- Endometrial hyperplasia
- Cancer of cervix and endometrium
- Endometrial polyps
- Hormonally active tumors (rare)
- Leiomyomata
- Vaginal tumors (rare)

TRAUMA
- Genital injury (accidental, coital trauma, sexual abuse)
- Foreign body
- Primary coagulation disorders

SYSTEMIC DISEASES
- Diabetes mellitus
- Thyroid dysfunction (hypothyroidism, hyperthyroidism)
- Severe organ disease (renal or liver failure)

IATROGENIC CAUSES
- Exogenous hormone use (oral contraceptives, menopausal hormone therapy)
- Medications with estrogenic activity
- Herbal preparation (ginseng)

Sources: American College of Nurse-Midwives (ACNM). (2002). Abnormal and dysfunctional uterine bleeding. ACNM Clinical Bulletin No. 6. *Journal of Midwifery and Women's Health, 47*(3), 207-213; Katz, V. (2007). Benign gynecologic lesions: Vulva, vagina, cervix, uterus, oviducts and ovary. In V. Katz, G. Lentz, R. Lobo, & D. Gershenson (Eds.). *Comprehensive gynecology* (5th ed.). Philadelphia: Mosby.

EVIDENCE-BASED PRACTICE

Heavy Menstrual Bleeding: Treatments to Improve Quality of Life

Pat Gingrich

ASK THE QUESTION

What treatments are available for women experiencing heavy menstrual bleeding? Is surgery or medicine the better treatment?

SEARCH FOR EVIDENCE

Search Strategies: Professional organization guidelines, metaanalyses, systematic reviews, randomized controlled trials, nonrandomized prospective studies, retrospective studies, and systematic reviews of qualitative research since 2006

Search Databases: Cumulative Index to Nursing and Allied Health Literature, Cochrane, Medline, National Guideline Clearinghouse, Turning Research Into Practice (TRIP) Database, and National Institute for Clinical Excellence (NICE)

CRITICALLY ANALYZE THE DATA

Heavy menstrual bleeding (HMB) is usually defined as anything more than 80 ml lost. A systematic review of qualitative research reported that women experiencing HMB find it to be physically, socially, and emotionally challenging to their quality of life (Garside, Britten, & Stein, 2008). The authors reported that uncertainty, embarrassment, feeling that concerns were minimized, difficulty with menstrual etiquette, and fears of anemia and cancer can cause women to experience stress and anxiety.

The range of treatments for HMB includes medication and surgical interventions. Danazol, a modified testosterone, has anti-estrogen and anti-progesterone properties. A metaanalysis of randomized controlled trials revealed that danazol was more effective than progesterone, nonsteroidal antiinflammatory drugs (NSAIDs), oral contraceptives (Beaumont et al., 2007), or tranexamic acid (Lethaby, Irvine, & Cameron, 2008). However, danazol may produce intolerable side effects of masculinization, menopause-like symptoms, weight gain, or acne. The recommendation statement of the National Institute for Health and Clinical Excellence (2007) lists the first-line drug as the levonorgestrel-releasing intrauterine system (an intrauterine device [IUD] that releases progesterone, preventing endometrial proliferation). Their second-line treatments include tranexamic acid, NSAIDs, and combined oral contraceptives. Third line includes oral and injected progesterones.

Surgically, HMB can be treated according to the severity of the symptoms and the woman's desire to preserve fertility. Hysterectomy is successful at stopping the bleeding, but it carries the most surgical risk. Endometrial ablation can use several mechanical and thermal techniques to destroy the uterine lining. This more conservative surgery can be performed on an outpatient basis and has reduced risk of postoperative complications. Both hysterectomy and endometrial ablation eliminate future pregnancies. If the bleeding is caused by a fibroid and the woman desires future pregnancies, the blood supply to the fibroid can be blocked using uterine artery embolization, or the tumor can be removed using a myomectomy. The NICE recommendation guidelines (2007) state that dilation and curettage for HMB is not recommended.

IMPLICATIONS FOR PRACTICE

Women experiencing HMB may delay in getting medical care because of embarrassment or uncertainty. Nurses should regularly ask their female patients about their menstrual cycle amount and duration, including clots. Evaluate for anemia. Concerns about bleeding should trigger a detailed focused menstrual history and pregnancy history, including the desire for future pregnancies. The nurse can explain normal parameters for duration and flow. Clots are usually an indicator of heavy flow. Once identified, nurses should ask women experiencing HMB about their concerns and fears. As the health care provider identifies the various options, the woman and her partner may need a sounding board and resource for answers to questions. In the event of loss of fertility, counseling and referral to a group such as Resolve (www.resolve.org) may provide support.

References:

Beaumont, H., Augood, C., Duckitt, K., & Lethaby, A. (2007). Danazol for heavy menstrual bleeding. In *The Cochrane Database of Systematic Reviews 2007*, Issue 3.

Garside, R., Britten, N., & Stein, K. (2008). The experience of heavy menstrual bleeding: A systematic review and meta-ethnography of qualitative studies. *Journal of Advanced Nursing, 63*(6), 550-562.

Lethaby, A., Irvine, G., & Cameron, I. (2008). Cyclical progesterones for heavy menstrual bleeding. In *The Cochrane Database of Systematic Reviews 2008*, Issue 1.

National Institute for Health and Clinical Excellence (NICE). (2007). *Heavy menstrual bleeding [NICE Clinical Guideline 44]*. Internet document available at www.nice.org.uk/Guidance/CG44 (accessed May 2, 2009).

CARE MANAGEMENT

Medical and nursing management have been discussed with each menstrual problem. Specific aspects of the nursing process are listed in the Nursing Process box.

INFECTIONS

Infections of the reproductive tract can occur throughout a woman's life and are often the cause of significant reproductive morbidity, including ectopic pregnancy and tubal factor infertility (Centers for Disease Control and Preven-

NURSING PROCESS *Menstrual Disorders*

ASSESSMENT

- Take a thorough menstrual, obstetric, sexual, and contraceptive history.
- Explore the woman's perceptions of her condition, cultural or ethnic influences, lifestyle, and patterns of coping.
- Evaluate the amount of pain or bleeding experienced and its effect on daily activities.
- Note any home remedies and prescriptions to relieve discomfort. A symptom diary, in which the woman records emotions, behaviors, physical symptoms, diet, and exercise and rest patterns, is a useful diagnostic tool.

NURSING DIAGNOSES

Nursing diagnoses include:

- *Risk for ineffective individual coping* related to:
  - Insufficient knowledge of the cause of the disorder
  - Emotional and physiologic effects of the disorder
- *Deficient knowledge* related to:
  - Self-management
  - Available therapy for the disorder
- *Risk for disturbed body image* related to:
  - Menstrual disorder
  - Sexual dysfunction
- *Risk for situational low self-esteem* related to:
  - Others' perception of her discomfort
  - Inability to conceive
- *Acute or chronic pain* related to:
  - Menstrual disorder

EXPECTED OUTCOMES OF CARE

Expected outcomes for the woman are that she will do the following:

- Verbalize her understanding of reproductive anatomy, cause of her disorder, medication regimen, and diary use.
- Verbalize her understanding and accept her emotional and physical responses to her menstrual cycle.
- Develop personal goals that benefit her emotionally and physically.
- Choose appropriate therapeutic measures for her menstrual problems.
- Adapt successfully to the condition, if cure is not possible.

PLAN OF CARE AND INTERVENTIONS

- Accept the woman's symptoms as valid.
- Correlate data from the daily diary of emotional status, subjective feelings, and physical state with physiologic changes.
- Encourage the woman to express her feelings about her symptoms.
- Provide information about therapeutic options (pharmacologic and nonpharmacologic) so that the woman (couple) makes choices considered best for her (them).
- Provide information about local support groups.

EVALUATION

Care has been effective when the woman reports improvement in the quality of her life, skill in self-management, and a positive self-concept and body image.

tion [CDC], 2007a). The direct economic costs of these infections can be substantial, and the indirect cost is equally overwhelming. Some consequences of maternal infection, such as infertility, last a lifetime. The emotional costs may include damaged relationships and lowered self-esteem.

Sexually Transmitted Infections

Sexually transmitted infections are infections or infectious disease syndromes transmitted primarily by sexual contact (Box 3-2). The term *sexually transmitted infection* includes more than 25 infectious organisms that are transmitted through sexual activity and the dozens of clinical syndromes that they cause. STIs are among the most common health problems in the United States today, with an estimated 19 million people in the United States being infected with STIs every year (CDC, 2007c). Later, this chapter discusses the most common STIs in women. Chapter 21 discusses effects on pregnancy and the fetus. Chapter 24 discusses neonatal effects.

Prevention

Preventing infection (primary prevention) is the most effective way of reducing the adverse consequences of STIs for women. Prompt diagnosis and treatment of current infections (secondary prevention) also can prevent personal complications and transmission to others. Preventing the spread of STIs requires that women at risk for transmitting or acquiring infections change their behavior. A critical first step is to include questions about a woman's sexual history, sexual risk behaviors, and drug-related risky behaviors as a part of her assessment (Box 3-3). When you identify risk factors or risky behaviors, you have an opportunity to provide prevention counseling. Techniques that are effective in providing prevention counseling include using open-ended questions, using understandable language, and reassuring the woman that treatment will be provided regardless of consideration such as ability to pay, language spoken, or lifestyle (CDC, 2006; Ravin, 2007). Prevention messages should include descriptions of specific actions to prevent contracting or transmitting STIs (e.g., refraining from sexual activity when STI-related symptoms are present), and should be individualized for each woman, giving attention to her specific risk factors.

To be motivated to take preventive actions, a woman must believe that catching a disease will be serious for her

Nursing Care Plan: Sexually Transmitted Infections

BOX 3-2

Sexually Transmitted Infections

BACTERIA
- Chlamydia
- Gonorrhea
- Syphilis
- Chancroid
- Lymphogranuloma venereum
- Genital mycoplasmas
- Group B streptococci

VIRUSES
- Human immunodeficiency virus
- Herpes simplex virus, types 1 and 2
- Cytomegalovirus
- Viral hepatitis A and B
- Human papillomavirus

PROTOZOA
- Trichomoniasis

PARASITES
- Pediculosis (may or may not be sexually transmitted)
- Scabies (may or may not be sexually transmitted)

BOX 3-3

Essential Areas of Assessment for a Woman at Risk for or Who Has a Sexually Transmitted Infection (STI)

CURRENT PROBLEM

What symptoms are present?
- Vaginal discharge
- Lesions
- Rash
- Dysuria
- Fever
- Itching, burning
- Dyspareunia
- Malaise

MEDICAL HISTORY
- History of STIs (self or partner)
- Allergies, especially to medications

MENSTRUAL HISTORY
- Last menstrual period (possibility of pregnancy)

PERSONAL AND SOCIAL HISTORY (SEXUAL HISTORY)
- Sexual preference (men, women, or both)
- Number of partners (past, 12 months; present, last 2 months)
- Types of sexual activity
- Frequency of sexual activity
- Use of protection against STIs, HIV

LIFESTYLE BEHAVIORS
- Intravenous drug use (or use by partner)
- Smoking
- Alcohol use
- Inadequate or poor nutrition
- High levels of stress, fatigue

HIV, Human immunodeficiency virus.

and that she is at risk for infection. Unfortunately, most individuals tend to underestimate their personal risk of infection in a given situation. Therefore many women may not perceive themselves as being at risk for contracting an STI. Although levels of awareness of STIs are generally high, widespread misconceptions or specific gaps in knowledge also exist. Therefore nurses have a responsibility to ensure that their patients have accurate, complete knowledge about transmission and symptoms of STIs and risky behaviors that place them at risk for contracting an infection.

Primary preventive measures are individual activities aimed at deterring infection. Risk-free options include complete abstinence from sexual activities that transmit semen, blood, or other body fluids or that allow for skin-to-skin contact (CDC, 2006). Alternatively, involvement in a mutually monogamous relationship with an uninfected partner also eliminates the risk of contracting STIs.

Risk-reduction measures. An essential component of primary prevention is counseling and educating women regarding risk-reduction practices, including knowledge of her partner, reduction in the number of partners, low risk sex, avoiding the exchange of body fluids, and vaccination (CDC, 2006).

No aspect of prevention is more important than knowing one's partner. Reducing the number of partners and avoiding partners who have had many previous sexual partners decreases a woman's chance of contracting an STI. Discussing each new partner's previous sexual history and exposure to STIs will augment other efforts to reduce risk; however, sexual partners are not always truthful about their sexual history.

Teach women about low risk sexual practices and which sexual practices to avoid. Mutual masturbation is low risk as long as bodily fluids come in contact only with intact skin. Caressing, hugging, body rubbing, massage, and hand-to-genital touching are low risk behaviors. Anal-genital intercourse, anal-oral contact, and anal digital activity are high risk sexual behaviors and should be avoided.

Currently the sole physical barrier promoted for the prevention of sexual transmission of STIs is the latex male condom. Encourage women to have sexual partners use condoms. Teach women the differences among condoms, price ranges, sizes, and where they can be purchased. Information to be discussed includes importance of using latex rather than natural skin condoms. Remind women to use only condoms with a current expiration date and to store them away from high heat. Women may choose to carry condoms safely in wallets, in shoes, or inside a bra. Chapter 4 has instructions for how to apply a condom. Remind women to use a condom only one time and with every sexual encounter.

The female condom–a lubricated polyurethane sheath with a ring on each end that is inserted into the vagina–has been shown in laboratory studies to be an effective mechanical barrier to viruses, including human immunodeficiency virus (HIV). A few clinical studies have been completed to evaluate the efficacy of female condoms in protecting against STIs. The CDC (2006) states that, when used correctly and consistently, the female condom may substantially reduce STI risk and recommends its use when a male condom cannot be used properly.

Evidence has shown that vaginal spermicides do not protect against certain STIs (e.g., chlamydia, cervical gonorrhea) and that frequent use of spermicides containing nonoxynol-9 has been associated with genital lesions and may increase HIV transmission. Condoms lubricated with nonoxynol-9 are not recommended (ACOG, 2008; CDC, 2006).

Vaccination is an effective method for the prevention of some STIs such as hepatitis B and human papillomavirus (HPV). Hepatitis B vaccine is recommended for women at high risk for STIs. A vaccine is available for HPV types 6, 11, 16, and 18 for girls and women 9 to 26 years of age (CDC, 2006).

Counsel women to watch out for situations that make it hard to talk about and practice risk reduction. These situations include romantic times when condoms are not available and when alcohol or drugs make it difficult to make wise decisions.

Bacterial Sexually Transmitted Infections

Chlamydial infection

Chlamydia trachomatis is the most common and fastest spreading STI in U.S. women (CDC, 2006). These infections are often silent and highly destructive; their sequelae and complications are very serious. In women, chlamydial infections are difficult to diagnose; the symptoms, if present, are nonspecific, and the organism is expensive to culture.

Acute salpingitis, or pelvic inflammatory disease, is the most serious complication of chlamydial infections. Past chlamydial infections are associated with an increased risk of ectopic pregnancy and tubal factor infertility. Furthermore, chlamydial infection of the cervix causes inflammation, resulting in microscopic cervical ulcerations that may increase risk of acquiring HIV infection.

Sexually active women younger than 20 years are the ones most likely to become infected with chlamydia. Women older than age 30 have the lowest rate of infection. Risky behaviors, including multiple partners and not using barrier methods of birth control, increase a woman's risk of chlamydial infection.

Screening and diagnosis. In addition to obtaining information regarding the presence of risk factors (e.g., women younger than 26 years old, older women who do not use barrier contraceptives, women with new or multiple partners), inquire about the presence of any symptoms (CDC, 2006). Although infection is usually asymptomatic, some women may experience spotting or postcoital bleeding, mucoid or purulent cervical discharge, or dysuria. Bleeding results from inflammation and erosion of the cervical columnar epithelium.

Laboratory diagnosis of chlamydia is by culture (expensive and labor intensive), DNA probe (relatively less expensive but less sensitive), enzyme immunoassay (also relatively less expensive but less sensitive), and nucleic acid amplification tests (expensive but has relatively higher sensitivity) (CDC, 2006).

Management. The CDC (2006) recommendations for the treatment of chlamydial infections include doxycycline (100 mg orally twice a day for 7 days) or azithromycin (1 g orally in a single dose). Azithromycin is often prescribed when compliance is a problem because only one dose is needed. Because chlamydia is often asymptomatic, caution the woman to take all medication prescribed. All exposed sexual partners should be treated. Woman treated with doxycycline or azithromycin do not need to be retested unless symptoms continue (CDC, 2006).

Gonorrhea

Gonorrhea is caused by the aerobic, gram-negative diplococci *Neisseria gonorrhoeae* and is the second most reported infection in the United States (CDC, 2006). Gonorrhea is almost exclusively transmitted by the contact of sexual activity. The principal means of communication is genital-to-genital contact; however, it is also spread by oral-to-genital and anal-to-genital contact. Gonorrhea can also be transmitted to the newborn in the form of ophthalmia neonatorum during birth by direct contact with gonococcal organisms in the cervix.

Age is probably the most important risk factor associated with gonorrhea. The majority of those contracting gonorrhea are younger than age 25 years. Other risk factors include early onset of sexual activity, multiple sexual partners, and drug use. Sexually active women who are considered at increased risk should be screened.

Women are often asymptomatic, but when they are symptomatic, they may have a greenish-yellow purulent endocervical discharge or may experience menstrual irregularities. Women may complain of pain, chronic or acute severe pelvic or lower abdominal pain, or menses that last longer or are more painful than normal. Gonococcal rectal infection may occur in women after anal intercourse. Individuals with rectal gonorrhea may be completely asymptomatic or, conversely, may experience severe symptoms with profuse purulent anal discharge, rectal pain, and blood in the stool. Rectal itching, fullness, pressure, and pain are also common symptoms, as is diarrhea. A diffuse vaginitis with vulvitis is the most common form of gonococcal infection in prepubertal girls. There may be few signs of infection, or vaginal discharge, dysuria, or swollen, reddened labia are sometimes present.

Screening and diagnosis. Gonococcal infection cannot be diagnosed reliably by clinical signs and symptoms alone. Cultures are considered the gold standard for diagnosis of gonorrhea. Cultures are obtained from the endocervix, rectum, and, when indicated, the pharynx. Thayer-Martin cultures are recommended to diagnose gonorrhea in women. Because STIs tend to coexist, any woman suspected of having gonorrhea should have a chlamydial culture and serologic test for syphilis and offered HIV testing (CDC, 2006).

Management. Management of gonorrhea is straightforward, and the cure is usually rapid with appropriate antibiotic therapy. Single-dose efficacy is a major consideration in selecting an antibiotic regimen for women with gonorrhea. Another important consideration is the high percentage (45%) of women with coexisting chlamydial infections. The recommended treatment is one dose of the following medications: ceftriaxone 125 mg single dose intramuscularly or cefixime 400 mg orally (CDC, 2007c). The CDC also suggests concomitant treatment for chlamydia if this infection is not ruled out (CDC, 2007c).

Gonorrhea is a highly communicable disease. Recent (previous 30 days) sexual partners should be examined, cultured, and treated with appropriate regimens. Most treatment failures result from reinfection; the woman needs to be informed of this possibility, as well as of the consequences of reinfection in terms of chronicity, complications (e.g., pelvic inflammatory disease), and potential infertility. Counsel women to have their partners use condoms. Offer all patients with gonorrhea confidential counseling and testing for HIV infection.

LEGAL TIP **Reporting a Communicable Disease**

Gonorrhea is a reportable communicable disease. Health care providers are legally responsible for reporting all cases to the health authorities, usually the local health department in the woman's county of residence. Inform women that the case will be reported, told why, and informed of the possibility of being contacted by a health department epidemiologist.

Syphilis

Treponema pallidum, a motile spirochete, causes syphilis. Transmission is by entry in the subcutaneous tissue through microscopic abrasions that can occur during sexual intercourse. The disease can also be transmitted through kissing, biting, or oral-genital sex. Transplacental transmission may occur at any time during pregnancy; the degree of risk is related to the quantity of spirochetes in the maternal bloodstream.

Rates of syphilis have increased among women since 2004. Between 2005 and 2006 the rate for African-Americans women increased by more than 11%, whereas the rate for other ethnic groups remained about the same (CDC, 2007a, 2007b).

Syphilis is a complex disease that can lead to serious systemic disease and even death if untreated. Infection manifests itself in distinct stages with different symptoms and clinical manifestations. Primary syphilis is characterized by a primary lesion, the chancre, that appears 5 to 90 days after infection; this lesion often begins as a painless papule at the site of inoculation and then erodes to form a nontender, shallow, indurated, clean ulcer several millimeters to centimeters in size (Fig. 3-2, *A*). Secondary syphilis, occurring 6 weeks to 6 months after the appearance of the chancre, is characterized by a widespread, symmetric maculopapular rash on the palms and soles and generalized lymphadenopathy. The infected individual also may experience fever, headache, and malaise. Condyloma lata (wartlike infectious lesions) may develop on the vulva, perineum, or anus (Fig. 3-2, *B*). If the woman is untreated, she enters a latent phase that is asymptomatic for most individuals. If left untreated, approximately one third of patients will develop tertiary syphilis. Neurologic and cardiovascular, musculoskeletal,

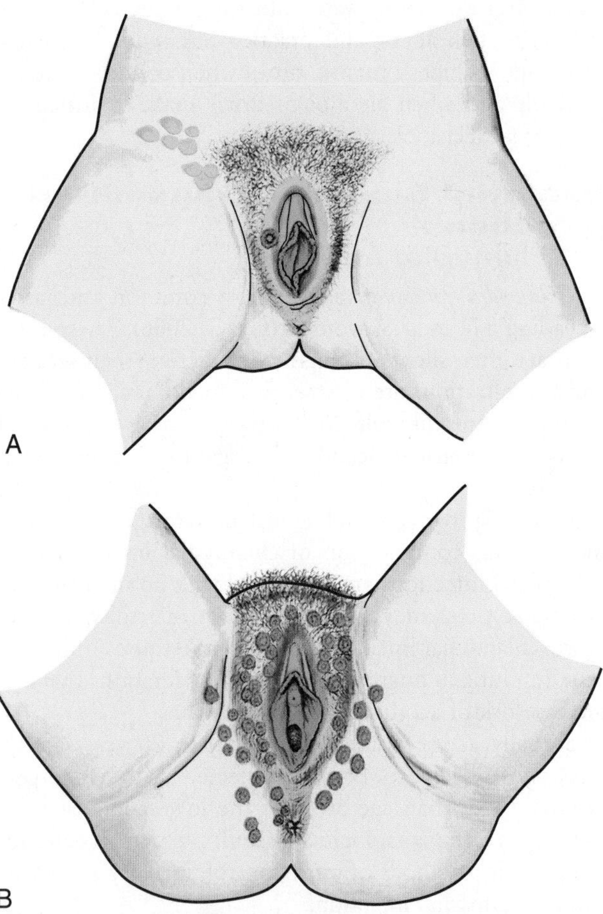

Fig. 3-2 Syphilis. **A,** Primary stage: chancre with inguinal adenopathy. **B,** Secondary stage: condyloma lata.

or multiorgan system complications can develop in this third stage.

Screening and diagnosis. Diagnosis is dependent on microscopic examination of primary and secondary lesion tissue and serologic testing during latency and late infection. Any test for antibodies may not be reactive in the presence of active infection because of the time needed for the body's immune system to develop antibodies to any antigens. Two types of serologic tests are used: nontreponemal and treponemal. Nontreponemal antibody tests such as the Venereal Disease Research Laboratory (VDRL) or rapid plasma reagin (RPR) are used as screening tests. False-positive results are not unusual, particularly when conditions such as acute infection, autoimmune disorders, malignancy, pregnancy, and drug addiction exist and after immunization or vaccination. The treponemal tests, fluorescent treponemal antibody absorbed (FTA-ABS) and microhemagglutination assays for antibody to *T. pallidum* (MHA-TP), are used to confirm positive results. Test results in patients with early primary or incubating syphilis are sometimes negative. Seroconversion usually takes place 6 to 8 weeks after exposure, so repeat testing in 1 to 2 months should be scheduled when a suspicious genital lesion exists. Positive nontreponemal tests usually become nonreactive after treatment, but most patients with positive treponemal antibody test results will remain positive for life, regardless of treatment or disease activity (CDC, 2006). Tests for chlamydia and gonorrhea are performed, and HIV testing is offered.

Management. Penicillin is the preferred medication for treating patients with all stages of syphilis (CDC, 2006). One intramuscular injection of benzathine penicillin G (2.4 million units) is the recommended dose.

NURSING ALERT Patients treated for syphilis may experience a Jarisch-Herxheimer reaction after antibiotic therapy, an acute febrile reaction often accompanied by headache, myalgias, and arthralgias that develop within the first 24 hours of treatment. This reaction may be treated symptomatically with analgesics and antipyretics.

Emphasize the necessity of long-term serologic testing at 6 and 12 months to assess the response to the treatment even in the absence of symptoms. Advise the patient to practice sexual abstinence until treatment is completed, all evidence of primary and secondary syphilis is gone, and serologic evidence of a cure is demonstrated. Tell women to notify all partners who may have been exposed. Inform them that the disease is reportable. Discuss preventive measures.

Pelvic inflammatory disease

Pelvic inflammatory disease (PID) is an infectious process that most commonly involves the uterine tubes (salpingitis), uterus (endometritis), and, more rarely, the ovaries and peritoneal surfaces. Multiple organisms cause PID, and most cases are associated with more than one organism. *C. trachomatis* causes one half of all cases of PID. In addition to gonorrhea and chlamydia, a wide variety of anaerobic and aerobic bacteria cause PID. Because a wide variety of infectious agents can cause PID and it encompasses a wide variety of pathologic processes, the infection can be acute, subacute, or chronic and has a wide range of symptoms.

Animation: Pelvic Inflammatory Disease

Most PID results from ascending spread of microorganisms from the vagina and endocervix to the upper genital tract. This spread most frequently happens at the end of or just after menses after reception of an infectious agent. PID also may develop after an elective abortion, pelvic surgery, or childbirth.

Risk factors for acquiring PID are those associated with the risk of contracting an STI–a history of PID or STIs, intercourse with a partner who has untreated urethritis, recent IUD insertion, and nulliparity.

Women who have had PID are at increased risk for ectopic pregnancy, infertility, and chronic pelvic pain. Other problems associated with PID include dyspareunia, pyosalpinx (pus in the uterine tubes), tuboovarian abscess, and pelvic adhesions.

The symptoms of PID vary, depending on whether the infection is acute, subacute, or chronic; however, pain is common to all types of infection. It may be dull, cramping, and intermittent (subacute) or severe, persistent, and incapacitating (acute). Women may also report one or more of the following: fever, chills, nausea and vomiting, increased vaginal discharge, symptoms of a urinary tract infection, and irregular bleeding. Abdominal pain is usually present (Eckert & Lentz, 2007b).

Screening and diagnosis. PID is difficult to diagnose because of the accompanying wide variety of symptoms. The CDC (2006) recommends treatment for PID in all sexually active young women and others at risk for STIs if the following criteria are present and no other cause or causes of the illness are found: lower abdominal tenderness, bilateral adnexal tenderness, and cervical motion tenderness. Other criteria for diagnosing PID include an oral temperature of 38.3° C or above, abnormal cervical or vaginal discharge, elevated erythrocyte sedimentation rate, elevated C-reactive protein, and laboratory documentation of cervical infection with *N. gonorrhoeae* or *C. trachomatis*.

Management. Perhaps the most important nursing intervention is prevention. Primary prevention includes education in preventing the acquisition of STIs, and secondary prevention involves preventing a lower genital tract infection from ascending to the upper genital tract. Instructing women in self-protective behaviors such as practicing risk reduction measures and using barrier methods is critical. Also important is the detection of asymptomatic gonorrheal and chlamydial infections through routine screening of women with risky behaviors or specific risk factors such as age.

Although treatment regimens vary with the infecting organism, a broad-spectrum antibiotic is generally used (CDC, 2006). Treatment for mild to moderately severe PID may be oral (e.g., ceftriaxone plus doxycycline with or without metronidazole) or parenteral (e.g., cefotetan or cefoxitin plus doxycycline [oral]), and regimens can be administered in inpatient or outpatient settings (CDC, 2007c). The woman with acute PID should be on bed rest in a semi-Fowler's position. Comfort measures include analgesics for pain and all other nursing measures applicable to a patient confined to bed. The woman should have as few pelvic examinations as possible during the acute phase of the disease. During the recovery phase, the woman should restrict her activity and make every effort to get adequate rest and a nutritionally sound diet. Follow-up laboratory work after treatment should include endocervical cultures for a test of cure.

Health education is central to effective management of PID. Explain to women the nature of their disease, and encourage them to comply with all therapy and prevention recommendations, emphasizing the necessity of taking all medication, even if symptoms disappear. Counsel women to refrain from sexual intercourse until their treatment is completed. Provide contraceptive counseling. Suggest that the woman select a barrier method such as condoms or a diaphragm. A woman with a history of PID should not choose an IUD as her contraceptive method (Mishell, 2007).

The potential or actual loss of reproductive capabilities can be devastating and can adversely affect a woman's self-concept. Because PID is so closely tied to sexuality, body image, and self-concept, the woman diagnosed with it will need supportive care. Referral to a support group or for counseling may be appropriate.

Viral Sexually Transmitted Infections

Human papillomavirus

Human papillomavirus (HPV) infection, also known as *condylomata acuminata* and *genital warts,* is the most common viral STI seen in ambulatory health care settings. An estimated 20 million Americans are infected with HPV, and approximately 6.2 million new infections occur every year (CDC, 2008a). HPV, a double-stranded DNA virus, has more than 30 serotypes that can be sexually transmitted. HPV types 6 and 11 are known to cause genital wart formation, and HPV types 16, 18, 31, 33, and 35 are thought to have oncogenic potential (CDC, 2006). HPV is the primary cause of cervical neoplasia (American Cancer Society [ACS], 2009b).

Genital warts in women are most commonly seen in the posterior part of the introitus (Fig. 3-3). However, lesions are also found on the buttocks, vulva, vagina, anus, and cervix. Typically, warts are small (2 to 3 mm in diameter and 10 to 15 mm in height), soft, papillary swellings occurring singularly or in clusters on the genital and anal-rectal region. Infections of long duration may appear as a cauliflower-like mass. In moist areas such as the vaginal introitus, the lesions may appear to have multiple, fine, finger-like projections. Vaginal lesions are often multiple. Flat-topped papules, 1 to 4 mm in diameter, occur most often on the cervix. In many instances, these lesions are visualized only under magnification. Warts are usually flesh colored or slightly darker on Caucasian women, black on African-American women, and brownish on Asian women. Condylomata acuminata are often painless but may also be uncomfortable, particularly when very large. They can become inflamed and ulcerated.

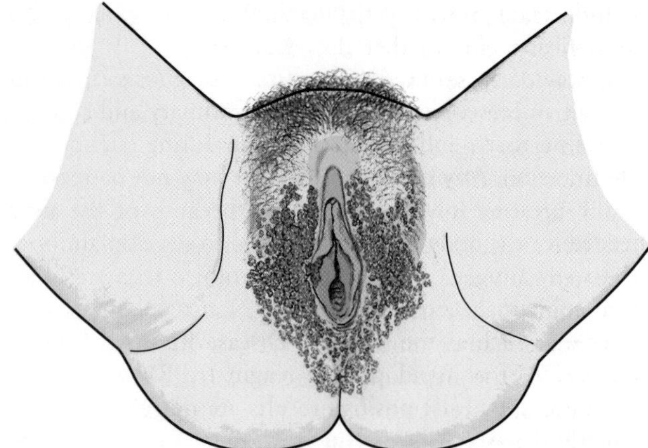

Fig. 3-3 Human papillomavirus infection.

Screening and diagnosis. Viral screening and typing for HPV is available but not standard practice. History, evaluation of signs and symptoms, Papanicolaou (Pap) test, and physical examination are used in making a diagnosis. The HPV-DNA test is used in women over the age of 30 in combination with the Pap test to test for types of HPV that are likely to cause cancer or in women with abnormal Pap test results (ACS, 2009b) (see Chapter 2). The only definitive diagnostic test for presence of HPV is histologic evaluation of a biopsy specimen.

Management. Untreated warts may resolve on their own in young women, given that their immune system may be strong enough to fight the HPV infection. If treatment is needed for external genital warts, a topical application such as podofilox 0.5% solution or gel or imiquimod 5% cream is used (CDC, 2006). Cryotherapy, electrocautery, and laser therapy may also be used. No one treatment is best, and no therapy has been shown to eliminate HPV. The goal of treatment is removal of warts and relief of signs and symptoms. The woman must often make multiple office visits, and she frequently tries many different treatments.

Women who are experiencing discomfort associated with genital warts may find that bathing with an oatmeal solution and drying the area with a cool hair dryer will provide some relief. Keeping the area clean and dry will also decrease growth of the warts. Cotton underwear and loose-fitting clothes that decrease friction and irritation also may decrease discomfort. Advise women to maintain a healthy lifestyle to aid the immune system. Counsel women regarding diet, rest, stress reduction, and exercise.

Patient counseling is essential. Women must understand the virus, how it is transmitted, that no immunity is conferred with infection, and that reinfection is likely with repeated contact. Encourage all sexually active women with multiple partners or a history of HPV to use latex condoms for intercourse to decrease acquisition or transmission of the infection. Semiannual or annual health examinations are recommended to assess disease recurrence and screening for cervical cancer. Women who have been treated for HPV infections should have at least annual Pap tests (CDC, 2006).

Genital herpes simplex virus

Unknown until the middle of the twentieth century, genital herpes simplex virus (HSV) is now one of the most common STIs in the United States, especially in women. HSV infection causes a painful vesicular eruption of the skin and mucosa of the genitals caused by two different antigen subtypes of HSV: herpes simplex virus 1 (HSV-1) and herpes simplex virus 2 (HSV-2). HSV-2 is usually transmitted sexually and HSV-1 nonsexually. Although HSV-1 is more commonly associated with gingivostomatitis and oral labial ulcers (fever blisters) and HSV-2 with genital lesions, neither type is exclusively associated with the respective sites.

Estimates suggest that at least 50 million people in the United States are infected with herpes (CDC, 2006). Women between ages 15 and 34 are most likely to become infected. Recurrent HSV infections are common. Prevalence is increased in women with multiple sex partners.

An initial herpetic infection characteristically has both systemic and local symptoms and lasts approximately 3 weeks. Women generally have a more severe clinical course than do men. In many instances the first symptoms after incubation are genital discomfort and neuralgic pain. Systemic symptoms appear early, peak 3 to 4 days after lesions appear, and then subside over 3 to 4 days (Fig. 3-4). Ulcerative lesions last 4 to 15 days before crusting over. New lesions may develop up to the tenth day of the course of the infection. Viral shedding and therefore infectivity may last 6 or 8 weeks.

Common systemic symptoms with the primary infection include fever, malaise, headache, and photophobia. Women with primary genital herpes have many lesions that progress from macules to papules, then vesicles, pustules, and ulcers that crust and heal without scarring. These ulcers are extremely tender, and primary infections may be bilateral. Women may also have itching, inguinal tenderness, and lymphadenopathy. Severe vulvar edema may develop, and women may have difficulty sitting. Cervicitis also is common with initial infections, and a heavy, watery

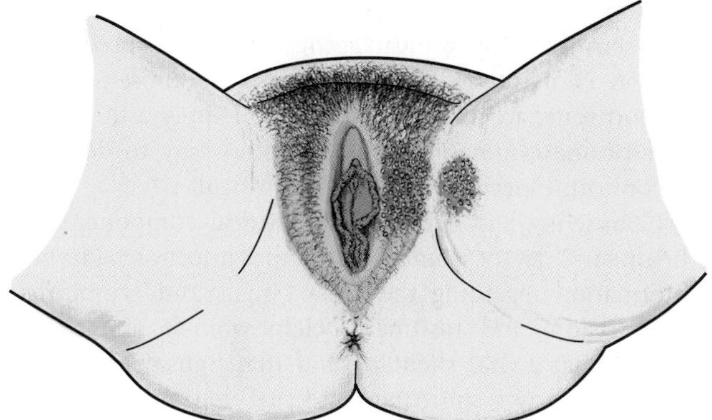

Fig. 3-4 Herpes genitalis.

to purulent vaginal discharge is common. Extragenital lesions are often present because of autoinoculation. Urinary retention and dysuria may occur secondary to autonomic involvement of the sacral nerve root.

Women experiencing recurrent episodes of HSV infections will often have only local symptoms, which are usually less severe than those associated with the initial infection. Systemic symptoms are usually absent, although the characteristic prodromal genital tingling is common. Recurrent lesions are unilateral, are less severe, and usually last 7 to 10 days without prolonged viral shedding. Lesions begin as vesicles and progress rapidly to ulcers. Very few women with recurrent disease have cervicitis.

Screening and diagnosis. Although a diagnosis of herpes infection may be suspected from the history and physical examination, it is confirmed by viral tissue cultures.

Management. Genital herpes is a chronic and recurring disease for which there is no known cure. Oral medications used for treating the first clinical HSV infection include acyclovir, famciclovir, and valacyclovir. These medications are considered for episodic or suppressive therapy for recurrent HSV. Intravenous acyclovir may be used for women with severe disease (CDC, 2006). Management is directed toward specific treatment during primary and recurrent infections, prevention, self-help measures, and psychologic support.

Cleaning lesions twice a day with saline will help prevent secondary infection. Bacterial infection must be treated with appropriate antibiotics. Measures that increase comfort for women when lesions are active include warm sitz baths with baking soda and keeping lesions warm and dry by blowing the area dry using a hair dryer set on cool or patting dry with a soft towel. Wearing cotton underwear and loose clothing, using drying aids such as hydrogen peroxide, Burrow's solution, or oatmeal baths and applying cool, wet black tea bags to lesions also aid comfort. Women can also apply compresses infused with cloves or peppermint oil and clove oil to lesions.

Analgesics such as aspirin or ibuprofen help relieve pain and systemic symptoms associated with initial infections.

Because the mucous membranes affected by herpes are very sensitive, any topical agents should be used with caution. Non-antiviral ointments, especially those containing cortisone, are avoided. Women can apply a thin layer of lidocaine ointment or an antiseptic spray to decrease discomfort, especially if walking is difficult.

Counseling and education are critical components of the nursing care of women with herpes infections. Provide information regarding the causes, signs and symptoms, transmission, and treatment. Help women understand asymptomatic viral shedding and that transmission to a partner is likely if this occurs and that they should refrain from sexual contact from the onset of prodrome until complete healing of lesions. Condoms may not prevent transmission, particularly male-to-female transmission; however, this does not mean that the partners should avoid all intimacy. Encourage women to maintain close contact with their partners while avoiding contact with lesions. Teach women how to look for herpetic lesions using a mirror and good light source to aid vision and a wet cloth or finger covered with a finger cot to rub lightly over the labia. Ensure that women understand that when lesions are active, they need to avoid sharing intimate articles (e.g., washcloth, wet towel) that come into contact with the lesions. Plain soap and water are all that is needed to clean hands that have come in contact with herpetic lesions.

Stress, menstruation, trauma, febrile illnesses, chronic illness, and ultraviolet light have all been found to trigger recurrences of genital herpes (Fraley, 2002). Women may wish to keep a diary to identify which stressors seem to be associated with recurrent herpes attacks so that they can then avoid those stressors when possible. Referral for stress-reduction therapy, yoga, or meditation classes may be provided when indicated. You can discuss the role of exercise in reducing stress. Avoiding excessive heat and sun and hot baths and using a lubricant during sexual intercourse to reduce friction is also helpful. Daily suppressive use of valacyclovir has been shown to decrease sexual transmission. The CDC recommends that therapy be discontinued after 12 months to see if the rate of recurrence has decreased (CDC, 2006).

The emotional effect of contracting an incurable STI such as herpes is considerable. At diagnosis, many emotions may surface–helplessness, anger, denial, guilt, anxiety, shame, or inadequacy. Women need the opportunity to discuss their feelings and help in learning to live with the disease. Herpes can affect a woman's sexuality, her sexual practices, and her current and future relationships. She may need help in raising the issue with her partner or with future partners.

Hepatitis

This section focuses on hepatitis A, B, and C viruses. Hepatitis D and E viruses, most common among users of intravenous drugs and recipients of multiple blood transfusions, are not included in this discussion.

Hepatitis A. Hepatitis A virus (HAV) infection is acquired primarily through a fecal-oral route by ingestion of contaminated food, particularly milk, shellfish, or polluted water, or via person-to-person contact. Influenza-like symptoms with malaise, fatigue, anorexia, nausea, pruritus, fever, and upper right quadrant pain characterize HAV infection. Serologic testing to detect the immunoglobulin M (IgM) antibody confirms acute infections. Because HAV infection is self-limited and does not result in chronic infection or chronic liver disease, treatment is usually supportive. Women who become dehydrated from nausea and vomiting or who have fulminating hepatitis A may need to be hospitalized. Medications that might cause liver damage or that are metabolized in the liver should be used with caution. No specific diet or activity restrictions are necessary. Hepatitis A vaccine and immune globulin (IG) for intramuscular administration are effective in preventing most hepatitis A infections (CDC, 2006).

Hepatitis B. Hepatitis B virus (HBV), a common STI, is much more contagious than HIV. It is caused by a large DNA virus and is associated with three antigens and their antibodies: hepatitis B surface antigen (HBsAg), HBV antigen (HBeAg), HBV core antigen (HBcAg), antibody to HBsAg (anti-HBs), antibody to HBeAg (anti-HBe), and antibody to HBcAg (anti-HBc). Screening for active or chronic disease or disease immunity is based on testing for these antigens and their antibodies.

Populations at risk include women of Asian, Pacific Island (Polynesian, Micronesian, Melanesian), or Alaskan Inuit descent and women born in Haiti or sub-Saharan Africa. Women with a history of acute or chronic liver disease, who work or receive treatment in a dialysis unit, or who have household or sexual contact with a hemodialysis patient are at increased risk. Women who work or live in institutions for the cognitively challenged are considered to be at risk, as are women with a history of multiple blood transfusions. Health care workers and public safety workers exposed to blood in the workplace are at risk. Behaviors such as having multiple sexual partners and a history of intravenous drug use increase the risk of contracting HBV infections.

HBsAg is found in blood, saliva, sweat, tears, vaginal secretions, and semen. Drug abusers who share needles are at risk, as are health care workers who are exposed to blood and needlesticks. Perinatal transmission most often occurs in mothers who have acute hepatitis infection late in the third trimester or during the intrapartum or postpartum period from exposure to HBsAg-positive vaginal secretions, blood, amniotic fluid, saliva, and breast milk. HBV has also been transmitted by artificial insemination. Although HBV can be transmitted via blood transfusion, the incidence of such infections has decreased significantly since testing of blood for HBsAg became routine.

Hepatitis B (HB) is a disease of the liver and is often a silent infection. In the adult, the course of the infection can be fulminating and the outcome fatal. Early symptoms include skin eruptions, urticaria, arthralgias, arthritis, lassitude, anorexia, nausea, vomiting, headache, fever, and mild abdominal pain. Later the patient may have clay-colored stools, dark urine, increased abdominal pain, and jaundice. Between 5% and 10% of individuals with HB have persistence of HBsAg and become chronic HBV carriers.

Screening and diagnosis. All women at high risk for contracting HB should be screened on a regular basis. The HBsAg screening test is usually performed, given that a rise in HBsAg occurs at the onset of clinical symptoms and usually indicates an active infection. If HBsAg persists in the blood, the woman is identified as a carrier. If the HBsAg test result is positive, further laboratory studies may be ordered: anti-HBe, anti-HBc, serum glutamic-oxaloacetic transaminase (SGOT), alkaline phosphatase, and liver panel.

Management. No specific treatment has been developed for HB. Recovery is usually spontaneous in 3 to 16 weeks. Advise women to increase bed rest; eat a high-protein, low-fat diet; and increase their fluid intake. They should avoid drugs and alcohol and medications metabolized in the liver. Women with a definite exposure to HBV should be given HB immune globulin (HBIG) and begin the HB vaccine series within 14 days of the most recent contact to prevent infection (CDC, 2006).

HB vaccination is the most effective means of preventing HBV infections. Vaccination is also recommended for all nonimmune women who have had multiple sex partners within the past 6 months, intravenous drug users, residents of correctional or long-term care facilities, persons seeking care for an STI, sex workers, women whose partners are intravenous drug users or bisexual, and women who work in high risk occupations. The vaccine is given in a series of three (some authorities recommend four) doses over a 6-month period, with the first two doses given at least 1 month apart and the first and third doses at least 4 months apart. The vaccine is given in the deltoid muscle in adults (CDC, 2006).

Patient education includes explaining the meaning of HBV infection, including transmission, state of infectivity, and sequelae. Also, explain the need for immunoprophylaxis for household members and sexual contacts. To decrease transmission of the virus, advise women with HB or who test positive for HBV to maintain a high level of personal hygiene: Wash hands after using the toilet, carefully dispose of tampons, pads, and bandages in plastic bags, and they should not share razor blades, toothbrushes, needles, and manicure implements. These women should have male partners use a condom if unvaccinated and without hepatitis, avoid sharing saliva through kissing, or sharing of silverware or dishes, and wipe up blood spills immediately with soap and water. They should inform all health care providers of their carrier state.

COMMUNITY ACTIVITY

Visit a physician's office or clinic in your community that is appropriate for referring the following women. Evaluate the resources in terms of access, costs (insurance), Medicare coverage, confidentiality, and follow-up care. Include the appropriateness of the information in relation to age, culture, and language. Evaluate whether the services are adequate, and if not, suggest what is needed.

A. A 30-year-old Latina (non–English speaking) woman with secondary dysmenorrhea
B. A 20-year-old woman who is sexually active and believes that she has a sexually transmitted infection
C. A 40-year-woman of Muslim culture who has never had a Pap test or breast examination and reports a lump in her breast

Hepatitis C. Hepatitis C virus (HCV) infection has become an important health problem as increasing numbers of persons acquire the disease. Hepatitis C is responsible for nearly 50% of the cases of chronic viral hepatitis. Risk factors include having STIs such as HB and HIV, multiple sexual partners, history of blood transmissions, and history of intravenous drug use. HCV is readily transmitted through exposure to blood and much less efficiently via semen, saliva, or urine.

Most patients with hepatitis C are asymptomatic or have general influenza-like symptoms similar to those of hepatitis A. HCV infection is confirmed by the presence of anti-C antibody during laboratory testing. Interferon-alpha alone or with ribavirin for 6 to 12 months is the main therapy for chronic HCV-related liver disease, although effectiveness of this treatment varies. Currently, no vaccine is available for hepatitis C.

Human immunodeficiency virus

Approximately 37,000 new HIV infections occur in the United States each year (CDC, 2008b). An estimated 26% of these new infections occur in women. African-American women are estimated to have 66% of these infections, Caucasian women are estimated to have 17%, Hispanic women, 14%, and Native American women less than 1% (CDC, 2008b).

Transmission of HIV, a retrovirus, occurs primarily through exchange of body fluids (semen, blood, vaginal secretions). Severe depression of the cellular immune system associated with HIV infection characterizes acquired immunodeficiency syndrome (AIDS). Although behaviors that place women at risk have been well documented, you should assess all women for the possibility of HIV exposure. The most commonly reported opportunistic diseases are *Pneumocystis carinii* pneumonia (PCP), *Candida* esophagitis, and wasting syndrome. Other viral infections such as HSV and cytomegalovirus infections seem to be more prevalent in women than men (CDC, 2006). PID is often more severe in HIV-infected women than in the general population, and rates of HPV and cervical dysplasia are sometimes higher in HIV-infected women. (Eckert & Lentz, 2007a). The clinical course of HPV infection in women with HIV infection is accelerated, and recurrence is more frequent in non–HIV-infected women.

Once HIV enters the body, seroconversion to HIV positivity usually occurs within 6 to 12 weeks. Although HIV seroconversion may be totally asymptomatic, it is usually accompanied by a viremic, influenza-like response. Symptoms include fever, headache, night sweats, malaise, generalized lymphadenopathy, myalgias, nausea, diarrhea, weight loss, sore throat, and rash.

Laboratory studies may reveal leukopenia, thrombocytopenia, anemia, and an elevated erythrocyte sedimentation rate. HIV has a strong affinity for surface-marker proteins on T lymphocytes. This affinity leads to significant T-cell destruction. Both clinical and epidemiologic studies have shown that declining CD_4 levels are strongly associated with increased incidence of AIDS-related diseases and death in many different groups of HIV-infected persons.

HIV testing and counseling. Screening, teaching, and counseling regarding HIV risk factors, indications for being tested, and testing are major roles for nurses caring for women today. A significant number of behaviors place women at risk for HIV infection, including intravenous drug use, high risk sex partners, multiple sex partners, and a previous history of multiple STIs. HIV infection is usually diagnosed by using HIV-1 and HIV-2 antibody tests. Antibody testing is first performed with a sensitive screening test such as the enzyme immunoassay (EIA). Reactive screening tests are confirmed by an additional test, such as the Western blot or an immunofluorescence assay. If a positive antibody test is confirmed by a supplemental test, it means that a woman is infected with HIV and is capable of infecting others. HIV antibodies are detectable in at least 95% of patients within 3 months after infection. Although a negative antibody test usually indicates that a person is not infected, antibody tests cannot exclude recent infection. Because HIV antibody crosses the placenta, a definite diagnosis of HIV in children younger than 18 months is based on laboratory evidence of HIV in blood or tissues by culture, nucleic acid, or antigen detection (CDC, 2006).

The U.S. FDA (2008a) has approved six rapid HIV antibody screening tests. These tests use a blood sample obtained by fingerstick or venipuncture, an oral fluid sample, or a urine sample to provide test results within 20 minutes, with sensitivity and specificity rates of more than 99%. If the results are reactive, further testing is necessary (Centers for Disease Control and Prevention, Divisions of HIV/AIDS Prevention, 2008). Quicker results mean that patients do not have to make extra visits for follow-up standard tests, and the oral test provides an option for patients who do not want to have a blood test.

The CDC (2006) guidelines recommend offering HIV testing to all women whose behavior places them at risk for HIV infection. On entry into the health care system, inform patients (orally or in writing) about the risk factors for the AIDS virus and to inform the nurse if she believes she is at risk. She should be told that she does not have to say why she may be at risk, only that she thinks she might be.

Counseling before and after HIV testing is standard nursing practice today. One of the nursing responsibilities is to assess a woman's understanding of the information such a test would provide and to be sure the woman thoroughly understands the emotional, legal, and medical implications of a positive or negative test result before she is ready to take an HIV test.

LEGAL TIP **HIV Testing**

If HIV test results are placed in the patient's chart—the appropriate place for all health information—they are available to all who have access to the chart. Inform the woman of this availability before testing. Informed consent must be obtained before an HIV test is performed. In some states, written consent is mandated. In many sites, HIV testing is performed unless patients decline (i.e., opt-out testing). Nurses must know what procedures are being used for informed consent in their facility.

Counseling associated with HIV testing has two components: pretest and posttest counseling. During pretest counseling, a personalized risk assessment is conducted, the meaning of positive and negative test results is explained, informed consent for HIV testing is obtained, and women are helped to develop a realistic plan for reducing risk and preventing infection. Posttest counseling includes informing the patient of the test results, reviewing the meaning of the results, and reinforcing prevention messages. Document all pretest and posttest counseling.

Unless rapid testing is performed, there is generally a 1- to 3-week waiting period after testing for HIV, which is an anxious time for the woman. The nurse should inform her that this time period between drawing blood and receiving test results is routine. Test results, whatever they are, must always be communicated in person, and women must be informed in advance that such is the procedure. Whenever possible, the person who provided the pretest counseling should also tell the woman her test results. Explore women's reactions to a negative test with the question "How do you feel?" HIV-negative result counseling sessions are another opportunity to provide education. You can place emphasis on ways in which a woman can remain HIV free and encourage her to stay negative. Remind her that if she has been exposed to HIV in the past 6 months, she should be retested and that if she continues high risk behaviors she should have ongoing testing.

When providing posttest counseling to an HIV-positive woman, privacy with no interruptions is essential. Make sure that the woman understands what a positive test means, and review the reliability of the test results. Reemphasize risk-reduction practices. Make referrals for appropriate medical evaluation and follow-up, and assess the need or desire for psychosocial or psychiatric referrals. You should also stress the importance of early medical evaluation so that a baseline assessment can be made and prophylactic medication begun.

Management. During the initial contact with an HIV-infected woman, establish what the woman knows about HIV infection. Ensure that the woman is being cared for by a medical practitioner or at a facility with expertise in caring for persons with HIV infections, including AIDS. Psychologic referral also may be indicated. Resources such as counseling for financial assistance, legal advocacy, suicide prevention, and death and dying may be appropriate. All women who are drug users should be referred to a substance abuse cessation program. A major focus of counseling involves preventing transmission of HIV to partners.

Nurses counseling seropositive women wishing contraceptive information may recommend oral contraceptives and latex condoms or tubal sterilization or vasectomy and latex condoms. For women who are HIV infected, the diaphragm is classified as having more risks than advantages; the IUD appears safe for selected patients (World Health Organization, 2004). Offer female condoms or abstinence to women whose male partners refuse to use condoms.

No cure is available for HIV infections at this time. Rare and unusual diseases are characteristic of HIV infections. Opportunistic infections and concurrent diseases are managed vigorously with treatment specific to the infection or disease. Routine gynecologic care for HIV-positive women should include a pelvic examination every 6 months. Thorough Pap screening is essential because of the greatly increased incidence of abnormal findings on examination (CDC, 2006). In addition, HIV-positive women should be screened for syphilis, gonorrhea, chlamydia, and other vaginal infections and treated if infections are present. General prevention strategies are an important part of care (e.g., smoking cessation, sound nutrition) as is antiretroviral therapy. Discussion of the medical care of HIV-positive women or women with AIDS is beyond the scope of this chapter because of the rapidly changing recommendations.

HIV in pregnancy. HIV counseling and testing should be offered to all women at their initial entry into prenatal care. Universal testing is recommended versus selective testing for maternal HIV because it results in a greater number of women being screened and treated (American Academy of Pediatrics Committee on Pediatric AIDS, 2008; Branson, et al., 2006). Perinatal transmission of HIV has decreased significantly in the past decade because of the administration of antiretroviral prophylaxis (e.g., zidovudine) to pregnant women in the prenatal and the perinatal periods. Treatment of HIV-infected women with the triple-drug antiviral therapy or highly active antiretroviral therapy (HAART) during pregnancy has been reported to decrease the mother-to-child transmission to 1% to 2% (Volmink, Siegfried, van der Merwe, & Brocklehurst, 2007).

All HIV-infected women should be treated with a combination of antiretroviral drugs (e.g., HAART) during pregnancy, regardless of their CD_4 cell counts (Perinatal HIV Guidelines Working Group, 2008). Antiviral therapy is administered orally and is usually started after the first trimester and continued throughout pregnancy. The major side effect of this drug is bone marrow suppression. Periodic hematocrit, white blood cell count, and platelet count assessments should be performed (Perinatal HIV Guidelines Working Group). Women who are HIV positive should also be vaccinated against HB, pneumococcal infection, *Haemophilus influenzae* type B, and viral influenza. To support any pregnant woman's immune system, appropriate counseling is provided about optimal nutrition, sleep, rest, exercise, and stress reduction. Use of condoms is encouraged to minimize further exposure to HIV if her partner is the source.

In the intrapartum period, antiretroviral therapy and cesarean birth are recommended to prevent vertical transmission of HIV (Perinatal HIV Guidelines Working Group, 2008). Women should be given the option of having a scheduled cesarean birth at 38 weeks of gestation to decrease this risk. A vaginal birth may be an option for HIV-infected women who have a viral load of less than 1000 copies/ml at 36 weeks, if a woman has ruptured membranes and labor is progressing rapidly, or if she declines a cesarean birth. Intravenous zidovudine is administered 3 hours before the scheduled cesarean birth and is continued until the baby is born. It should be given during labor and birth if the woman is having a vaginal birth (Perinatal HIV Guidelines Working Group). Fetal scalp electrode and scalp pH sampling should be avoided because these procedures may result in inoculation of the virus into the fetus. Similarly, the use of forceps or vacuum extractor should be avoided when possible. Infants should receive oral zidovudine for 6 weeks after birth. Avoidance of breastfeeding is recommended in the United States and most developed countries (American Academy of Pediatrics Committee on Pediatric AIDS, 2008).

Women who have HIV but who are without symptoms may have an unremarkable postpartum course. Immunosuppressed women with symptoms may be at increased risk for postpartum urinary tract infections (UTIs), vaginitis, postpartum endometritis, and poor wound healing. Good perineal hygiene should be stressed. Women who are HIV positive but who were not on antiretroviral drugs before pregnancy should be tested in the postpartum period to determine whether therapy that was initiated in pregnancy should be continued (Perinatal HIV Guidelines Working Group, 2008). After the initial bath the newborn can be with the mother. In planning for discharge, comprehensive care and support services will need to be arranged. After discharge the woman and her infant are referred to physicians who are experienced in the treatment of HIV and AIDS and associated conditions for intensive monitoring and follow-up (Lachat, Scott, & Relf, 2006).

Vaginal Infections

Vaginal discharge and itching of the vulva and vagina are among the most common reasons a woman seeks help from a health care provider. Indeed, more women complain of vaginal discharge than of any other gynecologic symptom. Vaginal discharge resulting from infection differs from normal secretions. Normal vaginal secretion or leukorrhea is clear to cloudy in appearance and may turn yellow after drying; the discharge is slightly slimy, is nonirritating, and has a mild inoffensive odor. Normal vaginal secretions are acidic, with a pH range of 4 to 5. The amount of leukorrhea present differs with phases of the menstrual cycle, with relatively greater amounts occurring at ovulation and just before menses. Leukorrhea is also increased during pregnancy. Normal vaginal secretions contain lactobacilli and epithelial cells. Women who have adequate endogenous or exogenous estrogen will have vaginal secretions.

The most common vaginal infections are bacterial vaginosis (BV), candidiasis, and trichomoniasis. Vulvovaginitis, or inflammation of the vulva and vagina, may be caused by vaginal infection or copious amounts of leukorrhea, which can cause maceration of tissues. Chemical irritants, allergens, and foreign bodies that produce inflammatory reactions can also cause vulvovaginitis.

Bacterial vaginosis

Bacterial vaginosis, formerly called *nonspecific vaginitis, Haemophilus vaginitis,* or *Gardnerella,* is the most common type of symptomatic vaginitis today (Eckert & Lentz, 2007a). BV is associated with preterm labor and birth. The exact cause of BV is unknown. It is a syndrome in which normal, hydrogen peroxide–producing lactobacilli are replaced with high concentrations of anaerobic bacteria (e.g., *Gardnerella, Mobiluncus*). With the increase of anaerobes, the level of vaginal amines is raised and the normal acidic pH of the vagina is altered. Epithelial cells slough, and numerous bacteria attach to their surfaces (clue cells). When the amines are volatilized, the characteristic odor of BV occurs.

Many women with BV complain of a characteristic "fishy odor." The odor may be noticed by the woman or her partner after heterosexual intercourse because semen releases the vaginal amines. When present, the BV discharge is usually profuse, thin, and white or gray, or milky, in appearance. Some women also may experience mild irritation or pruritus.

Screening and diagnosis. A focused history may help distinguish BV from other vaginal infections if the woman is symptomatic. Reports of fishy odor and increased thin vaginal discharge are most significant, and a report of increased odor after intercourse is also suggestive of BV. You should question women with previous occurrence of similar symptoms, diagnosis, and treatment because women with BV often have been treated incorrectly because of misdiagnosis.

Microscopic examination of vaginal secretions is always performed (Table 3-3). Both normal saline and 10% potassium hydroxide (KOH) smears are made. The presence of clue cells (vaginal epithelial cells coated with bacteria) on wet saline smear is highly diagnostic because the phenomenon is specific to BV. Test vaginal secretions for pH and amine odor. Nitrazine paper is sensitive enough to detect a pH of 4.5 or greater. The fishy odor of BV will be released when KOH is added to vaginal secretions on the lip of the withdrawn speculum.

Management. Treatment of BV with oral metronidazole (Flagyl) is most effective (CDC, 2006), although vaginal preparations (e.g., metronidazole gel, clindamycin cream) are also used. Side effects of metronidazole are numerous, including sharp, unpleasant metallic taste in the mouth, furry tongue, central nervous system reactions, and urinary tract disturbances. When the woman is taking oral metronidazole, advise her to avoid drinking alcoholic beverages, or she will experience the severe side effects of

TABLE 3-3

Wet Smear Tests for Vaginal Infections

INFECTION	TEST	POSITIVE FINDINGS
Trichomoniasis	Saline wet smear (vaginal secretions mixed with normal saline on a glass slide)	Presence of trichomonads (anaerobic flagellated protozoa)
Candidiasis	Potassium hydroxide (KOH) preparation (vaginal secretions mixed with KOH on a glass slide)	Presence of hyphae and pseudohyphae (buds and branches of yeast cells)
Bacterial vaginosis	Normal saline smear	Presence of clue cells (vaginal epithelial cells coated with bacteria)
	Whiff test (vaginal secretions mixed with KOH)	Release of fishy odor

abdominal distress, nausea, vomiting, and headache. Gastrointestinal symptoms are common whether alcohol is consumed or not. Treatment of sexual partners is not routinely recommended (CDC, 2006).

Candidiasis

Vulvovaginal candidiasis, or yeast infection, is the second most common type of vaginal infection in the United States. Although vaginal candidiasis infections are common in healthy women, those seen in women with HIV infection are often more severe and persistent by comparison. Genital candidiasis lesions are often painful, coalescing ulcerations necessitating continuous prophylactic therapy.

The most common organism is *Candida albicans;* estimates indicate that more than 90% of the yeast infections in women are caused by this organism. However, in the past 10 years, the incidence of non–*C. albicans* infections has risen steadily. Women with chronic or recurrent infections often are infected with these organisms (Eckert & Lentz, 2007a).

Numerous factors have been identified as predisposing a woman to yeast infections, including antibiotic therapy, particularly broad-spectrum antibiotics such as ampicillin, tetracycline, cephalosporins, and metronidazole. Some conditions, such as pregnancy, uncontrolled diabetes, and obesity, predispose women to yeast infections. Diets high in refined sugars or artificial sweeteners, use of corticosteroids and exogenous hormones, and immunosuppressed states also influence susceptibility. Clinical observations and research have suggested that tight-fitting clothing and underwear or pantyhose made of nonabsorbent materials create an environment in which vaginal fungus can grow.

The most common symptom of yeast infections is vulvar and possibly vaginal pruritus. The itching may be mild or intense, interfere with rest and activities, and may occur during or after intercourse. Some women report a feeling of dryness. Others may experience painful urination as the urine flows over the vulva, which usually occurs in women who have excoriations resulting from scratching. Most often the discharge has a thick, white, lumpy, and cottage cheese–like consistency. The discharge may be found in patches on the vaginal walls, cervix, and labia. Commonly, the vulva is red and swollen, as are the labial folds, vagina, and cervix. Although there is not a characteristic odor with yeast infections, sometimes a yeasty or musty smell can be detected.

Screening and diagnosis. In addition to a complete history of the woman's symptoms, their onset, and their course, the history is a valuable screening tool for identifying predisposing risk factors. Physical examination should include a thorough inspection of the vulva and vagina. A speculum examination is always performed. Commonly, health care practitioners will obtain saline and KOH wet smear and vaginal pH (see Table 3-3). Vaginal pH is normal (less than 4.5) with a yeast infection. The characteristic pseudohyphae (bud or branching of a fungus) may be seen on a wet smear performed with normal saline; however, they may be confused with other cells and artifacts (CDC, 2006).

Management. A sizable number of antifungal preparations are available for the treatment of *C. albicans* infection. Intravaginal agents include miconazole, clotrimazole, butoconazole, tioconazole, terconazole, and nystatin; fluconazole is an effective oral agent (CDC, 2006). Many of these vaginal medications (e.g., Monistat, Gyne-Lotrimin) are available OTC. Exogenous lactobacillus (in the form of dairy products [yogurt] or powder, tablet, capsule, or suppository supplements) and garlic have been suggested for prevention and treatment of vulvovaginal candidiasis, but research is inconclusive, and no recommendations have been developed for use in practice (Eckert & Lentz, 2007a). The first time a woman suspects that she may have a yeast infection, she should see a health care provider for confirmation of the diagnosis and treatment recommendation. If she experiences another infection, she may wish to purchase an OTC preparation and self-treat; if she chooses to do so, she should always be counseled regarding seeking care for numerous recurrent or chronic yeast infections. If vaginal discharge is extremely thick and copious, vaginal débridement with a cotton swab followed by application of vaginal medication is useful.

Women who have extensive irritation, swelling, and discomfort of the labia and vulva may find sitz baths helpful in decreasing inflammation and increasing comfort. Adding Aveeno powder to the bath may also increase the woman's comfort. Not wearing underpants to bed may help decrease symptoms and prevent recurrences. Completing the full course of treatment prescribed is essential to removing the pathogen. Instruct women to continue the medication even during menstruation. Explain that they should avoid using tampons during menses because the tampon will readily absorb the medication. If possible, women should avoid intercourse during treatment; if abstinence is not feasible, the woman's partner should use a condom to prevent the introduction of more organisms (see Patient Instructions for Self-Management box).

Trichomoniasis

Trichomonas vaginalis is almost always an STI and is also a common cause of vaginal infection (5% to 50% of all vaginitis) and discharge (Eckert & Lentz, 2007a).

Trichomoniasis is caused by *T. vaginalis,* an anaerobic, one-celled protozoan with characteristic flagella. Although trichomoniasis may be asymptomatic, women commonly experience characteristically yellowish to greenish, frothy, mucopurulent, copious, malodorous discharge. Inflammation of the vulva, vagina, or both may be present, and the woman may complain of irritation and pruritus. Dysuria and dyspareunia are often present. Typically the discharge worsens during and after menstruation. The cervix and

PATIENT INSTRUCTIONS FOR SELF-MANAGEMENT

Prevention of Genital Tract Infections

- Practice genital hygiene.
- Choose underwear or hosiery with a cotton crotch.
- Avoid tight-fitting clothing (especially tight jeans).
- Select cloth car seat covers instead of vinyl.
- Limit time spent in damp exercise clothes (especially swimsuits, leotards, and tights).
- Limit exposure to bath salts or bubble bath.
- Avoid colored or scented toilet tissue.
- If sensitive, discontinue use of feminine hygiene deodorant sprays.
- Use condoms.
- Void before and after intercourse.
- Decrease dietary sugar.
- Drink yeast-active milk and eat yogurt (with lactobacilli).
- Do not douche.

vaginal walls demonstrate characteristic "strawberry spots," or tiny petechiae in less than 10% of women, and the cervix may bleed on contact. In severe infections the vaginal walls, the cervix, and, occasionally, the vulva is acutely inflamed.

Screening and diagnosis. In addition to obtaining a history of current symptoms, obtain a thorough sexual history. Note any history of similar symptoms in the past and treatment used. Determine whether the woman's partner or partners were treated and if she has had subsequent relations with new partners.

A speculum examination is always performed, even though it may be uncomfortable for the woman. Any of the classic signs may or may not be seen on physical examination. The typical one-celled flagellate trichomonads are easily distinguished on a normal saline wet preparation (see Table 3-3). The pH of the discharge is greater than 5. Because trichomoniasis is an STI, once diagnosis is confirmed, the appropriate laboratory studies for other STIs should be carried out.

Management. The recommended treatment is metronidazole or tinadazole, 2 g orally in a single dose (CDC, 2006). Although the male partner is usually asymptomatic, he should receive treatment also because he often harbors the trichomonads in the urethra or prostate. Nurses need to discuss the importance of partner treatment with their patients. If partners are not treated, the infection will likely recur.

Women with trichomoniasis need to understand the sexual transmission of this disease. The woman should know that the organism can be present without symptoms, perhaps for several months, and that determining when she became infected is impossible.

Group B streptococci

Group B streptococci (GBS) may be considered normal vaginal flora in a woman who is not pregnant, and therefore no treatment is needed. GBS is a concern in pregnancy because of the increased risk for problems such as preterm labor and transmission to the newborn. For further discussion, see Chapters 21 and 24.

Infection Control

Infection-control measures are essential to protect care providers and to prevent nosocomial infection of patients, regardless of the infectious agent. The risk for occupational transmission varies with the disease. Even when the risk is low, as with HIV, the existence of any risk warrants reasonable precautions. Precautions against airborne disease transmission are available in all health care agencies. Box 3-4 lists Standard Precautions (precautions to use in the care of all persons for infection control) and additional precautions for labor and birth settings.

PROBLEMS OF THE BREAST

Benign Problems

Fibrocystic changes

Approximately 50% of women experience a breast problem at some point in their adult life. The most common benign breast problem is fibrocystic changes. Fibrocystic changes occur in varying degrees in breasts of healthy women. The etiologic agent responsible for these changes has not been found. One theory is that estrogen excess and progesterone deficiency in the luteal phase of the menstrual cycle may cause changes in breast tissue.

Fibrocystic changes are characterized by lumpiness, with or without tenderness, in both breasts (Valea & Katz, 2007). Single simple cysts may also occur. Symptoms usually develop approximately a week before menstruation begins and subside approximately a week after menstruation ends. Symptoms include dull heavy pain and a sense of fullness and tenderness often in the upper outer quadrants of the breasts. Physical examination may reveal excessive nodularity that many describe as feeling similar to a "plate of peas." Larger cysts are often described as feeling like water-filled balloons. Women in their twenties report the most severe pain. Women in their thirties have premenstrual pain and tenderness; small multiple nodules are usually present. Women in their forties usually do not report severe pain, but cysts will be tender and often regress in size (Crochetiere, 2005).

BOX 3-4

Standard Precautions

Medical history and examination cannot reliably identify all persons infected with human immunodeficiency virus (HIV) or other blood-borne pathogens. Standard Precautions should therefore be used consistently in the care of all persons. These precautions apply to blood, body fluids, and all secretions and excretions, except sweat, nonintact skin, and mucous membranes. The following infection-control practices should be applied during the delivery of health care to reduce the risk of transmission of microorganisms from known and unknown sources of infection (Seigel, Rhinehart, Jackson, Chiarello, & The Healthcare Infection Control Practices Advisory Committee, 2007):

1. *Hand hygiene.* During the delivery of health care, avoid unnecessary touching of surfaces in close proximity to the patient to prevent both contamination of clean hands from environmental surfaces and transmission of pathogens from contaminated hands to surfaces. Wash dirty or contaminated hands with either a non-antimicrobial or an antimicrobial soap and water. If hands are not visibly soiled, decontaminate hands with an alcohol-based hand rub, or hands may be washed with an antimicrobial soap and water. Perform hand hygiene (1) before having direct contact with patients, (2) after contact with blood, body fluids, or excretions, mucous membranes, nonintact skin, or wound dressings, (3) after contact with a patient's intact skin (e.g., when taking a pulse or blood pressure or lifting a patient), (4) if hands will be moving from a contaminated body site to a clean body site during patient care, (5) after contact with inanimate objects (including medical equipment) in the immediate vicinity of the patient, and (6) after removing gloves. Wash hands with non-antimicrobial soap and water or with antimicrobial soap and water if contact with spores (e.g., *Clostridium difficile* or *Bacillus anthracis*) is likely to have occurred. The physical action of washing and rinsing hands under such circumstances is recommended because alcohols, chlorhexidine, iodophors, and other antiseptic agents have poor activity against spores. Do not wear artificial fingernails or extenders if duties include direct contact with patients at high risk for infection and associated adverse outcomes.
2. Personal protective equipment (PPE). Observe the following principles of use:
   - *Gloves.* Wear gloves when a reasonably anticipated possibility exists that contact with blood or other potentially infectious materials, mucous membranes, nonintact skin, or potentially contaminated intact skin (e.g., of a patient incontinent of stool or urine) might occur. Gloves should be worn during infant eye prophylaxis, care of the umbilical cord, circumcision site, parenteral procedures, diaper changes, contact with colostrum, and postpartum assessments. Wear gloves with fit and durability appropriate to the task. Remove gloves after contact with a patient or the surrounding environment (including medical equipment) using proper technique to prevent hand contamination. Do not wear the same pair of gloves for the care of more than one patient. Change gloves during patient care if the hands will move from a contaminated body site (e.g., perineal area) to a clean body site (e.g., face).
   - *Gowns.* Wear a gown that is appropriate to the task to protect the skin and prevent soiling or contamination of clothing during procedures and patient-care activities when contact with blood, body fluids, secretions, or excretions is anticipated. Remove the gown and perform hand hygiene before leaving the patient's environment. Do not reuse gowns, even for repeated contacts with the same patient. Routine donning of gowns on entrance into a high risk unit (e.g., intensive care unit [ICU], neonatal intensive care unit [NICU]) is not indicated.
   - *Mouth, nose, eye protection.* Use PPE to protect the mucous membranes of the eyes, nose, and mouth during procedures and patient-care activities that are likely to generate splashes or sprays of blood, body fluids, secretions, and excretions. Select masks, goggles, face shields, and combinations of each according to the need anticipated by the task performed.
3. Respiratory hygiene and cough etiquette. Post signs at entrances and in strategic places (e.g., elevators, cafeterias) within ambulatory and inpatient settings with instructions to patients and other persons with symptoms of a respiratory infection to cover their mouth and nose when coughing or sneezing, use and dispose of tissues, and perform hand hygiene after hands have been in contact with respiratory secretions. Provide tissues and no-touch receptacles (e.g., foot pedal–operated lid or open, plastic-lined waste basket) for disposal of tissues. Provide resources and instructions for performing hand hygiene in or near waiting areas in ambulatory and inpatient settings; provide conveniently located dispensers of alcohol-based hand rubs and, where sinks are available, supplies for handwashing. During periods of increased prevalence of respiratory infections in the community, offer masks to coughing patients and other symptomatic persons (e.g., persons who accompany ill patients) on entry into the facility, and encourage them to maintain special separation, ideally a distance of at least 3 feet, from others in common waiting areas.
4. *Safe injection practices.* The following recommendations apply to the use of needles, cannulas that replace needles, and, where applicable, intravenous delivery systems:
   - Use aseptic technique to prevent contamination of sterile injection equipment. Needles, cannulae, and syringes are sterile, single-use items; they should not be reused for another patient. Use fluid infusion and administration sets (i.e., intravenous bags, tubing, and connectors) for one patient only, and dispose appropriately after use. Use single-dose vials for parenteral medications whenever possible. If multi-dose vials must be used, both the needle (or cannula) and the syringe used to access the multi-dose vial must be sterile. Do not keep multidose vials in the immediate patient treatment area, and store in accordance with the manufacturer's recommendations; discard if sterility is compromised or questionable.

Source: Seigel, J., Rhinehart, E., Jackson, M., Chiarello, L., & The Healthcare Infection Control Practices Advisory Committee. (2007). *2007 Guidelines for isolation precaution and preventing transmission of infectious agents in healthcare settings.* Internet document available at www.cdc.gov/ncidod/dhqp/gl_isolation.html (accessed May 1, 2009).

Steps in the work-up of a breast lump may begin with ultrasonography to determine whether it is fluid filled or solid. Fluid-filled cysts are aspirated, and the woman is monitored on a routine basis for the development of other cysts. If the lump is solid, a mammogram is obtained if the woman is older than age 50 years. A fine-needle aspiration (FNA) is performed, regardless of the woman's age, to determine the nature of the lump. In some cases a core biopsy may need to follow FNA to harvest adequate amounts of tissue for pathologic examination (Valea & Katz, 2007).

Management depends on the severity of the symptoms. Dietary changes and vitamin supplements are one management approach. Although research findings are contradictory, some practitioners advocate reducing consumption or eliminating methylxanthines (e.g., colas, coffee, tea, chocolate) and tobacco (Valea & Katz, 2007).

Women may report decreased symptoms with such measures as taking vitamin E supplements and decreasing sodium intake or taking mild diuretics shortly before menses. Other pain relief measures include taking analgesics or NSAIDs, wearing a supportive bra, and applying heat or cold to the breasts. Evening primrose oil may be effective for some women, although evidence is lacking (Crochetiere, 2005). Oral contraceptives, danazol, bromocriptine, and tamoxifen have also been used with varying degrees of success (Valea & Katz, 2007).

Nodules are surgically removed only in rare cases. In the presence of multiple nodules the surgical approach would involve multiple incisions and tissue manipulation and may not prevent the development of more nodules.

Fibroadenoma

The next most common benign condition of the breast is a **fibroadenoma.** It is the single most common type of tumor seen in the adolescent population, although it can also occur in women in their thirties. Fibroadenomas are discrete, usually solitary lumps less than 3 cm in diameter (Valea & Katz, 2007). Occasionally the woman with a fibroadenoma will experience tenderness in the tumor during the menstrual cycle. Fibroadenomas increase in size during pregnancy and decrease in size as the woman ages. The cause of fibroadenomas is unknown.

Diagnosis is made by reviewing patient history and physical examination. Mammography, ultrasound, or magnetic resonance imaging helps determine the cause of the lesion. FNA may be used to determine underlying pathologic conditions. Surgical excision may be necessary if the lump is suspicious or if the symptoms are severe. Periodic observation of masses by professional physical examination or mammography may be all that is necessary for those masses not needing surgical intervention. Breast self-examination can be practiced by the woman in between professional examinations (see Chapter 2).

Nipple discharge

Nipple discharge is a common occurrence that concerns many women. Although most nipple discharge is physiologic, evaluate each woman who has this problem thoroughly because a small percentage will be found to have a serious endocrine disorder or malignancy.

Another form of breast discharge not related to malignancy is galactorrhea–a bilaterally spontaneous, milky, sticky discharge. It is a normal finding in pregnancy. Galactorrhea can also occur as the result of elevated prolactin levels caused by a thyroid disorder, pituitary tumor, or chest wall surgery or trauma. Obtaining a complete medication history on each woman is essential. Some tranquilizers (e.g., tricyclic antidepressants), narcotics, and antihypertensive medications, as well as oral contraceptives, can precipitate galactorrhea in some women (Lobo, 2007c).

Diagnostic tests that may be indicated include a prolactin level, a microscopic analysis of the discharge from each breast, a thyroid profile, a pregnancy test, and a mammogram (Lobo, 2007c).

Mammary duct ectasia is an inflammation of the ducts behind the nipple. It occurs most often in perimenopausal women. In mammary duct ectasia, nipple discharge is thick, sticky, and colored white, brown, green, or purple. The woman frequently experiences a burning pain, an itching, or a palpable mass behind the nipple. The work-up includes a mammogram and aspiration and culture of fluid. Treatment is usually symptomatic; mild pain relievers, warm compresses applied to the breast, or wearing a supportive bra may provide relief. If a mass is present or an abscess occurs, treatment may include a local excision of the affected duct or ducts, provided that the woman has no future plans to breastfeed (Mayo Foundation for Education and Research, 2008).

Intraductal papilloma

Intraductal papilloma is a rare, benign condition that develops within the terminal nipple ducts. The cause is unknown. It usually occurs in women between ages 30 and 50. The papilloma is usually too small to be palpated, and the characteristic sign is nipple discharge that is serous, serosanguineous, or bloody. After eliminating the possibility of malignancy the affected segments of the ducts and breasts are surgically excised (Valea & Katz, 2007). Table 3-4 compares manifestations of benign breast diseases.

Collaborative care

The history should focus on risk factors for breast diseases, events related to the breast mass, and health maintenance practices. Risk factors for breast cancer are discussed later in this chapter. Information related to the breast mass should include how, when, and by whom the mass was discovered. The following patient information is documented: presence of pain, whether symptoms increase with menses, dietary habits, smoking habits, and use of oral contraceptives. The woman's emotional status, includ-

TABLE 3-4

Comparison of Common Manifestations of Benign Breast Masses

FIBROCYSTIC CHANGES	FIBROADENOMA	INTRADUCTAL PAPILLOMA	MAMMARY DUCT ECTASIA
Multiple lumps	Single lump	Single or multiple	Mass behind nipple
Nodular	Well delineated	Not well delineated	Not well delineated
Palpable	Palpable	Nonpalpable	Palpable
Movable	Movable	Nonmobile	Nonmobile
Round, smooth	Round, lobular	Small, ball-like	Irregular
Firm or soft	Firm	Firm or soft	Firm
Tenderness influenced by menstrual cycle	Usually asymptomatic	Usually nontender	Painful, burning, itching
Bilateral	Unilateral	Unilateral	Unilateral
May or may not have nipple discharge	No nipple discharge	Serous or bloody nipple discharge	Thick, sticky nipple discharge

ing her stress level, fears, and concerns, and her ability to cope, also should be assessed.

Physical examination may include assessment of the breasts for symmetry, masses (size, number, consistency, mobility), and nipple discharge.

Nursing actions might include the following:

- Discuss the intervals for and facets of breast screening, including professional examination and mammography (Table 3-5). Women with breast implants may need special views of the breast, and precautions might have to be taken to prevent rupturing the implant during mammography.
- Provide written educational materials.
- Encourage the verbalization of fears and concerns about treatment and prognosis.
- Provide specific information regarding the woman's condition and treatment, including dietary changes, drug therapy, comfort measures, stress management, and surgery.
- Demonstrate correct breast self-examination technique if the woman desires to practice it (see Chapter 2, p. 31).
- Describe pain-relieving strategies in detail, and collaborate with the primary health care provider to ensure effective pain control.
- Encourage discussion of feelings about body image.
- Refer to a support group or stress management resource if needed to cope with long-term consequences of benign breast conditions.

Cancer of the Breast

The United States has one of the highest rates of carcinoma in the world. One in eight American women will develop breast cancer in her lifetime (National Cancer Institute [NCI], 2006). No clear method for prevention has been formulated. The prognosis for and survival of the woman are improved with early detection. Therefore women must be educated about risk factors, early detection, and screening.

TABLE 3-5

Detection in Asymptomatic Women Recommended by the American Cancer Society

AGE (YR)	EXAMINATION	FREQUENCY
20-39	Clinical breast examination	Every 3 yr
40 and older	Clinical breast examination	Yearly
	Mammography	Yearly

Source: American Cancer Society. (2013). *Cancer facts and figures, 2013.* Atlanta, GA: American Cancer Society.

Although the exact cause of breast cancer is still unknown, researchers have identified certain factors that increase a woman's risk for developing a malignancy. Box 3-5 lists these factors. The most important predictor for breast cancer is age; the risk increases as the woman ages.

Case Study: Breast Cancer

Much discussion has taken place about possible links between breast cancer and hormonal therapy; several large research studies, including the Women's Health Initiative, have found that the risk of breast cancer increases when a woman is taking combined estrogen and progesterone (Rossouw et al., 2002). However, no consensus about possible links has been reached (Valea & Katz, 2007).

Studies that include a long-term study of breast implant patients implemented by the National Cancer Institute concluded that silicone breast implants did not increase the risk of breast cancer (Deapen, 2007; Nelson, 2000).

Nursing Care Plan: Breast Cancer

Although most breast cancers are not related to genetic factors, the identification of the BRCA1 and BRCA2 genes has demonstrated the role of heredity and genetic mutations in this disease. Only approximately 5% to 10% of all breast cancers are attributed to heredity. Women who have abnormalities in the BRCA1 and BRCA2 genes have up

BOX 3-5

Risk Factors for Breast Cancer*

Risks that are not modifiable:
- Age—risk increases with age
- Previous history of breast cancer
- Family history of breast cancer, especially a mother or sister (particularly significant if premenopausal)
- Inherited genetic mutations in BRCA1 and BRCA2 genes
- Previous history of ovarian, endometrial, colon, or thyroid cancer
- High breast tissue density
- Early menarche (before age 12)
- Late menopause (after age 55)
- Previous history of benign breast disease with epithelial hyperplasia
- Race (Caucasian women have highest incidence)

Lifestyle and modifiable risks:
- Nulliparity or first pregnancy after age 30
- Not breastfeeding
- Postmenopausal use of combined estrogen-progestin replacement therapy
- Obesity after menopause
- Alcohol consumption of more than one drink per day
- Sedentary lifestyle
- Vitamin D—low levels increase risk

Data from American Cancer Society (ACS). (2011). *Breast cancer 2011.* www.cancer.org; American Cancer Society (ACS). (2012). *Cancer facts and figures.* Atlanta: American Cancer Society.

*Risk factors are cumulative (i.e., the more risk factors that are present, the greater is the likelihood of breast cancer occurring).

BOX 3-6

Ethical Considerations for Genetic Testing

The ability to test for BRCA1 and BRCA2 has generated heated ethical debate within the health care community. Testing is expensive (approximately $2500 for the first person in the family to be tested [National Women's Health Resource Center, 2000]), and the test is often not covered by insurance. Who should be tested (usually not recommended for women without a family history of breast or ovarian cancer) and who should pay for it have not been addressed adequately. What to do when a positive result is discovered is not universally agreed on. Women and their families will most likely have increased anxiety after a positive finding. How often should screening be performed? Should prophylactic mastectomies be recommended? Will employment discrimination occur if this information is in a woman's medical record? Women requesting testing must be fully informed of the possible risks and benefits of testing before consenting to the procedure. Genetic counseling should include helping the woman determine how to inform other family members. Use of an ethical principle framework can guide approaches to solving ethical dilemmas about testing.

Sources: National Women's Health Resource Center. (2000). Genetic testing and women's health. *National Women's Health Report,* 22(6), 1-8; Quillin, J., & Lyckholm, L. (2006-2007). A principle-based approach to ethical issues in predictive genetic testing for breast cancer. *Breast Disease,* 27(1), 137-148; U.S. Preventive Health Services Task Force. (2005). *Genetic risk assessment and BRCA mutation testing for breast and ovarian cancer susceptibility.* Internet document available at www.ahrq.gov/Clinic/uspstf/uspsbrgen.htm (accessed May 1, 2009).

to an 80% chance of developing breast cancer (ACS, 2009a). Other genetic mutations that can cause breast cancer include mutations of the ATM gene, the p53 tumor suppressor gene, the PTEN gene, and the CHEK-2 gene (ACS) (Box 3-6).

Although the clinical applicability of risk factors has limits, screen women at increased risk at frequent intervals, and help these women consider changing risk factors that can be changed, such as losing weight if obese and limiting alcohol intake (ACS, 2009b).

Prevention

Chemoprevention is the use of medications to reduce cancer risk. Tamoxifen and raloxifene block the effect of estrogen on breast tissue. Studies have shown that these two drugs can reduce the risk of breast cancer, and the FDA has approved them for such use (ACS, 2009a) (see Medication Guides).

Surgical prophylaxis (bilateral mastectomy, oophorectomy) can also reduce the risk of breast cancer, but it should be considered only for persons at very high risk (ACS, 2009a).

Screening and diagnosis

Estimates indicate that 90% of all breast lumps are detected by the woman. Of this 90%, only 20% to 25% are malignant. More than half of all lumps are discovered in the upper outer quadrant of the breast. The most common presenting symptom is a lump or thickening of the breast. The lump may feel hard and fixed or soft and spongy. It may have well-defined or irregular borders. It may be fixed to the skin, thereby causing dimpling to occur. A nipple discharge that is bloody or clear also may be present.

Early detection and diagnosis reduce the risk of mortality because cancer is found when it is smaller, lesions are more localized, and the tendency is to have a lower percentage of positive nodes. However, cultural factors may influence a woman's decision to participate in breast cancer screening. Knowledge of these factors and use of culturally sensitive messages and materials that appeal to the unique concerns, beliefs, and reading abilities of target groups will assist the nurse in helping women overcome barriers to seeking care. For example, the ACS (2009b) reported that women who are African-American, Hispanic, or Native American were less likely to get mammograms than Caucasian or Asian-American women.

Clinical examination by a qualified health care provider and screening mammography (x-ray examination of the

Medication Guide

Tamoxifen (Nolvadex)

ACTION

- Antiestrogenic effects; attaches to hormone receptors on cancer cells and prevents natural hormones from attaching to the receptors

INDICATIONS

- For treatment of metastatic breast cancer; for treatment of breast cancer after breast cancer surgery and radiation therapy; to reduce the incidence of breast cancer in women at high risk

DOSAGE

- 20 to 40 mg orally, daily. Doses greater than 20 mg should be given in divided doses (morning and evening).

ADVERSE REACTIONS

- Common side effects include hot flashes, nausea, vomiting, vaginal bleeding or discharge, menstrual irregularities, and rash. Hair loss is an uncommon effect. Serious side effects include deep vein thrombosis, increased risk of endometrial cancer, and stroke.

NURSING CONSIDERATIONS

- The medication may be taken on an empty stomach or with food. Missed doses should be taken as soon as possible, but taking two doses at once is not recommended. A barrier or nonhormonal form of contraception is recommended in premenopausal women because tamoxifen may be harmful to the fetus.

Medication Guide

Raloxifene Hydrochloride (Evista)

ACTION

A selective estrogen receptor modulator, serving as an agonist and antagonist to estrogen receptor sites

INDICATIONS

Treatment and prevention of osteoporosis; reduction in the risk of invasive breast cancer in postmenopausal women with osteoporosis; reduction of risk of invasive breast cancer in postmenopausal women at high risk of invasive breast cancer

DOSAGE

60 mg orally, daily

ADVERSE REACTIONS

Common side effects include hot flashes, nausea, vomiting, peripheral edema, arthralgia, sweating. Serious and life-threatening side effects can occur from existing condition. Raloxifene is contraindicated in women with an active or past history of venous thromboembolism.

NURSING CONSIDERATIONS

The medication may be taken on an empty stomach or with food. Missed doses should be taken as soon as possible, but taking two doses at once is not recommended. Counsel woman to contact her physician if she experiences leg pain or a feeling of warmth in the lower legs, swelling of the hands and feet, sudden chest pain or shortness of breath, or sudden changes in vision. Calcium 1200 mg plus 400 to 800 IU of vitamin D daily are recommended.

breast) (Fig. 3-5) may aid in the early detection of breast cancers (see Table 3-5).

When a suspicious finding on a mammogram is noted or a lump is detected, the diagnosis is confirmed by needle aspiration, a core needle biopsy, or surgical excision (Fig. 3-6). Ultrasound may also be used to assess a specific area of abnormality found during a mammogram procedure (ACS, 2009b). Patients need specific information regarding advantages and disadvantages of these procedures in making a decision about which one is most appropriate for them.

Laboratory examination of breast tissue determines if cancer is present and, if so, the extent. Other tests performed to determine the spread of the cancer include chest x-ray examination, bone scan, computed tomography (CT), magnetic resonance imaging (MRI), and positron emission tomography (PET scan) (ACS, 2009a).

An important step in evaluating a breast cancer is to test for the presence of estrogen and progesterone receptors in the biopsied tissue. Cancer cells may contain one, both, or neither of these receptors. Breast cancers that contain estrogen receptors are often called *ER-positive* cancers, whereas those containing progesterone receptors are called *PR-positive* cancers. Women with hormone-positive tumors tend to respond better to treatment and have higher survival rates than the general population (ACS, 2009a).

A HER2/neu test also may be performed on the biopsied breast tissue. HER2/neu is a growth-promoting hormone, and in approximately 50% of breast cancers, excessive amounts of the hormone are present, causing the cancer to be more aggressive in spreading than other types of breast cancer. Treatment is often more effective if HER2/neu testing is performed (ACS, 2009a).

CARE MANAGEMENT

Medical management. Controversy continues regarding the best treatment of breast cancer. Nodal involvement, tumor size, receptor status, and aggressiveness are important variables for treatment selection. Many

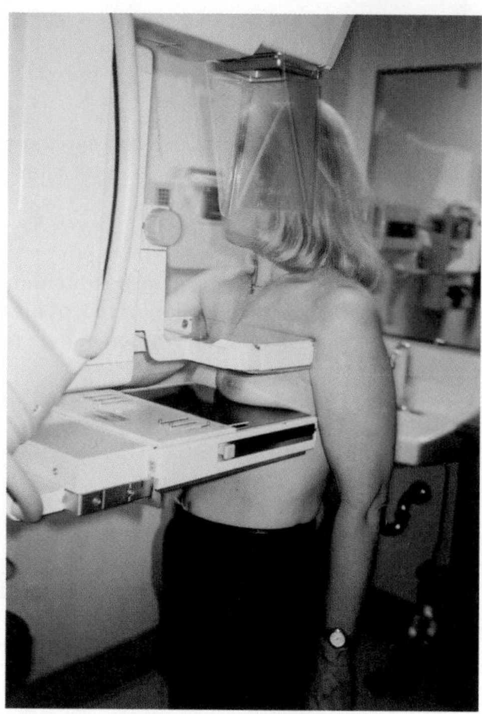

Fig. 3-5 Patient undergoing mammography. (Courtesy Shannon Perry, Phoenix, AZ.)

women face difficult decisions about the various treatment options. Box 3-7 lists questions that must be addressed in decision making. Most health care providers recommend that the malignant mass be removed, as well as the axillary nodes, specifically the sentinel node, for staging purposes (DiSaia & Creasman, 2007). The treatment can be conservative or more radical. The most frequently recommended surgical approaches for the treatment of breast cancer are lumpectomy and modified radical mastectomy. Breast-conserving surgery, such as a **lumpectomy** (Fig. 3-7, *A*) or quadrantectomy (Fig. 3-7, *B*) is the removal of the breast tumor and a small amount of surrounding tissue. Sampling of axillary lymph nodes usually occurs through a separate incision at the time of these procedures, and the surgery is usually followed by radiation therapy to the remaining breast tissue (DiSaia & Creasman). These procedures are for the primary treatment of women with early-stage (I or II) breast cancer. Lumpectomy offers survival equivalent to that with modified radical mastectomy (DiSaia & Creasman).

A **simple mastectomy** (see Fig. 3-7, *C*) is the removal of the breast containing the tumor. A **modified radical mastectomy** is the removal of the breast tissue, skin, and fascia of the pectoralis muscle and dissection of the axillary nodes. A **radical mastectomy,** although rarely performed, is the removal of the breast and underlying pectoralis muscles and complete axillary node dissection (see Fig. 3-7, *D*). After surgery, follow-up treatment may include radiation, chemo-

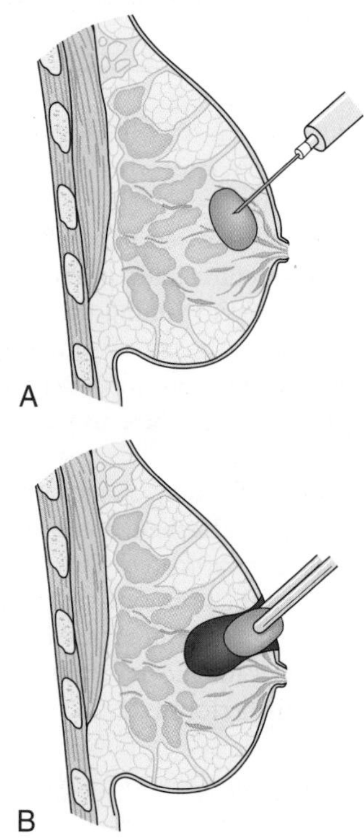

Fig. 3-6 Diagnosis. **A,** Needle aspiration. **B,** Open biopsy. (Redrawn from National Women's Health Resource Center. [1995]. Breast health. *National Women's Health Report, 13*[5], 3.)

BOX 3-7

Decision-Making Questions to Ask

1. What kind of breast cancer is it (invasive or noninvasive)?
2. What is the stage of the cancer (i.e., how extensive is the spread)?
3. Did the cancer test positive for hormone (estrogen)? (May be slower growing.)
4. What further tests are recommended?
5. What are the treatment options? (Pros and cons of each, including side effects.)
6. If surgery is recommended, what will the scar look like?
7. If a mastectomy is performed, can breast reconstruction be initiated (at the time of surgery or later)?
8. How long will the patient be in the hospital? What kind of postoperative care will the patient need?
9. How long will treatment last if radiation or chemotherapy is recommended? What effects can the patient expect from these treatments?
10. What community resources are available for support?

Source: American Cancer Society. (2009c). *Detailed guide: Breast cancer. What should you ask your doctor about breast cancer?* Internet document available at www.cancer.org/docroot/CRI/content/CRI_2_4_5X_What_should_you_ask_your_physician_about_breast_cancer_5.asp?sitearea= (accessed May 2, 2009).

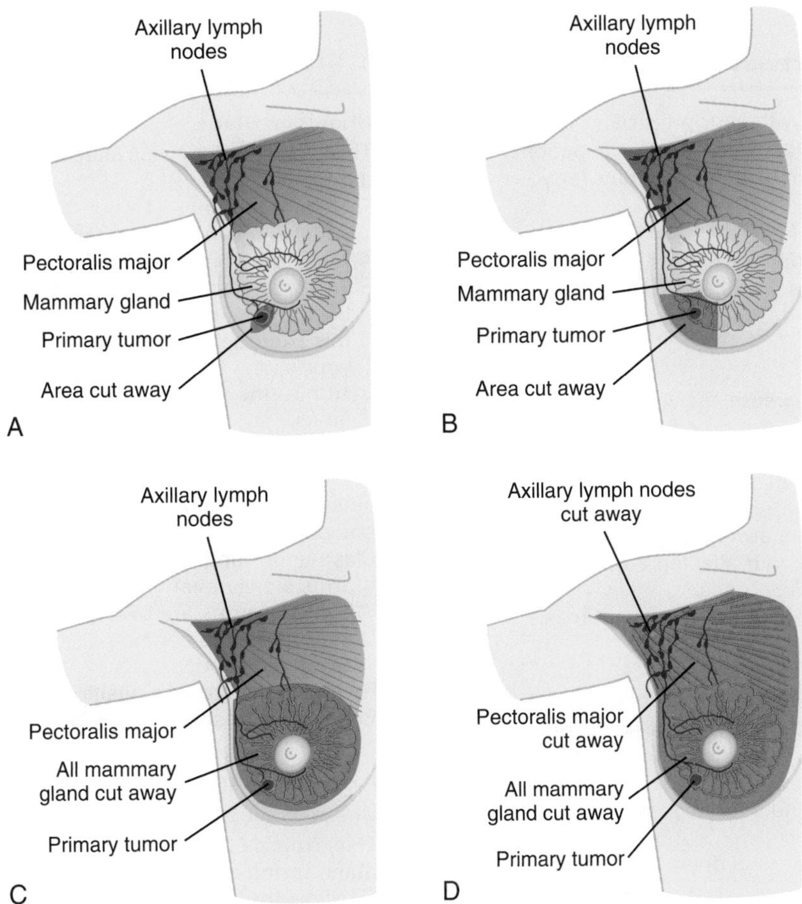

Fig. 3-7 Surgical alternatives for breast cancer. **A,** Lumpectomy (tylectomy). **B,** Quadrantectomy (segmental resection). **C,** Total (simple) mastectomy. **D,** Radical mastectomy.

therapy, or hormonal therapy (ACS, 2009a). The decision to include follow-up therapy is based on the stage of disease, age and menopausal status of the woman, the woman's preference, and her hormonal receptor status. Follow-up treatment is usually initiated to decrease the risk of recurrence in women who have no evidence of metastasis.

Radiation is usually recommended as follow-up therapy for women who have stage I or II cancer. Hormone therapy with tamoxifen, an estrogen agonist, is recommended for women over the age of 50 for at least 5 years (DiSaia & Creasman, 2007) (see Medication Guide). Chemotherapy is often given to premenopausal women who have positive nodes. Therapy for more advanced tumors usually includes surgery followed by chemotherapy, radiation, or both (Valea & Katz, 2007).

Nursing care. Surgery may be performed in an outpatient surgical setting or as an inpatient procedure, depending on what type of surgery is being performed. Nursing care and teaching are focused on the perioperative period. Preoperatively, assess the woman's psychologic readiness and specific teaching needs related to the procedure, as well as what to expect after surgery. A visit from a woman who has had a similar experience may be beneficial preoperatively, as well as postoperatively.

Discuss reconstruction surgery, including the risks and benefits before the surgery, if appropriate. Available options include autologous reconstruction (grafts of muscle and skin from the woman's back, abdomen, or hip) and silicone gel- or saline-filled breast implants (Djohan, Gage, & Bernard, 2008; FDA, 2006). Surgical reconstruction can be performed at the time if surgery or later. A discussion of partial and full external prostheses also may be appropriate, including where to purchase one and the types of bras that may be worn. Local American Cancer Society units can provide sources, and volunteers of Reach to Recovery can offer hints and suggestions for wearing apparel and coping with prostheses.

Postoperative nursing care focuses on recovery. Women who had surgery in an outpatient setting usually go home within a few hours after surgery. A 24- to 48-hour stay is usual after modified radical mastectomy. Try to avoid taking blood pressure, giving injections, or taking blood from the arm on the affected side. The woman may have drainage tubes from the incision site that you will need to assess and drain. Incision care may include dressing changes. If postoperative arm exercises are appropriate, initiate these during the early postoperative period (Box 3-8). The woman is usually discharged

BOX 3-8

Exercises after Breast Surgery

It is important to talk with your physician before starting any exercises. A physical therapist or occupational therapist can help design an exercise program for you.

EXERCISES IN THE LYING POSITION

These exercises should be performed on a bed or the floor while lying on your back with your knees and hips bent and feet flat.

Wand Exercise

This exercise helps increase the forward motion of the shoulders. You will need a broom handle, yardstick, or other similar object to perform this exercise.

Hold the wand in both hands with palms facing up.

Lift the wand up over your head (as far as you can) using your unaffected arm to help lift the wand until you feel a stretch in your affected arm.

Hold this position for 5 seconds.

Lower the arms and repeat five to seven times.

Elbow Winging

This exercise helps increase the mobility of the front of your chest and shoulder. Several weeks of regular exercise may be needed before your elbows will get close to the bed (or floor).

Clasp your hands behind your neck with your elbows pointing toward the ceiling.

Move your elbows apart and down toward the bed (or floor).

Repeat five to seven times.

EXERCISES IN THE SITTING POSITION

Shoulder Blade Stretch

This exercise helps increase the mobility of the shoulder blades.

Sit in a chair very close to a table with your back against the chair back.

Place the unaffected arm on the table with your elbow bent and palm down. Do not move this arm during the exercise.

Place the affected arm on the table, palm down with your elbow straight.

Without moving your trunk, slide the affected arm toward the opposite side of the table. You should feel your shoulder blade move as you slide your arm.

Relax your arm and repeat five to seven times.

Shoulder Blade Squeeze

This exercise also helps increase the mobility of the shoulder blade.

Facing straight ahead, sit in a chair in front of a mirror without resting on the back of the chair.

Arms should be at your sides with elbows bent.

Squeeze shoulder blades together, bringing your elbows behind you. Keep your shoulders level as you perform this exercise. Do not lift your shoulders up toward your ears.

Return to the starting position and repeat five to seven times.

Side Bending

This exercise helps increase the mobility of the trunk or body.

Clasp your hands together in front of you and lift your arms slowly over your head, straightening your arms.

When your arms are over your head, bend your trunk to the right while bending at the waist and keeping your arms overhead.

Return to the starting position and bend to the left.

Repeat five to seven times.

EXERCISES IN STANDING POSITION

Chest Wall Stretch

This exercise helps stretch the chest wall.

Stand facing a corner with toes approximately 8 to 10 inches from the corner.

Bend your elbows and place forearms on the wall, one on each side of the corner. Your elbows should be as close to shoulder height as possible.

Keep your arms and feet in position and move your chest toward the corner. You will feel a stretch across your chest and shoulders.

Return to starting position and repeat five to seven times.

Shoulder Stretch

This exercise helps increase the mobility in the shoulder.

Stand facing the wall with your toes approximately 8 to 10 inches from the wall.

Place your hands on the wall. Use your fingers to "climb the wall," reaching as high as you can until you feel a stretch.

Return to starting position and repeat five to seven times.

Source: American Cancer Society. (2008). *Exercises after breast surgery.* Internet document available at www.cancer.org/docroot/CRI/content/CRI_2_6x_Exercises_After_Breast_Surgery.asp?sitearea=CRI&viewmode=print& (accessed May 2, 2009).

to home after being given self-management instructions. Because teaching time is short, providing printed information gives the woman and her family something to refer to at home (see Patient Instructions for Self-Management box).

Concerns about appearance after breast surgery may affect the woman's self-concept. Before surgery the woman and her partner need information about the woman's postoperative appearance. Both the woman and her partner need to be able to discuss feelings and concerns about accepting the changes. Nurses can assist the couple to communicate these feelings and concerns. Information about community resources and support groups such as Reach to Recovery are often beneficial.

PATIENT INSTRUCTIONS FOR SELF-MANAGEMENT

Post-Mastectomy

- Wash hands well before and after touching incision area or drains.
- Empty surgical drains twice a day and as needed, recording the date, time, drain site (if more than one drain is present), and amount of drainage in milliliters in the diary you will take to each surgical checkup until your drains are removed. (Before discharge, you may receive a graduated container for emptying drains and measuring drainage.)
- Avoid driving, lifting more than 10 pounds, or reaching above your head until given permission by the surgeon.
- Take medications for pain as soon as the pain begins.
- Perform arm exercises as directed.
- Call the physician if inflammation of the incision or swelling of the incision or the arm occurs.
- Avoid tight clothing, tight jewelry, and other causes of decreased circulation in the affected arm.
- Until drains are removed, wear loose-fitting underwear (camisole or half-slip) and clothes, pinning surgical drains inside of clothing. (Health care worker will teach you how to do this safely.)
- After drains are removed and surgical sites are healing and still tender, wear a mastectomy bra or camisole with a cotton-filled, muslin temporary prosthesis. Temporary prostheses of this type are often available from Reach to Recovery.
- Avoid depilatory creams, strong deodorants, and shaving of affected chest area, axilla, and arm.
- Sponge bathe until drains are removed.
- Return to the surgeon's office for incision check, drain inspection, and possible drain removal as directed.
- Contact Reach to Recovery for assistance in obtaining an external prosthesis and lingerie when dressings, drains, and staples are removed and wound is healing and nontender.
- Contact the insurance company for information about coverage of a prosthesis and wig if needed. Obtain prescriptions for the prosthesis and wig to submit with receipts of purchase for these items to the insurance company. If insurance does not pay for these items, contact the hospital or agency social worker or the local American Cancer Society for assistance.
- Breast self-examination (BSE) of the unaffected side and affected surgical site and axilla can be performed.
- Encourage mother, sisters, and daughters (if applicable) to have annual professional breast examinations and mammography (if appropriate).
- Keep follow-up visits for professional examination, mammography, and testing to detect recurrent breast cancer.
- Expect decreased sensation and tingling at incision sites and in the affected arm for weeks to months after surgery.
- Resume sexual activities as desired.

KEY POINTS

- Menstrual disorders diminish the quality of life for affected women and their families.
- PMS is a disorder that begins in the luteal phase of the menstrual cycle and resolves with the onset of menses.
- PMS is a disorder with both psychologic and physiologic characteristics.
- Endometriosis is characterized by dysmenorrhea, infertility, and, less often, alterations in menstrual cycle bleeding and dyspareunia.
- Reduced risky sexual practices are key STI prevention strategies.
- HIV is transmitted through body fluids, primarily blood, semen, and vaginal secretions.
- Prevention of mother-to-newborn HIV transmission is most effective when the woman receives antiretroviral drugs during pregnancy and labor and birth and the infant also receives the drugs after the birth.
- HPV is the most common viral STI.
- Syphilis has reemerged as a common STI, affecting more African-American women than any other ethnic group.
- Chlamydia is the most common STI in U.S. women and the most common cause of PID.
- Young sexually active women who do not practice reduced-risk sexual behaviors and have multiple partners are at greatest risk for STIs and HIV infection.
- STIs are responsible for substantial morbidity and mortality, personal suffering, and a heavy economic burden in the United States.
- STIs and vaginitis are biologic events for which all individuals have a right to expect objective, compassionate, and effective health care.
- The development of breast neoplasms, whether benign or malignant, can have a significant physical and emotional effect on the woman and her family.
- The risk of U.S. women developing breast cancer is 1 in 8.
- Clinical breast examinations by a health care provider and routine screening mammograms are recommended for early detection of breast cancer.
- The primary therapy for most women with stage I or II breast cancer is breast-conserving surgery with axillary lymph node sampling followed by radiation therapy.
- Tamoxifen is a common adjuvant therapy for breast cancers that are estrogen-receptor positive.

Audio Chapter Summaries Access an audio summary of these Key Points on evolve

References

American Academy of Pediatrics Committee on Pediatric AIDS. (2008). HIV testing and prophylaxis to prevent mother-to-child transmission in the United States. *Pediatrics, 122*(5), 1127-1134.

American Cancer Society (ACS). (2009a). *Breast cancer.* Internet document available at www.cancer.org (accessed June 6, 2009).

American Cancer Society (ACS). (2009b). *Cancer facts and figures, 2009.* New York: ACS.

American College of Obstetricians and Gynecologists (ACOG). (2008). *ACOG patient education: How to prevent STDs.* Washington, DC: ACOG.

American College of Obstetricians and Gynecologists (ACOG). (2000). Premenstrual syndrome. *ACOG Practice Bulletin, No. 15.* Washington, DC: ACOG.

American College of Obstetricians and Gynecologists Committee on Adolescent Health Care. (2005). Endometriosis in adolescents. ACOG Committee Opinion No. 310. *Obstetrics and Gynecology, 105*(4), 921-927.

American Psychiatric Association (APA). (2000). *Diagnostic and statistical manual of mental disorders* (4th ed., text revision). Washington, DC: American Psychiatric Association Press.

Association of Women's Health, Obstetric and Neonatal Nurses (AWHONN). (2003). *Evidence-based clinical practice guideline: Nursing management for cyclic perimenstrual pain and discomfort.* Washington, DC: AWHONN.

Branson, B., Handsfield, H., Lampe, M., Janssen, R., Taylor, A., Lyss, S., Clark, J., & Centers for Disease Control and Prevention. (2006). Revised recommendations for HIV testing of adults, adolescents, and pregnant women in health-care settings. *Morbidity and Mortality Weekly Report Recommendations and Reports, 55*(RR14), 1-17.

Centers for Disease Control and Prevention (CDC). (2008a). *Genital HPV infection–CDC fact sheet.* Internet document available at www.cdc.gov/std/HPV/STD-fact-HPV.htm#common (accessed June 6, 2009).

Centers for Disease Control and Prevention (CDC). (2008b). *HIV/AIDS among women.* Internet document available at www.cdc.gov/hiv/topics/women/resources/factsheets/women.htm (accessed June 6, 2009).

Centers for Disease Control and Prevention (CDC). (2007a). *STD Surveillance 2006: racial and ethnic minorities.* Internet document available at www.cdc.gov/std/stats06/minorities.htm (accessed May 1, 2009).

Centers for Disease Control and Prevention (CDC). (2007b). *STD surveillance 2006: trends in reportable sexually transmitted diseases in the United States, 2006: National surveillance data for chlamydia, gonorrhea, and syphilis.* Internet document available at www.cdc.gov/std/stats07/trends.htm (accessed May 1, 2009).

Centers for Disease Control and Prevention (CDC). (2007c). *Updated recommended treatment regimens for gonococcal infections and associated conditions, United States, April, 2007.* Internet document available at www.cdc.gov/std/treatment/2006/GonUpdateApril2007.pdf (accessed May 1, 2009).

Centers for Disease Control and Prevention (CDC). (2006). Sexually transmitted diseases treatment guidelines 2006. *Morbidity and Mortality Weekly Report Recommendations and Reports, 55*(RR-11), 1-94.

Centers for Disease Control and Prevention Divisions of HIV/AIDS Prevention. (2008). *FDA-approved rapid HIV antibody screening tests.* Internet document available at www.cdc.gov/hiv/topics/testing/rapid/rt-comparison.htm (accessed June 6, 2009).

Collins Sharp, B., Taylor, D., Thomas, K., Killeen, M., & Dawood, M. (2002). Cyclic perimenstrual pain and discomfort: The scientific basis for practice. *AWHONN, 31*(6), 637-649.

Crochetiere, C. (2005). Breast pain: diagnosis & treatment. *AWHONN Lifelines, 9*(4), 298-304.

Dehlin, L., & Schuiling, K. (2006). Chronic pelvic pain. In K. Schuiling & F. Lokis (Eds.). *Women's gynecologic health.* Boston: Jones & Bartlett.

Deapen, D. (2007). Breast implants and breast carcinoma: Review of incidence, detection, mortality, and survival. *Plastic and Reconstructive Surgery, 120*(7 Suppl 1), 70S-80S.

DiSaia, P., & Creasman, W. (2007). *Clinical gynecologic oncology* (7th ed.). Philadelphia: Mosby.

Djohan, R., Gage, E., & Bernard, S. (2008). Breast reconstruction options following mastectomy. *Cleveland Clinical Journal of Medicine, 75*(Suppl 1), S17-S23.

Eckert L., & Lentz, G. (2007a). Infections of the lower genital tract. In V. Katz, G. Lentz, R. Lobo, & D. Gershenson (Eds.). *Comprehensive gynecology* (5th ed.). Philadelphia: Mosby.

Eckert L., & Lentz, G. (2007b). Infections of the upper genital tract. In V. Katz, G. Lentz, R. Lobo, & D. Gershenson (Eds.). *Comprehensive gynecology* (5th ed.). Philadelphia: Mosby.

Fraley, S. (2002). Psychosocial outcomes in individuals living with genital herpes. *Journal of Obstetric, Gynecologic, and Neonatal Nursing, 31*(5), 508-513.

Katz, V. (2007). Benign gynecologic lesions: Vulva, vagina, cervix, uterus, oviducts and ovary. In V. Katz, G. Lentz, R. Lobo, & D. Gershenson (Eds.). *Comprehensive gynecology* (5th ed.). Philadelphia: Mosby.

Lachat, M., Scott, C., & Relf, M. (2006). HIV and pregnancy: Considerations for nursing practice. *MCN the American Journal of Maternal/Child Nursing, 31*(4), 233-240.

Lebrun, C. (2007). The female athlete triad: What's a doctor to do? *Current Sports Medicine Reports, 6*(6), 397-404.

Lentz, G. (2007a). Differential diagnosis of major gynecologic problems by age group: Vaginal bleeding, pelvic pain, and pelvic mass. In V. Katz, G. Lentz, R. Lobo, & D. Gershenson (Eds.). *Comprehensive gynecology* (5th ed.). Philadelphia: Mosby.

Lentz, G. (2007b). Primary and secondary dysmenorrhea, premenstrual syndrome, and premenstrual dysphoric disorder: Etiology, diagnosis, and management. In V. Katz, G. Lentz, R. Lobo, & D. Gershenson (Eds.). *Comprehensive gynecology* (5th ed.). Philadelphia: Mosby.

Lobo, R. (2007a). Abnormal uterine bleeding: Ovulatory and anovulatory dysfunctional uterine bleeding: management of acute and chronic excessive bleeding. In V. Katz, G. Lentz, R. Lobo, & D. Gershenson (Eds.). *Comprehensive gynecology* (5th ed.). Philadelphia: Mosby.

Lobo, R. (2007b). Endometriosis. In V. Katz, G. Lentz, R. Lobo, & D. Gershenson (Eds.). *Comprehensive gynecology* (5th ed.). Philadelphia: Mosby.

Lobo, R. (2007c). Hyperprolactinemia, galactorrhea, and pituitary adenomas: Etiology, differential diagnosis, natural history, management. In V. Katz, G. Lentz, R. Lobo, & D. Gershenson (Eds.). *Comprehensive gynecology* (5th ed.). Philadelphia: Mosby.

Lobo, R. (2007d). Primary and secondary amenorrhea and precocious puberty. In V. Katz, G. Lentz, R. Lobo, & D. Gershenson (Eds.). *Comprehensive gynecology* (5th ed.). Philadelphia: Mosby.

Mayo Foundation for Medical Education and Research. (2008). *Mammary duct ectasia.* Internet document available at www.mayoclinic.com/health/mammary-duct-ectasia/DS00751 (accessed May 1, 2009).

Mishell, D. (2007). Family planning: Contraception, sterilization, and abortion. In V. Katz, G. Lentz, R. Lobo, & D. Gershenson (Eds.). *Comprehensive gynecology* (5th ed.). Philadelphia: Mosby.

National Cancer Institute (NCI). (2006). *Probability of breast cancer in American women.* Internet document available at http://cis.nci.nih.gov/fact/5_6.htm (accessed June 8, 2009).

Nelson, N. (2000). Silicone breast implants not linked to breast cancer risk. *Journal of the National Cancer Institute, 92*(21), 1714-1715.

Perinatal HIV Guidelines Working Group. (2008). *Public Health Service Task Force recommendations: Use of antiretroviral drugs in pregnant HIV-infected women for maternal health and interventions to reduce perinatal HIV transmission in the United States.* Internet document available at http://aidsinfo.nih.gov/contentfiles/PerinatalGL.pdf (accessed May 1, 2009).

Ravin, C. (2007). Preventing STIs: Ask the questions. *Nursing for Women's Health, 11*(1), 88-91.

Rossouw, J., Anderson, G., Prentice, R., LaCroix, A., Kooperberg, C., Stefanick, M., et al. (2002). Risks and benefits of estrogen plus progestin in health postmenopausal women: Principal results from the Women's Health Initiative randomized controlled trial. *Journal of the American Medical Association, 288*(3), 321-333.

Speroff, L., & Fritz, M. (2005). *Clinical gynecologic endocrinology and infertility* (7th ed.). Philadelphia: Lippincott Williams & Wilkins.

U.S. Food and Drug Administration (FDA). (2008a). *HIV testing.* Internet document available at www.fda.gov/oashi/aids/test.html (accessed May 1, 2009).

U.S. Food and Drug Administration (FDA). (2006). *FDA News: FDA approves silicone gel-filled breast implants after in-depth evaluation. Agency requiring 10 years of patient follow-up.* Internet document available at www.fda.gov/bbs/topics/news/2006/new01512.html (accessed May 1, 2009).

Valea, F. & Katz, V. (2007). Breast disease: Diagnosis and treatment of benign and malignant disease. In V. Katz, G. Lentz, R. Lobo, & D. Gershenson (Eds.). *Comprehensive gynecology* (5th ed.). Philadelphia: Mosby.

Volmink, J., Siegfried, N., van der Merwe, L., & Brocklehurst, P. (2006). Antiretrovirals for reducing the risk of mother-to-child transmission of HIV infection. *Cochrane Database of Systematic Reviews* Issue 2006 Art. No. CD003510.

World Health Organization (WHO). (2004). *Medical eligibility criteria for contraceptive use* (3rd ed.). Geneva: WHO.

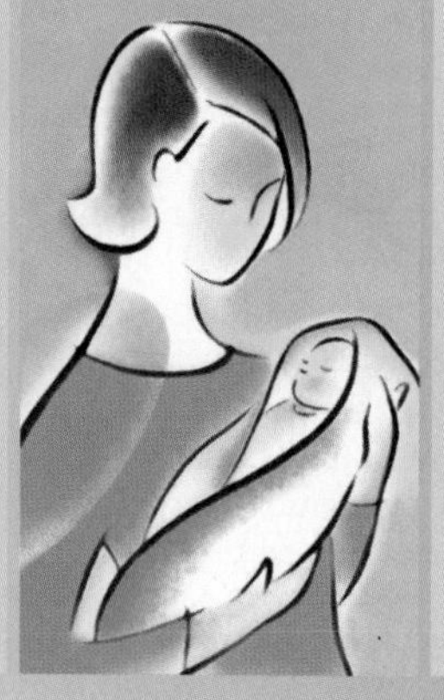

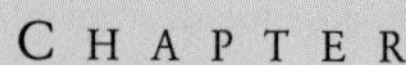

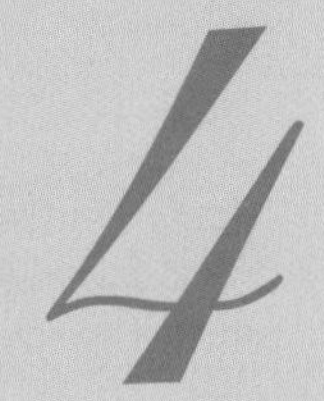

CHAPTER 4

Contraception, Abortion, and Infertility

DEITRA LEONARD LOWDERMILK

LEARNING OBJECTIVES

- *Compare the various methods of contraception.*
- *State the advantages and disadvantages of commonly used methods of contraception.*
- *Explain the common nursing interventions that facilitate contraceptive use.*
- *Recognize the various ethical, legal, cultural, and religious considerations of contraception.*
- *Describe the techniques used for medical and surgical interruption of pregnancy.*
- *Recognize the various ethical and legal considerations of elective abortion.*
- *List the common causes of infertility.*
- *Discuss the psychologic impact of infertility.*
- *Identify common diagnoses and treatments for infertility.*
- *Examine the various ethical and legal considerations of assisted reproductive therapies for infertility.*

KEY TERMS AND DEFINITIONS

assisted reproductive therapies (ARTs) Treatments for infertility, including in vitro fertilization procedures, embryo adoption, embryo hosting, and therapeutic insemination

basal body temperature (BBT) Lowest body temperature of a healthy person taken immediately after awakening and before getting out of bed

contraception The intentional prevention of pregnancy using a device or practice.

fertility awareness methods (FAMs) Methods of family planning that identify the beginning and end of the fertile period of the menstrual cycle

induced abortion Intentionally produced termination of pregnancy

infertility Impaired fertility, including a prolonged time to conceive and/or the inability to conceive.

natural family planning (NFP) Contraceptive methods in which a woman abstains from sexual intercourse during the fertile period of her menstrual cycle; no other form of birth control is used during this period

semen analysis Examination of semen specimen to determine liquefaction, volume, pH, sperm density, and normal morphologic features

sterilization Surgical contraceptive procedures intended to be permanent contraception

therapeutic donor insemination (TDI) Introduction of donor semen by instrument injection into the vagina or uterus for impregnation

WEB RESOURCES

Additional related content can be found on the companion website at evolve

http://evolve.elsevier.com/Lowdermilk/Maternity/

- NCLEX Review Questions
- Critical Thinking Exercise: Patient Teaching: Contraception
- Nursing Care Plan: Infertility
- Nursing Care Plan: Sexual Activity/ Contraception
- Spanish Guidelines: Contraception

The reproductive spectrum is the focus of this chapter, covering voluntary control of fertility, interruption of pregnancy, and impaired fertility. The nursing role in the care of women varies, depending on whether management of these fertility-related concerns is associated with assessment of needs, investigation of problems, or implementation of interventions.

CONTRACEPTION

Contraception is the intentional prevention of pregnancy during sexual intercourse. *Birth control* is the device or practice used to decrease the risk of conceiving, or bearing, offspring. Family planning is the conscious decision on when to conceive, or avoid pregnancy, throughout the reproductive years. With the wide assortment of birth control options available, a woman can use several different contraceptive methods at various stages throughout her fertile years. Nurses interact with the woman to compare and contrast available options, reliability, relative cost, the individual's comfort level, and partner's willingness to use a particular birth control method. Those who use contraception may still be at risk for pregnancy simply because their choice of contraceptive method is not perfect or is used inconsistently or incorrectly. Providing adequate instruction about how to use a contraceptive method, when to use a backup method, and when to use emergency contraception could decrease the risk of an unintended pregnancy (Stewart, Trussell, & Van Look, 2007).

CARE MANAGEMENT

Family, friends, media, partner or partners, religious affiliation, and health care professionals all influence a woman's perception of contraceptive choices. These external influences form a woman's unique view. The nurse assists in supporting the woman's decision based on the woman's individual situation (see Nursing Process box: Contraception).

Informed consent is a vital part in the education of the patient concerning contraception or sterilization. The nurse has the responsibility of documenting information provided and the understanding of that information by the patient. The acronym BRAIDED is often useful (see Legal Tip).

LEGAL TIP **Informed Consent**

B—Benefits: information about advantages and success rates
R—Risks: information about disadvantages and failure rates
A—Alternatives: information about other available methods
I—Inquiries: opportunity to ask questions
D—Decisions: opportunity to decide or to change mind
E—Explanations: information about method and how it is used
D—Documentation: information given and patient's understanding

To foster a safe environment for consultation, provide a private setting in which the woman can openly interact. Minimize any distractions, and have samples of birth control devices available for interactive teaching (Fig. 4-1). The ideal contraceptive is safe, easily available, economical, simple to use, and promptly reversible. Although no method may ever achieve all these objectives, significant advances in the development of new contraceptive technologies have occurred over the past 30 years (World Health Organization [WHO], 2004).

The contraceptive failure rate refers to the percentage of contraceptive users expected to have an unintended pregnancy during the first year, even when they use a method consistently and correctly. Contraceptive effectiveness varies from couple to couple and depends on both the properties of the method and the characteristics of the user (WHO, 2004). Failure rates decrease over time, either because a user gains experience by using a method more appropriately or because those for whom a method is less effective stop using it.

NURSING ALERT Make sure the woman has a backup method of birth control and emergency contraceptive pills (ECPs) readily available during the initial learning phase when she uses a new method of contraception to help prevent an unintentional conception.

Safety of a method depends on the woman's medical history. Barrier methods offer some protection from sexually transmitted infections (STIs), and oral contraceptives may reduce the incidence of breast, ovarian, and endometrial cancer but increase the risk of thromboembolic problems.

Nursing Care Plan: Sexual Activity/Contraception

Methods of Contraception

Coitus interruptus

Coitus interruptus (withdrawal or "pulling out") involves the male partner withdrawing the entire penis from the woman's vagina and moving away from her external genitalia before he ejaculates. In theory, the spermatozoa are unlikely to reach the ovum to cause fertilization. Although the effectiveness of coitus interruptus depends mostly on the man's disciplined capability to consistently ignore the powerful urge to continue thrusting, it has some concrete advantages over using no method. Adolescents and men with premature ejaculation often find this method difficult to use. This method is immediately available, costs nothing, and involves no hormonal alterations or chemicals. The effectiveness of this birth control technique is similar to that of barrier methods (Kowal, 2007). The percentage of women who will experience an unintended pregnancy

NURSING PROCESS *Contraception*

ASSESSMENT

- Determine the woman's knowledge about contraception and her sexual partner's commitment to any particular method.
- Collect data about the frequency of coitus, the number of sexual partners, the level of contraceptive involvement, and her or her partner's objections to any methods.
- Assess the woman's level of comfort and willingness to touch her genitals and cervical mucus.
- Identify any misconceptions, as well as religious and cultural factors. Pay close attention to the woman's verbal and nonverbal responses to hearing about the various available methods.
- Consider the woman's reproductive life plan.
- Complete a history (including menstrual, contraceptive, and obstetric), physical examination (including pelvic examination), and laboratory tests.

NURSING DIAGNOSES

Examples of nursing diagnoses related to contraception include the following:

- *Decisional conflict* related to:
  - Contraceptive alternatives
  - Partner's willingness to agree on contraceptive method
- *Fear* related to:
  - Contraceptive method side effects
- *Risk for infection* related to:
  - Unprotected sexual intercourse
  - Use of contraceptive method
  - Broken skin or mucous membrane after surgery or intrauterine device (IUD) insertion
- *Ineffective sexuality patterns* related to:
  - Fear of pregnancy
- *Acute pain* related to:
  - Postoperative recovery after sterilization
- *Risk for spiritual distress* related to:
  - Discrepancy between religious or cultural beliefs and choice of contraception

EXPECTED OUTCOMES OF CARE

The expected outcomes include that the woman or couple will do the following:

- Verbalize understanding about contraceptive methods.
- Verbalize understanding of all information necessary to give informed consent.
- State comfort and satisfaction with the chosen method.
- Use the contraceptive method correctly and consistently.
- Experience no adverse sequelae as a result of the chosen method of contraception.
- Prevent unplanned pregnancy or plan a pregnancy,

PLAN OF CARE AND INTERVENTIONS

- Implement the appropriate teaching for the specific contraceptive used.
- Have the woman perform a return demonstration to assess her understanding.
- Give written instructions and telephone numbers for questions.
- If the woman has difficulty understanding written instructions, offer her (and her partner, if available) graphic material and a telephone number to call as necessary.
- Offer the woman an opportunity to return for further instruction. See text for discussion of methods of contraception.

EVALUATION

Care is effective when the patient-centered expected outcomes have been achieved: the woman and her partner learn about the various methods of contraception; the couple achieves pregnancy only when planned; and they have no complications as a result of the chosen method of contraception.

Critical Thinking Exercise: Patient Teaching: Contraception

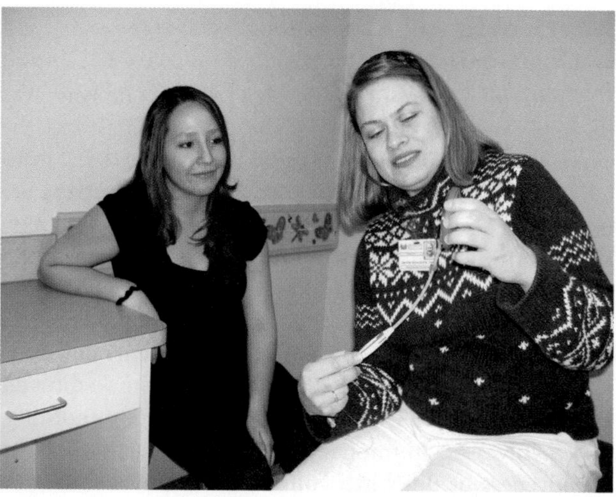

Fig. 4-1 Nurse counseling woman about contraceptive methods. (Courtesy Ed Lowdermilk, Chapel Hill, NC.)

within the first year of typical use (failure rate) of withdrawal is approximately 27% (Trussell, 2007). Some religions and cultures prohibit this technique. Coitus interruptus does not adequately protect against STIs or human immunodeficiency virus (HIV) infection.

Fertility awareness methods

Fertility awareness methods (FAMs) of contraception depend on identifying the beginning and end of the fertile period of the menstrual cycle. When educating women who want to use FAMs about the menstrual cycle, three phases should be identified:

1. Infertile phase: before ovulation
2. Fertile phase: approximately 5 to 7 days around the middle of the cycle, including several days before, during, and the day after ovulation
3. Infertile phase: after ovulation

Critical Thinking/Clinical Decision Making

Contraception

Jessica is a 20-year-old college student who has come to the student health clinic for contraception. She has a history of heavy periods that are somewhat irregular and she has "really bad" cramps the first day or two of her period. She thinks the "pill" would be a good choice because she has friends who take oral contraceptive pills (OCPs) and they do not have cramps. How should the nurse respond to this statement?

1. Evidence—Is the evidence sufficient to draw conclusions about what response the nurse should give?
2. Assumptions—Describe the underlying assumptions about the following issues:
   a. Personal considerations for choosing a birth control method
   b. Efficacy of methods of birth control
   c. Noncontraceptive benefits of OCPs
3. What implications and priorities for nursing care can be drawn at this time?
4. Does the evidence objectively support your conclusion?
5. Are there alternative perspectives to your conclusion?

Although ovulation is often unpredictable in many women, teaching the woman how to directly observe fertility patterns is empowering. FAMs consist of nearly a dozen categories. Each one uses a combination of charts, records, calculations, tools, observations, and either abstinence (natural family planning) or barrier methods of birth control during the fertile period in the menstrual cycle to prevent pregnancy (Jennings & Arevalo, 2007). Women can also use the charts and calculations associated with these methods to increase the likelihood of detecting the optimal timing of intercourse to achieve conception.

FAMs have many advantages, including low to no cost, absence of chemicals and hormones, and lack of alteration in the menstrual flow pattern. However, some disadvantages to using FAMs exist. For some people, keeping strict records and attending time-consuming training sessions to learn about the method may be difficult. FAMs also decrease the spontaneity of coitus. In addition, external influences such as illness can alter a woman's core body temperature and vaginal secretions. FAMs have decreased effectiveness in women with irregular cycles (particularly adolescents who have not established regular ovulatory patterns) (Jennings & Arevalo, 2007) (Box 4-1). FAMs do not protect against STIs or HIV infection. The typical failure rate for most FAMs is 25% during the first year of use (Trussell, 2007).

FAMs involve several techniques to identify high risk fertile days. The following discussion includes the most common techniques and some promising techniques for the future.

BOX 4-1

Potential Pitfalls of Using Fertility-Awareness Methods of Contraception

Potential pitfalls of using fertility awareness methods include the five Rs:

- Restriction on sexual spontaneity
- Rigorous daily monitoring
- Required training
- Risk of pregnancy during prolonged training period
- Risk of pregnancy high on unsafe days

Source: Zieman, M., Hatcher, R., Cwiak, C., Darney, P., Creinin, M., & Stosur, H. (2007). *A pocket guide to managing contraception, 2007-2009.* Tiger, GA: Bridging the Gap Foundation.

Natural family planning (NFP) provides contraception by using methods that rely on avoidance of intercourse during fertile periods. NFP methods are the only contraceptive practices acceptable to the Roman Catholic Church. NFP methods combine charting signs and symptoms of the menstrual cycle with the use of abstinence during fertile periods. Signs and symptoms most commonly used are menstrual bleeding, cervical mucus, and basal body temperature (see later discussions) (Jennings & Arevalo, 2007).

The human ovum can be fertilized no later than 16 to 24 hours after ovulation. Motile sperm have been recovered from the uterus and the oviducts as long as 60 hours after coitus. However, their ability to fertilize the ovum probably lasts no longer than 24 to 48 hours. Pregnancy is unlikely to occur if a couple abstains from intercourse for 4 days before and for 3 or 4 days after ovulation (fertile period). Unprotected intercourse on the other days of the cycle (safe period) should not result in pregnancy. However, this method presents two principal problems: (1) The exact time of ovulation cannot be predicted accurately, and (2) some couples have difficulty exercising restraint for several days before and after ovulation. Women with irregular menstrual periods have the greatest risk of failure with this form of contraception.

Calendar rhythm method. Practice of the calendar rhythm method is based on the number of days in each cycle counting from the first day of menses. With this method, the woman determines the fertile period after accurately recording the lengths of menstrual cycles for 6 months. The beginning of the fertile period is estimated by subtracting 18 days from the length of the shortest cycle. The end of the fertile period is determined by subtracting 11 days from the length of the longest cycle (Jennings & Arevalo, 2007). If the shortest cycle is 24 days and longest is 30 days, you apply the formula as follows:

Shortest cycle: 24 − 18 = sixth day
Longest cycle: 30 − 11 = nineteenth day

To prevent conception the couple would abstain during the fertile period–days 6 through 19. If the woman has very regular cycles of 28 days each, the fertile days would be as follows:

Shortest cycle: 28 − 18 = tenth day
Longest cycle: 28 − 11 = seventeenth day

To prevent pregnancy, the couple abstains from day 10 through 17 because ovulation occurs on day 14 plus or minus 2 days.

Standard days method. The *Standard Days Method* (SDM) is essentially a modified form of the calendar rhythm method that has a *fixed* number of days of fertility for each cycle–that is, days 8 to 19. The woman can purchase a CycleBeads necklace–a color-coded string of beads–as a concrete tool to track fertility (Fig. 4-2). Day 1 of the menstrual flow is the first day to begin the counting. Women who use this device avoid unprotected intercourse on days 8 to 19 (white beads on CycleBeads necklace). Although this method is useful to women whose cycles are 26 to 32 days long, it is unreliable to those who have longer or shorter cycles (CycleBeads, 2007). The typical failure rate for the SDM is 14% during the first year of use (Jennings & Arevalo, 2007).

TwoDay method of family planning. Based on monitoring and the recording of cervical secretions, the *TwoDay Algorithm* is used to identify the fertile window (Jennings & Arevalo, 2007). It appears to be simpler to teach, learn, and use than current natural methods. The woman needs to ask two questions each day: (1) "Did I note secretions today?" and (2) "Did I note secretions yesterday?" If the answer is yes to either question, she should avoid coitus or use a backup method of birth control. If the answer is no to both questions, her probability of getting pregnant is very low (Germano & Jennings, 2006).

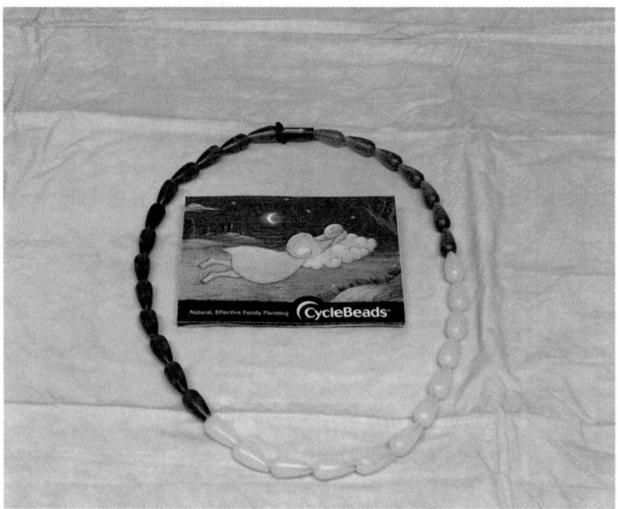

Fig. 4-2 CycleBeads. Red bead marks the first day of the menstrual cycle. White beads mark days that are likely to be fertile days; therefore unprotected intercourse should be avoided. Brown beads are days when pregnancy is unlikely and unprotected intercourse is permitted. (Courtesy Dee Lowdermilk, Chapel Hill, NC.)

Ovulation method. The cervical mucus ovulation-detection method (also called the Billings method and the Creighton model ovulation method) requires that the woman recognize and interpret the cyclic changes in the amount and consistency of cervical mucus that characterize her own unique pattern of changes (see Patient Instructions for Self-Management box). The cervical mucus that accompanies ovulation is necessary for viability and motility of sperm. It alters the pH environment, neutralizing the acidity, to be more compatible for sperm survival. Without adequate cervical mucus, coitus does not result in conception. Women check the quantity and character of mucus on the vulva or introitus with fingers or tissue paper each day for several months to learn the cycle. To ensure an accurate assessment of changes the cervical mucus should be free from semen, contraceptive gels or foams, and blood or discharge from vaginal infections for at least one full cycle. Other factors that create difficulty in identifying mucus changes include douches and vaginal deodorants, being in the sexually aroused state (which thins the mucus), and taking medications such as antihistamines (which dry up the mucus). Intercourse is considered safe without restriction beginning 4 days after the last day of wet, clear, slippery mucus (postovulation) (Jennings & Arevalo, 2007).

Symptothermal method. The symptothermal method is a tool that the woman uses to gain fertility awareness as she tracks the physiologic and psychologic symptoms that mark the phases of her cycle. This method combines at least two methods, usually cervical mucus changes with **basal body temperature (BBT)**, in addition to heightened awareness of secondary, cycle phase-related symptoms. Secondary symptoms include increased libido, midcycle spotting, mittelschmerz, pelvic fullness or tenderness, and vulvar fullness. The woman learns to palpate her cervix to assess for changes in texture, position, and dilation, which indicate ovulation. During the preovulatory and ovulatory periods the cervix softens, opens, rises in the vagina, and is more moist. During the postovulatory period the cervix drops, becomes firm, and closes. The woman notes the days on which coitus, changes in routine, illness, and so on have occurred (Fig. 4-3). Calendar calculations and cervical mucus changes help to estimate the onset of the fertile period, and changes in cervical mucus or the BBT help to estimate its end (see Patient Instructions for Self-Management: Assessing Basal Body Temperature).

Home predictor test kits for ovulation. All of the preceding methods discussed estimate the occurrence and approximate timing of ovulation, but none of

PATIENT INSTRUCTIONS FOR SELF-MANAGEMENT

Cervical Mucus Characteristics

SETTING THE STAGE

- Show charts of menstrual cycle along with changes in the cervical mucus.
- Have the woman practice with raw egg white.
- Supply her with a basal body temperature (BBT) log and graph if she does not already have one.
- Explain that assessment of cervical mucus characteristics is best when mucus is not mixed with semen, contraceptive jellies or foams, or discharge from infections. Tell her to refrain from douching before the assessment.

CONTENT RELATED TO CERVICAL MUCUS

- Explain to the woman (couple) how cervical mucus changes throughout the menstrual cycle.
  a. Postmenstrual mucus: scant
  b. Preovulation mucus: cloudy, yellow or white, sticky
  c. Ovulation mucus: clear, wet, sticky, slippery
  d. Postovulation fertile mucus: thick, cloudy, sticky
  e. Postovulation, postfertile mucus: scant
- Right before ovulation, the watery, thin, clear mucus becomes more abundant and thick (Fig. A). It feels similar to a lubricant and can be stretched 5+ cm between the thumb and forefinger; this quality of mucus is called spinnbarkeit (Fig. B), and its presence indicates the period of maximal fertility. Sperm deposited in this type of mucus can survive until ovulation occurs.

ASSESSMENT TECHNIQUE

- Stress that good handwashing is imperative to begin and end all self-assessment.
- Start observation from last day of menstrual flow.
- Assess cervical mucus several times a day for several cycles. Mucus can be obtained from vaginal opening; reaching into the vagina to the cervix is unnecessary.
- Record the findings on the same record on which the BBT is entered.

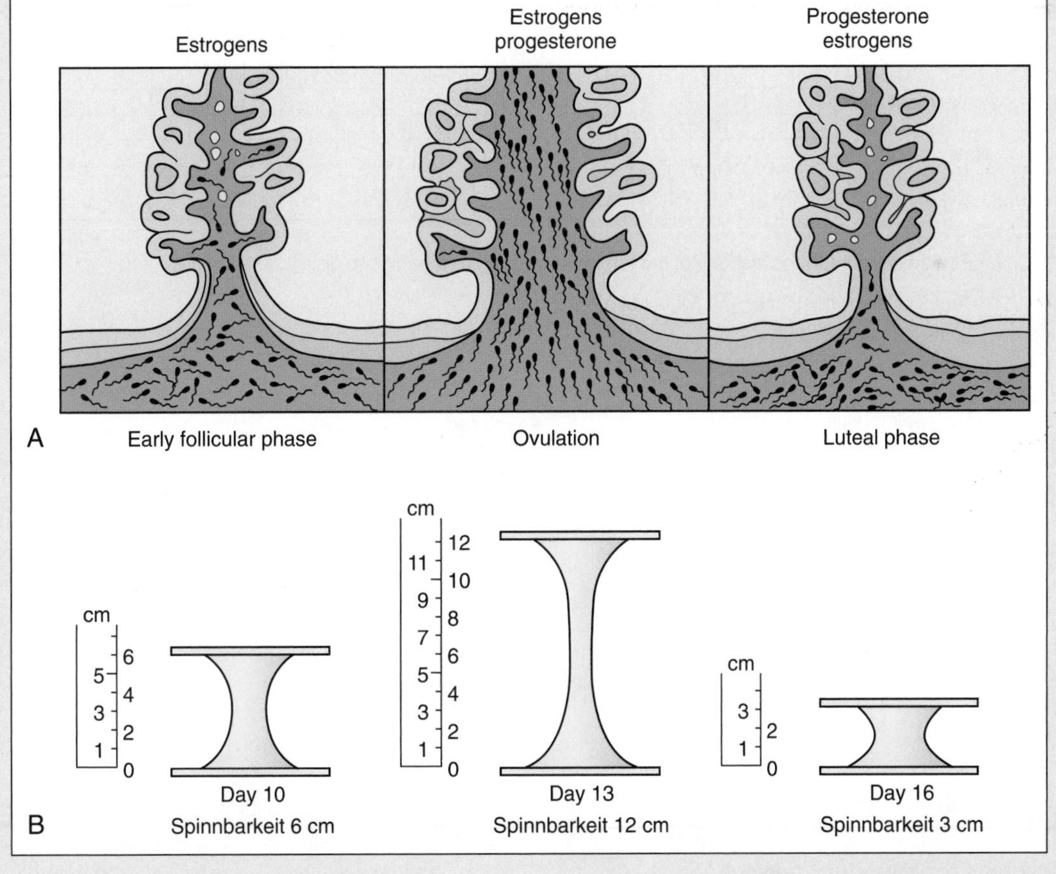

these methods can prove ovulation is occurring (Fig. 4-4). The urine predictor test for ovulation detects the sudden surge of luteinizing hormone (LH) that occurs approximately 12 to 24 hours before ovulation. Unlike BBT, illness, emotional upset, or physical activity do not affect the test. For home use, a test kit contains sufficient material for several days of testing during each cycle. An easy-to-read color change indicates a positive response or an LH surge. Directions for use of urine predictor test kits vary with the manufacturer. Saliva predictor tests for ovu-

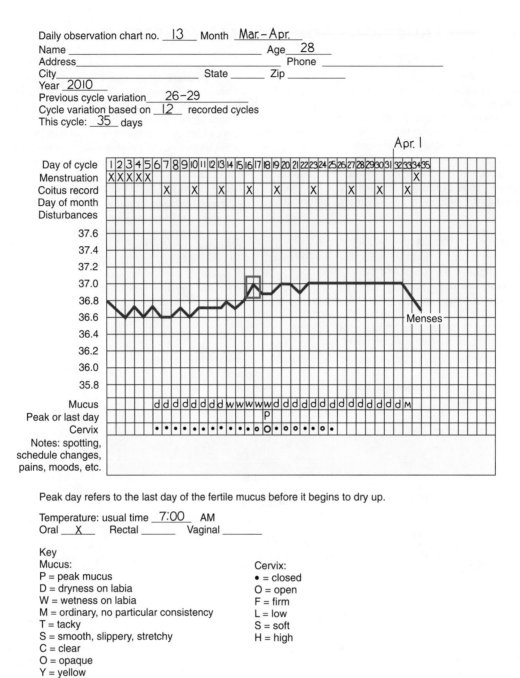

Daily observation chart no. 13 Month Mar.–Apr.
Name ______ Age 28
Address ______ Phone ______
City ______ State ______ Zip ______
Year 2010
Previous cycle variation 26–29
Cycle variation based on 12 recorded cycles
This cycle: 35 days

Apr. 1

Day of cycle	Menstruation	Coitus record	Mucus	Peak or last day	Cervix
1	X				
2	X				
3	X				
4	X				
5	X				
6			d		•
7		X	d		•
8			d		•
9			d		•
10		X	d		•
11			d		•
12			d		•
13		X	d		•
14			w		•
15			w		•
16		X	w		•
17			w		o
18			w	P	O
19		X	d		•
20			d		o
21			d		o
22			d		•
23		X	d		•
24			d		o
25			d		•
26			d		
27		X	d		
28			d		
29			d		
30		X	d		
31			d		
32			d		
33		X	M		
34	X				
35					

Day of month
Disturbances
37.6
37.4
37.2
37.0
36.8
36.6
36.4
36.2
36.0
35.8
Menses
Notes: spotting, schedule changes, pains, moods, etc.

Peak day refers to the last day of the fertile mucus before it begins to dry up.

Temperature: usual time 7:00 AM
Oral X Rectal ______ Vaginal ______

Key

Mucus:
P = peak mucus
D = dryness on labia
W = wetness on labia
M = ordinary, no particular consistency
T = tacky
S = smooth, slippery, stretchy
C = clear
O = opaque
Y = yellow

Cervix:
• = closed
O = open
F = firm
L = low
S = soft
H = high

Fig. 4-3 Example of a completed symptothermal chart. Note basal temperature shows drop and sharp rise at time of ovulation.

lation use dried, nonfoamy saliva as a tool to show fertility patterns. More research is needed to determine the efficacy of use of these tests for pregnancy prevention.

An electronic hormonal fertility-monitoring device, the ClearBlue Early Fertility Monitor (CEFM), is a handheld device that uses test strips to measure urinary metabolites of estrogen and LH. The monitor provides the user with *low, high,* and *peak* fertility readings. The CEFM method incorporates the use of the monitor as an aid to learning NFP and fertility awareness. It continues to be investigated for its effectiveness in helping couples prevent pregnancy (Fehring, Schneider, Raviele, & Barron, 2007).

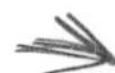

Barrier methods

Barrier contraceptives have gained in popularity not only as a contraceptive method, but also as a protective measure against the spread of STIs, such as human papillomavirus and herpes simplex virus (HSV). Some male condoms and female vaginal methods provide a physical barrier to several STIs, and some male condoms provide

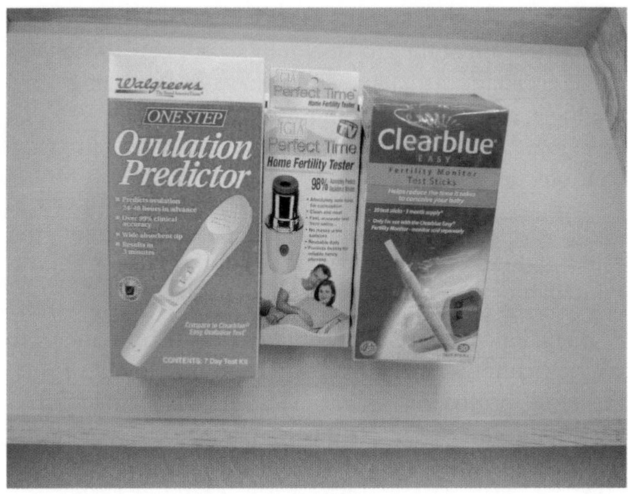

Fig. 4-4 Examples of ovulation prediction tests. (Courtesy Shannon Perry, Phoenix, AZ.)

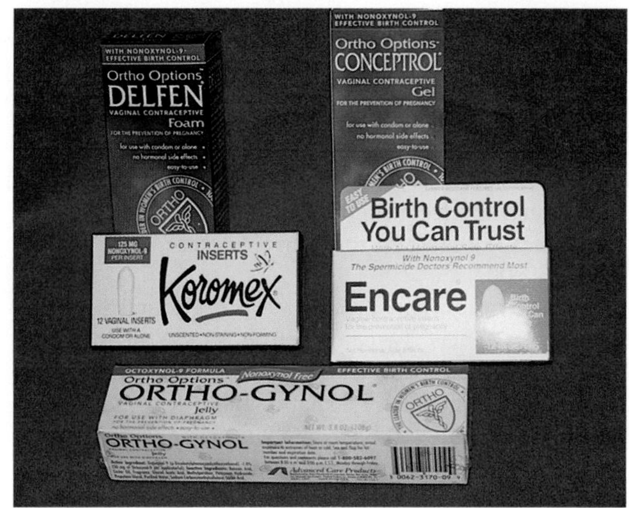

Fig. 4-5 Spermicides. (Courtesy Marjorie Pyle, RNC, Lifecircle, Costa Mesa, CA.)

PATIENT INSTRUCTIONS FOR SELF-MANAGEMENT

Basal Body Temperature (BBT)

- Take your BBT using a special calibrated thermometer every morning at the same time before you get out of bed.
- You may take your BBT orally, vaginally, or rectally, but always use the same site.
- Record your temperature daily on a graph and connect the dots (see Fig. 4-3).
- You may see a slight drop in temperature (0.05° C) about the time of ovulation but many women will not experience this change.
- Your temperature likely will rise 0.4° C to 0.8° C around the time of ovulation and stay elevated until just before the next menses.
- Avoid intercourse until 3 days of higher temperatures occur after 6 days of lower than baseline temperatures.
- Infection, fatigue, less than 3 hours sleep per night, awakening late, and anxiety may cause temperature fluctuations, altering the expected pattern.
- Jet lag, alcohol and antipyretic medications taken the evening before, or sleeping in a heated waterbed also must be noted on the chart because each factor affects the BBT.

Source: Jennings, V. & Arevalo, M. (2007). Fertility awareness-based methods. In R. Hatcher et al. (Eds.), *Contraceptive technology* (19th ed.). New York: Ardent Media.

COMMUNITY ACTIVITY

Contact the local obstetrics offices, health departments, school nurses, or clinics to obtain information related to family planning services in your community. Identify location, hours, access, and fee schedules for insured and uninsured patients. Are local, state, and federal funds available? Describe how health teaching is provided. What methods of contraception are available? What services provide Plan B as a back up? How are requests for Plan B managed if patients are not 18 years of age?

protection against HIV (Cates & Raymond, 2007; Warner, & Steiner, 2007). Spermicides serve as chemical barriers against the sperm.

Spermicides. Spermicides work by reducing the sperm's mobility; the chemicals attack the sperm flagella and body, thereby preventing the sperm from reaching the cervical os. Nonoxynol-9 (N-9), the most commonly used spermicidal chemical in the United States, is a surfactant that destroys the sperm cell membrane. However, data suggest that frequent use (more than two times a day) of N-9, or use as a lubricant during anal intercourse, may increase the transmission of HIV and can cause lesions (Cates & Raymond, 2007). Women with high risk behaviors that increase their likelihood of contracting HIV and other STIs need to avoid the use of spermicidal products containing N-9, including lubricated condoms, diaphragms, and cervical caps to which N-9 is added (WHO, 2004). Intravaginal spermicides are marketed and sold without a prescription as foams, tablets, suppositories, creams, films, and gels (Fig. 4-5). Preloaded, single-dose applicators small enough to be carried in a small purse are available. Effectiveness of spermicides depends on consistent and accurate use. Caution patients against misunderstanding terms: Contraceptive gel differs from fruit jelly, and cosmetics or hair products containing the nonspermicidal forms of nonoxynol are not adequate substitutes. The spermicide should be inserted high into the vagina so that it makes contact with the cervix. Some spermicides should be inserted at least 15 minutes before, but no longer than 1 hour before, sexual intercourse. Spermicide needs to be reapplied for each additional act of intercourse, even if using a barrier method. Studies have shown varying effectiveness rates for spermicidal use alone. The typical failure rate for spermicide use alone is 29% (Trussell, 2007).

Condoms. The male condom is a thin, stretchable sheath that covers the penis before genital, oral, or anal contact and is removed after the penis is withdrawn from the partner's orifice after ejaculation (Fig. 4-6, *A*). Condoms are made of latex rubber, polyurethane (strong, thin plastic), or natural membranes (animal tissue). In addition to providing a physical barrier for sperm, nonspermicidal latex condoms also provide a barrier for STIs (particularly gonorrhea, chlamydia, and trichomoniasis) and HIV transmission. Condoms lubricated with N-9 are not recommended for preventing STIs or HIV (Centers for Disease Control and Prevention, 2006). Latex condoms will break down with oil-based lubricants and should be used only with water-based or silicone lubricants (Warner, & Steiner, 2007). Because of the growing number of people with latex allergies, condom manufacturers have begun using polyurethane, which is thinner and stronger than latex. Research is ongoing to determine the effectiveness of polyurethane condoms to protect against STIs and HIV.

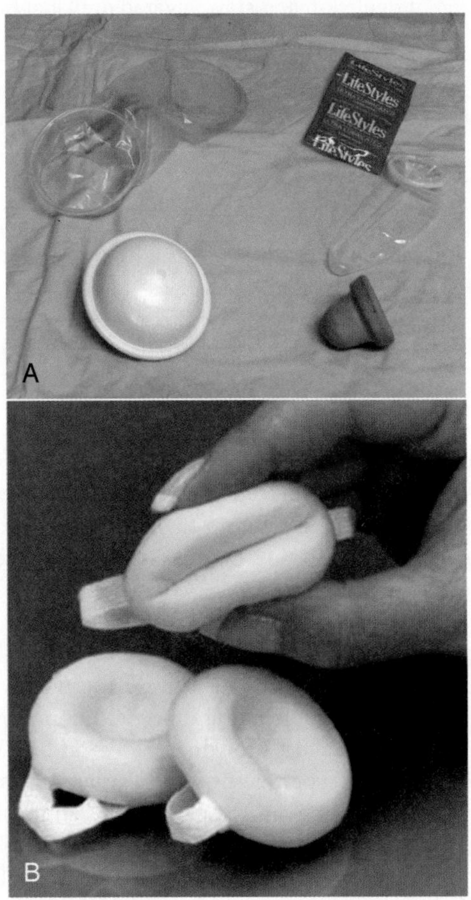

Fig. 4-6 **A,** Mechanical barriers. From the top left corner clockwise: female condom, male condom, cervical cap, diaphragm. **B,** Contraceptive sponge. (**A,** Courtesy Dee Lowdermilk, Chapel Hill, NC.; **B,** courtesy Allendale Pharmaceuticals, Inc., Allendale, NJ.)

NURSING ALERT Question all persons about the potential for latex allergy. Latex condom use is contraindicated for people with latex sensitivity.

A small percentage of condoms are made from the lamb cecum (natural skin). Natural skin condoms do not provide the same protection against STIs and HIV infection as latex condoms. Natural skin condoms contain small pores that could allow passage of viruses such as hepatitis B, HSV, and HIV. Condoms need to be discarded after each single use. They are available without a prescription.

A functional difference in condom shape is the presence or absence of a sperm-reservoir tip (see Fig. 4-6, *A*). To enhance vaginal stimulation, some condoms are contoured and rippled or have ribbed or roughened surfaces. Thinner construction increases heat transmission and sensitivity; a variety of colors and flavors increases condoms' acceptability and attractiveness (Trussell, 2007). A wet jelly or dry powder lubricates some condoms. Typical failure rate in the first year of male condom use is 15% (Trussell). To prevent unintended pregnancy and the spread of STIs, individuals must use condoms consistently and correctly. You can use instructions, such as those listed in Box 4-2, for patient teaching.

The female condom is a lubricated vaginal sheath made of polyurethane and has flexible rings at both ends (see Fig. 4-6, *A*). The closed end of the pouch is inserted into the vagina and is anchored around the cervix, and the open ring covers the labia. Women whose partner will not wear a male condom can use this as a protective mechanical barrier. Rewetting drops or oil- or water-based lubricants help decrease the distracting noise that is produced while penile thrusting occurs. The female condom is available in one size, intended for single use only, and is sold over the counter. Individuals should not use male condoms with the female condom, because the friction from both sheaths can increase the likelihood of either or both tearing (Female Health Company, 2008). Typical failure rate in the first year of female condom use is 21% (Trussell, 2007).

Diaphragms, cervical caps, and sponges. Diaphragms, cervical caps, and shields are soft latex or silicone barriers that cover the cervix and prevent the sperm from migrating to fertilize the ovum. These barriers are used with spermicidal jelly or cream as an additional method to prevent pregnancy.

Diaphragms. The contraceptive diaphragm is a shallow, dome-shaped latex or silicone device with a flexible rim that covers the cervix (see Fig. 4-6, *A*). Three types of diaphragms are available: coil spring, arcing spring, and wide seal rim. Available in many sizes, the diaphragm

BOX 4-2

Male Condoms

MECHANISM OF ACTION

A sheath is applied over the erect penis before insertion or loss of preejaculatory drops of semen. Used correctly, condoms prevent sperm from entering the cervix. Spermicide-coated condoms cause ejaculated sperm to be immobilized rapidly, thus increasing contraceptive effectiveness.

FAILURE RATE

- Typical users, 15%
- Correct and consistent users, 2%

ADVANTAGES

- Safe
- No side effects
- Readily available
- Premalignant changes in cervix prevented or ameliorated in women whose partners use condoms
- Method of male nonsurgical contraception

DISADVANTAGES

- Lovemaking must be interrupted to apply the sheath.
- Sensation may be altered.
- If condom is used improperly, spillage of sperm can result in pregnancy.
- Condoms may occasionally tear during intercourse.

PROTECTION AGAINST SEXUALLY TRANSMITTED INFECTIONS (STIs)

If a condom is used throughout the act of intercourse and no unprotected contact occurs with female genitals, a latex rubber condom, which is impermeable to viruses, can act as a protective measure against STIs.

NURSING CONSIDERATIONS

Teach men to do the following:

- Use a new condom (check expiration date) for each act of sexual intercourse or other acts between partners that involve contact with the penis.
- Place the condom after the penis is erect and before intimate contact.
- Place the condom on head of penis (Fig. A) and unroll it all the way to the base (Fig. B).
- Leave an empty space at the tip (Fig. A); remove any air remaining in the tip by gently pressing air out toward the base of the penis.
- If a lubricant is desired, use water-based products such as K-Y lubricating jelly. Do not use petroleum-based products because they can cause the condom to break.
- After ejaculation, carefully withdraw the still-erect penis from the vagina, holding onto condom rim; remove and discard the condom.
- Store unused condoms in a cool, dry place.
- Do not use condoms that are sticky, brittle, or obviously damaged.

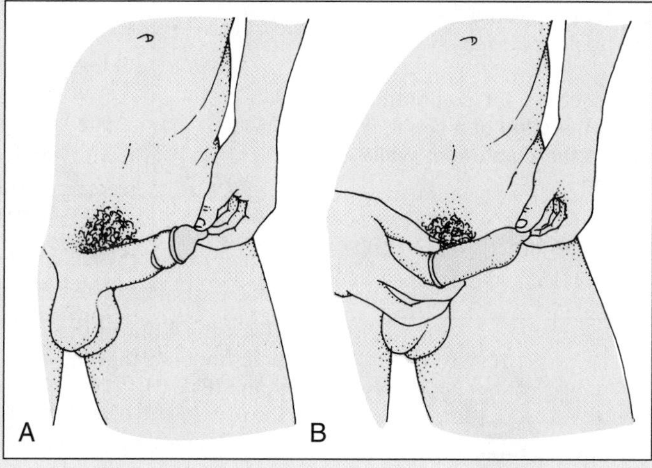

should be the largest size the woman can wear without her being aware of its presence. All diaphragms require a prescription, but over-the-counter products are being researched (Cates & Raymond, 2007). Typical failure rate of the diaphragm combined with spermicide is 16% in the first year of use (Trussell, 2007). Effectiveness of the diaphragm is less when used without spermicide (Trussell). Women at high risk for HIV should avoid use of N-9 spermicides with the diaphragm (Cates & Raymond).

Inform the woman that she needs an annual gynecologic examination to assess the fit of the diaphragm. The woman should inspect the device before every use and replace it at least every 2 years. It will need to be refitted for a 20% weight fluctuation, after any abdominal or pelvic surgery, and after every term pregnancy and miscarriage or abortion that occurs after 14 weeks of gestation (Planned Parenthood, 2008). Because various types of diaphragms are on the market, use the package insert for teaching the

PATIENT INSTRUCTIONS FOR SELF-MANAGEMENT

Use and Care of the Diaphragm

INSPECTION OF THE DIAPHRAGM

You must inspect your diaphragm carefully before each use. The best way to perform this inspection is as follows:

- Hold the diaphragm up to a light source. Carefully stretch the diaphragm at the area of the rim, on all sides, making sure there are no holes. Remember, sharp fingernails can puncture the diaphragm.
- Another way to check for pinholes is to fill the diaphragm with water carefully. If any problem develops, you will see it immediately.
- A diaphragm that is puckered, especially near the rim, could mean thin spots.
- If you see any of these problems, do not use the diaphragm and consult your health care provider.

PREPARATION OF THE DIAPHRAGM

Rinse off the cornstarch. Your diaphragm must always be used with a spermicidal lubricant to be effective. Pregnancy cannot be prevented effectively by the diaphragm alone.

Always empty your bladder before inserting the diaphragm. Place approximately 2 tsp of contraceptive jelly or contraceptive cream on the side of the diaphragm that will rest against the cervix (or whichever way you have been instructed). Spread it around to coat the surface and the rim. This measure aids in insertion and offers a more complete seal. Many women also spread some jelly or cream on the other side of the diaphragm (Fig. A).

POSITIONS FOR INSERTION OF THE DIAPHRAGM

Squatting: Squatting is the most commonly used position, and most women find it satisfactory.

Leg-up method: Another position is to raise the left foot (if right hand is used for insertion) on a low stool, and, while in a bending position, insert the diaphragm.

Chair method: Another practical method for diaphragm insertion is to sit far forward on the edge of a chair.

Reclining: You may prefer to insert the diaphragm while in a semireclining position in bed.

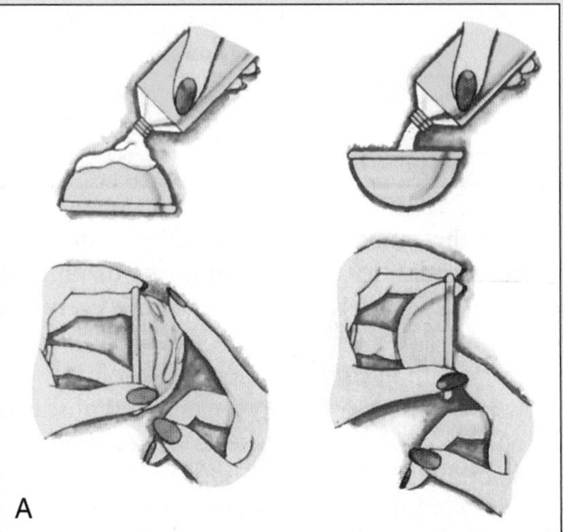
A

INSERTION OF THE DIAPHRAGM

The diaphragm can be inserted up to 6 hours before intercourse. Hold the diaphragm between your thumb and fingers. The dome can be either up or down, as directed by your health care provider. Place your index finger on the outer rim of the compressed diaphragm (Fig. B).

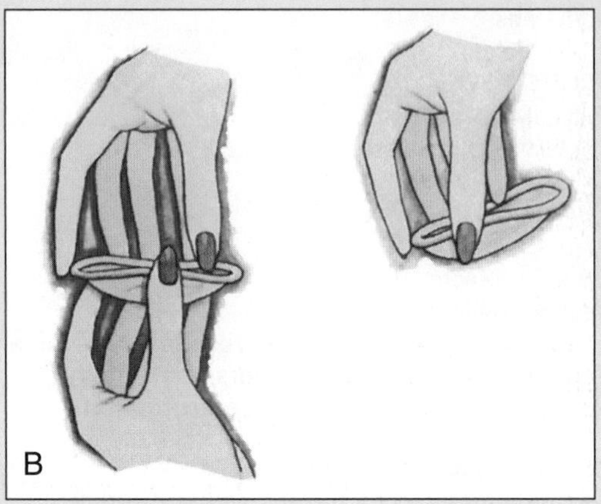
B

Use the fingers of the other hand to spread the labia (lips of the vagina). This action will assist in guiding the diaphragm into place.

Insert the diaphragm into the vagina. Direct it inward and downward as far as it will go to the space behind and below the cervix (Fig. C).

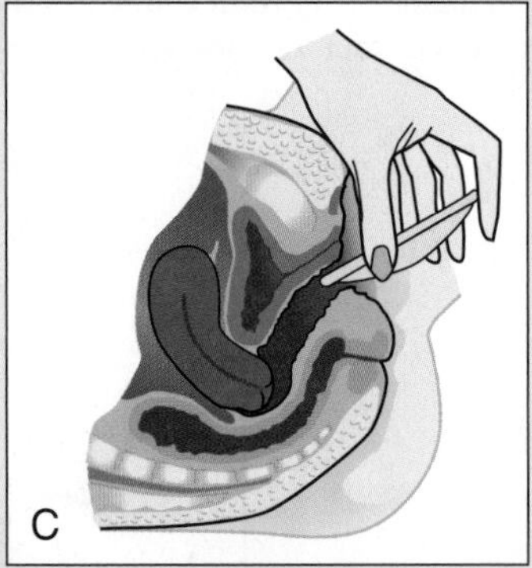
C

Tuck the front of the rim of the diaphragm behind the pubic bone so that the rubber hugs the front wall of the vagina (Fig. D).

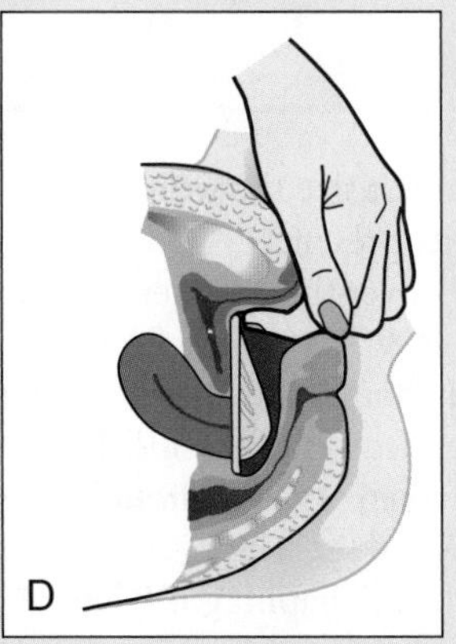
D

PATIENT INSTRUCTIONS FOR SELF-MANAGEMENT

Use and Care of the Diaphragm—cont'd

Feel for your cervix through the diaphragm to be certain it is properly placed and securely covered by the rubber dome (Fig. E).

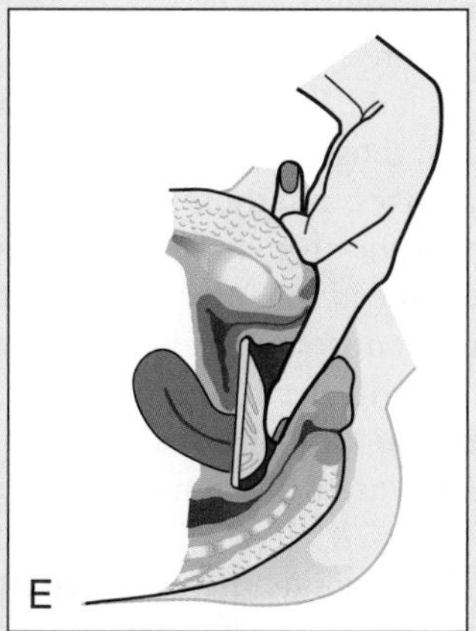

GENERAL INFORMATION

Regardless of the time of the month, you must use your diaphragm every time intercourse takes place. Your diaphragm must be left in place for at least 6 hours after the last intercourse. If you remove your diaphragm before the 6-hour period, you will greatly increase your chance of becoming pregnant. If you have repeated acts of intercourse, you must add more spermicide for each act of intercourse.

REMOVAL OF THE DIAPHRAGM

The only proper way to remove the diaphragm is to insert your forefinger up and over the top side of the diaphragm and slightly to the side.

Next, turn the palm of your hand downward and backward, hooking the forefinger firmly on top of the inside of the upper rim of the diaphragm, breaking the suction.

Pull the diaphragm down and out. This technique prevents tearing the diaphragm with the fingernails. You should not remove the diaphragm by trying to catch the rim from below the dome (Fig. F).

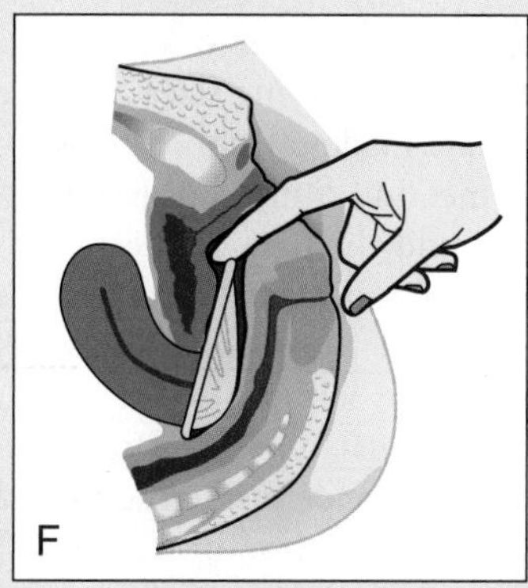

CARE OF THE DIAPHRAGM

When using a vaginal diaphragm, avoid using oil-based products, such as certain body lubricants, mineral oil, baby oil, vaginal lubricants, or vaginitis preparations. These products can weaken the rubber.

A little care means longer wear for your diaphragm. After each use, wash the diaphragm in warm water and mild soap. Do not use detergent soaps, cold-cream soaps, deodorant soaps, and soaps containing oil products because they can weaken the rubber.

After washing, dry the diaphragm thoroughly. Remove all water and moisture with a towel. Then dust the diaphragm with cornstarch. Do not use scented talc, body powder, baby powder, or similar products because they can weaken the rubber.

To clean the introducer (if one is used), wash with mild soap and warm water, rinse, and dry thoroughly.

Place the diaphragm back in the plastic case for storage. Do not store it near a radiator or heat source or in a location that is exposed to light for an extended period.

woman how to use and care for the diaphragm (see Patient Instructions for Self-Management).

Some women are reluctant to insert and remove the diaphragm. Although it can be inserted up to 6 hours before intercourse, a cold diaphragm and a cold gel temporarily reduce vaginal response to sexual stimulation if insertion of the diaphragm occurs immediately before intercourse. Some women or couples object to the messiness of the spermicide. These annoyances of diaphragm use, along with failure to insert the device once foreplay has begun, are the most common reasons for failures of this method. Side effects include irritation of tissues related to contact with spermicides. The diaphragm is not a good option for women with poor vaginal muscle tone or recurrent urinary tract infections. For proper placement, the diaphragm must rest behind the pubic symphysis and completely cover the cervix. To decrease the chance of exerting urethral pressure, the woman should empty her bladder before diaphragm insertion and immediately after intercourse. Diaphragms are contraindicated for women with pelvic relaxation (uterine prolapse) or a large cystocele. Women with a latex allergy should not use latex diaphragms.

Toxic shock syndrome (TSS), although reported in very small numbers, can occur in association with the use of the contraceptive diaphragm and cervical caps (Cates & Raymond, 2007). Instruct the woman about ways to reduce her risk for TSS. These measures include prompt removal of the diaphragm 6 to 8 hours after intercourse, not using the diaphragm or cervical caps during menses, and learning and watching for danger signs of TSS.

NURSING ALERT Be alert for signs of TSS in women who use a diaphragm or cervical cap as a contraceptive method. The most common signs include a sunburn-type rash, diarrhea, dizziness, faintness, weakness, sore throat, aching muscles and joints, sudden high fever, and vomiting (Planned Parenthood, 2008).

Cervical caps. Three types of cervical caps are available. Two types come in varying sizes and one type is one size fits all. They are made of rubber or latex-free silicone and have soft domes and firm brims (see Fig. 4-6, *A*). The cap fits snugly around the base of the cervix close to the junction of the cervix and vaginal fornices. The cap should remain in place no less than 6 hours and not more than 48 hours at a time. It is left in place at least 6 hours after the last act of intercourse. The seal provides a physical barrier to sperm; spermicide inside the cap adds a chemical barrier. The extended period of wear may be an added convenience for women.

Instructions for the actual insertion and use of the cervical cap closely resemble the instructions for the use of the contraceptive diaphragm. However, the cervical cap can be inserted hours before sexual intercourse without a need for additional spermicide later, and no additional spermicide is required for repeated acts of intercourse when the cap is used. In addition, the cervical cap requires less spermicide than the diaphragm when initially inserted. The angle of the uterus, the vaginal muscle tone, and the shape of the cervix may interfere with the cervical cap's ease of fitting and use. Correct fitting requires time, effort, and skill from both the woman and the clinician. The woman must check the cap's position before and after each act of intercourse (see Patient Instructions for Self-Management box).

Because of the potential risk of TSS associated with the use of the cervical cap, another form of birth control is recommended for use during menstrual bleeding and up to at least 6 weeks postpartum. Women should have the cap refitted after any gynecologic surgery or birth and after major weight losses or gains. Otherwise, the size should be checked at least once a year.

Women who are not good candidates for wearing the cervical cap include those with abnormal Papanicolaou (Pap) test results, those who cannot be fitted properly with the existing cap sizes, and those who find the insertion and removal of the device too difficult. Women with a history of TSS, vaginal or cervical infections, and those who experience allergic responses to the latex cap or spermicide are also not good candidates for cervical caps.

Contraceptive sponge. The vaginal sponge is a small, round, polyurethane sponge that contains N-9 spermicide (see Fig. 4-6, *B*). It is designed to fit over the cervix (one size fits all). The side that is placed next to the cervix is concave for better fit. The opposite side has a woven polyester loop to be used for removal of the sponge.

The woman moistens the sponge with water before insertion. It provides protection for up to 24 hours and for repeated instances of sexual intercourse. The sponge should be left in place for at least 6 hours after the last act of intercourse. Wearing longer than 24 to 30 hours may put the woman at risk for TSS (Cates & Raymond, 2007).

Failure rates for these barriers in the first year of use are 16% in nulliparas and 32% in multiparous women (Trussell, 2007).

Hormonal methods

More than 70 different contraceptive formulations are available in the United States today. Table 4-1 describes

PATIENT INSTRUCTIONS FOR SELF-MANAGEMENT

Use of the Cervical Cap

- Push the cap up into the vagina until it covers the cervix.
- Press the rim against the cervix to create a seal.
- To remove, push the rim toward the right or left hip to loosen from the cervix, and then withdraw.
- The woman can assume several positions to insert the cervical cap. See the four positions shown for inserting the diaphragm.

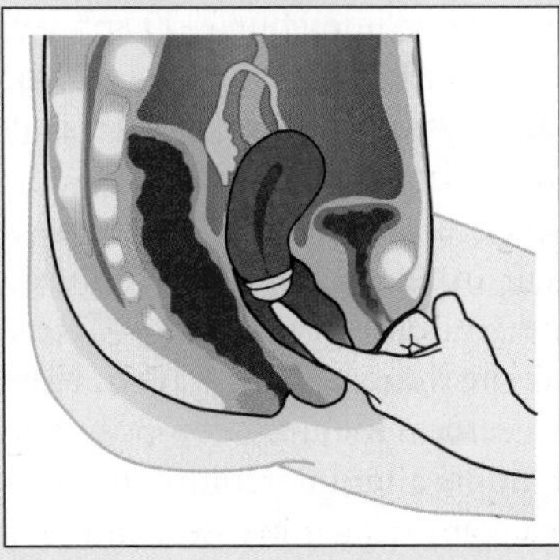

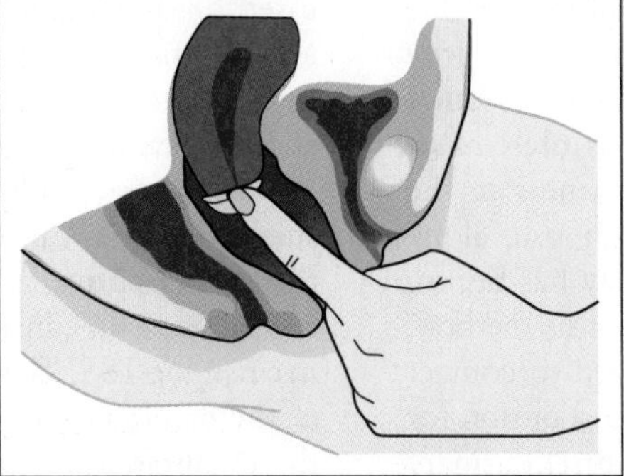

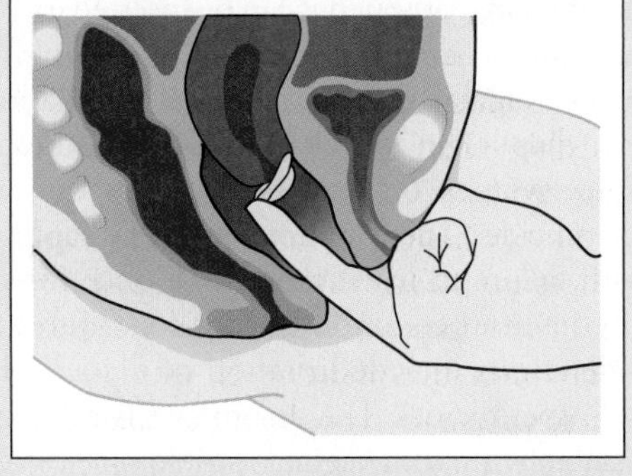

TABLE 4-1

Hormonal Contraception

COMPOSITION	ROUTE OF ADMINISTRATION	DURATION OF EFFECT
Combination estrogen and progestin (synthetic estrogens and progestins in varying doses and formulations)	Oral	24 hours; extended cycle—12 weeks
	Transdermal	7 days
	Vaginal ring insertion	3 weeks
Progestin only:		
Norethindrone, norgestrel	Oral	24 hours
Medroxyprogesterone acetate	Intramuscular injection; subcutaneous injection	3 months
Progestin; etonogestrel	Subdermal implant	Up to 3 years
Levonorgestrel	Intrauterine device	Up to 5 years

the general classes. Because of the wide variety of preparations available, the woman and nurse must read the package insert for information about specific products prescribed. Formulations include combined estrogen-progestin medications and progestational agents. The formulations are administered orally, transdermally, vaginally, by implantation, by injection, or via the intrauterine route.

Combined estrogen-progestin contraceptives

Oral contraceptives. The normal menstrual cycle is maintained by a feedback mechanism. The body secretes follicle-stimulating hormone (FSH) and LH in response to fluctuating levels of ovarian estrogen and progesterone. Regular ingestion of combined oral contraceptive pills (COCs) suppresses the action of the hypothalamus and anterior pituitary that inhibits production of FSH and LH; therefore follicles do not mature, suppressing ovulation.

Combined steroids induce other contraceptive effects. These substances alter maturation of the endometrium, making it a less favorable site for implantation. COCs also have a direct effect on the endometrium such that from 1 to 4 days after the last COC is taken the endometrium sloughs and bleeds as a result of hormone withdrawal. The withdrawal bleeding is usually less profuse than that of normal menstruation and may last only 2 to 3 days. Some women have no bleeding at all. The cervical mucus remains thick from the effect of the progestin (Nelson, 2007).

Cervical mucus under the effect of progesterone does not provide as suitable an environment for sperm penetration as does the thin, watery mucus at ovulation. The possible effect, if any, of altered tubal and uterine motility induced by COCs is not clear.

Monophasic pills provide fixed doses of estrogen and progestin. Multiphasic pills (e.g., biphasic and triphasic oral contraceptives) alter the amount of progestin and sometimes the amount of estrogen within each cycle. These preparations reduce the total dose of hormones in a single cycle without sacrificing contraceptive efficacy (Nelson, 2007). To maintain adequate hormonal levels for contraception and enhance compliance, women should take COCs at the same time each day.

Advantages. Because taking the pill does not relate directly to the sexual act, its acceptability may be increased. Improvement in sexual response may occur once the possibility of pregnancy is not an issue. For some women, knowing when to expect the next menstrual flow is convenient.

Evidence of noncontraceptive benefits of oral contraceptives is based on studies of high-dose pills (50 mg of estrogen). Few data exist on noncontraceptive benefits of low-dose oral contraceptives (less than 35 mg of estrogen) (Nelson, 2007). The noncontraceptive health benefits of COCs include decreased menstrual blood loss and decreased iron-deficiency anemia, regulation of menorrhagia and irregular cycles, and reduced incidence of dysmenorrhea and premenstrual syndrome (PMS). Oral contraceptives also offer protection against endometrial cancer and ovarian cancer, reduce the incidence of benign breast disease, and improve acne. They also protect against the development of functional ovarian cysts and salpingitis and decrease the risk of ectopic pregnancy. Oral contraceptives are considered a safe option for nonsmoking women until menopause. Perimenopausal women can benefit from regular bleeding cycles, a regular hormonal pattern, and the noncontraceptive health benefits of oral contraceptives (Nelson).

Women taking COCs are examined before the medication is prescribed and yearly thereafter. The examination includes medical and family history, weight, blood pressure, general physical and pelvic examinations, and screening cervical cytologic analysis (Pap test). Consistent monitoring by the health care provider is valuable in the detection of non–contraception-related disorders as well so that providers can initiate timely treatment. Most health care providers assess the woman 3 months after she begins COCs to detect any complications.

Oral hormonal contraceptives are initiated in three ways: (1) quick start–taking the first pill the same day as the clinic appointment and using a back-up method for 7 days, (2) first day start–taking the first pill on the first day of the menstrual cycle (menses), and (3) Sunday start–taking the first pill on the first Sunday after the start of their menstrual period (Nelson, 2007). Taken exactly as directed, COCs prevent ovulation, and pregnancy cannot occur; the overall effectiveness rate is almost 100%. Almost all failures (i.e., occurrence of pregnancy) are caused by omission of one or more pills during the regimen. The typical failure rate of COCs resulting from omission is 8% (Trussell, 2007).

COCs also can be taken using different patterns. Most are taken on a monthly cycle of 3 weeks of active pills followed by seven placebo pills. Some regimens now come with fewer placebo pills and more active pills, although research is still needed on the efficacy and safety of these regimens. Another pattern of use is the extended cycle–taking pills for longer times, which lessens the frequency of menstrual periods (i.e., withdrawal bleeding). The extended period can be short, such as for a special event like a vacation or honeymoon, or for more extended times. For example, a woman can take 2 months of active pills followed by seven placebo pills at the end of the second package or take a U.S. Food and Drug Administration (FDA)-approved extended-use pill. One such pill is levonorgestrel–ethinyl estradiol (Seasonale) that contains both estrogen and progestin, taken in 3-month cycles of 12 weeks of active pills followed by 1 week of inactive pills. Menstrual periods occur during the thirteenth week of the cycle. This active pill provides no protection from STIs, and risks are similar to those of COCs. Available only by prescription, women must take Seasonale on a daily schedule, regardless of the frequency of intercourse. Because users will have fewer menstrual flows, they should consider the possibility of pregnancy if they do not experience their thirteenth-week flow. Typical failure rate in the first year of Seasonale use is less than 5% (U.S. FDA, 2009).

Disadvantages and side effects. Since hormonal contraceptives have come into use, the amount of estrogen and progestational agent contained in each tablet has been reduced considerably. This factor is important because adverse effects are, to a degree, dose related.

You need to screen women for medical conditions that preclude the use of oral contraceptives. Contraindications for COC use include a history or presence of thromboembolic disorders, cerebrovascular or coronary artery disease, valvular heart disease, breast cancer or other estrogen-dependent tumors, impaired liver function, and liver tumor. Women older than 35 years of age who smoke (more than 15 cigarettes per day), or those with severe hypertension or who have headaches with focal neurologic symptoms should not use COCs. Surgery with prolonged immobilization or any surgery on the legs and diabetes mellitus (of more than 20 years' duration) with vascular disease also contraindicate COC use (Nelson, 2007).

Certain side effects of COCs are attributable to estrogen, progestin, or both. Serious adverse effects documented with high doses of estrogen and progesterone include stroke, myocardial infarction, thromboembolism, hypertension, gallbladder disease, and liver tumors. Common side effects of estrogen excess include nausea, breast tenderness, fluid retention, and chloasma. Side effects of estrogen deficiency include early spotting (days 1 to 14), hypomenorrhea, nervousness, and atrophic vaginitis leading to painful intercourse (dyspareunia). Side effects of progestin excess include increased appetite, tiredness, depression, breast tenderness, vaginal yeast infection, oily skin and scalp, hirsutism, and postpill amenorrhea. Side effects of progestin deficiency include late spotting and breakthrough bleeding (days 15 to 21), heavy flow with clots, and decreased breast size. One of the most common side effects of combined COCs is bleeding irregularities (Nelson, 2007).

In the presence of side effects, especially those that are bothersome to the woman, a different product, different drug content, or another method of contraception may be required. The "right" product for a woman contains the lowest dose of hormones that prevents ovulation and that has the fewest and least harmful side effects. Predicting the right dose for any particular woman is impossible. Issues to consider in prescribing oral contraceptives include history of oral contraceptive use, side effects during past use, menstrual history, and drug interactions (Nelson, 2007).

The following medications, when taken simultaneously with oral contraceptives, can reduce the effectiveness of contraceptives (Nelson, 2007).

- Anticonvulsants: barbiturates, oxcarbazepine, phenytoin, phenobarbital, felbamate, carbamazepine, primidone, and topiramate
- Systemic antifungals: griseofulvin
- Antituberculosis drugs: rifampicin and rifabutin
- Anti-HIV protease inhibitors

NURSING ALERT Over-the-counter medications, as well as some herbal supplements (e.g., St John's wort), can alter the effectiveness of COCs. Ask women about their use when COCs are being considered for contraception.

No strong pharmacokinetic evidence exists that shows a relationship between broad-spectrum antibiotic use and altered hormonal levels among oral contraceptive users, although potential antibiotic interaction can occur (Nelson, 2007). A meta-analysis of studies on the incidence of breast cancer in current or past COC users ages 35 to 64 has not found a significant increase of breast cancer in women who use COCs (Marchbanks et al., 2002).

After discontinuation of oral contraception, return to fertility usually happens quickly (Nelson, 2007). Many women ovulate the next month after stopping oral contraceptives. Women who discontinue oral contraception for a planned pregnancy commonly ask whether they should wait before attempting to conceive. Studies indicate that these infants have no greater chance of being born with any type of birth defect than do infants born to women in the general population, even if conception occurred in the first month after the medication was discontinued. However, women should begin folic acid supplements at least 3 months before discontinuing the pill (Nelson).

Nursing considerations. Many different preparations of oral hormonal contraceptives are available. Review the prescribing information in the package insert with the woman. Because of the wide variations, make sure each woman is clear about the unique dose regimen for the preparation prescribed for her. Directions for care after missing one or two tablets also vary (Fig. 4-7).

Withdrawal bleeding tends to be short and scanty when some combination pills are taken. A woman may see no fresh blood at all. A drop of blood or a brown smudge on a tampon or the underwear counts as a menstrual period.

Approximately 68% of women who start taking oral contraceptives are still taking them after 1 year (Trussell, 2007). The nurse should therefore recommend and instruct the woman with a second method of birth control and make sure she is comfortable with this backup method. Most women stop taking oral contraceptives for nonmedical reasons.

The nurse also reviews the signs of potential complications associated with the use of oral contraceptives (see Signs of Potential Complications box). Oral contraceptives do not protect a woman against STIs or HIV. A barrier method such as condoms and spermicide should be used for protection.

Transdermal contraceptive system. Available by prescription only, the contraceptive transdermal patch delivers continuous levels of norelgestromin (progesterone) and ethinyl estradiol. The patch is applied to intact skin of the upper outer arm, upper torso (front and back, excluding the breasts), lower abdomen, or buttocks (Fig. 4-8). Application is on the same day once a week for 3 weeks followed by a week without the patch. Withdrawal bleeding occurs during the "no patch" week. A transient skin reaction at the site of the application is common; site rotation is suggested. Patches can be worn during bathing showering, swimming, and exercise (Nanda, 2007). Mechanism of action, efficacy, contraindications, skin reactions, and side effects are similar to those of COCs. A potential serious health concern is the possible increased risk of venous thrombophlebotic conditions because total serum estrogen levels may be higher than with COCs (Courtney, 2006). The typical failure rate during the first year of use is 8% (Trussell, 2007).

signs of POTENTIAL COMPLICATIONS

Oral Contraceptives

Alert the woman who experiences any of the following symptoms to stop taking the pill and to report any of these symptoms to her health care provider immediately. The mnemonic ACHES helps in retention of this list (Nelson, 2007):

A—Abdominal pain may indicate a problem with the liver or gallbladder.
C—Chest pain or shortness of breath may indicate possible clot problem within the lungs or heart.
H—Headaches (sudden or persistent) may be caused by a cardiovascular accident or hypertension.
E—Eye problems may indicate a vascular accident or hypertension.
S—Severe leg pain may indicate a thromboembolic process.

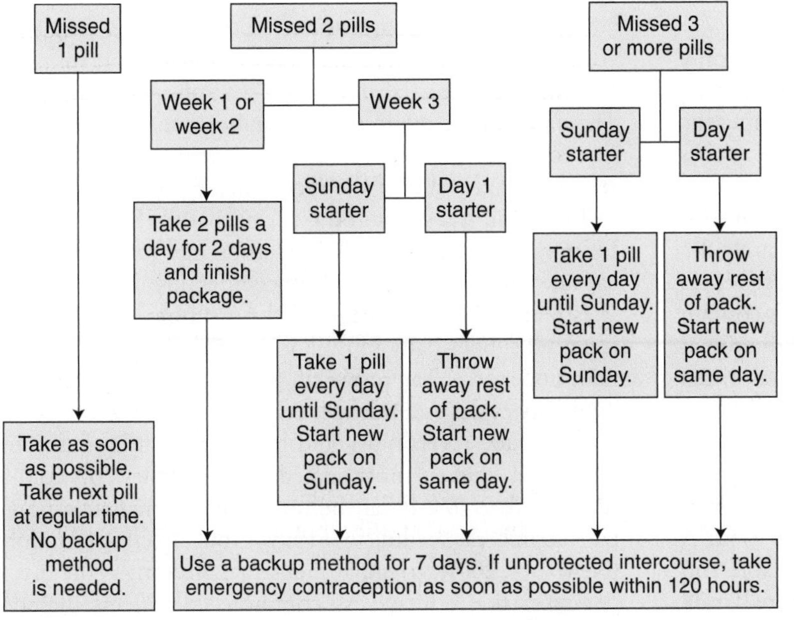

Fig. 4-7 Flowchart for missed contraceptive pills (2008). (Courtesy Patsy Huff, PharmD, Chapel Hill, NC.)

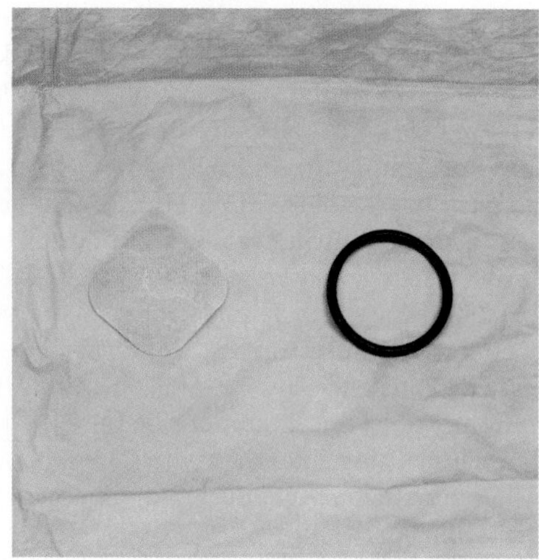

Fig. 4-8 Hormonal contraceptive transdermal patch and vaginal ring. (Courtesy Dee Lowdermilk, Chapel Hill, NC.)

Vaginal contraceptive ring. Available only with a prescription, the vaginal contraceptive ring is a flexible ring (made of ethylene vinyl acetate copolymer) worn in the vagina to deliver continuous levels of etonorgestrel (progesterone) and ethinyl estradiol (see Fig. 4-9). The woman wears the vaginal ring for 3 weeks followed by a week without the ring. The ring can also be used for extended cycles of 49 to 364 days (with changes every 21 days). The ring is inserted by the woman and does not have to be fitted. Some wearers may experience vaginitis, leukorrhea, and vaginal discomfort (Nanda, 2007). Withdrawal bleeding occurs during the "no ring" week. If the woman or partner notices discomfort during coitus, the ring should not be removed from the vagina for longer than 3 hours for it to still be effective for the rest of the 3-week period. Mechanism of action, efficacy, contraindications, and side effects are similar to those of COCs. The typical failure rate of the vaginal contraceptive ring is 8% during the first year of use (Trussell, 2007).

Progestin-only contraceptives. Progestin-only methods impair fertility by inhibiting ovulation, thickening and decreasing the amount of cervical mucus, thinning the endometrium, and altering cilia in the uterine tubes (Raymond, 2007).

Oral progestins (minipill). Failure rate of progestin-only pills (POPs) for typical users is approximately 8% in the first year of use (Trussell, 2007). Effectiveness increases if POPs are taken correctly. Because POPs contain such a low dose of progestin, women must take the pill at the same time every day (Raymond, 2007). Users often complain of irregular vaginal bleeding.

Injectable progestins. Depot medroxyprogesterone acetate (DMPA or Depo-Provera), 150 mg, is given intramuscularly in the deltoid or gluteus maximus muscle. A 21- to 23-gauge needle, 2.5 to 4 cm long, is used. A subcutaneous formulation of DMPA is also available and can be given in the anterior thigh or abdominal wall. DMPA is initiated during the first 5 days of the menstrual cycle and administered every 12 weeks or 3 months.

NURSING ALERT When administering an intramuscular injection of progestin (e.g., Depo-Provera), do not massage the site after the injection because this action can hasten the absorption and shorten the period of effectiveness.

Advantages of DMPA include a contraceptive effectiveness comparable to that of COCs, long-lasting effects, requirement of injections only four times a year. DMPA may be used by breastfeeding women, but how soon after the birth it is administered continues to be a controversial issue (Goldberg & Grimes, 2007). Side effects at the end of a year include decreased bone mineral density, weight gain, lipid changes, increased risk of venous thrombosis and thromboembolism, irregular vaginal spotting, decreased libido, and breast changes. Other disadvantages include a lack of protection against STIs (including HIV). A delay in return to fertility may be as long as 6 to 12 months after discontinuing DMPA (Goldberg & Grimes). Typical failure rate is 3% in the first year of use (Trussell, 2007).

NURSING ALERT Women who use DMPA may lose significant bone mineral density with increasing duration of use. This loss appears to be reversible with discontinuation of use. Whether DMPA use during adolescence or early adulthood will reduce peak bone mass and increase the risk of osteoporotic fracture in later life is unknown. DMPA should not be used as a long-term birth control method (e.g., longer than 2 years) unless other birth control methods are inadequate. Women at high risk for osteoporosis may not be good candidates for DMPA use. Counsel women who receive DMPA about calcium intake and exercise (Goldberg & Grimes, 2007).

Implantable progestins. Contraceptive implants consist of one or more nonbiodegradable flexible tubes or rods that are inserted under the skin of a woman's arm. These implants contain a progestin hormone and are effective for contraception for at least 3 years. They must be removed at the end of the recommended time.

Implanon is a single-rod implant that is FDA approved for use in the United States. Insertion and removal of the capsule are minor surgical procedures involving a local anesthetic, a small incision, and no sutures. The capsule is placed subdermally in the inner aspect of the nondominant upper arm. The progestin prevents some, but not all, ovulatory cycles and thickens cervical mucus. Other advantages include reversibility and long-term continuous contraception that is not related to frequency of coitus (Raymond, 2007). It can be implanted immediately postpartum in breastfeeding women without affecting lactation (Newberry, 2007). Irregular menstrual bleeding is the most common side effect. Less common side effects include headaches, nervousness, nausea, skin changes, and vertigo (Fischer, 2008). Implanon does not protect against STIs; thus condoms should be used for protection. Typical failure rates for the first year of use are 0.05% (Trussell, 2007).

Emergency contraception

Emergency contraception (EC) offers protection against pregnancy after intercourse occurs in instances such as broken condoms, sexual assault, dislodged cervical cap, disruption of use of any other method, or any other case of unprotected intercourse. Methods that are available in the United States that could provide postcoital contraception include:

- Ella (Ulipristal): single 30-mg pill containing an antiprogestin
- Plan B One-Step: single progestin-only pill containing 1.5 mg levonorgestrel
- Next Choice: two levonorgestrel 0.75-mg tablets taken orally 12 hours apart or both together
- Combined oral: estrogen-progestin contraceptive pills (e.g., 100-mcg ethinyl estradiol plus 0.5 mg levonorgestrel); two doses given 12 hours apart (Yuzpe regimen)
- Copper intrauterine device (IUD) insertion within 120 hours of intercourse

Plan B One-Step and Next Choice are approved by the FDA for over-the-counter sale to women ages 17 and older with proof of age. Adolescents 16 years and under require a prescription. Ella is available only with a prescription. States vary in the ability of pharmacists to dispense EC, and some states have implemented refusal legislation (Guttmacher Institute, 2012b).

In general, for the most effectiveness, EC should be taken by a woman as soon as possible but within 72 hours of unprotected intercourse or a birth control mishap (e.g., broken condom, dislodged ring or cervical cap, missed oral contraceptive pills, late for injection) to prevent unintended pregnancy (Fritz and Speroff, 2011a). Research has shown a moderate amount of effectiveness between 72 and 120 hours but no data are available for effectiveness after 120 hours (Trussell and Schwartz, 2011).

If taken before ovulation, EC prevents ovulation by inhibiting follicular development. If taken after ovulation occurs, there is little effect on ovarian hormone production or the endometrium. To minimize the side effect of nausea that occurs with high doses of estrogen and progestin (Yuzpe regimen), the woman can be advised to take an over-the-counter antiemetic 1 hour before each dose. Nausea is not as common with the Plan B (One-Step, Next Choice) regimen. Women with contraindications for estrogen use should use progestin-only EC. No medical contraindications for EC exist, except pregnancy and undiagnosed abnormal vaginal bleeding (Trussell and Schwarz, 2011). If the woman does not begin menstruation within 21 days after taking the pills, she should be evaluated for pregnancy (Trussell and Schwarz, 2011). EC is ineffective if the woman is pregnant since the pills do not disturb an implanted pregnancy. Risk of pregnancy is reduced by as much as 75% and 89% if the woman takes EC pills (Trussell and Schwarz, 2011).

TABLE 4-2

Oral Emergency Contraceptives

BRAND NAMES	FIRST DOSE*	SECOND DOSE (12 HR LATER)
PROGESTIN ONLY		
Plan B One-Step	1 white tablet	
Next Choice 2-dose regimen	1 white tablet	1 white tablet
ULIPRISTAL ACETATE		
Ella	1 white tablet	
COMBINED ORAL CONTRACEPTIVES		
Ogestrel	2 white tablets	2 white tablets
Cryselle	4 white tablets	4 white tablets
Jolessa	4 pink tablets	4 pink tablets
Portia	4 pink tablets	4 pink tablets
Seasonale	4 pink tablets	4 pink tablets
Lo/Ovral	4 white tablets	4 white tablets
Low-Ogestrel	4 white tablets	4 white tablets
Enpresse	4 orange tablets	4 orange tablets
Nordette	4 light orange tablets	4 light orange tablets
Levora	4 white tablets	4 white tablets
Quasense	4 white tablets	4 white tablets
Trivora	4 yellow tablets	4 yellow tablets
Seasonique	4 light blue-green tablets	4 light blue-green tablets
Lessina	5 pink tablets	5 pink tablets
Aviane	5 orange tablets	5 orange tablets
LoSeasonique	5 orange tablets	5 orange tablets
Syronx	5 white tablets	5 white tablets
Lutera	5 white tablets	5 white tablets
Lybel	6 yellow tablets	6 yellow tablets

*First dose should be taken as soon as possible after unprotected intercourse but within 120 hours.
†Antinausea medications needed for any of the combined oral contraceptives.
Sources: American College of Obstetricians and Gynecologists. (2010). Emergency contraception: ACOG Practice Bulletin No. 112. *Obstetrics and Gynecology, 115*(5), 1100-1109; Emergency Contraception. (2010). *Emergency contraception pills.* Available at http://ec.princeton.edu/questions/dose/html#dose. Accessed May 29, 2013; Trussell, J., & Schwarz, E. (2011). Emergency contraception. In R. Hatcher, J. Trussell, A. Nelson, W. Cates, F.D. Kowal, & M. Policar (Eds.). *Contraceptive technology* (20th rev. ed.). Atlanta, GA: Ardent Media.

NURSING ALERT Emergency contraception will not protect the woman against pregnancy if she engages in unprotected intercourse in the days or weeks that follow treatment. Because ingestion of ECPs may delay ovulation, caution the woman that she needs to establish a reliable form of birth control so as to prevent unintended pregnancy (Trussell & Schwarz, 2011). Information about emergency contraception method options and access to providers are available on the web at www.not-2-late.com or by calling 1-888-NOT-2-LATE.

IUDs containing copper (see later discussion) provide another emergency contraception option. The IUD should be inserted within 8 days of unprotected intercourse (Trussell & Schwarz, 2011). This method is only for women who wish to have the benefit of long-term contraception. The risk of pregnancy is reduced by as much as 99% with emergency insertion of the copper-releasing IUD.

Provide contraceptive counseling to all women requesting emergency contraception, including a discussion of modification of risky sexual behaviors to prevent STIs and unwanted pregnancy (Lever, 2005).

Intrauterine devices

An IUD is a small, T-shaped device with bendable arms for insertion through the cervix (Fig. 4-9). Once the trained health care provider inserts the IUD against the uterine fundus, the arms open near the uterine tubes to maintain position of the device and to adversely affect sperm motility and irritate the lining of the uterus. Two strings hang from the base of the stem through the cervix and protrude into the vagina for the woman to feel to assure that the device has not been dislodged (Grimes, 2007). The woman should have had a negative pregnancy test, treatment for dysplasia, cervical cultures to rule out STIs, and a consent form signed before IUD insertion. Advantages to choosing this method of contraception include long-term protection from pregnancy and immediate return to fertility when removed. Disadvantages include increased risk of pelvic inflammatory disease (PID) shortly after placement, unintentional expulsion of the device, infection, and possible uterine perforation. IUDs offer no protection against HIV or other STIs. Nulliparity is related to an increased risk for expulsion (Grimes).

Two IUDs have been approved by the FDA. The ParaGard T-380A (copper IUD) is made of radiopaque polyethylene and fine solid copper and is approved for 10 years of use. The copper serves primarily as a spermicide and inflames the endometrium, preventing fertilization (Grimes, 2007). Women sometimes experience more bleeding and cramping within the first year after insertion, but women can take nonsteroidal antiinflammatory drugs (NSAIDs) for pain relief. The typical failure rate in the first year of use of the copper IUD is approximately 0.8% (Trussell, 2007).

Mirena is a hormonal intrauterine system that releases levonorgestrel from its vertical reservoir. Effective for 5 years or more, it impairs sperm motility, irritates the lining of the uterus, and has some anovulatory effects (Grimes, 2007). Uterine cramping and uterine bleeding are usually improved with this device, although irregular spotting is common in the first few months after insertion. The typical failure rate in the first year of use is approximately 0.2% (Trussell, 2007).

Nursing considerations. Teach the woman to check for the presence of the IUD strings after menstruation to rule out expulsion of the device. If pregnancy occurs with the IUD in place, an ultrasound will confirm that it is not ectopic. Early removal of the IUD helps decrease the risk of spontaneous miscarriage or preterm labor. The woman should report any signs of influenza-like illness, which may indicate a septic miscarriage (Grimes, 2007). In some women who are allergic to copper, a rash develops, necessitating the removal of the copper-bearing IUD. Teach women the signs of potential complications listed in the Signs of Potential Complications box.

Sterilization

Sterilization refers to surgical procedures intended to render a person infertile and is the most commonly used method of contraception in the United States (Pollack, Thomas, & Barone, 2007). Most procedures involve the occlusion of the passageways for the ova and sperm (Fig. 4-10). For the woman, the uterine tubes are occluded; for the man, both of the vas deferens are occluded. Only surgical removal of the ovaries (oophorectomy) or the uterus (hysterectomy) or both will result in absolute sterility for the woman. Most other sterilization procedures have a less than 1% failure rate (Trussell, 2007).

Female sterilization. Female sterilization (bilateral tubal ligation [BTL]) (see Fig. 4-10, *A*) is usually performed immediately after childbirth (within 48 hours), concomitant with abortion, or as an interval procedure (during any phase of the menstrual cycle). Approximately one half of all female sterilization procedures in the United States are performed immediately after childbirth. If sterilization is performed as an interval procedure, the health

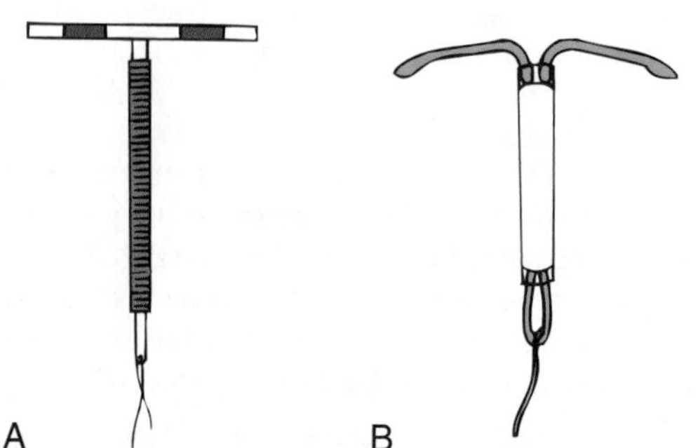

Fig. 4-9 Intrauterine devices (IUDs). **A,** Copper T-380A. **B,** Levonorgestrel-releasing IUD.

signs of POTENTIAL COMPLICATIONS

Intrauterine Devices

- Severe abdominal pain, pain with intercourse
- A late or missed period; abnormal spotting or bleeding
- Abnormal vaginal discharge
- Not feeling well, fever, or chills
- String missing, shorter or longer
- Presence of the device outside the cervix or in the vagina

EVIDENCE-BASED PRACTICE

An Ideal Solution: The Intrauterine Device

Pat Gingrich

ASK THE QUESTION

What are the advantages and disadvantages for women using the intrauterine device (IUD) for contraception? Which IUD is best?

SEARCH FOR EVIDENCE

Search Strategies: Professional organization guidelines, meta-analyses, systematic reviews, randomized controlled trials, nonrandomized prospective studies, and retrospective studies since 2006.

Search Databases: CINAHL, Cochrane, Medline, National Guideline Clearinghouse, TRIP Database and websites for Association of Women's Health, Obstetric, and Neonatal Nurses and Royal College of Obstetrics & Gynaecology.

CRITICALLY ANALYZE THE DATA

The IUD is a safe, cost-effective, highly reliable and reversible method of contraception. It may be an ideal option for many women, but it remains underused. Copper-covered IUDs have been the gold standard for decades, with the longest duration of action (approved for 10 years) and the most effectiveness (Kulier, Gülmezoglu, Hofmeyr, Cheng, & Campana, 2007). Although several designs are offered in Europe, the copper IUD approved for use in the United States is the CuT380A. Its mechanism of action is primarily by the prevention of fertilization. More recently the levonorgestrel intrauterine system (LNG-IUS), which delivers low levels of progestin, has become very popular both as a contraceptive and a treatment for heavy menstrual bleeding or severe dysmenorrhea (Royal College of Obstetrics & Gynaecology Faculty of Sexual and Reproductive Health Care, 2007). The action of the LNG-IUS is primarily through hormonally affecting the endometrium, preventing implantation. The LNG-IUS is approved for 5 years of use before it must be replaced.

The IUD can be recommended to women regardless of parity, age, or history of ectopic pregnancy or pelvic inflammatory disease. According to the guidelines of the Royal College of Obstetricians and Gynaecologists (2007), the copper IUD is the first choice for women with diabetes, breast cancer, and cardiovascular disease and those at risk for thrombophlebitis. The LNG-IUS is the best choice for women with anemia, thalassemia, sickle cell disease, or heavy bleeding. Insertion can occur anytime, as long as the woman is not pregnant.

The copper IUD is also recommended as an effective form of emergency contraception. Inserted shortly after unprotected intercourse, it works by preventing implantation. It can then be left in place to provide ongoing contraception (Cheng, Gülmezoglu, Piaggo, Ezcurra, & Van Look, 2008).

IMPLICATIONS FOR PRACTICE

For many women the IUD would be the ideal method of contraception throughout their childbearing years, but many women do not know much about it. Any doubts about its safety have been long dispelled. The IUD could benefit teens who have a notoriously difficult time with contraception. Either type of IUD can be inserted at 4 weeks postpartum and provides reversible contraception to aid with age spacing between children. At 40 years of age a woman can get a copper IUD, or at 45 she can get a LNG-IUS, which will then provide contraception for the woman through menopause. The nurse should counsel the woman about its mode of action and obtain a thorough health history. Women should know that a very small (2 out of 1000) risk exists of perforation on insertion. Having accurate, evidence-based information allows women to make the best choice of contraception for themselves and their families.

References:

Cheng, L., Gülmezoglu, A., Piaggo, G., Ezcurra, E., & Van Look, P. (2008). Interventions for emergency contraception. In *The Cochrane Database of Systematic Reviews 2008,* Issue 1. Art No. CD001324.

Kulier, R., O'Brien P., Helmerhorst, F., Usher-Patel, M., & d'Arcangues, C. (2007). Copper containing, framed intra-uterine devices for contraception. In *The Cochrane Database of Systematic Reviews 2007,* Issue 3. Art No. CD005347.

Royal College of Obstetrics & Gynaecology Faculty of Sexual and Reproductive Healthcare. (2007). *Clinical guidance: Intrauterine contraception.* Internet document available at www.fsrh.org/admin/uploads/CEUGuidanceIntrauterineContraceptionNov07.pdf (accessed June 9, 2009).

care provider must be certain that the woman is not pregnant (Pollack et al., 2007). Sterilization procedures can be safely performed on an outpatient basis.

Options for approach and occlusion methods. Two approaches for female sterilization are transabdominal and transcervical. A transabdominal procedure, the most common approach in the United States, is performed through a mini-laparotomy or laparoscopy. The mini-laparotomy is most commonly used after vaginal birth. The laparoscopic approach is the most common interval procedure and is performed on an outpatient basis. The transcervical approach uses hysteroscopic techniques.

Tubal occlusion methods include tubal ligation alone or combined with resection of the tubes, tubal electrocoagulation (bipolar cautery), the application of bands (Silastic: Fallope ring or Yoon Band) or clips (Hulka-Clemens spring clip or Filshie clip), and injection of occlusion devices into the tubes (Pollack et al., 2007).

For the mini-laparotomy or laparoscopic approach the woman takes nothing by mouth after midnight before the procedure. Preoperative sedation is given. The procedure may be carried out with a local anesthetic, regional, or general anesthetic. For the mini-laparoscopy, the provider makes a small incision in the abdominal wall below the umbilicus. Two small incisions are made if laparoscopy is used–a small one under the umbilicus for the laparoscope and one above the symphysis pubis to occlude or ligate the tubes. The woman may experience sensations of tugging but no pain, and the operation is completed within 20 minutes. She is often discharged several hours later after she has recovered from anesthesia if the procedure is performed on an outpatient basis and usually the next day if performed postpartum. Any abdominal discomfort usually can be controlled with a mild analgesic (e.g., acetaminophen). Within days the scar is almost invisible (see Patient Instructions for Self-Management box). As with any surgery, a possibility of complications of anesthesia, infection, hemorrhage, and trauma to other organs always exists.

Still considered experimental, hysteroscopic techniques are used to inject occlusion agents into the uterine tubes. One FDA-approved device is the Essure System, an interval sterilization method (not intended for the postpartum period). A trained health care professional inserts a small catheter holding the polyester fibers through the vagina and cervix and places the small metallic implants into each uterine tube. The device works by stimulating the woman's own scar tissue formation to occlude the uterine tubes and prevent conception (Pollack et al., 2007). Advantages include the nonhormonal nature of the contraception and the ability to insert the device during an office procedure without anesthesia. Analgesia is recommended to decrease mild to moderate discomfort associated with tubal spasm. Particularly convenient for obese women or those with abdominal adhesions, the transcervical approach eliminates the need for abdominal surgery. Because the procedure is not immediately effective, the woman and her partner must use another form of contraception until tubal blockage is proven (Theroux, 2008). Up to 3 months may be needed for tubal occlusion to occur fully, and a hysterosalpingogram will confirm success. Other disadvantages include expulsion and perforation. Typical failure rate during the first year of use of the Essure System is less than 1% (Essure, 2009). Long-term efficacy and safety rates are unknown (Pollack).

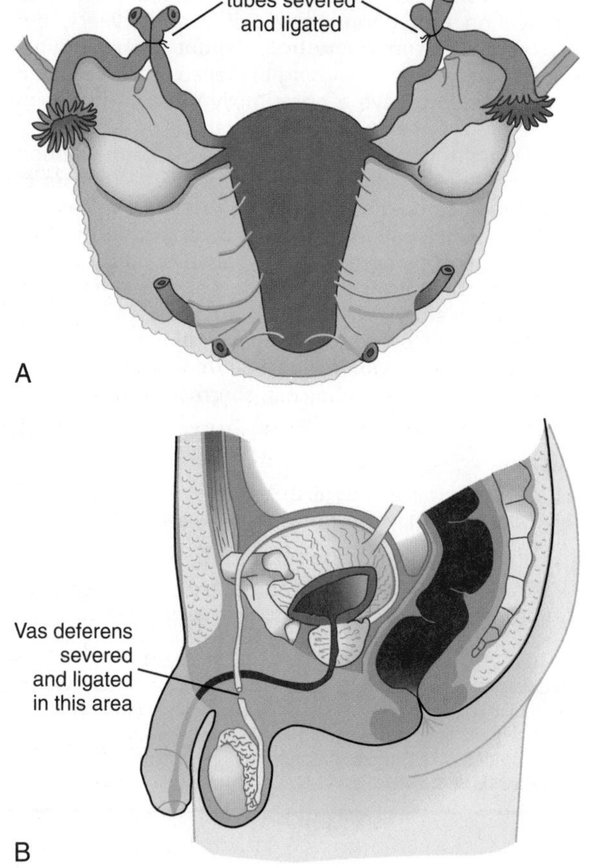

Fig. 4-10 Sterilization. **A,** Uterine tubes severed and ligated (tubal ligation). **B,** Sperm duct severed and ligated (vasectomy).

Tubal reconstruction. Restoration of tubal continuity (reanastomosis) and function is technically feasible except after laparoscopic tubal electrocoagulation. Sterilization reversal, however, is costly, difficult (requiring microsurgery), and uncertain. The success rate varies with the extent of tubal destruction and removal. The risk of ectopic pregnancy after tubal reanastomosis ranges from 1% to 7% (Pollack et al., 2007).

Male sterilization. Vasectomy is the sealing, tying, or cutting of each vas deferens so that the sperm cannot travel from the testes to the penis (FDA, 2009). It is considered the easiest and most commonly used operation for male sterilization. Vasectomy can be carried out with local anesthesia on an outpatient basis. Pain, bleeding, infection, and other postsurgical complications are the disadvantages to the surgical procedure (FDA). It is considered a permanent method of sterilization because reversal is generally unsuccessful.

Two methods are used for scrotal entry: conventional and no-scalpel vasectomy. The surgeon identifies and immobilizes the vas deferens through the scrotum. Then

PATIENT INSTRUCTIONS FOR SELF-MANAGEMENT

What to Expect after Tubal Ligation

- You should expect no change in hormones and their influence.
- Your menstrual period will be about the same as it was before the sterilization.
- You may feel pain at ovulation.
- The ovum disintegrates within the abdominal cavity.
- It is highly unlikely that you will become pregnant.
- You should not have a change in sexual functioning; you may enjoy sexual relations more because you will not be concerned about becoming pregnant.
- Sterilization offers no protection against sexually transmitted infections; therefore you may need to use condoms.

each vas is ligated or cauterized (see Fig. 4-10, *B*). Surgeons vary in their techniques to occlude the vas deferens: ligation with sutures, division, cautery, application of clips, excision of a segment of the vas, fascial interposition, or some combination of these methods (Pollack et al., 2007).

Postoperatively, instruct the man in self-care to promote a safe return to routine activities. To reduce swelling and relieve discomfort, the man should apply ice packs to the scrotum intermittently for a few hours after surgery. A scrotal support will decrease discomfort as well. Moderate inactivity for approximately 2 days is advisable because of local scrotal tenderness. Sexual intercourse may be resumed as desired; however, sterility is not immediate. Some sperm will remain in the proximal portions of the sperm ducts after vasectomy. Generally, several months are required to clear the ducts of sperm; therefore counsel men to use some form of contraception for 12 weeks. Semen analysis is also recommended (Pollack et al., 2007).

A vasectomy has no effect on potency (the ability to achieve and maintain erection) or volume of ejaculate. Endocrine production of testosterone continues so that secondary sex characteristics are not affected. Sperm production continues, but sperm are unable to leave the epididymis and are lysed by the immune system. Complications after vasectomy are uncommon and usually not serious. They include hematoma, bruising, wound infection, epididymitis, or adverse reaction to anesthetic agent (Pollack et al., 2007). Less common are painful granulomas from accumulation of sperm. Typical failure rate in the first year for male sterilization is 0.15% (Trussell, 2007).

Vasectomy reversal. Microsurgery to reanastomose (restore tubal continuity) the sperm ducts can be accomplished successfully (i.e., sperm in the ejaculate) in 75% to 100% of cases; however, the fertility rate is only approximately 38% to 89% (Pollack et al., 2007). The rate of success decreases as the time since the procedure increases.

Laws and regulations. All states have strict regulations for informed consent. Many states permit voluntary sterilization of any mature, rational woman without reference to her marital or pregnancy status. Although the law does not require the partner's consent, encourage the woman to discuss the situation with the partner, and health care providers may request the partner's consent. Most states restrict the sterilization of minors or mentally incompetent individuals and often require the approval of a board of eugenicists or other court-appointed individuals (see Legal Tip).

LEGAL TIP **Female Sterilization**

- If federal funds are used for sterilization, the person must be aged 21 years or older.
- Informed consent must include an explanation of the risks, benefits, and alternatives; a statement that describes sterilization as a permanent, irreversible method of birth control; and a statement that mandates a 30-day waiting period between giving consent and the sterilization.
- Informed consent must be in the person's native language, or a translator must be provided to read the consent form to the person.

Nursing considerations. Nurses play an important role in assisting people with decision making so that all requirements for informed consent are met. You will also provide information about alternatives to sterilization, such as contraception. Nurses act as a "sounding board" for people who are exploring the possibility of choosing sterilization and their feelings about and motivation for this choice. You record this information, which is often the basis for referral to a family-planning clinic, a psychiatric social worker, or another professional health care provider.

Give information about what occurs in various procedures, how much discomfort or pain to expect, and what type of care is needed. Many individuals fear sterilization procedures because of the imagined effect on their sex life. They need reassurance concerning the hormonal and psychologic basis for sexual function and that uterine tube occlusion or vasectomy has no biologic sequelae in terms of sexual adequacy (Pollack et al., 2007).

Preoperative care includes a health assessment, which includes a psychologic assessment, physical examination, and laboratory tests. The nurse assists with the health assessment, answers questions, and confirms the patient's understanding of printed instructions (e.g., nothing by mouth after midnight). Report ambivalence and extreme fear of the procedure to the physician.

Postoperative care depends on the procedure performed (e.g., laparoscopy, laparotomy, or vasectomy). General care includes recovery after anesthesia, vital signs, fluid and electrolyte balance (intake and output, laboratory values), prevention of or early identification and treatment for infection or hemorrhage, control of discomfort, and assessment of emotional response to the procedure and recovery.

Discharge planning depends on the type of procedure performed. In general, give the patient written instructions about observing for and reporting symptoms and signs of complications, the type of recovery to expect, and the date and time for a follow-up appointment.

Breastfeeding: Lactational amenorrhea method

The *Lactational Amenorrhea Method* (LAM) is a highly effective, temporary method of birth control. It is more popular in underdeveloped countries and traditional societies where breastfeeding is used to prolong birth intervals. The method has seen limited use in the United States because only approximately one half of new mothers initiate breastfeeding, and most American women do not establish breastfeeding patterns that provide maximal protection against pregnancy (Kennedy & Trussell, 2007).

When the infant suckles at the breast, the woman's body releases a surge of prolactin hormone, which inhibits estrogen production and suppresses ovulation and the return of menses. LAM works best if the mother is exclusively or almost exclusively breastfeeding, if the woman has not had a menstrual flow since giving birth, and if the infant is under 6 months of age. Frequent feedings at intervals of less than 4 hours during the day and no more than 6 hours during the night, long duration of each feeding, and no bottle supplementation or limited supplementation by spoon or cup enhance effectiveness. The typical failure rate is 2% (Kennedy & Trussell, 2007).

NURSING ALERT Counsel the woman that disruption of the breastfeeding pattern or supplementation can increase the risk of pregnancy.

Future trends

Contraceptive options are more limited in the United States and Canada than in some other industrialized countries. Lack of funding for research, governmental regulations, conflicting values about contraception, and low interest in contraceptive development by drug companies are obstacles to new and improved methods. Existing methods of contraception are being improved, however, and a variety of new methods are being developed.

Lower-dose COCs (15 mcg of ethinyl estradiol) are available in Europe. Female barrier methods (new female condoms, patient-fitted diaphragms and caps, and new vaginal sponges) are being tested. Vaginal hormonal methods including progestin-only vaginal rings and progesterone daily suppositories are under investigation. Researchers are also evaluating two new IUDs and spermicidal microbicides. Male hormonal methods also are being investigated, including hormonal injections (testosterone), gonadotropin-releasing hormone (GnRH) antagonists, antisperm compounds, immunologic methods, and contraceptive vaccines (Gabelnick, Schwartz, & Darrock, 2007).

INDUCED ABORTION

Induced abortion is the purposeful interruption of a pregnancy before 20 weeks of gestation. (Chapter 21 discusses spontaneous abortion [miscarriage].) Abortion that is requested by the woman is called an elective abortion. If the abortion is performed for reasons of maternal or fetal health or disease, the procedure is called a therapeutic abortion. Many factors contribute to a woman's decision to have an abortion. Indications include (1) preservation of the life or health of the mother, (2) genetic disorders of the fetus, (3) rape or incest, and (4) the pregnant woman's request. The control of birth, dealing as it does with human sexuality and the question of life and death, is one of the most emotional components of health care and has been a controversial social issue since the mid-twentieth century. Regulations exist to protect the mother from the complications of abortion.

Abortion is regulated in most countries, including the United States. Before 1970, legal abortion was not widely available in the United States. However, in January 1973 the U.S. Supreme Court set aside previous antiabortion laws and legalized abortion. This decision established a trimester approach to abortion. In the first trimester, abortion is permissible, the decision is between the woman and her health care provider, and a state has little right to interfere (Paul & Stewart, 2007). In the second trimester, abortion was left to the discretion of the individual states to regulate procedures as long as they are reasonably related to the woman's health. In the third trimester, abortions may be limited or even prohibited by state regulation unless the restriction interferes with the life or health of the pregnant woman (Paul & Stewart).

In 1992 the U.S. Supreme Court made another landmark ruling, this time allowing states to restrict early abortion services as long as the restrictions did not place an "undue burden" on the woman's ability to choose abortion. Since then, many bills have been introduced to limit access to and funds for women seeking abortion.

The laws for abortion in Canada have changed over the last 35 years as well. Before 1969, abortion was permitted only to save the life of the woman. Between 1969 and 1988 the laws became more liberal in interpretation of the health of the woman. In 1988 this law was struck down, and Canada is now one of the only countries in the world without abortion regulation. Abortion is available throughout pregnancy (Santoro, 2004).

LEGAL TIP **Induced Abortion**

Nurses need to know the laws regarding abortion in their state of practice before they offer abortion counseling or nursing care to a woman choosing an abortion. Many states enforce a mandatory delay or state-directed counseling before a woman may legally obtain an abortion.

Incidence

The reported number of abortions performed in the United States in 2005 was 1.2 million (Jones, Zolna, Henshaw, & Finer, 2008). Approximately 88% of all abortions are performed in the first trimester, with approximately 60% of these in the first 8 weeks after the last menstrual period. Most women who are having an elective abortion are Caucasian, younger than 24 years of age, and unmarried. More than 60% have had at least one previous live birth (Jones et al., 2008). In 2005, there were 97,254 abortions reportedly performed in Canada (Statistics Canada, 2008).

Decision to Have an Abortion

A woman who is deciding whether or not to have an abortion is often ambivalent. She needs information and an opportunity to discuss her feelings about pregnancy, abortion, and the impact of either choice on her future. She needs to make her decision without feeling coercion about her choice (Simmonds & Likis, 2005).

Nurses and other health care providers often struggle with the same values and moral convictions as those of the pregnant woman. Projecting your own conflicts and doubts on women who are already anxious and overly sensitive is relatively easy. Regardless of your personal views on abortion, when providing care to women seeking abortion, you have a responsibility to counsel women about their options or to make appropriate referrals (Simmonds & Likis, 2005).

The Association of Women's Health, Obstetric and Neonatal Nurses (AWHONN) (1999) continues to support a nurse's right to choose to participate in abortion procedures in keeping with his or her "personal, moral, ethical, or religious beliefs." AWHONN also advocates that "nurses have a professional obligation to inform their employers, at the time of employment, of any attitudes and beliefs that may interfere with essential job functions."

LEGAL TIP Refusal to Give Care Based on Moral, Religious, and Ethical Reasons

Nurses' rights and responsibilities related to abortion as described by AWHONN (1999) should be protected through institutional policies that are written to address how the institution will make "reasonable accommodations" for the nurse's moral or ethical beliefs and what the nurse should do to give notice in such situations to avoid patient abandonment. Nurses should know what policies are in place in their institutions and encourage such policies to be written if they are not available (The Joint Commission, 2009).

Critical Thinking/Clinical Decision Making

Abortion

Caroline is a 19-year-old college student who engaged in unprotected intercourse with her date after attending a party. She has missed a period and at the clinic today learns that she is approximately 9 weeks pregnant. She has requested an appointment for an abortion. She has many questions about the choices she has and what she can expect during the procedure and afterward. How should the nurse respond?

1. Evidence—Is evidence sufficient to draw conclusions about what response the nurse should give?
2. Assumptions—Describe underlying assumptions about the following issues:
   a. Physical response related to termination of pregnancy with vacuum aspiration
   b. Psychologic and emotional response
   c. Future childbearing
3. What implications and priorities for nursing care can be drawn at this time?
4. Does the evidence objectively support your conclusion?
5. Are there alternative perspectives to your conclusion?

First-Trimester Abortion

Methods for performing early abortion (less than 9 weeks of gestation) include surgical (aspiration) and medical methods (mifepristone with misoprostol and methotrexate with misoprostol).

Aspiration

Aspiration (vacuum or suction curettage) is the most common procedure in the first trimester (Strauss et al., 2007). Aspiration abortion is usually performed using local anesthesia in the physician's office, the clinic, or the hospital. The suction procedure for performing an early elective abortion (ideal time is 8 to 12 weeks since the last menstrual period) usually requires less than 5 minutes.

Preabortion procedures include history taking, clinical examination, and laboratory tests as needed (e.g., pregnancy test, Rho[D] determination, hematocrit). Mild oral or intravenous sedation is administered. A bimanual examination occurs before the procedure to assess uterine size and position. The provider inserts a speculum and anesthetizes the cervix with a local anesthetic agent. The cervix is dilated if necessary, and a cannula connected to suction is inserted into the uterine cavity. The products of conception are evacuated from the uterus (Paul & Stewart, 2007).

During the procedure the nurse or physician keeps the woman informed about what to expect next (e.g., menstrual-like cramping, sounds of the suction machine). The nurse assesses the woman's vital signs. The aspirated uterine contents must be carefully inspected to ascertain whether all fetal parts and adequate placental tissue have been evacuated. After the abortion the woman rests on the table until she is ready to stand. She then remains in the recovery area or waiting room for 1 to 3 hours for detection of excessive cramping or bleeding; she is then discharged.

Normally, bleeding after the operation is approximately the equivalent of a heavy menstrual period, and cramps are rarely severe. Excessive vaginal bleeding and infection, such as endometritis or salpingitis, are the most common complications of elective abortion. Retained products of conception are the primary cause of vaginal bleeding. Evacuation of the uterus, uterine massage, and administration of oxytocin or methylergonovine (Methergine) or both may be necessary. Prophylactic antibiotics to decrease the risk of infection are commonly prescribed (Paul & Stewart, 2007). Postabortion pain may be relieved with NSAIDs such as ibuprofen.

Postabortion instructions differ among health care providers (e.g., not using tampons for at least 3 days or for up to 3 weeks and resuming sexual intercourse within 1 week or 2 weeks). The woman may shower daily. Give instruc-

signs of POTENTIAL COMPLICATIONS

Induced Abortion

Call your health care provider if you have any of the following signs:

- Fever greater than 38° C (100.4° F)
- Chills
- Bleeding greater than two saturated pads in 2 hours or heavy bleeding lasting a few days
- Foul-smelling vaginal discharge
- Severe abdominal pain, cramping, or backache
- Abdominal tenderness (when pressure applied)
- No return of menstrual period within 6 weeks

Source: Paul, M., & Stewart, F. (2007). Abortion. In R. Hatcher et al. (Eds.), *Contraceptive technology* (19th ed.). New York: Ardent Media Inc.

tion to watch for excessive bleeding and other signs of complications (see Signs of Potential Complications box) and to avoid douches of any type. The woman can expect her menstrual period to resume 4 to 6 weeks from the day of the procedure. Offer information about the birth control method the woman prefers if this has not been done previously during the counseling interview that usually precedes the decision to have an abortion. Some methods, such as an IUD insertion, can be initiated immediately. Hormonal methods may be started immediately or within a week (Paul & Stewart, 2007). Strongly encourage the woman to return for her follow-up visit so that complications can be detected.

Medical abortion

Early medical abortion has been popular in Canada and Europe for more than 15 years, but it is a relatively new procedure in the United States. Medical abortions are available for use in the United States for up to 9 weeks after the last menstrual period. Methotrexate, misoprostol, and mifepristone are the drugs used in the current regimens to induce early abortion. All are considered safe and effective, with combined drugs being more effective than single agents (Kulier, Gülmezoglu, Hofmeyr, Cheng, & Compana, 2004). Approximately 13% of all reported abortion procedures in the United States in 2005 were medical procedures (Jones et al., 2008).

Methotrexate is a cytotoxic drug that causes early abortion by blocking folic acid in fetal cells so that they cannot divide. Misoprostol (Cytotec) is a prostaglandin analog that acts directly on the cervix to soften and dilate and on the uterine muscle to stimulate contractions. Mifepristone, formerly known as RU-486, was approved by the FDA in 2000. It works by binding to progesterone receptors and blocking the action of progesterone, which is necessary for maintaining pregnancy (National Abortion Federation [NAF], 2008; Paul & Stewart, 2007).

Methotrexate and misoprostol. Although no standard protocol has been established, methotrexate is given intramuscularly or orally in the clinic up to 7 weeks after the woman's last menstrual period. Vaginal placement of misoprostol by the woman at home follows in 3 to 7 days (NAF, 2008). The woman returns for a follow-up visit to confirm the abortion is complete. If it is not, the woman is offered an additional dose of misoprostol, or vacuum aspiration is performed if the woman prefers it. Further follow-up is scheduled if needed (Paul & Stewart, 2007).

Mifepristone and misoprostol. Mifepristone can be taken up to 8 weeks after the last menstrual period. The FDA-approved regimen is that the woman takes 600 mg of mifepristone orally; 48 hours later, she returns to the office and takes 400 mcg of misoprostol orally (unless abortion has already occurred and been confirmed). Two weeks after the administration of mifepristone the woman must return to the office for a clinical examination or ultrasound to confirm that the pregnancy has been terminated. If not, surgical abortion (aspiration) is needed (NAF, 2008).

An alternative regimen can be given up to 9 weeks after the last menstrual period and includes administration of 200 mg mifepristone orally followed by misoprostol 800 mcg vaginally in 6 to 72 hours. The woman can perform this vaginal insertion at home. Buccal administration by the woman is also an option. A follow-up visit to the office or clinic is needed to determine abortion outcome (NAF, 2008; Paul & Stewart, 2007).

With any medical abortion regimen, the woman will usually experience bleeding and cramping. Side effects of the medications include nausea, vomiting, diarrhea, headache, dizziness, fever, and chills. These side effects are attributed to misoprostol and usually subside in a few hours after administration. Mild analgesics (e.g., acetaminophen, ibuprofen) may be taken for pain relief (Paul & Stewart, 2007). Signs of complications should be reported immediately to the health care provider (see Signs of Potential Complications box on induced abortion). All women who are Rho(D) negative will receive Rho(D) immune globulin.

Second-Trimester Abortion

Second-trimester abortion is associated with more complications and costs than first-trimester abortion. Dilation and evacuation (D&E) accounts for almost all second-trimester procedures performed in the United States. Induction of uterine contractions with hypertonic solutions (e.g., saline, urea) injected directly into the uterus, and uterotonic agents (e.g., misoprostol, dinoprostone) account for only approximately 0.6% of all reported abortions (Strauss et al., 2007).

Dilation and evacuation

D&E can be performed at up to 20 weeks of gestation, although it is most commonly performed between 13 and

COMMUNITY ACTIVITY

Locate the facilities (freestanding and hospital based) that offer abortion counseling and procedures in your community. Describe the types of counseling offered. Are alternatives included in the counseling? Describe the types of procedures performed. Determine if follow-up care includes both physical and psychologic needs. Investigate the laws in your state related to informed consent and treatment of minors who request an abortion.

16 weeks of gestation (Paul & Stewart, 2007). The cervix requires more dilation because the products of conception are larger. Often, osmotic dilators (e.g., laminaria) are inserted several hours or several days before the procedure, or misoprostol is applied to the cervix. The procedure is similar to vaginal aspiration except a larger cannula is used and other instruments may be needed to remove the fetus and placenta. Nursing care includes monitoring vital signs, providing emotional support, administering analgesics, and using postoperative monitoring. All women who are Rho(D) negative will receive Rho(D) immune globulin. Disadvantages of D&E may include possible long-term harmful effects on the cervix (Paul & Stewart).

Nursing considerations. The woman will need help exploring the meaning of the various alternatives and consequences to herself and her significant others. A woman often has difficulty expressing her true feelings (e.g., what abortion means to her now and in the future and what support or regret her friends and peers may demonstrate). A calm, matter-of-fact approach on the part of the nurse is helpful (e.g., "Yes, I know you are pregnant. I am here to help. Let's talk about alternatives."). Listening to what the woman has to say and encouraging her to speak are essential. Neutral responses such as "Oh," "Uh-huh," and "Umm" and nonverbal encouragement such as nodding, maintaining eye contact, and use of touch are helpful in setting an open, accepting environment. Clarifying, restating, and reflecting statements, open-ended questions, and feedback are useful communication techniques that maintain a realistic focus on the situation and bring the woman's problems into the open. Once the woman has made a decision, she needs reassurance of continued support. You will need to give her information about various procedures, how much discomfort or pain to expect, and what type of care is necessary. You will also need to discuss the various feelings a woman might experience after the abortion, including depression, guilt, regret, and relief. Information about community resources for postabortion counseling is sometime necessary (Simmonds & Likis, 2005). If family or friends cannot be involved, scheduling time for nursing personnel to give the necessary support is an essential component of the care plan.

After the abortion, studies have indicated that most women report relief, but some have temporary distress or mixed emotions. Guilt and anxiety may occur more with young women, women with poor social support, multiparous women, and women with a history of psychiatric illness. Because symptoms can vary among women who have had abortions, assess women for grief reactions, and facilitate the grieving process through active listening and nonjudgmental support and care (Paul & Stewart, 2007).

Critical Thinking/Clinical Decision Making

Infertility

Diane is a 39-year-old accountant who has recently married for the first time. Charles is 41 and has two children from a previous marriage. Diane has a history of amenorrhea when she was in college and a member of the track team. Currently, her menstrual periods are irregular. Diane wants to have a baby "before it's too late," and she and Charles have been having unprotected sex for almost a year. They have come to the fertility clinic today for an evaluation. Diane tells the nurse that she has heard a lot about the success of in vitro fertilization (IVF) and wants to know if she will be able to have it performed. How should the nurse respond to Diane's comments and questions?

1. Evidence—Is evidence sufficient to draw conclusions about what response the nurse should give?
2. Assumptions—Describe underlying assumptions about the following issues:
   a. Age and fertility
   b. Infertility as a major life stressor
   c. Success rates for IVF pregnancy and birth
   d. Causes of female infertility
3. What implications and priorities for nursing care can be drawn at this time?
4. Does the evidence objectively support your conclusion?
5. Are there alternative perspectives to your conclusion?

INFERTILITY

Infertility is a serious medical concern that affects quality of life and is a problem for 10% to 15% of reproductive-age couples (American Society for Reproductive Medicine [ASRM], 2009a; Nelson & Marshall, 2007). The term *infertility* implies subfertility, a prolonged time to conceive, as opposed to *sterility*, which means the inability to conceive. Normally a fertile couple has approximately a 20% chance of conception in each ovulatory cycle. Primary infertility applies to a woman who has never been pregnant; secondary infertility applies to a woman who has been pregnant in the past.

The prevalence of infertility is relatively stable among the overall population but increases with the age of the woman, particularly in those older than 40 years (Lobo, 2007). Probable causes include the trend toward delaying pregnancy until later in life, when fertility decreases naturally and the prevalence of diseases such as endometriosis and ovulatory dysfunction increases. Some controversy has surfaced regarding whether an increase in male infertility has occurred or whether male infertility is easier to identify because of improvements in diagnosis.

Diagnosis and treatment of infertility require considerable physical, emotional, and financial investment over an extended period. Men and women often perceive infertility differently, with women having more stress from tests and treatments. The attitude, sensitivity, and caring nature of individuals who are involved in the assessment and treatment of infertility lay the foundation for patients' ability to cope with the many tests and treatments they must undergo.

Factors Associated with Infertility

Many factors, in both men and women, contribute to normal fertility. A normally developed reproductive tract in both the male and female partner is essential. Normal functioning of an intact hypothalamic-pituitary-gonadal axis supports gametogenesis–the formation of sperm and ova. Although sperm cells remain viable in the female's reproductive tract for 48 hours or more, probably only a few retain fertilization potential for more than 24 hours. Ova remain viable for approximately 24 hours, but the optimal time for fertilization may be no more than 1 to 2 hours (Cunningham, Leveno, Blooms, Hauth, Gilstrap, & Wenstrom, 2005); thus the timing of intercourse becomes critical.

After fertilization the conceptus must travel down the patent uterine tube to the uterus and implant within 7 to 10 days in a hormone-prepared endometrium. The conceptus must develop normally, reach viability, and be born in good condition for extrauterine life.

An alteration in one or more of these structures, functions, or processes results in some degree of impaired fertility. In general, approximately 20% of couples will have unexplained or idiopathic causes of infertility. Among the 80% of couples who have an identifiable cause of infertility, approximately 40% to 55% are related to factors in the female partner, 30% to 40% are related to factors in the male partner, and 15% to 20% are related to unexplained or unusual factors (Lobo, 2007; Nelson & Marshall, 2007). Boxes 4-3 and 4-4 list factors affecting female and male infertility.

BOX 4-3

Factors Affecting Female Fertility

OVARIAN FACTORS

- Developmental anomalies
- Anovulation, primary
- Pituitary or hypothalamic hormone disorder
- Adrenal gland disorder
- Congenital adrenal hyperplasia
- Anovulation, secondary
- Disruption of hypothalamic-pituitary-ovarian axis
- Amenorrhea after discontinuing oral contraceptive pills
- Premature ovarian failure
- Increased prolactin levels

UTERINE, TUBAL, AND PERITONEAL FACTORS

- Developmental anomalies
- Tubal motility reduced
- Inflammation within the tube
- Tubal adhesions
- Endometrial and myometrial tumors
- Asherman syndrome (uterine adhesions or scar tissue)
- Endometriosis
- Chronic cervicitis
- Hostile or inadequate cervical mucus

OTHER FACTORS

- Nutritional deficiencies (e.g., anemia)
- Thyroid dysfunction
- Idiopathic condition

CARE MANAGEMENT

Some of the data needed to investigate impaired fertility are of a sensitive, personal nature. Some patients view obtaining these data an invasion of privacy. The tests and examinations are occasionally painful and intrusive and can take the romance out of lovemaking. Patients require a high level of motivation to endure the investigation. Religious, cultural, and ethnic considerations are important factors because they may place restrictions on tests and treatments (Box 4-5).

Because multiple factors involving both partners are common, the investigation of impaired fertility is conducted systematically and simultaneously for both male and female partners. Both partners must be interested in the solution to the problem. The medical investigation requires time (3-4 months) and considerable financial expense, and it causes emotional distress and strain on the couple's interpersonal relationship (ASRM, 2009b) (see Nursing Process box: Infertility and Nursing Care Plan box).

Diagnosis

The basic infertility survey of the woman involves evaluation of the cervix, uterus, tubes, and peritoneum and documentation of ovulation. Diagnostic tests include serum progesterone concentration, urinary LH excretion, hysterosalpingography, transvaginal ultrasound examination, endometrial biopsy, and laparoscopy (Lobo, 2007; Nelson & Marshall, 2007; Speroff & Fritz, 2005). You can alleviate some of the anxiety associated with diagnostic testing by explaining to patients the timing and rationale for each test (Table 4-3). Box 4-6 summarizes test findings that are favorable to fertility.

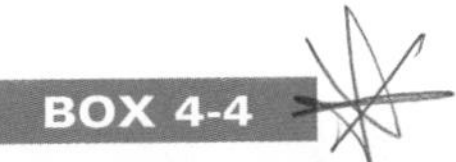

BOX 4-4

Factors Affecting Male Fertility

STRUCTURAL OR HORMONAL DISORDERS
- Undescended testes ✓
- Hypospadias
- Varicocele
- Obstructive lesions of the vas deferens or epididymis
- Low testosterone levels ✓
- Hypopituitarism
- Endocrine disorders
- Testicular damage caused by mumps
- Retrograde ejaculation

OTHER FACTORS
- Sexually transmitted infections
- Exposure to workplace hazards such as radiation or toxic substances
- Exposure of scrotum to high temperatures
- Nutritional deficiencies
- Antisperm antibodies
- Substance abuse
- Changes in sperm—cigarette smoke, heroin, marijuana, amyl nitrate, butyl nitrate, ethyl chloride, methaqualone
- Decrease in libido—heroin, methadone, selective serotonin reuptake inhibitors, and barbiturates
- Impotence—alcohol, antihypertensive medications
- Idiopathic condition

BOX 4-5

Religious and Cultural Considerations of Fertility

RELIGIOUS CONSIDERATIONS

Civil laws and religious proscriptions about sex must always be kept in mind by the health care provider.

Conservative and reform Jewish couples are accepting of most infertility treatment; however, the Orthodox Jewish husband and wife may face infertility investigation and management problems because of religious laws that govern marital relations. For example, according to Jewish law, the Orthodox couple may not engage in marital relations during menstruation and through the following 7 "preparatory days." The wife is then immersed in a ritual bath (mikvah) before relations can resume. Fertility problems can arise when the woman has a short cycle (i.e., a cycle of 24 days or fewer; when ovulation would occur on day 10 or earlier).

The Roman Catholic Church regards the embryo as a human being from the first moment of existence and regards as unacceptable technical procedures such as in vitro fertilization, therapeutic donor insemination, and freezing of embryos.

Other religious groups may have ethical concerns about infertility tests and treatments. For example, most Protestant denominations and Muslims usually support infertility management as long as in vitro fertilization (IVF) is performed with the husband's sperm, the number of fetuses is not reduced, and insemination is performed with the husband's sperm. These groups are less supportive of surrogacy and use of donor sperm and eggs. Christian Scientists do not permit surgical procedures or IVF but do permit insemination with husband and donor sperm.

Care providers should seek to understand the woman's spirituality and how it affects her perception of health care, especially in relation to infertility. Women may wish to seek infertility treatment but have questions about proposed diagnostic and therapeutic procedures because of religious proscriptions. Providers should encourage these women to consult their minister, rabbi, priest, or other spiritual leader for advice.

CULTURAL CONSIDERATIONS

Worldwide cultures continue to use symbols and rites that celebrate fertility. One fertility rite that persists today is the custom of throwing rice at the bride and groom. Other fertility symbols and rites include passing out of congratulatory cigars, candy, or pencils by a new father and baby showers held in anticipation of a child's birth.

In many cultures, the responsibility for infertility is usually attributed to the woman. A woman's inability to conceive may be a result of her sins, of evil spirits, or of the fact that she is an inadequate person. The virility of a man in some cultures remains in question until he demonstrates his ability to reproduce by having at least one child.

Source: D'Avanzo, C. (2008). *Mosby's pocket guide to cultural health assessment* (4th ed.). St. Louis: Mosby.

The basic test for male infertility is the **semen analysis.** A complete semen analysis, study of the effects of cervical mucus on sperm for motility and survival, and evaluation of the sperm's ability to penetrate an ovum provide basic information. Semen is collected by ejaculation into a clean container or a plastic sheath that does not contain a spermicidal agent. The specimen is usually collected by masturbation after 2 to 5 days of abstinence from ejaculation. The semen is taken to the laboratory in a sealed container within 2 hours of ejaculation. Avoid exposure to excessive heat or cold. Box 4-7 lists commonly accepted values based on the WHO criteria for semen characteristics. If results are in the fertile range, no further sperm evaluation is necessary. If not within this range, the test is repeated. If

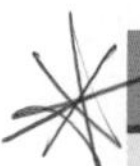

NURSING PROCESS *Infertility*

ASSESSMENT

Assessment of female infertility:

- Complete a history that includes duration of infertility, past obstetric events, a detailed menstrual and sexual history, medical and surgical conditions, exposure to reproductive hazards in the home and workplace, use of alcohol and other drugs, and emotional stresses
- A specific assessment of the reproductive tract follows a complete general physical examination.
- Obtain data from routine urine and blood tests along with results of other diagnostic tests (see text).

Assessment of male infertility:

- Complete a thorough history that includes nutritional deficiency; debilitating or chronic disease; trauma; exposure to environmental hazards such as radiation, heat, and toxic substances; use of tobacco, alcohol, and marijuana
- Complete a physical examination.
- Diagnostic assessment starts with noninvasive tests such as the semen analysis and ultrasound examination (see text).

NURSING DIAGNOSES

Examples of nursing diagnoses related to impaired fertility include the following:

- *Anxiety* related to:
  - Unknown outcome of diagnostic workup
- *Disturbed body image* or *situational low self-esteem* related to:
  - Impaired fertility
- *Risk for ineffective individual coping* related to:
  - Methods used in the investigation of impaired fertility
  - Alternatives to therapy: child-free living or adoption
- *Interrupted family processes* related to:
  - Unmet expectations for pregnancy
- *Acute pain* related to:
  - Effects of diagnostic tests (or surgery)
- *Ineffective sexuality patterns* related to:
  - Loss of libido secondary to medically imposed restrictions
- *Deficient knowledge* related to:
  - Preconception risk factors
  - Factors surrounding ovulation
  - Factors surrounding fertility

EXPECTED OUTCOMES OF CARE

Expected outcomes include that the couple will do the following:

- Verbalize understanding of the anatomy and physiology of the reproductive system.
- Verbalize understanding of treatment for any abnormalities identified through various tests and examinations (e.g., infections, blocked uterine tubes, sperm allergy, varicocele) and be able to make an informed decision about treatment.
- Verbalize understanding of their potential to conceive.
- Resolve guilt feelings and not need to focus blame.
- Conceive or, failing to conceive, decide on an alternative acceptable to both of them (e.g., child-free living, adoption).

PLAN OF CARE AND INTERVENTIONS

- Assist couples to express feelings about their infertility.
- Provide explanations or reinforcement or both about diagnostic tests and results of tests.
- Provide supportive care during diagnostic and treatment phases.
- Implement treatment interventions as ordered.
- Teach and encourage use of stress reducing activities.
- Provide information about community resources available.
- Refer for counseling or follow-up as needed.

EVALUATION

Evaluation of the effectiveness of care of the couple experiencing impaired fertility is based on the previously stated outcomes (see Nursing Care Plan).

results are still in the subfertile range, further evaluation is needed to identify the problem (Nelson & Marshall, 2007).

Other tests are performed as needed and include hormone analyses for testosterone, gonadotropin, FSH, and LH, the sperm penetration assay to evaluate the ability of sperm to penetrate an egg, and testicular biopsy (Nelson & Marshall, 2007).

The postcoital test (PCT) has been a traditional test for identifying cervical factor infertility, but evidence is lacking that the PCT is a valid clinical tool and thus is not necessary for most couples (Nelson & Marshall, 2007; Speroff & Fritz 2005).

Interventions

The management of patients with infertility problems includes psychosocial, nonmedical, medical, and surgical interventions. Assisted reproductive therapies may be indicated. Nursing interventions are an important aspect of care.

Psychosocial. Within the United States, feelings connected to impaired fertility are numerous and complex. The origins of some of these feelings are myths, superstitions, and misinformation about the causes of infertility. Other feelings arise from the need to undergo many tests and examinations and from being different from others.

Infertility is a major life stressor that can affect self-esteem and relations with the spouse, family, and friends, and careers. Couples often need assistance in separating their concepts of success and failure related to treatment for infertility from personal success and failure. Recognizing the significance of infertility as a loss and resolving these feelings are crucial to putting infertility into perspective, even if treatment is successful (Forbus, 2005; Paterno, 2008).

NURSING CARE PLAN Infertility

NURSING DIAGNOSIS Deficient knowledge related to lack of understanding of the reproductive process with regard to conception as evidenced by patient questions

Expected Outcome *Woman and partner will verbalize understanding of the components of the reproductive process, common problems leading to infertility, usual infertility testing, and the importance of completing testing in a timely manner.*

Nursing Interventions/*Rationales*

- Assess the woman's current level of understanding of the factors promoting conception *to identify gaps or misconceptions in her knowledge base.*
- Provide information in a supportive manner regarding factors promoting conception, including common factors leading to infertility of either partner, *to raise the woman's awareness and promote trust in her caregiver.*
- Identify and describe the basic infertility tests and the rationale for precise scheduling *to enhance completion of the diagnostic phase of the infertility workup.*

NURSING DIAGNOSIS Ineffective individual coping related to inability to conceive as evidenced by woman and partner statements

Expected Outcome *Woman and partner will identify situational stressors and positive coping methods to deal with testing and unknown outcomes.*

Nursing Interventions/*Rationales*

- Provide opportunities through therapeutic communication to discuss feelings and concerns *to identify common feelings and perceived stressors.*
- Evaluate the couple's support system, including support of each other during this process, *to identify any barriers to effective coping.*
- Identify support groups and refer as needed *to enhance coping by sharing experiences with other couples experiencing similar problems.*

NURSING DIAGNOSIS Hopelessness related to inability to conceive as evidenced by woman's and partner's statements

Expected Outcome *Woman and partner will verbalize a realistic plan to decrease feelings of hopelessness.*

Nursing Interventions/*Rationales*

- Provide support for the couple while grieving for the loss of fertility *to allow the couple to work through their feelings.*
- Assess for behaviors indicating possible depression, anger, and frustration *to prevent an impending crisis.*
- Refer to support groups *to promote a common bond with other couples during their expression of feelings and concerns.*

TABLE 4-3

General Tests for Impaired Fertility

TEST OR EXAMINATION	TIMING (MENSTRUAL CYCLE DAYS)	RATIONALE
Hysterosalpingogram (HSG) (uterine abnormalities, tubal patency)	7-10	Late follicular, early proliferative phase; will not disrupt a fertilized ovum; may open uterine tubes before time of ovulation
Chlamydia immunoglobulin G antibodies (tubal patency)	Variable	Negative antibody test may indicate tubal patency assessment (HSG); not needed in low risk women
Hysterosalpingo-contrast sonography (uterine abnormalities, tubal patency)	7-10	Late follicular, early proliferative phase; will not disrupt a fertilized ovum; evaluates tubal patency, uterine cavity, and myometrium
Serum progesterone (ovulation)	7 days before expected menses	Midluteal-phase progesterone levels; check adequacy of corpus luteum progesterone production
Assessment of cervical mucus (ovulation)	Variable, ovulation	Cervical mucus should have low viscosity, high spinnbarkeit (ability to stretch) during ovulation
Basal body temperature (ovulation)	Chart entire cycle	Elevation occurs in response to progesterone; documents ovulation
Urinary ovulation predictor kit (ovulation)	Variable, ovulation	Detects timing of lutein hormone surge before ovulation
Semen analysis (male factor)	2 to 7 days after abstinence	Detects ability of sperm to fertilize egg
Sperm penetration assay (male factor)	After 2 days but ≤1 wk of abstinence	Evaluation of ability of sperm to penetrate egg
Follicle-stimulating hormone (FSH) level (ovarian reserve)	Day 3	High FSH levels (>20) indicate that pregnancy will not occur with woman's own eggs; value <10 indicates adequate ovarian reserve
Clomiphene citrate challenge test (CCCT) (ovarian reserve)	Administer clomiphene 100 mg days 3 through 10	Assess FSH on days 3 and 10 in presence of clomiphene stimulation; high FSH levels (>20) indicate that pregnancy will not occur with woman's own eggs; FSH <15 suggestive of adequate ovarian reserve

BOX 4-6

Summary of Findings Favorable to Fertility

1. Follicular development, ovulation, and luteal development are supportive of pregnancy:
   a. Basal body temperature (BBT) (presumptive evidence of ovulatory cycles) is biphasic, with temperature elevation that persists for 12 to 14 days before menstruation.
   b. Cervical mucus characteristics change appropriately during phases of the menstrual cycle.
   c. Laparoscopic visualization of the pelvic organs verifies follicular and luteal development.
2. The luteal phase is supportive of pregnancy:
   a. Levels of plasma progesterone are adequate.
   b. Findings from endometrial biopsy samples are consistent with the day of the cycle.
3. Cervical factors are receptive to sperm during the expected time of ovulation:
   a. The cervical os is open.
   b. The cervical mucus is clear, watery, abundant, and slippery and demonstrates good spinnbarkeit and arborization (fern pattern).
   c. Cervical examination does not reveal lesions or infections.
   d. Postcoital test findings are satisfactory (adequate number of live, motile, normal sperm present in cervical mucus).
   e. No immunity to sperm is demonstrated.
4. The uterus and uterine tubes are supportive of pregnancy:
   a. Uterine and tubal patency are documented by:
      (1) Spillage of dye into the peritoneal cavity
      (2) Outlines of the uterine and tubal cavities that are of adequate size and shape, with no abnormalities
   b. Laparoscopic examination verifies the normal development of the internal genitals and the absence of adhesions, infections, endometriosis, and other lesions.
5. The male partner's reproductive structures are normal:
   a. No evidence of developmental anomalies of penis, testicular atrophy, or varicocele (varicose veins on the spermatic vein)
   b. No evidence of infection in prostate, seminal vesicles, and urethra
   c. Testes: 4 cm in the largest diameter
6. Semen is supportive of pregnancy:
   a. Sperm (number per milliliter) are adequate in ejaculate.
   b. Most sperm show normal morphologic features.
   c. Most sperm are motile, forward moving.
   d. No autoimmunity exists.
   e. Seminal fluid is normal.

Psychologic responses to a diagnosis of infertility may tax a couple's giving and receiving of physical and sexual closeness. The prescriptions and proscriptions for achieving conception may add tension to a couple's sexual functioning. Couples may report decreased desire for intercourse, orgasmic dysfunction, or midcycle erectile disorders.

BOX 4-7

Semen Analysis

- Semen volume at least 1.5 L
- Semen pH 7.2 or higher
- Sperm density greater than 15 million/mL
- Total sperm count greater than 39 million per ejaculate
- Normal morphologic features greater than 4% (normal oval)
- Motility (important consideration in sperm evaluation)—percentage of forward-moving sperm estimated with respect to abnormally motile and nonmotile sperm, 40%
- Liquification—usually within 15 minutes but no longer than 60 minutes

NOTE: These values are not absolute but are only relative to final evaluation of the couple as a single reproductive unit. Values also differ according to source used as a reference.

Source: World Health Organization (WHO): *Laboratory manual for the examination of human semen,* ed 5, Geneva, 2010, WHO.

To be able to deal comfortably with a couple's sexuality, you must be comfortable with your own sexuality so that you can better help couples understand why the private act of lovemaking must be shared with health care professionals. You need up-to-date factual knowledge about human sexual practices and must be able to accept the preferences and activities of others without being judgmental. You must be skilled in interviewing and in therapeutic use of self, sensitive to the nonverbal cues of others, and knowledgeable regarding each couple's sociocultural and religious beliefs.

Explore support systems of the couple with impaired fertility. This exploration should include persons available to assist, their relationship to the couple, their ages, their availability, and the cultural or religious support that is available. Mental health professionals experienced in infertility treatment also may be helpful to the couple (ASRM, 2009b).

If the couple conceives, you need to be aware that the concerns and problems of the previously infertile couple may not be over. Many couples are overjoyed with the pregnancy; however, some are not. Some couples rearrange their lives, sense of self, and personal goals within their acceptance of their infertile state. The couple may believe that those who worked with them to identify and treat impaired fertility expect them to be happy with the pregnancy. Some couples are shocked to find that they themselves feel resentment because the pregnancy, once a cherished dream, now necessitates another change in goals, aspirations, and identities. They may perceive the normal ambivalence toward pregnancy as a change from the original choice to become parents. The couple might choose to abort the pregnancy at this time. Other couples worry about miscarriage. If the couple wishes to continue with the pregnancy, they will need the care that other expectant couples need. In addition, a history of impaired fertility is considered to be a risk factor for pregnancy.

If the couple does not conceive, assess them regarding their desire to be referred for help with adoption, therapeutic intrauterine insemination, and other reproductive alternatives or with choosing a child-free state. The couple may find a list of agencies, support groups such as RESOLVE (www.resolve.org) and other resources in their community helpful.

Nonmedical. Simple changes in lifestyle may be effective in the treatment of subfertile men. Couples should use only water-soluble lubricants during intercourse because many commonly used lubricants contain spermicides or have spermicidal properties. Daily hot tub bathing or saunas can keep the testes at temperatures too high for efficient spermatogenesis.

Treatment is available for women who have immunologic reactions to sperm. The use of condoms during genital intercourse for 6 to 12 months will reduce female antibody production in most women who have elevated antisperm antibody titers. After the serum reaction subsides, condoms are used at all times except at the expected time of ovulation. Approximately one third of couples with this problem conceive by following this course of action.

Changes in nutrition and habits may increase fertility for both men and women. For example, a well-balanced diet, exercise, decreased alcohol intake, not smoking or abusing drugs, and stress management also are effective.

Herbal alternative measures. Most herbal remedies have not been proven clinically to promote fertility or to be safe in early pregnancy. Women should take these only when prescribed by a physician or nurse-midwife who has expertise in herbology. Relaxation, osteopathy, stress management (e.g., aromatherapy, yoga), and nutritional and exercise counseling have increased pregnancy rates in some women (Tiran & Mack, 2000). Herbal remedies that reportedly promote fertility in general include red clover flowers, nettle leaves, dong quai, St. John's wort, chasteberry, and false unicorn root (Dennehy, 2006; Weed, 1986). Vitamin C, calcium, and magnesium may promote fertility and conception (Tiran & Mack). Vitamins E and C, glutathione, and coenzyme Q10 are antioxidants that have proven beneficial effects for male infertility (Sheweita, Tilmisany, & Al-Sawaf, 2005). Herbs to avoid while trying to conceive include licorice root, yarrow, wormwood, ephedra, fennel, goldenseal, lavender, juniper, flaxseed, pennyroyal, passionflower, wild cherry, cascara, sage, thyme, and periwinkle (Sampey, Bourque, & Wren, 2004).

Medical. Pharmacologic therapy for female infertility is often directed at treating ovulatory dysfunction either by stimulating ovulation or by enhancing ovulation so that more oocytes mature. The most common medications include clomiphene citrate, human menopausal gonadotropin (hMG), FSH, human chorionic gonadotropin (hCG), and GnRH (Lobo, 2007; Nelson & Marshall, 2007). Metformin (an insulin sensitizing agent) is used for anovulatory cycling women who have polycystic ovarian disease. Bromocriptine is used to treat anovulation associated with hyperprolactinemia. Thyroid-stimulating hormone is indicated if the woman has hypothyroidism. Combined oral contraceptives, GnRH agonists, or danazol may be used to treat endometriosis; progesterone may be used to treat luteal phase defects. (ASRM, 2006b; Lobo; Nelson & Marshal). Table 4-4 describes common medications used for treating infertility.

Drug therapy may be indicated for male infertility. Problems with the thyroid or adrenal glands are corrected with appropriate medications. Infections are treated promptly with antimicrobials. FSH, hMG, and clomiphene are sometimes used to stimulate spermatogenesis in men with hypogonadism (Nelson & Marshall, 2007).

The primary care provider is responsible for informing patients fully about the prescribed medications. However, be ready to answer patients' questions and to confirm their understanding of the drug, its administration, potential side effects, and expected outcomes.

Surgical. Several surgical procedures treat problems that cause female infertility. Ovarian tumors must be excised. When possible, functional ovarian tissue is left intact. Scar tissue adhesions caused by chronic infections may cover much or all of the ovary. These adhesions usually necessitate surgery to free and expose the ovary so that ovulation can occur.

Hysterosalpingography (Fig. 4-11) is useful for the identification of tubal obstruction and for the release of blockage. During laparoscopy, delicate adhesions may be divided and removed, and endometrial implants may be destroyed by electrocoagulation or laser (Fig. 4-12). Laparotomy and even microsurgery is sometimes required to perform extensive repair of the damaged tube. Prognosis depends on the degree to which tubal patency and function can be restored.

Surgical removal of tumors or fibroids involving the endometrium or uterus often improves the woman's chance of conceiving and maintaining the pregnancy to viability. Surgical treatment of uterine tumors or maldevelopment that results in successful pregnancy usually requires birth by cesarean surgery near term gestation to prevent uterine rupture as a result of weakness of the area of surgical healing.

Surgical procedures are also used for problems that cause male infertility. Surgical repair of a varicocele (varicosity in the network of veins that drain the testicles) has been relatively successful in increasing sperm counts but not fertility rates.

Reproductive alternatives

Assisted reproductive therapies. Although remarkable developments have occurred in reproductive medicine, assisted reproductive therapies (ARTs) account for less than 1% of all U.S. births (Wright, Chang, Jeng,

TABLE 4-4

Selected Infertility Medications

DRUG	INDICATION	MECHANISM OF ACTION	DOSAGE	COMMON SIDE EFFECTS
Clomiphene citrate	Ovulation induction, treatment of luteal-phase inadequacy	Thought to bind to estrogen receptors in the pituitary, blocking them from detecting estrogen	Tablets, starting with 50 mg/day by mouth for 5 days beginning on fifth day of menses; if ovulation does not occur, may increase dose next cycle; variable dosage	Vasomotor flushes, abdominal discomfort, nausea and vomiting, breast tenderness, ovarian enlargement
Menotropins (human menopausal gonadotropins)	Ovarian follicular growth and maturation	LH and FSH in 1:1 ratio, direct stimulation of ovarian follicle; given sequentially with hCG to induce ovulation	IM injections; dosage regimen variable based on ovarian response Initial dose is 75 International Units of FSH and 75 International Units of LH (1 ampule) daily for 7-12 days followed by 10,000 International Units hCG	Ovarian enlargement, ovarian hyperstimulation, local irritation at injection site, multifetal gestations
Follitropins (purified FSH)	Treatment of polycystic ovarian disease; follicle stimulation for assisted reproductive techniques	Direct action on ovarian follicle	Subcutaneous or IM injections; dosage regimen variable	Ovarian enlargement, ovarian hyperstimulation, local irritation at injection site, multifetal gestations
Human chorionic gonadotropin (hCG)	Ovulation induction	Direct action on ovarian follicle to stimulate meiosis and rupture of the follicle	5000-10,000 International Units IM 1 day after last dose of menotropins; dosage regimen variable	Local irritation at injection site; headaches, irritability, edema, depression, fatigue

GnRH agonists (nafarelin acetate, leuprolide acetate)	Treatment of endometriosis, uterine fibroids	Desensitization and downward regulation of GnRH receptors of pituitary, resulting in suppression of LH, FSH, and ovarian function	Nafarelin, 200 mcg (1 spray) intranasally twice daily for 6 months; leuprolide acetate 3.75 mg IM every month for 3 to 6 months	Nafarelin—irritation, nosebleeds Both nafarelin and leuprolide— hot flashes, vaginal dryness, myalgia and arthralgia, headaches, mild bone loss (usually reversible within 12-18 months after treatment)
Progesterone	Treatment of luteal-phase inadequacy	Direct stimulation of endometrium	Vaginal gel 8%, 1 prefilled applicator per day; after ovulation induction, continue through 10-12 weeks of pregnancy	Breast tenderness, local irritation, headaches
GnRH antagonists (ganirelix acetate, cetrorelix acetate)	Controlled ovarian stimulation for infertility treatment	Suppress gonadotropin secretion, inhibit premature LH surges in women undergoing ovarian hyperstimulation	250 mcg daily subcutaneously, usually in the early to midfollicular phase of the menstrual cycle; usually followed by hCG administration	Abdominal pain, headache, vaginal bleeding, irritation at the injection site
Metformin	Restores cyclic ovulation and menses in many women with polycystic ovary disease	Induces ovulation through reducing insulin resistance, thus affecting gonadotropins and androgens; simulates the ovary	Initial dose is 500 mg and titrated up over several weeks to 1500 mg/day; administered orally	Nausea, vomiting, diarrhea, lactic acidosis, liver dysfunction
Letrozole	Ovulation induction	Aromatase inhibitor that inhibits E_2 production, which causes an increase in LH:FHS ratio	2.5- to 5-mg tablets administered orally for 5 days beginning on cycle day 3 to 5	Hot flashes, headaches, breast tenderness; may increase risk of congenital anomalies

Data from American Society for Reproductive Medicine (ASRM). (2012). *Medications for inducing ovulation: A patient guide.* www.asrm.org/Factsheetsandbooklets/; Facts and Comparisons. (2013). *A to Z drug facts.* www.factsandcomparisons.com; and Lobo, R. (2012). Infertility: Etiology, diagnostic evaluation, management, prognosis. In G. Lentz, R. Lobo, D. Gershenson, V. Katz. (Eds.). *Comprehensive gynecology.* (6th ed.). Philadelphia: Mosby.

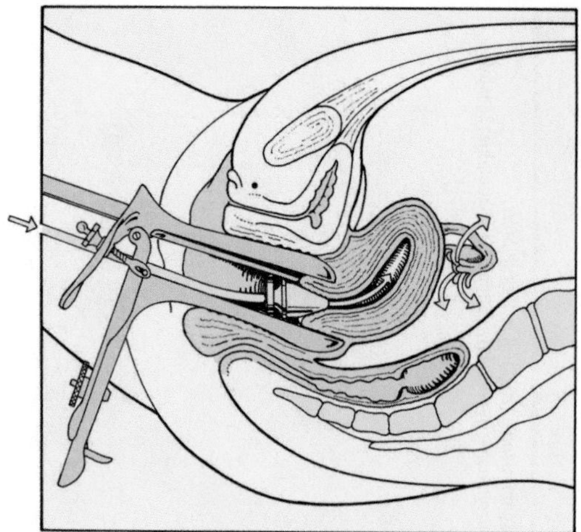

Fig. 4-11 Hysterosalpingography. Note that contrast medium flows through intrauterine cannula and out through the uterine tube.

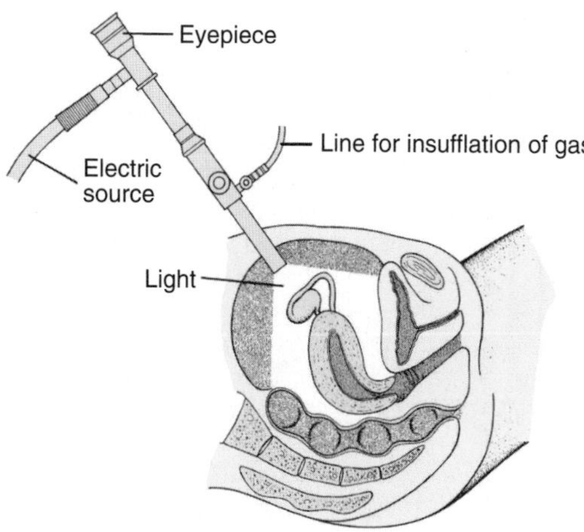

Fig. 4-12 Laparoscopy.

Macaluso, & CDC, 2008) and less than 3% of infertility treatment (ASRM, 2009a). They are associated with many ethical and legal issues (Box 4-8). The lack of information or misleading information about success rates and the risks and benefits of treatment alternatives prevents couples from making informed decisions. You can provide information so that couples have an accurate understanding of their chances for a successful pregnancy and live birth. In 2005 the success rate for pregnancy with ART transfer procedures was 42%, whereas the success rate for live births was 35% (Wright et al., 2008).

Some of the ARTs for treatment of infertility include in vitro fertilization procedures: in vitro fertilization-embryo transfer (IVF-ET), gamete intrafallopian transfer (GIFT) (Fig. 4-13), zygote intrafallopian transfer (ZIFT), ovum transfer (oocyte donation), embryo adoption, embryo hosting, surrogate mothering, **therapeutic donor insemination (TDI)**, intracytoplasmic sperm injection, and assisted hatching. Table 4-5 describes these procedures and the possible indications for the ARTs.

BOX 4-8

Issues to Be Addressed by Infertile Couples before Treatment

- Maximum embryos to be implanted
- Risks of multiple gestation
- Possible need for multifetal reduction
- Possible need for donor oocytes, sperm, or embryos or gestational carrier (surrogate mother)
- Freezing of embryos for later use
- Possible risks of long-term effects of medications and treatment on women, children, and families

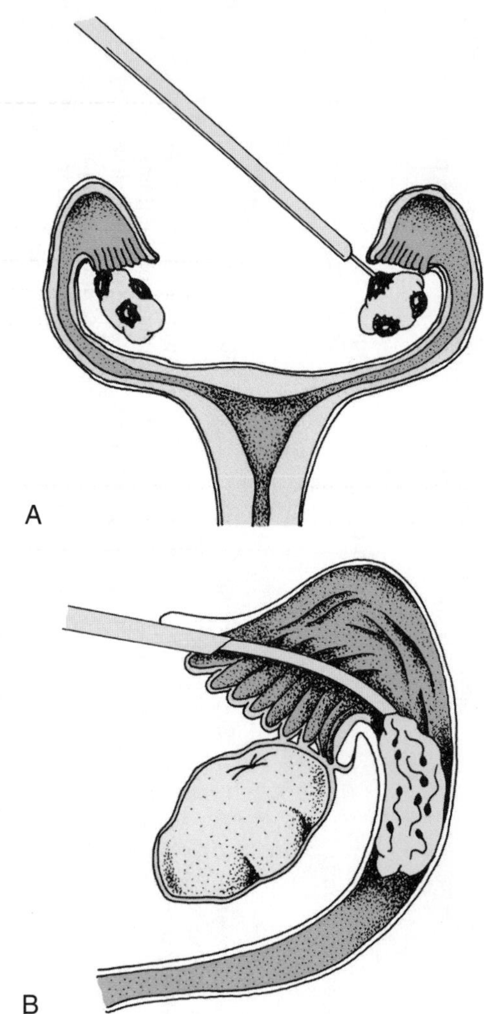

Fig. 4-13 Gamete intrafallopian transfer (GIFT). **A,** Through laparoscopy, a ripe follicle is located and fluid containing the egg is removed. **B,** The sperm and egg are placed separately in the uterine tube, where fertilization occurs.

LEGAL TIP **Cryopreservation of Human Embryos**

Couples who have excess embryos frozen for later transfer must be fully informed before consenting to the procedure to make decisions regarding the disposal of embryos in the event of (1) death, (2) divorce, or (3) the decision that the couple no longer wants the embryos at a later time.

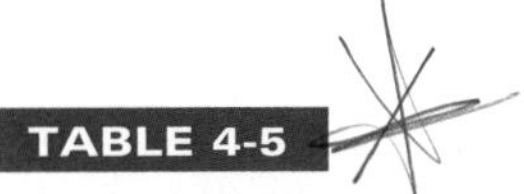

TABLE 4-5

Assisted Reproductive Therapies

PROCEDURE	DEFINITION	INDICATIONS
In vitro fertilization–embryo transfer (IVF-ET)	A woman's eggs are collected from her ovaries, fertilized in the laboratory with sperm, and transferred to her uterus after normal embryo development has occurred.	Tubal disease or blockage; severe male infertility; endometriosis; unexplained infertility; cervical factor; immunologic infertility
Gamete intrafallopian transfer (GIFT)	Oocytes are retrieved from the ovary, placed in a catheter with washed motile sperm, and immediately transferred into the fimbriated end of the uterine tube. Fertilization occurs in the uterine tube.	Same as for IVF-ET, except for the following: normal tubal anatomy, patency, and absence of previous tubal disease in at least one uterine tube
IVF-ET and GIFT with donor sperm	This process is the same as described above except in cases in which the male partner's fertility is severely compromised and donor sperm can be used; if donor sperm are used, the woman must have indications for IVF and GIFT.	Severe male infertility; azoospermia; indications for IVF-ET or GIFT
Zygote intrafallopian transfer (ZIFT)	This process is similar to IVF-ET; after in vitro fertilization the ova are placed in one uterine tube during the zygote stage.	Same as for GIFT
Donor oocyte	Eggs are donated by an IVF procedure, and the donated eggs are inseminated. The embryos are transferred into the recipient's uterus, which is hormonally prepared with estrogen/progesterone therapy.	Early menopause; surgical removal of ovaries; congenitally absent ovaries; autosomal or sex-linked disorders; lack of fertilization in repeated IVF attempts because of subtle oocyte abnormalities or defects in oocyte-spermatozoa interaction
Donor embryo (embryo adoption)	A donated embryo is transferred to the uterus of an infertile woman at the appropriate time (normal or induced) of the menstrual cycle.	Infertility not resolved by less-aggressive forms of therapy; absence of ovaries; male partner is azoospermic or is severely compromised
Gestational carrier (embryo host); surrogate mother	A couple undertakes an IVF cycle, and one or more embryos are transferred to the uterus of another woman (the carrier) who has contracted with the couple to carry the baby to term. The carrier has no genetic investment in the child. Surrogate motherhood is a process by which a woman is inseminated with semen from the infertile woman's partner and then carries the baby until birth.	Congenital absence or surgical removal of uterus; a reproductively impaired uterus, myomas, uterine adhesions, or other congenital abnormalities; a medical condition that might be life-threatening during pregnancy, such as diabetes, immunologic problems, or severe heart, kidney, or liver disease
Therapeutic donor insemination (TDI)	Donor sperm are used to inseminate the female partner.	Male partner is azoospermic or has a very low sperm count; couple has a genetic defect; male partner has antisperm antibodies
Intracytoplasmic sperm injection	Selection of one sperm cell that is injected directly into the egg to achieve fertilization. Used with IVF.	Same as TDI
Assisted hatching	The zona pellucida is penetrated chemically or manually to create an opening for the dividing embryo to hatch and implant into uterine wall.	Recurrent miscarriages; to improve implantation rate in women with previously unsuccessful IVF attempts; advanced age

Sources: American Society for Reproductive Medicine (ASRM). (2009a). *Frequently asked questions about infertility.* Internet document available at www.asrm.org (accessed Sept 12, 2009; Lobo, R. (2007). Infertility: Etiology, diagnostic evaluation, management, prognosis. In V. Katz, G. Lentz, R. Lobo, & D. Gershenson (Eds.), *Comprehensive gynecology* (5th ed.). Philadelphia: Mosby.

COMMUNITY ACTIVITY

Investigate any reproductive alternatives that are available in your community. Identify the methods used to diagnose infertility. Explore the psychologic, medical, and nonmedical treatments and modalities with a health care provider. Determine if support groups are available in the community. Describe the state Medicare program eligibility related to infertility. What options are available for adoption?

Complications. Other than the established risks associated with laparoscopy and general anesthesia, few risks are associated with IVF-ET, GIFT, and ZIFT. The more common transvaginal needle aspiration requires only local or intravenous analgesia. Congenital anomalies occur no more frequently than among naturally conceived embryos. Multiple gestations are more likely and are associated with increased risks for both the mother and infants (Wright et al., 2008). Ectopic pregnancies occur more often as well, and these carry a significant maternal risk. TDI causes no increase in maternal or perinatal complications; the same frequencies of anomalies (approximately 5%) and obstetric complications (between 5% and 10%) that accompany natural insemination (through sexual intercourse) apply also to TDI.

Preimplantation genetic diagnosis. Preimplantation genetic diagnosis (PGD) is a form of early genetic testing designed to identify embryos with serious genetic defects before implantation through one of the ARTs and to prevent couples from facing the risk of later termination of the pregnancy for genetic reasons. It can also improve conception chances using ART in couples with a poor prognosis. Couples need to be counseled about their options and choices, as well as the implications of their choices, when genetic analysis is considered (Kuliev, & Verlinsky, 2008).

Adoption. Some couples choose to build their family by adopting children who are not their own biologically. However, with increased availability of birth control and abortion and increasing numbers of single mothers keeping their babies, the adoption of Caucasian infants is extremely limited. Minority infants, infants with special needs, older children, and foreign adoptions are other options.

Couples who decide to adopt a child have decided that being a parent and having a child is more important than the actual process of birthing the child. The birth process is a small aspect of having a baby and becoming a parent. Sometimes so much emphasis is placed on being pregnant and having a child with one's own genetic makeup that the focus of the reason to have a child becomes cloudy. Adoption places importance on having and rearing the child. The question couples who are considering adoption need to answer is, "What is important to you–that you become parents or that you go through the experience of pregnancy and birth?" Nurses should have information on options for adoption available for couples or refer them to community resources for further assistance (ASRM, 2006a).

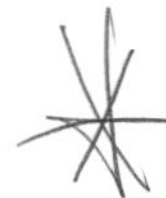

KEY POINTS

- A variety of contraceptive methods are available with various effectiveness rates, advantages, and disadvantages.
- Nurses need to help couples choose the contraceptive method or methods best suited to them.
- Effective contraceptives are available through both prescription and nonprescription sources.
- A variety of techniques are available to enhance the effectiveness of periodic abstinence in motivated couples that prefer this natural method.
- Hormonal contraception includes both precoital and postcoital prevention through various modalities and requires thorough patient education.
- Emergency contraceptive methods should be initiated as soon as possible after unprotected intercourse but no later than 120 hours.
- Barrier methods—diaphragm and cervical cap—provide safe and effective contraception for women or couples motivated to use them consistently and correctly.
- Proper use of latex condoms provides protection against STIs.
- Tubal ligations and vasectomies are permanent sterilization methods that have become two of the most widely used methods of contraception.
- Elective abortion performed in the first trimester is safer than an abortion performed in the second trimester.
- The most common complications of elective abortion include infection, retained products of conception, and excessive vaginal bleeding.
- Major psychologic sequelae of elective abortion are rare.
- Infertility is the inability to conceive and carry a child to term gestation at a time the couple has chosen to do so.
- Infertility affects between 10% and 15% of otherwise healthy adults. Infertility increases in women older than 40 years.
- In the United States, 80% of infertility has an identified cause related to factors involving the man and the woman, and 20% of infertility is related to unexplained causes.
- Common etiologic factors of infertility include decreased sperm production, ovulation disorders, tubal occlusion, and endometriosis.
- Reproductive alternatives for family building include IVF-ET, GIFT, ZIFT, oocyte donation, embryo donation, TDI, surrogate motherhood, and adoption.

Audio Chapter Summaries Access an audio summary of these Key Points on evolve

GIFT, Gamete intrafallopian transfer; *IVF-ET*, in vitro fertilization-embryo transfer; *TDI*, therapeutic donor insemination; *ZIFT*, zygote intrafallopian transfer.

References

American Society for Reproductive Medicine (ASRM). (2006a). *Adoption: A guide for patients.* Internet document available at www.asrm.org (accessed June 9, 2009).

American Society for Reproductive Medicine (ASRM). (2006b). *Medications for inducing ovulation: A patient guide.* Internet document available at www.asrm.org (accessed June 9, 2009).

American Society for Reproductive Medicine. (2009a). *Frequently asked questions about infertility.* Internet document available at www.asrm.org (accessed Sept 12, 2009).

American Society for Reproductive Medicine (ASRM). (2009b). *Frequently asked questions: The psychological component of infertility.* Internet document available at www.asrm.org (accessed June 9, 2009).

Association of Women's Health, Obstetric and Neonatal Nurses (AWHONN). (1999). *Nurses' rights and responsibilities related to abortion and sterilization. Policy position statement.* Internet document available at www. awhonn.org (accessed June 9, 2009).

Cates, W., & Raymond, E. (2007). Vaginal barriers and spermicides. In R. Hatcher, J. Trussell, A. Nelson, W. Cates, F. Stewart, & D. Kowal. (Eds.), *Contraceptive technology* (19th ed.). New York: Ardent Media.

Centers for Disease Control and Prevention. (2006). Sexually transmitted disease treatment guidelines, 2006. *Morbidity and Mortality Weekly Report, 55*(RR-11), 1-94.

Courtney, K. (2006). The contraceptive patch: Latest developments. *AWHONN Lifelines, 10*(3), 250-254.

Cunningham, F., Leveno, K., Blooms, S., Hauth, J., Gilstrap, L., & Wenstrom, K. (2005). *Williams obstetrics* (22nd ed.). New York: McGraw-Hill.

CycleBeads. (2007). *Frequently asked questions.* Internet document available at http://cyclebeads.com/ (accessed June 9, 2009).

Dennehy, C. (2006). The use of herbs and dietary supplements in gynecology: An evidenced-based review. *Journal of Midwifery & Women's Health, 51*(6), 402-409.

Essure. (2009). *Risks and benefits of the Essure procedure.* Internet document available at www.essure.com (accessed June 9, 2009).

Female Health Company. (2008). *Female condom: The product.* Internet document available at www.femalehealth.com/theproduct.html (accessed June 9, 2009).

Fehring, R., Schneider, M., Raviele, K., & Barron, M. (2007). Efficacy of cervical mucus observations plus electronic hormonal fertility monitoring as a method of natural family planning. *Journal of Obstetric, Gynecologic, and Neonatal Nursing, 36*(2), 152-160.

Fischer, M. (2008). Implanon: A new contraceptive implant. *Journal of Obstetric, Gynecologic, and Neonatal Nursing, 37*(3), 361-368.

Forbus, S. (2005). Age-related infertility: Tuning in to the ticking clock. *AWHONN Lifelines 9*(2), 127-132.

Gabelnick, H., Schwartz, J., & Darrock, J. (2007). Contraceptive research and development. In R. Hatcher et al. (Eds.), *Contraceptive technology* (19th ed.). New York: Ardent Media.

Germano, E., & Jennings, V. (2006). New approaches to fertility awareness-based methods: Incorporating the Standard Days and Two Day methods into practice. *Journal of Midwifery & Women's Health, 51*(5), 471-477.

Goldberg, A., & Grimes, D. (2007). Injectable contraceptives. In R. Hatcher et al. (Eds.), *Contraceptive technology* (19th ed.). New York: Ardent Media.

Grimes, D. (2007). Intrauterine devices (IUDs). In R. Hatcher et al. (Eds.), *Contraceptive technology* (19th ed.). New York: Ardent Media.

Guttmacher Institute: Emergency contraception. (2012). www.guttmacher.org/statecenter/spibs/spib_EC.pdf.

Jennings, V., & Arevalo, M. (2007). Fertility awareness-based methods. In R. Hatcher et al. (Eds.), *Contraceptive technology* (19th ed.). New York: Ardent Media.

Joint Commission. (2009). Human resources. In *Comprehensive accreditation manual for hospitals: The official handbook.* Oakbrook Terrace, IL: Joint Commission.

Jones, R., Zolna, M., Henshaw, S., & Finer, L. (2008). Abortion in the United States: Incidence and access to services, 2005. *Journal of Perspectives in Sexual and Reproductive Health, 40*(1), 6-16.

Kennedy, K., & Trussell, J. (2007). Postpartum contraception and lactation. In R. Hatcher et al. (Eds.), *Contraceptive technology* (19th ed.). New York: Ardent Media.

Kowal, D. (2007). Coitus interruptus (withdrawal). In R. Hatcher et al. (Eds.), *Contraceptive technology* (19th ed.). New York: Ardent Media.

Kulier, R., Gülmezoglu, M., Hofmeyr, G., Cheng, L., & Campana, A. (2004). Medical versus surgical methods for first trimester termination of pregnancy (Cochrane Review). In *The Cochrane Database of Systematic Reviews, 2004* Issue 1. Art No. CD002855.

Kuliev, A, & Verlinsky, Y. (2008). Preimplantation genetic diagnosis: Technological advances to improve accuracy and range of applications. *Reproductive Biomedicine Online, 16*(4), 532-538.

Lever, K. (2005). Emergency contraception: Nurses can empower women. *AWHONN Lifelines, 9*(3), 218-227.

Lobo, R. (2007). Infertility: Etiology, diagnostic evaluation, management, prognosis. In V. Katz, G. Lentz, R. Lobo, & D. Gershenson (Eds.), *Comprehensive gynecology* (5th ed.). Philadelphia: Mosby.

Marchbanks, P., McDonald, J., Wilson, H., Folger, S., Mandel, M., Daling, J., et al. (2002). Oral contraceptives and the risk of breast cancer. *New England Journal of Medicine, 346*(26), 2025-2032.

Nanda, K. (2007). Contraceptive patch and vaginal contraceptive ring. In R. Hatcher et al. (Eds.), *Contraceptive technology* (19th ed.). New York: Ardent Media.

National Abortion Federation. (2008). *Clinical policy guidelines.* Washington, DC: National Abortion Federation.

Nelson, A. (2007). Combined oral contraceptives. In R. Hatcher et al. (Eds.), *Contraceptive technology* (19th ed.). New York: Ardent Media.

Nelson, A., & Marshall, J. (2007). Impaired fertility. In R. Hatcher et al. (Eds.), *Contraceptive technology* (19th ed.). New York: Ardent Media.

Newberry, Y. (2007). Implanon: A new implantable contraceptive. *Nursing for Women's Health, 11*(6), 607-611.

Office of Population Research and Association of Reproductive Health Professionals. (2009). *Questions and answers about emergency contraception.* Internet document available at www.not-2-late.com (accessed Sept 12, 2009).

Paterno, M. (2008). Families of two: Meeting the needs of couples experiencing male infertility. *Nursing for Women's Health, 12*(4), 300-306.

Paul, M., & Stewart, F. (2007). Abortion. In R. Hatcher et al. (Eds.), *Contraceptive technology* (19th ed.). New York: Ardent Media.

Planned Parenthood. (2008). *Diaphragms.* Internet document available at www.plannedparenthood.org/health-topics/birth-control/diaphragm-4244.htm (accessed May 14, 2009).

Pollack, A., Thomas, L., & Barone, M. (2007). Female and male sterilization. In R. Hatcher et al. (Eds.), *Contraceptive technology* (19th ed.). New York: Ardent Media.

Raymond, E. (2007). Progestin-only pills. In R. Hatcher et al. (Eds.), *Contraceptive technology* (19th ed.). New York: Ardent Media.

Sampey, A., Bourque, J., & Wren, K. (2004). Learning scope: Herbal medicines. *Advance for Nurses*, *6*(25), 13-19.

Santoro, D. (2004). *A short summary of the criminal law surrounding abortion*. Internet document available at www.ncln.ca/articles.php?id=2&article=55 (accessed May 14, 2009).

Sheweita, S., Tilmisany, A., & Al-Sawaf, H. (2005). Mechanisms of male infertility: Role of antioxidants. *Current Drug Metabolism*, *6*(5), 495-501.

Simmonds, K., & Likis, F. (2005). Providing options: Counseling women with unwanted pregnancies. *Journal of Obstetric, Gynecologic, and Neonatal Nursing*, *34*(3), 373-379.

Speroff, L., & Fritz, M. (2005). *Clinical gynecologic endocrinology and infertility* (7th ed.). Philadelphia: Lippincott Williams & Wilkins.

Statistics Canada. (2008). *Induced abortions by province and territory of report*. Internet document available at www40.statcan.ca/l01/cst01/health40a-eng.htm (accessed May 14, 2009).

Strauss, L., Gamble, S. Parker, W., Cook, D., Zane, S., Hamdan, S., & Centers for Disease Control and Prevention (CDC). (2007). Abortion surveillance–United States, 2004. *Morbidity and Mortality Weekly Report, Surveillance Summary*, *56*(9), 1-33.

Theroux, T. (2008). The hysteroscopic approach to sterilization. *Journal of Obstetric, Gynecologic, and Neonatal Nursing*, *37*(3), 356-360.

Tiran, D., & Mack, S. (2000). *Complementary therapies for pregnancy and childbirth*. Edinburgh: Bailliere Tindall.

Trussell, J. (2007). Contraceptive efficacy. In R. Hatcher et al. (Eds.), *Contraceptive technology* (19th ed.). New York: Ardent Media.

Trussell, J., Schwarz, E. (2011). Emergency contraception. In R.A. Hatcher, J. Trussell, A.L. Nelson (Eds.). *Contraceptive technology*. Atlanta: Ardent Media.

U.S. Food and Drug Administration (FDA). (2009). *Birth control guide*. Internet document available at www.fda.gov/womens/healthinformation/birthcontrol.html (accessed June 9, 2009).

Warner, L., & Steiner M. (2007). Male condoms. In R. Hatcher et al. (Eds.), *Contraceptive technology* (19th ed.). New York: Ardent Media.

Weed, S. (1986). *Wise woman herbal for the childbearing years*. Woodstock, NY: Ash Tree Publishing.

World Health Organization (WHO) Department of Reproductive Health and Research. (2004). *Medical criteria for contraceptive use* (3rd ed.). Geneva: WHO.

Wright, V., Chang, J., Jeng, G., Macaluso, M., & CDC. (2008). Assisted reproductive technology surveillance–United States, 2005. *Morbidity and Mortality Weekly Report Surveillance Summaries*, *57*(5), 1-23.

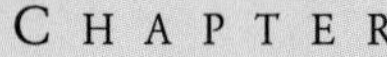
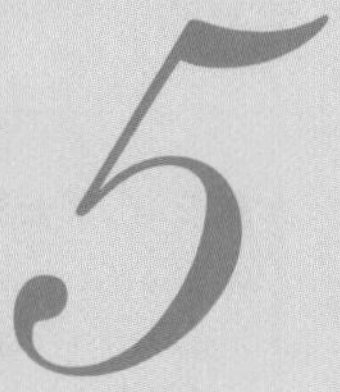
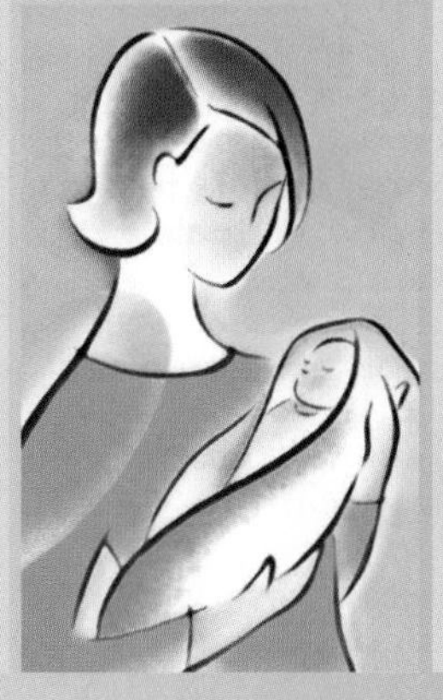

CHAPTER 5

Genetics, Conception, and Fetal Development

SHANNON E. PERRY

LEARNING OBJECTIVES

- *Explain the key concepts of basic human genetics.*
- *Discuss the purpose, key findings, and potential outcomes of the Human Genome Project.*
- *Describe expanded roles for nurses in genetics and genetic counseling.*
- *Examine the ethical dimensions of genetic screening.*
- *Discuss the current status of gene therapy (gene transfer).*
- *Summarize the process of fertilization.*
- *Describe the development, structure, and functions of the placenta.*
- *Describe the composition and functions of the amniotic fluid.*
- *Identify three organs or tissues arising from each of the three primary germ layers.*
- *Summarize the significant changes in growth and development of the embryo and fetus.*
- *Identify the potential effects of teratogens during vulnerable periods of embryonic and fetal development.*

KEY TERMS AND DEFINITIONS

blastocyst Stage in development of a mammalian embryo, occurring after the morula stage, that consists of an outer layer, or trophoblast, and a hollow sphere of cells enclosing a cavity

chorionic villi Tiny vascular protrusions on the chorionic surface that project into the maternal blood sinuses of the uterus and that help form the placenta and secrete human chorionic gonadotropin

chromosomes Elements within the cell nucleus carrying genes and composed of deoxyribonucleic acid (DNA) and proteins

conception Union of the sperm and ovum resulting in fertilization; formation of the one-celled zygote

decidua basalis Maternal aspect of the placenta made up of uterine blood vessels, endometrial stroma, and glands that shed in lochial discharge after birth

embryo Conceptus from day 15 of development until approximately the eighth week after conception

fertilization Union of an ovum and a sperm

fetal membranes Amnion and chorion surrounding the fetus

fetus Developing human in utero from approximately the ninth week after conception until birth

gamete Mature male or female germ cell; the mature sperm or ovum

genetics Study of single gene or gene sequences and their effects on living organisms

genome Complete copy of genetic material in an organism

genomics Study of the entire DNA structure of all of an organism's genes, including functions and interactions of genes

implantation Embedding of the fertilized ovum in the uterine mucosa; nidation

karyotype Schematic arrangements of the chromosomes within a cell to demonstrate their numbers and morphologic features

lanugo very fine hairs that appear first at 12 weeks and by 20 weeks cover the entire body of the fetus

meiosis Process by which germ cells divide and decrease their chromosomal numbers by one half

mitosis Process of somatic cell division in which a single cell divides, but both of the new cells have the same number of chromosomes as the first

monosomy Chromosomal aberration characterized by the absence of one chromosome from the normal diploid complement

KEY TERMS AND DEFINITIONS—cont'd

morula Developmental stage of the fertilized ovum characterized by a solid mass of cells resembling a mulberry

mosaicism Condition in which some somatic cells are normal, whereas others show chromosomal aberrations

nutrigenetics Study of the effect of genetic variations on diet and health with implications for susceptible subgroups

nutrigenomics Study of the effect of nutrients on health through alteration of genome, proteome, and metabolome and noting changes in physiologic features that result

pharmacogenetics/pharmacogenomics Study of inherited variations in drug metabolism and response

sex chromosomes Chromosomes associated with determination of sex: the X (female) and Y (male) chromosomes; the normal female having two X chromosomes and the normal male having one X and one Y chromosome

teratogens Environmental substances or exposures that result in functional or structural disability

vernix caseosa White, cheesy vernix caseosa, the material that protects the skin of the fetus

zygote Cell formed by the union of two reproductive cells or gametes; the fertilized ovum resulting from the union of a sperm and an ovum

WEB RESOURCES

Additional related content can be found on the companion website at evolve

http://evolve.elsevier.com/Lowdermilk/Maternity/

- NCLEX Review Questions
- Animation: Fertilization and Implantation
- Animation: First Trimester, Fetal Development
- Animation: Male Reproductive Ducts
- Animation: Male Accessory Sex Glands
- Animation: Male External Genitalia
- Animation: Maternal and Fetal Circulation
- Animation: Oogenesis and Meiosis
- Animation: Pathway of Ovum
- Animation: Pathway of Sperm
- Animation: Second Trimester, Fetal Development
- Animation: Spermatogenesis
- Animation: Spermatozoa
- Animation: Testes
- Animation: Third Trimester, Fetal Development
- Critical Thinking Exercise: Genetic Counseling
- Nursing Care Plan: The Family with an Infant Who Has Down Syndrome

This chapter presents a brief discussion of genetics and an overview of the process of fertilization and of the development of the normal embryo and fetus.

GENETICS

Genetics, the study of a single gene or gene sequences and their effects on living organisms, is a contributing factor in virtually all human illnesses. In maternity care, genetics issues occur before, during, and after pregnancy. With growing public interest in genetics, increasing commercial pressures, and web-based opportunities for individuals, families, and communities to participate in the direction and design of their genetic health care, genetic services are rapidly becoming an integral part of routine health care.

For most genetic conditions, therapeutic or preventive measures do not exist or are very limited. Consequently, the most useful means of reducing the incidence of these disorders is by preventing their transmission. It is standard practice to assess all pregnant women for heritable disorders to identify potential problems.

Genetic disorders affect people of all ages, from all socioeconomic levels, and from all racial and ethnic backgrounds. Genetic disorders affect not only individuals, but also families, communities, and society. Advances in genetic testing and genetically based treatments have altered the care provided to affected individuals. Improvements in diagnostic capability have resulted in earlier diagnosis and enabled individuals who previously would have died in childhood to survive into adulthood. The genetic aberrations that lead to disease are present at birth but may not develop clinically for many years, possibly never.

Some disorders appear more often in ethnic groups. Examples include Tay-Sachs disease in Ashkenazi Jews, French Canadians of the Eastern St. Lawrence River valley area of Quebec, Cajuns from Louisiana, and the Amish in Pennsylvania; beta thalassemia in Mediterranean, Middle Eastern, Transcaucasus, Central Asian, Indian, and Far Eastern groups, as well as those of African heritage; sickle cell anemia in African-Americans; alpha thalassemia in those from Southeast Asia, South China, the Philippine Islands, Thailand, Greece, and Cyprus; lactase deficiency in adult Chinese and Thailanders; neural tube defects in

Cultural Considerations

Parental Occupation, Hispanic Ethnicity, and Risk of Selected Congenital Malformations in Offspring

Brender, Suarez, and Langlois (2008) examined the effect of parental occupation of Hispanic parents on risk of birth defects in a case-control study among Texas births. A random sample of live births without congenital malformations served as a comparison group. The occupation of mothers as a cook or nurse was associated with oral clefts and neural tube defects among births to Hispanic mothers but not with births to non-Hispanic white mothers. Chromosomal anomalies, especially trisomy 18, were more common in offspring of Hispanic fathers who were electricians than in non-Hispanic white fathers. Risk estimates were different by Hispanic ethnicity for oral clefts and the father's occupation as electronic equipment operator, farm worker, janitor, police officer, and printer. Further study of risks is recommended with other Hispanic populations.

Source: Brender, J. D., Suarez, L., & Langlois, P. H. (2008). Parental occupation, Hispanic ethnicity, and risk of selected congenital malformations in offspring. *Ethnicity and Disease, 18*(2), 218-224.

Irish, Scots, and Welsh; phenylketonuria (PKU) in Irish, Scots, Scandinavians, Icelanders, and Polish; cystic fibrosis (CF) in Caucasians, Ashkenazi Jews, and Hispanics; and Niemann-Pick disease type A, in Ashkenazi Jews (Hamilton & Wynshaw-Boris, 2009; Solomon, Jack, & Feero, 2008) (Cultural Considerations box).

Genomics

Genomics addresses the functions and interactions of all the genes in an organism. It is the study of the entire DNA structure. New fields incorporating genomic knowledge are emerging, for example, **nutrigenetics,** the study of the effect of genetic variations on diet and health with implications for susceptible subgroups; **nutrigenomics,** the study of the effect of nutrients on health through alteration of **genome,** proteome, and metabolome and noting changes in physiology that result; and **pharmacogenetics/pharmacogenomics,** the study of inherited variations in drug metabolism and response to the drug. Genomic health care incorporates assessment, diagnosis, and treatment that use information about gene function. It is highly individualized because treatment options are based on the phenotypic responses of an individual. Genetic information includes personal data, as well as information about blood relatives.

Genetics and Nursing

Genetic disorders span every clinical practice specialty and site, including school, clinic, office, hospital, mental health agency, and community health settings. Because the potential impact on families and the community is significant (Box 5-1), genetic information, technology, and testing must be integrated into health care services, and genetics must be integrated into nursing education and practice.

BOX 5-1

Potential Impact of Genetic Disease on Family and Community

- Financial cost to family
- Decrease in planned family size
- Loss of geographic mobility
- Decreased opportunities for siblings
- Loss of family integrity
- Loss of career opportunities and job flexibility
- Social isolation
- Lifestyle alterations
- Reduction in contributions by families to their community
- Disruption of husband-wife or partner relationship
- Threatened family self-concept
- Coping with intolerant public attitudes
- Psychologic effects
- Stresses and uncertainty of treatment
- Physical health problems
- Loss of dreams and aspirations
- Cost to society of institutionalization or home or community care
- Cost to society because of additional problems and needs of other family members
- Cost of long-term care
- Housing and living arrangement changes

Source: Lashley, F. (2005). *Clinical genetics in nursing practice* (3rd ed.). New York: Springer.

Although diagnosis and treatment of genetic disorders requires medical skills, nurses with advanced preparation are assuming important roles in counseling people about genetically transmitted or genetically influenced conditions. Nurses with expertise in genetics and genomics function in many areas of maternity and women's health nursing. Examples include preconception counseling and preimplantation diagnosis for patients at risk for the transmission of a genetic disorder, prenatal screening and testing, prenatal care for women with psychiatric disorders that have a genetic component such as bipolar disorder and schizophrenia, newborn screening and testing, the care of families who have lost a fetus or a child affected by a genetic condition, the identification and care of children with genetic conditions and their families, and care of women with genetic conditions who require specialized care during pregnancy.

Nurses are usually the ones who provide follow-up care and maintain contact with the patients. Community health nurses can identify groups within populations that are at high risk for illness, as well as provide care to individuals, families, and groups. These nurses provide a vital link in follow-up for newborns who may need newborn screening (http://genes-r-us.uthscsa.edu).

Referral to appropriate agencies is an essential part of the follow-up management. Many organizations and foundations (e.g., the Cystic Fibrosis Foundation, the Muscular Dystrophy Association) help provide services and equipment for affected children. Numerous parent groups exist in which the family can share experiences and derive mutual support from other families with similar problems.

Probably the most important of all nursing functions is providing emotional support to the family during all aspects of the counseling process. Feelings that are generated under the real or imagined threat posed by a genetic disorder are as varied as the people being counseled. Responses may include a variety of stress reactions such as apathy, denial, anger, hostility, fear, embarrassment, grief, and loss of self-esteem.

In 2005 a panel of more than 50 nursing leaders from clinical, research, and academic settings developed and came to consensus on a document, "Essential Nursing Competencies and Curricula Guidelines for Genetics and Genomics." The competencies in the document reflect the minimal amount of genetic and genomic competency expected of all nurses. The competencies are not intended to replace or recreate current standards of practice. The document is available online at www.nursingworld.org/MainMenuCategories/EthicsStandards/Genetics_1.aspx. Examples of competencies in the professional practice domain include that the registered nurse:

- Demonstrates an understanding of the relationship of genetics and genomics to health, prevention, screening, diagnostics, prognostics, selection of treatment, and monitoring of treatment effectiveness
- Demonstrates ability to elicit a minimum of three-generation family health history information
- Constructs a pedigree from collected family history information using standardized symbols and terminology
- Collects personal, health, and developmental histories that consider genetic, environmental, and genomic influences and risks
- Assesses patients' knowledge, perceptions, and responses to genetic and genomic information
- Develops a plan of care that incorporates genetic and genomic assessment information

Genetics-related activities that all nurses should be able to provide are further delineated in *Genetics/Genomics Nursing: Scope and Standards of Practice* (2nd ed.) (International Society of Nurses in Genetics [ISONG] and American Nurses Association [ANA], 2006). This document includes standards and levels of practice for genetics nursing that were established cooperatively by ISONG and ANA. These activities are not limited to particular practice settings, nor are they limited to specific specialty areas.

Critical Thinking Exercise: Genetic Counseling

Genetic History-Taking and Genetic Counseling Services

Determining whether a heritable disorder exists in a couple or in anyone in either of their families is standard practice in obstetrics. The goal of screening is to detect or define risk for disease in low risk populations and identify those for whom diagnostic testing may be appropriate. Obtaining a complete three-generation medical history that includes ethnicity information is the best genetic "test" applicable to preconception care (Solomon Jack, & Feero, 2008). The U.S. Surgeon General Family History Initiative has posted My Family Health Portrait at https://familyhistory.hhs.gov/fhh-web/home.action. Nurses can recommend to their patients that they complete a family history using this website. In addition, nurses can obtain a genetic history using a questionnaire or a checklist such as the one in Fig. 5-1.

Individuals and families seek out, or are referred for, genetic counseling for a wide variety of reasons and at all stages of their lives. Some seek preconception or prenatal information; others are referred after the birth of a child with a birth defect or a suspected genetic condition; still others seek information because they have a family history of a genetic condition. Regardless of the setting or the individual and family's stage of life, genetic counseling should be offered and available to all individuals and families who have questions about genetics and their health.

Genetic counseling that follows may occur in the office, or referral to a geneticist may be necessary. The most efficient counseling services are associated with the larger universities and major medical centers. These facilities are also where support services are available (e.g., biochemistry and cytology laboratories), usually from a group of specialists under the leadership of a physician trained in medical genetics. Health professionals should become familiar with people who provide genetic counseling and the places that offer counseling services in their area of practice.

Estimation of risk

Most families with a history of genetic disease want an answer to the following question: What is the chance that our future children will have this disease? Because the answer to this question may have profound implications for individual family members and the family as a whole, health care professionals must be able to answer this question as accurately as they can in a timely manner.

If a couple has not yet had children, but they are known to be at risk for having children with a genetic disease, they will be given an *occurrence* risk. Once the mating of a couple has produced one or more children with a genetic disease, the couple will be given a *recurrence* risk. Both occurrence and recurrence risks are determined by the mode of inheritance for the genetic disease in question. For genetic diseases caused by a factor that segregates during cell division (genes and chromosomes), risk can be estimated with a high degree of accuracy by application of mendelian principles.

In an autosomal dominant disorder, both the occurrence and recurrence risk is 50%, or one in two, that a subsequent offspring will be affected. The recurrence

Risk Factors for Genetic Disorders

Answer the following questions about risk factors. If you answer "yes" to any of them, you may be at increased risk for having a baby with a genetic disorder.

_____Will you be age 35 years or older when your baby is due?

_____Will the baby's father be age 50 years or older when your baby is due?

_____If you or the baby's father are of Mediterranean or Asian descent, do either of you or does anyone in your families have thalassemia?

_____Is there a family history of neural tube defects?

_____Have you or the baby's father ever had a child with a neural tube defect?

_____Is there a family history of congenital heart defects?

_____Is there a family history of Down syndrome?

_____Have you or the baby's father ever had a child with Down syndrome?

_____If you or the baby's father are of Eastern European Jewish, French Canadian, or Cajun descent, is there a family history of Tay-Sachs disease?

_____If you or your partner are of Eastern European Jewish descent, is there a family history of Canavan disease or any other genetic disorders?

_____If you or your partner are African-American, is there a family history of sickle cell disease or sickle cell trait?

_____Is there a family history of hemophilia?

_____Is there a family history of muscular dystrophy?

_____Is there a family history of cystic fibrosis?

_____Is there a family history of Huntington's disease?

_____Does anyone in your family or the family of the baby's father have cystic fibrosis?

_____Is anyone in your family or the family of the baby's father's mentally retarded?

_____If so, was that person tested for fragile X syndrome?

_____Do you, the baby's father, anyone in your families, or any of your children have any other genetic diseases, chromosomal disorders, or birth defects?

_____Do you have a metabolic disorder such as diabetes or phenylketonuria?

_____Do you have a history of pregnancy issues (miscarriage or stillbirth)?

Fig. 5-1 Questionnaire for identifying couples having increased risk for offspring with genetic disorders. (Courtesy American College of Obstetricians and Gynecologists. [2010]. *Your pregnancy and childbirth month to month* [5th ed.]. Washington, DC: Author.)

risk for autosomal recessive disorders is 25%, or one in four. For X-linked disorders, recurrence is related to the child's sex. Translocation chromosomes have a high risk of recurrence.

The risk of recurrence for multifactorial conditions can be estimated empirically. An empiric risk is based not on genetics theory but rather on experience and observation of the disorder in other families. Recurrence risks are determined by applying the frequency of a similar disorder in other families to the case under consideration.

Disorders in which a subsequent pregnancy would carry no more risk than the risk for pregnancy alone (estimated at 1 in 30) include those resulting from isolated incidences not likely to be present in another pregnancy. These disorders include maternal infections (e.g., rubella, toxoplasmosis), maternal ingestion of drugs, most chromosomal abnormalities, and a disorder determined to be the result of a fresh mutation.

Interpretation of Risk

The guiding principle for genetics counselors is the principle of *nondirectiveness.* According to this principle, the individual who is providing genetic counseling respects the right of the individual or family being counseled to make autonomous decisions. Counselors using a nondirective approach avoid making recommendations, and they try to communicate genetics information in an unbiased manner. The first step in providing nondirective counseling is becoming aware of one's own values and beliefs. Another important step is recognizing how one's values and beliefs can influence or interfere with the communication of genetics information.

Counselors explain the risk estimates and provides appropriate information about the nature of the disorder, the extent of the risks in the specific case, the probable consequences, and (if appropriate) alternative options available. The final decision to become pregnant or to continue a pregnancy must be left to the family. An important nursing role is reinforcing the information the families are given and continuing to interpret this information at their level of understanding.

It must be emphasized to families is that *each pregnancy is an independent event.* For example, in monogenic disorders, in which the risk factor is one in four that the child will be affected, the risk remains the same no matter how many affected children are already in the family. Families may make the erroneous assumption that the presence of one affected child ensures that the next three will be free of the disorder. However, "chance has no memory." The risk is one in four for *each* pregnancy. On the other hand, in a family with a child who has a disorder with multifactorial causes, the risk increases with each subsequent child born with the disorder.

Ethical Considerations

Learning about conditions that might affect the pregnancy in the preconception period is ideal (Solomon et al., 2008). Individuals can then make informed reproductive decisions that might include adoption, surrogacy, or use of donor sperm. However, most genetic testing is offered prenatally so as to identify genetic disorders in fetuses (Wapner, Jenkins, & Khalek, 2009). When an affected fetus is identified, parents can be prepared for birth of such an infant. Termination of the pregnancy is also an option. Other requests for genetic testing occur for sex selection or for late-onset disorders. An ethic of social responsibility should guide genetic counselors in their interactions with patients while recognizing that people make their choices by integrating personal values and beliefs with their new knowledge of genetic risk and medical treatments.

Other ethical issues relate to autonomy, privacy, and confidentiality. Should genetic testing be performed when no treatment is available for the disease? When should family members at risk for inherited diseases be warned? When should presymptomatic testing be performed? Some who might benefit from genetic testing choose not to have it, fearing discrimination based on the risk of a genetic disorder. Several states have prohibitions against insurance discrimination; other states are expected to follow their lead. Until guidelines for genetic testing are created, caution should be exercised. The benefits of testing should be weighed carefully against the potential for harm. The American Academy of Pediatrics (2001) and the Canadian College of Medical Geneticists (2003) recommend against genetic testing of children for disorders that have a late-onset and for which no treatment exists.

Preimplantation genetic screening (PGS) is available in a limited number of centers. In this procedure, embryos are tested before implantation by in vitro fertilization (IVF) (Wapner et al., 2009). PGS has the potential to eliminate specific disorders in pregnancies conceived by IVF. Work is ongoing to test fetal cells and nucleic acid retrieved from the maternal blood samples as means of noninvasive prenatal diagnosis (Wapner et al.).

The Human Genome Project

The Human Genome Project was a publicly funded international effort coordinated by the National Institutes of Health (NIH) and the U.S. Department of Energy. Not only was the Human Genome Project responsible for a long list of amazing genetics discoveries, but it also stimulated and facilitated the work of thousands of scientists worldwide. Within 24 hours after a piece of DNA had been sequenced by Human Genome Project scientists the results were posted on a public database (www.ncbi.nlm.nih.gov/genome/guide/human); no restrictions on its use or redistribution have been enacted.

Two key findings from initial efforts to sequence and analyze the human genome are that (1) all human beings are 99.9% identical at the DNA level, and (2) approximately 30,000 to 40,000 genes (pieces or sequences of DNA that contain information needed to make proteins) make up the human genome (International Human Genome Sequencing Consortium, 2001). The finding that human beings are 99.9% identical at the DNA level should help to discourage the use of science as a justification for drawing precise racial boundaries around certain groups of people. The vast majority of the 0.1% genetic variations are found within and not among populations. The finding that humans have 30,000 to 40,000 genes, which is only twice as many as roundworms (18,000) and flies (13,000), was unexpected. Scientists had estimated the human genome contained 80,000 to 150,000 genes. The assumption was that humans are more evolved and more highly sophisticated than other species because they have more genes.

Initial efforts to sequence and analyze the human genome have proven invaluable in the identification of genes involved in disease and in the development of genetic tests. More than 100 genes involved in diseases such as Huntington disease (HD), breast cancer, colon cancer, Alzheimer disease, achondroplasia, and CF have been identified. Genetic tests for 1672 inherited conditions are commercially available; of these, 1379 are clinical tests and 293 are research tests (www.genetics.org).

Genetic testing

Genetic testing involves the analysis of human DNA, ribonucleic acid (RNA), **chromosomes** (threadlike packages of genes and other DNA in the nucleus of a cell), or proteins to detect abnormalities related to an inherited condition. Genetic tests can be used to examine directly the DNA and RNA that make up a gene (direct or molecular testing), look at markers that are coinherited with a gene that causes a genetic condition (linkage analysis), examine the protein products of genes (biochemical testing), or examine chromosomes (cytogenetic testing).

Most of the genetic tests now being offered in clinical practice are tests for single-gene disorders in patients with

EVIDENCE-BASED PRACTICE

Genetic Risk Assessment for Breast Cancer

Pat Gingrich

ASK THE QUESTION

Is genetic risk assessment for breast cancer beneficial for women? Now that women are able to determine if they have the BRCA1 or 2 mutations, what can they do with that information?

SEARCH FOR EVIDENCE

Search Strategies: Professional organization guidelines, meta-analyses, systematic reviews, randomized controlled trials, nonrandomized prospective studies, and retrospective studies since 2006.

Databases Searched: CINAHL, Cochrane, Medline, National Guideline Clearinghouse, Agency for Healthcare Research and Quality Database and websites for the Association of Women's Health, Obstetric, and Neonatal Nurses and the American Cancer Society.

CRITICALLY ANALYZE THE DATA

Women seeking a risk assessment for breast cancer now have a new and powerful tool: genetic testing. The BRCA1 mutation can predispose a woman to breast cancer, whereas the BRCA2 can increase the risk for breast or ovarian cancer or both. An accurate reflection of risks could lead to greater psychologic well-being and less worry. In a meta-analysis reported in the Cochrane database, women who received genetic risk assessment reported less distress, a more accurate perceived risk, and increased knowledge about breast cancer and genetics (Sivell, Iredale, Gray, & Coles, 2007).

Women with a high risk of breast or ovarian cancer have the choice of risk-reducing surgery or more frequent screening. A study of 517 women, cancer-free but positive for BRCA1 or BRCA2, found that women were more likely to have prophylactic mastectomy and oophorectomy if they have a close family history with breast or ovarian cancer (Metcalfe, Foulkes, Kim-Sing, Ainsworth, Rosen, Armel, et al., 2008). A smaller study of 272 female carriers of the gene noted that predictors for prophylactic surgery were age less than 60 years and previous history of breast or ovarian cancer and that most made their decision within a median of 4 months (Beattie, Crawford, Lin, Vittinghoff, & Ziegler, 2009).

Women who have already had breast cancer can now assess their risk for recurrence. In a study by the Hereditary Breast Cancer Clinical Study Group an international cohort of 927 women with hereditary breast cancer were much more likely to undergo prophylactic mastectomy in North America than in Europe (Metcalfe, Lubinski, Ghadirian, Lynch, Kim-Sing, Friedman, et al., 2008). Similarly, the same study revealed that older women and women who chose mastectomy over breast-conserving surgery at the time of original diagnosis were more likely to choose the prophylactic contralateral mastectomy.

IMPLICATIONS FOR PRACTICE

Women at risk for breast and ovarian cancer can have genetic risk assessments that can aid their decision making and improve their psychologic well-being. The regional differences in the decision for prophylactic mastectomy and oophorectomy may indicate a difference in medical opinion, cultural preference, or available medical care and expense. The role that age played in the decision-making process was unclear. Perhaps young women at high genetic risk might choose to screen frequently, nurse their children, and then undergo the risk-reducing surgery. Much more evidence and ethical guidance are needed to assist women in deciding if and when to be tested for the gene.

References:

Beattie, M. S., Crawford, B., Lin, F., Vittinghoff, E., & Ziegler, J. (2009). Uptake, time course, and predictors of risk-reducing surgeries in BRCA carriers. *Genetic Testing and Molecular Biomarkers, 13*(1), 51-56.

Metcalfe, K. A., Foulkes, W. D., Kim-Sing, C., Ainsworth, P., Rosen, B., Armel, S., et al. (2008). Family history as a predictor of uptake of cancer preventive procedures by women with a BRCA1 or BRCA2 mutation. *Clinical Genetics, 73*(5), 479-499.

Metcalfe, K. A., Lubinski, J., Ghadirian, P., Lynch, H., Kim-Sing, C., Friedman, E., et al. (2008). Predictors of contralateral prophylactic mastectomy in women with a BRCA1 or BRCA2 mutation: The Hereditary Breast Cancer Clinical Group Study Group. *Journal of Clinical Oncology, 26*(7), 1093-1097.

Sivell, S., Iredale, R., Gray, J., & Coles, B. (2007). Cancer genetic risk assessment for individuals at risk of familial cancer. In *The Cochrane Database of Systematic Reviews, 2007,* Issue 2, CD 003721.

clinical symptoms or who have a family history of a genetic disease. Some of these genetic tests are prenatal tests or tests used to identify the genetic status of a pregnancy at risk for a genetic condition. Current prenatal testing options include maternal serum screening (a blood test used to see if a pregnant woman is at increased risk for carrying a fetus with a neural tube defect or a chromosomal abnormality such as Down syndrome) and invasive procedures (amniocentesis and chorionic villus sampling) (see Chapter 19). Other tests are carrier screening tests, which are used to identify individuals who have a gene mutation for a genetic condition but do not show symptoms of the condition because it is a condition that is inherited in an autosomal recessive form (e.g., CF, sickle cell disease, and Tay-Sachs disease) (Peach & Hopkin, 2007).

Predictive testing is used to clarify the genetic status of asymptomatic family members. Predictive testing is presymptomatic or predispositional. In presymptomatic testing, if the gene mutation is present, symptoms are certain to appear if the individual lives long enough (e.g., HD). Predispositional testing differs from presymptomatic testing in that a positive result indicating that a mutation is present (e.g., BRCA-1) does not indicate a 100% risk of developing the condition (breast cancer).

In addition to using genetic tests to test for single-gene disorders, genetic tests are being used for population-based screening, for example, state-mandated newborn screening for PKU and other inborn errors of metabolism (IEMs), and for testing for common complex diseases such as cancer and cardiovascular conditions. Genetic tests also are being used to determine paternity, identify victims of war and other tragedies, and profile criminals.

Pharmacogenomics

One of the most immediate clinical applications of the Human Genome Project may be pharmacogenomics, or the use of genetic information to individualize drug therapy. There is speculation that pharmacogenomics may become part of standard practice for a large number of disorders and drugs by 2020. The expectation is that by identifying common variants in genes that are associated with the likelihood of a good or bad response to a specific drug, drug prescriptions can be individualized based on the individual's unique genetic makeup. A primary benefit of pharmacogenomics is the potential to reduce adverse drug reactions.

Gene therapy (gene transfer)

The aim of gene therapy is to correct defective genes that are responsible for disease development. The most common technique is to insert a normal gene in a location within the genome to replace a gene that is nonfunctional. In the early 1990s a great deal of optimism existed about the possibility of using genetic information to provide quick solutions to a long list of health problems. Although the early optimism about gene therapy was probably never fully justified, the development of safer and more effective methods for gene delivery will likely ensure a significant role for gene therapy in the treatment of some diseases. Major challenges include targeting the right gene to the right location in the right cells, expressing the transferred gene at the right time, and minimizing adverse reactions. No human gene therapy product has yet been approved by the U.S. Food and Drug Administration for sale. Current research includes treatment for inherited blindness, lung cancer tumors, melanoma, myeloid disorders, deafness, sickle cell disease, and other blood disorders.

Ethical, legal, and social implications

Because of widespread concern about misuse of the information gained through genetics research, 5% of the Human Genome Project budget was designated for the study of the Ethical, Legal, and Social Implications (ELSIs) of human genome research.

Two large ELSI programs were created to identify, analyze, and address the ELSIs of human genome research at the same time that the basic science issues were being studied. The two ELSI programs are separate but complementary. During the past decade, issues of high priority for these programs have been privacy and fairness in the use and interpretation of genetic information; clinical integration of new genetics technologies; issues surrounding genetics research, such as possible discrimination and stigmatization; and education for professionals and the general public about genetics, genetics health care, and ELSIs of human genome research. Both ELSI programs have excellent websites that include vast amounts of educational information, as well as links to other informative sites.

The ELSI programs address the potential that genetic information may be used to discriminate against individuals or for eugenic purposes. Informed consent is very difficult to ensure when some of the outcomes, benefits, and risks of genetic testing remain unknown. Some ethical considerations include: What is normal or a disability, and who decides? Do disabilities or diseases exist that need to be prevented or cured? Who will have access to these expensive therapies, and who will pay for them? Continued awareness of and vigilance against misuse of information is the collective responsibility of health care providers, ethicists, and society.

Factors Influencing the Decision to Undergo Genetic Testing

The decision to undergo genetic testing is seldom an autonomous decision based solely on the needs and preferences of the individual being tested. Instead, a decision is often based on feelings of responsibility and commitment to others. For example, a woman who is receiving treatment for breast cancer may undergo BRCA1/BRCA2 mutation testing not because she wants to find out if she carries a BRCA1 or BRCA2 mutation, but because her two unaffected sisters have asked her to be tested, and she feels a sense of responsibility and commitment to them. A female airline pilot with a family history of HD, who has no desire to find out if she has the gene mutation associated with HD, may undergo mutation analysis for HD because she believes she has an obligation to her family, her employer, and the people who fly with her.

Decisions about genetic testing are shaped, and in many instances constrained, by factors such as social norms, where care is received, and socioeconomic status. Most pregnant women in the United States now have at least one ultrasound examination, many undergo some type of multiple-marker screening, and a growing number undergo other types of prenatal testing. The range of prenatal testing options available to a pregnant woman and her family may vary significantly, based on where the pregnant woman receives prenatal care and her socioeconomic status. Certain types of prenatal testing may not be available in smaller communities and rural settings (e.g., chorionic villus sampling and FISH analysis [fluorescent in situ hybridization]). In addition, certain types of genetic testing may not be offered in conservative medical communities (e.g., preimplantation diagnosis). Some types of genetic testing are expensive and typically not covered by health insurance. Because of this, these tests may be available only to a relatively small number of individuals and families: those who can afford to pay for them.

Cultural and ethnic differences also have a significant impact on decisions about genetic testing. When prenatal diagnosis was first introduced, the principal constituency was a self-selected group of Caucasian, well-informed, middle to upper-class women. Today the widespread use of genetic testing has introduced prenatal testing to new groups of women, women who had not previously considered genetics services. The fact that many of the women currently undergoing prenatal testing may not share mainstream U.S. views about the role of medicine and prenatal care, the meaning of disability, or how to respond to scientific risks and uncertainties further amplifies the complexity of ethical issues associated with prenatal testing.

Critical Thinking/Clinical Decision Making

Ultrasound Dating of Pregnancy

Monica believes she is 8 weeks pregnant, but her midwife believes she is closer to 12 weeks of gestation. Monica has come to the clinic for an ultrasound examination for dating. She has many questions for the nurse: How can they tell the length of gestation? What would the fetus look like at this time if she is at 8 weeks of gestation? If she is at 12 weeks of gestation? What fetal structures would be apparent on ultrasound if she is 8 weeks pregnant? If she is 12 weeks pregnant? Would any structural anomalies be apparent at 8 weeks? At 12 weeks? Why is it important to date a pregnancy accurately?

What information should the nurse provide Monica?

1. Evidence—Is evidence sufficient to draw conclusions about what information the nurse should provide Monica?
2. Assumptions—What assumptions can be made about the following factors:
   a. Monica's motivation to learn about fetal development
   b. Monica's understanding of fetal development
   c. Monica's knowledge about ultrasound examinations
   d. Why dating the pregnancy is important
3. What implications and priorities for nursing care can be drawn at this time?
4. Does the evidence objectively support your conclusion?
5. Are there alternative perspectives to your conclusion?

Clinical Genetics

Genetic transmission

Human development is a complicated process that depends on the systematic unraveling of instructions found in the genetic material of the egg and the sperm. Development from conception to birth of a normal, healthy baby occurs without incident in most cases; occasionally, however, some anomaly in the genetic code of the embryo creates a birth defect or disorder. The science of genetics seeks to explain the underlying causes of congenital disorders (disorders present at birth) and the patterns in which inherited disorders are passed from generation to generation.

Genes and Chromosomes

The hereditary material carried in the nucleus of each somatic (body) cell determines an individual's physical characteristics. This material–DNA–forms threadlike strands known as **chromosomes.** Each chromosome is composed of many smaller segments of DNA referred to as *genes.* Genes or combinations of genes contain coded information that determines an individual's unique characteristics. The code consists of the specific linear order of the molecules that combine to form the strands of DNA. Genes never act in isolation; they always interact with other genes and the environment.

All normal human somatic cells contain 46 chromosomes arranged as 23 pairs of homologous (matched) chromosomes; one chromosome of each pair is inherited from each parent. There are 22 pairs of autosomes, which control most traits in the body, and one pair of **sex chromosomes,** which determines sex and some other traits. The large female chromosome is called the X; the tiny male chromosome is the Y. When one X chromosome and one Y chromosome are present, the embryo develops as a male. When two X chromosomes are present, the embryo develops as a female.

Homologous chromosomes (except the X and Y chromosomes in males) have the same number and arrangement of genes. In other words, if an autosome has a gene for hair color, its partner also has a gene for hair color–in the same location on the chromosome. Although both genes code for hair color, they may not code for the same hair color. Genes at corresponding loci on homologous chromosomes that code for different forms or variations of the same trait are called *alleles*. An individual with two copies of the same allele for a given trait is *homozygous* for that trait. With two different alleles, the person is *heterozygous* for the trait.

The term *genotype* is typically used to refer to the genetic makeup of an individual when discussing a specific gene pair, but at times, genotype is used to refer to an individual's entire genetic makeup or all the genes that the individual can pass on to future generations. *Phenotype* refers to the observable expression of an individual's genotype, such as physical features, a biochemical or molecular trait, and even a psychologic trait. A trait or disorder is considered *dominant* if it is expressed or phenotypically apparent when only one copy of the gene is present. It is considered *recessive* if it is expressed only when two copies of the gene are present.

Chromosomal Abnormalities

The incidence of chromosomal aberrations is estimated to be 0.6% in newborns. Approximately 62% of miscarriages and 10% of stillbirths and perinatal deaths are caused by chromosomal abnormalities (Hamilton & Wynshaw-Boris, 2009). Errors resulting in chromosomal abnormalities can occur in mitosis or meiosis. These errors occur in either the autosomes or the sex chromosomes. Even without the presence of obvious structural malformations, small deviations in chromosomes can cause problems in fetal development.

The pictorial analysis of the number, form, and size of an individual's chromosomes is known as a **karyotype**. Cells from any nucleated, replicating body tissue (except red blood cells, nerves, or muscles) can be used. The most commonly used tissues are white blood cells and fetal cells in amniotic fluid. The cells are grown in a culture and arrested when they are in metaphase, and then the cells are dropped onto a slide. This process breaks the cell membranes and spreads the chromosomes, making them easier to visualize. The cells are stained with special stains (e.g., Giemsa stain) that create striping or "banding" patterns. These patterns aid in the analysis because they are consistent from person to person. Once the chromosome spreads are photographed or scanned by a computer, they are cut out and arranged in a specific numeric order according to their length and shape. The chromosomes are numbered from largest to smallest, 1 to 22, and the sex chromosomes are designated by the letter X or Y. Each chromosome is divided into two "arms" designated by p (short arm) and q (long arm). A female karyotype is designated as 46, XX and a male karyotype is designated as 46, XY. Fig. 5-2 illustrates the chromosomes in a body cell and a karyotype. Karyotypes can be used to determine the sex of a child and the presence of any gross chromosomal abnormalities.

Autosomal abnormalities

Autosomal abnormalities involve differences in the number or structure of autosomal chromosomes (pairs 1-22) resulting from unequal distribution of the genetic material during **gamete** (egg and sperm) formation.

Abnormalities of chromosome number. Euploidy denotes the correct number of chromosomes. Deviations from the correct number of chromosomes or

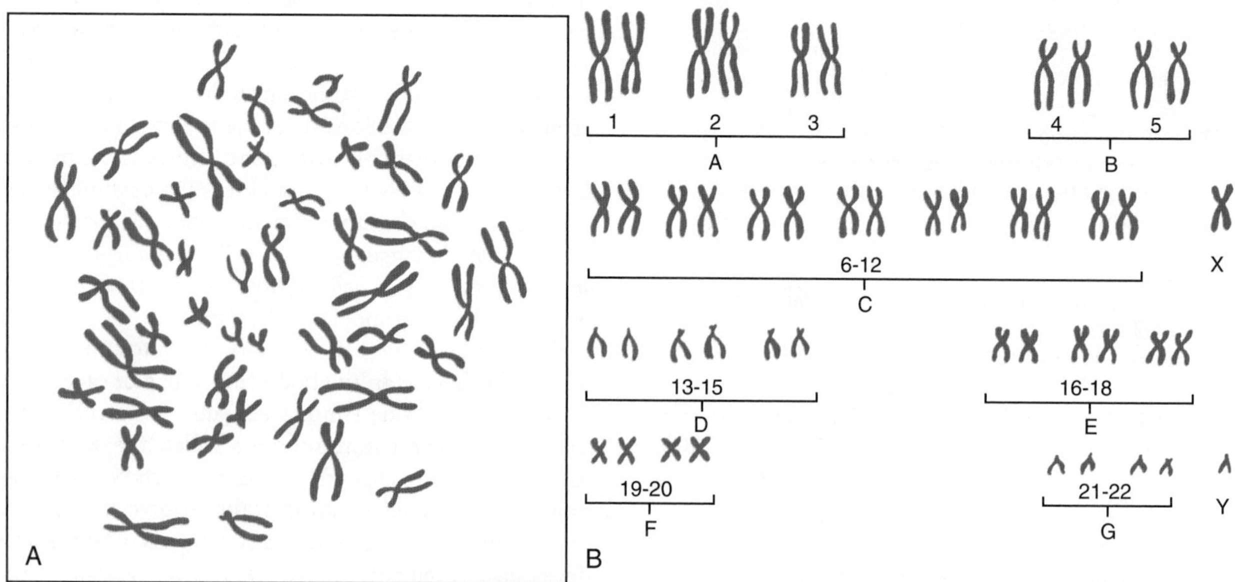

Fig. 5-2 Chromosomes during cell division. **A,** Example of photomicrograph. **B,** Chromosomes arranged in karyotype; female and male sex-determining chromosomes.

the diploid number (2N, 46 chromosomes) can be one of two types: (1) *polyploidy,* in which the deviation is an exact multiple of the haploid number of chromosomes or one chromosome set (23 chromosomes); or (2) *aneuploidy,* in which the numerical deviation is not an exact multiple of the haploid set. A *triploid* (3N) cell is an example of a polyploidy. It has 69 chromosomes. A *tetraploid* (4N) cell, also an example of a polyploidy, has 92 chromosomes.

Aneuploidy is the most commonly identified chromosome abnormality in humans. Aneuploidy occurs in at least 5% of all clinically recognized pregnancies, and it is the leading known cause of pregnancy loss. Aneuploidy is also the leading genetic cause of mental retardation. The two most common aneuploid conditions are monosomies and trisomies. A **monosomy** is the product of the union between a normal gamete and a gamete that is missing a chromosome. Monosomic individuals have only 45 chromosomes in each of their cells. Limited data are available concerning the origin of monosomies because when an embryo is missing an autosomal chromosome, the embryo never survives.

The product of the union of a normal gamete with a gamete containing an extra chromosome is a trisomy. Trisomies are more common than monosomies. Trisomic individuals have 47 chromosomes in each of their cells. Most trisomies are caused by nondisjunction during the first meiotic division. That is, one pair of chromosomes fails to separate. One of the resulting cells contains two chromosomes, and the other contains none.

The most common trisomal abnormality is Down syndrome, or trisomy 21 (47, XX+21, female with Down syndrome; or 47, XY+21, male with Down syndrome). Although the risk of having a child with Down syndrome increases with maternal age (incidence is approximately 1 in 1200 for a 25-year-old woman, 1 in 350 for a 35-year-old woman, and 1 in 30 for a 45-year-old woman), children with Down syndrome can be born to mothers of any age. Eighty percent of children with Down syndrome are born to mothers younger than 35 years (National Down Syndrome Society, 2006) (Nursing Care Plan).

Other autosomal trisomies that have been identified are trisomy 18 (Edwards syndrome) and trisomy 13 (Patau syndrome). Infants with trisomy 18 and trisomy 13 are usually severely to profoundly retarded. Although both conditions have a very poor prognosis, with the vast majority of affected infants dying within the first few days of life, a significant percentage of these infants will survive the first 6 months to 1 year of life; some children with trisomy 18 and trisomy 13 have lived beyond age 10 years.

Nondisjunction can also occur during mitosis. If it occurs early in development, when cell lines are forming, the individual has a mixture of cells, some with a normal number of chromosomes and others either missing a chromosome or containing an extra chromosome. This condition is known as **mosaicism.** Mosaicism in autosomes is most commonly seen as another form of Down syndrome. Approximately 1% to 2% of individuals with Down syndrome have mosaic Down syndrome.

Abnormalities of chromosome structure. Structural abnormalities can occur in any chromosome. Types of structural abnormalities include translocation, duplication, deletion, microdeletion, and inversion. Translocation occurs when an exchange of chromosomal material occurs between two chromosomes. Exposure to certain drugs, viruses, and radiation can cause translocations, but they often arise for no apparent reason. Thus instead of two normal pairs of chromosomes, the individual has one normal chromosome of each pair and a third chromosome that is a fusion of the other two chromosomes. As long as all genetic material is retained in the cell, the individual is unaffected but is a carrier of a balanced translocation. In an unbalanced translocation, the gamete receives one of the two normal chromosomes and the fused version. The resulting offspring will have an extra copy of one of the chromosomes with often serious clinical effects.

Whenever a portion of a chromosome is deleted from one chromosome and added to another the gamete produced may have either extra copies of genes or too few copies. The clinical effects produced may be mild or severe, depending on the amount of genetic material involved. Two of the more common conditions are the deletion of the short arm of chromosome 5 (cri du chat syndrome) and the deletion of the long arm of chromosome 18.

Sex chromosome abnormalities

Several sex chromosome abnormalities are caused by nondisjunction during gametogenesis in either parent. The most common deviation in females is Turner syndrome, or monosomy X (45, X). The affected female exhibits juvenile external genitalia with undeveloped ovaries. She is usually short in stature with webbing of the neck. Intelligence may be impaired. Most affected embryos miscarry spontaneously.

The most common deviation in males is Klinefelter syndrome, or trisomy XXY. The affected male has poorly developed secondary sexual characteristics and small testes. He is infertile, usually tall, and effeminate, and he may be slow to learn. Males who have mosaic Klinefelter syndrome may be fertile.

Patterns of Genetic Transmission

Heritable characteristics are those that can be passed on to offspring. The patterns by which genetic material is transmitted to the next generation are affected by the number of genes involved in the expression of the trait. Many phenotypic characteristics result from two or more genes on different chromosomes acting together *(multifactorial inheritance)*; others are controlled by a single gene *(unifactorial inheritance)*. Defects at the gene level cannot be determined by conventional laboratory methods such as

NURSING CARE PLAN *The Family with an Infant Who Has Down Syndrome*

NURSING DIAGNOSIS Risk for interrupted family processes related to birth of a neonate with an inherited disorder

Expected Outcome *The couple will verbalize accurate information about Down syndrome, including implications for future pregnancies.*

Nursing Interventions/*Rationales*

- Assess knowledge base of couple regarding the clinical signs and symptoms of Down syndrome and inheritance patterns *to correct any misconceptions and establish basis for teaching plan.*
- Provide information throughout the genetics evaluation regarding risk status and clinical signs and symptoms of Down syndrome *to give couple a realistic picture of neonate's defects and assist with decision making for future pregnancies.*
- Use therapeutic communication during discussions with the couple *to provide opportunity for expression of concern.*
- Refer to support groups, social services, or counseling *to assist with family cohesive actions and decision making.*
- Refer to child development specialist *to provide family with realistic expectations regarding cognitive and behavioral differences of child with Down syndrome.*

NURSING DIAGNOSIS Situational low self-esteem related to diagnosis of inherited disorder, as evidenced by parents' statements of guilt and shame

Expected Outcome *The parents will express an increased number of positive statements regarding the birth of a neonate with Down syndrome.*

Nursing Interventions/*Rationales*

- Assist parents to list strengths and coping strategies that have been helpful in past situations *to promote use of appropriate strategies during this situational crisis.*
- Encourage expression of feelings using therapeutic communication *to provide clarification and emotional support.*
- Clarify and provide information regarding Down syndrome *to decrease feelings of guilt and gradually increase feelings of positive self-esteem.*
- Refer for further counseling as needed *to provide more in-depth and ongoing support.*

NURSING DIAGNOSIS Risk for impaired parenting related to birth of neonate with Down syndrome

Expected Outcome *Parents demonstrate competent skills in parenting a child with Down syndrome and willingness to care for neonate.*

Nursing Interventions/*Rationales*

- Assist parents to see and describe normal aspects of infant *to promote bonding.*
- Encourage and assist with breastfeeding if that is parents' choice of feeding method *to facilitate closeness with infant and provide benefits of breast milk.*
- Assure parents that information regarding the neonate will remain confidential *to assist the parents to maintain some situational control and allow for time to work through their feelings.*
- Discuss and role play with parents ways of informing family and friends of infant's diagnosis and prognosis *to promote positive aspects of infant and decrease potential isolation from social interactions.*
- Provide anticipatory guidance about what to expect as infant develops *to assist family in preparing for behavior problems or mental deficits.*

NURSING DIAGNOSIS Spiritual distress related to situational crisis of child born with Down syndrome

Expected Outcome *Parents seek appropriate support persons (family members, priest, minister, rabbi) for assistance.*

Nursing Interventions/*Rationales*

- Listen for cues indicative of parents' feelings ("Why did God do this to us?") *to identify messages indicating spiritual distress.*
- Acknowledge parents' spiritual concerns and encourage expression of feelings *to help build a therapeutic relationship.*
- Facilitate visits from clergy and provide privacy during visits *to demonstrate respect for the parents' relationship with their clergy.*
- Encourage parents to discuss concerns with clergy to use expert spiritual care resources *to help the parents.*
- Facilitate interaction with family members and other support persons *to encourage expressions of concern and seeking comfort.*

NURSING DIAGNOSIS Risk for social isolation related to full-time caretaking responsibilities for a neonate with Down syndrome

Expected Outcome *Parents will describe a plan to use resources to prevent social isolation.*

Nursing Interventions/*Rationales*

- Provide opportunity for parents to express feelings about caring for a neonate with Down syndrome *to facilitate effective communication and trust.*
- Discuss with parents their expectations about caring for the neonate *to identify potential areas of concern.*
- Assist parents to identify potential caregiving resources *to permit parents to return to a routine at home.*
- Identify appropriate referrals for home care *to provide continuity of care.*
- Refer to support groups of parents of children with Down Syndrome *to enlist support, understanding, and strategies for coping.*

COMMUNITY ACTIVITY

Select a disorder that has a genetic basis. Search the Internet for resources on this disorder. Are these resources for parents or for professionals (or for both)?

Compare and contrast the appearance, the readability, and the information contained in the sites.

- To whom would you recommend these sites?
- Is the information culturally relevant?
- What information would parents need?
- How could you as a nurse use this information?

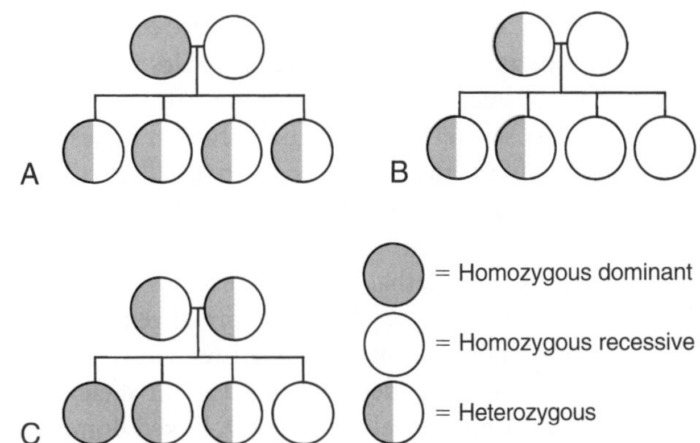

Fig. 5-3 Possible offspring in three types of matings. **A,** Homozygous-dominant parent and homozygous-recessive parent. Children: all heterozygous, displaying dominant trait. **B,** Heterozygous parent and homozygous-recessive parent. Children: 50% heterozygous, displaying dominant trait; 50% homozygous, displaying recessive trait. **C,** Both parents heterozygous. Children: 25% homozygous, displaying dominant trait; 25% homozygous, displaying recessive trait; 50% heterozygous, displaying dominant trait.

karyotyping. Instead, specialists in genetics (e.g., geneticists, genetic counselors, and nurses with advanced expertise in genetics) predict the probability of the presence of an abnormal gene from the known occurrence of the trait in the individual's family and the known patterns by which the trait is inherited.

Multifactorial Inheritance

Most common congenital malformations, such as cleft lip and palate and neural tube defects, result from multifactorial inheritance, a combination of genetic and environmental factors. Each malformation may range from mild to severe, depending on the number of genes for the defect present or the amount of environmental influence. Multifactorial disorders tend to occur in families. A neural tube defect may range from spina bifida, a bony defect in the lumbar region of the vertebrae with little or no neurologic impairment, to anencephaly, the absence of brain development, which is always fatal. Some malformations occur more often in one sex than the other. For example, pyloric stenosis and cleft lip are more common in males, and cleft palate is more common in females.

Unifactorial inheritance

If a single gene controls a particular trait, disorder, or defect, its pattern of inheritance is called *unifactorial mendelian* or *single-gene inheritance.* The number of unifactorial abnormalities far exceeds the number of chromosomal abnormalities. Potential patterns of inheritance for single-gene disorders include autosomal dominant, autosomal recessive, and X-linked dominant and recessive modes of inheritance (Fig. 5-3).

Autosomal dominant inheritance. Autosomal dominant inheritance disorders are those in which only one copy of a variant allele is needed for phenotypic expression. The variant allele may appear as a result of a mutation, a spontaneous and permanent change in the normal gene structure. In this case the disorder occurs for the first time in the family. Usually an affected individual comes from multiple generations having the disorder (see Fig. 5-3, *B* and *C*). A vertical pattern of inheritance can be seen (no skipping of generations occurs; if an individual has an autosomal dominant disorder such as HD, so must one of his or her parents). Males and females are equally affected.

Autosomal dominant disorders are not always expressed with the same severity of symptoms. For example, a woman who has an autosomal dominant disorder may show few symptoms and may not become aware of her diagnosis until after she gives birth to a severely affected child. Predicting whether an offspring will have a minor or severe abnormality is not possible. Examples of common autosomal dominant disorders are Marfan syndrome, neurofibromatosis, myotonic dystrophy, Stickler syndrome, Treacher Collins syndrome, and achondroplasia (dwarfism).

Autosomal recessive inheritance. Autosomal recessive inheritance disorders are those in which both genes of a pair must be abnormal for the disorder to be expressed. Heterozygous individuals have only one variant allele and are unaffected clinically because their normal gene overshadows the variant allele. They are known as carriers of the recessive trait. Because these recessive traits are inherited by generations of the same family, an increased incidence of the disorder occurs in consanguineous matings (closely related parents). For the trait to be expressed, two carriers must each contribute a variant allele to the offspring (Fig. 5-3, *C*). The chance of the trait occurring in each child is 25%. A clinically normal offspring may be a carrier of the gene. Autosomal recessive disorders have a horizontal pattern of inheritance, rather than the vertical pattern seen with autosomal dominant disorders. That is, autosomal recessive disorders are usually observed in one or more siblings, but not in earlier generations. Males and females are equally affected. Most IEMs, such as PKU, galactosemia, maple syrup urine disease, Tay-Sachs disease, sickle cell anemia, and CF, are autosomal recessive inherited disorders.

X-linked dominant inheritance. X-linked dominant inheritance disorders occur in males and heterozygous females. Because of X inactivation, affected females are usually less severely affected than affected males, and they are more likely to transmit the variant allele to their offspring. Heterozygous females have a 50% chance of transmitting the variant allele to each offspring. The variant allele is often lethal in affected males given that, unlike affected females, they have no normal gene. Mating of an affected male and an unaffected female is uncommon as a result of the tendency for the variant allele to be lethal in affected males. Relatively few X-linked dominant disorders have been identified. Two examples are vitamin D–resistant rickets and fragile X syndrome.

X-linked recessive inheritance. Abnormal genes for X-linked recessive inheritance disorders are carried on the X chromosome. Females may be heterozygous or homozygous for traits carried on the X chromosome because they have two X chromosomes. Males are hemizygous because they have only one X chromosome carrying genes, with no alleles on the Y chromosome. Therefore X-linked recessive disorders most often occur in the male with the abnormal gene on his single X chromosome. Hemophilia, color blindness, and Duchenne muscular dystrophy are all X-linked recessive disorders.

The male receives the disease-associated allele from his carrier mother on her affected X chromosome. Female carriers (those heterozygous for the trait) have a 50% probability of transmitting the disease-associated allele to each offspring. An affected male can pass the disease-associated allele to his daughters but not to his sons. The daughters will be carriers of the trait if they receive a normal gene on the X chromosome from their mother. They will be affected only if they receive a disease-associated allele on the X chromosome from both their mother and their father.

Inborn errors of metabolism

More than 350 IEMs have been recognized. Individually, IEMs are relatively rare, but collectively, they are common (1 in 5000 live births). As noted previously, most IEMs are inherited in an autosomal recessive pattern. IEMs occur when a gene mutation reduces the efficiency of encoded enzymes to a level at which normal metabolism cannot occur. Defective enzyme action interrupts the normal series of chemical reactions from the affected point onward. The result may be an accumulation of a damaging product, such as phenylalanine in PKU, or the absence of a necessary product, such as the lack of melanin in albinism caused by lack of tyrosinase. Diagnostic and carrier testing is available for a growing number of IEMs. In addition, many states in the United States have started screening for specific IEMs as part of their expanded newborn screening programs using tandem mass spectrometry. However, many of the deaths caused by IEMs are the result of enzyme variants not currently screened for in many of the newborn screening programs. (See Table 17-3 for screening tests for inborn errors of metabolism.)

Nongenetic Factors Influencing Development

Not all congenital disorders are inherited. Congenital means that the condition was present at birth. Some congenital malformations may be the result of **teratogens**, that is, environmental substances or exposures that result in functional or structural disability. In contrast to other forms of developmental disabilities, disabilities caused by teratogens are, in theory, totally preventable. Known human teratogens are drugs and chemicals, infections, exposure to radiation, and certain maternal conditions such as diabetes and PKU (Box 5-2). A teratogen has the greatest effect on the organs and parts of an embryo during its periods of rapid differentiation. This occurs during the embryonic period, specifically from days 15 to 60. During the first 2 weeks of development, teratogens either have little or no effect on the embryo or have effects so severe that they cause miscarriage. Brain growth and development continue during the fetal period, and teratogens can severely affect mental development throughout gestation (Fig. 5-4).

BOX 5-2

Etiology of Human Malformations

ETIOLOGY	MALFORMED LIVE BIRTHS (%)
Environmental	10
Maternal conditions: alcoholism, diabetes, endocrinopathies, phenylketonuria, smoking, nutritional problems	4
Infectious agents: rubella, toxoplasmosis, syphilis, herpes simplex, cytomegalic inclusion disease, varicella, Venezuelan equine encephalitis	3
Mechanical problems (deformations): amniotic band constrictions, umbilical cord constraint, disparity in uterine size and uterine contents	2
Chemicals, drugs, radiation, hyperthermia	1
Genetic: single-gene disorders; chromosomal abnormalities	20-25
Unknown:	65-70
Polygenic or multifactorial (gene-environment interactions)	
"Spontaneous" errors of development	
Other unknowns	

Source: Hudgins, L. & Cassidy, S. (2006). Congenital anomalies. In A. Fanaroff, R. Martin, & M. C. Walsh (Eds.), *Fanaroff and Martin's neonatal-perinatal medicine: Diseases of the fetus and infant* (8th ed.). St. Louis: Mosby.

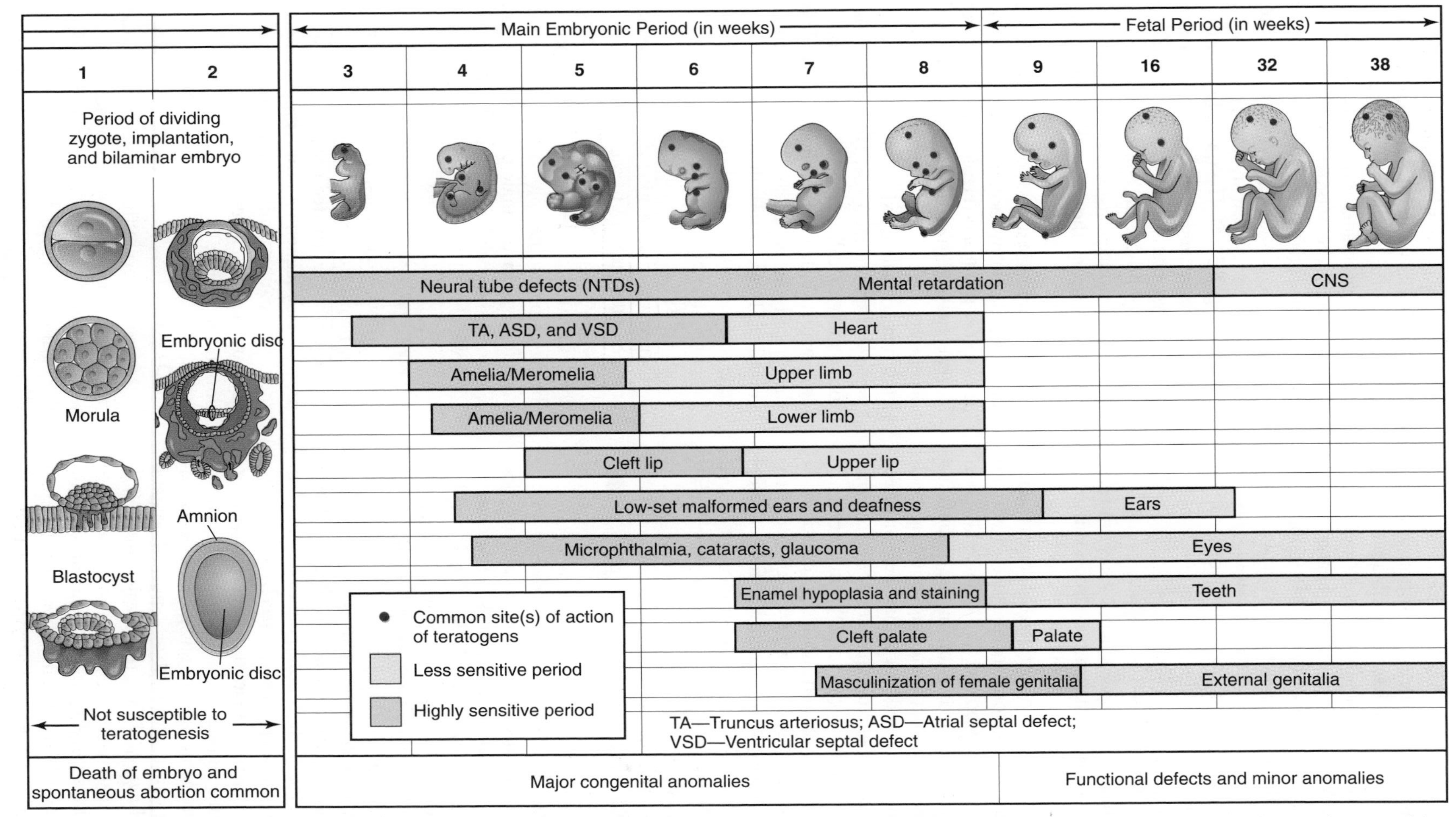

Fig. 5-4 Sensitive, or critical, periods in human development. Dark color denotes highly sensitive periods; light color indicates stages that are less sensitive to teratogens. (From Moore, K. & Persaud, T. [2008]. *Before we are born: Essentials of embryology and birth defects* [7th ed.]. Philadelphia: Saunders.) *Amelia,* Lacking one or more limbs; *meromelia,* lacking one or more arms or legs (hand or foot is present).

In addition to genetic makeup and the influence of teratogens, the adequacy of maternal nutrition influences development. The embryo and fetus must obtain the nutrients they need from the mother's diet; they cannot tap the maternal reserves. Malnutrition during pregnancy produces low-birth-weight newborns susceptible to infection. Malnutrition also affects brain development during the latter half of gestation and may result in learning disabilities in the child. Inadequate folic acid is associated with neural tube defects.

Behavioral genetics

The field of human behavioral genetics seeks to understand genetic and environmental influences on variations in human behavior (McInerney, 2008). Behavior involves multiple genes. Study of behavior and genes requires analysis of families and populations to compare those who have the trait with those who do not. The result is an estimate of the amount of variation in the population attributable to genetic factors. The findings of this research have significant political and social implications. For example, what are the social consequences of determining a genetic diagnosis of traits such as intelligence, criminality, or homosexuality? Caution must be exercised in accepting discoveries in behavioral genetics until substantial scientific corroboration is obtained. For further information, OMIM–Online Mendelian Inheritance in Man, a large database involving genes, genetic traits, and hereditary disorders–can be consulted.

Animation: Spermatogenesis

CONCEPTION

Cell Division

Cells are reproduced by two different methods: mitosis and meiosis. In **mitosis** the body cells replicate to yield two cells with the same genetic makeup as the parent cell. First the cell makes a copy of its DNA; then it divides, with each daughter cell receiving one copy of the genetic material. Mitotic division facilitates growth and development or cell replacement.

Animation: Oogenesis and Meiosis

Meiosis, the process by which germ cells divide and decrease their chromosomal number by half, produces gametes (eggs and sperm). Each homologous pair of chromosomes contains one chromosome received from the mother and one from the father; thus meiosis results in cells that contain one of each of the 23 pairs of chromosomes. Because these germ cells contain 23 single chromosomes, half of the genetic material of a normal somatic cell, they are called *haploid.* When the female gamete (egg or ovum) and the male gamete (spermatozoon) unite to form the zygote, the diploid number of human chromosomes (46, or 23 pairs) is restored.

Animation: Pathway of Ovum

Gametogenesis

Oogenesis, the process of ovum formation, begins during fetal life of the female. All the cells that may undergo meiosis in a woman's lifetime are contained in her ovaries at birth. The majority of the estimated 2 million primary oocytes (the cells that undergo the first meiotic division) degenerate spontaneously. Only 400 to 500 ova will mature during the approximately 35 years of a woman's reproductive lifetime. The primary oocytes begin the first meiotic division (i.e., they replicate their DNA) during fetal life, but remain suspended at this stage until puberty (Fig. 5-5, *A*). Then, usually monthly, one primary oocyte matures and completes the first meiotic division, yielding two unequal cells: the secondary oocyte and a small polar body. Both contain 22 autosomes and one X sex chromosome.

At ovulation the second meiotic division begins. However, the ovum does not complete the second meiotic division unless fertilization occurs. At fertilization, a second polar body and the **zygote** (the united egg and sperm) are produced (Fig. 5-5, *C*). The three polar bodies degenerate. If fertilization does not occur, the ovum also degenerates.

When a male reaches puberty, his testes begin the process of spermatogenesis. The cells that undergo meiosis in the male are called *spermatocytes.* The primary spermatocyte, which undergoes the first meiotic division, contains the diploid number of chromosomes. The cell has already copied its DNA before division, so four alleles for each gene are present. Because the copies are bound together (i.e., one allele plus its copy on each chromosome) the cell is still considered diploid.

During the first meiotic division, two haploid secondary spermatocytes are formed. Each secondary spermatocyte contains 22 autosomes and one sex chromosome; one contains the X chromosome (plus its copy) and the other the Y chromosome (plus its copy). During the second meiotic division the male produces two gametes with an X chromosome and two gametes with a Y chromosome, all of which will develop into viable sperm (Fig. 5-5, *B*).

Conception

Conception, defined as the union of a single egg and sperm, marks the beginning of a pregnancy. Conception occurs not as an isolated event but as part of a sequential process. This sequential process includes **gamete** (egg and sperm) formation, ovulation (release of the egg), union of the gametes (which results in an embryo), and implantation in the uterus.

Ovum

Meiosis occurs in the female in the ovarian follicles and produces an egg, or ovum. Each month, one ovum matures with a host of surrounding supportive cells. At ovulation the ovum is released from the ruptured ovarian follicle. High estrogen levels increase the motility of the uterine tubes so that their cilia are able to capture the ovum and propel it through the tube toward the uterine cavity. An ovum cannot move by itself.

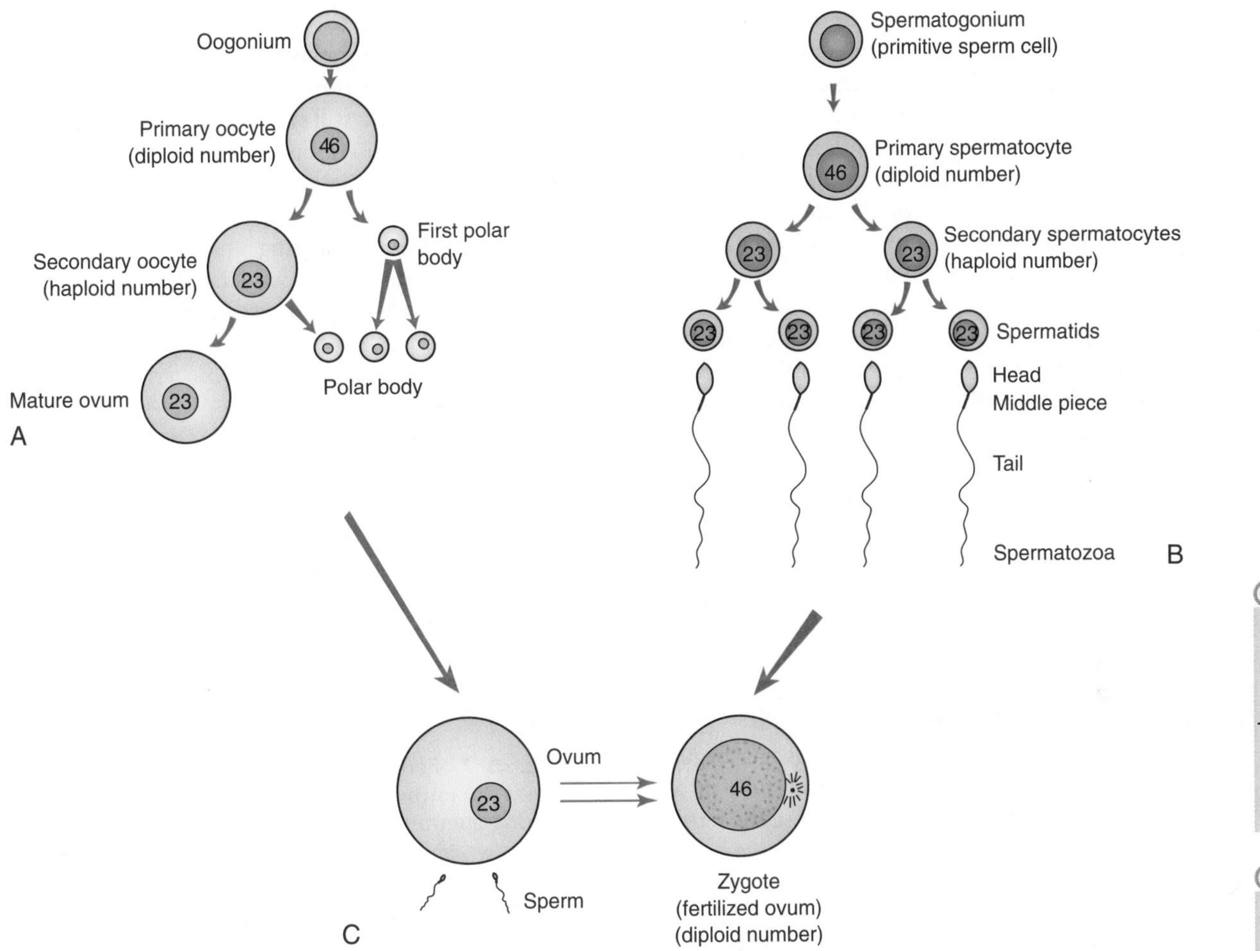

Oogonium
Primary oocyte (diploid number)
46
Secondary oocyte (haploid number)
23
First polar body
Mature ovum
23
Polar body
A

Spermatogonium (primitive sperm cell)
Primary spermatocyte (diploid number)
46
Secondary spermatocytes (haploid number)
23
Spermatids
Head
Middle piece
Tail
Spermatozoa
B

Ovum
23
46
Sperm
Zygote (fertilized ovum) (diploid number)
C

Fig. 5-5 Gametogenesis. **A,** Oogenesis. Gametogenesis in the female produces one mature ovum and three polar bodies. Note relative difference in overall size between ovum and sperm. **B,** Spermatogenesis. Gametogenesis in the male produces four mature gametes, the sperm. **C,** Fertilization results in the single-cell zygote and restoration of the diploid number of chromosomes.

Animation: Spermatozoa

Animation: Testes

Animation: Male Reproductive Ducts

Animation: Pathway of Sperm

Two protective layers surround the ovum (Fig. 5-6). The inner layer is a thick, acellular layer called the zona pellucida. The outer layer, called the corona radiata, is composed of elongated cells.

Ova are considered fertile for approximately 24 hours after ovulation. If unfertilized by a sperm the ovum degenerates and is reabsorbed.

Sperm

Ejaculation during sexual intercourse normally propels almost a teaspoon of semen containing as many as 200 to 500 million sperm into the vagina. The sperm swim by means of the flagellar movement of their tails. Some sperm can reach the site of fertilization within 5 minutes, but average transit time is 4 to 6 hours. Sperm remain viable within the woman's reproductive system for an average of 2 to 3 days. Most sperm are lost in the vagina, within the cervical mucus, or in the endometrium; or they enter the tube that contains no ovum.

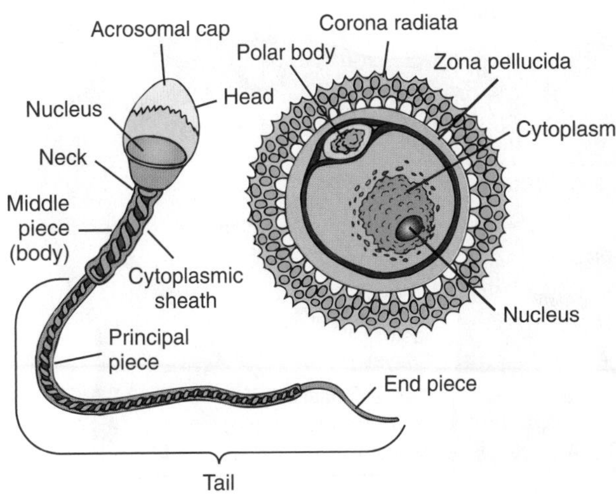

Fig. 5-6 Sperm and ovum.

Animation: Male External Genitalia

As sperm travel through the female reproductive tract, enzymes are produced to aid in their capacitation. Capacitation is a physiologic change that removes the protective coating from the heads of the sperm. Small perforations then form in the acrosome (a cap on the sperm) and allow enzymes (e.g., hyaluronidase) to escape (see Fig. 5-6). These enzymes are necessary for the sperm to penetrate the protective layers of the ovum before fertilization.

Animation: Male Accessory Sex Glands

Fertilization

Fertilization takes place in the ampulla (the outer third) of the uterine tube. When a sperm successfully penetrates the membrane surrounding the ovum, both sperm and ovum are enclosed within the membrane, and the membrane becomes impenetrable to other sperm; this process is termed the *zona reaction*. The second meiotic division of the secondary oocyte is then completed, and the ovum nucleus becomes the female pronucleus. The head of the sperm enlarges to become the male pronucleus, and the tail degenerates. The nuclei fuse and the chromosomes combine, restoring the diploid number (46) (Fig. 5-7). Conception, the formation of the zygote (the first cell of the new individual), has been achieved.

Mitotic cellular replication, called cleavage, begins as the zygote travels the length of the uterine tube into the uterus. This voyage takes 3 to 4 days. Because the fertilized egg divides rapidly with no increase in size, successively smaller cells, called blastomeres, are formed with each division. A 16-cell **morula**, a solid ball of cells, is produced within 3 days and is still surrounded by the protective zona pellucida (Fig. 5-8, *A*). Further development occurs as the morula floats freely within the uterus. Fluid passes through the zona pellucida into the intercellular spaces between the blastomeres, separating them into two parts: the trophoblast (which gives rise to the placenta) and the embryoblast (which gives rise to the embryo). A cavity

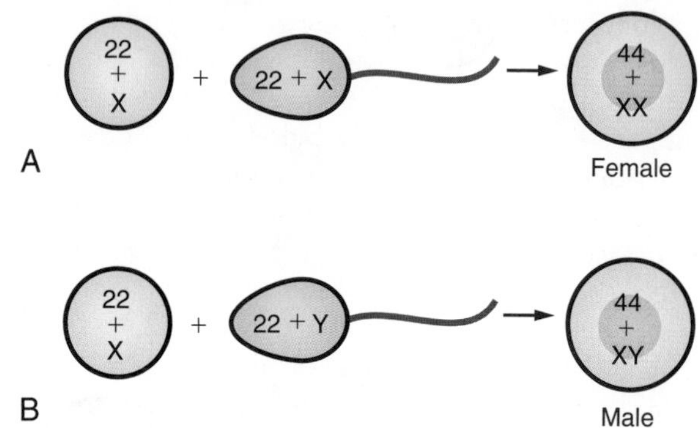

Fig. 5-7 Fertilization. **A,** Ovum fertilized by X-bearing sperm to form female zygote. **B,** Ovum fertilized by Y-bearing sperm to form male zygote.

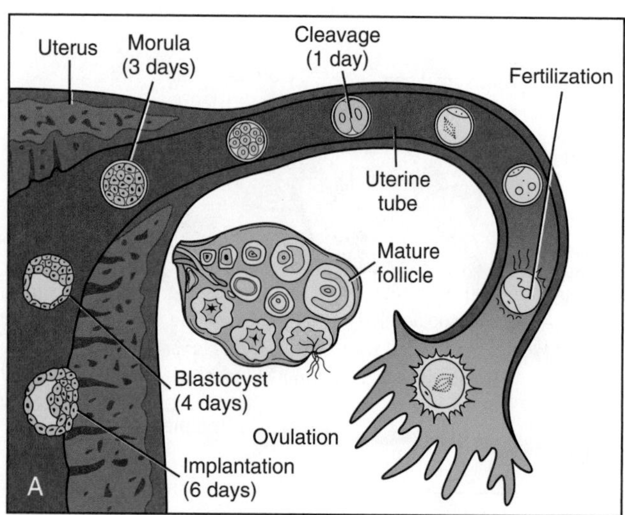

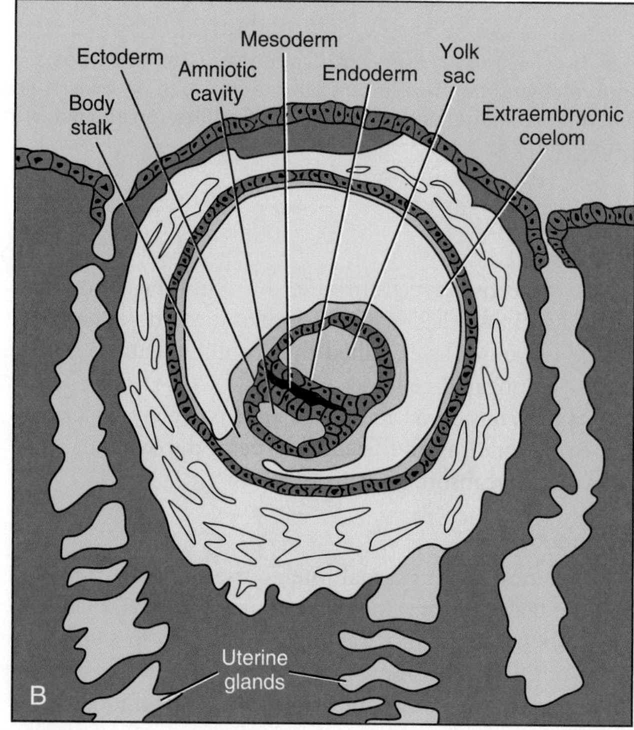

Fig. 5-8 **A,** First weeks of human development. Follicular development in ovary, ovulation, fertilization, and transport of early embryo down uterine tube and into uterus, where implantation occurs. **B,** Blastocyst embedded in endometrium. Germ layers forming. (**A,** From Carlson, B. [2009]. *Human embryology and developmental biology.* [4th ed.]. St. Louis: Mosby. **B,** Adapted from Langley, L., Telford, I. R., & Christenson, J. B. [1980]. *Dynamic human anatomy and physiology* [5th ed.]. New York: McGraw-Hill.)

forms within the cell mass as the spaces come together, forming a structure called the **blastocyst** cavity. When the cavity becomes recognizable, the whole structure of the developing embryo is known as the blastocyst. Stem cells are derived from the inner cell mass of the blastocyst. The outer layer of cells surrounding the cavity is the trophoblast.

Implantation

The zona pellucida degenerates, and the trophoblast attaches itself to the uterine endometrium, usually in the anterior or posterior fundal region. Between 6 and 10 days after conception the trophoblast secretes enzymes that enable it to burrow into the endometrium until the entire blastocyst is covered (Fig. 5-8, *B*). This process is known as **implantation.** Endometrial blood vessels erode, and some women experience slight implantation bleeding (slight spotting and bleeding during the time of the first missed menstrual period). **Chorionic villi,** or finger-like projections, develop out of the trophoblast and extend into the blood-filled spaces of the endometrium. These villi are vascular processes that obtain oxygen and nutrients from the maternal bloodstream and dispose of carbon dioxide and waste products into the maternal blood.

After implantation the endometrium is called the *decidua.* The portion directly under the blastocyst, where the chorionic villi tap into the maternal blood vessels, is the **decidua basalis.** The portion covering the blastocyst is the decidua capsularis, and the portion lining the rest of the uterus is the decidua vera (Fig. 5-9).

THE EMBRYO AND FETUS

Animation: Fertilization and Implantation

Pregnancy lasts approximately 10 lunar months, 9 calendar months, 40 weeks, or 280 days. Length of pregnancy is computed from the first day of the last menstrual period (LMP) until the day of birth. However, conception occurs approximately 2 weeks after the first day of the LMP. Thus the postconception age of the fetus is 2 weeks less, for a total of 266 days or 38 weeks. Postconception age is used in the discussion of fetal development.

Intrauterine development is divided into three stages: ovum (preembryonic stage), embryo, and fetus (see Fig. 5-4). The stage of the ovum lasts from conception until day 14. This period covers cellular replication, blastocyst formation, initial development of the embryonic membranes, and establishment of the primary germ layers.

Primary Germ Layers

During the third week after conception the embryonic disk differentiates into three primary germ layers: the *ectoderm, mesoderm,* and *endoderm* (or entoderm) (see Fig. 5-8, *B*). All tissues and organs of the embryo develop from these three layers.

The ectoderm, or upper layer of the embryonic disk, gives rise to the epidermis, glands (anterior pituitary, cutaneous, and mammary), nails and hair, central and peripheral nervous systems, lens of the eye, tooth enamel, and floor of the amniotic cavity.

The mesoderm, or middle layer, develops into the bones and teeth, muscles (skeletal, smooth, and cardiac),

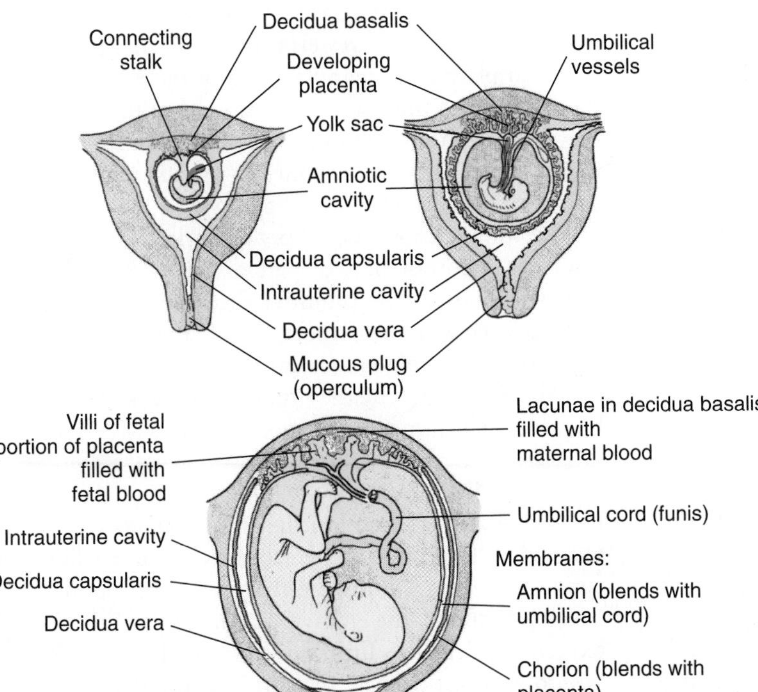

Fig. 5-9 Development of fetal membranes. Note gradual obliteration of intrauterine cavity as decidua capsularis and decidua vera meet. Also note thinning of uterine wall. Chorionic and amnionic membranes are in apposition to each other but may be peeled apart.

dermis and connective tissue, cardiovascular system and spleen, and urogenital system.

The endoderm, or lower layer, gives rise to the epithelium lining the respiratory tract and digestive tract, including the oropharynx, liver and pancreas, urethra, bladder, and vagina. The endoderm forms the roof of the yolk sac.

Development of the Embryo

The stage of the **embryo** lasts from day 15 until approximately 8 weeks after conception, when the embryo measures approximately 3 cm from crown to rump. The embryonic stage is the most critical time in the development of the organ systems and the main external features. Developing areas with rapid cell division are the most vulnerable to malformation by environmental teratogens. At the end of the eighth week, all organ systems and external structures are present, and the embryo is unmistakably human (see Fig. 5-4 and The Visible Embryo, www.visembryo.com, for a pictorial view of normal and abnormal development).

Membranes

At the time of implantation, two **fetal membranes** that will surround the developing embryo begin to form. The chorion develops from the trophoblast and contains the chorionic villi on its surface. The villi burrow into the decidua basalis and increase in size and complexity as the vascular processes develop into the placenta. The chorion becomes the covering of the fetal side of the placenta. It contains the major umbilical blood vessels that branch out over the surface of the placenta. As the embryo grows, the decidua capsularis stretches. The chorionic villi on this side atrophy and degenerate, leaving a smooth chorionic membrane.

The inner cell membrane, the amnion, develops from the interior cells of the blastocyst. The cavity that develops between this inner cell mass and the outer layer of cells (trophoblast) is the amniotic cavity (see Fig. 5-8, *B*). As it grows larger, the amnion forms on the side opposite the developing blastocyst (see Fig. 5-8, *B*, and Fig. 5-9). The developing embryo draws the amnion around itself to form a fluid-filled sac. The amnion becomes the covering of the umbilical cord and covers the chorion on the fetal surface of the placenta. As the embryo grows larger, the amnion enlarges to accommodate the embryo or fetus and the surrounding amniotic fluid. The amnion eventually comes in contact with the chorion surrounding the fetus.

Amniotic Fluid

At first the amniotic cavity derives its fluid by diffusion from the maternal blood. The amount of fluid increases weekly, and 800 to 1200 ml of transparent liquid are normally present at term. The volume of amniotic fluid changes constantly. The fetus swallows fluid, and fluid flows into and out of the fetal lungs. The fetus urinates into the fluid, greatly increasing its volume.

The amniotic fluid serves many functions for the embryo and fetus. Amniotic fluid helps maintain a constant body temperature. It serves as a source of oral fluid and as a repository for waste. It cushions the fetus from trauma by blunting and dispersing outside forces. It allows freedom of movement for musculoskeletal development. The fluid keeps the embryo from tangling with the membranes, facilitating symmetric growth of the fetus. If the embryo does become tangled with the membranes, amputations of extremities or other deformities can occur from constricting amniotic bands.

The volume of amniotic fluid is an important factor in assessing fetal well-being. Having less than 300 ml of amniotic fluid (oligohydramnios) is associated with fetal renal abnormalities. Having more than 2 L of amniotic fluid (hydramnios) is associated with gastrointestinal and other malformations.

Amniotic fluid contains albumin, urea, uric acid, creatinine, lecithin, sphingomyelin, bilirubin, fructose, fat, leukocytes, proteins, epithelial cells, enzymes, and lanugo hair. Study of fetal cells in amniotic fluid through amniocentesis yields much information about the fetus. Genetic studies (karyotyping) provide knowledge about the sex of the fetus and the number and structure of chromosomes. Other studies such as the lecithin/sphingomyelin (L/S) ratio determine the health or maturity of the fetus.

Yolk Sac

At the same time the amniotic cavity and amnion are forming, another blastocyst cavity forms on the other side of the developing embryonic disk (see Fig. 5-8, *B*). This cavity becomes surrounded by a membrane, forming the yolk sac. The yolk sac aids in transferring maternal nutrients and oxygen, which have diffused through the chorion, to the embryo. Blood vessels form to aid transport. Blood cells and plasma are manufactured in the yolk sac during the second and third weeks. At the end of the third week, the primitive heart begins to beat and circulate the blood through the embryo, connecting stalk, chorion, and yolk sac.

The folding in of the embryo during the fourth week results in incorporation of part of the yolk sac into the embryo's body as the primitive digestive system. Primordial germ cells arise in the yolk sac and move into the embryo. The shrinking remains of the yolk sac degenerate (see Fig. 5-8, *B*), and by the fifth or sixth week, the remnant has separated from the embryo.

Umbilical Cord

By day 14 after conception the embryonic disk, amniotic sac, and yolk sac are attached to the chorionic villi by the connecting stalk. During the third week the blood vessels develop to supply the embryo with maternal nutrients and oxygen. During the fifth week, the embryo has curved inward on itself from both ends bringing the connecting stalk to the ventral side of the embryo. The connecting stalk becomes compressed from both sides by the amnion and forms the narrower umbilical cord (see Fig. 5-9). Two arteries carry blood from the embryo to the chorionic villi, and one vein returns blood to the embryo. Approximately 1% of umbilical cords contain only two vessels: one artery and one vein. This occurrence is sometimes associated with congenital malformations.

The cord rapidly increases in length. At term the cord is 2 cm in diameter and ranges from 30 to 90 cm in length (with an average of 55 cm). It twists spirally on itself and loops around the embryo or fetus. A true knot is rare, but false knots occur as folds or kinks in the cord and may jeopardize circulation to the fetus. Connective tissue called *Wharton jelly* prevents compression of the blood vessels and ensures continued nourishment of the embryo or fetus. Compression can occur if the cord lies between the fetal head and the pelvis or is twisted around the fetal body. When the cord is wrapped around the fetal neck, it is called a *nuchal cord.*

Because the placenta develops from the chorionic villi, the umbilical cord is usually located centrally. A peripheral location is less common and is known as a *battledore placenta.* The blood vessels are arrayed out from the center to all parts of the placenta (Fig. 5-10, *B*).

Placenta

Structure

The placenta begins to form at implantation. During the third week after conception the trophoblast cells of the chorionic villi continue to invade the decidua basalis. As the uterine capillaries are tapped, the endometrial spiral arteries fill with maternal blood. The chorionic villi grow into the spaces with two layers of cells: the outer syncytium and the inner cytotrophoblast. A third layer develops into anchoring septa, dividing the projecting decidua into separate areas called *cotyledons.* In each of the 15 to 20 cotyledons, the chorionic villi branch out, and a complex system of fetal blood vessels forms. Each cotyledon is a functional unit. The whole structure is the placenta (Fig. 5-10).

The maternal-placental-embryonic circulation is in place by day 17, when the embryonic heart starts beating. By the end of the third week, embryonic blood is circulating between the embryo and the chorionic villi. In the intervillous spaces, maternal blood supplies oxygen and nutrients to the embryonic capillaries in the villi (Fig. 5-11). Waste products and carbon dioxide diffuse into the maternal blood.

The placenta functions as a means of metabolic exchange. Exchange is minimal at this time because the two cell layers of the villous membrane are too thick. Permeability increases as the cytotrophoblast thins and disappears; by the fifth month, only the single layer of syncytium is left between the maternal blood and the fetal capillaries. The syncytium is the functional layer of the placenta. By the eighth week, genetic testing can be per-

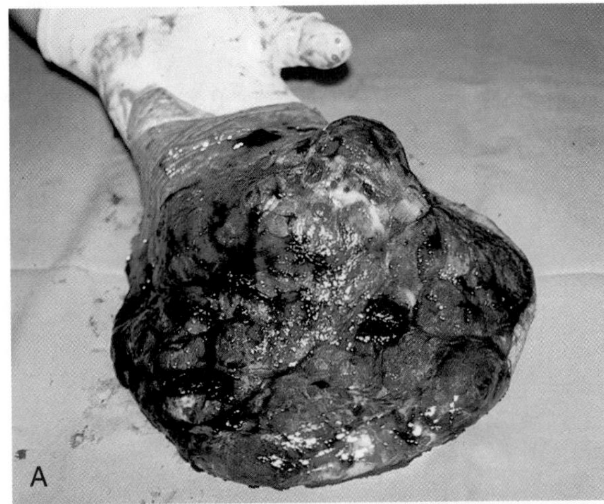

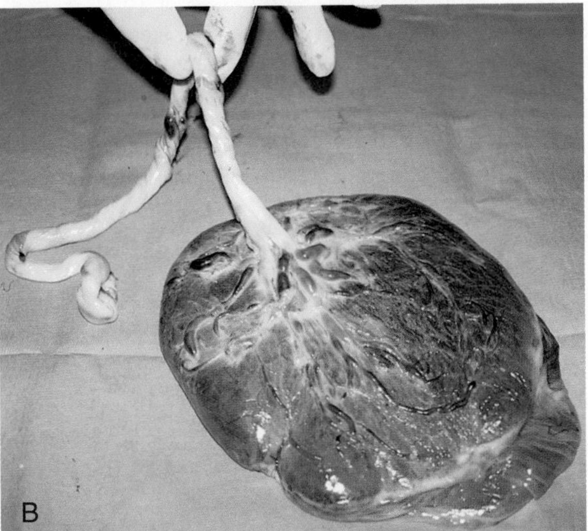

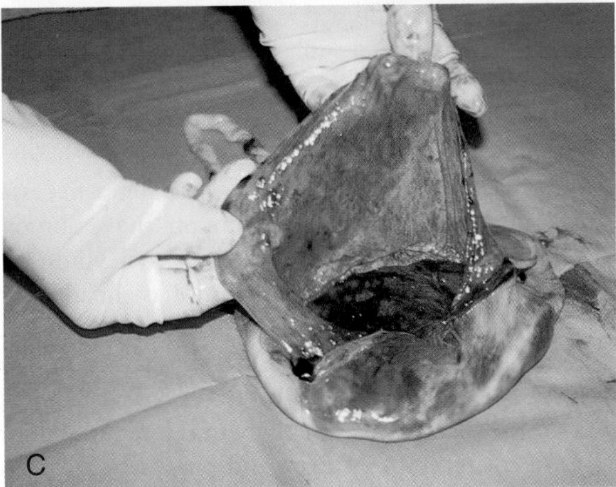

Fig. 5-10 Full-term placenta. **A,** Maternal (or uterine) surface, showing cotyledons and grooves. **B,** Fetal (or amniotic) surface, showing blood vessels running under amnion and converging to form umbilical vessels at attachment of umbilical cord. **C,** Amnion and smooth chorion are arranged to show that they are (1) fused and (2) continuous with margins of placenta. (Courtesy Marjorie Pyle, RNC, Lifecircle, Costa Mesa, CA.)

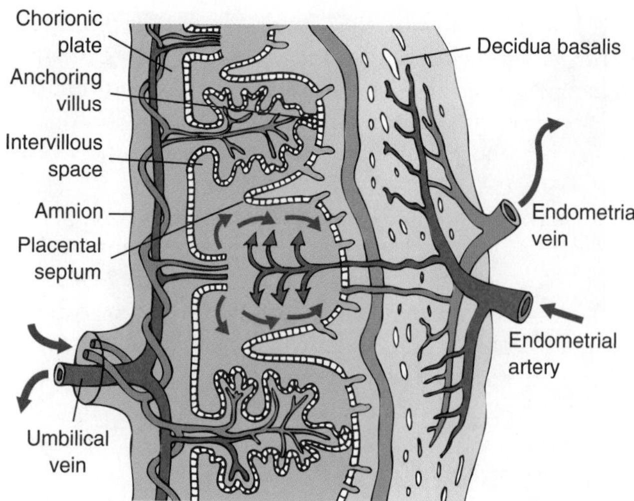

Fig. 5-11 Schematic drawing of the placenta illustrating how it supplies oxygen and nutrition to the embryo and removes its waste products. Deoxygenated blood leaves the fetus through the umbilical arteries and enters the placenta, where it is oxygenated. Oxygenated blood leaves the placenta through the umbilical vein, which enters the fetus via the umbilical cord.

formed on a sample of chorionic villi obtained by aspiration biopsy; however, limb defects have been associated with chorionic villus sampling performed before 10 weeks. The structure of the placenta is complete by the twelfth week. The placenta continues to grow wider until 20 weeks, when it covers approximately one half of the uterine surface. It then continues to grow thicker. The branching villi continue to develop within the body of the placenta, increasing the functional surface area.

Functions

One of the early functions of the placenta is as an endocrine gland that produces four hormones necessary to maintain the pregnancy and support the embryo or fetus. The hormones are produced in the syncytium.

The protein hormone human chorionic gonadotropin (hCG) can be detected in the maternal serum by 7 to 10 days after conception, shortly after implantation. This hormone is the basis for pregnancy tests. The hCG preserves the function of the ovarian corpus luteum, ensuring a continued supply of estrogen and progesterone needed to maintain the pregnancy. Miscarriage occurs if the corpus luteum stops functioning before the placenta can produce sufficient estrogen and progesterone. The hCG reaches its maximum level at 50 to 70 days, then begins to decrease.

The other protein hormone produced by the placenta is human chorionic somatomammotropin (hCS) or human placental lactogen (hPL). This substance is similar to a growth hormone and stimulates maternal metabolism to supply needed nutrients for fetal growth. This hormone increases the resistance to insulin, facilitates glucose transport across the placental membrane, and stimulates breast development to prepare for lactation.

The placenta eventually produces more of the steroid hormone progesterone than the corpus luteum does during the first few months of pregnancy. Progesterone maintains the endometrium, decreases the contractility of the uterus, and stimulates maternal metabolism and development of breast alveoli.

By 7 weeks after fertilization the placenta is producing most of the maternal estrogens, which are steroid hormones. The major estrogen secreted by the placenta is estriol, whereas the ovaries produce mostly estradiol. Measuring estriol levels is a clinical assay for placental functioning. Estrogen stimulates uterine growth and uteroplacental blood flow. It causes a proliferation of the breast glandular tissue and stimulates myometrial contractility. Placental estrogen production increases greatly toward the end of pregnancy. One theory for the cause of the onset of labor is the decrease in circulating levels of progesterone and the increased levels of estrogen.

The metabolic functions of the placenta are respiration, nutrition, excretion, and storage. Oxygen diffuses from the maternal blood across the placental membrane into the fetal blood, and carbon dioxide diffuses in the opposite direction. In this way the placenta functions as a lung for the fetus.

Carbohydrates, proteins, calcium, and iron are stored in the placenta for ready access to meet fetal needs. Water, inorganic salts, carbohydrates, proteins, fats, and vitamins pass from the maternal blood supply across the placental membrane into the fetal blood, supplying nutrition. Water and most electrolytes with a molecular weight less than 500 readily diffuse through the membrane. Hydrostatic and osmotic pressures aid in the flow of water and some solutions. Facilitated and active transport assist in the transfer of glucose, amino acids, calcium, iron, and substances with higher molecular weights. Amino acids and calcium are transported against the concentration gradient between the maternal blood and fetal blood.

The fetal concentration of glucose is lower than the glucose level in the maternal blood because of its rapid metabolism by the fetus. This fetal requirement demands larger concentrations of glucose than simple diffusion can provide. Therefore maternal glucose moves into the fetal circulation by active transport.

Pinocytosis is a mechanism used for transferring large molecules such as albumin and gamma globulins across the placental membrane. This mechanism conveys the maternal immunoglobulins that provide early passive immunity to the fetus.

Metabolic waste products of the fetus cross the placental membrane from the fetal blood into the maternal blood. The maternal kidneys then excrete them. Many viruses can cross the placental membrane and infect the fetus. Some bacteria and protozoa first infect the placenta and then infect the fetus. Drugs can also cross the placen-

BOX 5-3

Developmentally Toxic Exposures in Humans

- Aminopterin
- Androgens
- Angiotensin-converting enzyme inhibitors
- Carbamazepine
- Cigarette smoke
- Cocaine
- Coumarin anticoagulants
- Cytomegalovirus
- Diethylstilbestrol
- Ethanol (>1 drink/day)
- Etretinate
- Hyperthermia
- Iodides
- Ionizing radiation (>10 rad)
- Isotretinoin
- Lead
- Lithium
- Methimazole
- Methyl mercury
- Parvovirus B19
- Penicillamine
- Phenytoin
- Radioiodine
- Rubella
- Syphilis
- Tetracycline
- Thalidomide
- Toxoplasmosis
- Trimethadione
- Valproic acid
- Varicella

tal membrane and may harm the fetus. Caffeine, alcohol, nicotine, carbon monoxide, and other toxic substances in cigarette smoke, as well as prescription and recreational drugs (e.g., marijuana, cocaine), readily cross the placenta (Box 5-3).

Although no direct link exists between the fetal blood in the vessels of the chorionic villi and the maternal blood in the intervillous spaces, only one cell layer separates them. Breaks occasionally occur in the placental membrane. Fetal erythrocytes then leak into the maternal circulation, and the mother can develop antibodies to the fetal red blood cells. This development is often the way the Rh-negative mother becomes sensitized to the erythrocytes of her Rh-positive fetus (see the discussion of isoimmunization in Chapter 24).

Placental function depends on the maternal blood pressure supplying the circulation. Maternal arterial blood, under pressure in the small uterine spiral arteries, spurts into the intervillous spaces (see Fig. 5-11). As long as rich arterial blood continues to be supplied, pressure is exerted on the blood already in the intervillous spaces, pushing it toward drainage by the low-pressure uterine veins. At term gestation, 10% of the maternal cardiac output goes to the uterus.

If interference with the circulation to the placenta occurs the placenta cannot supply the embryo or fetus. Vasoconstriction, such as that caused by hypertension or cocaine use, diminishes uterine blood flow. Decreased maternal blood pressure or decreased cardiac output also diminishes uterine blood flow.

When a woman lies on her back with the pressure of the uterus compressing the vena cava, blood return to the right atrium is diminished (see Fig. 11-5). Excessive maternal exercise that diverts blood to the muscles away from the uterus compromises placental circulation. Optimal circulation is achieved when the woman is lying at rest on her side. Decreased uterine circulation may lead to intrauterine growth restriction of the fetus and infants who are small for gestational age.

Braxton Hicks contractions seem to enhance the movement of blood through the intervillous spaces, aiding placental circulation. However, prolonged contractions or too-short intervals between contractions during labor can reduce the blood flow to the placenta.

Fetal Maturation

The stage of the fetus lasts from 9 weeks (when the embryo becomes recognizable as a human being) until the pregnancy ends. Changes during the fetal period are not as dramatic because refinement of structure and function is taking place. The fetus is less vulnerable to teratogens, except for those that affect central nervous system functioning.

Viability refers to the capability of the fetus to survive outside the uterus. In the past the earliest age at which fetal survival could be expected was 28 weeks after conception. With modern technology and advances in maternal and neonatal care, viability is now possible approximately 20 weeks after conception (22 weeks since LMP; fetal weight of 500 g or more). The limitations on survival outside the uterus are based on central nervous system function and oxygenation capability of the lungs.

Respiratory system

The respiratory system begins development during embryonic life and continues through fetal life and into childhood. The development of the respiratory tract begins in week 4 and continues through week 17 with formation of the larynx, trachea, bronchi, and lung buds. Between 16 and 24 weeks the bronchi and terminal bronchioles enlarge, and vascular structures and primitive alveoli are formed. Between 24 weeks and term birth, more alveoli form. Specialized alveolar cells, type I and type II cells, secrete pulmonary surfactants to line the interior of the alveoli. After 32 weeks, sufficient surfactant is present in developed alveoli to provide infants with a good chance of survival.

Pulmonary surfactants. The detection of the presence of pulmonary surfactants (surface-active phospholipids) in amniotic fluid has been used to determine the degree of fetal lung maturity, or the ability of the lungs to function after birth. Lecithin (L) is the most critical alveolar surfactant required for postnatal lung expansion. It is detectable at approximately 21 weeks and increases in amount after week 24. Another pulmonary phospholipid, sphingomyelin (S), remains constant in amount. Therefore the measure of lecithin in relation to sphingomyelin, or the L/S ratio, is used to determine fetal lung maturity. When the L/S ratio reaches 2 : 1, the lungs are considered to be mature, which occurs at approximately 35 weeks of gestation.

Certain maternal conditions that cause decreased maternal placental blood flow, such as maternal hypertension, placental dysfunction, infection, or corticosteroid use, accelerate lung maturity. This process is apparently caused by the resulting fetal hypoxia, which stresses the fetus and increases the blood levels of corticosteroids that accelerate alveolar and surfactant development.

Conditions such as gestational diabetes and chronic glomerulonephritis can retard fetal lung maturity. The use of intrabronchial synthetic surfactant in the treatment of respiratory distress syndrome in the newborn has greatly improved the chances of survival for preterm infants.

Fetal respiratory movements have been seen on ultrasound as early as the eleventh week. These fetal respiratory movements may aid in development of the chest wall muscles and regulate lung fluid volume. The fetal lungs produce fluid that expands the air spaces in the lungs. The fluid drains into the amniotic fluid or is swallowed by the fetus.

Before birth, secretion of lung fluid decreases. The normal birth process squeezes out approximately one third of the fluid. Infants of cesarean births do not benefit from this squeezing process; therefore they may have more respiratory difficulty at birth. The fluid remaining in the lungs at birth is usually reabsorbed into the infant's bloodstream within 2 hours of birth.

Fetal circulatory system

Animation: Maternal and Fetal Circulation

The cardiovascular system is the first organ system to function in the developing human. Blood vessel and blood cell formation begins in the third week and supplies the embryo with oxygen and nutrients from the mother. By the end of the third week the tubular heart begins to beat, and the primitive cardiovascular system links the embryo, connecting stalk, chorion, and yolk sac. During the fourth and fifth weeks the heart develops into a four-chambered organ. By the end of the embryonic stage, the heart is developmentally complete.

The fetal lungs do not function for respiratory gas exchange, so a special circulatory pathway, the ductus arteriosus, bypasses the lungs. Oxygen-rich blood from the placenta flows rapidly through the umbilical vein into the fetal abdomen (Fig. 5-12). When the umbilical vein reaches the liver, it divides into two branches. One branch circulates some oxygenated blood through the liver. Most of the blood passes through the ductus venosus into the inferior vena cava. There it mixes with the deoxygenated blood from the fetal legs and abdomen on its way to the right atrium. Most of this blood passes straight through the right atrium and through the foramen ovale, an opening into the left atrium. There it mixes with the small amount of deoxygenated blood returning from the fetal lungs through the pulmonary veins.

The blood flows into the left ventricle and is squeezed out into the aorta, where the arteries supplying the heart, head, neck, and arms receive most of the oxygen-rich blood. This pattern of supplying the highest levels of oxygen and nutrients to the head, neck, and arms enhances the cephalocaudal (head-to-rump) development of the embryo and fetus.

Deoxygenated blood returning from the head and arms enters the right atrium through the superior vena cava. This blood is directed downward into the right ventricle, where it is squeezed into the pulmonary artery. A small amount of blood circulates through the resistant lung tissue, but the majority follows the path with less resistance through the ductus arteriosus into the aorta, distal to the point of exit of the arteries supplying the head and arms with oxygenated blood. The oxygen-poor blood flows through the abdominal aorta into the internal iliac arteries, where the umbilical arteries direct most of it back through the umbilical cord to the placenta. There the blood gives up its wastes and carbon dioxide in exchange for nutrients and oxygen. The blood remaining in the iliac arteries flows through the fetal abdomen and legs, ultimately returning through the inferior vena cava to the heart.

The following three special characteristics enable the fetus to obtain sufficient oxygen from the maternal blood:

- Fetal hemoglobin carries 20% to 30% more oxygen than maternal hemoglobin.
- The hemoglobin concentration of the fetus is approximately 50% greater than that of the mother.
- The fetal heart rate (FHR) is 110 to 160 beats/min, making the cardiac output per unit of body weight higher than that of an adult.

Hematopoietic system

Hematopoiesis, the formation of blood, occurs in the yolk sac (see Fig. 5-8, *B*) beginning in the third week. Hematopoietic stem cells seed the fetal liver during the fifth week, and hematopoiesis begins there during the sixth week. This development accounts for the relatively large size of the liver between the seventh and ninth weeks. Stem cells seed the fetal bone marrow, spleen and thymus, and lymph nodes between weeks 8 and 11 (for more information about stem cells, see http://stemcells.nih.gov/index.asp).

The antigenic factors that determine blood type are present in the erythrocytes soon after the sixth week. For this reason the Rh-negative woman is at risk for isoimmunization in any pregnancy that lasts longer than 6 weeks after fertilization.

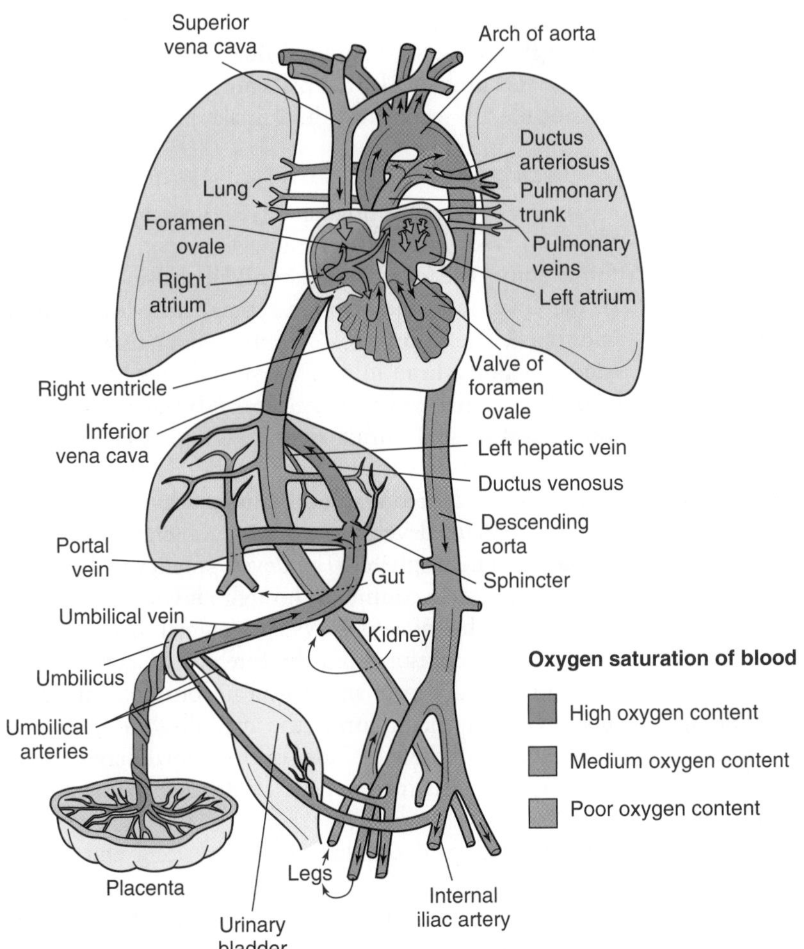

Fig. 5-12 Schematic illustration of fetal circulation. The *colors* indicate the oxygen saturation of the blood, and the *arrows* show the course of the blood from the placenta to the heart. The organs are not drawn to scale. Observe that three shunts permit most of the blood to bypass the liver and lungs: (1) ductus venosus, (2) foramen ovale, and (3) ductus arteriosus. A small amount of highly oxygenated blood from the inferior vena cava remains in the right atrium and mixes with poorly oxygenated blood from the superior vena cava. This medium oxygenated blood then passes into the right ventricle. The poorly oxygenated blood returns to the placenta for oxygen and nutrients through the umbilical arteries. (From Moore, K.L., Persaud, T.V.N., Torchia, M.G. [2013]. *Before we are born: essentials of embryology and birth defects* [8th ed.]. Philadelphia: Saunders.)

Hepatic system

The liver and biliary tract develop from the foregut during the fourth week of gestation. Hematopoiesis begins during the sixth week and requires that the liver be large. The embryonic liver is prominent, occupying most of the abdominal cavity. Bile, a constituent of meconium, begins to form in the twelfth week.

Glycogen is stored in the fetal liver beginning at week 9 or 10. At term, glycogen stores are twice those of the adult. Glycogen is the major source of energy for the fetus and for the neonate stressed by in utero hypoxia, extrauterine loss of the maternal glucose supply, the work of breathing, or cold stress. Iron is also stored in the fetal liver. If maternal intake is sufficient, the fetus can store enough iron to last for 5 months after birth.

During fetal life the liver does not have to conjugate bilirubin for excretion because the unconjugated bilirubin is cleared by the placenta. Therefore the glucuronyl transferase enzyme needed for conjugation is present in the fetal liver in amounts less than those required after birth. This circumstance predisposes the neonate, especially the preterm infant, to hyperbilirubinemia.

Coagulation factors II, VII, IX, and X cannot be synthesized in the fetal liver because of the lack of vitamin K synthesis in the sterile fetal gut. This coagulation deficiency persists after birth for several days and is the rationale for the prophylactic administration of vitamin K to the newborn.

Gastrointestinal system

During the fourth week the shape of the embryo changes from almost straight to a C shape as both ends fold in toward the ventral surface. A portion of the yolk sac is incorporated into the body from head to tail as the primitive gut (digestive system).

The foregut produces the pharynx, part of the lower respiratory tract, the esophagus, the stomach, the first half of the duodenum, the liver, the pancreas, and the gallbladder. These structures evolve during the fifth and sixth weeks. Malformations that can occur in these areas include esophageal atresia, hypertrophic pyloric stenosis, duodenal stenosis or atresia, and biliary atresia.

The midgut becomes the distal half of the duodenum, the jejunum and ileum, the cecum and appendix, and the proximal half of the colon. The midgut loop projects into the umbilical cord between weeks 5 and 10. A malformation, omphalocele (see Table 24-10), results if the midgut fails to return to the abdominal cavity, causing the intestines to protrude from the umbilicus. Meckel diverticulum is the most common malformation of the midgut. It occurs when a remnant of the yolk stalk that has failed to degenerate attaches to the ileum, leaving a blind sac.

The hindgut develops into the distal half of the colon, the rectum and parts of the anal canal, the urinary bladder, and the urethra. Anorectal malformations are the most common abnormalities of the digestive system.

The fetus swallows amniotic fluid beginning in the fifth month. Gastric emptying and intestinal peristalsis occur. Fetal nutrition and elimination are functions of the placenta. As the fetus nears term, fetal waste products accumulate in the intestines as dark green to black, tarry meconium. Normally this substance is passed through the rectum within 24 hours of birth. Sometimes, with a breech presentation or fetal hypoxia, meconium is passed in utero into the amniotic fluid. The failure to pass meconium after birth may indicate atresia somewhere in the digestive tract, an imperforate anus (see Table 24-10), or meconium ileus, in which a firm meconium plug blocks passage (seen in infants with CF).

The metabolic rate of the fetus is relatively low, but the infant has great growth and development needs. Beginning in week 9 the fetus synthesizes glycogen for storage in the liver. Between 26 and 30 weeks the fetus begins to lay down stores of brown fat in preparation for extrauterine cold stress. Thermoregulation in the neonate requires increased metabolism and adequate oxygenation.

The gastrointestinal system is mature by 36 weeks. Digestive enzymes (except pancreatic amylase and lipase) are present in sufficient quantity to facilitate digestion. The neonate cannot digest starches or fats efficiently. Little saliva is produced.

Renal system

The kidneys form during the fifth week and begin to function approximately 4 weeks later. Urine is excreted into the amniotic fluid and forms a major part of the amniotic fluid volume. Oligohydramnios is indicative of renal dysfunction. Because the placenta acts as the organ of excretion and maintains fetal water and electrolyte balance the fetus does not need functioning kidneys while in utero. At birth, however, the kidneys are required immediately for excretory and acid-base regulatory functions.

A fetal renal malformation can be diagnosed in utero. Corrective or palliative fetal surgery may treat the malformation successfully, or plans can be made for treatment immediately after birth.

At term the fetus has fully developed kidneys. However, the glomerular filtration rate is low, and the kidneys lack the ability to concentrate urine. This circumstance makes the newborn more susceptible to both overhydration and dehydration.

Most newborns void within 24 hours of birth. With the loss of the swallowed amniotic fluid and the metabolism of nutrients provided by the placenta, voidings for the first days of life are scant until fluid intake increases.

Neurologic system

The nervous system originates from the ectoderm during the third week after fertilization. The open neural tube forms during the fourth week. It initially closes at what will be the junction of the brain and spinal cord, leaving both ends open. The embryo folds in on itself lengthwise at this time, forming a head fold in the neural tube at this junction. The cranial end of the neural tube closes, then the caudal end closes. During week 5, different growth rates cause more flexures in the neural tube, delineating three brain areas: the forebrain, midbrain, and hindbrain.

The forebrain develops into the eyes (cranial nerve II) and cerebral hemispheres. The development of all areas of the cerebral cortex continues throughout fetal life and into childhood. The olfactory system (cranial nerve I) and thalamus also develop from the forebrain. Cranial nerves III and IV (oculomotor and trochlear) form from the midbrain. The hindbrain forms the medulla, the pons, the cerebellum, and the remainder of the cranial nerves. Brain waves can be recorded on an electroencephalogram by week 8.

The spinal cord develops from the long end of the neural tube. Another ectodermal structure, the neural crest, develops into the peripheral nervous system. By the eighth week, nerve fibers traverse throughout the body. By week 11 or 12 the fetus makes respiratory movements, moves all extremities, and changes position in utero. The fetus can suck his or her thumb, swim in the amniotic fluid pool, turn somersaults, and sometimes such fetal movements result in a knot in the umbilical cord. Sometime between 16 and 20 weeks, when the movements are strong enough to be perceived by the mother as "the baby moving," quickening has occurred. The perception of movement occurs earlier in the multipara than in the primipara. The mother also becomes aware of the sleep and wake cycles of the fetus.

Sensory awareness. Purposeful movements of the fetus have been demonstrated in response to a firm touch transmitted through the mother's abdomen. Because it can feel, the fetus requires anesthesia when invasive intrauterine procedures are performed.

Fetuses respond to sound by 24 weeks. Different types of music evoke different movements. The fetus can be soothed by the sound of the mother's voice. Acoustic stimulation can be used to evoke an FHR response. The fetus becomes accustomed (habituates) to noises heard repeatedly. Hearing is fully developed at birth.

The fetus is able to distinguish taste. By the fifth month, when the fetus is swallowing amniotic fluid, a sweetener added to the fluid causes the fetus to swallow faster. The fetus also reacts to temperature changes. A cold solution placed into the amniotic fluid can cause fetal hiccups.

The fetus can see. Eyes have both rods and cones in the retina by the seventh month. A bright light shone on the mother's abdomen in late pregnancy causes abrupt fetal movements. During sleep time, rapid eye movements (REMs) have been observed similar to those occurring in children and adults while dreaming.

At term the fetal brain is approximately one fourth the size of an adult brain. Neurologic development continues. Stressors on the fetus and neonate (e.g., chronic poor nutrition or hypoxia, drugs, environmental toxins, trauma, disease) cause damage to the central nervous system long after the vulnerable embryonic time for malformations in other organ systems. Neurologic insult can result in cerebral palsy, neuromuscular impairment, mental retardation, and learning disabilities.

Endocrine system

The thyroid gland develops along with structures in the head and neck during the third and fourth weeks. The secretion of thyroxine begins during the eighth week. Maternal thyroxine does not readily cross the placenta; therefore the fetus that does not produce thyroid hormones will be born with congenital hypothyroidism. If untreated, hypothyroidism can result in severe mental retardation. Screening for hypothyroidism is typically included in the testing when screening for PKU after birth.

The adrenal cortex is formed during the sixth week and produces hormones by the eighth or ninth week. As term approaches, the fetus produces more cortisol. This hormone is believed to aid in initiation of labor by decreasing the maternal progesterone and stimulating production of prostaglandins.

The pancreas forms from the foregut during the fifth through eighth weeks. The islets of Langerhans develop during the twelfth week. Insulin is produced by the twentieth week. In infants of mothers with uncontrolled diabetes, maternal hyperglycemia produces fetal hyperglycemia, stimulating hyperinsulinemia and islet cell hyperplasia. This results in a macrosomic (large-sized) fetus. The hyperinsulinemia also blocks lung maturation, placing the neonate at risk for respiratory distress and hypoglycemia when the maternal glucose source is lost at birth. Control of the maternal glucose level before and during pregnancy minimizes problems for the fetus and infant.

Reproductive system

Sex differentiation begins in the embryo during the seventh week. Female and male external genitalia are indistinguishable until after the ninth week. Distinguishing characteristics appear around the ninth week and are fully differentiated by the twelfth week. When a Y chromosome is present, testes are formed. By the end of the embryonic period, testosterone is being secreted and causes formation of the male genitalia. By week 28 the testes begin descending into the scrotum. After birth, low levels of testosterone continue to be secreted until the pubertal surge.

The female, with two X chromosomes, forms ovaries and female external genitalia. By the sixteenth week, oogenesis has been established. At birth the ovaries contain the female's lifetime supply of ova. Most female hormone production is delayed until puberty. However, the fetal endometrium responds to maternal hormones, and withdrawal bleeding or vaginal discharge (pseudomenstruation) may occur at birth when these hormones are lost. The high level of maternal estrogen also stimulates mammary engorgement and secretion of fluid ("witch's milk") in newborn infants of both sexes.

Musculoskeletal system

Bones and muscles develop from the mesoderm by the fourth week of embryonic development. At that time the cardiac muscle is already beating. The mesoderm next to the neural tube forms the vertebral column and ribs. The parts of the vertebral column grow toward each other to enclose the developing spinal cord. Ossification, or bone formation, begins. If the bony fusion has a defect, various forms of spina bifida may occur. A large defect affecting several vertebrae may allow the membranes and spinal cord to pouch out from the back, producing neurologic deficits and skeletal deformity.

The flat bones of the skull develop during the embryonic period, and ossification continues throughout childhood. At birth, connective tissue sutures exist where the bones of the skull meet. The areas where more than two bones meet (called *fontanels*) are especially prominent. The sutures and fontanels allow the bones of the skull to mold, or move during birth, enabling the head to pass through the birth canal.

The bones of the shoulders, arms, hips, and legs appear in the sixth week as a continuous skeleton with no joints. Differentiation occurs, producing separate bones and joints. Ossification will continue through childhood to allow growth. Beginning in the seventh week, muscles contract spontaneously. Arm and leg movements are visible on ultrasound, although the mother does not perceive them until sometime between 16 and 20 weeks.

Integumentary system

The epidermis begins as a single layer of cells derived from the ectoderm at 4 weeks. By the seventh week, two layers of cells have formed. The cells of the superficial layer are sloughed and become mixed with the sebaceous gland secretions to form the white, cheesy *vernix caseosa*, the material that protects the skin of the fetus. The vernix is thick at 24 weeks but becomes scant by term.

The basal layer of the epidermis is the germinal layer, which replaces lost cells. Until 17 weeks the skin is thin and wrinkled, with blood vessels visible underneath. The skin thickens, and all layers are present at term. After 32 weeks, as subcutaneous fat is deposited under the dermis, the skin becomes less wrinkled and red in appearance.

By 16 weeks the epidermal ridges are present on the palms of the hands, the fingers, the bottom of the feet, and the toes. These handprints and footprints are unique to that infant.

Hairs form from hair bulbs in the epidermis that project into the dermis. Cells in the hair bulb keratinize to form the hair shaft. As the cells at the base of the hair shaft proliferate, the hair grows to the surface of the epithelium. Very fine hairs, called *lanugo*, appear first at 12 weeks on the eyebrows and upper lip. By 20 weeks they cover the entire body. At this time the eyelashes, eyebrows, and scalp hair are beginning to grow. By 28 weeks the scalp hair is longer than the lanugo, which thins and may disappear by term gestation.

Fingernails and toenails develop from thickened epidermis at the tips of the digits beginning during the tenth week. They grow slowly. Fingernails usually reach the fingertips by 32 weeks, and toenails reach the toe tips by 36 weeks.

Immunologic system

During the third trimester, albumin and globulin are present in the fetus. The only immunoglobulin (Ig) that crosses the placenta, IgG, provides passive acquired immunity to specific bacterial toxins. The fetus produces IgM immunoglobulins by the end of the first trimester. These immunoglobulins are produced in response to blood group antigens, gram-negative enteric organisms, and some viruses. IgA immunoglobulins are not produced by the fetus; however, colostrum, the precursor to breast milk, contains large amounts of IgA and can provide passive immunity to the neonate who is breastfed.

The normal-term neonate can fight infection, but not as effectively as an older child. The preterm infant is at much greater risk for infection.

Table 5-1 provides a summary of embryonic and fetal development.

Multifetal Pregnancy

Twins

The incidence of twinning is 1 in 43 births (Benirschke, 2009). The number of multiple births has steadily risen since 1973. This increase is attributed to increasing maternal age at childbirth and the use of assistive reproductive technologies.

Dizygotic Twins. When two mature ova are produced in one ovarian cycle, both have the potential to be fertilized by separate sperm. This results in two zygotes, or dizygotic twins (Fig. 5-13). In every instance, there are two amnions, two chorions, and two placentas that may be fused together. These dizygotic or fraternal twins may be the same sex or different sexes and are genetically no more alike than siblings born at different times. Dizygotic twinning occurs in families, is more common among African-American women than Caucasian women, and is least common among Asian-American women. Dizygotic twinning increases in frequency with maternal age up to 35 years, with parity, and with the use of fertility drugs.

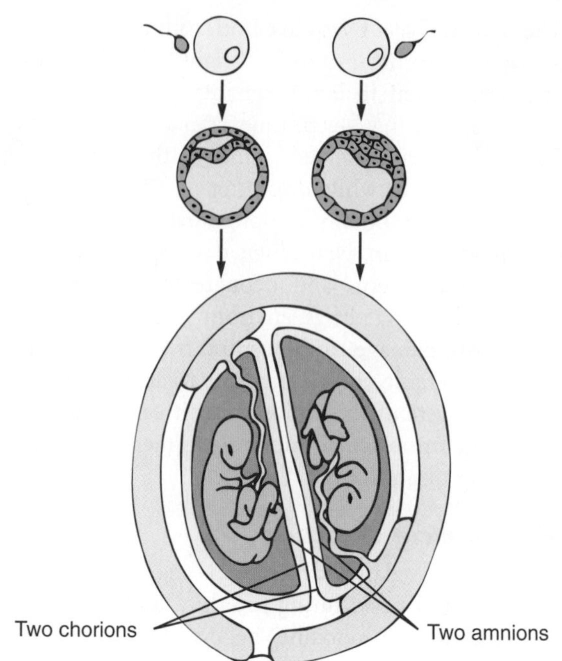

Fig. 5-13 Formation of dizygotic twins showing fertilization of two ova, two implantations, two placentas, two chorions, and two amnions.

Monozygotic twins. Identical or monozygotic twins develop from one fertilized ovum, which then divides (Fig. 5-14). They are the same sex and have the same genotype. If division occurs soon after fertilization, two embryos, two amnions, two chorions, and two placentas that may be fused will develop. Most often, division occurs between 4 and 8 days after fertilization, leaving two embryos, two amnions, one chorion, and one placenta. Rarely, division occurs after the eighth day after fertilization. In this case, two embryos are within a common amnion and a common chorion with one placenta. This often causes circulatory problems because the umbilical cords may tangle together, and one or both fetuses may die. If division occurs very late, cleavage may not be complete, and conjoined or "Siamese" twins could result (Fig. 5-14, *C*). Monozygotic twinning rate is between 3.5 and 4 per 1000 births (Benirschke, 2009). No association with race, heredity, maternal age, or parity has been found. Use of fertility drugs increases the incidence of monozygotic twinning.

Other multifetal pregnancies

The occurrence of multifetal pregnancies with three or more fetuses has increased with the use of fertility drugs and IVF. Triplets occur in approximately 1 of 1341 pregnancies (Benirschke, 2009). They can occur from the division of one zygote into two, with one of the two dividing again, producing identical triplets. Triplets can also be produced from two zygotes, one dividing into a set of identical twins and the second zygote a single fraternal sibling, or from three zygotes. Quadruplets, quintuplets, sextuplets, and so on have similar possible derivations.

TABLE 5-1

Milestones in Human Development before Birth since Last Menstrual Period

4 WEEKS	8 WEEKS	12 WEEKS
EXTERNAL APPEARANCE		
Body flexed, C shaped; arm and leg buds present; head at right angles to body 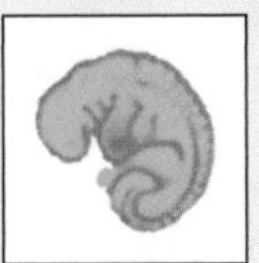	Body fairly well formed; nose flat, eyes far apart; digits well formed; head elevating; tail almost disappeared; eyes, ears, nose, and mouth recognizable 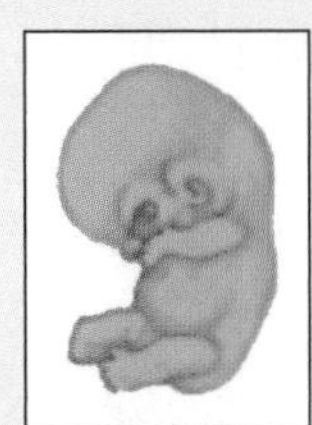	Nails appearing; resembles a human; head erect but disproportionately large; skin pink, delicate 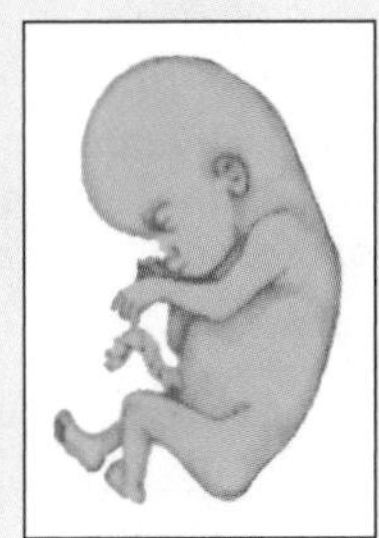
CROWN-TO-RUMP MEASUREMENT; WEIGHT		
0.4-0.5 cm; 0.4 g	2.5-3 cm; 2 g	6-9 cm; 19 g
GASTROINTESTINAL SYSTEM		
Stomach at midline and fusiform; conspicuous liver; esophagus short; intestine a short tube	Intestinal villi developing; small intestines coil within umbilical cord; palatal folds present; liver very large	Bile secreted; palatal fusion complete; intestines have withdrawn from cord and assume characteristic positions
MUSCULOSKELETAL SYSTEM		
All somites present	First indication of ossification—occiput, mandible, and humerus; fetus capable of some movement; definitive muscles of trunk, limbs, and head well represented	Some bones well outlined, ossification spreading; upper cervical to lower sacral arches and bodies ossify; smooth muscle layers indicated in hollow viscera
CIRCULATORY SYSTEM		
Heart develops, double chambers visible, begins to beat; aortic arch and major veins completed	Main blood vessels assume final plan; enucleated red cells predominate in blood	Blood forming in marrow
RESPIRATORY SYSTEM		
Primary lung buds appear	Pleural and pericardial cavities forming; branching bronchioles; nostrils closed by epithelial plugs	Lungs acquire definite shape; vocal cords appear
RENAL SYSTEM		
Rudimentary ureteral buds appear	Earliest secretory tubules differentiating; bladder-urethra separates from rectum	Kidney able to secrete urine; bladder expands as a sac
NERVOUS SYSTEM		
Well-marked midbrain flexure; no hindbrain or cervical flexures; neural groove closed	Cerebral cortex begins to acquire typical cells; differentiation of cerebral cortex, meninges, ventricular foramina, cerebrospinal fluid circulation; spinal cord extends entire length of spine	Brain structural configuration almost complete; cord shows cervical and lumbar enlargements; fourth ventricle foramina are developed; sucking present
SENSORY ORGANS		
Eye and ear appearing as optic vessel and otocyst	Primordial choroid plexuses develop; ventricles large relative to cortex; development progressing; eyes converging rapidly; internal ear developing; eyelids fuse	Earliest taste buds indicated; characteristic organization of eye attained
GENITAL SYSTEM		
Genital ridge appears (fifth week)	Testes and ovaries distinguishable; external genitalia sexless but begin to differentiate	Sex recognizable; internal and external sex organs specific

Animation: First Trimester, Fetal Development

Continued

TABLE 5-1

Milestones in Human Development before Birth since Last Menstrual Period—cont'd

Animation: Second Trimester, Fetal Development

16 WEEKS	20 WEEKS	24 WEEKS
EXTERNAL APPEARANCE		
Head still dominant; face looks human; eyes, ears, and nose approach typical appearance on gross examination; arm/leg ratio proportionate; scalp hair appears	Vernix caseosa appears; lanugo appears; legs lengthen considerably; sebaceous glands appear	Body lean but fairly well proportioned; skin red and wrinkled; vernix caseosa present; sweat glands forming
CROWN-TO-RUMP MEASUREMENT; WEIGHT		
11.5-13.5 cm; 100 g	16-18.5 cm; 300 g	23 cm; 600 g
GASTROINTESTINAL SYSTEM		
Meconium in bowel; some enzyme secretion; anus open	Enamel and dentine depositing; ascending colon recognizable	—
MUSCULOSKELETAL SYSTEM		
Most bones distinctly indicated throughout body; joint cavities appear; muscular movements can be detected	Sternum ossifies; fetal movements strong enough for mother to feel	—
CIRCULATORY SYSTEM		
Heart muscle well developed; blood formation active in spleen	—	Blood formation increases in bone marrow and decreases in liver
RESPIRATORY SYSTEM		
Elastic fibers appears in lungs; terminal and respiratory bronchioles appear	Nostrils reopen; primitive respiratory-like movements begin	Alveolar ducts and sacs present; lecithin begins to appear in amniotic fluid (weeks 26 to 27)
RENAL SYSTEM		
Kidney in position; attains typical shape and plan	—	—
NERVOUS SYSTEM		
Cerebral lobes delineated; cerebellum assumes some prominence	Brain grossly formed; cord myelination begins; spinal cord ends at level of first sacral vertebra (S1)	Cerebral cortex layered typically; neuronal proliferation in cerebral cortex ends
SENSORY ORGANS		
General sense organs differentiated	Nose and ears ossify	Can hear
GENITAL SYSTEM		
Testes in position for descent into scrotum: vagina open	—	Testes at inguinal ring in descent to scrotum

TABLE 5-1

Milestones in Human Development before Birth since Last Menstrual Period—cont'd

28 WEEKS	30-31 WEEKS	36 AND 40 WEEKS
EXTERNAL APPEARANCE		
Lean body, less wrinkled and red; nails appear	Subcutaneous fat beginning to collect; more rounded appearance; skin pink and smooth; has assumed birth position	36 weeks: skin pink, body rounded; general lanugo disappearing; body usually plump 40 weeks: skin smooth and pink; scant vernix caseosa; moderate to profuse hair; lanugo on shoulders and upper body only; nasal and alar cartilage apparent
CROWN-TO-RUMP MEASUREMENT; WEIGHT		
27 cm; 1100 g	31 cm; 1800-2100 g	36 weeks: 35 cm; 2200-2900 g 40 weeks: 40 cm; 32001 g
MUSCULOSKELETAL SYSTEM		
Astragalus (talus, ankle bone) ossifies; weak, fleeting movements, minimum tone	Middle fourth phalanxes ossify; permanent teeth primordia seen; can turn head to side	36 weeks: distal femoral ossification centers present; sustained, definite movements; fair tone; can turn and elevate head 40 weeks: active, sustained movement; good tone; may lift head
RESPIRATORY SYSTEM		
Lecithin forming on alveolar surfaces	L/S ratio = 1.2:1	36 weeks: L/S ratio = 2:1 40 weeks: pulmonary branching only two thirds complete
RENAL SYSTEM		
	—	36 weeks: formation of new nephrons ceases
NERVOUS SYSTEM		
Appearance of cerebral fissures, convolutions rapidly appearing; indefinite sleep-wake cycle; cry weak or absent; weak suck reflex	—	36 weeks: end of spinal cord at level of third lumbar vertebra (L3); definite sleep-wake cycle 40 weeks: myelination of brain begins; patterned sleep-wake cycle with alert periods; cries when hungry or uncomfortable; strong suck reflex
SENSORY ORGANS		
Eyelids reopen; retinal layers completed, light receptive; pupils capable of reacting to light	Sense of taste present; aware of sounds outside mother's body	—
GENITAL SYSTEM		
—	Testes descending to scrotum	40 weeks: testes in scrotum; labia majora well developed

L/S, Lecithin/sphingomyelin.

Animation: Third Trimester, Fetal Development

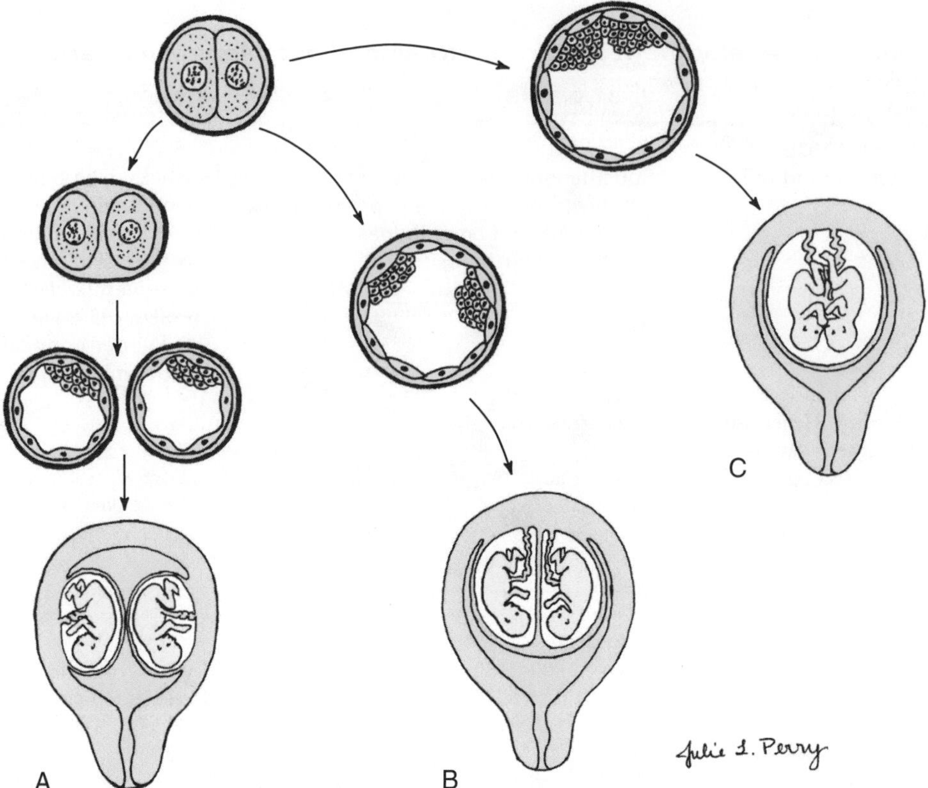

Fig. 5-14 Formation of monozygotic twins. **A,** One fertilization: blastomeres separate, resulting in two implantations, two placentas, and two sets of membranes. **B,** One blastomere with two inner cell masses, one fused placenta, one chorion, and separate amnions. **C,** One blastomere with incomplete separation of cell mass resulting in conjoined twins.

KEY POINTS

- Genetic disease affects people of all ages, from all socioeconomic levels, and from all racial and ethnic backgrounds.
- Genetic disorders span every clinical practice specialty.
- Nurses with advanced preparation are assuming important roles in genetic counseling.
- Genes are the basic units of heredity, responsible for all human characteristics. They make up 23 pairs of chromosomes: 22 pairs of autosomes and one pair of sex chromosomes.
- Genetic disorders follow mendelian inheritance patterns of dominance, segregation, and independent assortment of normal genetic transmission.
- Multifactorial inheritance includes both genetic and environmental contributions.
- Mitosis is the process by which body cells replicate for growth and development and cell replacement of the organism.
- Meiosis is the process by which gametes are formed for reproduction of the organism.
- Human gestation is approximately 280 days after the LMP, or 266 days after conception.
- Fertilization occurs in the uterine tube within 24 hours of ovulation. The zygote undergoes mitotic divisions, creating a 16-cell morula.
- Implantation begins 6 days after fertilization.
- The organ systems and external features develop during the embryonic period, that is, the third to the eighth week after fertilization.
- Refinement of structure and function occurs during the fetal period, and the fetus becomes capable of extrauterine survival.
- Critical periods occur in human development during which the embryo or fetus is vulnerable to environmental teratogens.
- The incidence of multiple births has increased since 1973.

Audio Chapter Summaries: Access an audio summary of these Key Points on evolve

References

American Academy of Pediatrics. (2001). Ethical issues with genetic testing in pediatrics. *Pediatrics, 107*(6), 1451-1455.

American Nurses Association (ANA) (2006). *Essential nursing competencies and curricula guidelines for genetics and genomics.* Silver Spring, MD: ANA.

Benirschke, K. (2009). Multiple gestation. The biology of twinning. In R. Creasy, R. Resnik, J. Iams, C. J. Lockwood, & T. R. Moore (Eds.). *Creasy and Resnik's Maternal-fetal medicine: Principles and practice* (6th ed.). Philadelphia: Saunders.

Canadian College of Medical Geneticists. (2003). Guidelines for genetic testing of healthy children. *Paediatrics & Child Health, 8*(1), 42-45.

Hamilton, B., & Wynshaw-Boris, A. (2009). Basic genetics and patterns of inheritance. In R. Creasy, R. Resnik, J. Iams, C. J. Lockwood, & T. R. Moore (Eds.). *Creasy and Resnik's maternal-fetal medicine: Principles and practice* (6th ed.). Philadelphia: Saunders.

International Human Genome Sequencing Consortium. (2001). Initial sequencing and analysis of the human genome. *Nature, 409* (6822), 860-921.

International Society of Nurses in Genetics (ISONG). (2006). *Genetics/genomics nursing: Scope and standards of practice* (2nd ed.). Washington, DC: American Nurses Association.

Lashley, F. (2005). *Clinical genetics in nursing practice* (3rd ed.). New York: Springer.

McInerney, J. (2008). *Behavioral genetics.* Internet document available at www.ornl.gov/sci/techresources/Human_Genome/elsi/behavior.shtml (accessed June 21, 2009).

National Down Syndrome Society. (2006). *About Down syndrome. Incidences and maternal age.* Internet document available at www.ndss.org/index.php?option=com_content&view=category&id=35&itemid=57 (accessed June 20, 2009).

Peach, E. & Hopkin, R. (2007). Advances in prenatal genetic testing: Current options, benefits, and limitations. *Newborn & Infant Nursing Reviews, 7*(4), 205-210.

Solomon, B. D., Jack, B. W., & Feero, G. (2008). The clinical content of preconception care: Genetics and genomics. *American Journal of Obstetrics & Gynecology, 199*, (6 Suppl 2), S340-S344.

Wapner, R. J., Jenkins, T. M., & Khalek, N. (2009). Prenatal diagnosis of congenital disorders. In R. Creasy, R. Resnik, J. Iams, C. J. Lockwood, & T. R. Moore (Eds.), *Creasy and Resnik's maternal-fetal medicine: Principles and practice* (6th ed.). Philadelphia: Saunders.

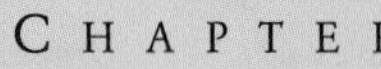
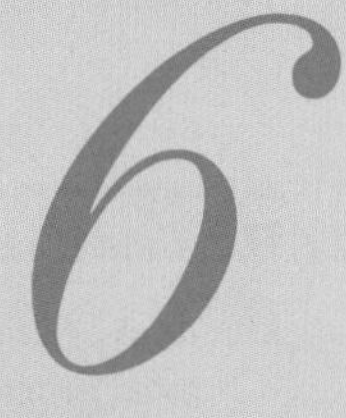
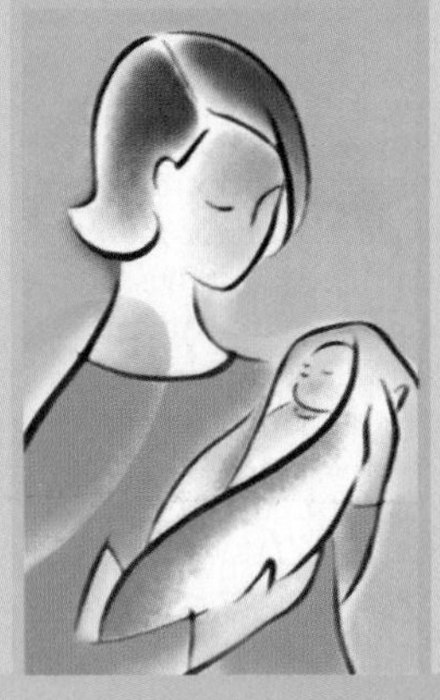

CHAPTER 6

Anatomy and Physiology of Pregnancy

DEITRA LEONARD LOWDERMILK

LEARNING OBJECTIVES

- *Determine gravidity and parity by using the five- and two-digit systems.*
- *Describe the various types of pregnancy tests, including the timing of tests and interpretation of results.*
- *Explain the expected maternal anatomic and physiologic adaptations to pregnancy for each body system.*
- *Differentiate among presumptive, probable, and positive signs of pregnancy.*
- *Compare normal adult laboratory values with values for pregnant women.*
- *Identify the maternal hormones produced during pregnancy, their target organs, and their major effects on pregnancy.*
- *Compare the characteristics of the abdomen, vulva, and cervix of the nullipara and multipara.*

KEY TERMS AND DEFINITIONS

ballottement Diagnostic technique using palpation; a floating fetus, when tapped or pushed, moves away and then returns to touch the examiner's hand

Braxton Hicks sign Mild, intermittent, painless uterine contractions that occur during pregnancy; occurring more frequently as pregnancy advances but not representing true labor; however, they should be distinguished from preterm labor

carpal tunnel syndrome Syndrome in which edema compresses the median nerve beneath the carpal ligament of the wrist; causing tingling, burning, or numbness in the inner half of one or both hands

Chadwick sign Violet color of vaginal mucous membrane that is visible from approximately the fourth week of pregnancy; caused by increased vascularity

chloasma Increased pigmentation over the bridge of the nose and cheeks of pregnant women and some women taking oral contraceptives; also known as the *mask of pregnancy*

colostrum Fluid in the acini cells of the breasts present from early pregnancy into the early postpartal period; rich in antibodies, which provide protection to the breastfed newborn from many diseases; high in protein, which binds bilirubin; and laxative acting, which speeds the elimination of meconium and helps loosen mucus

diastasis recti abdominis Separation of the two rectus muscles along the median line of the abdominal wall; often seen in women with repeated childbirths or with a multiple gestation (e.g., triplets)

epulis Tumor-like benign lesion of the gingiva seen in pregnant women

funic souffle Soft, muffled, blowing sound produced by blood rushing through the umbilical vessels and synchronous with the fetal heart sounds

Goodell sign Softening of the cervix, a probable sign of pregnancy, occurring during the second month

Hegar sign Softening of the lower uterine segment that is classified as a probable sign of pregnancy, may be present during the second and third months of pregnancy, and is palpated during bimanual examination

human chorionic gonadotropin (hCG) Hormone that is produced by chorionic villi; the biologic marker in pregnancy tests

leukorrhea White or yellowish mucus discharge from the cervical canal or the vagina that may be normal physiologically or caused by pathologic states of the vagina and endocervix

lightening Sensation of decreased abdominal distention produced by uterine descent into the pelvic cavity as the fetal presenting part settles into the pelvis; usually occurs 2 weeks before the onset of labor in nulliparas

KEY TERMS AND DEFINITIONS—cont'd

linea nigra Line of darker pigmentation seen in some women during the latter part of pregnancy that appears on the middle of the abdomen and extends from the symphysis pubis toward the umbilicus

Montgomery tubercles Small, nodular prominences (sebaceous glands) on the areolas around the nipples of the breasts that enlarge during pregnancy and lactation

operculum Plug of mucus that fills the cervical canal during pregnancy

palmar erythema Rash on the surface of the palms sometimes seen in pregnancy

ptyalism Excessive salivation

pyrosis Burning sensation in the epigastric and sternal region from stomach acid (heartburn)

quickening Maternal perception of fetal movement; usually occurs between weeks 16 and 20 of gestation

striae gravidarum "Stretch marks"; shining reddish lines caused by stretching of the skin, often found on the abdomen, thighs, and breasts during pregnancy; these streaks turn to a fine pinkish white or silver tone in time in fair-skinned women and brownish in darker-skinned women

uterine souffle Soft, blowing sound made by the blood in the arteries of the pregnant uterus and synchronous with the maternal pulse

WEB RESOURCES

Additional related content can be found on the companion website at evolve

http://evolve.elsevier.com/Lowdermilk/Maternity/

- NCLEX Review Questions

The goal of maternity care is a healthy pregnancy with a physically safe and emotionally satisfying outcome for mother, infant, and family. Consistent health supervision and surveillance are of utmost importance in achieving this outcome. However, many maternal adaptations are unfamiliar to pregnant women and their families. Helping the pregnant woman recognize the relationship between her physical status and the plan for her care assists her in making decisions and encourages her to participate in her own care.

GRAVIDITY AND PARITY

An understanding of the terms that are used to describe pregnancy and the pregnant woman is essential to the study of maternity care. Box 6-1 describes these terms.

Gravidity and parity information is obtained during history-taking interviews. Obtaining and documenting this information accurately is important in making a plan of care for the pregnant woman.

NURSING ALERT Information may be recorded in patient records in a variety of ways because no one standardized system is in place. Until such a system is in place, the nurse should understand the documentation system used by the health care facility.

Two commonly used systems of summarizing the obstetrical history are discussed here. Gravidity and parity may be described with only two digits: The first digit represents the number of pregnancies the woman has had, including the present one; and parity is the number of pregnancies that have reached 20 or more weeks of gestation. For example, if the woman had twins at 36 weeks with her first pregnancy, parity would still be counted as one birth (gravida [G] 1, para [P]1) (Cunningham, Leveno, Bloom, Hauth, Gilstrap, & Wenstrom, 2005). If she becomes pregnant a second time, she would be G2 P1 until she gives birth at 38 weeks when she would then become G2 P2. Another system, which consists of five digits separated with hyphens, is commonly used in maternity centers. This system provides more information about the woman's obstetric history, although it may not provide accurate information about parity since it provides information about births and not pregnancies reaching 20 weeks of gestation (Beebe, 2005). The first digit represents gravidity, the second digit represents the total number of term births, the third indicates the number of preterm births, the fourth identifies the number of abortions (miscarriage or elective termination of pregnancy), and the fifth is the number of children currently living. The acronym *GTPAL* (gravidity, term, preterm, abortions, living children) may be helpful in remembering this system of notation. For example, if a woman pregnant only once gives birth at week 34 and the infant survives, the abbreviation that represents this information is *1-0-1-0-1.* During her next pregnancy, the abbreviation is *2-0-1-0-1.* Additional examples are given in Table 6-1.

BOX 6-1

Definitions Related to Gravidity and Parity

- *Gravida:* a woman who is pregnant
- *Gravidity:* pregnancy
- *Multigravida:* a woman who has had two or more pregnancies
- *Multipara:* a woman who has completed two or more pregnancies to 20 weeks of gestation or more
- *Nulligravida:* a woman who has never been pregnant
- *Nullipara:* a woman who has not completed a pregnancy with a fetus or fetuses beyond 20 weeks of gestation
- *Parity:* the number of pregnancies in which the fetus or fetuses have reached 20 weeks of gestation when they are born, not the number of fetuses (e.g., twins) born. Whether the fetus is born alive or is stillborn (fetus who shows no signs of life at birth) does not affect parity.
- *Postdate* or *postterm:* a pregnancy that goes beyond 42 weeks of gestation
- *Preterm:* a pregnancy that has reached 20 weeks of gestation but before completion of 37 weeks of gestation
- *Primigravida:* a woman who is pregnant for the first time
- *Primipara:* a woman who has completed one pregnancy with a fetus or fetuses who have reached 20 weeks of gestation
- *Term:* a pregnancy from the completion of week 37 of gestation to the end of week 42 of gestation
- *Viability:* capacity to live outside the uterus; there are no clear limits of gestational age or weight but it is rare for a fetus to survive before 22 to 24 weeks of gestation and weighing less than 500 grams

Sources: Cunningham, F., Leveno, K., Bloom, S., Hauth, J., Gilstrap, L., & Wenstrom, K. (2005). *Williams obstetrics* (22nd ed.). New York: McGraw-Hill; Katz, V. (2007). Spontaneous and recurrent abortions. In V. Katz, G. Lentz, R. Lobo, & D. Gershenson (Eds.). *Comprehensive gynecology* (5th ed.). Philadelphia: Mosby.

TABLE 6-1

Obstetric History Using Five-Digit (GTPAL) System and Two-Digit (G/P)System

Condition	G (Gravidity)	T (Term births)	P (Preterm births)	A (Abortions and miscarriages)	L (Living children)	G/P (Gravidity/ parity)
Jamilla is pregnant for the first time.	1	0	0	0	0	1/0
She carries the pregnancy to 35 weeks, and the neonate survives.	1	0	1	0	1	1/1
She becomes pregnant again.	2	0	1	0	1	2/1
Her second pregnancy ends in miscarriage at 12 weeks.	2	0	1	1	1	2/1
During her third pregnancy, she gives birth at 39 weeks.	3	1	1	1	2	3/2
Jamilla is pregnant for the fourth time and gives birth at 36 weeks to twins.	4	1	2	1	4	4/3

PREGNANCY TESTS

Early detection of pregnancy allows early initiation of care. **Human chorionic gonadotropin (hCG)** is the earliest biochemical marker for pregnancy, and pregnancy tests are based on the recognition of hCG or a beta (β) subunit of hCG. Production of β-hCG begins as early as the day of implantation and can be detected as early as 7 to 10 days after conception (Blackburn, 2007). The level of hCG increases until it peaks at approximately 60 to 70 days of gestation and then declines until about 80 days of pregnancy. It remains stable until approximately 30 weeks and then gradually increases until term. Higher than normal levels of hCG may indicate abnormal gestation (e.g., fetus with Down syndrome), or multiple gestation; an abnormally slow increase or a decrease in hCG levels may indicate impending miscarriage (Cunningham et al., 2005).

Serum and urine pregnancy tests are performed in clinics, offices, women's health centers, and laboratory settings, and urine pregnancy tests may be performed at home. Both serum and urine tests can provide accurate results. A 7- to 10-ml sample of venous blood is collected for serum testing. Most urine tests require a first-voided morning urine specimen because it contains levels of hCG approximately the same as those in serum. Random urine samples usually have lower levels. Urine tests are less expensive and provide more immediate results than do serum tests.

Many different pregnancy tests are available (Fig. 6-1). The wide variety of tests precludes discussion of each. The nurse should read the manufacturer's directions for the test that is to be used.

Enzyme-linked immunosorbent assay (ELISA) testing is the most popular method of testing for pregnancy. It uses a specific monoclonal antibody (anti-hCG) with enzymes to bond with hCG in urine. ELISA technology is the basis for most over-the-counter home pregnancy tests. With these one-step tests the woman usually applies urine to a strip or absorbent tipped applicator and reads the results. The test kits come with directions for collection of the specimen, the testing procedure, and reading of the results. A positive test result is indicated by a simple color change reaction or a digital reading. Most manufacturers of the kits provide a toll-free telephone number to call if users have concerns and questions about test procedures or results (see Teaching Guidelines). The most common error in performing home pregnancy tests is performing the test too early in pregnancy (Pagana & Pagana, 2006).

Interpreting the results of pregnancy tests requires some judgment. The type of pregnancy test and its degree of sensitivity (ability to detect low levels of a substance) and specificity (ability to discern the absence of a substance) must be considered in conjunction with the woman's history. This history includes the date of her last normal menstrual period (LNMP), her usual cycle length, and results of previous pregnancy tests. Knowing if the woman is a substance abuser and what medications she is taking is important because medications such as anticonvulsants and tranquilizers can cause false-positive results, whereas diuretics and promethazine can cause false-negative results (Pagana & Pagana, 2006). Improper collection of the specimen, hormone-producing tumors, and laboratory errors also may cause false results.

Depending on the specific test, levels of hCG as low as 6.3 milli-international units/ml can be detected as early as the first day of a missed menstrual period as reported by Cole, Sutton-Riley, Khanlian, Borkovskaya, Rayburn, & Rayburn (2005). These researchers found that most of the over-the-counter pregnancy tests in the study were less sensitive (25 to 100 milli-international units/ml) and detected only a small percentage of pregnancies on the first day of a missed period even though most products claimed to be 99% accurate. Tomlinson, Marshall, and Ellis (2008) found that digital readings of low hCG levels (i.e., 25 milli-international units/ml) were more accurately interpreted by consumers than nondigital tests.

Women who use a home pregnancy test should be advised about the variations in accuracy reporting and to use caution when interpreting results. Whenever any question arises, further evaluation or retesting is appropriate.

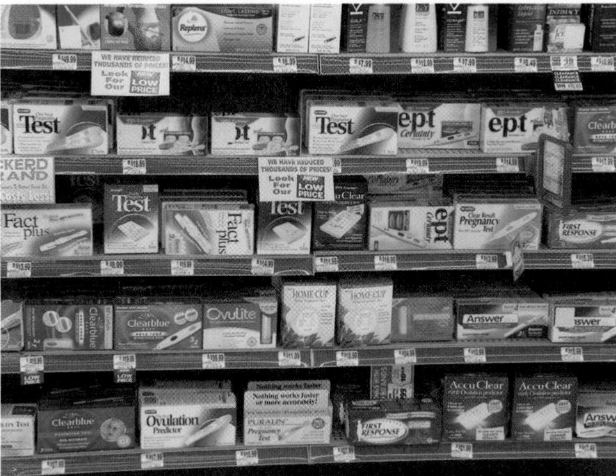

Fig. 6-1 Many pregnancy test products are available over the counter. (Courtesy Dee Lowdermilk, Chapel Hill, NC.)

TEACHING GUIDELINES

Home Pregnancy Testing

- Follow the manufacturer's instructions carefully. Do not omit steps.
- Review the manufacturer's list of foods, medications, and other substances that can affect the test results.
- Use a first-voided morning urine specimen.
- If the test performed at the time of your missed period is negative, repeat the test in 1 week if you still have not had a period.
- If you have questions about the test, contact the manufacturer.
- Contact your health care provider for follow-up if the test result is positive or if the test result is negative and you still have not had a period.

ADAPTATIONS TO PREGNANCY

Maternal physiologic adaptations are attributed to the hormones of pregnancy and to mechanical pressures arising from the enlarging uterus and other tissues. These adaptations protect the woman's normal physiologic functioning, meet the metabolic demands pregnancy imposes on her body, and provide a nurturing environment for fetal development and growth. Although pregnancy is a normal phenomenon, problems can occur.

Signs of Pregnancy

Some of the physiologic adaptations are recognized as signs and symptoms of pregnancy. Three commonly used categories of signs and symptoms of pregnancy are *presumptive* (specific changes felt by the woman–e.g., amenorrhea, fatigue, nausea and vomiting, breast changes), *probable* (changes observed by an examiner–e.g., Hegar sign, ballottement, pregnancy tests), and *positive* (signs that are attributable only to the presence of the fetus–e.g., hearing fetal heart tones, visualization of the fetus, palpating fetal movements). Table 6-2 summarizes these signs of pregnancy in relation to when they might occur and other causes for their occurrence.

Reproductive System and Breasts

Uterus

Changes in size, shape, and position. The phenomenal uterine growth in the first trimester is stimulated by high levels of estrogen and progesterone. Early uterine enlargement results from increased vascularity and dilation of blood vessels, hyperplasia (production of new muscle fibers and fibroelastic tissue) and hypertrophy (enlargement of preexisting muscle fibers and fibroelastic tissue), and development of the decidua. By 7 weeks of gestation the uterus is the size of a large hen's egg, by 10 weeks of gestation, it is the size of an orange (twice its nonpregnant size), and by 12 weeks of gestation, it is the size of a grapefruit. After the third month, the continuing

TABLE 6-2
Signs of Pregnancy

TIME OF OCCURRENCE (GESTATIONAL AGE)	SIGN	OTHER POSSIBLE CAUSE
PRESUMPTIVE SIGNS		
3-4 wk	Breast changes	Premenstrual changes, oral contraceptives
4 wk	Amenorrhea	Stress, vigorous exercise, early menopause, endocrine problems, malnutrition
4-14 wk	Nausea, vomiting	Gastrointestinal virus, food poisoning
6-12 wk	Urinary frequency	Infection, pelvic tumors
12 wk	Fatigue	Stress, illness
16-20 wk	Quickening	Gas, peristalsis
PROBABLE SIGNS		
5 wk	Goodell sign	Pelvic congestion
6-8 wk	Chadwick sign	Pelvic congestion
6-12 wk	Hegar sign	Pelvic congestion
4-12 wk	Positive result of pregnancy test (serum)	Hydatidiform mole, choriocarcinoma
6-12 wk	Positive result of pregnancy test (urine)	False-positive results may be caused by pelvic infection, tumors
16 wk	Braxton Hicks contractions	Myomas, other tumors
16-28 wk	Ballottement	Tumors, cervical polyps
POSITIVE SIGNS		
5-6 wk	Visualization of fetus by real-time ultrasound examination	No other causes
6 wk	Fetal heart tones detected by ultrasound examination	No other causes
16 wk	Visualization of fetus by radiographic study	No other causes
8-17 wk	Fetal heart tones detected by Doppler ultrasound stethoscope	No other causes
17-19 wk	Fetal heart tones detected by fetal stethoscope	No other causes
19-22 wk	Fetal movements palpated	No other causes
Late pregnancy	Fetal movements visible	No other causes

uterine enlargement is primarily the result of mechanical pressure of the growing fetus.

As the uterus enlarges, it also changes in shape and position. At conception the uterus is shaped like an upside-down pear. During the second trimester, as the muscular walls strengthen and become more elastic, the uterus becomes spherical or globular. Later, as the fetus lengthens, the uterus becomes larger and more ovoid and rises out of the pelvis into the abdominal cavity.

The pregnancy may "show" after the fourteenth week, although this depends to some degree on the woman's height and weight. Abdominal enlargement may be less apparent in the nullipara with good abdominal muscle tone (Fig. 6-2). Posture also influences the type and degree of abdominal enlargement that occurs. In normal pregnancies, the uterus enlarges at a predictable rate. As the uterus grows, it may be palpated above the symphysis pubis some time between the twelfth and fourteenth weeks of pregnancy (Fig. 6-3). The uterus rises gradually to the level of the umbilicus at about 22 weeks of gestation and nearly reaches the xiphoid process at term. Between weeks 38 and 40, fundal height drops as the fetus begins to descend and engage in the pelvis (**lightening**) (see Fig. 6-3, *dashed line*). Generally, lightening occurs in the nullipara approximately 2 weeks before the onset of labor and at the start of labor in the multipara.

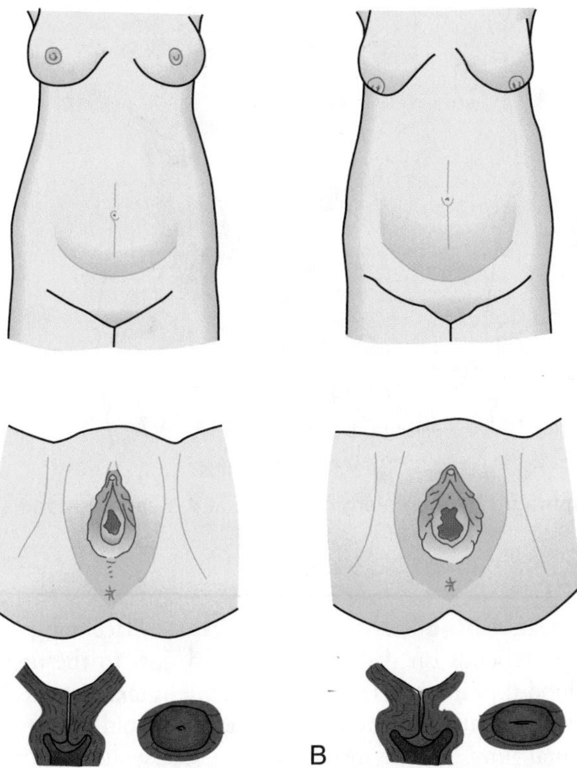

Fig. 6-2 Comparison of abdomen, vulva, and cervix in nullipara **(A)** and multipara **(B)** at the same stage of pregnancy.

Uterine enlargement is determined by measuring fundal height, a measurement commonly used to estimate the duration of pregnancy. However, variation in the position of the fundus or the fetus, variations in the amount of amniotic fluid present, the presence of more than one fetus, maternal obesity, and variation in examiner techniques can reduce the accuracy of this estimation of the duration of pregnancy.

The uterus normally rotates to the right as it elevates, probably because of the presence of the rectosigmoid colon on the left side, but the extensive hypertrophy (enlargement) of the round ligaments keeps the uterus in the midline. Eventually the growing uterus touches the anterior abdominal wall and displaces the intestines to either side of the abdomen (Fig. 6-4). Whenever a pregnant woman is standing, most of her uterus rests against the anterior abdominal wall, and this contributes to altering her center of gravity.

At approximately 6 weeks of gestation, softening and compressibility of the lower uterine segment (the uterine isthmus) occur (**Hegar sign**) (Fig. 6-5). This change results in exaggerated uterine anteflexion during the first 3 months of pregnancy. In this position, the uterine fundus presses on the urinary bladder, causing the woman to have urinary frequency.

Changes in contractility. Soon after the fourth month of pregnancy, uterine contractions can be felt through the abdominal wall. These contractions are known as the **Braxton Hicks sign.** Braxton Hicks contractions are irregular and painless and occur intermittently throughout pregnancy. These contractions facilitate uterine blood flow

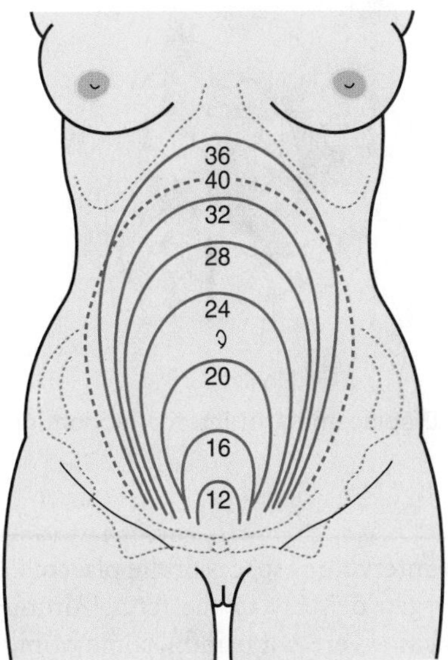

Fig. 6-3 Height of fundus by weeks of normal gestation with a single fetus. *Dashed line,* height after lightening. (From Seidel, H., Ball, J., Dains, J., & Benedict, G. [2006]. *Mosby's guide to physical examination* [6th ed.]. St. Louis: Mosby.)

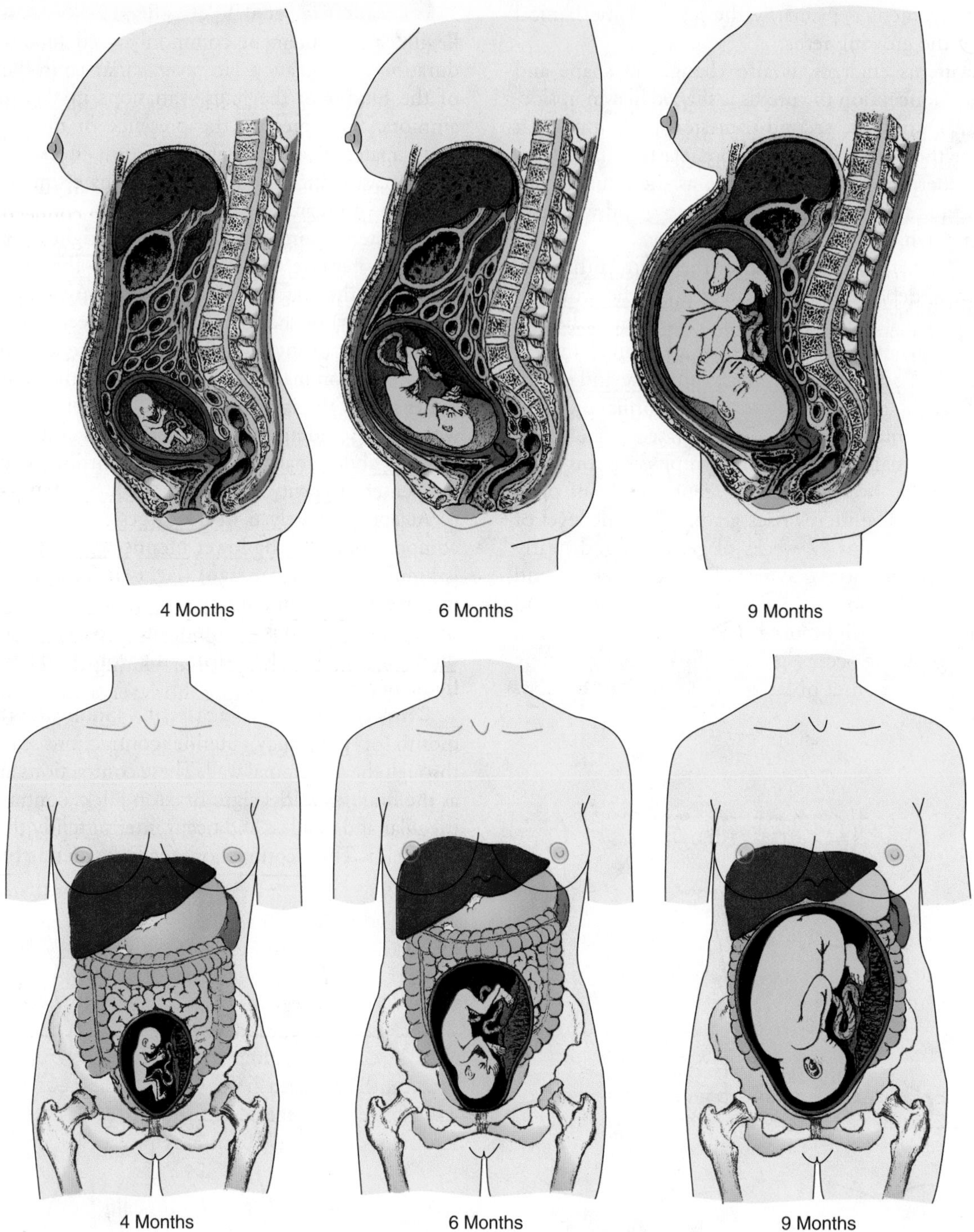

Fig. 6-4 Displacement of internal abdominal structures and diaphragm by the enlarging uterus at 4, 6, and 9 months of gestation.

through the intervillous spaces of the placenta and thereby promote oxygen delivery to the fetus. Although Braxton Hicks contractions are not painful, some women complain that they are annoying. After the twenty-eighth week, these contractions become much more definite, but they usually cease with walking or exercise. Braxton Hicks contractions can be mistaken for true labor; however, they do not increase in intensity or frequency or cause cervical dilation.

Uteroplacental blood flow. Placental perfusion depends on the maternal blood flow to the uterus. Blood flow increases rapidly as the uterus increases in size. Although uterine blood flow increases 20-fold the fetoplacental unit grows more rapidly. Consequently, more oxygen is extracted from the uterine blood during the latter part of pregnancy (Cunningham et al., 2005). In a normal term pregnancy, one sixth of the total maternal blood volume is within the uterine vascular system. The rate of blood flow through the uterus averages 500 ml/min, and oxygen consumption of the gravid uterus increases to meet fetal needs. A low maternal arterial pressure, contractions of the uterus, and maternal supine position are three factors known to decrease blood flow. Estrogen stimulation may increase uterine blood flow. Doppler ultrasound examination can be used to measure uterine blood flow velocity, especially in pregnancies at risk because of conditions associated with decreased placental perfusion such as hypertension, intrauterine growth restriction, diabetes mellitus, and multiple gestation (Blackburn, 2007). By using an ultrasound device or a fetal stethoscope, the health care provider may hear the **uterine souffle** (sound made by blood in the uterine arteries that is synchronous with the maternal pulse) or the **funic souffle** (sound made by blood rushing through the umbilical vessels and synchronous with the fetal heart rate).

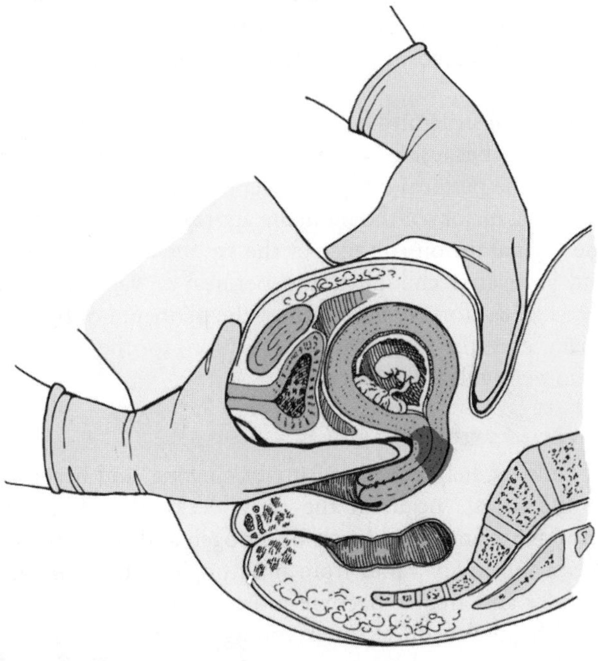

Fig. 6-5 Hegar sign. Bimanual examination for assessing compressibility and softening of the isthmus (lower uterine segment) while the cervix is still firm.

Cervical changes. A softening of the cervical tip called Goodell sign may be observed at approximately the beginning of the sixth week in a normal, unscarred cervix. This sign is brought about by increased vascularity, slight hypertrophy, and hyperplasia (increase in the number of cells) of the muscle and its collagen-rich connective tissue, which becomes loose, edematous, highly elastic, and increased in volume. The glands near the external os proliferate beneath the stratified squamous epithelium, giving the cervix the velvety appearance characteristic of pregnancy. *Friability* is increased and may cause slight bleeding after coitus with deep penetration or after vaginal examination. Pregnancy also can cause the squamocolumnar junction, the site for obtaining cells for cervical cancer screening, to be located away from the cervix. Because of all these changes, evaluation of abnormal Papanicolaou (Pap) tests during pregnancy can be complicated. A careful assessment of all pregnant women is important, however, because approximately 3% of all cervical cancers are diagnosed during pregnancy (Copeland & Landon, 2007).

The cervix of the nullipara is rounded. Lacerations of the cervix almost always occur during the birth process. With or without lacerations, however, after childbirth, the cervix becomes more oval in the horizontal plane, and the external os appears as a transverse slit (see Fig. 6-2).

Changes related to the presence of the fetus. Passive movement of the unengaged fetus is called ballottement and can be identified generally between the sixteenth and eighteenth week. Ballottement is a technique of palpating a floating structure by bouncing it gently and feeling it rebound. In the technique used to palpate the fetus, the examiner places a finger in the vagina and taps gently upward, causing the fetus to rise. The fetus then sinks, and a gentle tap is felt on the finger (Fig. 6-6).

The first recognition of fetal movements, or "feeling life," by the multiparous woman may occur as early as the fourteenth to sixteenth week. The nulliparous woman may not notice these sensations until the eighteenth week or later. Quickening is commonly described as a flutter and

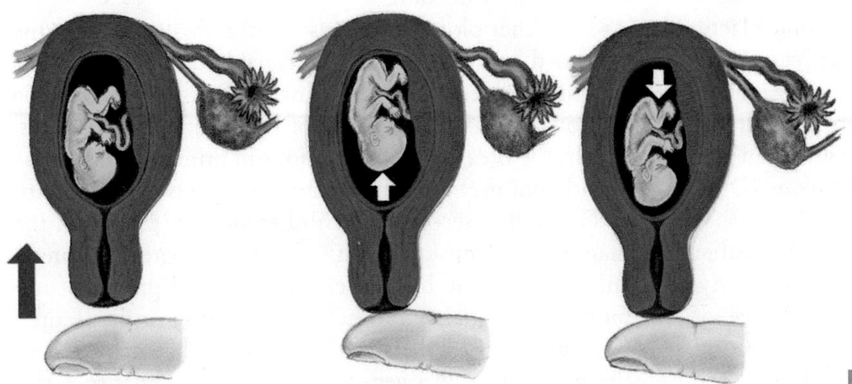

Fig. 6-6 Internal ballottement (18 weeks).

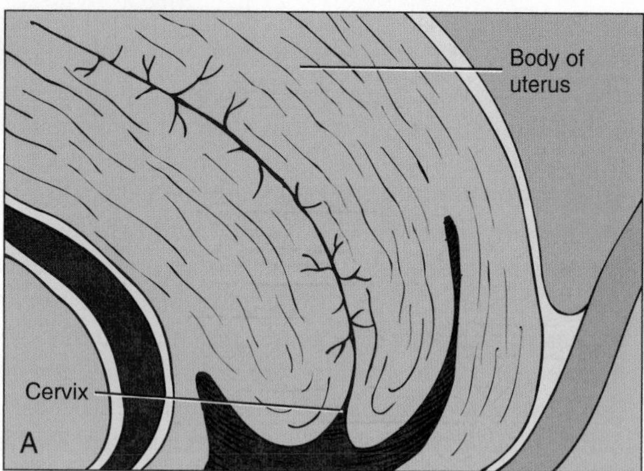

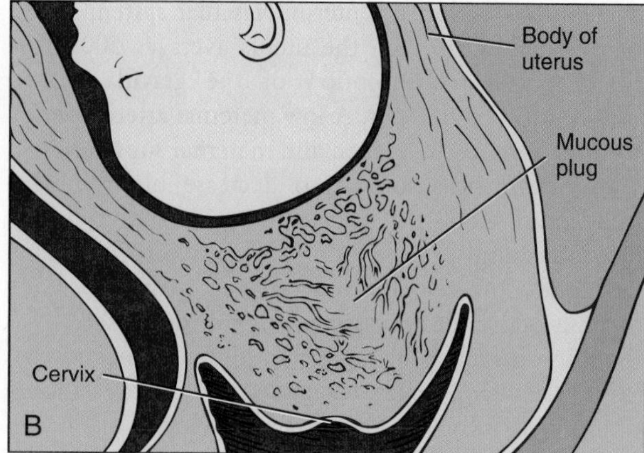

Fig. 6-7 **A,** Cervix in nonpregnant woman. **B,** Cervix during pregnancy.

is difficult to distinguish from peristalsis. Fetal movements gradually increase in intensity and frequency. The week when quickening occurs provides a tentative clue in dating the duration of gestation.

Vagina and vulva

Pregnancy hormones prepare the vagina for stretching during labor and birth by causing the vaginal mucosa to thicken, the connective tissue to loosen, the smooth muscle to hypertrophy, and the vaginal vault to lengthen. Increased vascularity results in a violet-bluish color of the vaginal mucosa and cervix. The deepened color, termed the **Chadwick sign,** may be evident as early as the sixth week but is easily noted at the eighth week of pregnancy (Blackburn, 2007).

Leukorrhea is a white or slightly gray mucoid discharge with a faint musty odor. This copious mucoid fluid occurs in response to cervical stimulation by estrogen and progesterone. The fluid is whitish because of the presence of many exfoliated vaginal epithelial cells caused by the hyperplasia of normal pregnancy. This vaginal discharge is never pruritic or blood stained. The mucus fills the endocervical canal, resulting in the formation of the mucous plug **(operculum)** (Fig. 6-7). The operculum acts as a barrier against bacterial invasion during pregnancy.

During pregnancy the pH of vaginal secretions is more acidic than normal (ranging from approximately 3.5 to 6 [normal 4 to 7]) because of increased production of lactic acid (Cunningham et al., 2005). Although this acidic environment provides more protection from some organisms, the pregnant woman is more vulnerable to other infections, especially yeast infections because the glycogen-rich environment is more susceptible to *Candida albicans* (Duff, Sweet, & Edwards, 2009).

The increased vascularity of the vagina and other pelvic viscera results in a marked increase in sensitivity. The increased sensitivity may lead to a high degree of sexual interest and arousal, especially during the second trimester of pregnancy. The increased congestion plus the relaxed walls of the blood vessels and the heavy uterus may result in edema and varicosities of the vulva. The edema and varicosities usually resolve during the postpartum period.

External structures of the perineum are enlarged during pregnancy because of an increase in vasculature, hypertrophy of the perineal body, and deposition of fat (Fig. 6-8). The labia majora of the nullipara approximate and obscure the vaginal introitus; those of the parous woman separate and gape after childbirth and perineal or vaginal injury. (See Fig. 6-2 for a comparison of the perineum of the nullipara and the multipara in relation to the pregnant abdomen, vulva, and cervix.)

Breasts

Fullness, heightened sensitivity, tingling, and heaviness of the breasts begin in the early weeks of gestation in response to increased levels of estrogen and progesterone. Breast sensitivity varies from mild tingling to sharp pain. Nipples and areolae become more pigmented, secondary pinkish areolae develop, extending beyond the primary areolae, and nipples become more erectile. Hypertrophy of the sebaceous (oil) glands embedded in the primary areolae, called **Montgomery tubercles** (see Fig. 2-6), may be seen around the nipples. These sebaceous glands may have a protective role in that they keep the nipples lubricated for breastfeeding.

The richer blood supply causes the vessels beneath the skin to dilate. Once barely noticeable, the blood vessels become visible, often appearing in an intertwining blue network beneath the surface of the skin. Venous congestion in the breasts is more obvious in primigravidas. Striae gravidarum may appear at the outer aspects of the breasts.

During the second and third trimesters, growth of the mammary glands accounts for the progressive breast enlargement. The high levels of luteal and placental hormones in pregnancy promote proliferation of the lactiferous ducts and lobule-alveolar tissue so that palpation of the breasts reveals a generalized, coarse nodularity. Glan-

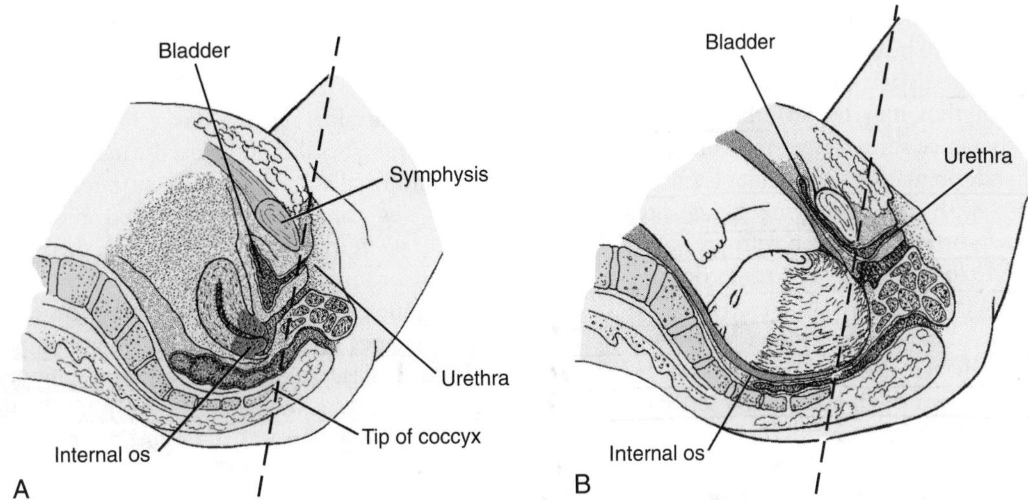

Fig. 6-8 **A,** Pelvic floor in nonpregnant woman. **B,** Pelvic floor at end of pregnancy. Note marked hypertrophy and hyperplasia below dotted line joining tip of coccyx and inferior margin of symphysis. Note elongation of bladder and urethra as a result of compression. Fat deposits are increased.

dular tissue displaces connective tissue, and as a result, the tissue becomes softer and looser.

Although development of the mammary glands is functionally complete by the middle of the pregnancy, lactation is inhibited until a decrease in estrogen level occurs after the birth. A thin, clear, viscous secretory material (precolostrum) can be found in the acini cells by the third month of gestation. Colostrum, the creamy, white-to-yellowish to orange premilk fluid, may be expressed from the nipples as early as 16 weeks of gestation (Blackburn, 2007). See Chapter 18 for discussion of lactation.

General Body System Changes

Cardiovascular system

Maternal adjustments to pregnancy involve extensive changes in the cardiovascular system, both anatomic and physiologic. Cardiovascular adaptations protect the woman's normal physiologic functioning, meet the metabolic demands pregnancy imposes on her body, and provide for fetal developmental and growth needs.

Slight cardiac hypertrophy (enlargement) is probably secondary to the increased blood volume and cardiac output that occurs. The heart returns to its normal size after childbirth. As the diaphragm is displaced upward by the enlarging uterus, the heart is elevated upward and rotated forward to the left (Fig. 6-9). The apical impulse, a point of maximal intensity (PMI), is shifted upward and laterally approximately 1 to 1.5 cm. The degree of shift depends on the duration of pregnancy and the size and position of the uterus.

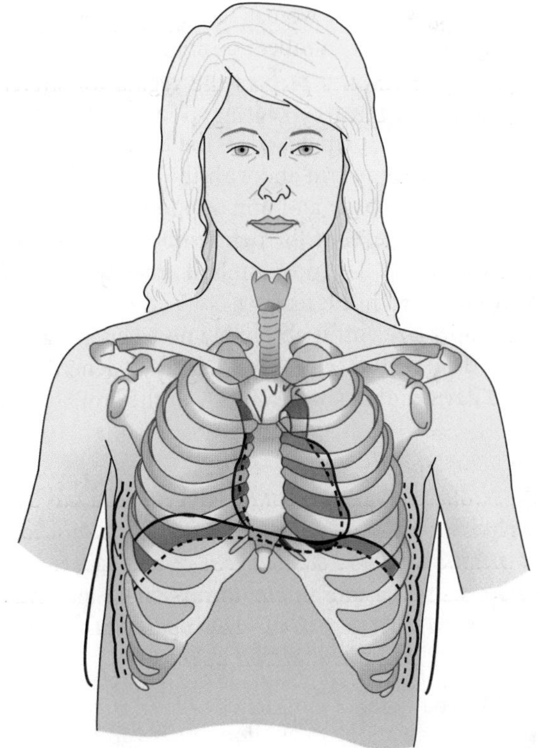

Fig. 6-9 Changes in position of heart, lungs, and thoracic cage in pregnancy. *Broken line,* nonpregnant; *solid line,* change that occurs in pregnancy.

The changes in heart size and position and increases in blood volume and cardiac output contribute to auscultatory changes common in pregnancy. A more audible splitting of heart sounds (S) S_1 and S_2 is heard, and S_3 may be readily heard after 20 weeks of gestation. In addition, systolic and diastolic murmurs may be heard over the pulmonic area. These sounds are transient and disappear shortly after the woman gives birth (Cunningham et al., 2005).

Between 14 and 20 weeks of gestation, the pulse increases approximately 10 to 15 beats/min, which then persists to term. Palpitations may occur. In twin gestations near term, the maternal heart rate increases up to 40% over the nonpregnant rate (Blackburn, 2007).

The cardiac rhythm may be disturbed. The pregnant woman may experience sinus arrhythmia, premature atrial contractions, and premature ventricular systole. In the healthy woman with no underlying heart disease, no therapy is needed; however, women with preexisting heart disease will need close medical and obstetric supervision during pregnancy (see Chapter 20).

Blood pressure. Arterial blood pressure (brachial artery) is affected by age, activity level, presence of health problems, and circadian rhythm, Other factors include use of alcohol, smoking, and pain. Additional factors must be considered during pregnancy. These factors include maternal anxiety, maternal position, and size and type of blood pressure apparatus (Pickering et al., 2005).

Maternal anxiety can elevate readings. If an elevated reading is found, the woman is given time to rest, and the reading is repeated.

Maternal position affects readings. Brachial blood pressure is highest when the woman is sitting, lowest when she is lying in the lateral recumbent position, and intermediate when she is supine, except for some women who experience supine hypotensive syndrome (see discussion later). Therefore at each prenatal visit the reading should be obtained in the same arm and with the woman in a seated position with her back and arm supported and with her upper arm at the level of the right atrium (Pickering et al., 2005; Sibai, 2007). The position and arm used should be recorded along with the reading.

The proper-size cuff is absolutely necessary for accurate readings. The cuff should have a bladder length that is 80% and a width that is at least 40% of the arm circumference. For example, an adult size cuff (16 × 30 cm) should be used for an arm circumference of 27 to 34 cm. Too small a cuff yields a false high reading; too large a cuff yields a false low reading (Pickering et al., 2005).

Caution also should be used when comparing auscultatory and oscillatory blood pressure readings, because discrepancies can occur. Automated monitors may give inaccurate readings in women with hypertensive conditions (Gordon, 2007).

Systolic blood pressure usually remains the same as the prepregnancy level but may decrease slightly as pregnancy advances. Diastolic blood pressure begins to decrease in the first trimester, continues to drop until 24 to 32 weeks, then gradually increases and returns to prepregnancy levels by term (Blackburn, 2007).

Calculating the *mean arterial pressure* (MAP) (mean of the blood pressure in the arterial circulation) can increase the diagnostic value of the findings. Normal MAP readings in the nonpregnant woman are 86.4 mm Hg ± 7.5 mm Hg. MAP readings for a pregnant woman are slightly higher (Gordon, 2007). One way to calculate an MAP is illustrated in Box 6-2.

Some degree of compression of the vena cava occurs in all women who lie flat on their backs during the second half of pregnancy (see Fig. 12-5). Some women experience a decrease in their systolic blood pressure of more than 30 mm Hg. After 4 to 5 minutes a reflex bradycardia is noted, cardiac output is reduced by one half, and the woman feels faint. This condition is known as *supine hypotensive syndrome* (Cunningham et al., 2005).

Compression of the iliac veins and inferior vena cava by the uterus causes increased venous pressure and reduced blood flow in the legs (except when the woman is in the lateral position). These alterations contribute to the dependent edema, varicose veins in the legs and vulva, and hemorrhoids that develop in the latter part of term pregnancy (Fig. 6-10).

Blood volume and composition. The degree of blood volume expansion varies considerably. Blood volume increases by approximately 1500 ml, or 40% to 45% above nonpregnancy levels (Cunningham et al., 2005). This increase consists of 1000 ml plasma plus 450 ml red blood cells (RBCs). The blood volume starts to increase at approximately the tenth to twelfth week,

Critical Thinking/Clinical Decision Making

Blood Pressure Monitoring in Pregnancy

You are the nurse educator for the prenatal clinic where you have been assigned to develop a protocol for blood pressure monitoring for pregnant patients. What information is important to include in such a document?

1. Evidence—Is there sufficient evidence to draw conclusions about what information you should include in the protocol?
2. Assumptions
   a. Differences in types of blood pressure apparatus
   b. Effects of cuff size and accuracy of readings
   c. Effects of maternal positioning and other factors on monitoring
3. What are the implications and priorities for developing and implementing the protocol?
4. Does the evidence objectively support your conclusion?
5. Do alternative perspectives to your conclusion exist?

BOX 6-2

Calculation of Mean Arterial Pressure

Blood pressure: 106/70 mm Hg
Formula:
(systolic) + 2(diastolic) ÷ 3
(106) + 2(70) ÷ 3
106 + 140 ÷ 3
246 ÷ 3 = 82 mm Hg

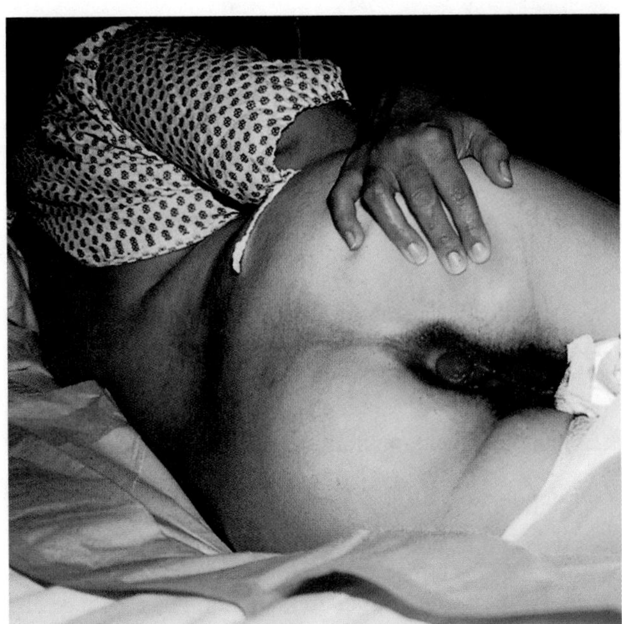

Fig. 6-10 Hemorrhoids. (Courtesy Marjorie Pyle, RNC, Lifecircle, Costa Mesa, CA.)

peaks at approximately the thirty-second to thirty-fourth week and then decreases slightly at the fortieth week. The increase in volume of a multiple gestation is greater than that for a pregnancy with a single fetus (Blackburn, 2007). Increased volume is a protective mechanism. It is essential for meeting the blood volume needs of the hypertrophied vascular system of the enlarged uterus, for adequately hydrating fetal and maternal tissues when the woman assumes an erect or supine position, and for providing a fluid reserve to compensate for blood loss during birth and the puerperium. Peripheral vasodilation maintains a normal blood pressure despite the increased blood volume in pregnancy.

During pregnancy, production of RBCs is accelerated (normal, 4.2 to 5.4 million cells/mm^3). The percentage of increase depends on the amount of iron available. The RBC mass increases by approximately 20% to 30% (Blackburn, 2007).

Because the plasma increase exceeds the increase in RBC production, a decrease occurs in normal hemoglobin values (12 to 16 g/dl blood [non-pregnant]) and hematocrit values (37% to 47% [non-pregnant]). This state of hemodilution is termed *physiologic anemia.* The decrease is more noticeable during the second trimester than at other times, when rapid expansion of blood volume takes place faster than RBC production. A hemoglobin value that drops below 11 g/dl should be considered abnormal and often is due to iron deficiency anemia (Samuels, 2007). The total white cell count increases during the second trimester and peaks during the third trimester. This increase is primarily in the granulocytes; the lymphocyte count stays approximately the same throughout pregnancy. Table 6-3 lists the laboratory values during pregnancy.

Cardiac output. Cardiac output increases from 30% to 50% over the nonpregnant rate by the thirty-second week of pregnancy; it declines to approximately a 20% increase at 40 weeks of gestation. This elevated cardiac output is largely a result of increased stroke volume and heart rate and occurs in response to increased tissue demands for oxygen (Blackburn, 2007). Cardiac output in late pregnancy is appreciably higher when the woman is in the lateral recumbent position than when she is supine. In the supine position the large, heavy uterus often impedes venous return to the heart and affects blood pressure. Cardiac output increases with any exertion, such as labor and birth. Table 6-4 summarizes cardiovascular changes in pregnancy.

Circulation and coagulation times. The circulation time decreases slightly by week 32. It returns to near normal by near term. The blood tends to coagulate (clot) during pregnancy because of increases in various clotting factors (factors VII, VIII, IX, X, and fibrinogen). This change, combined with the fact that fibrinolytic activity (the splitting up or the dissolving of a clot) is depressed during pregnancy and the postpartum period, provides a protective function to decrease the chance of bleeding, but it also makes the woman more vulnerable to thrombosis, especially after cesarean birth.

Respiratory system

Structural and ventilatory adaptations occur during pregnancy to provide for maternal and fetal needs. Maternal oxygen requirements increase in response to the acceleration in the metabolic rate and the need to add to the tissue mass in the uterus and breasts. In addition the fetus requires oxygen and a way to eliminate carbon dioxide.

Elevated levels of estrogen cause the ligaments of the rib cage to relax, permitting increased chest expansion (see Fig. 6-9). The transverse diameter of the thoracic cage increases by approximately 2 cm, and the circumference increases by 6 cm (Cunningham et al., 2005). The costal angle increases, and the lower rib cage appears to flare out. The chest may not return to its prepregnant state after birth (Seidel, Ball, Dains, & Benedict, 2006).

The diaphragm is displaced by as much as 4 cm during pregnancy. As pregnancy advances, thoracic (costal) breathing replaces abdominal breathing, and the diaphragm becomes less able to descend with inspiration. Thoracic breathing is accomplished primarily by the diaphragm rather than by the costal muscles (Blackburn, 2007).

The upper respiratory tract becomes more vascular in response to elevated levels of estrogen. As the capillaries become engorged, edema and hyperemia develop within the nose, pharynx, larynx, trachea, and bronchi. This congestion within the tissues of the respiratory tract gives rise to several conditions commonly seen during pregnancy,

TABLE 6-3

Laboratory Values for Pregnant and Nonpregnant Women

VALUES	NONPREGNANT	PREGNANT
HEMATOLOGIC		
Complete Blood Count (CBC)		
Hemoglobin (g/dl)	12-16*	>11*
Hematocrit, PCV (%)	37-47	>33*
Red blood cell (RBC) volume (per ml)	1400	1650
Plasma volume (per ml)	2400	40%-60% increase
RBC count (million per mm^3)	4.2-5.4	5.0-6.25
White blood cells (total per mm^3)	5000-10,000	5000-15,000
Neutrophils (%)	55-70	60-85
Lymphocytes (%)	20-40	15-40
Erythrocyte sedimentation rate (mm/hr)	20	Elevated in second and third trimesters
Mean corpuscular hemoglobin concentration (MCHC) (g/dl packed RBCs)	32-36	No change
Mean corpuscular hemoglobin (MCH) (pg)	27-31	No change
Mean corpuscular volume (MCV), per mm^3	80-95	No change
Blood coagulation and fibrinolytic activity†		
Factor VII	65-140	Increase in pregnancy, return to normal in early puerperium
Factor VIII	55-145	Increases during pregnancy and immediately after birth
Factor IX	60-140	Same as Factor VII
Factor X	45-155	Same as Factor VII
Factor XI	65-135	Decrease in pregnancy
Factor XII	50-150	Same as Factor VII
Prothrombin time (PT) (sec)	11-12.5	Slight decrease in pregnancy
Partial thromboplastin time (PTT) (sec)	60-70	Slight decrease in pregnancy and decrease during second and third stage of labor (indicates clotting at placental site)
Bleeding time (min)	1-9 (Ivy)	No appreciable change
Coagulation time (min)	6-10 (Lee/White)	No appreciable change
Platelets per (mm^3)	150,000-400,000	No significant change until 3-5 days after birth and then a rapid increase (may predispose woman to thrombosis) and gradual return to normal
Fibrinolytic activity	Normal	Decreases in pregnancy and then abruptly returns to normal (protection against thromboembolism)
Fibrinogen (mg/dl)	200-400	Increased levels late in pregnancy
Mineral and vitamin concentrations		
Vitamin B_{12}, folic acid, ascorbic acid	Normal	Moderate decrease
Serum proteins		
Total (g/dl)	6.4-8.3	5.5-7.5
Albumin (g/dl)	3.5-5	Slight increase
Globulin, total (g/dl)	2.3-3.4	3.0-4.0
Blood glucose		
Fasting (mg/dl)	70-105	Decreases
2-hr postprandial (mg/dl)	<140	<140 after a 100-g carbohydrate meal is considered normal
Acid-base values in arterial blood		
Po_2 (mm Hg)	80-100	104-108 (increased)
Pco_2 (mm Hg)	35-45	27-32 (decreased)
Sodium bicarbonate (HCO_3) (mEq/L)	21-28	18-31 (decreased)
Blood pH	7.35-7.45	7.40-7.45 (slightly increased, more alkaline)

TABLE 6-3

Laboratory Values for Pregnant and Nonpregnant Women—cont'd

VALUES	NONPREGNANT	PREGNANT
HEPATIC		
Bilirubin, total (mg/dl)	≤1	Unchanged
Serum cholesterol (mg/dl)	120-200	Increases from 16-32 weeks of pregnancy; remains at this level until after birth
Serum alkaline phosphatase, units/L	30-120	Increases from week 12 of pregnancy to 6 weeks after birth
Serum albumin (g/dl)	3.5-5.0	Slight increase
RENAL		
Bladder capacity (ml)	1300	1500
Renal plasma flow (RPF) (ml/min)	490-700	Increase by 25%-30%
Glomerular filtration rate (GFR) (ml/min)	88-128	Increase by 30%-50%
Nonprotein nitrogen (NPN) (mg/dl)	25-40	Decreases
Blood urea nitrogen (BUN) (mg/dl)	10-20	Decreases
Serum creatinine (mg/dl)	0.5-1.1	Decreases
Serum uric acid (mg/dl)	2.7-7.3	Decreases but returns to prepregnancy level by end of pregnancy
Urine glucose	Negative	Present in 20% of pregnant women
Intravenous pyelogram (IVP)	Normal	Slight-to-moderate hydroureter and hydronephrosis; right kidney larger than left kidney

Sources: Blackburn, S. (2007). *Maternal, fetal, & neonatal physiology: A clinical perspective* (3rd ed.). St. Louis: Saunders; Gordon, M. (2007). Maternal physiology. In S. Gabbe, J. Niebyl, & J. Simpson (Eds.), *Obstetrics: Normal and problem pregnancies* (5th ed.). Philadelphia: Churchill Livingstone; Pagana, K., & Pagana, T. (2006). *Mosby's manual of diagnostic and laboratory tests* (3rd ed.). St. Louis: Mosby.

*At sea level. Permanent residents of higher altitudes (e.g., Denver) require higher levels of hemoglobin.

†Pregnancy represents a hypercoagulable state.

dl, Deciliter; *mm³*, cubic millimeter; *ng*, nanogram; *pg*, picogram; *PVC*, packed cell volume.

TABLE 6-4

Cardiovascular Changes in Pregnancy

Heart rate	Increases 10-15 beats/min
Blood pressure	Systolic: Slight or no decrease from prepregnancy levels Diastolic: Slight decrease to midpregnancy (24-32 weeks) and gradually returns to prepregnancy levels by the end of pregnancy
Blood volume	Increases by 1500 ml or 40%-50% above prepregnancy level
Red blood cell mass	Increases 17%
Hemoglobin	Decreases
Hematocrit	Decreases
White blood cell count	Increases in second and third trimesters
Cardiac output	Increases 30%-50%

including nasal and sinus stuffiness, epistaxis (nosebleed), changes in the voice, and a marked inflammatory response that can develop into a mild upper respiratory infection.

Increased vascularity of the upper respiratory tract can also cause the tympanic membranes and eustachian tubes to swell, giving rise to symptoms of impaired hearing, earaches, or a sense of fullness in the ears.

Pulmonary function. Respiratory changes in pregnancy are related to the elevation of the diaphragm and to chest wall changes. Changes in the respiratory center result in a lowered threshold for carbon dioxide. The actions of progesterone and estrogen are presumed responsible for the increased sensitivity of the respiratory center to carbon dioxide. In addition, pregnant women become more aware of the need to breathe; many complain of nasal stuffiness, and some have epistaxis (Gordon, 2007). (Table 6-5 summarizes respiratory changes in pregnancy.) Although pulmonary function is not impaired by pregnancy, diseases of the respiratory tract may be more serious during this time (Cunningham et al., 2005). One important factor responsible for this circumstance may be the increased oxygen requirement.

TABLE 6-5

Respiratory Changes in Pregnancy

Respiratory rate	Unchanged or slightly increased
Tidal volume	Increased 30%-40%
Vital capacity	Unchanged
Inspiratory capacity	Increased
Expiratory volume	Decreased
Total lung capacity	Unchanged to slightly decreased
Oxygen consumption	Increased 20%-40%

Source: Gordon, M. (2007). Maternal physiology. In S. Gabbe, J. Niebyl, & J. Simpson (Eds.), *Obstetrics: Normal and problem pregnancies* (5th ed.). Philadelphia: Churchill Livingstone.

Basal metabolic rate. The basal metabolic rate (BMR) increases during pregnancy. This increase varies considerably, depending on the prepregnancy nutritional status of the woman and fetal growth (Blackburn, 2007). The BMR returns to nonpregnant levels by 5 to 6 days after birth. The elevation in BMR during pregnancy reflects increased oxygen demands of the uterine-placental-fetal unit and greater oxygen consumption because of increased maternal cardiac work. Peripheral vasodilation and acceleration of sweat gland activity help dissipate the excess heat resulting from the increased BMR during pregnancy. Pregnant women may experience heat intolerance, which is annoying to some women. Lassitude and fatigability after only slight exertion are experienced by many women in early pregnancy. These feelings, along with a greater need for sleep, may persist and may be caused in part by the increased metabolic activity.

Acid-base balance. By about the tenth week of pregnancy, the partial pressure of carbon dioxide (PCO_2) decreases by approximately 5 mm Hg. Progesterone may be responsible for increasing the sensitivity of the respiratory center receptors such that tidal volume is increased, PCO_2 decreases, the base excess (bicarbonate [HCO_3]) decreases, and pH increases slightly. These alterations in acid-base balance indicate that pregnancy is a state of compensatory respiratory alkalosis (Gordon, 2007). These changes also facilitate the transport of carbon dioxide from the fetus and oxygen release from the mother to the fetus (see Table 6-3).

Renal system

The kidneys are responsible for maintaining electrolyte and acid-base balance, regulating extracellular fluid volume, excreting waste products, and conserving essential nutrients.

Anatomic changes. Changes in renal structure during pregnancy result from hormonal activity (estrogen and progesterone), pressure from an enlarging uterus, and an increase in blood volume. As early as the tenth week of pregnancy, the renal pelves and the ureters dilate. Dilation of the ureters is more pronounced above the pelvic brim, in part because they are compressed between the uterus and the pelvic brim. In most women, the ureters below the pelvic brim are of normal size. The smooth-muscle walls of the ureters undergo hyperplasia, hypertrophy, and muscle tone relaxation. The ureters elongate, become tortuous, and form single or double curves. In the latter part of pregnancy the renal pelvis and ureter are dilated more on the right side than on the left because the heavy uterus is displaced to the right by the sigmoid colon.

Because of these changes a larger volume of urine is held in the pelves and ureters, and urine flow rate is slowed. The resulting urinary stasis or stagnation has the following consequences:

- A lag occurs between the time urine is formed and when it reaches the bladder. Therefore clearance test results may reflect substances contained in glomerular filtrate several hours before.
- Stagnated urine is an excellent medium for the growth of microorganisms. In addition, the urine of pregnant women contains more nutrients, including glucose, thereby increasing the pH (making the urine more alkaline). This makes pregnant women more susceptible to urinary tract infection.

Bladder irritability, nocturia, and urinary frequency and urgency (without dysuria) are commonly reported in early pregnancy. Near term, bladder symptoms may return, especially after lightening occurs.

Urinary frequency results initially from increased bladder sensitivity and later from compression of the bladder (see Fig. 6-8). In the second trimester the bladder is pulled up out of the true pelvis into the abdomen. The urethra lengthens to 7.5 cm as the bladder is displaced upward. The pelvic congestion that occurs in pregnancy is reflected in hyperemia of the bladder and urethra. This increased vascularity causes the bladder mucosa to be traumatized and bleed easily. Bladder tone may decrease, which increases the bladder capacity to 1500 ml. At the same time, the bladder is compressed by the enlarging uterus, resulting in the urge to void even if the bladder contains only a small amount of urine.

Functional changes. In normal pregnancy, renal function is altered considerably. The glomerular filtration rate (GFR) and renal plasma flow (RPF) increase early in pregnancy (Cunningham et al., 2005). These changes are caused by pregnancy hormones, an increase in blood volume, the woman's posture, physical activity, and nutritional intake. The woman's kidneys must manage the increased metabolic and circulatory demands of the maternal body and the excretion of fetal waste products. Renal function is most efficient when the woman lies in the lateral recumbent position and least efficient when the woman assumes a supine position. A side-lying position increases renal perfusion, which increases urinary output and decreases edema. When the pregnant woman is lying supine, the heavy uterus compresses the vena cava and the

COMMUNITY ACTIVITY

Visit the first in a series of childbirth class offerings in your community. What concepts related to body system changes during pregnancy were discussed in the class? Were concepts discussed in detail at the woman's level of understanding? What teaching materials were used to explain the concepts? Were printed materials available in several languages and written in a way that participants could understand? How did instructors validate that participants understood the materials?

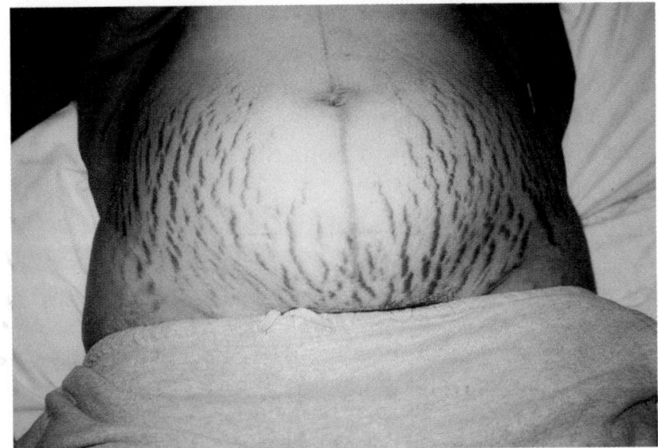

Fig. 6-11 Striae gravidarum and linea nigra in a dark-skinned person. (Courtesy Shannon Perry, Phoenix, AZ.)

aorta, and cardiac output decreases. As a result, blood flow to the brain and heart is continued at the expense of other organs, including the kidneys and uterus.

Fluid and electrolyte balance. Selective renal tubular reabsorption maintains sodium and water balance regardless of changes in dietary intake and losses through sweat, vomitus, or diarrhea. From 500 to 900 mEq of sodium is normally retained during pregnancy to meet fetal needs. To prevent excessive sodium depletion, the maternal kidneys undergo a significant adaptation by increasing tubular reabsorption. Because of the need for increased maternal intravascular and extracellular fluid volume, additional sodium is needed to expand fluid volume and to maintain an isotonic state. As efficient as the renal system is, it can be overstressed by excessive dietary sodium intake or restriction or by use of diuretics. Severe hypovolemia and reduced placental perfusion are two consequences of using diuretics during pregnancy.

The capacity of the kidneys to excrete water during the early weeks of pregnancy is more efficient than it is later in pregnancy. As a result, some women feel thirsty in early pregnancy because of the greater amount of water loss. The pooling of fluid in the legs in the latter part of pregnancy decreases renal blood flow and GFR. This pooling of blood in the lower legs is sometimes called *physiologic edema* or dependent edema and requires no treatment. The normal diuretic response to the water load is triggered when the woman lies down, preferably on her side, and the pooled fluid reenters general circulation.

Normally the kidney reabsorbs almost all of the glucose and other nutrients from the plasma filtrate. In pregnant women, however, tubular reabsorption of glucose is impaired such that glycosuria occurs at varying times and to varying degrees. Normal values range from 0 to 20 mg/dl, meaning that during any day, the urine is sometimes positive and sometimes negative. In nonpregnant women, blood glucose levels must be at 160 to 180 mg/dl before glucose is "spilled" into the urine (not reabsorbed). During pregnancy, glycosuria occurs when maternal glucose levels are lower than 160 mg/dl. Why glucose, as well as other nutrients such as amino acids, is wasted during pregnancy is not understood, nor has the exact mechanism been discovered. Although glycosuria may be found in normal pregnancies (2+ levels may be seen with increased anxiety states), the possibility of diabetes mellitus and gestational diabetes must be kept in mind.

Proteinuria usually does not occur in normal pregnancy except during labor or after birth (Cunningham et al., 2005). However, the increased amount of amino acids that must be filtered may exceed the capacity of the renal tubules to absorb it; thus small amounts of protein are then lost in the urine. The amount of protein excreted is not an indication of the severity of renal disease, nor does an increase in protein excretion in a pregnant woman with known renal disease necessarily indicate a progression in her disease. However, a pregnant woman with hypertension and proteinuria must be carefully evaluated because she may be at greater risk for an adverse pregnancy outcome (Gordon, 2007) (see Table 6-3).

Integumentary system

Alterations in hormonal balance and mechanical stretching are responsible for several changes in the integumentary system during pregnancy. Hyperpigmentation is stimulated by the anterior pituitary hormone melanotropin, which is increased during pregnancy. Darkening of the nipples, areolae, axillae, and vulva occurs at approximately the sixteenth week of gestation. Facial melasma, also called **chloasma**, or the mask of pregnancy, is a blotchy, brownish hyperpigmentation of the skin over the cheeks, nose, and forehead, especially in dark-complexioned pregnant women. Chloasma appears in 50% to 70% of pregnant women, beginning after the sixteenth week and increasing gradually until term. The sun intensifies this pigmentation in susceptible women. Chloasma caused by normal pregnancy usually fades after birth.

The **linea nigra** (Fig. 6-11) is a pigmented line extending from the symphysis pubis to the top of the fundus in the midline; this line is known as the *linea alba* before hormone-induced pigmentation. In primigravidas the extension of the linea nigra, beginning in the third month, keeps pace with the rising height of the fundus; in multigravidas, the entire line often appears earlier than the third month. Not all pregnant women develop linea nigra, and some women notice hair growth along the line with or without the change in pigmentation.

Striae gravidarum, or stretch marks (seen over lower abdomen in Fig. 6-11), which appear in 50% to 90% of pregnant women during the second half of pregnancy, may be caused by action of adrenocorticosteroids. Striae reflect separation within the underlying connective (collagen) tissue of the skin. These slightly depressed streaks tend to occur over areas of maximal stretch (i.e., abdomen, thighs, and breasts). The stretching sometimes causes a sensation that resembles itching. The tendency to develop striae may be familial. After birth they usually fade, although they never disappear completely. Color of striae varies depending on the pregnant woman's skin color. The striae appear pinkish on a woman with light skin and are lighter than surrounding skin in dark-skinned women. In the multipara, in addition to the striae of the present pregnancy, glistening silvery lines (in light-skinned women) or purplish lines (in dark-skinned women) are commonly seen. These lines represent the scars of striae from previous pregnancies.

Angiomas are commonly called *vascular spiders.* They are tiny, star-shaped or branched, slightly raised and pulsating end-arterioles usually found on the neck, thorax, face, and arms. They occur as a result of elevated levels of circulating estrogen. The spiders are bluish in color and do not blanch with pressure. Vascular spiders appear during the second to the fifth month of pregnancy in almost 65% of Caucasian women and 10% of African-American women. The spiders usually disappear after birth (Blackburn, 2007).

Pinkish-red, diffuse mottling or well-defined blotches are seen over the palmar surfaces of the hands in approximately 60% of Caucasian women and 35% of African-American women during pregnancy (Blackburn, 2007). These color changes, called palmar erythema, are related primarily to increased estrogen levels.

NURSING ALERT Because integumentary system changes vary greatly among women of different racial backgrounds, the color of a woman's skin should be noted along with any changes that may be attributed to pregnancy when performing physical assessments.

Some dermatologic conditions have been identified as unique to pregnancy or as having an increased incidence during pregnancy. Mild pruritus (pruritus gravidarum) is a relatively common dermatologic symptom in pregnancy. The goal of management is to relieve the itching. Topical steroids and emollients are the usual treatments. The problem usually resolves in the postpartum period (Papoutsis & Kroumpouzos, 2007). Systemic diseases can also cause pruritus, but these causes are uncommon or rare (Cappell, 2007) (Box 6-3). Preexisting skin diseases may complicate pregnancy or be improved. (See Chapter 20 for further discussion.)

BOX 6-3

Prevalence of Dermatologic Disorders of Pregnancy

Pruritic urticarial papules and plaques of pregnancy (PUPPP): 1:130 to 1:300
Prurigo of pregnancy (PP): 1:300 to 1:450
Herpes gestationis (HG): 1:50,000
Pruritic folliculitis of pregnancy (PFP): very rare; approximately 30 cases

Source: Papoutsis, J. & Kroupouzos, G. (2007). Dermatologic disorders. In S. Gabbe, J. Niebyl, & J. Simpson (Eds.), *Obstetrics: Normal and problem pregnancies* (5th ed.). Philadelphia: Churchill Livingstone.

NURSING ALERT Women with severe acne taking isotretinoin (Accutane) should avoid pregnancy while receiving the treatment because it is teratogenic and is associated with major malformations.

Gum hypertrophy may occur. An epulis (gingival granuloma gravidarum) is a red, raised nodule on the gums that bleeds easily. This lesion may develop around the third month and usually continues to enlarge as pregnancy progresses. It is usually managed by preventing trauma to the gums (e.g., using a soft toothbrush). An epulis usually regresses spontaneously after birth.

Nail growth may be accelerated. Some women may notice thinning and softening of the nails. Oily skin and acne vulgaris may occur during pregnancy. For some women, the skin clears and looks radiant. Hirsutism, the excessive growth of hair or growth of hair in unusual places, is commonly reported. An increase in fine hair growth may occur but tends to disappear after pregnancy; however, growth of coarse or bristly hair does not usually disappear. The rate of scalp hair loss slows during pregnancy, while increased hair loss may be noted in the postpartum period.

Increased blood supply to the skin leads to increased perspiration. Women feel hotter during pregnancy, a condition possibly related to a progesterone-induced increase in body temperature and the increased BMR.

Musculoskeletal system

The gradually changing body and increasing weight of the pregnant woman cause noticeable alterations in her posture (Fig. 6-12) and the way she walks. The great abdominal distention that gives the pelvis a forward tilt, decreased abdominal muscle tone, and increased weight bearing require a realignment of the spinal curvature late

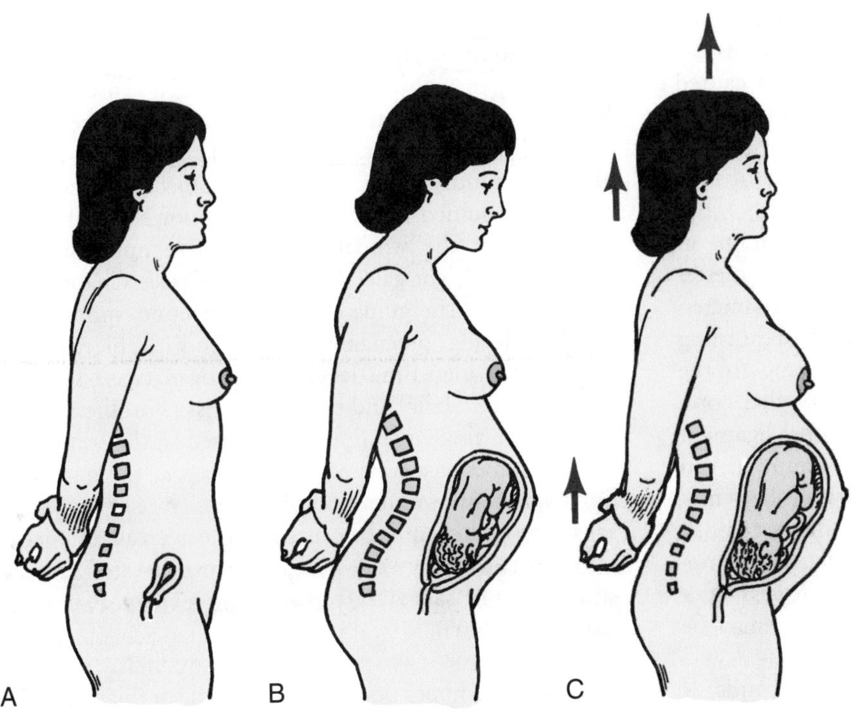

Fig. 6-12 Postural changes during pregnancy. **A,** Nonpregnant. **B,** Incorrect posture. **C,** Correct posture during pregnancy.

in pregnancy. The woman's center of gravity shifts forward. An increase in the normal lumbosacral curve (lordosis) develops, and a compensatory curvature in the cervicodorsal region (exaggerated anterior flexion of the head) develops to help her maintain her balance. Aching, numbness, and weakness of the upper extremities may result. Large breasts and a stoop-shouldered stance will further accentuate the lumbar and dorsal curves. Walking is more difficult, and the waddling gait of the pregnant woman, called "the proud walk of pregnancy" by Shakespeare, is well known. The ligamentous and muscular structures of the middle and lower spine may be severely stressed. These and related changes often cause musculoskeletal discomfort, especially in older women or those with a back disorder or a faulty sense of balance.

Slight relaxation and increased mobility of the pelvic joints are normal during pregnancy. They are secondary to the exaggerated elasticity and softening of connective and collagen tissue caused by increased circulating steroid sex hormones, especially estrogen. Relaxin, an ovarian hormone, assists in this relaxation and softening. These adaptations permit enlargement of pelvic dimensions to facilitate labor and birth. The degree of relaxation varies, but considerable separation of the symphysis pubis and the instability of the sacroiliac joints may cause pain and difficulty in walking. Obesity and multifetal pregnancy tend to increase the pelvic instability. Peripheral joint laxity also increases as pregnancy progresses, but the cause is not known (Cunningham et al., 2005).

The muscles of the abdominal wall stretch and ultimately lose some tone. During the third trimester, the rectus abdominis muscles may separate (Fig. 6-13), allowing abdominal contents to protrude at the midline. The umbilicus flattens or protrudes. After birth, the muscles gradually regain tone; however, separation of the muscles (**diastasis recti abdominis**) may persist.

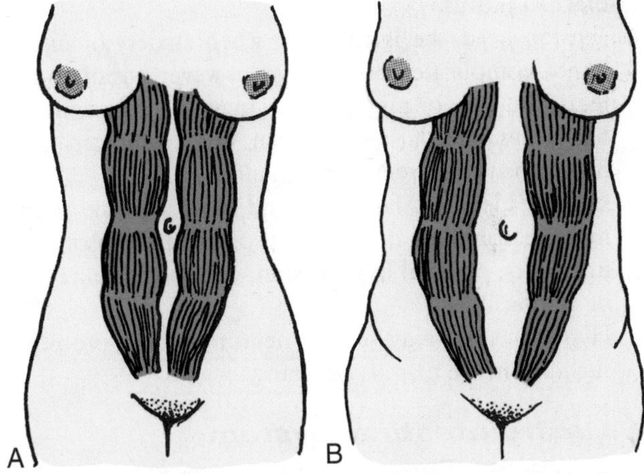

Fig. 6-13 Possible change in rectus abdominis muscles during pregnancy. **A,** Normal position in nonpregnant woman. **B,** Diastasis recti abdominis in pregnant woman.

Neurologic system

Little is known regarding specific alterations in function of the neurologic system during pregnancy, aside from hypothalamic-pituitary neurohormonal changes. Specific physiologic alterations resulting from pregnancy may cause the following neurologic or neuromuscular symptoms:

- Compression of pelvic nerves or vascular stasis caused by enlargement of the uterus may result in sensory changes in the legs.
- Dorsolumbar lordosis may cause pain because of traction on nerves or compression of nerve roots.
- Edema involving the peripheral nerves may result in **carpal tunnel syndrome** during the last trimester (Samuels & Niebyl, 2007). The syndrome is characterized by paresthesia (abnormal sensation such as burning or tingling) and pain in the hand, radiating to the elbow. The sensations are caused by edema that compresses the median nerve beneath the carpal ligament of the wrist. Smoking and alcohol consumption can impair the microcirculation and may worsen the symptoms. The dominant hand is usually affected most, although as many as 80% of women experience symptoms in both hands. Symptoms usually regress after pregnancy. In some cases, surgical treatment may be necessary (Samuels & Niebyl).
- Acroesthesia (numbness and tingling of the hands) is caused by the stoop-shouldered stance (see Fig. 6-12, *B*) assumed by some women during pregnancy. The condition is associated with traction on segments of the brachial plexus.
- Tension headache is common when anxiety or uncertainty complicates pregnancy. However, vision problems, sinusitis, or migraine also may be responsible for headaches. Headaches also can be a symptom of a hypertensive disorder of pregnancy.
- Light-headedness, faintness, and even syncope (fainting) are common during early pregnancy. Vasomotor instability, postural hypotension, or hypoglycemia may be responsible.
- Hypocalcemia may cause neuromuscular problems such as muscle cramps or tetany.

Gastrointestinal system

Appetite. During pregnancy, the woman's appetite and food intake fluctuate. Early in pregnancy, some women have nausea with or without vomiting (morning sickness), possibly in response to increasing levels of hCG and altered carbohydrate metabolism (Gordon, 2007). Morning sickness or nausea and vomiting of pregnancy (NVP) appears at approximately 4 to 6 weeks of gestation and usually subsides by the end of the third month (first trimester) of pregnancy. Severity varies from mild distaste for certain foods to more severe vomiting. The condition may be triggered by the sight or odor of various foods. By the end of the second trimester, the appetite increases in response to increasing metabolic needs. Rarely does NVP have harmful effects on the embryo, fetus, or the woman. Whenever the vomiting is severe or persists beyond the first trimester, or when it is accompanied by fever, pain, or weight loss, further evaluation is necessary, and medical intervention is likely (see Chapter 21).

Women may also have changes in their sense of taste, leading to cravings and changes in dietary intake. Some women have nonfood cravings (called *pica*), such as for ice, clay, and laundry starch. Usually the subjects of these cravings, if consumed in moderation, are not harmful to the pregnancy if the woman has adequate nutrition with appropriate weight gain (Gordon, 2007) (see Chapter 8).

Mouth. The gums become hyperemic, spongy, and swollen during pregnancy. They tend to bleed easily because the increasing levels of estrogen cause selective increased vascularity and connective tissue proliferation (a nonspecific gingivitis). Epulis (discussed in the section on the integumentary system) may develop at the gum line. Some pregnant women complain of **ptyalism** (excessive salivation), which may be caused by the decrease in unconscious swallowing by the woman when nauseated or from stimulation of salivary glands by eating starch (Cunningham et al., 2005).

Esophagus, stomach, and intestines. Herniation of the upper portion of the stomach (hiatal hernia) occurs after the seventh or eighth month of pregnancy in approximately 15% to 20% of pregnant women. This condition results from upward displacement of the stomach, which causes the hiatus of the diaphragm to widen. It occurs more often in multiparas and older or obese women.

Increased estrogen production causes decreased secretion of hydrochloric acid; therefore peptic ulcer formation or flare-up of existing peptic ulcers is uncommon during pregnancy and may improve (Gordon, 2007).

Increased progesterone production causes decreased tone and motility of smooth muscles, resulting in esophageal regurgitation, slower emptying time of the stomach, and reverse peristalsis. As a result, the woman may experience "acid indigestion" or heartburn (**pyrosis**) beginning as early as the first trimester and intensifying through the third trimester.

Iron is absorbed more readily in the small intestine in response to increased needs during pregnancy. Even when the woman is deficient in iron, it will continue to be absorbed in sufficient amounts for the fetus to have a normal hemoglobin level.

Increased progesterone (causing loss of muscle tone and decreased peristalsis) results in an increase in water absorption from the colon and may cause constipation. Constipation also may result from hypoperistalsis (sluggishness of the bowel), food choices, lack of fluids, iron supplementation, decreased activity level, abdominal distention by the pregnant uterus, and displacement and compression of the intestines. If the pregnant woman has hemorrhoids (see Fig. 6-10) and is constipated, then the hemorrhoids may become everted or may bleed during straining at stool.

Gallbladder and liver. The gallbladder is quite often distended because of its decreased muscle tone during pregnancy. Increased emptying time and thickening of bile caused by prolonged retention are typical changes. These features, together with slight hypercholesterolemia from increased progesterone levels, may account for the development of gallstones during pregnancy.

Hepatic function is difficult to appraise during pregnancy; however, only minor changes in liver function develop. Occasionally, intrahepatic cholestasis (retention and accumulation of bile in the liver caused by factors within the liver) occurs late in pregnancy in response to placental steroids and may result in pruritus gravidarum (severe itching) with or without jaundice. These distressing symptoms are difficult to treat during pregnancy and may be associated with fetal risks. However, symptoms subside after birth (Cappell, 2007).

Abdominal discomfort. Intraabdominal alterations that can cause discomfort include pelvic heaviness or pressure, round ligament tension, flatulence, distention and bowel cramping, and uterine contractions. In addition to displacement of intestines, pressure from the expanding uterus causes an increase in venous pressure in the pelvic organs. Although most abdominal discomfort is a consequence of normal maternal alterations, the health care provider must be constantly alert to the possibility of disorders such as bowel obstruction or an inflammatory process.

Appendicitis may be difficult to diagnose in pregnancy because the appendix is displaced upward and laterally, high and to the right, away from the McBurney point (Fig. 6-14).

Endocrine system

Profound endocrine changes are essential for pregnancy maintenance, normal fetal growth, and postpartum recovery.

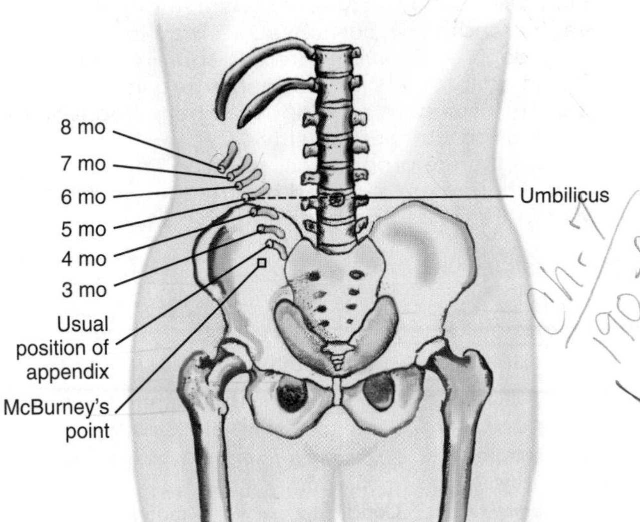

Fig. 6-14 Change in position of appendix in pregnancy. Note the McBurney point.

Pituitary and placental hormones. During pregnancy, the elevated levels of estrogen and progesterone (produced first by the corpus luteum in the ovary until approximately 14 weeks of gestation and then by the placenta) suppress secretion of follicle-stimulating hormone (FSH) and luteinizing hormone (LH) by the anterior pituitary. The maturation of a follicle and ovulation do not occur. Although the majority of women have amenorrhea (absence of menses), at least 20% have some slight, painless spotting during early gestation. Implantation bleeding and bleeding after intercourse related to cervical friability can occur. Most of the women experiencing slight gestational bleeding continue to term and have normal infants; however, all instances of bleeding should be reported and evaluated.

After implantation, the fertilized ovum and the chorionic villi produce hCG, which maintains the production by the corpus luteum of estrogen and progesterone until the placenta takes over production (Burton, Sibley, & Jauniaux, 2007).

Progesterone is essential for maintaining pregnancy by relaxing smooth muscles, resulting in decreased uterine contractility and prevention of miscarriage. Progesterone and estrogen cause fat to deposit in subcutaneous tissues over the maternal abdomen, back, and upper thighs. This fat serves as an energy reserve for both pregnancy and lactation. Estrogen also promotes the enlargement of the genitals, uterus, and breasts and increases vascularity, causing vasodilation. Estrogen causes relaxation of pelvic ligaments and joints. It also alters metabolism of nutrients by interfering with folic acid metabolism, increasing the level of total body proteins, and promoting retention of sodium and water by kidney tubules. Estrogen may decrease secretion of hydrochloric acid and pepsin, which may be responsible for digestive upsets such as nausea.

Serum prolactin produced by the anterior pituitary begins to increase early in the first trimester and increases progressively to term. It is responsible for initial lactation; however, the high levels of estrogen and progesterone inhibit lactation by blocking the binding of prolactin to breast tissue until after birth (Gordon, 2007).

Oxytocin is produced by the posterior pituitary in increasing amounts as the fetus matures. This hormone can stimulate uterine contractions during pregnancy, but high levels of progesterone prevent contractions until near term. Oxytocin also stimulates the let-down or milk-ejection reflex after birth in response to the infant's sucking at the mother's breast.

Human chorionic somatomammotropin (hCS), previously called human placental lactogen and produced by the placenta, has been suggested to act as a growth hormone and contribute to breast development. It also may decrease the maternal metabolism of glucose and increase the amount of fatty acids for metabolic needs (Burton et al., 2007).

Thyroid gland. During pregnancy, gland activity and hormone production increase. The increased activity is reflected in a moderate enlargement of the thyroid gland caused by hyperplasia of the glandular tissue and increased vascularity (Cunningham et al., 2005). Thyroxine-binding globulin (TBG) increases as a result of increased estrogen levels. This increase begins at approximately 20 weeks of gestation. The level of total (free and bound) thyroxine (T_4) increases between 6 and 9 weeks of gestation and plateaus at 18 weeks of gestation. Free T_4 and free triiodothyronine (T_3) return to nonpregnant levels after the first trimester. Despite these changes in hormone production, hyperthyroidism usually does not develop in the pregnant woman (Cunningham et al.).

Parathyroid gland. Parathyroid hormone controls calcium and magnesium metabolism. Pregnancy induces a slight hyperparathyroidism, a reflection of increased fetal requirements for calcium and vitamin D. The peak level of parathyroid hormone occurs between 15 and 35 weeks of gestation, when the needs for growth of the fetal skeleton are greatest. Levels return to normal after birth.

Pancreas. The fetus requires significant amounts of glucose for its growth and development. To meet its need for fuel, the fetus not only depletes the store of maternal glucose but also decreases the mother's ability to synthesize glucose by siphoning off her amino acids. Maternal blood glucose levels decrease. Maternal insulin does not cross the placenta to the fetus. As a result, in early pregnancy the pancreas decreases its production of insulin.

As pregnancy continues, the placenta grows and produces progressively greater amounts of hormones (i.e., hCS, estrogen, progesterone). Cortisol production by the adrenals also increases. Estrogen, progesterone, hCS, and cortisol collectively decrease the mother's ability to use insulin. Cortisol stimulates increased production of insulin but also increases the mother's peripheral resistance to insulin (i.e., the tissues cannot use the insulin). Decreasing the mother's ability to use her own insulin is a protective mechanism that ensures an ample supply of glucose for the needs of the fetoplacental unit. The result is an added demand for insulin by the mother that continues to increase at a steady rate until term. The normal beta cells of the islets of Langerhans in the pancreas can meet this demand for insulin.

Adrenal glands. The adrenal glands change little during pregnancy. Secretion of aldosterone is increased, resulting in reabsorption of excess sodium from the renal tubules. Cortisol levels also are increased (Blackburn, 2007).

KEY POINTS

- The biochemical, physiologic, and anatomic adaptations that occur during pregnancy are profound and revert to the nonpregnant state after birth and lactation.
- Maternal adaptations are attributed to the hormones of pregnancy and to mechanical pressures exerted by the enlarging uterus and other tissues.
- ELISA testing, with monoclonal antibody technology, is the most popular method of pregnancy testing and is the basis for most over-the-counter home pregnancy tests.
- Presumptive, probable, and positive signs of pregnancy aid in the diagnosis of pregnancy; only positive signs (identification of a fetal heartbeat, verification of fetal movements, and visualization of the fetus) can establish the diagnosis of pregnancy.
- Adaptations to pregnancy protect the woman's normal physiologic functioning, meet the metabolic demands pregnancy imposes, and provide for fetal development and growth needs.
- Although the pH of the pregnant woman's vaginal secretions is acidic, she is still vulnerable to some vaginal infections, especially yeast infections.
- Increased vascularity and sensitivity of the vagina and other pelvic viscera may lead to a high degree of sexual interest and arousal.
- Some adaptations to pregnancy result in discomforts such as fatigue, urinary frequency, nausea, and breast sensitivity.
- As pregnancy progresses, balance and coordination are affected by changes in the woman's joints and her center of gravity.

Audio Chapter Summaries Access an audio summary of these Key Points on evolve

References

Beebe, K. (2005). The perplexing parity puzzle. AWHONN *Lifelines*, *9*(5), 394-399.

Blackburn, S. (2007). *Maternal, fetal, & neonatal physiology: A clinical perspective* (3rd ed.). St. Louis: Saunders.

Burton, G., Sibley, C., & Jauniaux, E. (2007). Placental anatomy and physiology. In S. Gabbe, J. Niebyl, & J. Simpson (Eds.), *Obstetrics: Normal and problem pregnancies* (5th ed.). Philadelphia: Churchill Livingstone.

Cappell, M. (2007). Hepatic and gastrointestinal diseases. In S. Gabbe, J. Niebyl, & J. Simpson (Eds.), *Obstetrics: Normal and problem pregnancies* (5th ed.). Philadelphia: Churchill Livingstone.

Cole, L., Sutton-Riley, J., Khanlian, S., Borkovskaya, M., Rayburn, B., & Rayburn, W. (2005). Sensitivity of over-the-counter pregnancy tests: Comparison of utility and marketing messages. *Journal of the American Pharmacists Association*, *45*(5), 608-615.

Copeland, L., & Landon, M. (2007). Malignant diseases and pregnancy. In S. Gabbe, J. Niebyl, & J. Simpson (Eds.), *Obstetrics: Normal and problem pregnancies* (5th ed.). Philadelphia: Churchill Livingstone.

Cunningham, F., Leveno, K., Bloom, S., Hauth, J., Gilstrap, L., & Wenstrom, K. (2005). *Williams obstetrics* (22nd ed.). New York: McGraw-Hill.

Duff, W., Sweet, R., & Edwards, R. (2009). Maternal and fetal infections. In R. Creasy, R. Resnik, & J. Iams (Eds.), *Creasy & Resnik's maternal-fetal medicine: Principles and practice* (6th ed.). Philadelphia: Saunders.

Gordon, M. (2007). Maternal physiology. In S. Gabbe, J. Niebyl, & J. Simpson (Eds.), *Obstetrics: Normal and problem pregnancies* (5th ed.). Philadelphia: Churchill Livingstone.

Pagana, K., & Pagana, T. (2006). *Mosby's manual of diagnostic and laboratory tests* (3rd ed.). St. Louis: Mosby.

Papoutsis, J., & Kroumpouzos, G. (2007). Dermatologic disorders In S. Gabbe, J. Niebyl, & J. Simpson (Eds.), *Obstetrics: Normal and problem pregnancies* (5th ed.). Philadelphia: Churchill Livingstone.

Pickering, T., Hall, J., Appel, L., Falkner, B., Graves, J., Hill, M. et al. (2005). Recommendations for blood pressure measurement in humans and experimental animals: Part 1: Blood pressure measurement in Humans: A statement for professionals from the Subcommittee of Professional and Public Education of the American Heart Association Council on High Blood Pressure Research. *Hypertension 45*(1), 142-161.

Samuels. P. (2007). Hematologic complications of pregnancy. In S. Gabbe, J. Niebyl, & J. Simpson (Eds.), *Obstetrics: Normal and problem pregnancies* (5th ed.). Philadelphia: Churchill Livingstone.

Samuels, P., & Niebyl, J. (2007). Neurologic disorders. In S. Gabbe, J. Niebyl, & J. Simpson (Eds.), *Obstetrics: Normal and problem pregnancies* (5th ed.). Philadelphia: Churchill Livingstone.

Seidel, H., Ball, J., Dains, J., & Benedict, G. (2006). *Mosby's guide to physical examination* (6th ed.). St. Louis: Mosby.

Sibai, B. (2007). Hypertension. In S. Gabbe, J. Niebyl, & J. Simpson (Eds.), *Obstetrics: Normal and problem pregnancies* (5th ed.). Philadelphia: Churchill Livingstone.

Tomlinson, C., Marshall, J., & Ellis, J. (2008). Comparison of accuracy and certainty of results of six home pregnancy tests available over-the-counter. *Current Medical Research and Opinion, 24*(6), 1645-1649.

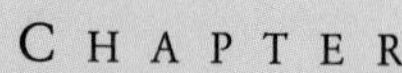
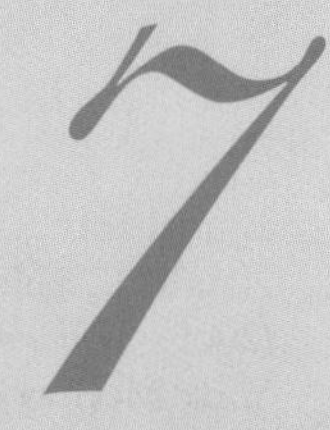
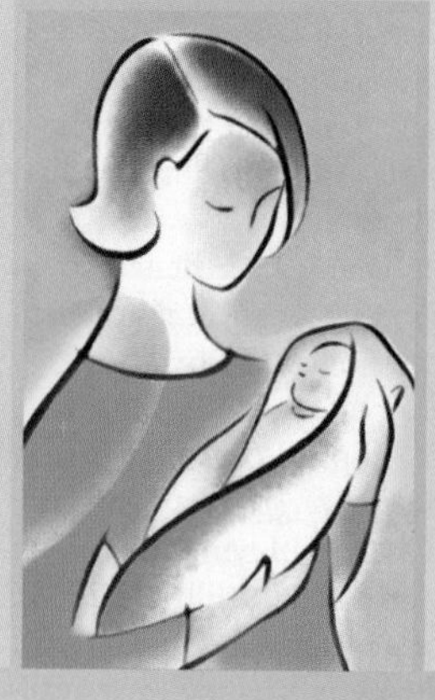

CHAPTER 7

Nursing Care of the Family during Pregnancy

DEITRA LEONARD LOWDERMILK

LEARNING OBJECTIVES

- *Describe the process of confirming pregnancy and estimating the date of birth.*
- *Summarize the physical, psychosocial, and behavioral changes that usually occur as the mother and other family members adapt to pregnancy.*
- *Discuss the benefits of prenatal care and problems of accessibility for some women.*
- *Outline the patterns of health care used to assess maternal and fetal health status at the initial and follow-up visits during pregnancy.*
- *Identify the typical nursing assessments, diagnoses, interventions, and methods of evaluation in providing care for the pregnant woman.*
- *Discuss education needed by pregnant women to understand physical discomforts related to pregnancy and to recognize signs and symptoms of potential complications.*
- *Examine the impact of culture, age, parity, and number of fetuses on the response of the family to the pregnancy and on the prenatal care provided.*

KEY TERMS AND DEFINITIONS

birth plan A tool by which parents can explore their childbirth options and choose those that are most important to them

couvade syndrome The phenomenon of expectant fathers' experiencing pregnancy-like symptoms

cultural prescriptions Practices that are expected or acceptable

cultural proscriptions Forbidden; taboo practices

doula Trained assistant hired to give the woman support during pregnancy, labor and birth, and postpartum

home birth Planned birth of the child at home, usually performed under the supervision of a midwife

morning sickness Nausea and vomiting that affect some women during the first few months of their pregnancy; may occur at any time of day

multifetal pregnancy Pregnancy in which more than one fetus is in the uterus at the same time; multiple gestation

Nägele's rule One method for calculating the estimated date of birth, or "due date"

pelvic tilt (rock) Exercise used to help relieve low back discomfort during menstruation and pregnancy

pinch test Determines whether nipples are everted or inverted by placing thumb and forefinger on areola and pressing inward; the nipple will stand erect or will invert

supine hypotension Drop in blood pressure caused by impaired venous return when the gravid uterus presses on the ascending vena cava, when woman is lying flat on her back; vena cava syndrome

trimesters One of three periods of approximately 3 months each into which pregnancy is divided

WEB RESOURCES

Additional related content can be found on the companion website at evolve
http://evolve.elsevier.com/Lowdermilk/Maternity/

- NCLEX Review Questions
- Assessment Videos: Chest wall, breast, abdomen/fundal height, fetal heart rate
- Case Study: First Trimester
- Case Study: Second Trimester
- Case Study: Third Trimester
- Critical Thinking Exercise: Discomforts of Pregnancy
- Critical Thinking Exercise: Teenage Pregnancy
- Nursing Care Plan: Adolescent Pregnancy
- Nursing Care Plan: Discomforts of Pregnancy and Warning Signs
- Spanish Guidelines: Assessment of Respiratory Symptoms
- Spanish Guidelines: Prenatal Interview
- Spanish Guidelines: Prenatal Physical Examination

The prenatal period is a time of physical and psychologic preparation for birth and parenthood. Becoming a parent is one of the milestones of adult life, and as such, it is a time of intense learning for both parents and those close to them. The prenatal period provides a unique opportunity for nurses and other members of the health care team to influence family health. During this period, essentially healthy women seek regular care and guidance. The nurse's health-promotion interventions can affect the well-being of the woman, her unborn child, and the rest of her family for many years.

Regular prenatal visits, ideally beginning soon after the first missed menstrual period, offer opportunities to ensure the health of the expectant mother and her fetus. Prenatal health care permits diagnosis and treatment of preexisting maternal disorders and any disorder that may develop during the pregnancy. Prenatal care is designed to monitor the growth and development of the fetus and to identify any abnormalities that will interfere with the course of normal labor. Prenatal care also provides education and support for self-management and parenting.

Pregnancy spans 9 months, but health care providers do not use the familiar monthly calendar to determine fetal age or discuss the pregnancy. Instead, they use lunar months, which last 28 days, or 4 weeks. According to the lunar calendar, normal pregnancy lasts approximately 10 lunar months, which is the same as 40 weeks or 280 days. Health care providers also refer to early, middle, and late pregnancy as **trimesters**. The first trimester lasts from weeks 1 through 13; the second, from weeks 14 through 26; and the third, from weeks 27 through 40. A pregnancy is considered at term if it advances to the completion of 37 weeks.

The focus of this chapter is on meeting the health needs of the expectant family over the course of pregnancy, or the *prenatal period.*

DIAGNOSIS OF PREGNANCY

Women may suspect pregnancy when they miss a menstrual period. Many women come to the first prenatal visit after a positive home pregnancy test; however, the clinical diagnosis of pregnancy before the second missed period is difficult in some women. Physical variations, obesity, or tumors, for example, may confuse even the experienced examiner. Accuracy is important, however, because emotional, social, medical, or legal consequences of an inaccurate diagnosis, either positive or negative, can be extremely serious. A correct date for the *last (normal) menstrual period* (LMP or LNMP) and for the date of intercourse and a basal body temperature (BBT) record are of great value in the accurate diagnosis of pregnancy (see Chapter 4).

Signs and Symptoms

Great variability is possible in the subjective and objective signs and symptoms of pregnancy; therefore the diagnosis of pregnancy is often uncertain for a time. Many of the indicators of pregnancy are clinically useful in the diagnosis of pregnancy. They are classified as presumptive, probable, or positive (see Table 6-2).

The presumptive indicators of pregnancy can be caused by conditions other than gestation. For example, illness or excessive exercise can cause amenorrhea, anemia or infection can be the cause of fatigue, a tumor may cause enlargement of the abdomen, and a gastrointestinal (GI) upset or food allergy may cause nausea or vomiting. Therefore these signs alone are not reliable for diagnosis.

Estimating Date of Birth

After the diagnosis of pregnancy, the woman's first question usually concerns when she will give birth. This date has traditionally been termed the *estimated date of confinement* (EDC), although *estimated date of delivery* (EDD) is also used. However, the term *estimated date of birth* (EDB) promotes a more positive perception of both pregnancy and birth. Because the precise date of conception is generally unknown, several formulas can be used for calculating the EDB. None of these guides is infallible, but Nägele's rule is reasonably accurate and is usually used (Johnson, Gregory, & Niebyl, 2007).

LMP = last menstrual period

BOX 7-1

Use of Nägele's Rule

July 10, 2009, is the first day of the last menstrual period (LMP).

	Month	Day	Year
LMP	7	10	2009
	−3	+7	
Estimated day of birth:	4	17	2010

The estimated date of birth (EDB) is April 17, 2010.

Nägele's rule is as follows: After determining the first day of the LMP, subtract 3 calendar months and add 7 days; or alternatively, add 7 days to the LMP and count forward 9 calendar months. Box 7-1 demonstrates use of Nägele's rule. Nägele's rule assumes that the woman has a 28-day menstrual cycle and that pregnancy occurred on the fourteenth day. Obtaining an accurate menstrual history is important as well in using this method of dating.

ADAPTATION TO PREGNANCY

Case Study: First Trimester

Pregnancy affects all family members, and each family member must adapt to the pregnancy and interpret its meaning in light of his or her own needs. This process of family adaptation to pregnancy takes place within a cultural environment influenced by societal trends. Dramatic changes have occurred in Western society in recent years, and the nurse needs to be prepared to support single-parent families, reconstituted families, dual-career families, and alternative families, as well as traditional families, in the childbirth experience.

Much of the research on family dynamics during pregnancy in the United States and Canada has focused on Caucasian, middle-class nuclear families. Hence the findings do not always apply to families that do not fit the traditional North American model. Adaptation of terms is appropriate to avoid embarrassment to the nurse and offense to the family. Additional research is needed on a variety of families to determine if study findings generated in traditional families are applicable to others.

Maternal Adaptation

Women of all ages use the months of pregnancy to adapt to the maternal role, a complex process of social and cognitive learning. Early in pregnancy, nothing seems to be happening, and a woman may spend much time sleeping. With the perception of fetal movement in the second trimester, the woman turns her attention inward to her pregnancy and to relationships with her mother and other women who have been or who are pregnant.

Pregnancy is a maturational milestone that is often stressful but also rewarding as the woman prepares for a new level of caring and responsibility. Her self-concept changes in readiness for parenthood as she prepares for her new role. She moves gradually from being self-contained and independent to being committed to a lifelong concern for another human being. This growth requires mastery of certain developmental tasks: accepting the pregnancy, identifying with the role of mother, reordering the relationships between herself and her mother and between herself and her partner, establishing a relationship with the unborn child, and preparing for the birth experience (Lederman, 1996). The partner's emotional support is an important factor in the successful accomplishment of these developmental tasks. Single women with limited support may have difficulty making this adaptation.

Accepting the Pregnancy

The first step in adapting to the maternal role is accepting the idea of pregnancy and assimilating the pregnant state into the woman's way of life. Mercer (1995) described this process as *cognitive restructuring* and credited Reva Rubin (1984) as the nurse theorist who pioneered our understanding of maternal role attainment. The degree of acceptance is reflected in the woman's emotional responses. Many women are upset initially at finding themselves pregnant, especially if the pregnancy is unintended. Eventual acceptance of pregnancy parallels the growing acceptance of the reality of a child. However, do not equate nonacceptance of the pregnancy with rejection of the child; a woman may dislike being pregnant but feel love for the unborn child.

Women who are happy and pleased about their pregnancy often view it as biologic fulfillment and part of their life plan. They have high self-esteem and tend to be confident about outcomes for themselves, their babies, and other family members. Despite a general feeling of well-being, many women are surprised to experience emotional lability, or rapid and unpredictable changes in mood. These swings in emotions and increased sensitivity to others are disconcerting to the expectant mother and those around her. Increased irritability, explosions of tears and anger, and feelings of great joy and cheerfulness alternate, apparently with little or no provocation.

Profound hormonal changes that are part of the maternal response to pregnancy are responsible for mood changes. Other reasons such as concerns about finances and changed lifestyle contribute to this seemingly erratic behavior.

Most women have ambivalent feelings during pregnancy whether the pregnancy was intended or not. Ambivalence–having conflicting feelings simultaneously–is a normal response for people preparing for a new role. For example, during pregnancy, some women feel great pleasure that they are fulfilling a lifelong dream, but they also feel great regret that life as they now know it is ending.

Even women who are pleased to be pregnant may experience feelings of hostility toward the pregnancy or unborn child from time to time. Such incidents as a partner's chance remark about the attractiveness of a slim, nonpregnant woman or news of a colleague's promotion can give rise to ambivalent feelings. Body sensations, feelings of dependence, or the realization of the responsibilities of child care also can generate such feelings.

Intense feelings of ambivalence that persist through the third trimester may indicate an unresolved conflict with the motherhood role (Mercer, 1995). After the birth of a healthy child, memories of these ambivalent feelings are usually dismissed. If the child is born with a defect, however, a woman may look back at the times when she did not want the pregnancy and feel intensely guilty. She may believe that her ambivalence caused the birth defect. She will then need assurance that her feelings were not responsible for the problem.

Identifying with the mother role

The process of identifying with the mother role begins early in each woman's life when she is being mothered as a child. Her social group's perception of the feminine role can subsequently influence her toward choosing between motherhood or a career, being married or single, being independent rather than interdependent, or being able to manage multiple roles. Practice roles, such as playing with dolls, baby-sitting, and taking care of siblings, increase her understanding of what being a mother involves.

Many women have always wanted a baby, liked children, and looked forward to motherhood. Their high motivation to become a parent promotes acceptance of pregnancy and eventual prenatal and parental adaptation. Other women apparently have not considered in any detail what motherhood means to them. During pregnancy, these women must resolve conflicts such as not wanting the pregnancy and child-related or career-related decisions.

Reordering personal relationships

Close relationships of the pregnant woman undergo change during pregnancy as she prepares emotionally for the new role of mother. As family members learn their new roles, periods of tension and conflict may occur. An understanding of the typical patterns of adjustment can help the nurse to reassure the pregnant woman and explore issues related to social support. Promoting effective communication patterns between the expectant mother and her own mother and between the expectant mother and her partner are common nursing interventions provided during the prenatal visits.

The woman's own relationship with her mother is significant in adaptation to pregnancy and motherhood. Important components in the pregnant woman's relationship with her mother are the mother's availability (past and present), her reactions to the daughter's pregnancy, respect for her daughter's autonomy, and the willingness to reminisce (Mercer, 1995).

The mother's reaction to the daughter's pregnancy signifies her acceptance of the grandchild and of her daughter. If the mother is supportive, the daughter has an opportunity to discuss pregnancy, labor, and her feelings with a knowledgeable and accepting woman (Fig. 7-1). Reminiscing about the pregnant woman's early childhood and sharing the prospective grandmother's account of her childbirth experience help the daughter to anticipate and prepare for labor and birth.

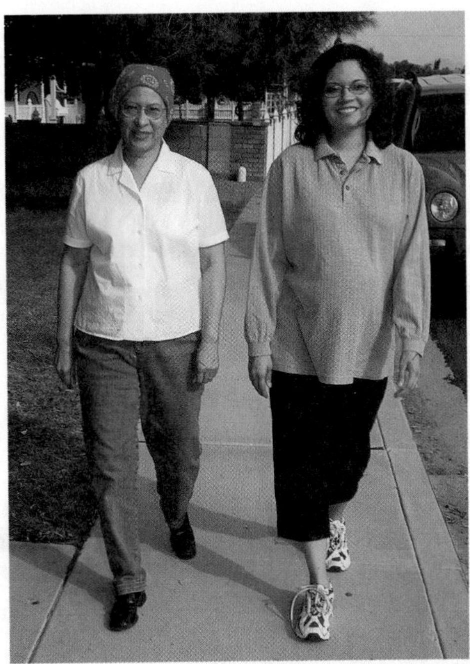

Fig. 7-1 A pregnant woman and her mother enjoying their walk together. (Courtesy Michael S. Clement, MD, Mesa, AZ.)

Although the woman's relationship with her mother is significant in considering her adaptation in pregnancy, the most important person to the pregnant woman is usually the father of her child. Women express two major needs within this relationship during pregnancy: feeling loved and valued and having the child accepted by the partner.

The marital or committed relationship is not static but evolves over time. The addition of a child changes forever the nature of the bond between partners. This is often a time when couples grow closer, and the pregnancy has a maturing effect on the partners' relationship as they assume new roles and discover new aspects of one another. Partners who trust and support each other are able to share mutual-dependency needs (Mercer, 1995).

Sexual expression during pregnancy is highly individualized. Physical, emotional, and interactional factors, including misinformation about sex during pregnancy, sexual dysfunction, and physical changes in the woman, affect the sexual relationship. Many women and their partners express anxiety about the presence of the fetus as a third party in lovemaking. An individual may also believe that anomalies, mental retardation, and other injuries to the fetus and mother occur during sexual relations in pregnancy. Some couples fear that the birth process will drastically change the woman's genitals. Some couples do not express their concerns to the health care provider because of embarrassment or because they do not want to appear foolish.

As pregnancy progresses, changes in body shape, body image, and levels of discomfort influence both partners' desire for sexual expression. During the first trimester, the woman's sexual desire often decreases, especially if she has breast tenderness, nausea, fatigue, or sleepiness. As she progresses into the second trimester, however, her sense of well-being combined with the increased pelvic congestion that occurs at this time may increase her desire for sexual release. In the third trimester, somatic complaints and physical bulkiness increase physical discomfort and again diminish interest in sex. As a woman's pregnancy progresses, her enlarging gravid abdomen may limit the use of the man-on-top position for intercourse. Therefore other positions (e.g., side to side or the woman on top) may allow intercourse and minimize pressure on the woman's abdomen (Westheimer & Lopater, 2005).

Partners need to feel free to discuss their sexual responses during pregnancy with each other and with their health care provider. Their sensitivity to each other and willingness to share concerns can strengthen their sexual relationship. Partners who do not understand the rapid physiologic and emotional changes of pregnancy can become confused by the other's behavior. By talking to each other about the changes they are experiencing, couples can define problems and then offer the needed support. Nurses can facilitate communication between partners by talking to expectant couples about possible changes in feelings and behaviors they will experience as pregnancy progresses (see later discussion).

Establishing a relationship with the fetus

Emotional attachment–feelings of being tied by affection or love–begins during the prenatal period as women use fantasizing and daydreaming to prepare themselves for motherhood (Rubin, 1975). They think of themselves as mothers and imagine maternal qualities they would like to possess. Expectant parents desire to be warm, loving, and close to their child. They try to anticipate changes that the child will bring in their lives and wonder how they will react to noise, disorder, reduced freedom, and caregiving activities. The mother-child relationship progresses through pregnancy as a developmental process that unfolds in three phases.

In phase 1 the woman accepts the biologic fact of pregnancy. She needs to be able to state, "I am pregnant" and incorporate the idea of a child into her body and self-image. The woman's thoughts center on herself and the reality of her pregnancy. The child is viewed as part of herself, not a separate and unique person.

In phase 2 the woman accepts the growing fetus as distinct from herself, usually accomplished by the fifth month. She can now say, "I am going to have a baby." This differentiation of the child from the woman's self permits the beginning of the mother-child relationship that involves not only caring, but also responsibility. Planned pregnancies usually enhance attachment of a mother to her child, and the attachment increases when ultrasound examination and quickening confirm the reality of the fetus.

With acceptance of the reality of the child (hearing the heartbeat and feeling the child move) and an overall feeling of well-being the woman enters a quiet period and becomes more introspective. Fantasies about the child become precious to the woman. As the woman seems to withdraw and to concentrate her interest on the unborn child, her partner sometimes feels left out. If other children are in the family, they may become more demanding in their efforts to redirect the mother's attention to themselves.

During phase 3 of the attachment process, the woman prepares realistically for the birth and parenting of the child. She expresses the thought, "I am going to be a mother" and defines the nature and characteristics of the child. She may, for example, speculate about the child's personality traits based on patterns of fetal activity.

Although the mother alone experiences the child within, both parents and siblings believe the unborn child responds in a very individualized, personal manner. Family members may interact a great deal with the unborn child by talking to the fetus and stroking the mother's abdomen, especially when the fetus shifts position (Fig. 7-2). The fetus may even have a nickname used by family members.

Preparing for childbirth

Many women actively prepare for birth by reading books, viewing films, attending parenting classes, and talking to other women. They seek the best caregiver possible for advice, monitoring, and caring. The multiparous woman has her own history of labor and birth, which influences her approach to preparation for this childbirth experience.

Anxiety can arise from concern about a safe passage for herself and her child during the birth process (Mercer, 1995; Rubin, 1975). Some women do not express this concern overtly, but they give cues to the nurse by making plans for care of the new baby and other children in case "anything should happen." These feelings persist despite statistical evidence about the safe outcome of pregnancy for mothers and their infants. Many women fear the pain of childbirth or mutilation because they do not understand anatomy and the birth process. Education can alleviate many of these fears. Women also express concern over what behaviors are appropriate during the birth process and whether caregivers will accept them and their actions.

Toward the end of the third trimester, breathing is difficult, and fetal movements become vigorous enough to disturb the woman's sleep. Backaches, frequency and

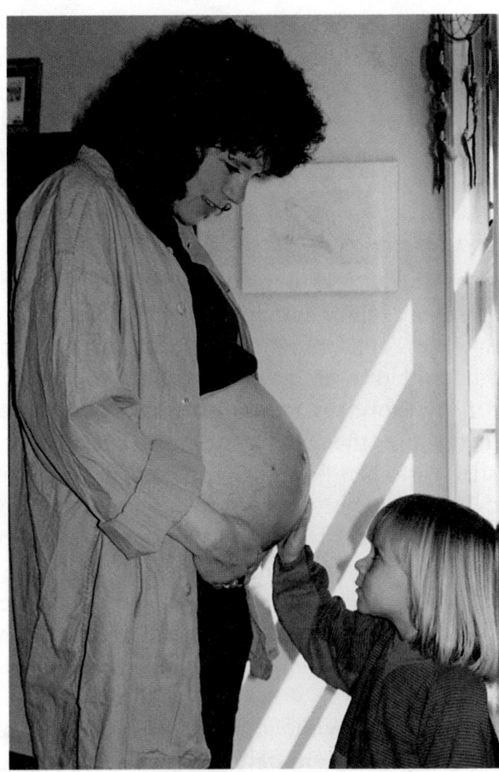

Fig. 7-2 Sibling feeling movement of fetus. (Courtesy Kim Molloy, Knoxville, IA.)

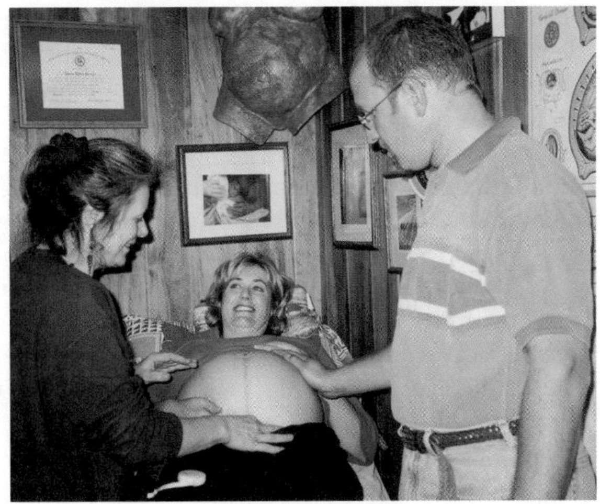

Fig. 7-3 Father participating in prenatal visit. Nurse-midwife discusses feeling fetal movement while father puts hand on mother's abdomen. (Courtesy Shannon Perry, Phoenix, AZ.)

urgency of urination, constipation, and varicose veins are often troublesome. The bulkiness and awkwardness of her body makes caring for other children, routine work-related duties, and sleep difficult. By this time, most women become impatient for labor to begin, whether the birth is anticipated with joy, dread, or a mixture of both. A strong desire to see the end of pregnancy, to be over and done with it, makes women at this stage ready to move on to childbirth.

Paternal Adaptation

The father's beliefs and feelings about the ideal mother and father and his cultural expectation of appropriate behavior during pregnancy affect his response to his partner's need for him. One man may engage in nurturing behavior. Another may feel lonely and alienated as the woman focuses her physical and emotional attention on the unborn child. He may seek comfort and understanding outside the home or become interested in a new hobby or involved with his work. Some men view pregnancy as proof of their masculinity and their dominant role. To others, pregnancy has no meaning in terms of responsibility to either mother or child. However, for most men, pregnancy is a time of preparation for the parental role with intense learning.

Accepting the pregnancy

The ways fathers adjust to the parental role has been the subject of considerable research. In older societies the man enacted the ritual couvade; that is, he behaved in specific ways and respected taboos associated with pregnancy and giving birth so the man's new status was recognized and endorsed. Now, some men experience pregnancy-like symptoms, such as nausea, weight gain, and other physical symptoms. This phenomenon is known as the **couvade syndrome**. Changing cultural and professional attitudes have encouraged fathers' participation in the birth experience in the last 30 years (Fig. 7-3).

The man's emotional responses to becoming a father, his concerns, and his informational needs change during the course of pregnancy. Phases of the developmental pattern become apparent. May (1982) described three phases characterizing the developmental tasks experienced by the expectant father:

- The announcement phase may last from a few hours to a few weeks. The developmental task is to accept the biologic fact of pregnancy. Men react to the confirmation of pregnancy with joy or sadness, depending on whether the pregnancy is desired or unplanned or unwanted. Ambivalence in the early stages of pregnancy is common.
- If pregnancy is unplanned or unwanted, some men find the alterations in life plans and lifestyles difficult to accept. Some men engage in extramarital affairs for the first time during their partner's pregnancy. Others batter their wives for the first time or escalate the frequency of battering episodes (Krieger, 2008). Chapter 2 provides information about violence against women and offers guidance on assessment and intervention.
- The second phase, the moratorium phase, is the period when he adjusts to the reality of pregnancy. The developmental task is to accept the pregnancy. Men appear to put conscious thought of the pregnancy aside for a time. They become more introspective and engage in many discussions about their philosophy of life,

religion, childbearing, and childrearing practices and their relationships with family members, particularly with their father. Depending on the man's readiness for the pregnancy, this phase may be relatively short or persist until the last trimester.

- The third phase, the focusing phase, begins in the last trimester and is characterized by the father's active involvement in both the pregnancy and his relationship with his child. The developmental task is to negotiate with his partner the role he is to play in labor and to prepare for parenthood. In this phase the man concentrates on his experience of the pregnancy and begins to think of himself as a father.

Identifying with the father role

Each man brings to pregnancy attitudes that affect the way in which he adjusts to the pregnancy and parental role. His memories of the fathering he received from his own father, the experiences he has had with child care, and the perceptions of the male and father roles within his social group will guide his selection of the tasks and responsibilities he will assume. Some men are highly motivated to nurture and love a child. Some are excited and pleased about the anticipated role of father. Others are more detached or even hostile to the idea of fatherhood.

Reordering personal relationships

The partner's main role in pregnancy is to nurture and respond to the pregnant woman's feelings of vulnerability. The partner must also deal with the reality of the pregnancy. The partner's support indicates involvement in the pregnancy and preparation for attachment to the child.

Some aspects of a partner's behavior indicate rivalry, and it is especially evident during sexual activity. For example, men may protest that fetal movements prevent sexual gratification or that they are being watched by the fetus during sexual activity. However, feelings of rivalry are often unconscious and not verbalized, but they are expressed in subtle behaviors.

The woman's increased introspection may cause her partner to feel uneasy as she becomes preoccupied with thoughts of the child and of her motherhood, with her growing dependence on her physician or midwife, and with her reevaluation of the couple's relationship.

Establishing a relationship with the fetus

The father-child attachment can be as strong as the mother-child relationship, and fathers can be as competent as mothers in nurturing their infants. The father-child attachment also begins during pregnancy. A father may rub or kiss the maternal abdomen, try to listen, talk, or sing to the fetus, or play with the fetus as he notes movement. Calling the unborn child by name or nickname helps to confirm the reality of pregnancy and promote attachment.

Men prepare for fatherhood in many of the same ways as women do for motherhood–by reading and by fantasizing about the baby. Daydreaming about their role as father is common in the last weeks before the birth; men rarely describe their thoughts unless they are reassured that such daydreams are normal.

Preparing for childbirth

The days and weeks immediately before the expected day of birth are full of anticipation and anxiety. Boredom and restlessness are common as the couple focuses on the birth process. However, during the last 2 months of pregnancy, many expectant fathers experience a surge of creative energy at home and on the job. They may become dissatisfied with their present living space. If possible, they tend to act on the need to alter the environment (remodeling, painting, etc.). This activity is their way of sharing in the childbearing experience. They are able to channel the anxiety and other feelings experienced during the final weeks before birth into productive activities. This behavior earns recognition and compliments from friends, relatives, and their partners.

Major concerns for the man are getting the woman to a medical facility in time for the birth and not appearing ignorant. Many men want to be able to recognize labor and determine when it is appropriate to leave for the hospital or call the physician or nurse-midwife. They may fantasize different situations and plan what they will do in response to them, or they may rehearse taking various routes to the hospital, timing each route at different times of the day.

Some prospective fathers have questions about the labor suite's furniture, nursing staff, and location, as well as the availability of the physician and anesthesiologist. Others want to know what is expected of them when their partners are in labor. The man may also have fears concerning safe passage of his child and partner and the possible death or complications of his partner and child. He should verbalize these fears, otherwise he cannot help his mate deal with her own unspoken or spoken apprehension.

With the exception of childbirth preparation classes, a man has few opportunities to learn ways to be an involved and active partner in this rite of passage into parenthood. Mothers often sense the tensions and apprehensions of the unprepared, unsupportive father, and it often increases their fears.

The same fears, questions, and concerns may affect birth partners who are not the biologic fathers. Nurses need to keep birth partners informed, supported, and included in all activities in which the mother desires their participation. The nurse can do much to promote pregnancy and birth as a family experience.

Sibling Adaptation

Sharing the spotlight with a new brother or sister may be the first major crisis for a child. The older child often

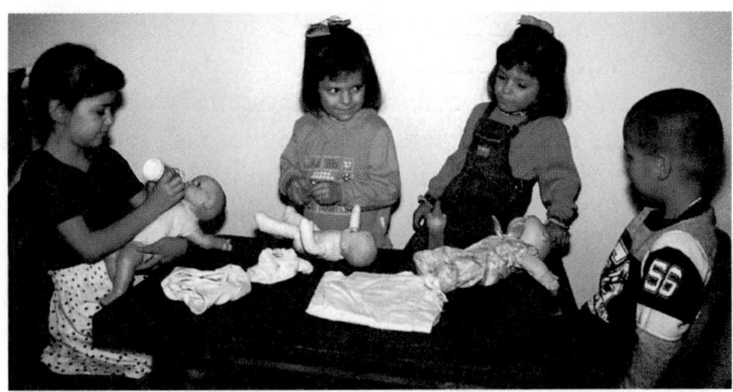

Fig. 7-4 A sibling class of preschoolers learns infant care using dolls. (Courtesy Marjorie Pyle, RNC, Lifecircle, Costa Mesa, CA.)

experiences a sense of loss or feels jealous at being "replaced" by the new sibling. Some of the factors that influence the child's response are age, the parents' attitudes, the role of the father, the length of separation from the mother, the hospital's visitation policy, and the way the child has been prepared for the change.

A mother with other children must devote time and effort to reorganizing her relationships with them. She needs to prepare siblings for the birth of the child (Fig. 7-4 and Box 7-2) and begin the process of role transition in the family by including the children in the pregnancy and being sympathetic to older children's concerns about losing their places in the family hierarchy. No child willingly gives up a familiar position.

Siblings' responses to pregnancy vary with their age and dependency needs. The 1-year-old infant seems largely unaware of the process, but the 2-year-old child notices the change in his or her mother's appearance and may comment that "Mommy's fat." The toddlers' need for sameness in the environment makes the children aware of any change. They may exhibit more clinging behavior and sometime regress in toilet training or eating.

By age 3 or 4 years, children like to hear the story of their own beginning and to hear how their development compares with that of the present pregnancy. They like to listen to the fetal heartbeat and feel the baby moving in utero (see Fig. 7-2). Sometimes they worry about how the baby is being fed and what it wears.

School-age children take a more clinical interest in their mother's pregnancy. They may want to know in more detail, "How did the baby get in there?" and "How will it get out?" Children in this age group notice pregnant women in stores, churches, and schools and sometimes seem shy if they need to approach a pregnant woman directly. On the whole, they look forward to the new baby, see themselves as "mothers" or "fathers," and enjoy buying baby supplies and preparing a place for the baby. Because they still think in concrete terms and base judgments on the here and now, they respond positively to their mother's current good health.

Early and middle adolescents preoccupied with the establishment of their own sexual identity may have difficulty accepting the overwhelming evidence of the sexual activity of their parents. They reason that if they are too young for such activity, certainly their parents are too old. They seem to take on a critical parental role and may ask, "What will people think?" or "How can you let yourself get so fat?" or "How can you let yourself get pregnant?" Many pregnant women with teenage children will confess that the attitudes of their teenagers are the most difficult aspect of their current pregnancy.

Late adolescents do not appear to be unduly disturbed. They are busy making plans for their own lives and realize that they will soon be gone from home. Parents usually

BOX 7-2

Tips for Sibling Preparation

PRENATAL
- Take your child on a prenatal visit. Let the child listen to the fetal heartbeat and feel the baby move.
- Involve the child in preparations for the baby, such as helping decorate the baby's room.
- Move the child to a bed (if still sleeping in a crib) at least 2 months before the baby is due.
- Read books, show videos, and take child to sibling preparation classes, including a hospital tour.
- Answer your child's questions about the coming birth, what babies are like, and any other questions.
- Take your child to the homes of friends who have babies so that the child has realistic expectations of what babies are like.

DURING THE HOSPITAL STAY
- Have someone bring the child to the hospital to visit you and the baby (unless you plan to have the child attend the birth).
- Do not force interactions between the child and the baby. The child will often be more interested in seeing you and being reassured of your love.
- Help the child explore the infant by showing how and where to touch the baby.
- Give the child a gift (from you or you, the father, and baby).

GOING HOME
- Leave the child at home with a relative or baby-sitter.
- Have someone else carry the baby from the car so that you can hug the child first.

ADJUSTMENT AFTER THE BABY IS HOME
- Arrange for a special time with the child alone with each parent.
- Do not exclude the child during infant feeding times. The child can sit with you and the baby and feed a doll or drink juice or milk with you or sit quietly with a game.
- Prepare small gifts for the child so that when the baby gets gifts the sibling will not feel left out. The child can also help open the baby gifts.
- Praise the child for acting age appropriately (so that being a baby does not seem better than being older).

report they are comforting and act more as other adults than as children.

Grandparent Adaptation

Every pregnancy affects all family relationships. For expectant grandparents, a first pregnancy in a child is undeniable evidence that they are growing older. Many think of a grandparent as old, white-haired, and becoming feeble of mind and body; however, some people face grandparenthood while still in their thirties or forties. Some individuals react negatively to the news that they will be grandparents, indicating that they are not ready for the new role.

In some family units, expectant grandparents are nonsupportive and inadvertently decrease the self-esteem of the parents-to-be. Mothers may talk about their terrible pregnancies, fathers may discuss the endless cost of rearing children, and mothers-in-law may complain that their sons are neglecting them because their concern is now directed toward the pregnant daughters-in-law.

However, most grandparents are delighted at the prospect of a new baby in the family. It reawakens the feelings of their own youth, the excitement of giving birth, and their delight in the behavior of the parents-to-be when they were infants. They set up a memory store of the child's first smiles, first words, and first steps, which they can use later for "claiming" the newborn as a member of the family. These behaviors provide a link between the past and present for the parents- and grandparents-to-be.

In addition, the grandparent is the historian who transmits the family history, a resource who shares knowledge based on experience, a role model, and a support person. The grandparent's presence and support can strengthen family systems by widening the circle of support and nurturance (Fig. 7-5).

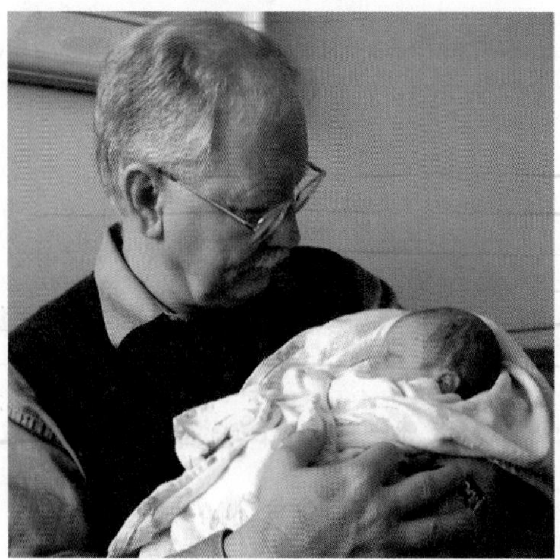

Fig. 7-5 Grandfather getting to know his grandson. (Courtesy Sharon Johnson, Petaluma, CA.)

CARE MANAGEMENT

The purpose of prenatal care is to identify existing risk factors and other deviations from normal in order to enhance pregnancy outcomes (Johnson, Gregory, & Niebyl, 2007). Major emphasis is placed on preventive aspects of care, primarily to motivate the pregnant woman to practice optimal self-management and to report unusual changes early so as to minimize or prevent problems. In holistic care, nurses provide information and guidance about not only the physical changes, but also the psychosocial impact of pregnancy on the woman and members of her family. The goals of prenatal nursing care, therefore, are to foster a safe birth for the infant and to promote satisfaction of the mother and family with pregnancy and the birth experience.

Advances have occurred in the number of women in the United States who receive adequate prenatal care. In 2005, almost 84% of all women received care in the first trimester. African-American, Hispanic, and Native-American women were two times as likely to get late prenatal care or no care at all than Caucasian women (Martin et al., 2008). Although women of middle or high socioeconomic status routinely seek prenatal care, women living in poverty or who lack health insurance are not always able to use public medical services or gain access to private care. Lack of culturally sensitive care providers and barriers in communication resulting from differences in language also interfere with access to care (Darby, 2007). Similarly, immigrant women who come from cultures in which prenatal care is not emphasized may not know to seek routine prenatal care. Birth outcomes in these populations are less positive, with higher rates of maternal and fetal or newborn complications. Problems with low birth weight (LBW; less than 2500 g) and infant mortality have in particular been associated with lack of adequate prenatal care.

Barriers to obtaining health care during pregnancy include lack of transportation, unpleasant clinic facilities or procedures, inconvenient clinic hours, child care problems and personal attitudes (American College of Obstetricians and Gynecologists Committee on Health Care for Underserved Women, 2006; Daniels, Noe, & Mayberry, 2006; Johnson, Hatcher, et al., 2007). The increasing use of advanced practice nurses in collaborative practice with physicians can help improve the availability and accessibility of prenatal care. A regular schedule of home visiting by nurses during pregnancy has also proven effective (Dawley & Beam, 2005).

The current model for provision of prenatal care has been used for more than a century. The initial visit usually occurs in the first trimester, with visits every four weeks through week 28 of pregnancy. Thereafter, visits are scheduled every 2 weeks until week 36 and then every week until birth (American Academy of Pediatrics and American College of Obstetricians and Gynecologists [2007])

BOX 7-3

Prenatal Visit Schedule

TRADITIONAL*	CENTERINGPREGNANCY®†
First visit within the first trimester (12 weeks)	First visit within the first trimester (12 weeks)
Every 4 weeks from week 16-28	Every 4 weeks—week 16-28
Every two weeks from week 29-36	Every 2 weeks—week 29-40
Weekly visits week 36 to birth	

*Frequency of visits may be decreased in low risk women and increased in women with high risk pregnancies.
†Additional individual visits may be added as needed.

(Box 7-3). Research supports a model of fewer prenatal visits, and in some practices there is a growing tendency to have fewer visits with women who are at low risk for complications (Villar, Carroli, Khan-Neelofur, Piaggio, & Gulmezoglu, 2001; Walker, McCully, & Vest, 2001).

CenteringPregnancy® is a care model that is gaining in popularity. This model is one of group prenatal care in which authority is shifted from the provider to the woman and other women who have similar due dates. The model creates an atmosphere that facilitates learning, encourages discussion, and develops mutual support. Most care takes place in the group setting after the first visit and continues for 10 2-hour sessions scheduled throughout the pregnancy (Moos, 2006) (see Box 7-3). At each meeting the first 30 minutes is spent in completing assessments (by self and by provider), and the rest of the time is spent in group discussion of specific issues such as discomforts of pregnancy and preparation for labor and birth. Families and partners are encourage to participate (Massey, Rising, & Ickovics, 2006; Reid, 2007).

Prenatal care is ideally a multidisciplinary activity in which nurses work with physicians or midwives, nutritionists, social workers, and others. Collaboration among these individuals is necessary to provide holistic care. The case management model, which makes use of care maps and critical pathways, is one system that promotes comprehensive care with limited overlap in services. To emphasize the nursing role, care management for the initial visit and follow-up visits is organized around the central elements of the nursing process: assessment, nursing diagnoses, expected outcomes, plan of care and interventions, and evaluation (see Nursing Process box).

Initial Assessment

The initial evaluation includes a comprehensive health history emphasizing the current pregnancy, previous pregnancies, the family, a psychosocial profile, a physical assessment, diagnostic testing, and an overall risk assessment. A prenatal history form (paper or electronic) is often used to document information obtained. The pregnant woman and family members who may accompany the woman for her care need to know that the first prenatal visit is more lengthy and detailed than future visits. In some clinics and offices, women may have the diagnostic tests done first and have the prenatal history and physical examination at the next visit.

Interview

The therapeutic relationship between the nurse and the woman is established during the initial assessment interview. Two types of data are collected: the woman's subjective appraisal of her health status and the nurse's objective observations.

One or more family members will often accompany the pregnant woman. With her permission, include those accompanying the woman in the initial prenatal interview. The observations and information about the woman's family are then included in the database. For example, if the woman has small children with her the nurse can ask about her plans for child care during the time of labor and birth. Note any special needs at this time (e.g., wheelchair access, assistance in getting on and off the examining table, and cognitive deficits).

Reason for seeking care

Although pregnant women are scheduled for "routine" prenatal visits, they often come to the health care provider seeking information or reassurance about a particular concern. The woman's chief concerns are recorded in her own words; this helps other personnel identify the priority of needs as identified by the woman. At the initial visit the desire for information about what is normal in the course of pregnancy is typical.

Current pregnancy

The presumptive signs of pregnancy may be of great concern to the woman. A review of symptoms she is experiencing and how she is coping with them helps to establish a database to develop a plan of care. The nurse can provide some early teaching at this time.

Obstetric and gynecologic history

Data are gathered on the woman's age at menarche, menstrual history, and contraceptive history; the nature of any infertility or gynecologic conditions; her history of any sexually transmitted infections (STIs); her sexual history; and a detailed history of all her pregnancies, including the present pregnancy, and their outcomes. Note the date of the last Papanicolaou (Pap) test and the result. Obtain the date of her LMP to establish the EDB.

Medical history

The medical history includes specific medical or surgical conditions that may affect the pregnancy or that may be affected by the pregnancy. For example, a pregnant

NURSING PROCESS *Prenatal Care*

ASSESSMENT

The assessment process begins at the initial prenatal visit and continues throughout the pregnancy. Assessment techniques include the interview, physical examination, and laboratory tests. Because the initial visit and follow-up visits are distinctly different in content and process, they are described separately (see text).

NURSING DIAGNOSES

The following are examples of the nursing diagnoses that may be appropriate in the prenatal period:

- *Anxiety* related to:
  - Physical discomforts of pregnancy
  - Ambivalent and labile emotions
  - Changes in family dynamics
  - Fetal well-being
  - Ability to manage anticipated labor
- *Constipation* related to:
  - Progesterone relaxation of gastrointestinal smooth muscle
  - Dietary behaviors
- *Imbalanced nutrition: less than body requirements* related to:
  - Morning sickness (nausea and vomiting)
  - Fatigue
- *Disturbed body image* related to:
  - Anatomic and physiologic changes of pregnancy
  - Changes in the couple relationship
- *Disturbed sleep patterns* related to:
  - Discomforts of late pregnancy
  - Anxiety about approaching labor

EXPECTED OUTCOMES OF CARE

Measured outcomes of prenatal care include not only physical outcomes, but also developmental and psychosocial outcomes. Examples of expected outcomes are that the pregnant woman will achieve the following:

- Verbalize decreased anxiety about the health of her fetus and herself.
- Verbalize improved family dynamics.
- Show appropriate weight gain patterns per trimester.
- Report increasing acceptance of changes in body image.
- Demonstrate knowledge for self-management.
- Seek clarification of information about pregnancy and birth.
- Report signs and symptoms of complications.
- Describe appropriate measures taken to relieve physical discomforts.
- Develop a realistic birth plan.

PLAN OF CARE AND INTERVENTIONS

A variety of educational materials are available to enhance the learning of the pregnant woman and her family. The following four topics are discussed in detail in the text (see detailed discussion starting on p. 208).

- Education about maternal and fetal changes
- Education for self-management
- Sexual counseling
- Psychosocial support

EVALUATION

Evaluation of the effectiveness of care of the woman during pregnancy is based on the previously stated outcomes (see Nursing Care Plan on pp. 222 and 223).

woman who has diabetes, hypertension, or epilepsy requires special care. Because most women are anxious during the initial interview, pay attention to cues, such as a MedicAlert bracelet, and prompt the woman to explain allergies, chronic diseases, or medications being taken (e.g., cortisone, insulin, anticonvulsants).

The woman should also describe the nature of previous surgical procedures. If a woman has undergone uterine surgery or extensive repair of the pelvic floor, then a cesarean birth may be necessary; appendectomy rules out appendicitis as a cause of right lower quadrant pain in pregnancy; and spinal surgery may contraindicate the use of spinal or epidural anesthesia. Note any injury involving the pelvis.

Women who have chronic or handicapping conditions often forget to mention them during the initial assessment because they have become so adapted to them. Special shoes or a limp may indicate the existence of a pelvic structural defect, which is an important consideration in pregnant women. The nurse who observes these special characteristics and inquires about them sensitively can obtain individualized data that will provide the basis for a comprehensive nursing care plan (Smeltzer, 2007).

Nutritional history

The woman's nutritional history is an important component of the prenatal history because her nutritional status has a direct effect on the growth and development of the fetus. A dietary assessment will reveal special diet practices, food allergies, eating behaviors, the practice of pica, and other factors related to her nutritional status. Pregnant women are usually motivated to learn about good nutrition and respond well to nutritional advice generated by this assessment. (See Chapter 8 for further discussion.)

History of drug and herbal preparations use

A woman's past and present use of legal (over-the-counter [OTC] and prescription medications, herbal preparations, caffeine, alcohol, nicotine) and illegal (marijuana, cocaine, heroin) drugs is assessed. This assessment is needed because many substances cross the placenta and may harm the developing fetus. Periodic urine toxicologic screening tests are often recommended during the pregnancies of women who have a history of illegal drug use. In some states of the United States, these test results have been used for criminal prosecution, which violates the patient-provider relationship and ethical responsibilities to the patient (Harris & Paltrow, 2003). To preserve constitutional rights and the ethical patient-provider relationship, drug-testing policies should encourage open communication between patient and physician, emphasize the availability of treatment options, and advocate for the health of woman and child.

LEGAL TIP **Informed Consent for Drug Testing**

Hospitals must obtain informed consent from a pregnant woman before she can be tested for drug use (Kehringer, 2003).

Family history

The family history provides information about the woman's immediate family, including her parents, siblings, and children. Information about the immediate family of the father of the baby is also important. These data help identify familial or genetic disorders or conditions that could affect the present health status of the woman or her fetus.

Social, experiential, and occupational history

Situational factors such as the family's ethnic and cultural background and socioeconomic status can be assessed over several encounters. Explore the woman's perception of this pregnancy by asking her questions such as the following:

- Is this pregnancy planned or not, wanted or not?
- Is the woman pleased, displeased, accepting, or nonaccepting?
- What problems related to finances, career, or living accommodations will occur as a result of the pregnancy?

Determine the family support system by asking:

- What primary support is available to her?
- Are changes needed to promote adequate support?
- What are the existing relationships among the mother, father or partner, siblings, and in-laws?
- What preparations is she making for her care and that of dependent family members during labor and for the care of the infant after birth?
- Does she need financial, educational, or other support from the community?
- What are the woman's ideas about childbearing, her expectations of the infant's behavior, and her outlook on life and the female role?

Other such questions to ask include the following:

- What does the woman think it will be like to have a baby in the home?
- How is her life going to change by having a baby?
- What plans does having a baby interrupt?

During interviews throughout the pregnancy the nurse should remain alert to the appearance of potential parenting problems, such as depression, lack of family support, and inadequate living conditions. The nurse needs to assess the woman's attitude toward health care, particularly during childbearing, her expectations of health care providers, and her view of the relationship between herself and the nurse.

Coping mechanisms and patterns of interacting are identified. Early in the pregnancy the nurse should determine the woman's knowledge of pregnancy, maternal changes, fetal growth, self-management, and care of the newborn, including feeding. Asking about attitudes toward unmedicated or medicated childbirth and about her knowledge of the availability of parenting skills classes is important. Before planning for nursing care the nurse needs information about the woman's decision-making abilities and living habits (e.g., exercise, sleep, diet, diversional interests, personal hygiene, clothing). Common stressors during childbearing include the baby's welfare, labor and birth process, behaviors of the newborn, the woman's relationship with the baby's father and her family, changes in body image, and physical symptoms.

Explore attitudes concerning the range of acceptable sexual behavior during pregnancy by asking questions such as the following: What has your family (partner, friends) told you about sex during pregnancy? Give more emphasis to the woman's sexual self-concept by asking questions such as the following: How do you feel about the changes in your appearance? How does your partner feel about your body now? How do you feel about wearing maternity clothes?

History of physical abuse

All women should be assessed for a history or risk of physical abuse, particularly because the likelihood of abuse increases during pregnancy. Although a woman's appearance or behavior may suggest the possibility of abuse, do not limit questioning to only those women who fit the supposed profile of the battered woman. Identification of abuse and immediate clinical intervention that includes information about safety will help prevent future abuse and increase the safety and well-being of the woman and her infant (Krieger, 2008) (see Fig. 2-11).

During pregnancy the target body parts change during abusive episodes. Women report physical blows directed to the head, breasts, abdomen, and genitalia. Sexual assault is common.

Battering and pregnancy in teenagers constitute a particularly difficult situation. Some adolescents are trapped in the abusive relationship because of their inexperience.

Many professionals and the adolescents themselves ignore the violence because it may not be believable, because relationships are transient, and because the jealous and controlling behavior is interpreted as love and devotion. Routine screening for abuse and sexual assault is recommended for pregnant adolescents. (Family Violence Prevention Fund, 2009). Because pregnancy in young adolescent girls is commonly the result of sexual abuse, assess the desire to maintain the pregnancy.

Review of systems

During this portion of the interview, ask the woman to identify and describe preexisting or concurrent problems in any of the body systems. Assess her mental status as well. Question the woman about physical symptoms she has experienced, such as shortness of breath or pain. Pregnancy affects and is affected by all body systems; therefore information on the present status of the body systems is important in planning care. For each sign or symptom described, obtain the following additional data: body location, quality, quantity, chronology, aggravating or alleviating factors, and associated manifestations (onset, character, course) (Seidel, Ball, Dains, & Benedict, 2006).

Physical examination

The initial physical examination provides the baseline for assessing subsequent changes. The examiner should determine the woman's needs for basic information regarding reproductive anatomy and provide this information, along with a demonstration of the equipment that may be used and an explanation of the procedure itself. The interaction requires an unhurried, sensitive, and gentle approach with a straightforward attitude.

The physical examination begins with assessment of vital signs, including height and weight (for calculation of body mass index [BMI]) and blood pressure (BP). The bladder should be empty before pelvic examination. A urine specimen may be obtained to test for protein, glucose, or leukocytes or for other urine tests.

Each examiner develops a routine for proceeding with the physical examination; most choose the head-to-toe progression. The examiner evaluates heart and lung sounds, and examines extremities. Distribution, amount, and quality of body hair are of particular importance because the findings reflect nutritional status, endocrine function, and attention to hygiene. The examiner assesses the thyroid gland thoroughly. The height of the fundus is noted if the first examination is performed after the first trimester of pregnancy. During the examination the examiner needs to remain alert to cues that indicate a potential threatening condition, such as supine hypotension–low BP that occurs while the woman is lying on her back, causing feelings of faintness. See Chapter 2 for a detailed description of the physical examination.

Whenever a pelvic examination is performed, the examiner assesses the tone of the pelvic musculature and the woman's knowledge of Kegel exercises. Particular attention is paid to the size of the uterus because this assessment provides useful information on gestational age. One vaginal examination during early pregnancy is recommended, but another is usually not performed unless medically indicated.

Assessment Video: Chest Wall

Assessment Video: Breast

Assessment Video: Prenatal Interview

Spanish Guidelines: Prenatal Interview

Laboratory tests

The laboratory data yielded by the analysis of the specimens obtained during the examination provide important information concerning the symptoms of pregnancy and the woman's health status.

Specimens are collected at the initial visit so that the cause of any abnormal findings can be treated. Blood is drawn for a variety of tests (Table 7-1). A sickle cell screen is recommended for women of African, Asian, or Middle Eastern descent, and testing for antibody to the human immunodeficiency virus (HIV) is strongly recommended for all pregnant women (Box 7-4). In addition, pregnant women and fathers with a family history of cystic fibrosis and of Caucasian ethnicity may want to have blood drawn for testing to determine if they are a cystic fibrosis carrier (Fries, Bashford, & Nunes (2005). Urine specimens are usually tested by dipstick; culture and sensitivity tests are ordered as necessary. During the pelvic examination, cervical and vaginal smears may be obtained for cytologic studies and for diagnosis of infection (e.g., *Chlamydia*, gonorrhea, group B *Streptococcus* [GBS]).

The finding of risk factors during pregnancy may indicate the need to repeat some tests at other times. For example, exposure to tuberculosis or an STI would necessitate repeat testing. STIs are common in pregnancy and may have negative effects on mother and fetus. Thorough assessment and screening are essential.

Follow-Up Visits

In traditional prenatal care, monthly visits are scheduled routinely during the first and second trimesters, although patients can make additional appointments as the need arises. During the third trimester, however, the possibility for complications increases, and closer monitoring is necessary. Starting with week 28, maternity visits are scheduled every 2 weeks until week 36 and then every week until birth, unless the health care provider individualizes the schedule. Visits can occur more or less frequently, often depending on individual needs, complications, and risks of the pregnant woman. The pattern of interviewing the woman first and then assessing physical changes and performing laboratory tests continues.

In prenatal care models that use a reduced frequency screening schedule or in CenteringPregnancy®, the timing of follow-up visits will be different, but assessments and care will be similar.

Interview

Follow-up visits are less intensive than the initial prenatal visit. At each of these follow-up visits, ask the woman

TABLE 7-1

Recommended Laboratory Tests in Prenatal Period

LABORATORY TEST	PURPOSE
Hemoglobin, hematocrit, WBC, differential	Detects anemia; detects infection
Hemoglobin electrophoresis	Identifies women with hemoglobinopathies (e.g., sickle cell anemia, thalassemia)
Blood type, Rh, and irregular antibody	Identifies fetuses at risk for developing erythroblastosis fetalis or hyperbilirubinemia in neonatal period
Rubella titer	Determines immunity to rubella
Tuberculin skin testing; chest film after 20 weeks of gestation in women with reactive tuberculin tests	Screens for exposure to tuberculosis
Urinalysis, including microscopic examination of urinary sediment; pH, specific gravity, color, glucose, albumin, protein, RBCs, WBCs, casts, acetone; hCG	Identifies women with unsuspected diabetes mellitus, renal disease, hypertensive disease of pregnancy, infection, occult hematuria
Urine culture	Identifies women with asymptomatic bacteriuria
Renal function tests: BUN, creatinine, electrolytes, creatinine clearance, total protein excretion	Evaluates level of possible renal compromise in women with a history of diabetes, hypertension, or renal disease
Pap test	Screens for cervical intraepithelial neoplasia, herpes simplex type 2, and HPV
Vaginal or rectal smear for *Neisseria gonorrhoeae, Chlamydia,* HPV, GBS	Screens high risk population for asymptomatic infection; GBS test performed at 35-37 weeks
RPR, VDRL, or FTA-ABS	Identifies women with untreated syphilis
HIV antibody, hepatitis B surface antigen, toxoplasmosis	Screen for infections
MSAFP/Quad Screen	Screen for Down syndrome, NTDs; performed at 15 to 20 weeks
1-hr glucose tolerance	Screens for gestational diabetes; performed at initial visit for women with risk factors; performed at 24-28 weeks for all pregnant women who are not already known to be diabetic
3-hr glucose tolerance	Screens for diabetes in women with elevated glucose level after 1-hr test; must have two elevated readings for diagnosis of gestational diabetes
Cardiac evaluation: ECG, chest x-ray film, and echocardiogram	Evaluates cardiac function in women with a history of hypertension or cardiac disease

BUN, Blood urea nitrogen; *ECG,* electrocardiogram; *FTA-ABS,* fluorescent treponemal antibody absorption test; *GBS,* group B *Streptococcus; hCG,* human chorionic gonadotropin; *HIV,* human immunodeficiency virus; *HPV,* human papillomavirus; *NTD,* neural tube defects; *RBC,* red blood cell; *RPR,* rapid plasma reagin; *VDRL,* Venereal Disease Research Laboratory; *WBC,* white blood cell.

BOX 7-4

HIV Screening

- Pregnant women are ethically obligated to seek reasonable care during pregnancy and to avoid causing harm to the fetus. Women's health nurses should be advocates for the fetus while accepting of the pregnant woman's decision regarding testing and/or treatment for HIV.
- The incidence of perinatal transmission from an HIV-positive mother to her fetus ranges from 16% to 25%. Triple drug antiviral or highly active antiretroviral therapy (HAART) during pregnancy decreases perinatal transmission to as low as 1% to 2% (Burr, 2011).
- The CDC (2010) recommends testing for HIV infections for all pregnant women as early as possible in pregnancy and a second test in the third trimester, ideally before 36 weeks. This is especially important for women known to be at high risk for HIV infection.
- Testing has the potential to identify HIV-positive women who can then be treated. Health care providers have an obligation to ensure that pregnant women are well informed about HIV symptoms, testing, and methods of decreasing maternal-fetal transmission. The Centers for Disease Control and Prevention (CDC) and the American College of Obstetricians and Gynecologists (ACOG) recommend universal opt-out screening, which means that all pregnant women are offered HIV screening but have the opportunity to opt out if desired (ACOG Committee on Obstetric Practice, 2011; CDC, 2010). The Association of Women's Health, Obstetric and Neonatal Nurses (AWHONN, 2008) supports this system of HIV screening that allows all pregnant women to be offered screening.

Data from American College of Obstetricians and Gynecologists Committee on Obstetric Practice: Committee Opinion No. 418. (2011). Prenatal and perinatal human immunodeficiency virus testing—expanded recommendations. *Obstetrics and Gynecology,* 104(5 Part 1),1119-1124; AWHONN. (2008). *HIV screening procedures for pregnant women and newborns—policy position statement,* Washington: DC; Burr, C. (2011). Reducing maternal-infant HIV transmission. In S. Coffey (Ed.). *Guide for HIV/AIDS clinical care.* Rockville: MD; U.S. Department of Health and Human Services, Health Resources and Services Administration, http://hab. hrsa.gov/deliverhivaidscare/clinicalguide11/cg-402_pmtct.html; Centers for Disease Control and Prevention. (2010). Sexually transmitted diseases treatment guidelines. *MMWR Morbidity and Mortality Weekly Report 59*(RR12), 1-110.

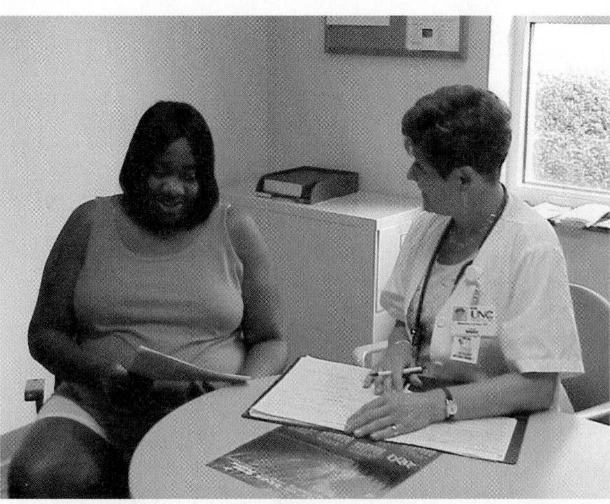

Fig. 7-6 Prenatal interview. (Courtesy Dee Lowdermilk, Chapel Hill, NC.)

EMERGENCY

Supine Hypotension

SIGNS AND SYMPTOMS

- Pallor
- Dizziness, faintness, breathlessness
- Tachycardia
- Nausea
- Clammy (damp, cool) skin; sweating

INTERVENTIONS

- Position woman on her side until her signs and symptoms subside and vital signs stabilize within normal limits (WNL).

Spanish Guidelines: Prenatal Interview

to summarize relevant events that have occurred since the previous visit (Fig. 7-6). Also inquire about her general emotional and physiologic well-being, complaints or problems, and questions she may have. Identify and explore any personal and family needs.

Emotional changes are common during pregnancy, and therefore asking whether the woman has experienced any mood swings, reactions to changes in her body image, bad dreams, or worries is reasonable. Note any positive feelings (her own and those of her family). Record the reactions of family members to the pregnancy and the woman's emotional changes.

During the third trimester, assess current family situations and their effect on the woman. For example, assess siblings' and grandparents' responses to the pregnancy and the coming child. In addition, make the following assessments of the woman and her family: warning signs of emergencies, signs of preterm and term labor, the labor process and concerns about labor, and fetal development and methods to assess fetal well-being. The nurse should ask if the woman is planning to attend childbirth preparation classes and what she knows about pain management during labor.

Spanish Guidelines: Prenatal Physical Examination

A review of the woman's physical systems is appropriate at each prenatal visit, and any suspicious signs or symptoms are assessed in depth. Identify any discomforts reflecting adaptations to pregnancy.

Physical examination

Reevaluation is a constant aspect of a pregnant woman's care. Each woman reacts differently to pregnancy. As a result, careful monitoring of the pregnancy and her reactions to care is vital. The database is updated at each time of contact with the pregnant woman. Physiologic changes are documented as the pregnancy progresses and reviewed for possible deviations from normal progress.

At each visit, physical parameters are measured. Ideally the BP is taken by using the same arm at every visit, with the woman sitting, using a cuff of appropriate size (which is noted on her chart). Her weight is assessed, and the appropriateness of the gestational weight gain is evaluated in relationship to her BMI. Urine may be checked by dipstick, and the presence and degree of edema are noted. For examination of the abdomen, the woman lies on her back with her arms by her side and head supported by a pillow. The bladder should be empty. First an abdominal inspection is performed, followed by a measurement of the height of the fundus. While the woman lies on her back, be alert for the occurrence of supine hypotension (see Emergency box). When a woman is lying in this position, the weight of abdominal contents may compress the vena cava and aorta, causing a decrease in BP and a feeling of faintness.

The findings revealed during the interview and physical examination reflect the status of maternal adaptations. When any of the findings is suspicious, perform an in-depth examination. For example, careful interpretation of BP is important in the risk factor analysis of all pregnant women. BP is evaluated based on absolute values and the length of gestation and is interpreted in consideration of modifying factors.

NURSING ALERT Individuals whose systolic BP (SBP) is 120 to 139 mm Hg or whose diastolic BP (DBP) is 80 to 89 mm Hg are considered prehypertensive. To prevent cardiovascular disease, they require health-promoting lifestyle modifications (National High Blood Pressure Education Program, 2003).

An absolute SBP of 140 to 159 mm Hg and a DBP of 90 to 99 mm Hg suggests the presence of stage 1 hypertension. An SBP at or above 160 mm Hg or a DBP at or above 100 mm Hg is indicative of stage 2 hypertension (National High Blood Pressure Education Program, 2003). See Chapter 21 for an in-depth discussion of problems associated with hypertension.

Monitor the pregnant woman at each visit for a range of signs and symptoms that indicate potential complications in addition to hypertension (see Signs of Potential Complications box).

signs of POTENTIAL COMPLICATIONS

First, Second, and Third Trimesters

Signs and Symptoms	Possible Causes
FIRST TRIMESTER	
Severe vomiting	Hyperemesis gravidarum
Chills, fever	Infection
Burning on urination	Infection
Diarrhea	Infection
Abdominal cramping; vaginal bleeding	Miscarriage, ectopic pregnancy
SECOND AND THIRD TRIMESTERS	
Persistent, severe vomiting	Hyperemesis gravidarum, hypertension, preeclampsia
Sudden discharge of fluid from vagina before 37 wk	Premature rupture of membranes (PROM)
Vaginal bleeding, severe abdominal pain	Miscarriage, placenta previa, abruptio placentae
Chills, fever, burning on urination, diarrhea	Infection
Severe backache or flank pain	Kidney infection or stones; preterm labor
Change in fetal movements: absence of fetal movements after quickening, any unusual change in pattern or amount	Fetal jeopardy or intrauterine fetal death
Uterine contractions; pressure; cramping before 37 wk	Preterm labor
Visual disturbances: blurring, double vision, or spots	Hypertensive conditions, preeclampsia
Swelling of face or fingers and over sacrum	Hypertensive conditions, preeclampsia
Headaches: severe, frequent, or continuous	Hypertensive conditions, preeclampsia
Muscular irritability or convulsions	Hypertensive conditions, eclampsia
Epigastric or abdominal pain (perceived as severe stomachache, heartburn)	Hypertensive conditions, preeclampsia, abruptio placentae
Glycosuria, positive glucose tolerance test reaction	Gestational diabetes mellitus

Fetal assessment

Toward the end of the first trimester, before the uterus is an abdominal organ, the fetal heart tones (FHTs) are audible with an ultrasound fetoscope or an ultrasound stethoscope. To hear the FHTs, place the instrument in the midline, just above the symphysis pubis, and apply firm pressure. Offer the woman and her family the opportunity to listen to the FHTs (see Fig. 7-8, *A*) Assess the health status of the fetus at each visit for the remainder of the pregnancy.

Fundal height

During the second trimester, the uterus becomes an abdominal organ. The fundal height, measurement of the height of the uterus above the symphysis pubis, is one indicator of fetal growth. The measurement also provides a gross estimate of the duration of pregnancy. From approximately gestational weeks (GWs) 18 to 32, the height of the fundus in centimeters is approximately the same as the number of weeks of gestation (±2 GWs), with an empty bladder at the time of measurement (Cunningham, Leveno, Bloom, Hauth, Gilstrap, & Wenstrom, 2005). For example, a woman of 28 GWs, with an empty bladder would measure from 26 to 30 cm. In addition, fundal height measurement may aid in the identification of high risk factors. A stable or decreased fundal height may indicate the presence of intrauterine growth restriction (IUGR); an excessive increase could indicate the presence of multifetal gestation (more than one fetus) or hydramnios.

Typically a paper tape is used to measure fundal height. To increase the reliability of the measurement the same person examines the pregnant woman at each of her prenatal visits, but this is often not possible. All clinicians who examine a particular pregnant woman should be consistent in their measurement technique. Ideally, an established method should be used for the health care setting in which the measurement technique is explicitly set forth, and the woman's position on the examining table, the measuring device, and method of measurement used are specified. Also describe conditions under which the measurements are taken in the woman's records, including whether the bladder was empty and whether the uterus was relaxed or contracted at the time of measurement.

Various positions for measuring fundal height have been described. The woman can be supine, have her head elevated, have her knees flexed, or have both her head elevated and knees flexed. Measurements obtained with the woman in the various positions differ, making the task of standardizing the fundal height measurement technique even more important.

Placement of the tape measure also can vary. The tape can be placed in the middle of the woman's abdomen and the measurement made from the upper border of the symphysis pubis to the upper border of the fundus with the tape measure held in contact with the skin for the

Assessment Video: Fetal Heart Rate

Assessment Video: Abdomen/Fundal Height

entire length of the uterus (Fig. 7-7, *A*). In another measurement technique the upper curve of the fundus is not included in the measurement. Instead, hold one end of the tape measure at the upper border of the symphysis pubis with one hand, and place the other hand at the upper border of the fundus. The tape is placed between the middle and index fingers of the other hand, and the point where these fingers intercept the tape measure is taken as the measurement (Fig. 7-7, *B*).

Gestational age

In an uncomplicated pregnancy, fetal gestational age is estimated after determining the duration of pregnancy and the EDB. Fetal gestational age is determined from the menstrual history, contraceptive history, pregnancy test result, and the following findings obtained during the clinical evaluation:

- First uterine evaluation: date, size
- Fetal heart (FH) first heard: date, method (Doppler stethoscope, fetoscope)
- Date of quickening
- Current fundal height, estimated fetal weight (EFW)
- Current week of gestation by history of LMP or ultrasound examination or both
- Ultrasound examination: date, week of gestation, biparietal diameter (BPD)
- Reliability of dates

Quickening ("feeling of life") refers to the mother's first perception of fetal movement. It usually occurs between weeks 16 and 20 of gestation and is initially experienced as a fluttering sensation. Record the mother's report. Multiparas often perceive fetal movement earlier than primigravidas.

Routine use of ultrasound examination (also called a *sonogram*) in early pregnancy has been recommended, and many health care providers have this equipment available in the office. This procedure may be used to establish the duration of pregnancy if the woman cannot give a precise date for her LMP or if the size of the uterus does not conform to the EDB as calculated by Nägele's rule. Ultrasound also provides information about the well-being of the fetus (see Chapter 19 for further discussion).

Health status

The assessment of fetal health status includes consideration of fetal movement. The nurse instructs the mother to note the extent and timing of fetal movements and to report immediately if the pattern changes or if movement ceases. Regular movement has been found to be a reliable indicator of fetal health (Cunningham et al., 2005). There are numerous methods for assessing fetal movement. One method is for the woman to count fetal movements after a meal. Four or more kick counts in an hour is reassuring. See Chapter 19 for further discussion.

Once the FHR is audible, it is checked on routine visits (Fig. 7-8). Early in the second trimester the heartbeat may be heard with the Doppler stethoscope (Fig. 7-8, *B*). To detect the heartbeat before the fetus can be palpated by Leopold maneuvers (see procedure, p. 347), move the scope around the abdomen until the heartbeat is heard. Each nurse develops a set pattern for searching the abdomen for the heartbeat–for example, starting first in the midline approximately 2 to 3 cm above the symphysis, then moving to the left lower quadrant, and so on. You count the heartbeat for 1 minute and note the quality and rhythm. Later in the second trimester, you can determine the FHR with the fetoscope or Pinard fetoscope (Fig. 7-8, *A* and *C*). A normal rate and rhythm are other good indicators of fetal health. Once the heartbeat is heard, its absence is cause for immediate investigation.

Investigate fetal health status intensively if any maternal or fetal complications arise (e.g., gestational hypertension, IUGR, premature rupture of membranes [PROM], irregular or absent FHR, absence of fetal movements after quickening). Careful, precise, and concise recording of patient responses and laboratory results contributes to the

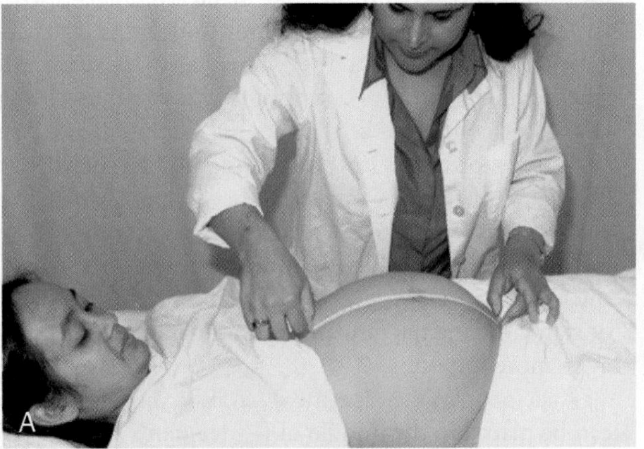

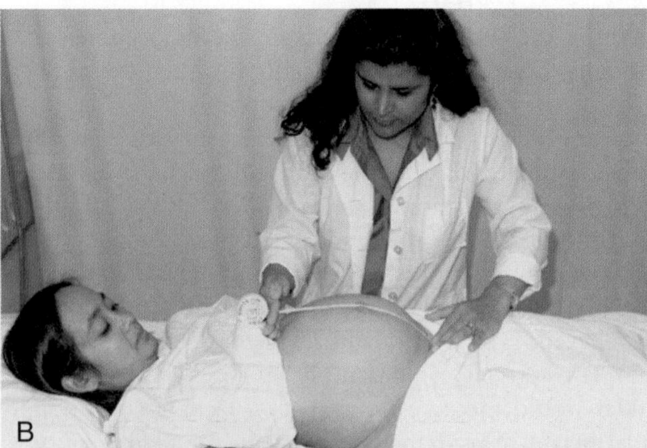

Fig. 7-7 Measurement of fundal height from symphysis that **(A)** includes the upper curve of the fundus and **(B)** does not include the upper curve of the fundus. Note position of hands and measuring tape. (Courtesy Chris Rozales, San Francisco, CA.)

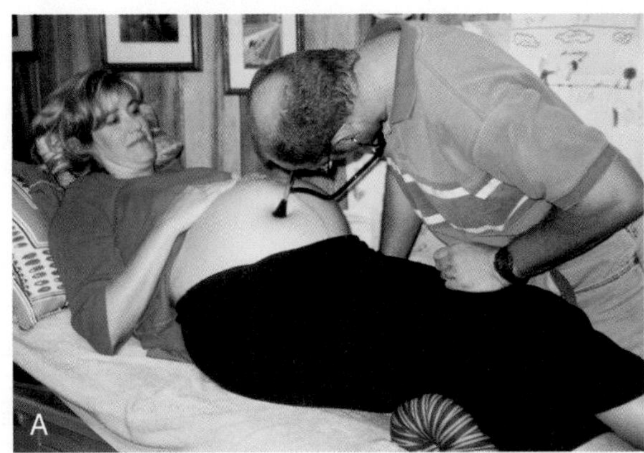

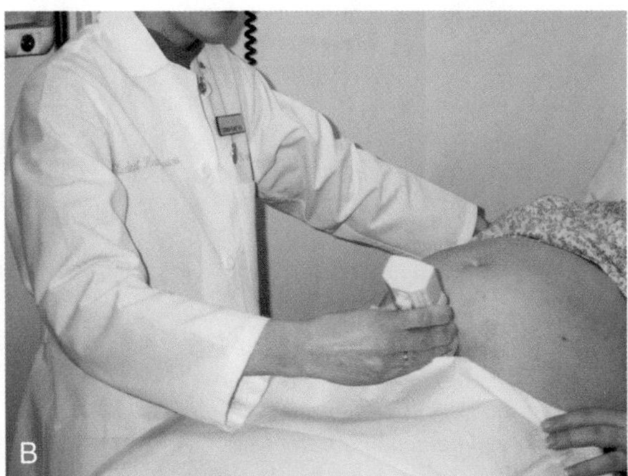

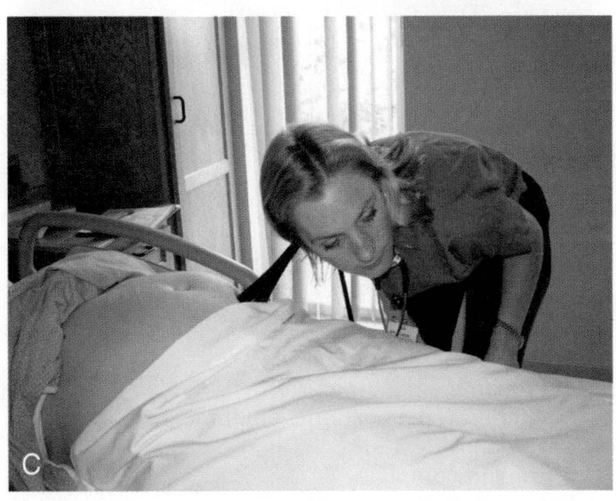

Fig. 7-8 Detecting fetal heart rate. **A,** Father can listen to the fetal heart with a fetoscope (first detectable around 18 to 20 weeks). **B,** Doppler ultrasound stethoscope (fetal heartbeat detectable at 12 weeks). **C,** Pinard fetoscope. Note: Hands should not touch fetoscope while listening. (**A,** Courtesy Shannon Perry, Phoenix, AZ. **B,** Courtesy Dee Lowdermilk, Chapel Hill, NC. **C,** Courtesy Julie Perry Nelson, Loveland, CO.)

continuous supervision vital to ensuring the well-being of the mother and fetus.

Laboratory tests

The number of routine laboratory tests performed during follow-up visits in pregnancy is limited for the low-risk pregnant woman. A clean-catch urine specimen may be obtained to test for glucose, protein, nitrites, and leukocytes at each visit; however, urine dips for glycosuria and proteinuria are not supported by evidence (Alto, 2005). Urine specimens for culture and sensitivity, as well as blood samples, are obtained only if signs and symptoms warrant.

First-trimester screening for chromosomal abnormalities is offered as a option between 11 and 14 weeks. This multiple marker screen includes sonographic evaluation of nuchal translucency (NT) and biochemical markers–pregnancy-associated placental protein (PAPP-A) and free beta-human chorionic gonadotrophin (β-hCG).

The maternal serum alpha-fetoprotein (MSAFP) screening or quadruple screening (MSAFP, hCG, unconjugated estriol, and inhibin-A) is recommended between 15 and 20 weeks of gestation, ideally between 16 and 18 weeks. These tests screen for neural tube defects, Down syndrome, and other chromosomal abnormalities. Abnormal levels are followed by ultrasonography for more in-depth investigation (Johnson, Gregory, & Niebyl, 2007). See Chapter 19 for further discussion. A glucose challenge is usually performed between 24 and 28 weeks of gestation. GBS testing is performed between 35 and 37 weeks of gestation; cultures collected earlier will not accurately predict GBS status at time of birth (Himmelberger, 2002).

Other diagnostic tests are available to assess the health status of both the pregnant woman and the fetus. Ultrasonography, for example, helps determine the status of the pregnancy and confirm gestational age of the fetus. Amniocentesis, a procedure used to obtain amniotic fluid for analysis, is necessary to evaluate the fetus for genetic disorders or gestational maturity. Chapter 19 describes these and other tests that determine health risks for the mother and infant.

Collaborative Care

Care Paths

Because a large number of health care professionals are often involved in care of the expectant mother, unintentional gaps or overlaps in care may occur. Care paths help improve the consistency of care and reduce costs. Although the Care Path on p. 208 focuses only on prenatal education, it is one example of the type of form developed to guide health care providers in carrying out the appropriate assess-

CARE PATH Prenatal Care Pathway

PRENATAL EDUCATION CLINICAL PATHWAY

INITIAL VISIT AND ORIENTATION: ______ SOCIAL SERVICE: ______ DIETITIAN: ______

I. EARLY PREGNANCY (WEEKS 1-20) (INITIAL AND DATE AFTER EDUCATION GIVEN)

Fetal growth and development ______
Maternal changes ______
Lifestyle:
- Exercise/stress/nutrition ______
  - Drugs, OTC, tobacco, alcohol ______
  - STIs ______
- Psychologic/social adjustments:
  - FOB involved/accepts baby for adoption ______

Testing: Labs____ Ultrasound: _____
Possible complications:
- a. Threatened miscarriage ______
- b. Diabetes ______
- c. ______ ______

Introduction to breastfeeding ______
Acceptance of pregnancy and childbirth preparation ______
Dietary follow-up ______

II. MIDPREGNANCY (WEEKS 21-27) (INITIAL AND DATE AFTER EDUCATION GIVEN)

Fetal growth and development ______
Maternal changes ______
Daily fetal movement ______
Possible complications:
- a. Preterm labor prevention ______
- b. Preeclampsia symptoms ______
- c. ______ ______

Breastfeeding or bottle feeding ______
Birth plan initiated ______
Childbirth preparation ______
Dietary follow-up ______

III. LATE PREGNANCY (WEEKS 28-40) (INITIAL AND DATE AFTER EDUCATION GIVEN)

Fetal growth and development ______
Fetal evaluation:
- Daily movement______ NSTs ____
- Kick counts______ BPPs____

Maternal changes ______
Possible complications:
- a. Preterm labor prevention ______
- b. Preeclampsia symptoms ______
- c. ______ ______

Breastfeeding preparation:
- Nipple assessment ______
- Dietary follow-up ______

Childbirth preparation:
- S/S of labor; labor process ______
- Pain management: natural childbirth, medications, epidural ______
- Cesarean; VBAC ______
- Birth plan complete ______
- Review hospital policies ______

Parenting preparation:
- Pediatrician ______ Childcare ______
- Siblings ______ Immunizations ___
- Car seat/safety ______

Postpartum
- PP care and checkup ______
- Emotional changes ______
- BC options ______
- Safer sex and STIs ______

Signature: ______

BC, Birth control; *BPP*, biophysical profile; *FOB*, father of baby; *NST*, nonstress test; *OTC*, over the counter; *PP*, postpartum; *S/S*, signs and symptoms; *STI*, sexually transmitted infection; *VBAC*, vaginal birth after cesarean.

ments and interventions in a timely way. Use of care paths also may contribute to improved satisfaction of families with the prenatal care provided, and members of the health care team may function more efficiently and effectively.

Education about maternal and fetal changes

Expectant parents are typically curious about the growth and development of the fetus and the subsequent changes that occur in the mother's body. Mothers in particular are sometimes more tolerant of the discomforts related to the continuing pregnancy if they understand the underlying causes. Educational literature that describes the fetal and maternal changes is available and can be used in explaining changes as they occur. The nurse's familiarity with any material shared with pregnant families is essential to effective patient education. Educational material includes electronic and written materials appropriate to the pregnant woman's or couple's literacy level and experience and the agency's resources. Available educational materials should reflect the pregnant woman's or couple's ethnicity, culture, and literacy level to be most effective.

COMMUNITY ACTIVITY

Interview both a pregnant woman and a nurse in a community clinic to determine what is perceived as significant physical and psychologic changes that happen during pregnancy. Discuss these changes in relation to each trimester. Describe what teaching and support is available to assist women in adapting to these changes. Share this information in a clinical post-conference.

The expectant mother needs information about many subjects. Many times, printed literature can supplement the individualized teaching the nurse provides, and women often avidly read books and pamphlets related to their own experience. In addition, the pregnant woman or couple may have questions from their Internet reviews. Nurses may also share recommended electronic sites from reliable sources. The following sections discuss selected topics that cause concerns in pregnant women.

Nutrition. Good nutrition is important for the maintenance of maternal health during pregnancy and the provision of adequate nutrients for embryonic and fetal development (American Dietetic Association [ADA], 2008). Assessing a woman's nutritional status and providing information on nutrition are part of the nurse's responsibilities in providing prenatal care. This includes assessment of weight gain during pregnancy as well as prenatal nutrition. Teaching may include discussion about foods high in iron, encouragement to take prenatal vitamins, and recommendations to limit caffeine intake. In some settings a registered dietitian conducts classes for pregnant women on the topics of nutritional status and nutrition during pregnancy or interviews them to assess their knowledge of these topics. Nurses can refer women to a registered dietitian if a need is revealed during the nursing assessment. (For detailed information concerning maternal and fetal nutritional needs and related nursing care, see Chapter 8.)

Personal hygiene. During pregnancy the sebaceous (sweat) glands are highly active because of hormonal influences, and women often perspire freely. Reassure them that the increase is normal and that their previous patterns of perspiration will return after the postpartum period. Baths and warm showers are therapeutic because they relax tense and tired muscles, help counter insomnia, and make the pregnant woman feel fresh. Tub bathing is permitted even in late pregnancy because little water enters the vagina unless under pressure. However, late in pregnancy, when the woman's center of gravity lowers, she is at risk for falling. Tub bathing is contraindicated after rupture of the membranes.

Prevention of urinary tract infections. Because of physiologic changes that occur in the renal system during pregnancy (see Chapter 6), urinary tract infections are common, but they may be asymptomatic. Instruct women to inform their health care provider if blood or pain occurs with urination. These infections pose a risk to the mother and fetus; therefore the prevention or early treatment of these infections is essential.

Assess the woman's understanding and use of good handwashing techniques before and after urinating and of the importance of wiping the perineum from front to back. Soft, absorbent toilet tissue that is white and unscented is suggested for use; harsh, scented, or printed toilet paper may cause irritation. Women should avoid bubble bath or other bath oils because these may irritate the urethra. Women should wear cotton crotch underpants and panty hose and avoid wearing tight-fitting slacks or jeans for long periods; anything that allows a buildup of heat and moisture in the genital area may foster the growth of bacteria.

Some women do not consume enough fluid. After discovering her preferences, advise the woman to drink at least 2 L (eight glasses) of liquid, preferably water, a day to maintain an adequate fluid intake that ensures frequent urination. Pregnant women should not limit fluids in an effort to reduce the frequency of urination. Women need to know that if urine appears dark (concentrated), they must increase their fluid intake. The consumption of yogurt and acidophilus milk may also help prevent urinary tract and vaginal infections. The nurse should review healthy urination practices with the woman. Tell women not to ignore the urge to urinate because holding urine lengthens the time bacteria are in the bladder and allows them to multiply. Women should plan ahead when they are faced with situations that may normally require them to delay urination (e.g., a long car ride). They always should urinate before going to bed at night. Bacteria can be introduced during intercourse; therefore advise women to urinate before and after intercourse, and then drink a large glass of water to promote additional urination. Although frequently recommended, evidence is conflicting regarding the effectiveness of cranberry juice and in particular the effective dose in the prevention of urinary tract infections (Jepson & Craig, 2008).

Kegel exercises. Kegel exercises, deliberate contraction and relaxation of the pubococcygeus muscle, strengthen the muscles around the reproductive organs and improve muscle tone. Many women are not aware of the muscles of the pelvic floor and that these muscles used during urination and sexual intercourse can be consciously controlled. The muscles of the pelvic floor encircle the vaginal outlet, and they need to be exercised because an exercised muscle can then stretch and contract readily at the time of birth. Practice of pelvic muscle exercises during pregnancy also results in fewer complaints of urinary incontinence in late pregnancy and postpartum (see Teaching Guidelines on p. 55 in Chapter 2).

Preparation for breastfeeding. Pregnant women are usually eager to discuss their plans for feeding the newborn. Breast milk is the food of choice, in part because breastfeeding is associated with a decreased incidence of perinatal morbidity and mortality. The American Academy of Pediatrics recommends breastfeeding for at least a year. However, an intense dislike for breastfeeding on the part of the woman or partner, the woman's need for certain medications or use of street drugs, and certain life-threatening illnesses and medical complications, such as HIV infection, are contraindications to breastfeeding (Lawrence & Lawrence, 2005).

Many women make the decision about the method of infant feeding before pregnancy; therefore the education of women of childbearing age about the benefits of breastfeeding is essential. If the pregnant woman is undecided, she and her partner are given information about the advantages and disadvantages of bottle feeding and breastfeeding so they can make an informed choice. Health care providers support their decisions and provide any needed teaching; see Chapter 18 for further discussion.

Women with inverted nipples need special consideration if they are planning to breastfeed. A **pinch test** is performed to determine whether the nipple is everted or inverted (Fig. 7-9). The woman is shown how to perform the pinch test. It involves having the woman place her thumb and forefinger on her areola and gently press inward. This action will cause her nipple either to stand erect or to invert. Most nipples will stand erect.

Exercises to break the adhesions that cause the nipple to invert do not work and may cause uterine contractions (Lawrence & Lawrence, 2005). The use of breast shells, small plastic devices that fit over the nipples, is recommended for women who have flat or inverted nipples (Fig. 7-10). Breast shells work by exerting a continuous, gentle pressure around the areola that pushes the nipple through a central opening in the inner shield. The woman should wear breast shells for 1 to 2 hours daily during the last trimester of pregnancy. They should be worn for gradually increasing lengths of time (Lawrence & Lawrence). Breast stimulation is contraindicated in women at risk for preterm labor; therefore the decision to suggest the use of breast shells to women with flat or inverted nipples must be made judiciously.

Teach the woman to cleanse the nipples with warm water to keep the ducts from being blocked with dried colostrum. She should not apply soap, ointments, alcohol, and tinctures because they remove protective oils that keep the nipples supple. The use of these substances may cause the nipples to crack during early lactation (Lawrence & Lawrence, 2005).

The woman who plans to breastfeed should purchase a nursing bra that will accommodate her increased breast size during the last few months of pregnancy and during lactation. If her breasts are very heavy, or if the woman feels uncomfortable with the weight unsupported, she should wear the bra day and night.

Dental care. Dental care during pregnancy is especially important because nausea during pregnancy may lead to poor oral hygiene, allowing dental caries to develop. The woman should use a fluoride toothpaste daily. Inflammation and infection of the gingival and periodontal tissues may occur (Russell & Mayberry, 2008). Research links periodontal disease with preterm births and LBW and an increased risk for preeclampsia (Bogess & Edelstein, 2006; Dasanayake, Gennaro, Hendricks-Munoz, & Chhun, 2008).

Because calcium and phosphorus in the teeth are fixed in enamel, the old adage "for every child a tooth" is not true. No scientific evidence has been found to support the belief that filling teeth or even dental extraction involving the administration of local or nitrous oxide–oxygen anesthesia precipitates miscarriage or premature labor. Emergency dental surgery is not contraindicated during pregnancy. However, explain the risks and benefits of dental surgery to the woman. The American Dental Association (2009) recommends that elective dental treatment not be scheduled in the first trimester or last half of the third trimester. The woman will be most comfortable during the second trimester because the uterus is now

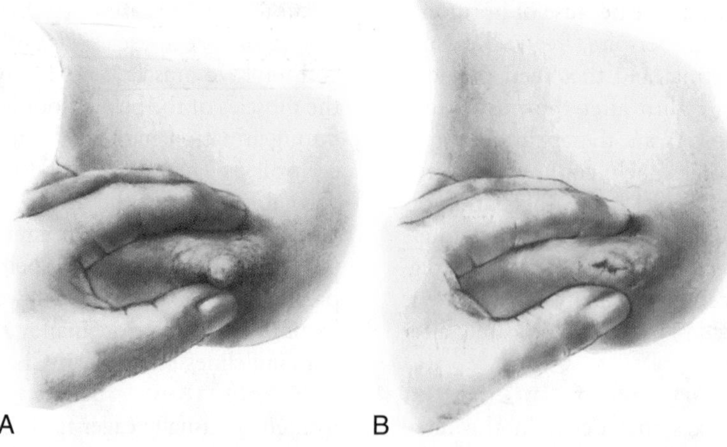

Fig. 7-9 **A,** Normal nipple everts with gentle pressure. **B,** Inverted nipple inverts with gentle pressure. (Modified from Lawrence, R. & Lawrence, R. [2005]. *Breastfeeding: A guide for the medical profession* [6th ed.]. Philadelphia: Mosby.)

outside the pelvis but not so large as to cause discomfort while she sits in a dental chair (Russell & Mayberry, 2008).

Physical activity. Physical activity promotes a feeling of well-being in the pregnant woman. It improves circulation, promotes relaxation and rest, and counteracts boredom, as it does in the nonpregnant woman (American College of Obstetricians and Gynecologists [ACOG], 2002). The Patient Instructions for Self-Management box (p. 212) presents detailed exercise tips for pregnancy. Fig. 7-11 demonstrates exercises that help relieve the low back pain that often arises during the second trimester because of the increased weight of the fetus.

Posture and body mechanics. Skeletal and musculature changes and hormonal changes (relaxin) in pregnancy may predispose the woman to backache and possible injury. As pregnancy progresses the pregnant woman's center of gravity changes, pelvic joints soften and relax, and stress is placed on abdominal musculature. Poor posture and body mechanics contribute to the discomfort and potential for injury. To minimize these problems, women can learn good body posture and body mechanics (Fig. 7-12). The Patient Instructions for Self-Management box on p. 213 presents strategies to prevent or relieve backache.

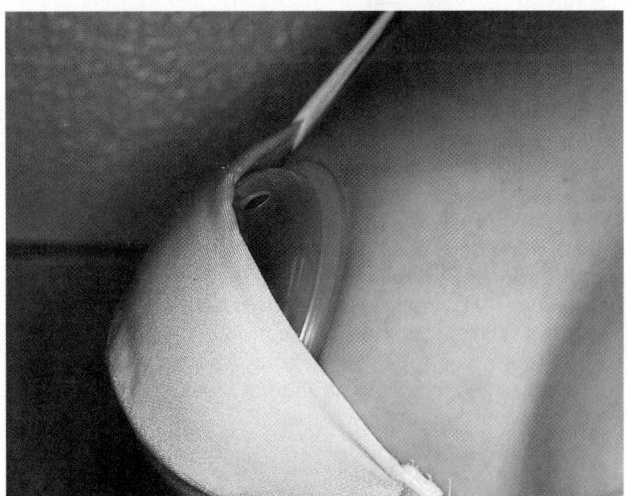

Fig. 7-10 Breast shell in place inside bra to evert nipple. (Courtesy Michael S. Clement, MD, Mesa, AZ.)

Rest and relaxation. The nurse encourages the pregnant woman to plan regular rest periods, particularly as pregnancy advances. The side-lying position is recommended because it promotes uterine perfusion and fetoplacental oxygenation by eliminating pressure on the ascending vena cava and descending aorta, which can lead to supine hypotension (Fig. 7-13). Show the mother how to rise slowly from a side-lying position to prevent placing strain on the back and to minimize the orthostatic hypotension caused by changes in position common in the latter part of pregnancy. To stretch and rest back muscles at home or work the nurse can show the woman the way to perform the following exercises:

- Stand behind a chair. Support and balance self by using the back of the chair (Fig. 7-14). Squat for 30 seconds; stand for 15 seconds. Repeat six times, several times per day, as needed.
- While sitting in a chair, lower head to knees for 30 seconds. Raise head. Repeat six times, several times per day, as needed.

Conscious relaxation is the process of releasing tension from the mind and body through deliberate effort and practice. The ability to relax consciously and intentionally is beneficial for the following reasons:

- To relieve the normal discomforts related to pregnancy
- To reduce stress and therefore diminish pain perception during the childbearing cycle
- To heighten self-awareness and trust in one's own ability to control responses and functions
- To help cope with stress in everyday life situations, whether the woman is pregnant or not

Case Study: Second Trimester

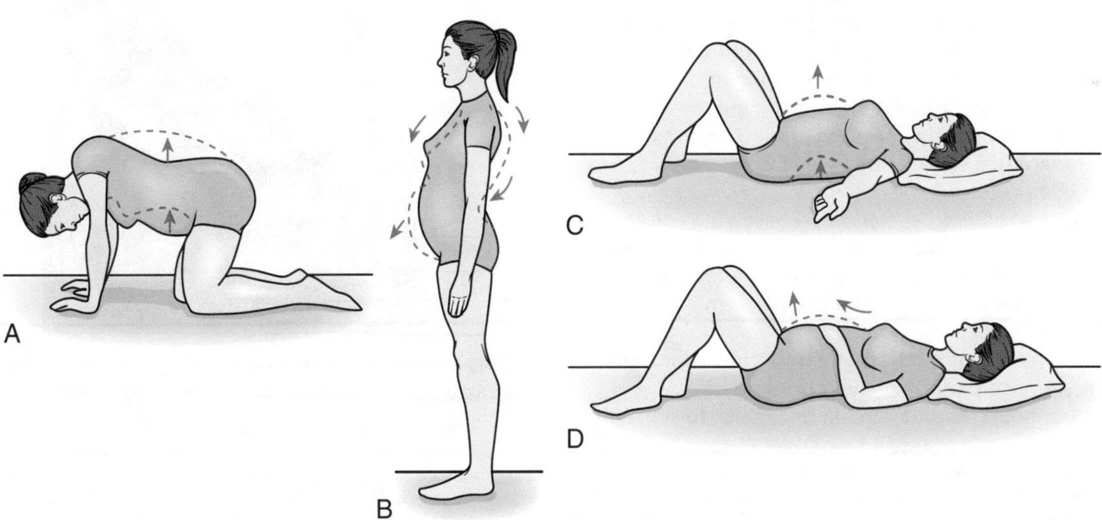

Fig. 7-11 Exercises. **A-C,** Pelvic rocking relieves low backache (excellent for relief of menstrual cramps as well). **D,** Abdominal breathing aids relaxation and lifts abdominal wall off uterus.

PATIENT INSTRUCTIONS FOR SELF-MANAGEMENT

Exercise Tips for Pregnant Women

Consult your health care provider when you know or suspect you are pregnant. Discuss your medical and obstetric history, your current exercise regimen, and the exercises you would like to continue throughout pregnancy.

Seek help in determining an exercise routine that is well within your limit of tolerance, especially if you have not been exercising regularly.

Consider decreasing weight-bearing exercises (jogging, running) and concentrating on non–weight-bearing activities such as swimming, cycling, or stretching. If you are a runner, starting in your seventh month, you may wish to walk instead.

Avoid risky activities such as surfing, mountain climbing, skydiving, and racquetball because such activities that require precise balance and coordination may be dangerous. Avoid activities that require holding your breath and bearing down (Valsalva maneuver). Avoid jerky, bouncy motions as well.

Exercise regularly every day if possible, as long as you are healthy, to improve muscle tone and increase or maintain your stamina. Exercising sporadically may put undue strain on your muscles. Thirty minutes of moderate physical exercise is recommended. This activity can be broken up into shorter segments with rest in between. For example, exercise for 10 to 15 minutes, rest for 2 to 3 minutes, then exercise for another 10 to 15 minutes.

Decrease your exercise level as your pregnancy progresses. The normal alterations of advancing pregnancy, such as decreased cardiac reserve and increased respiratory effort, may produce physiologic stress if you exercise strenuously for a long time.

Take your pulse every 10 to 15 minutes while you are exercising. If it is more than 140 beats/min, slow down until it returns to a maximum of 90 beats/min. You should be able to converse easily while exercising. If you cannot, then you need to slow down.

Avoid becoming overheated for extended periods. Avoid exercising for more than 35 minutes, especially in hot, humid weather. As your body temperature rises, the heat is transmitted to your fetus. Prolonged or repeated elevation of fetal temperature may result in birth defects, especially during the first 3 months. Your temperature should not exceed 38° C.

Avoid the use of hot tubs and saunas.

Warm-up and stretching exercises prepare your joints for more strenuous exercise and lessen the likelihood of strain or injury to your joints. After the fourth month of gestation, you should not perform exercises flat on your back.

A cool-down period of mild activity involving your legs after an exercise period will help bring your respiration, heart, and metabolic rates back to normal and prevent the pooling of blood in the exercised muscles.

Rest for 10 minutes after exercising, lying on your side. As the uterus grows, it puts pressure on a major vein in your abdomen, which carries blood to your heart. Lying on your side removes the pressure and promotes return circulation from your extremities and muscles to your heart, thereby increasing blood flow to your placenta and fetus. You should rise gradually from the floor to prevent dizziness or fainting (orthostatic hypotension).

Drink two or three 8-oz glasses of water after you exercise to replace the body fluids lost through perspiration. While exercising, drink water whenever you feel the need.

Increase your caloric intake to replace the calories burned during exercise and provide the extra energy needs of pregnancy. (Pregnancy alone requires an additional 300 kcal/day.) Choose such high-protein foods as fish, milk, cheese, eggs, and meat.

Take your time. This is not the time to be competitive or train for activities requiring speed or long endurance.

Wear a supportive bra. Your increased breast weight may cause changes in posture and put pressure on the ulnar nerve.

Wear supportive shoes. As your uterus grows, your center of gravity shifts and you compensate for this by arching your back. These natural changes may make you feel off balance and more likely to fall.

Stop exercising immediately if you experience shortness of breath, dizziness, numbness, tingling, pain of any kind, more than four uterine contractions per hour, decreased fetal activity, or vaginal bleeding, and consult your health care provider.

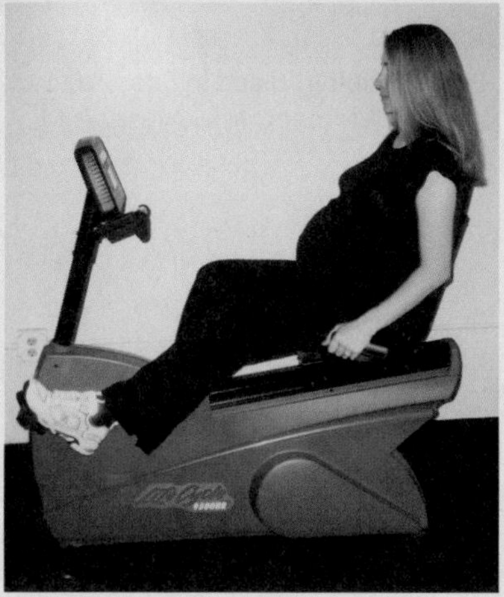

Riding a recumbent bicycle provides exercise while supplying back support. (Courtesy Shannon Perry, Phoenix, AZ.)

Sources: American College of Obstetricians and Gynecologists (ACOG). (2002). Exercise during pregnancy and the postpartum period. ACOG Committee Opinion No. 267. *Obstetrics & Gynecology*, 77(1), 79-81; Kramer, M., & McDonald, S. (2006). Aerobic exercise for women during pregnancy. In *The Cochrane Database of Systematic Reviews* 2006, Issue 2, CD 000180; Morris, S., & Johnson, N. (2005). Exercise in pregnancy: A critical appraisal of the literature. *Journal of Reproductive Medicine*, 50(3), 181-188.

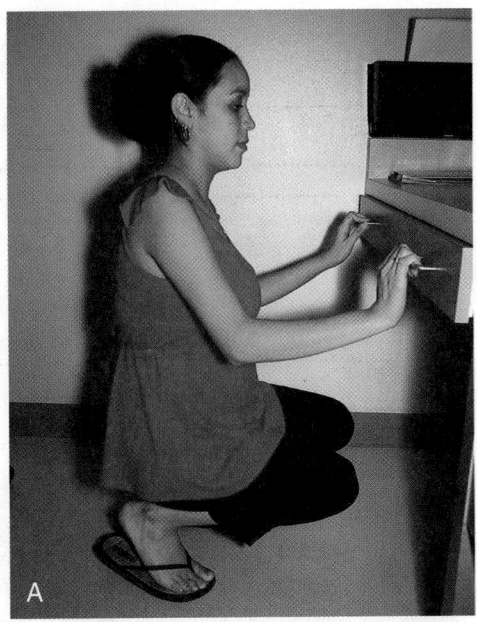

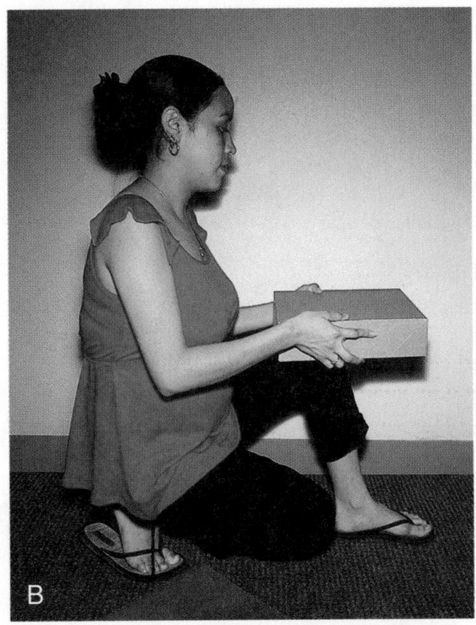

Fig. 7-12 Correct body mechanics. **A,** Squatting. **B,** Lifting. (Courtesy Michael S. Clement, MD, Mesa, AZ.)

PATIENT INSTRUCTIONS FOR SELF-MANAGEMENT

Posture and Body Mechanics

TO PREVENT OR RELIEVE BACKACHE

Do pelvic tilt:

- **Pelvic tilt (rock)** on hands and knees (see Fig. 7-11, *A*) and while sitting in straight-back chair.
- Pelvic tilt (rock) in standing position against a wall, or lying on floor (see Fig. 7-11, *B* and *C*).
- Perform abdominal muscle contractions during pelvic tilt while standing, lying, or sitting to help strengthen rectus abdominis muscle (see Fig. 7-11, *D*).
- Use good body mechanics.
- Use leg muscles to reach objects on or near floor. Bend at the knees, not from the back. Bend knees to lower body to squatting position. Keep feet 12 to 18 inches apart to provide a solid base to maintain balance (see Fig. 7-12, *A*).
- Lift with the legs. To lift heavy objects (e.g., young child), place one foot slightly in front of the other, and keep it flat as you lower yourself onto one knee. Lift the weight holding it close to your body and never higher than the chest. To stand up or sit down, place one leg slightly behind the other as you raise or lower yourself (see Fig. 7-12, *B*).

TO RESTRICT THE LUMBAR CURVE

- For prolonged standing (e.g., ironing, employment), place one foot on low footstool or box; change positions often.
- Move car seat forward so that knees are bent and higher than hips. If needed, use a small pillow to support low back area.
- Sit in chairs low enough to allow both feet to be placed on floor, preferably with knees higher than hips.

TO PREVENT ROUND LIGAMENT PAIN AND STRAIN ON ABDOMINAL MUSCLES

Implement suggestions given in Table 7-2.

The techniques for conscious relaxation are numerous and varied. Box 7-5 gives some guidelines.

Employment. Employment of pregnant women usually has no adverse effects on pregnancy outcomes. Job discrimination that is based strictly on pregnancy is illegal. However, some job environments pose potential risk to the fetus (e.g., dry-cleaning plants, chemistry laboratories, parking garages). Excessive fatigue is usually the deciding factor in the termination of employment. The Patient Instructions for Self-Management box on p. 214 describes strategies to improve safety during pregnancy.

Women with sedentary jobs need to walk around at intervals to counter the usual sluggish circulation in the legs. They also should neither sit nor stand in one position for long periods, and they should avoid crossing their legs at the knees because all these activities can foster the development of varices and thrombophlebitis. Standing for long periods also increases the risk of preterm labor. The pregnant woman's chair should provide adequate back support. Use of a footstool can prevent pressure on veins, relieve strain on varicosities, minimize edema of feet, and prevent backache.

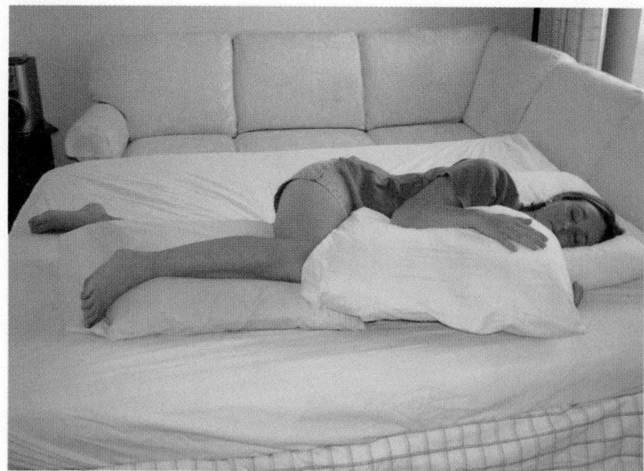

Fig. 7-13 Side-lying position for rest and relaxation. Some women prefer to support upper part of leg with pillows. (Courtesy Julie Perry Nelson, Loveland, CO.)

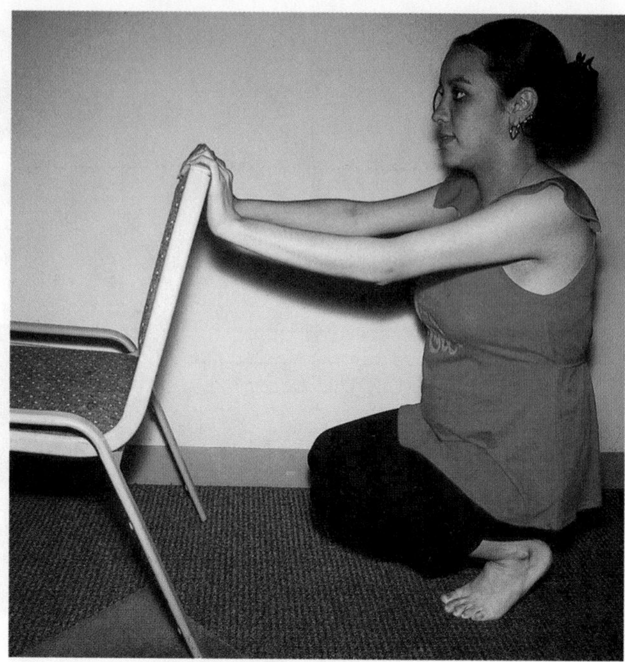

Fig. 7-14 Squatting for muscle relaxation and strengthening and for keeping leg and hip joints flexible. (Courtesy Michael S. Clement, MD, Mesa, AZ.)

BOX 7-5

Conscious Relaxation Tips

Preparation: Loosen clothing, assume a comfortable sitting or side-lying position, with all parts of body well supported with pillows.

Beginning: Allow yourself to feel warm and comfortable. Inhale and exhale slowly, and imagine peaceful relaxation coming over each part of the body, starting with the neck and working down to the toes. People who learn conscious relaxation often speak of feeling relaxed even if some discomfort is present.

Maintenance: Use imagery (fantasy or daydream) to maintain the state of relaxation. Using active imagery, imagine yourself moving or doing some activity and experiencing its sensations. Using passive imagery, imagine yourself watching a scene, such as a lovely sunset.

Awakening: Return to the wakeful state gradually. Slowly begin to take in stimuli from the surrounding environment.

Further retention and development of the skill: Practice regularly for some periods each day, for example, at the same hour for 10 to 15 minutes each day, to feel refreshed, revitalized, and invigorated.

PATIENT INSTRUCTIONS FOR SELF-MANAGEMENT

Safety during Pregnancy

Changes in the body resulting from pregnancy include relaxation of joints, alteration to center of gravity, faintness, and discomforts. Problems with coordination and balance are common. Therefore the woman should follow these guidelines:

- Use good body mechanics.
- Use safety features on tools and vehicles (seat belts, shoulder harnesses, headrests, goggles, helmets) as specified.
- Avoid activities requiring coordination, balance, and concentration.
- Take rest periods; reschedule daily activities to meet rest and relaxation needs.

Embryonic and fetal development is vulnerable to environmental teratogens. Many potentially dangerous chemicals are present in the home, yard, and workplace: cleaning agents, paints, sprays, herbicides, and pesticides. The soil and water supply may be unsafe. Therefore the woman should follow these guidelines:

- Read all labels for ingredients and proper use of product.
- Ensure adequate ventilation with clean air.
- Dispose of wastes appropriately.
- Wear gloves when handling chemicals.
- Change job assignments or workplace as necessary.
- Avoid high altitudes (not in pressurized aircraft), which could jeopardize oxygen intake.

EVIDENCE-BASED PRACTICE

Exercise and Work in Pregnancy

Pat Gingrich

ASK THE QUESTION

What sorts of work and leisure activities are safe for pregnant women?

SEARCH FOR EVIDENCE

Search Strategies: Professional organization guidelines, meta-analyses, systematic reviews, randomized controlled trials, nonrandomized prospective studies, and retrospective studies since 2006.

Databases Searched: CINAHL, Cochrane, Medline, National Guideline Clearinghouse, TRIP Database Plus, and the websites for American College of Gynecologists; Association of Women's Health, Obstetric, and Neonatal Nurses; and the Centers for Disease Control and Prevention.

CRITICALLY ANALYZE THE EVIDENCE

Historically, health care providers worried that exercise during pregnancy might lead to poor uteroplacental perfusion or increased inflammatory response, resulting in low birth weight, gestational hypertension, or prematurity. These concerns lead to restrictions on activity. However, exercise has been shown to have many physiologic and psychologic benefits. For example, in a randomized clinical trial of women with prior preeclampsia, walking and stretching promoted antioxidants and decreased recurrence of gestational hypertension (Yeo, Davidge, Ronis, Antonakos, Hayashi, & O'Leary, 2008).

In a review, Gavard and Atal (2008) found that healthy women benefited from exercising, with no difference in birth weights or gestational age at birth when compared with sedentary women. Moderate leisure and work activity conferred a protective effect against preeclampsia and gestational diabetes, especially if the exercise predated the pregnancy. Even vigorous exercise such as running, bicycling, lap swimming, or racquetball did not show any change in the outcomes of birthweight nor gestational age. For a small group of very intense exercisers, birth weight decreased 200 to 400 grams, which may reflect insufficient calories. Even previously sedentary women initiated exercise during pregnancy, with no change in gestational age (Barakat, Stirling, & Lucia, 2008).

Occupational activities of prolonged hours, shift work, lifting, standing and heavy physical work are not statistically associated with the outcomes of preterm birth: low birth weight, or gestational hypertension, according to a systematic review by Bonzini, Coggon, and Palmer (2007). The authors caution, however, that this activity does not confer any protective benefits, and they recommend decreasing work hours, standing time, and physical labor in the third trimester.

IMPLICATIONS FOR PRACTICE

- The nurse can encourage healthy pregnant and nonpregnant patients to incorporate moderate exercise, such as brisk walking, for 30 minutes a day, most days of the week. Benefits of regular exercise in pregnancy include weight control, psychologic well-being, and a protective effect against gestational hypertension and diabetes. The benefits are greater if she begins exercise before pregnancy, but even sedentary women can safely take up exercise during pregnancy. No evidence has been found to suggest that moderate cardiovascular exercise leads to prematurity or low birth weight.
- Women who exercise strenuously or those whose job requires heavy labor, prolonged hours, and shift work may need to consider modifying their activity in late pregnancy. This precaution might be of particular interest to pregnant nurses, whose jobs can involve long hours and physical labor.

References:

Barakat, R., Stirling, J. R., & Lucia, A. (2008). Does exercise training during pregnancy affect gestational age? A randomized, controlled trial. *British Journal of Sports Medicine, 42*(8):674-678 (Epub 2008 Jun 14).

Bonzini, M., Coggon, D., & Palmer, K. T. (2007). Risk of prematurity, low birthweight, and pre-eclampsia in relation to working hours and physical activities: A systematic review. *Occupational and Environmental Medicine, 67*, 228-243.

Gavard, J. A. & Artal, R. (2008). Effect of exercise on pregnancy outcome. *Clinical Obstetrics and Gynecology, 51*(2), 467-480.

Yeo, S., Davidge, S., Ronis, D. L., Antonakos, C. L., Hayashi, R., & O'Leary, S. (2008). A comparison of walking versus stretching exercises to reduce the incidence of preeclampsia: a randomized clinical trial. *Hypertension in Pregnancy, 27*(2), 113-130.

Clothing. Some women continue to wear their usual clothes during pregnancy as long as they fit and feel comfortable. If a woman needs maternity clothing, outfits may be purchased new or found at thrift shops or garage sales in good condition. Comfortable, loose clothing is recommended. Women should avoid tight bras and belts, stretch pants, garters, tight-top knee socks, panty girdles, and other constrictive clothing because tight clothing over the perineum encourages vaginitis and miliaria (heat rash), and impaired circulation in the legs can cause varicosities.

Maternity bras accommodate the increased breast weight, chest circumference, and the size of breast tail tissue (under the arm). These bras also have drop-flaps over the nipples to facilitate breastfeeding. A good bra can help prevent neck ache and backache.

Maternal support hose give considerable comfort and promote greater venous emptying in women with large varicose veins. Ideally, women should put on support stockings before getting out of bed in the morning. Fig. 7-15 demonstrates a position for resting the legs and reducing swelling and varicosities.

Comfortable shoes that provide firm support and promote good posture and balance are also advisable. Very high heels and platform shoes are not recommended because of the changes in the pregnant woman's center of gravity, and the hormone relaxin, which softens pelvic joints in later pregnancy, all of which can cause her to lose

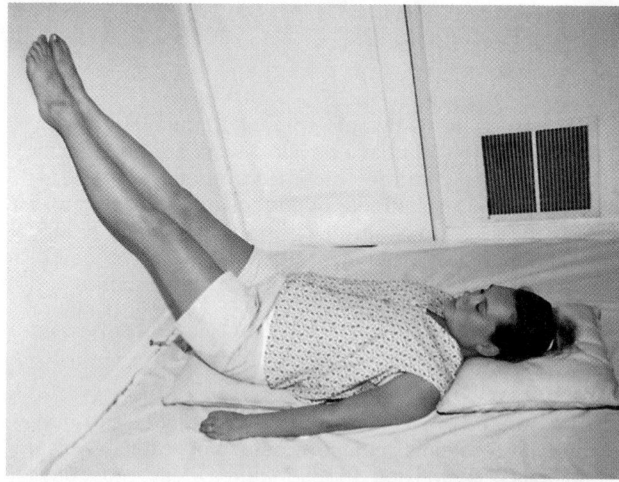

Fig. 7-15 Position for resting legs and for reducing edema and varicosities. Encourage woman with vulvar varicosities to include pillow under her hips. (Courtesy Dale Ikuta, San Jose, CA.)

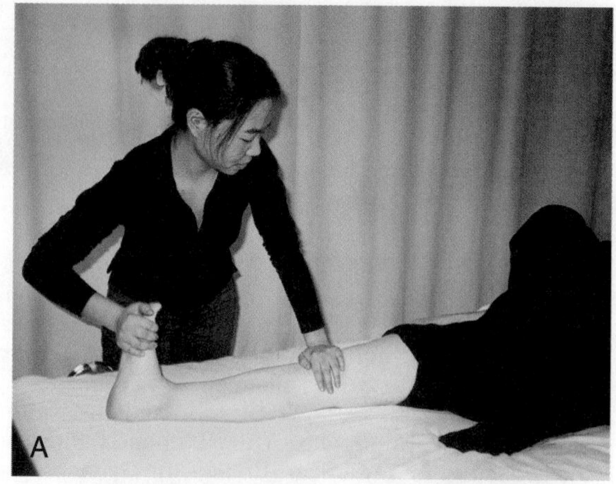

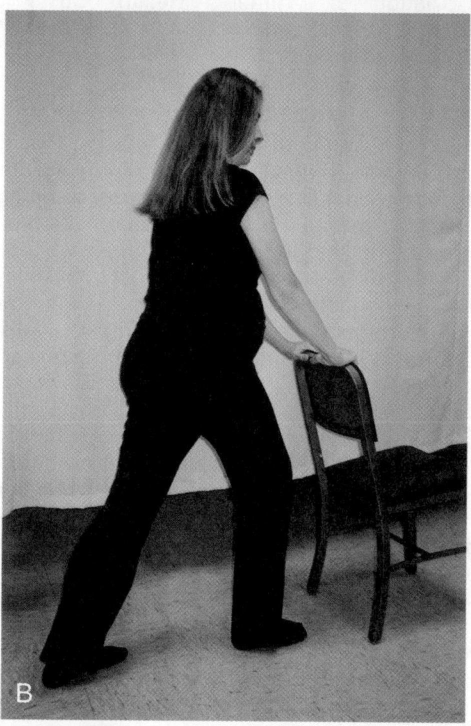

Fig. 7-16 Relief of muscle spasm (leg cramps). **A,** Another person dorsiflexes foot with knee extended. **B,** Woman stands and leans forward, thereby dorsiflexing foot of affected leg. (Courtesy Shannon Perry, Phoenix, AZ.)

her balance. In addition, in the third trimester the woman's pelvis tilts forward, and her lumbar curve increases. Nonsupportive shoes will aggravate the resulting leg aches and cramps (Fig. 7-16).

Travel. Travel is not contraindicated in low risk pregnant women. However, women with high risk pregnancies are advised to avoid long-distance travel in the later months of the pregnancy to prevent possible economic and psychologic consequences of giving birth to a preterm infant far from home. These women should avoid travel to areas in which medical care is poor, water is untreated, or malaria is prevalent. Women who contemplate foreign travel should be aware that many health insurance carriers do not cover a birth in a foreign setting or even hospitalization for preterm labor. In addition, some vaccinations for foreign travel are contraindicated during pregnancy.

Pregnant women who travel for long distances should schedule periods of activity and rest. While sitting, the woman can practice deep breathing, foot circling, and alternately contracting and relaxing different muscle groups. She should avoid becoming fatigued. Although travel in itself is not a cause of adverse outcomes such as miscarriage or preterm labor, certain precautions should be kept in mind while traveling in a car. For example, women riding in a car should wear automobile restraints and stop and walk every hour. A combination lap belt and shoulder harness is the most effective automobile restraint (Fig. 7-17). The woman should wear the lap belt worn low across the pelvic bones and as snug as is comfortable. The shoulder harness should be above the pregnant abdomen and crossing the body between the breasts. The pregnant woman should sit upright. The headrest should be used to prevent a whiplash injury. Airbags, if present, should remain engaged, but the steering wheel should be tilted upwards away from the abdomen and the seat moved back way from the steering wheel as much as possible (Cesario, 2007).

Pregnant women traveling in high-altitude regions have lowered oxygen levels that may cause fetal hypoxia, especially if the pregnant woman is anemic. However, the current information on this condition is limited, and recommendations are not standardized.

Airline travel in large commercial jets usually poses little risk to the pregnant woman, but policies vary from airline to airline. The pregnant woman should inquire about restrictions or recommendations from her carrier. Most health care providers allow air travel up to 36 weeks of gestation in women without medical or pregnancy complications. Because the cabins of commercial airlines maintain

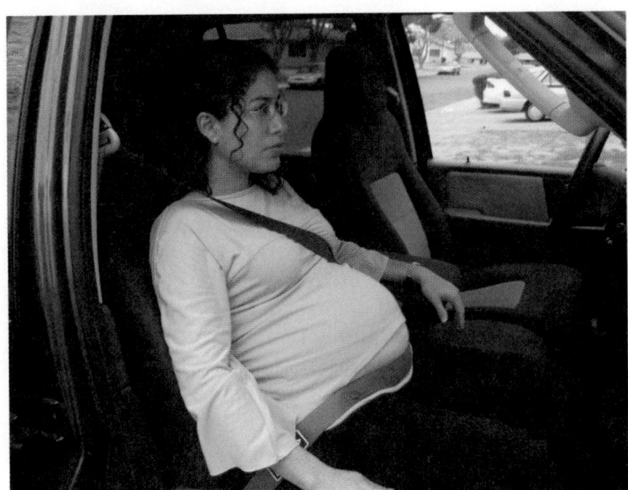

Fig. 7-17 Proper use of seat belt and headrest. (Courtesy Brian and Mayannyn Sallee, Las Vegas, NV.)

humidity at 8%, the woman may have some water loss; she should therefore drink plenty of water under these conditions. Sitting in the cramped seat of an airliner for prolonged periods may increase the risk of superficial and deep thrombophlebitis; therefore encourage pregnant women to take a 15-minute walk around the aircraft during each hour of travel to minimize this risk. Metal detectors used at airport security checkpoints are not harmful to the fetus.

Medications and herbal preparations. Although research has revealed much in recent years about fetal drug toxicity the possible teratogenicity of many medications, both prescription and OTC, is still unknown. This fact is especially true for new medications and combinations of drugs. Moreover, certain subclinical errors or deficiencies in intermediate metabolism in the fetus may cause an otherwise harmless drug to be converted into a hazardous one. The greatest danger of drug-caused developmental defects in the fetus extends from the time of fertilization through the first trimester, a time when the woman may not realize she is pregnant. The use of all drugs, including OTC medications, herbs, and vitamins, should be limited, and a record should be kept and discussed with the health care provider.

NURSING ALERT Although complementary and alternative medications (CAM) may benefit the woman during pregnancy, some practices should be avoided because they may cause miscarriage or preterm labor. Asking the woman what therapies she may be using is important.

Immunizations. Some individuals have raised concern over the safety of various immunization practices during pregnancy. Immunization with live or attenuated live viruses is contraindicated during pregnancy because of its potential teratogenicity but should be part of postpartum care. Live-virus vaccines include those for measles (rubeola and rubella), chickenpox, and mumps, as well as the Sabin (oral) poliomyelitis vaccine (no longer used in the United States). Vaccines consisting of killed viruses may be used. Vaccines that can be administered during pregnancy include tetanus, diphtheria, recombinant hepatitis B, and influenza (inactivated) vaccines (Centers for Disease Control and Prevention, 2008, www.cdc.gov/vaccines).

Alcohol, cigarette smoke, caffeine, and drugs. A safe level of alcohol consumption during pregnancy has not been established. Although the consumption of occasional alcoholic beverages is not always harmful to the mother or her developing embryo or fetus, complete abstinence is best. Maternal alcoholism is associated with high rates of miscarriage and fetal alcohol syndrome (March of Dimes Birth Defects Foundation, 2008). Considerably less alcohol use is reported among pregnant women than in nonpregnant women, but a high prevalence of some alcohol use among pregnant women still exists. Such a finding underscores the need for more systematic public health efforts to educate women about the hazards of alcohol consumption during pregnancy.

Cigarette smoking or continued exposure to secondhand smoke (even if the mother does not smoke) is associated with intrauterine fetal growth restriction and an increase in perinatal and infant morbidity and mortality. Smoking is associated with an increased frequency of preterm labor, PROM, abruptio placentae, placenta previa, and fetal death, possibly resulting from decreased placental perfusion. Smoking cessation activities should be incorporated into routine prenatal care (ACOG, 2005) (see Box 2-3).

Strongly encourage all women who smoke to quit or at least reduce the number of cigarettes they smoke. Pregnant women need to know about the negative effects of even secondhand smoke on the fetus and be encouraged to avoid such environments (Kleigman, 2006).

Most studies of human pregnancy have revealed no association between caffeine consumption and birth defects or LBW, but an increased risk for miscarriage with caffeine intake greater than 200 mg/day has been reported (Weng, Odouli, & Li, 2008). Because other effects are unknown, however, pregnant women need to limit their caffeine intake, particularly coffee intake, because it has a high caffeine content per unit of measure.

Any drug or environmental agent that enters the pregnant woman's bloodstream has the potential to cross the placenta and harm the fetus. Marijuana, heroin, and cocaine are common examples of such substances. Although the problem of substance abuse in pregnancy is a major public health concern, comprehensive care of drug-addicted women improves maternal and neonatal outcomes (see Chapters 20 and 24).

Normal discomforts. Pregnant women have physical symptoms that would be abnormal in the nonpregnant state. Women pregnant for the first time have an increased need for explanations of the causes of the discomforts and for advice on ways to relieve the discomforts. The discomforts of the first trimester are fairly specific. Table 7-2 gives information about the physiology

TABLE 7-2

Discomforts Related to Pregnancy

DISCOMFORT	PHYSIOLOGY	EDUCATION FOR SELF-MANAGEMENT
FIRST TRIMESTER		
Breast changes, new sensation: pain, tingling, tenderness	Hypertrophy of mammary glandular tissue and increased vascularization, pigmentation, and size and prominence of nipples and areolae caused by hormonal stimulation	Wear supportive maternity bras with pads to absorb discharge during the day and at night; wash with warm water and keep dry; breast tenderness may interfere with sexual expression or foreplay but is temporary
Urgency and frequency of urination	Vascular engorgement and altered bladder function caused by hormones; bladder capacity reduced by enlarging uterus and fetal presenting part	Empty bladder regularly; perform Kegel exercises; limit fluid intake before bedtime; wear perineal pad; report pain or burning sensation to primary health care provider
Languor and malaise; fatigue (early pregnancy, most commonly)	Unexplained; may be caused by increasing levels of estrogen, progesterone, and hCG or by elevated BBT; psychologic response to pregnancy and its required physical and psychologic adaptations	Rest as needed; eat well-balanced diet to prevent anemia
Nausea and vomiting, **morning sickness**—occurs in 50%-75% of pregnant women; starts between first and second missed periods and lasts until approximately fourth missed period; may occur any time during day; fathers also may have symptoms	Cause unknown; may result from hormonal changes, possibly hCG; may be partly emotional, reflecting pride in, ambivalence about, or rejection of pregnant state	Avoid empty or overloaded stomach; maintain good posture—give stomach ample room; stop smoking; eat dry carbohydrate on awakening; remain in bed until feeling subsides, or alternate dry carbohydrate every other hour with fluids such as hot herbal decaffeinated tea, milk, or clear coffee until feeling subsides; eat five to six small meals per day; avoid fried, odorous, spicy, greasy, or gas-forming foods; consult primary health care provider if intractable vomiting occurs
Ptyalism (excessive salivation) may occur starting 2 to 3 weeks after first missed period	Possibly caused by elevated estrogen levels; may be related to reluctance to swallow because of nausea	Use astringent mouth wash, chew gum, eat hard candy as comfort measures
Gingivitis and epulis (hyperemia, hypertrophy, bleeding, tenderness of the gums); condition will disappear spontaneously 1 to 2 months after birth	Increased vascularity and proliferation of connective tissue from estrogen stimulation	Eat well-balanced diet with adequate protein and fresh fruits and vegetables; brush teeth gently, and observe good dental hygiene; avoid infection; see dentist
Nasal stuffiness; epistaxis (nosebleed)	Hyperemia of mucous membranes related to high estrogen levels	Use humidifier; avoid trauma; normal saline nose drops or spray may be used
Leukorrhea: often noted throughout pregnancy	Hormonally stimulated cervix becomes hypertrophic and hyperactive, producing abundant amount of mucus	Not preventable; do not douche; wear perineal pads; perform hygienic practices such as wiping front to back; report to primary health care provider if accompanied by pruritus, foul odor, or change in character or color
Psychosocial dynamics, mood swings, mixed feelings	Hormonal and metabolic adaptations; feelings about female role, sexuality, timing of pregnancy, and resultant changes in life and lifestyle	Participate in pregnancy support group; communicate concerns to partner, family, and health care provider; request referral for supportive services if needed

TABLE 7-2

Discomforts Related to Pregnancy—cont'd

DISCOMFORT	PHYSIOLOGY	EDUCATION FOR SELF-MANAGEMENT
SECOND TRIMESTER		
Pigmentation deepens; acne, oily skin	Melanocyte-stimulating hormone (from anterior pituitary)	Not preventable; usually resolves during puerperium
Spider nevi (angiomas) appear over neck, thorax, face, and arms during second or third trimester	Focal networks of dilated arterioles (end arteries) from increased concentration of estrogens	Not preventable; they fade slowly during late puerperium; rarely disappear completely
Pruritus (noninflammatory)	Unknown cause; various types as follows: nonpapular; closely aggregated pruritic papules	Keep fingernails short and clean; contact primary health care provider for diagnosis of cause
	Increased excretory function of skin and stretching of skin possible factors	Not preventable; use comfort measures for symptoms such as Keri baths; distraction; tepid baths with sodium bicarbonate or oatmeal added to water; lotions and oils; change of soaps or reduction in use of soap; loose clothing; see health care provider if mild sedation is needed
Palpitations	Unknown; should not be accompanied by persistent cardiac irregularity	Not preventable; contact primary health care provider if accompanied by symptoms of cardiac decompensation
Supine hypotension (vena cava syndrome) and bradycardia	Induced by pressure of gravid uterus on ascending vena cava when woman is supine; reduces uteroplacental and renal perfusion	Side-lying position or semisitting posture, with knees slightly flexed (see supine hypotension, p. 204)
Faintness and, rarely, syncope (orthostatic hypotension) may persist throughout pregnancy	Vasomotor lability or postural hypotension from hormones; in late pregnancy may be caused by venous stasis in lower extremities	Moderate exercise, deep breathing, vigorous leg movement; avoid sudden changes in position and warm crowded areas; move slowly and deliberately; keep environment cool; avoid hypoglycemia by eating five or six small meals per day; wear support hose; sit as necessary; if symptoms are serious, contact primary health care provider
Food cravings	Cause unknown; craving influenced by culture or geographic area	Not preventable; satisfy craving unless it interferes with well-balanced diet; report unusual cravings to primary health care provider
Heartburn (pyrosis or acid indigestion): burning sensation, occasionally with burping and regurgitation of a little sour-tasting fluid	Progesterone slows GI tract motility and digestion, reverses peristalsis, relaxes cardiac sphincter, and delays emptying time of stomach; stomach displaced upward and compressed by enlarging uterus	Limit or avoid gas-producing or fatty foods and large meals; maintain good posture; sip milk for temporary relief; hot herbal tea; primary health care provider may prescribe antacid between meals; contact primary health care provider for persistent symptoms
Constipation	GI tract motility slowed because of progesterone, resulting in increased resorption of water and drying of stool; intestines compressed by enlarging uterus; predisposition to constipation because of oral iron supplementation	Drink six to eight glasses of water per day; include roughage in diet; moderate exercise; maintain regular schedule for bowel movements; use relaxation techniques and deep breathing; do not take stool softener, laxatives, mineral oil, other drugs, or enemas without first consulting primary health care provider
Flatulence with bloating and belching	Reduced GI motility because of hormones, allowing time for bacterial action that produces gas; swallowing air	Chew foods slowly and thoroughly; avoid gas-producing foods, fatty foods, large meals; exercise; maintain regular bowel habits

Continued

TABLE 7-2

Discomforts Related to Pregnancy—cont'd

DISCOMFORT	PHYSIOLOGY	EDUCATION FOR SELF-MANAGEMENT
Varicose veins (varicosities): may be associated with aching legs and tenderness; may be present in legs and vulva; hemorrhoids are varicosities in perianal area	Hereditary predisposition; relaxation of smooth-muscle walls of veins because of hormones, causing tortuous dilated veins in legs and pelvic vasocongestion; condition aggravated by enlarging uterus, gravity, and bearing down for bowel movements; thrombi from leg varices rare but may occur in hemorrhoids	Avoid obesity, lengthy standing or sitting, constrictive clothing, and constipation and bearing down with bowel movements; moderate exercise; rest with legs and hips elevated (see Fig. 7-15); wear support stockings; thrombosed hemorrhoid may be evacuated; relieve swelling and pain with warm sitz baths, local application of astringent compresses
Leukorrhea: often noted throughout pregnancy	Hormonally stimulated cervix becomes hypertrophic and hyperactive, producing abundant amount of mucus	Not preventable; do not douche; maintain good hygiene; wear perineal pads; report to primary health care provider if accompanied by pruritus, foul odor, or change in character or color
Headaches (through week 26)	Emotional tension (more common than vascular migraine headache); eye strain (refractory errors); vascular engorgement and congestion of sinuses resulting from hormone stimulation	Conscious relaxation; contact primary health care provider for constant "splitting" headache, to assess for preeclampsia
Carpal tunnel syndrome (involves thumb, second, and third fingers, lateral side of little finger)	Compression of median nerve resulting from changes in surrounding tissues; pain, numbness, tingling, burning; loss of skilled movements (typing); dropping of objects	Not preventable; elevate affected arms; splinting of affected hand may help; regressive after pregnancy; surgery is curative
Periodic numbness, tingling of fingers (acrodysesthesia); occurs in 5% of pregnant women	Brachial plexus traction syndrome resulting from drooping of shoulders during pregnancy; occurs especially at night and early morning	Maintain good posture; wear supportive maternity bra; condition will disappear if lifting and carrying baby does not aggravate it
Round ligament pain (tenderness)	Stretching of ligament caused by enlarging uterus	Not preventable; rest, maintain good body mechanics to prevent overstretching ligament; relieve cramping by squatting or bringing knees to chest; sometimes heat helps
Joint pain, backache, and pelvic pressure; hypermobility of joints	Relaxation of symphyseal and sacroiliac joints because of hormones, resulting in unstable pelvis; exaggerated lumbar and cervicothoracic curves caused by change in center of gravity resulting from enlarging abdomen	Maintain good posture and body mechanics; avoid fatigue; wear low-heeled shoes; abdominal supports may be useful; conscious relaxation; sleep on firm mattress; apply local heat or ice; get back rubs; perform pelvic tilt exercises; rest; condition will disappear 6 to 8 wk after birth
THIRD TRIMESTER		
Shortness of breath and dyspnea occur in 60% of pregnant women	Expansion of diaphragm limited by enlarging uterus; diaphragm is elevated about 4 cm; some relief after lightening	Good posture; sleep with extra pillows; avoid overloading stomach; stop smoking; contact health care provider if symptoms worsen to rule out anemia, emphysema, and asthma
Insomnia (later weeks of pregnancy)	Fetal movements, muscle cramping, urinary frequency, shortness of breath, or other discomforts	Reassurance; conscious relaxation; back massage or effleurage; support of body parts with pillows; warm milk or warm shower before retiring

ⓔ Spanish Guidelines: Assessment of Respiratory System

TABLE 7-2

Discomforts Related to Pregnancy—cont'd

DISCOMFORT	PHYSIOLOGY	EDUCATION FOR SELF-MANAGEMENT
Psychosocial responses: mood swings, mixed feelings, increased anxiety	Hormonal and metabolic adaptations; feelings about impending labor, birth, and parenthood	Reassurance and support from significant other and health care providers; improved communication with partner, family, and others
Urinary frequency and urgency return	Vascular engorgement and altered bladder function caused by hormones; bladder capacity reduced by enlarging uterus and fetal presenting part	Empty bladder regularly, Kegel exercises; limit fluid intake before bedtime; reassurance; wear perineal pad; contact health care provider for pain or burning sensation
Perineal discomfort and pressure	Pressure from enlarging uterus, especially when standing or walking; multifetal gestation	Rest, conscious relaxation, and good posture; contact health care provider for assessment and treatment if pain is present
Braxton Hicks contractions	Intensification of uterine contractions in preparation for work of labor	Reassurance; rest; change of position; practice breathing techniques when contractions are bothersome; effleurage; before 37 weeks it is important to contact health care provider to differentiate from preterm labor
Leg cramps (gastrocnemius spasm), especially when reclining	Compression of nerves supplying lower extremities because of enlarging uterus; reduced level of diffusible serum calcium or elevation of serum phosphorus; aggravating factors: fatigue, poor peripheral circulation, pointing toes when stretching legs or when walking, drinking more than 1 L (1 qt) of milk per day	Check for Homans sign; if negative, use massage and heat over affected muscle; dorsiflex foot until spasm relaxes (see Fig. 7-16, *A*); stand on cold surface; oral supplementation with calcium carbonate or calcium lactate tablets; aluminum hydroxide gel, 30 ml, with each meal removes phosphorus by absorbing it (consult primary health care provider before taking these remedies)
Ankle edema (nonpitting) to lower extremities	Edema aggravated by prolonged standing, sitting, poor posture, lack of exercise, constrictive clothing, or hot weather	Ample fluid intake for natural diuretic effect; put on support stockings before arising; rest periodically with legs and hips elevated (see Fig. 7-15), exercise moderately; contact health care provider if generalized edema develops; diuretics are contraindicated

BBT, Basal body temperature; *GI*, gastrointestinal; *hCG*, human chorionic gonadotropin.

and prevention of and self-management for discomforts experienced during the three trimesters. Box 7-6 lists alternative and complementary therapies and why a woman would use these in pregnancy (Fig. 7-18). Nurses can do much to allay a first-time mother's anxiety about such symptoms by telling her about them in advance and using terminology that the woman (or couple) can understand. Understanding the rationale for treatment promotes their participation in their care. Nurses should individualize interventions, with attention given to the woman's lifestyle and culture. See the Nursing Care Plan: Discomforts of Pregnancy and Warning Signs.

Recognizing potential complications. One of the most important responsibilities of care providers is to alert the pregnant woman to signs and symptoms that indicate a potential complication of pregnancy. The woman needs to know how and to whom to report such warning signs. Therefore reassure the pregnant woman and

Critical Thinking/Clinical Decision Making

Nausea in Pregnancy

Meka is 10 weeks pregnant with her first baby. She is complaining of nausea every morning. She has heard that ginger is good for nausea and want to know if she should take it. What is your response?

1. Evidence—Is evidence sufficient to draw conclusions about the effectiveness of ginger on nausea and vomiting of pregnancy?
2. Assumptions—Describe the underlying assumptions for each of the following issues:
   a. Causes of nausea and vomiting of pregnancy
   b. Self-medicating during pregnancy
   c. Evidence for herbal use in pregnancy
3. What implications and priorities for nursing care can be drawn at this time?
4. Does the evidence objectively support your conclusion?
5. Do alternative perspectives to your conclusion exist?

NURSING CARE PLAN *Discomforts of Pregnancy and Warning Signs*

FIRST TRIMESTER

NURSING DIAGNOSIS Anxiety related to deficient knowledge about schedule of prenatal visits throughout pregnancy, as evidenced by woman's questions and concerns

Expected Outcome *Woman will verbalize correct appointment schedule for the duration of the pregnancy and feelings of being "in control."*

Nursing Interventions/*Rationales*

- Provide information regarding schedule of visits, tests, and other assessments and interventions that will be provided throughout the pregnancy *to empower the patient to function in collaboration with the caregiver and diminish anxiety.*
- Allow woman time to describe level of anxiety *to establish a basis for care.*
- Provide information to woman regarding prenatal classes and labor area tours *to decrease feelings of anxiety about the unknown.*

NURSING DIAGNOSIS Imbalanced nutrition: less than body requirements, related to nausea and vomiting, as evidenced by woman's report and weight loss

Expected Outcome *Woman will gain 1 to 2.5 kg during the first trimester.*

Nursing Interventions/*Rationales*

- Verify prepregnant weight *to plan a realistic diet according to individual woman's nutritional needs.*
- Obtain diet history *to identify current meal patterns and foods that may be implicated in nausea.*
- Advise the woman to consume small frequent meals and avoid having an empty stomach *to prevent further nausea episodes.*
- Suggest that woman eat a simple carbohydrate such as dry crackers before arising in the morning *to avoid an empty stomach and decrease the incidence of nausea and vomiting.*
- Advise the woman to call health care provider if vomiting is persistent and severe *to identify the possible incidence of hyperemesis gravidarum.*

NURSING DIAGNOSIS Fatigue related to hormonal changes in the first trimester as evidenced by woman's complaints

Expected Outcome *Woman will report a decreased number of episodes of fatigue.*

Nursing Interventions/*Rationales*

- Rest as needed *to avoid increasing feeling of fatigue.*
- Eat a well-balanced diet *to meet increased metabolic demands and avoid anemia.*
- Discuss the use of support systems to help with household responsibilities *to decrease workload at home and decrease fatigue.*
- Reinforce to the woman the transitory nature of first trimester fatigue *to provide emotional support.*
- Explore with the woman a variety of techniques to prioritize roles *to decrease family expectations.*

SECOND TRIMESTER

NURSING DIAGNOSIS Constipation related to progesterone influence on gastrointestinal tract, as evidenced by the woman's report of altered patterns of elimination

Expected Outcome *Woman will report a return to normal bowel elimination pattern after implementation of interventions.*

Nursing Interventions/*Rationales*

- Provide information to woman regarding pregnancy-related causes—progesterone slowing gastrointestinal motility, growing uterus compressing intestines, and influence of iron supplementation—*to provide basic information for self-management during pregnancy.*
- Assist woman to plan a diet that will promote regular bowel movements, such as increasing amount of oral fluid intake to at least six to eight glasses of water a day, increasing the amount of fiber in daily diet, and maintaining moderate exercise program *to promote self-management.*
- Reinforce for the woman that she should avoid taking any laxatives, stool softeners, or enemas without first consulting the health care provider *to prevent any injuries to the woman or fetus.*

NURSING DIAGNOSIS Anxiety related to deficient knowledge about the course of the first pregnancy, as evidenced by woman's questions regarding possible complications of second and third trimesters

Expected Outcome *Woman will correctly list signs of potential complications that can occur during the second and third trimesters and exhibit no overt signs of stress.*

Nursing Interventions/*Rationales*

- Provide information concerning the potential complications or warning signs that can occur during the second and third trimesters, including possible causes of signs and the importance of calling the health care provider immediately *to ensure identification and treatment of problems in a timely manner.*
- Provide a written list of complications *to have a reference list for emergencies.*

THIRD TRIMESTER

NURSING DIAGNOSIS Fear related to deficient knowledge regarding the onset of labor and the processes of labor related to inexperience, as evidenced by woman's questions and statement of concerns

Expected Outcome *Woman will verbalize basic understanding of signs of labor onset and when to call the health care provider, identify resources for childbirth education, and express increasing confidence in readiness to cope with labor.*

Nursing Interventions/*Rationales*

- Provide information regarding signs of labor onset, when to call the health care provider, and give written

NURSING CARE PLAN Discomforts of Pregnancy and Warning Signs—cont'd

information regarding local childbirth education classes *to empower and promote self-management.*

- Promote ongoing effective communication with health care provider *to promote trust and decrease fear of the unknown.*
- Provide the woman with decision-making opportunities *to promote effective coping.*
- Provide opportunity for woman to verbalize fears regarding childbirth *to assist in decreasing fear through discussion.*

NURSING DIAGNOSIS Disturbed sleep patterns related to discomforts or insomnia of third trimester, as evidenced by the woman's report of inadequate rest

Expected Outcome *The woman will report an improvement of quality and quantity of rest and sleep.*

Nursing Interventions/*Rationales*

- Assess current sleep pattern and review need for increased requirement during pregnancy *to identify the need for change in sleep patterns.*
- Suggest change of position to side-lying with pillows between legs or to semi-Fowler position *to increase support and decrease any problems with dyspnea or heartburn.*
- Reinforce the possibility of the use of various sleep aides such as relaxation techniques, reading, and decreased activity before bedtime *to decrease the possibility of anxiety or physical discomforts before bedtime.*

NURSING DIAGNOSIS Ineffective sexuality patterns related to changes in comfort level and fatigue

Expected Outcome *Woman will verbalize feelings regarding changes in sexual desire.*

Nursing Interventions/*Rationales*

- Assess couple's usual sexuality patterns to determine how patterns have been altered by pregnancy.
- Provide information regarding expected changes in sexuality patterns during pregnancy *to correct any misconceptions.*
- Allow the couple to express feelings in a nonjudgmental atmosphere *to promote trust.*
- Refer the couple for counseling as appropriate *to assist the couple in coping with sexuality pattern changes.*
- Suggest alternative sexual positions *to decrease pressure on enlarging abdomen of woman and increase sexual comfort and satisfaction of couple.*

GI, Gastrointestinal.

BOX 7-6

Complementary and Alternative Therapies Used in Pregnancy

MORNING SICKNESS AND HYPEREMESIS

- Acupuncture
- Acupressure (see Fig. 7-18)
- Shiatzu
- Herbal remedies*
  - Peppermint
  - Spearmint
  - Ginger root

RELAXATION AND MUSCLE-ACHE RELIEF

- Yoga
- Biofeedback
- Reflexology
- Therapeutic touch
- Massage

Sources: Born, D., & Barron, M. (2005). Herb use in pregnancy: What nurses should know. *MCN-American Journal of Maternal/Child Nursing,* 30(3), 201-208; Smith, C., Crowther, C., Willson, K., Hotham, N., & McMillian, V. (2004). A randomized controlled trial of ginger to treat nausea and vomiting in pregnancy. *Obstetrics & Gynecology,* 103(4), 639-645; Tiran, D. & Mack, S. (2000). *Complementary therapies for pregnancy and childbirth* (2nd ed.). Edinburgh: Baillière Tindall.

*Some herbs can cause miscarriage, preterm labor, or fetal or maternal injury. Pregnant women should discuss use with pregnancy health care provider, as well as an expert qualified in the use of the herb.

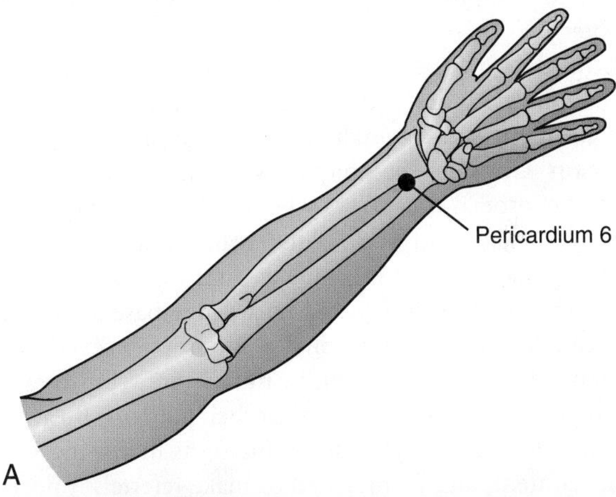

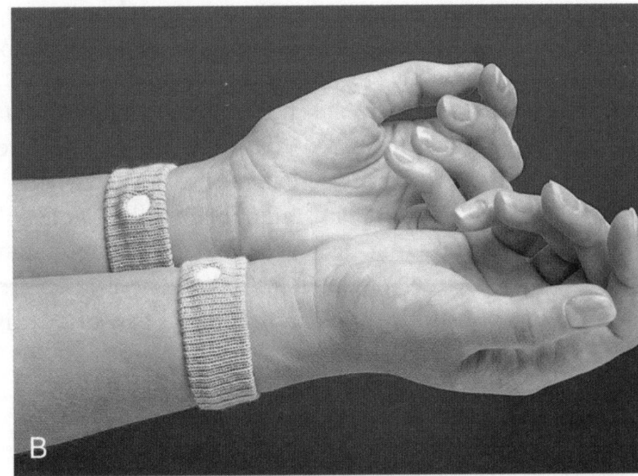

Fig. 7-18 **A,** Pericardium 6 (p6) acupressure point for nausea. **B,** Sea-Bands used for stimulation of acupressure point p6. (**B,** Courtesy Sea-Band International, Newport, RI.)

her family by giving them a printed form, listing the signs and symptoms that necessitate an investigation and the telephone numbers to call with questions or in an emergency. Make sure the form is appropriate for the patient's literacy level, language, and culture.

The nurse must answer questions honestly as they arise during pregnancy. Pregnant women often have difficulty deciding when to report signs and symptoms. Encourage the mother to refer to the printed list of potential complications and to listen to her body. If she senses that something is wrong, she should call her care provider. Several signs and symptoms must be discussed more extensively, including vaginal bleeding, alteration in fetal movements, symptoms of gestational hypertension, rupture of membranes, and preterm labor (see Signs of Potential Complications box on p. 205). See Chapters 20 and 21 for further discussion of complications of pregnancy.

Recognizing preterm labor. Teaching each expectant mother to recognize preterm labor is necessary for early diagnosis and treatment. Preterm labor occurs after the twentieth week but before the thirty-seventh week of pregnancy and consists of uterine contractions that, if untreated, cause the cervix to open earlier than normal and result in preterm birth. Warning signs and symptoms of preterm labor are discussed in Chapter 22.

Sexual counseling. Sexual counseling of expectant couples includes countering misinformation, providing reassurance of normality, and suggesting alternative behaviors. Consider the uniqueness of each couple within a biopsychosocial framework (see the Patient Instructions for Self-Management box). Nurses can initiate discussion about sexual adaptations to make during pregnancy, but they themselves need a sound knowledge base about the physical, social, and emotional responses to sex during pregnancy. Not all maternity nurses are comfortable dealing with the sexual concerns of their patients. Be aware of your personal strengths and limitations in dealing with sexual content, and be prepared to make referrals if necessary (Westheimer & Lopater, 2005).

Many women merely need permission to be sexually active during pregnancy. Many other women, however, need information about the physiologic changes that occur during pregnancy and to have the myths that are associated with sex during pregnancy dispelled. Many women also need to participate in open discussions of intercourse positions that decrease pressure on the gravid abdomen (Westheimer & Lopater, 2005). These tasks are the nurse's responsibility and are an integral part of health care.

Some couples will need a referral for sex therapy or family therapy. Couples with long-standing problems with sexual dysfunction that are intensified by pregnancy are candidates for sex therapy. Whenever a sexual problem is a symptom of a more serious relationship problem the couple would benefit from family therapy.

Countering misinformation. Many myths and much of the misinformation related to sex and pregnancy are masked by seemingly unrelated issues. For example, a discussion about the baby's ability to hear and see in utero may be prompted by questions about the baby being an "unseen observer" of the couple's lovemaking. Be extremely sensitive to the questions behind such questions when counseling in this highly charged emotional area.

Suggesting alternative behaviors. Research has not demonstrated conclusively that coitus and orgasm are contraindicated at any time during pregnancy for the obstetrically and medically healthy woman (Cunningham et al., 2005). However, a history of more than one miscarriage, a threatened miscarriage in the first trimester, impending miscarriage in the second trimester, and PROM, bleeding, or abdominal pain during the third trimester make caution necessary when coitus and orgasm are involved.

Couples can use solitary and mutual masturbation and oral-genital intercourse as alternatives to penile-vaginal intercourse. Partners who enjoy cunnilingus (oral stimulation of the clitoris or vagina) may feel "turned off" by the normal increase in the amount and odor of vaginal discharge during pregnancy. Caution couples who practice cunnilingus against the blowing of air into the vagina, particularly during the last few weeks of pregnancy when the cervix may be slightly open. An air embolism can occur if air is forced between the uterine wall and the fetal membranes and enters the maternal vascular system through the placenta.

Showing the woman or couple pictures of possible variations of coital position is often helpful (Fig. 7-19). The female-superior, side-by-side, rear-entry, and side-lying positions are possible alternative positions to the traditional male-superior position. The woman astride (superior position) allows her to control the angle and depth of penile penetration, as well as to protect her breasts and abdomen. Some women prefer the side-by-side position or any position that places less pressure on the pregnant abdomen and requires less energy during the third trimester.

Multiparous women sometimes have significant breast tenderness in the first trimester. Recommend a coital position that avoids direct pressure on the woman's breasts and decreased breast fondling during love play to such couples. Also, reassure the woman that this condition is normal and temporary.

Some women complain of lower abdominal cramping and backache after orgasm during the first and third trimesters. A back rub can often relieve some of the discomfort and provide a pleasant experience. A tonic uterine contraction, often lasting up to a minute, replaces the rhythmic contractions of orgasm during the third trimester. Changes in the FHR without fetal distress also have been reported.

PATIENT INSTRUCTIONS FOR SELF-MANAGEMENT

Sexuality in Pregnancy

- Be aware that maternal physiologic changes, such as breast enlargement, nausea, fatigue, abdominal changes, perineal enlargement, leukorrhea, pelvic vasocongestion, and orgasmic responses, may affect sexuality and sexual expression.
- Discuss responses to pregnancy with your partner.
- Keep in mind that cultural prescriptions ("dos") and proscriptions ("don'ts") may affect your responses.
- Although your libido may be depressed during the first trimester, it often increases during the second and third trimesters.
- Discuss and explore the following with your partner:
  - Alternative behaviors (e.g., mutual masturbation, foot massage, cuddling)
  - Alternative positions (e.g., female superior, side-lying) for sexual intercourse
- Intercourse is safe as long as it is not uncomfortable. No correlation exists between intercourse and miscarriage, but observe the following precautions:
  - Abstain from intercourse if you experience uterine cramping or vaginal bleeding; report the event to your caregiver as soon as possible.
  - Abstain from intercourse (or any activity that results in orgasm) if you have a history of cervical incompetence until the problem is corrected.
- Continue to use risk reducing behaviors. Women at risk for acquiring or conveying STIs are encouraged to use condoms during sexual intercourse throughout pregnancy.

STI, Sexually transmitted infection.

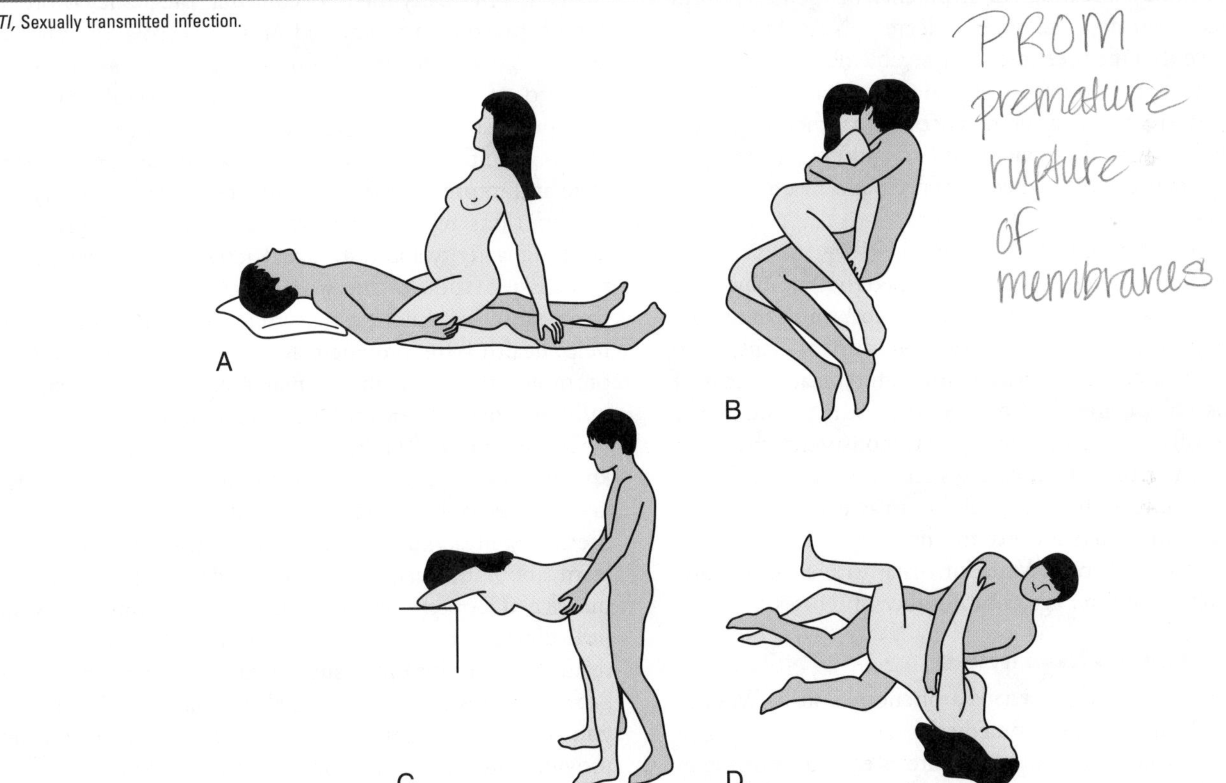

Fig. 7-19 Positions for sexual intercourse during pregnancy. **A,** Female superior. **B,** Side by side. **C,** Rear entry. **D,** Side-lying, facing each other.

The objective of risk-reduction measures is to provide prophylaxis against the acquisition and transmission of STIs (e.g., herpes simplex virus [HSV], HIV). Because these diseases may be transmitted to the woman and her fetus the use of condoms is recommended throughout pregnancy if the woman is at risk for acquiring an STI.

Well-informed nurses who are comfortable with their own sexuality and the sexual counseling needs of expectant couples can offer information and advice in this important but often neglected area. They can establish an open environment in which couples can feel free to introduce their concerns about sexual adjustment and seek support and guidance.

Psychosocial support

Esteem, affection, trust, concern, consideration of cultural and religious responses, and listening are all components of the emotional support given to the pregnant woman and her family. The woman's satisfaction with her relationships–partner and familial–and their support, her feeling of competence, and her sense of being in control are important issues to address in the third trimester. A discussion of fetal responses to stimuli, such as sound and light, as well as patterns of sleeping and waking, is helpful. Other issues of concern that may arise for the pregnant woman and couple include fear of pain, loss of control, and possible birth of the infant before reaching the hospital. Couples often have anxieties about parenthood and parental concerns about the safety of the mother and unborn child or about siblings and their acceptance of the new baby. Some other parental concerns include social and economic responsibilities and parental concerns arising from conflicts in cultural, religious, or personal value systems. In addition, the father's or partner's commitment to the pregnancy and to the couple's relationship and concerns about sexuality and its expression are topics for discussion for many couples. Providing the prospective mother and father with an opportunity to discuss their concerns and validating the normality of their responses can meet their needs to varying degrees. Nurses must also recognize that men feel more vulnerable during their partner's pregnancy. Anticipatory guidance and health promotion strategies can help partners cope with their concerns. Health care providers can stimulate and encourage open dialogue between the expectant father and mother.

Variations in prenatal care

The course of prenatal care described thus far may seem to suggest that the experiences of childbearing women are similar and that nursing interventions are uniformly consistent across all populations. Although typical patterns of response to pregnancy are easy to recognize and many aspects of prenatal care indeed are consistent, pregnant women enter the health care system with individual concerns and needs. The nurse's ability to assess unique needs and to tailor interventions to the individual is key to providing quality care. Variations that influence prenatal care include culture, age, and number of fetuses.

Cultural Influences

Prenatal care as we know it is a phenomenon of Western medicine. In the U.S. biomedical model of care, women are encouraged to seek prenatal care as early as possible in their pregnancy by visiting a physician, a nurse-midwife, or both. Such visits are usually routine and follow a systematic sequence as previously described. This model not only is unfamiliar but also seems strange to women of other cultures.

Many cultural variations can be found in prenatal care. Even if the prenatal care described is familiar to a woman, some practices may conflict with the beliefs and practices of a subculture group to which she belongs. Because of these and other factors, such as lack of money, lack of transportation, and language barriers, women from diverse cultures do not participate in the prenatal care system, for instance, by keeping prenatal appointments.

A concern for modesty is also a reason why many women avoid prenatal care. For some women, exposing body parts, especially to a man, is a major violation of their modesty. For many women, invasive procedures, such as a vaginal examination, are so threatening that they cannot even discuss them with their own husbands; therefore many women prefer a female health care provider. Too often, health care providers assume women lose this modesty during pregnancy and labor, but actually, most women value and appreciate efforts to maintain their modesty.

For many cultural groups a physician is appropriate only in times of illness. Because pregnancy is considered a normal process and the woman is in a state of health, the services of a physician are considered inappropriate. Even if what are considered problems with pregnancy by standards of Western medicine do develop, other cultural groups may not perceive these as problems.

Although many people consider pregnancy normal, certain practices are expected of women of all cultures to ensure a good outcome. **Cultural prescriptions** tell women what to do, and **cultural proscriptions** establish taboos. The purposes of these practices are to prevent maternal illness resulting from a pregnancy-induced imbalanced state and to protect the vulnerable fetus. Prescriptions and proscriptions regulate the woman's emotional response, clothing, activity and rest, sexual activity, and dietary practices. Exploration of the woman's beliefs, perceptions of the meaning of childbearing, and health care practices may help health care providers foster her self-actualization, promote attainment of the maternal role, and positively influence her relationship with her spouse.

To provide culturally sensitive care, you need to be knowledgeable about practices and customs, although knowing everything about every culture and subculture or the many lifestyles that exist is not possible. You should learn about the varied cultures in which specific nurses practice (Cooper, Grywalski, Lamp, Newhouse, & Studlien, 2007). When exploring cultural beliefs and practices related to childbearing, support and nurture those that promote physical or emotional adaptation. However, if you identify potentially harmful beliefs or activities, provide education and propose modifications.

Emotional responses

Virtually all cultures emphasize the importance of maintaining a socially harmonious and agreeable environment for a pregnant woman. An absence of stress is important in ensuring a successful outcome for the mother and baby. Harmony with other people must be fostered, and visits from extended family members may be required to demonstrate pleasant and noncontroversial relationships. If discord exists in a relationship, it is usually managed in culturally prescribed ways.

Besides proscriptions regarding food, other proscriptions involve forms of magic. For example, some Mexicans believe that pregnant women should not witness an eclipse of the moon because it may cause a cleft palate in the infant. They also believe that exposure to an earthquake may precipitate preterm birth, miscarriage, or even a breech presentation. In some cultures a pregnant woman must not ridicule someone with an affliction for fear her child might be born with the same handicap. A mother should not hate a person lest her child resemble that person, and dental work should not be performed because it may cause a baby to have a "harelip." A widely held folk belief in some cultures is that the pregnant woman should refrain from raising her arms above her head because such movement ties knots in the umbilical cord and may cause it to wrap around the baby's neck. Another belief is that placing a knife under the bed of a laboring woman will "cut" her pain.

Clothing

Although most cultural groups do not prescribe specific clothing to wear during pregnancy, modesty is an expectation of many. Some Mexican women of the Southwest wear a cord beneath the breasts and knotted over the umbilicus. This cord, called a *muñeco,* is thought to prevent morning sickness and ensure a safe birth. Some wear amulets, medals, and beads as protection against evil spirits.

Physical activity and rest

Norms that regulate the physical activity of mothers during pregnancy vary tremendously. Many groups, including Native Americans and some Asian groups, encourage women to be active, to walk, and to engage in normal, although not strenuous, activities to ensure that the baby is healthy and not too large. Conversely, other groups such as Filipinos believe that any activity is dangerous, and others willingly take over the work of the pregnant woman. Some Filipinos believe that this inactivity protects the mother and child. The mother is encouraged only to produce the succeeding generation. If health care providers do not know of this belief, they could misinterpret this behavior as laziness or noncompliance with the desired prenatal health care regimen. The nurse needs to find out the way each pregnant woman views activity and rest.

Sexual activity

In most cultures, sexual activity is not prohibited until the end of pregnancy. Some Latinos view sexual activity as necessary to keep the birth canal lubricated. Conversely, some Vietnamese may have definite proscriptions against sexual intercourse, requiring abstinence throughout the pregnancy because they believe that sexual intercourse may harm the mother and fetus.

Diet

Nutritional information given by Western health care providers may also be a source of conflict for many cultural groups, but many health care providers do not know such a conflict exists unless they understand the dietary beliefs and practices of the people for whom they are caring. For example, Muslims have strict regulations regarding preparation of food, and if meat cannot be prepared as prescribed, they may leave out meats from their diets. Many cultures permit pregnant women to eat only warm foods.

Age Differences

The age of the childbearing couple may have a significant influence on their physical and psychosocial adaptation to pregnancy. Normal developmental processes that occur in both very young and older mothers are interrupted by pregnancy and require a different type of adaptation to pregnancy than that of the woman of typical childbearing age. Although nurses need to recognize the individuality of each pregnant woman regardless of age, special needs exist for expectant mothers 15 years of age or younger or those 35 years of age or older.

Adolescents

Critical Thinking Exercise: Teenage Pregnancy

Teenage pregnancy is a worldwide problem. Approximately 1 million adolescents in the United States, or 4 out of every 10 girls, become pregnant each year. Most of the pregnancies are unintended. Adolescents are responsible for almost 450,000 births in the United States annually. Hispanic adolescents currently have the highest birth rate, although the rate for African-American adolescents is also high (Martin et al., 2008). Most of these young women are unmarried, and many are not ready for the emotional, psychosocial, and financial responsibilities of parenthood.

Despite these alarming statistics and the fact that the United States has the highest adolescent birth rate in the industrialized world the birth rate for adolescents steadily declined from 1991 to 2005 but rose 3% in 2006 (Martin et al., 2008). Numerous adolescent pregnancy-prevention programs have had varying degrees of success. Characteristics of programs that make a difference are those that have sustained commitment to adolescents over a long time, involve the parents and other adults in the community, promote abstinence and personal responsibility, and assist adolescents to develop a clear strategy for reaching future goals such as a college education or a career.

When adolescents do become pregnant and decide to give birth, they are much less likely than older women to receive adequate prenatal care, with many receiving no care at all. These young women also are more likely to smoke and less likely to gain adequate weight during pregnancy. As a result of these and other factors, babies born to adolescents are at greatly increased risk of LBW, of serious and long-term disability, and of dying during the first year of life (Chedraui, 2008).

Delayed entry into prenatal care is often the result of late recognition of pregnancy, denial of pregnancy, or confusion about the available services. Such a delay in care may leave an inadequate time before birth to attend to correctable problems. The very young pregnant adolescent

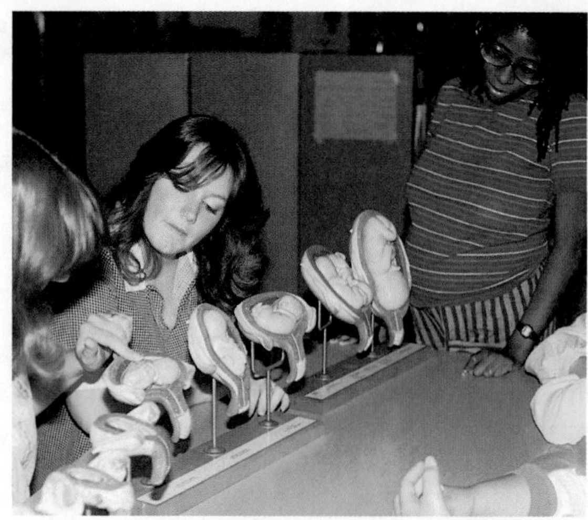

Fig. 7-20 Pregnant adolescents reviewing fetal development. (Courtesy Marjorie Pyle, RNC, Lifecircle, Costa Mesa, CA.)

is at higher risk for each of the variables associated with poor pregnancy outcomes (e.g., socioeconomic factors) and for conditions associated with a first pregnancy regardless of age (e.g., gestational hypertension). The role of the nurse in reducing the risks and consequences of adolescent pregnancy is very important as adolescents often see the nurse as trustworthy and someone who will keep their confidence, as well as provide them with accurate information. Therefore effective communication is essential in providing care to the pregnant adolescent (King-Jones, 2008) (Fig. 7-20) (Nursing Care Plan).

Women older than 35 years

Two groups of older parents have emerged in the population of women having a child late in their childbearing years. One group consists of women who have many children or who have an additional child during the menopausal period. The other group consists of women who have deliberately delayed childbearing until their late thirties or early forties.

Multiparous women. Multiparous women may have never used contraceptives because of personal choice or lack of knowledge concerning contraceptives. They may also be women who have used contraceptives successfully during the childbearing years, but as menopause approaches, they may cease menstruating regularly or stop using contraceptives and consequently become pregnant. The older multiparous woman may believe that pregnancy separates her from her peer group and that her age is a hindrance to close associations with young mothers. Other parents welcome the unexpected infant as evidence of continuing maternal and paternal roles.

Primiparous women. The number of first-time pregnancies in women between the ages of 35 and 40 years has increased significantly over the last three decades (Martin et al., 2007). Seeing women in their late thirties or forties during their first pregnancy is no longer unusual for health care providers. Reasons for delaying pregnancy include a desire to obtain advanced education, career priorities, and use of better contraceptive measures. Women who are infertile do not delay pregnancy deliberately but may become pregnant at a later age as a result of fertility studies and therapies.

These women choose parenthood. They are often successfully established in a career and a lifestyle with a partner that includes time for self-attention, the establishment of a home with accumulated possessions, and freedom to travel. When asked the reason they chose pregnancy later in life, many reply, "Because time is running out."

The dilemma of choice includes the recognition that being a parent will have positive and negative consequences. Couples should discuss the consequences of childbearing and childrearing before committing themselves to this lifelong venture. Partners in this group seem to share the preparation for parenthood, planning for a family-centered birth, and desire to be loving and competent parents; however, the reality of child care may prove difficult for such parents.

First-time mothers older than 35 years select the "right time" for pregnancy. Their awareness of the increasing possibility of infertility or of genetic defects in the infants of older women often influence their timing. Such women seek information about pregnancy from books, friends, and electronic resources. They actively try to prevent fetal disorders and are careful in searching for the best possible maternity care. They identify sources of stress in their lives. They have concerns about having enough energy and stamina to meet the demands of parenting and their new roles and relationships.

If older women become pregnant after treatment for infertility, they may suddenly have negative or ambivalent feelings about the pregnancy. They may experience a multifetal pregnancy that may create emotional and physical problems. Adjusting to parenting two or more infants requires adaptability and additional resources.

During pregnancy, parents explore the possibilities and responsibilities of changing identities and new roles. They must prepare a safe and nurturing environment during pregnancy and after birth. They must integrate the child into an established family system and negotiate new roles (parent roles, sibling roles, grandparent roles) for family members.

Adverse perinatal outcomes are more common in older primiparas than in younger women, even when they receive good prenatal care. Suplee, Dawley, and Bloch (2007) reported that women aged 35 years and older are more likely than younger primiparas to have LBW infants, premature birth, and multiple births. The occurrence of these complications is quite stressful for the new parents, and nursing interventions that provide information and psychosocial support are needed, as well as care for physical needs. In addition, women age 35 years or older have

NURSING CARE PLAN Pregnant Adolescent

NURSING DIAGNOSIS Imbalanced nutrition: less than body requirements related to intake insufficient to meet metabolic needs of fetus and adolescent patient

Expected Outcomes *Pregnant adolescent will gain weight as prescribed by age, take prenatal vitamins and iron as prescribed, and maintain normal hematocrit and hemoglobin.*

Nursing Interventions/*Rationales*

- Assess current diet history and intake *to determine prescriptions for additions or changes in present dietary pattern.*
- Compare prepregnancy weight with current weight *to determine if pattern is consistent with appropriate fetal growth and development.*
- Provide information concerning food prescriptions for appropriate weight gain, considering preferences for "fast food" and peer influences *to correct any misconceptions and increase chances for compliance with the diet.*
- Include pregnant adolescent's immediate family or support system during instruction *to ensure that person preparing family meals receives information.*

NURSING DIAGNOSIS Risk for injury, maternal or fetal, related to inadequate prenatal care and screening

Expected Outcomes *Pregnant adolescent will experience uncomplicated pregnancy and deliver a healthy fetus at term.*

Nursing Interventions/*Rationales*

- Provide information using therapeutic communication and confidentiality *to establish a helpful relationship and build trust.*
- Discuss importance of ongoing prenatal care and possible risks to adolescent patient and fetus *to reinforce that ongoing assessment is crucial to health and well-being of patient and fetus, even if she feels well.* The pregnant adolescent is at greater risk for certain complications that are manageable or preventable if prenatal visits are maintained.
- Discuss risks of alcohol, tobacco, and recreational drug use during pregnancy *to minimize risks to pregnant adolescent and fetus, because adolescent patient has a higher abuse rate than the rest of the pregnant population.*
- Assess for evidence of sexually transmitted infection (STI) and provide information regarding safer sexual practice *to minimize the risk to the patient and fetus because the adolescent is at greater risk for STIs.*
- Screen for preeclampsia on an ongoing basis *to minimize risk because the adolescent population is at greater risk for preeclampsia.*

NURSING DIAGNOSIS Social isolation related to body image changes of pregnant adolescent, as evidenced by patient statements and concerns

Expected Outcomes *Pregnant adolescent will identify support systems and report decreased feelings of social isolation.*

Nursing Interventions/*Rationales*

- Establish a therapeutic relationship *to listen objectively and establish trust.*
- Discuss with pregnant adolescent changes in relationships that have occurred as a result of the pregnancy *to determine extent of isolation from family, peers, and father of the baby.*
- Provide referrals and resources appropriate for developmental stage of adolescent *to give information for patient support.*
- Provide information regarding parenting classes, breastfeeding classes, and childbirth-preparation classes *to give further information and group support, which lessens social isolation.*

NURSING DIAGNOSIS Interrupted family processes related to adolescent pregnancy

Expected Outcome *Pregnant adolescent will reestablish relationship with her mother and the father of baby.*

Nursing Interventions/*Rationales*

- Encourage communication with mother *to clarify roles and relationships related to birth of infant.*
- Encourage communication with father of baby (if she desires continued contact) *to determine the level of support to be expected of the father of the baby.*
- Refer to support group *to learn more effective ways of problem solving and reducing conflict within the family.*

NURSING DIAGNOSIS Disturbed body image related to situational crisis of pregnancy

Expected Outcome *Pregnant adolescent will verbalize positive comments regarding her body image during the pregnancy.*

Nursing Interventions/*Rationales*

- Assess pregnant adolescent's perception of self related to pregnancy *to provide basis for further interventions.*
- Give information regarding expected body changes occurring during pregnancy *to provide a realistic view of these temporary changes.*
- Provide opportunity to discuss personal feelings and concerns *to promote trust and support.*

NURSING DIAGNOSIS Risk for impaired parenting related to immaturity and lack of experience in new role of adolescent mother

Expected Outcome *Parents will demonstrate parenting roles with confidence.*

Nursing Interventions/*Rationales*

- Provide information on growth and development *to enhance knowledge so that adolescent mother can have basis for caring for her infant.*
- Refer to parenting classes *to enhance knowledge and obtain support for providing appropriate care to the newborn and infant.*
- Initiate discussion of child care *to assist adolescent in problem solving for future needs.*
- Assess parenting abilities of the adolescent mother and father *to provide a baseline for education.*
- Provide information on parenting classes that are appropriate for parents' developmental stage *to give opportunity to share common feelings and concerns.*
- Assist parents *to identify pertinent support systems to give assistance with parenting as needed.*

an increased risk of maternal mortality. Pregnancy-related deaths result from hemorrhage, infection, embolisms, hypertensive disorders of pregnancy, cardiomyopathy, and strokes (Johnson, Gregory, & Niebyl, 2007).

Multifetal pregnancy

When the pregnancy involves more than one fetus, **multifetal pregnancy**, both the mother and fetuses are at increased risk for adverse outcomes. The maternal blood volume increases, resulting in an increased strain on the maternal cardiovascular system. Anemia often develops because of a greater demand for iron by the fetuses. Marked uterine distention and increased pressure on the adjacent viscera and pelvic vasculature and diastasis of the two rectus abdominis muscles (see Fig. 6-13, *B*) may occur. Placenta previa develops more commonly in multifetal pregnancies because of the large size or placement of the placentas (Gilbert, 2007). Premature separation of the placenta may occur before the second and any subsequent fetuses are born.

Twin pregnancies often end in prematurity. Spontaneous rupture of membranes before term is common. Congenital malformations are twice as common in monozygotic twins as in singletons, although no increase has been noted in the incidence of congenital anomalies in dizygotic twins. In addition, two-vessel cords–that is, cords with a vein and a single umbilical artery instead of two–occur more often in twins than in singletons, but this abnormality is most common in monozygotic twins. The clinical diagnosis of multifetal pregnancy is accurate in approximately 90% of cases. The likelihood of a multifetal pregnancy increases if any one or a combination of the following factors is present:

- History of dizygous twins in the female lineage
- Use of fertility drugs
- More rapid uterine growth for the number of weeks of gestation
- Hydramnios
- Palpation of more than the expected number of small or large parts
- Asynchronous fetal heartbeats or more than one fetal electrocardiographic tracing
- Ultrasonographic evidence of more than one fetus

The diagnosis of multifetal pregnancy can come as a shock to many expectant parents, and many need additional support and education to help them cope with the changes they face. The mother needs nutrition counseling so that she gains more weight than that needed for a singleton birth, counseling that maternal adaptations will probably be more uncomfortable, and information about the possibility of a preterm birth.

If the presence of more than three fetuses is diagnosed, then the parents may receive counseling regarding selective reduction of the pregnancies to reduce the incidence of premature birth and improve the opportunities for the remaining fetuses to grow to term gestation (Cleary-Goldman, Chitkara, & Berkowitz, 2007). This situation may pose an ethical dilemma for many couples, especially those who have worked hard to overcome problems with infertility and have strong values regarding right to life. Initiating a discussion to identify what resources can help the couple (e.g., a minister, priest, or mental health counselor) to make the decision is important because the decision-making process and the procedure itself may be stressful. Most women will have feelings of guilt anger and sadness but most will come to terms with the loss and will bond with the remaining fetus or fetuses (Cleary-Goldman et al.).

The prenatal care given to women with multifetal pregnancies includes changes in the pattern of care and modifications in other aspects such as the amount of weight gained and the nutritional intake necessary. These women often have prenatal visits at least every 2 weeks in the second trimester and weekly thereafter. Ultrasound evaluations are scheduled at 18 to 20 weeks and then every 3 to 4 weeks to monitor the fetal growth and amniotic fluid volume (Cleary-Goldman et al., 2007). In twin gestations the recommended weight gain is 16 to 20 kg. Iron and vitamin supplementation is desirable. As preeclampsia and eclampsia increase in multifetal pregnancies, nurses work intensively to prevent, identify, and treat these complications of pregnancy.

The considerable uterine distention involved can cause the backache commonly experienced by pregnant women to be even worse. Women can wear maternal support hose to control leg varicosities. If risk factors such as premature dilation of the cervix or bleeding are present, abstinence from orgasm and nipple stimulation during the last trimester helps prevent preterm labor. Some practitioners recommend bed rest beginning at 20 weeks in women carrying multiple fetuses to prevent preterm labor. Other practitioners question the value of prolonged bed rest. If bed rest is recommended, then the mother assumes a lateral position to promote increased placental perfusion. If birth is delayed until after the thirty-sixth week, the risk of morbidity and mortality decreases for the neonates.

Multiple newborns will likely place a strain on finances, space, workload, and the woman and family's coping capability. Lifestyle changes are often necessary. Parents will need assistance in making realistic plans for the care of the babies (e.g., whether to breastfeed and whether to raise them as "alike" or as separate persons). Refer parents to national and local organizations such as Parents of Twins and Triplets (www.potato.org), Mothers of Twins (www.nomot.org), and the La Leche League (lalecheleague.org) for further support.

CHILDBIRTH AND PERINATAL EDUCATION

The goal of childbirth and perinatal education is to assist individuals and their family members to make informed, safe decisions about pregnancy, birth, and early parenthood. This objective is also intended to assist them in comprehending the long-lasting potential that empowering birth experiences have in the lives of women and that early experiences have on the development of children and the family. The perinatal education program is an expansion of the earlier childbirth education movement that originally offered a set of classes in the third trimester of pregnancy to prepare parents for birth. Today, perinatal education programs consist of a menu of class series and activities from preconception through the early months of parenting.

Health-promoting education should be provided in a context that emphasizes how a healthy body is best able to adapt to the changes that accompany pregnancy. Without this context of health, routine care and testing for risks may contribute to a mindset of families that pregnancy is a pathologic as opposed to a healthy mind-body-spirit event.

Some of the decisions the childbearing family must consider are the decision to have a baby, followed by choices of a care provider and type of care (a midwifery model [natural oriented] versus a medical [intervention oriented] model), the place for birth (hospital, birthing center, home), and the type of infant feeding (breast or bottle) and infant care. If a woman has had a previous cesarean birth, she may consider having a vaginal birth. Perinatal education can provide information to help childbearing families make informed decisions about these issues.

Previous pregnancy and childbirth experiences are important elements that influence current learning needs. The woman's (and the support person's) age, cultural background, personal philosophy with regard to childbirth, socioeconomic status, spiritual beliefs, and learning styles are assessed to develop the best plan to help the woman meet her needs.

For the most part, the pregnant woman and her partner attend childbirth education classes, although sometimes a friend, teenage daughter, or parent is the designated support person (Fig. 7-21). In addition, classes for grandparents and siblings can help to prepare them for their attendance at birth and the arrival of the baby (see Fig. 7-4). Siblings often see a film about birth and learn ways they can help welcome the baby. They also learn to cope with changes that include a reduction in parental time and attention. Grandparents learn about current child care practices and how to help their adult children adapt to parenting in a supportive way.

Childbirth Education Programs

Childbirth, when one is prepared and well supported, presents to women a unique and powerful opportunity to find their core strength in a manner that forever changes their self-perception. Expectant parents and their families have different interests and information needs as the pregnancy progresses.

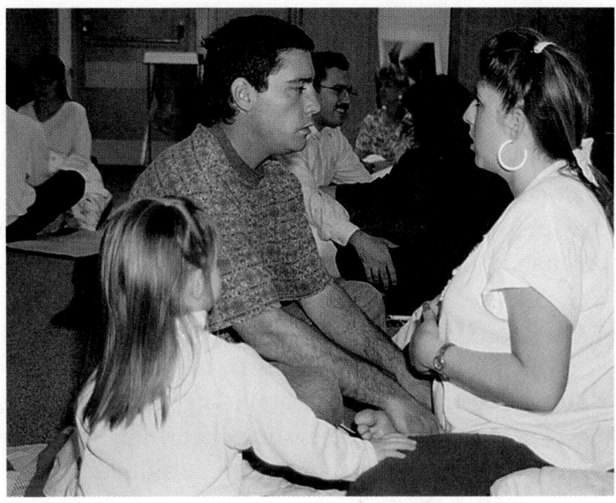

Fig. 7-21 Learning relaxation exercises with the whole family. (Courtesy Marjorie Pyle, RNC, Lifecircle, Costa Mesa, CA.)

Early pregnancy ("early bird") classes provide fundamental information. Classes are developed around the following areas: (1) early fetal development, (2) physiologic and emotional changes of pregnancy, (3) human sexuality, and (4) the nutritional needs of the mother and fetus. These classes often address environmental and workplace hazards. Exercises, nutrition, warning signs, drugs, and self-medication also are topics of interest and concern.

Midpregnancy classes emphasize the woman's participation in self-management. Classes provide information on preparation for breastfeeding and formula feeding, infant care, basic hygiene, common complaints and simple safe remedies, infant health, parenting, and updating and refining the birth plans.

Late pregnancy classes emphasize labor and birth. Different methods of coping with labor and birth can be used, and these methods are often the basis for various prenatal classes, including Lamaze, Bradley, and Dick-Read. These classes usually include a hospital tour.

Current practices in childbirth education

A variety of approaches to childbirth education have evolved as childbirth educators attempt to meet learning needs. In addition to classes designed specifically for pregnant adolescents, their partners, or parents, classes exist for other groups with special learning needs. These classes include those for first-time mothers over age 35, single women, adoptive parents, and parents of multiples or women with handicaps such as those who are visually impaired or deaf. Refresher classes for parents with children not only review coping techniques for labor and birth, but also help couples prepare for sibling reactions and adjustments to a new baby. Cesarean birth classes are available for couples that have this kind of birth scheduled because of breech position or other risk factors. Other classes focus on vaginal birth after cesarean (VBAC), because many women can successfully give birth vaginally after previous cesarean birth.

Throughout the series of classes is a discussion of support systems that people can use during pregnancy and after birth. Such support systems help parents function independently and effectively. During all the classes the open expression of feelings and concerns about any aspect of pregnancy, birth, and parenting is welcomed.

Pain management

Fear of pain in labor is a key issue for pregnant women and the reason many give for attending childbirth education classes. Numerous studies show that women who have received childbirth preparation later report no less pain but do report greater ability to cope with the pain during labor and birth and increased birth satisfaction than unprepared women. Therefore, although pain-management strategies are an essential component of childbirth education, total pain eradication is neither the primary source of birth satisfaction nor a goal. Eliminating suffering is a realistic goal. Control in childbirth, meaning participation in decision making, has repeatedly been the primary source of birth satisfaction.

Couples need information about the advantages and disadvantages of pain medication and about other techniques for coping with labor. An emphasis on nonpharmacologic pain management strategies helps couples manage the labor and birth with dignity and increased comfort. Most instructors teach a flexible approach, which helps couples learn and master many techniques to use during labor. Couples learn techniques such as massage, pressure on the palms or soles of the feet, hot compresses to the perineum, perineal massage, applications of heat or cold, breathing patterns, and focusing of attention on visual or other stimuli as ways to increase coping and decrease the distress from labor pain (see Chapter 10 for further discussion).

Perinatal care choices

The first decision the woman makes often involves who will be her primary health care provider for the pregnancy and birth. This decision is doubly important because it usually affects where the birth will take place.

The Coalition to Improve Maternity Services (CIMS) (2000), a group of more than 50 nursing and maternity care–oriented organizations, produced a document to assist women in selecting their perinatal care. Women are encouraged to ask potential care providers the following questions:

- Who can be with me during labor and birth?
- What happens during a normal labor and birth in your setting?
- How do you allow for differences in culture and beliefs?
- Can I walk and move around during labor? What position do you suggest for birth?
- How do you make sure everything goes smoothly when my nurse, physician, nurse-midwife, or agency work with one another?
- What things do you normally do to a woman in labor?
- How do you help mothers stay as comfortable as they can be? Besides drugs, how do you help mothers relieve the pain of labor?
- What if my baby is born early or has special problems?
- Do you circumcise babies?
- How do you help mothers who want to breastfeed?

Options for care providers

Physicians. Physicians (obstetricians, family practice physicians) attend 91.6% of births in the United States and Canada (Martin et al., 2007). They see low and high risk patients. Care often includes pharmacologic and medical management of problems as well as use of technologic procedures. Family practice physicians may need backup by obstetricians if a specialist is needed for a problem (e.g., a cesarean birth). Most physicians manage births in a hospital setting.

Nurse-midwives. Nurse-midwives are registered nurses with advanced training in care of obstetric patients. They provide care for more than 8% of the births in the United States and Canada (Martin et al., 2007). Certified nurse-midwives (CNMs) may practice with physicians or independently with a contracted health care provider agency for physician backup. They usually see low risk obstetric patients. Care is often noninterventionist, and they often encourage the woman and her family to be active participants in the care. Nurse-midwives refer patients to physicians for complications. Most births (approximately 94%) are managed in hospital settings or alternative birth centers; a small number are managed in a home setting.

Direct-entry midwives. *Direct-entry midwives* (also called certified professional midwives) are trained through self-study, apprenticeship, midwifery schools, or universities as a profession distinct from nursing. However, their certification process is administered by the American College of Nurse-Midwives. They manage slightly less than 1% of births in the United States; they also refer the patients in whom problems develop to physicians. A majority (61%) of births attended by these midwives take place in the home setting. Because of underreporting of direct-entry midwife–attended births, these data should be considered lower estimates of actual numbers of midwife-attended births.

Independent midwives. Independent midwives, who may also be called *lay midwives,* are nonprofessional caregivers. Their training varies greatly, from formal training to self-teaching. Most births are managed in the home setting.

Doulas. A doula is professionally trained to provide labor support, including physical, emotional, and informational support to women and their partners during labor and birth. The doula does not become involved with clinical tasks (Doulas of North America [DONA], 2008). Today, many couples, no matter which type of childbirth classes they take, also employ a doula for labor support. A Cochrane synopsis of 16 trials involving 13,391 women found that "continuous labor support like that provided by doulas reduces a woman's likelihood of having pain medication, increases her satisfaction and chances for spontaneous birth, and has no known risks" (Hodnett, Gates, Hofmeyr, & Sakala, 2007).

A doula typically meets with the woman and her husband or partner before labor. At this meeting, she ascertains the woman's expectations and desires for the birth experience. With this information as her guide during labor and birth the doula focuses her efforts on assisting the woman to achieve her goals. Doulas work collaboratively with other health care providers and the husband or other supportive individuals, but their primary goal is assisting the woman.

Doulas may be found through community contacts, other health care providers, or childbirth educators; several organizations offer information or referral services. The expectant mother should be comfortable with the doula who will be attending her. Box 7-7 lists questions to ask when arranging for a doula. Doulas of North America (DONA) is an organization that certifies doulas (www.dona.com). Although the doula role originally developed as an assistant during labor, some women benefit from assistance during the postpartum period. The number of postnatal doulas who provide assistance to the new mother as she develops competence with infant care, feeding, and other maternal tasks is small but growing.

BOX 7-7

Questions to Ask When Choosing a Doula

To discover the specific training, experience, and services offered by anyone who provides labor support, potential patients, nursing supervisors, physicians, midwives, and others should ask the following questions of that person:

- What training have you had?
- Tell me about your experience with birth, personally and as a doula.
- What is your philosophy about childbirth and supporting women and their partners through labor?
- May we meet to discuss our birth plans and the role you will play in supporting me through childbirth?
- May we call you with questions or concerns before and after the birth?
- When do you try to join women in labor? Do you come to our home or meet us at the hospital?
- Do you meet with us after the birth to review the labor and answer questions?
- Do you work with one or more backup doulas for times when you are not available? May we meet them?
- What is your fee?

Source: Doulas of North America (DONA). (2008). *Doulas of North America position paper: The doula's contribution to modern maternity care.* Internet document available at www.dona.org/PDF/QuestionsToAskADoula.pdf (accessed May 20, 2009).

Birth plans

Once the maternity care provider is chosen, numerous other decisions must to be made over the course of the perinatal year. Many prenatal care providers and childbirth educators encourage expectant parents to develop a birth plan to identify their options and set priorities. The **birth plan** is a natural evolution of a contemporary wellness-oriented lifestyle in which patients assume a level of responsibility for their own health. For some people, beginning this approach to perinatal care will influence their approach to health care throughout their lives. The birth plan is a tool with which parents can explore their childbirth options and choose those that are most important to them. The plan must be viewed as tentative since the realities of what is feasible may change as the actual labor and birth unfold. It is understood to be a preference list based on a best-case scenario (see further discussion in Chapter 12).

Case Study: Third Trimester

Birth setting choices

With careful thought, the concept of natural or family- or woman-centered maternity care can be implemented in any setting. The three primary options for birth settings today are the hospital, birth center, and home. Women consider several factors in choosing a setting for childbirth, including the preference of their health care provider, characteristics of the birthing unit, and preference of their third-party payer. Approximately 99% of all births in the United States take place in a hospital setting (Martin et al., 2007). However, the types of labor and birth services vary greatly, from the traditional labor and delivery rooms with separate postpartum and newborn units to in-hospital birthing centers where all or almost all care takes place in a single unit.

Labor, delivery, recovery, and postpartum (birthing) rooms. Labor, delivery, and recovery (LDR) and labor, delivery, recovery, and postpartum (LDRP) rooms offer families a comfortable, private space for childbirth (Fig. 7-22). Women are admitted to LDR units, labor and give birth, and spend the first 1 to 2 hours postpartum there for immediate recovery and to have time with their families to bond with their newborns. After this period of recovery the mothers and newborns move to a postpartum unit and nursery or mother-baby unit for the duration of their stay.

In LDRP units the same nursing staff usually provides total care from admission through postpartum discharge. The woman and her family may stay in this unit for 6 to 48 hours after giving birth. The units are furnished to provide a homelike atmosphere, as LDR units are, but have accommodations for family members to stay overnight.

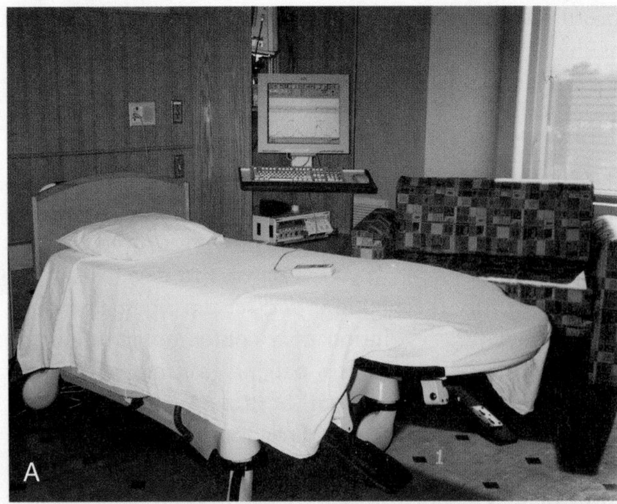

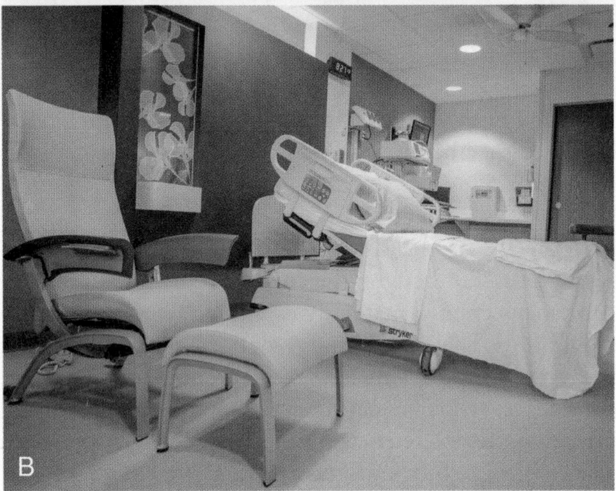

Fig. 7-22 Labor, delivery, recovery, and postpartum (LDRP) units. (*A*, Courtesy Dee Lowdermilk, Chapel Hill, NC. *B*, Courtesy Mercy Hospital, St. Louis, MO.)

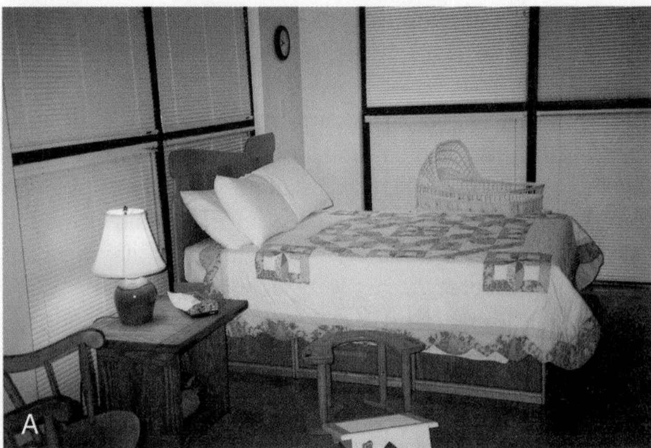

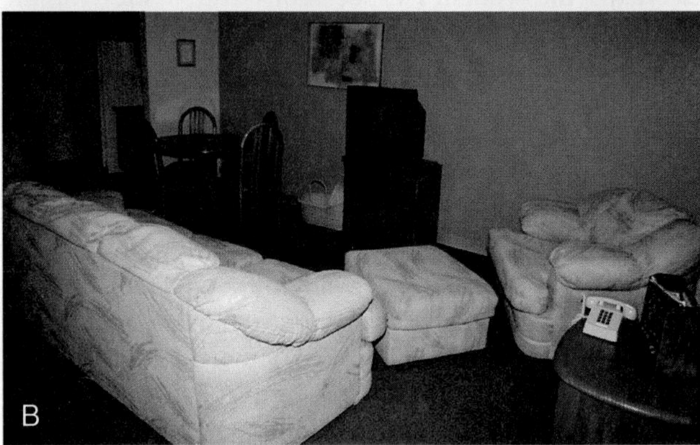

Fig. 7-23 Birth center. **A**, Note double bed, baby crib, and birthing stool. **B**, Lounge and kitchen. (**A**, Courtesy Dee Lowdermilk, Chapel Hill, NC. Photo location: The Women's Birth and Wellness Center; **B**, courtesy Michael S. Clement, MD, Mesa, AZ. Photo location: Bethany Birth Center, Phoenix, AZ.)

Both units have fetal monitors, emergency resuscitation equipment for both mother and newborn, and heated cribs or warming units for the newborn. This equipment is often out of sight in cabinets or closets when it is not being used.

Birth centers. Freestanding birth centers are usually built in locations separate from the hospital but are often located nearby in case transfer of the woman or newborn is needed. These birth centers offer families a safe and cost-effective alternative to hospital or home birth. Approximately 27% of the out-of-hospital births are in birthing centers (Martin et al., 2007). The centers are usually staffed by nurse-midwives or physicians who also have privileges at the local hospital. Only women at low risk for complications are included for care. Attendance at childbirth and parenting classes is required of all patients. The family is admitted to the birth center for labor and birth and will remain there until discharge, which often takes place within 6 hours of the birth.

Birth centers typically have homelike accommodations, including a double bed for the couple and a crib for the newborn (Fig. 7-23, *A*). Emergency equipment and drugs are usually in cabinets, out of view but easily accessible. Private bathroom facilities are incorporated into each birth unit. The facility may have an early labor lounge or a living room and small kitchen (Fig. 7-23, *B*).

Services provided by the freestanding birth centers include those necessary for safe management during the childbearing cycle. Patients must understand that some situations require transfer to a hospital, and they must agree to abide by those guidelines.

Birth centers, as well as a hospital with a comprehensive birthing program, may have resources for parents such as a lending library that includes books and videotapes; reference files on related topics; recycled maternity clothes, baby clothes, and equipment; and supplies and reference materials for childbirth educators. The centers may also have referral files for community resources that offer services relating to childbirth and early parenting, including support groups (e.g., for single parents, for postbirth support, for parents of twins), genetic counseling, women's issues, and consumer action.

When birth occurs in a birth center or a home setting, it should be located close to a major hospital so that quick transfer to that institution is possible if necessary. Ambulance service and emergency procedures must be readily available. Fees vary with the services provided but are typically less than or equal to those charged by local hospitals. Some base fees on the ability of the family to pay (a reduced-fee sliding scale). Several third-party payers, as well as Medicaid and the Civilian Health and Medical Programs of the Uniformed Services (TRICARE/CHAMPUS), recognize and reimburse these centers.

Home birth. Home birth has always been popular in certain countries, such as Sweden and The Netherlands. In developing countries, hospitals or adequate lying-in facilities often are unavailable to most pregnant women, and home birth is a necessity. In North America, home births account for approximately 65% of the less than 1% of births outside of the hospital setting (Martin et al., 2007).

Although home births are considered countercultural by many people in the United States, no evidence base has been found to discourage low risk couples who desire a carefully planned out-of-the-hospital birth (Johnson & Daviss, 2005). National groups supporting home birth are the Home Oriented Maternity Experience (HOME) and the National Association of Parents for Safe Alternatives in Childbirth (NAPSAC) (www.napsac.org). These groups work to foster more humane childbearing practices at all levels, integrating the alternatives for childbirth to meet the needs of the total population.

One advantage of home birth is that the family is in control of the experience. Another is that the birth may be more physiologically normal in familiar surroundings. The mother may be more relaxed than she would be in the hospital environment. Care providers who participate in home births tend to be more support oriented and less intervention oriented. The family can assist in and be a part of the happy event, and contact with the newborn is immediate and sustained. In addition, home birth may be less expensive than a hospital confinement. Serious infection may be less likely, assuming strict aseptic principles are followed, because people generally are relatively immune to their own home bacteria. A disadvantage of home birth is that if complications occur during labor or birth, timely transfer of care to a hospital setting may be problematic.

KEY POINTS

- The prenatal period is a preparatory one both physically, in terms of fetal growth and parental adaptations, and psychologically, in terms of anticipation of parenthood.
- Pregnancy affects parent-child, sibling-child, and grandparent-child relationships.
- Discomforts and changes of pregnancy can cause anxiety to the woman and her family and require sensitive attention and a plan for teaching self-management measures.
- Education about healthy ways of using the body (e.g., exercise, body mechanics) is essential given maternal anatomic and physiologic responses to pregnancy.
- Important components of the initial prenatal visit include detailed and carefully recorded findings from the interview, a comprehensive physical examination, and selected laboratory tests.
- Even in normal pregnancy the nurse must remain alert to hazards such as supine hypotension, warning signs and symptoms, and signs of family maladaptations.
- BP is evaluated based on absolute values and length of gestation and interpreted in light of modifying factors.
- Each pregnant woman needs to know how to recognize and report preterm labor.
- Childbirth education is a process designed to help parents make the transition from the role of expectant parents to the role and responsibilities of parents of a new baby.
- The likelihood of physical abuse increases during pregnancy.
- Nurses must be knowledgeable about practices and customs related to childbearing to provide culturally sensitive care.
- Cultural prescriptions and proscriptions influence responses to pregnancy and to the health care delivery system.
- Childbirth education teaches tuning into the body's inner wisdom and coping strategies that enhance women's ability to know how to give birth.
- Childbirth education strives to promote healthier pregnancies and family lifestyles.

Audio Chapter Summaries Access an audio summary of these Key Points on evolve

References

Alto, W. (2005). No need for glycosuria/proteinuria screen in pregnant women. *Journal of Family Practice*, *54*(11), 978-983.

American Academy of Pediatrics and American College of Obstetricians and Gynecologists. (2007). *Guidelines for perinatal care* (6th ed.). Washington, DC: Author.

American College of Obstetricians and Gynecologists (ACOG). (2002). Exercise during pregnancy and the postpartum period. ACOG Committee on Obstetric Practice Opinion No. 267. *Obstetrics & Gynecology*, *77*(1), 79-81.

American College of Obstetricians and Gynecologists Committee on Health Care for Underserved Women. (2006). Psychosocial risk factors: Perinatal screening and intervention. ACOG Committee Opinion No. 343. *Obstetrics & Gynecology*, *108*(2), 469-477.

American College of Obstetricians and Gynecologists Committee on Obstetric Practice. (2005). Smoking cessation during pregnancy. ACOG Committee Opinion No. 316, October 2005. *Obstetrics and Gynecology*, *106*(4), 883-888.

American College of Obstetricians and Gynecologists Committee on Obstetric Practice. (2004). Prenatal and perinatal human immunodeficiency virus testing: expanded recommendations. ACOG Committee Opinion No. 304. *Obstetrics and Gynecology*, *104*(5 Part 1), 1119-1124.

American Dental Association. (2009). *Oral health topics: Pregnancy*. Internet document available at www.ada.org/public/topics/pregnancy.asp (accessed June 22, 2009).

American Dietetic Association. (2008). Position of the American Dietetic Association: Nutrition and lifestyle for a healthy pregnancy outcome. *Journal of the American Dietetic Association*, *108*(3), 553-561.

Association of Women's Health, Obstetric and Neonatal Nurses. (2008). *HIV screening procedures for pregnant women and infants. Policy Position Statement*. Washington, DC: AWHONN. Also available at www.awhonn.org (accessed June 22, 2009).

Boggess, K., & Edelstein, B. (2006). Oral health in women during preconception and pregnancy: Implications for birth outcomes and infant oral health. *Maternal Child Health Journal*, *10*(5 supp), S169-S174.

Cesario, S. (2007). Seat belt use in pregnancy: History, misconceptions, and the need for education. *Nursing for Women's Health*, *11*(5), 474-481.

Centers for Disease Control and Prevention. (2008). ACIP: *Guidance for vaccine recommendations in pregnant and breastfeeding women*. Internet document available at www.cdc.gov/vaccines (accessed January 6, 2009).

Chedraui, P. (2008). Pregnancy among young adolescents: trends, risk factors, and maternal-perinatal outcome. *Journal of Perinatal Medicine*, *36*(3), 256-259.

Cleary-Goldman, J., Chitkara, U., & Berkowitz, R. (2007). Multiple gestation. In S. Gabbe, J. Niebyl, & J. Simpson (Eds.), *Obstetrics: Normal and problem pregnancies* (5th ed.). Philadelphia: Churchill Livingstone.

Coalition to Improve Maternity Services. (2000). *Having a baby? Ten questions to ask*. Internet document available at www.motherfriendly.org (accessed June 22, 2009).

Cooper, M., Grywalski, M., Lamp, J., Newhouse, L., & Studlien, R. (2007). Enhancing cultural competence: A model for nurses. *Nursing for Women's Health*, *11*(2), 148-159.

Cunningham, F., Leveno, K., Bloom, S., Hauth, J., Gilstrap, L., & Wenstrom, K. (2005). *Williams obstetrics* (22nd ed.). New York: McGraw-Hill.

Daniels, P., Noe, G., & Mayberry, R. (2006). Barriers to prenatal care among Black women of low socioeconomic status. *American Journal of Health Behavior*, *30*(2), 188-198.

Darby, S. (2007). Pre- and perinatal care of Hispanic families. *Nursing for Women's Health*, *11*(2), 160-169.

Dasanayake, A., Gennaro, S., Hendricks-Munoz, K., & Chhun, N. (2008). Maternal periodontal disease, pregnancy, and neonatal outcomes. *MCN The American Journal of Maternal Child Nursing*, *33*(1), 45-49.

Dawley, K., & Beam, R. (2005). "My nurse taught me how to have a healthy baby and be a good mother." Nurse home visiting with pregnant women 1888 to 2005. *Nursing Clinics of North America*, *40*(4), 803-815.

Doulas of North America (DONA). (2008). Doulas of North America Position Paper: *The doula's contribution to modern maternity care*. Internet document available at www.dona.org (accessed January 6, 2009).

Family Violence Prevention Fund. (2009). *The facts on teens and dating violence*. Internet document available at http://www.endabuse.org/userfiles/file/Teens/teens_facts.pdf (accessed June 20, 2009).

Fries, M., Bashford, M., & Nunes, M. (2005). Implementing prenatal screening for cystic fibrosis in routine obstetric practice. *American Journal of Obstetrics and Gynecology*, *192*(2), 527-534.

Gilbert, E. (2007). *Manual of high risk pregnancy & delivery* (4th ed.). St. Louis: Mosby.

Harris L., & Paltrow, L. (2003). The status of pregnant women and fetuses in U.S. criminal law. *Journal of the American Medical Association*, *289*(13), 1697-1699.

Himmelberger, S. (2002). Preventing group B strep in newborns. *AWHONN Lifelines*, *6*(4), 339-342.

Hodnett, E., Gates, S., Hofmeyr, G., & Sakala, C. (2007). Continuous support for women during childbirth. In *The Cochrane Database of Systematic Reviews* 2007, Issue 3, CD 003766.

Jepson, R., & Craig, J. (2008). Cranberries for preventing urinary tract infections (Cochrane Review). In *The Cochrane Database of Systematic Reviews* 2008, Issue 1, CD 001231.

Johnson, K., & Daviss, B. (2005). Outcomes of planned home births and certified professional midwives: Large prospective study in North America. *British Medical Journal*, *330*(7505), 1416.

Johnson, T., Gregory, K., & Niebyl, J. (2007). Preconception and prenatal care: Part of the continuum. In S. Gabbe, J. Niebyl, & J. Simpson (Eds.), *Obstetrics: Normal and problem pregnancies* (5th ed.). Philadelphia: Churchill Livingstone.

Johnson, A., Hatcher, B., El-Khorazaty, M., Milligan, R., Bhakar, B., Rodan, M., et al. (2007). Determinants of inadequate prenatal care utilization by African American women. *Journal of Health Care for the Poor and Underserved*, *18*(3), 620-636.

Kehringer, K. (2003). Informed consent: Hospitals must obtain informed consent prior to drug testing pregnant patients. *The Journal of Law, Medicine, & Ethics*, *32*(3), 455-457.

King-Jones, T. (2008). Caring for the pregnant adolescent: Perils and pearls of communication. *Nursing for Women's Health*, *12*(2), 114-119.

Kliegman, R. (2006). Intrauterine growth restriction. In R. Martin, A. Fanaroff, & M. Walsh (Eds.). *Fanaroff and Martins's neonatal-perinatal medicine: Diseases of the fetus and infant*. Philadelphia: Mosby.

Kramer, M., & McDonald, S. (2006). Aerobic exercise for women during pregnancy. In *The Cochrane Database of Systematic Reviews* 2006, Issue 2, CD 000180.

Krieger, C. (2008). Intimate partner violence: A review for nurses. *Nursing for Women's Health*, *12*(3), 224-234.

Lawrence, R., & Lawrence, R. (2005). *Breastfeeding: A guide for the medical profession* (6th ed.). Philadelphia: Mosby.

Lederman, R. (1996). *Psychosocial adaptation in pregnancy* (2nd ed.). New York: Springer.

March of Dimes Birth Defects Foundation. (2008). *Drinking alcohol during pregnancy*. Internet document available at www.marchofdimes.com (accessed June 22, 2009).

Martin, J., Hamilton, B., Sutton, P., Ventura, S., Menacker, F., Kirmeyer, S., et al. (2007). Births: Final data for 2005. *National vital statistics reports*, *56*(6). Hyattsville, MD: National Center for Health Statistics.

Martin, J., Kung, H., Mathews, T., Hoyert, D., Strobino, D., Guyer, B., et al. (2008). Annual summary of vital statistics–2006. *Pediatrics*, *121*(4), 788-801.

Massey, Z., Rising, S., & Ickovics, J. (2006). Centering Pregnancy group prenatal care: Promoting relationship-centered care. *Journal of Obstetric, Gynecologic, and Neonatal Nursing, 35*(2), 286-294.

May, K. (1982). Three phases of father involvement in pregnancy. *Nursing Research, 31*(6), 337-342.

Mercer, R. (1995). *Becoming a mother.* New York: Springer.

Moos, M. (2006). Prenatal care: Limitations and opportunities. *Journal of Obstetric, Gynecologic, and Neonatal Nursing, 35*(2), 278-285.

National High Blood Pressure Education Program. (2003). *Seventh Report of the Joint National Committee on Prevention, Detection, Evaluation, and Treatment of High Blood Pressure*, Bethesda, MD: U.S. Department of Health and Human Services, National Institutes of Health, National Heart, Lung, & Blood Institute.

Reid, J. (2007). CenteringPregnancy®: A model for group prenatal care. *Nursing for Women's Health, 11*(4), 382-388.

Rubin, R. (1975). Maternal tasks in pregnancy. *Maternal-Child Nursing Journal, 4*(3), 143-153.

Rubin, R. (1984). *Maternal identity and the maternal experience.* New York: Springer.

Russell, S., & Mayberry, L. (2008). Pregnancy and oral health: A review and recommendation to reduce gaps in practice and research. *MCN The American Journal of Maternal/Child Nursing, 33*(1), 32-37.

Seidel, H., Ball, J., Dains, J., & Benedict, G. (2006). *Mosby's guide to physical examination* (6th ed.). St. Louis: Mosby.

Smeltzer, S. (2007). Pregnancy in women with physical disabilities. *Journal of Obstetric, Gynecologic, and Neonatal Nursing, 36*(1), 88-96.

Suplee, P., Dawley, K., & Bloch, J. (2007). Tailoring peripartum nursing care for women of advanced maternal age. *Journal of Obstetric, Gynecologic, and Neonatal Nursing, 36*(6), 616-623.

Villar, J., Carroli, G., Khan-Neelofur, D., Piaggio, G., & Gulmezoglu, M. (2001). Patterns of routine antenatal care for low-risk pregnancy. In *The Cochrane Database of Systematic Reviews* 2001, Issue 4, CD 000934.

Walker, D., McCully, L., & Vest, V. (2001). Evidence-based prenatal care visits: When less is more. *Journal of Midwifery and Women's Health, 46*(3), 146-151.

Weng, X., Odouli, R., & Li, D. (2008). Maternal caffeine consumption during pregnancy and the risk of miscarriage: A prospective cohort study. *American Journal of Obstetrics and Gynecology, 198*(3), 279e-1 279e-8.

Westheimer, R., & Lopater, S. (2005). *Human sexuality: A psychosocial perspective* (2nd ed.). Philadelphia: Lippincott Williams & Wilkins.

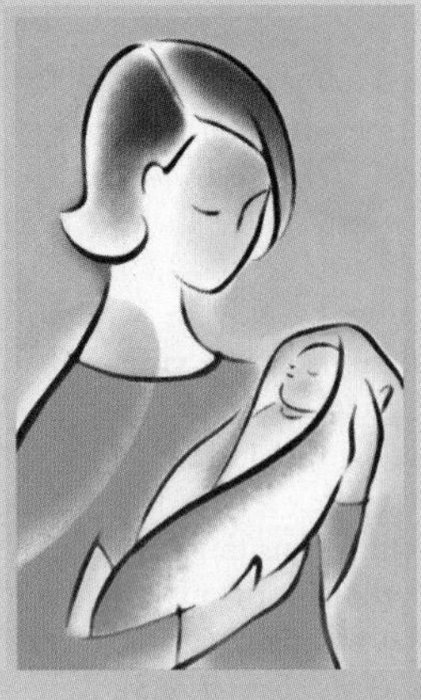

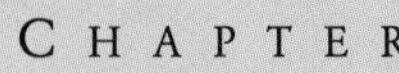

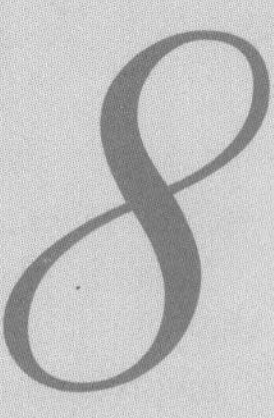

Chapter 8 Maternal and Fetal Nutrition

SHANNON E. PERRY

LEARNING OBJECTIVES

- *Delineate recommended components of nutrition and dietary supplements in the preconception period.*
- *Explain recommended maternal weight gain during pregnancy.*
- *Compare the recommended level of intake of energy sources, protein, and key vitamins and minerals during pregnancy and lactation.*
- *Give examples of the food sources that provide the nutrients required for optimal maternal nutrition during pregnancy and lactation.*
- *Examine the role of nutrition supplements during pregnancy.*
- *List five nutritional risk factors during pregnancy.*
- *Compare the dietary needs of adolescent and mature pregnant women.*
- *Analyze examples of cultural food patterns and possible dietary problems for two ethnic groups or for two alternative eating patterns.*
- *Assess nutritional status during pregnancy.*

KEY TERMS AND DEFINITIONS

Adequate Intakes (AIs) Recommended nutrient intakes estimated to meet the needs of almost all healthy people in the population; provided for nutrients or age-group categories for which the available information is not sufficient to warrant establishing recommended dietary allowances

anthropometric measurements Body measurements, such as height and weight

body mass index (BMI) Method of calculating appropriateness of weight for height (BMI = weight/height^2)

Dietary Reference Intakes (DRIs) Nutritional recommendations for the United States, consisting of the recommended dietary allowances, adequate intakes, and tolerable upper intake levels; the upper limit of intake associated with low risk in almost all members of a population

intrauterine growth restriction (IUGR) Fetal undergrowth from any cause

kcal Kilocalorie; unit of heat content or energy equal to 1000 small calories

lactose intolerance Inherited absence of the enzyme lactase

physiologic anemia Relative excess of plasma leading to a decrease in hemoglobin concentration and hematocrit; normal adaptation during pregnancy

pica Unusual oral craving during pregnancy (e.g., for laundry starch, dirt, red clay)

pyrosis A burning sensation in the epigastric and sternal region from stomach acid (heartburn)

Recommended Dietary Allowances (RDAs) Recommended nutrient intakes estimated to meet the needs of almost all (97%-98%) of the healthy people in the population

WEB RESOURCES

Additional related content can be found on the companion website at evolve
http://evolve.elsevier.com/Lowdermilk/Maternity/

- NCLEX Review Questions
- Critical Thinking Exercise: Nutrition Education
- Nursing Care Plan: Nutrition During Pregnancy
- Spanish Guidelines: Diet and Nutrition

Maternal nutritional status at the time of conception is a significant determinant of embryonic and fetal growth (Gardiner et al., 2008) and is one of the many factors that influence the outcome of pregnancy (Fig. 8-1). Nutrition is potentially alterable, and good nutrition before and during pregnancy is an important preventive measure for a variety of problems. These problems include birth of low-birth-weight (LBW; birth weight of 2500 g or less) and preterm infants (those born before 37 weeks of gestation). The 2% of infants born very preterm (less than 32 weeks of gestation) accounted for more than one half of all infant deaths in the United States in 2005. The infant mortality rate for late preterm infants (those born between 34 0/7 and 36 6/7weeks) was more than three times that for term infants (37 to 41 weeks) (Mathews & MacDorman, 2008). Evidence is growing that the mother's nutrition and lifestyle affect the long-term health of her children (Gardiner et al.). Thus the importance of good nutrition must be emphasized to all women of childbearing potential. Key components of nutrition care during the preconception period and pregnancy include:

- Nutrition assessment that includes appropriate weight for height and adequacy and quality of dietary intake and habits
- Diagnosis of nutrition-related problems or risk factors such as diabetes, phenylketonuria (PKU), and obesity
- Intervention based on an individual's dietary goals and plan to promote appropriate weight gain, ingestion of a variety of foods, appropriate use of dietary supplements, and physical activity
- Evaluation as an integral part of the nursing care provided to women during the preconception period and pregnancy, with referral to a nutritionist or dietitian as necessary (Gardiner et al.)

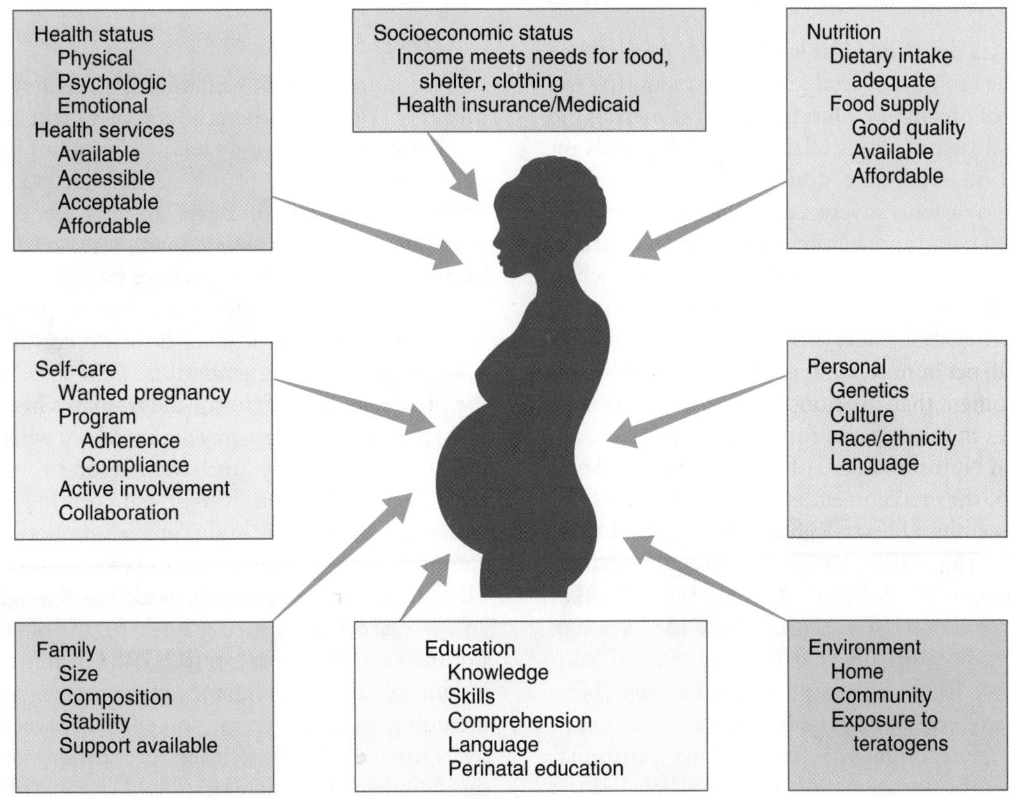

Fig. 8-1 Factors that affect the outcome of pregnancy.

NUTRIENT NEEDS BEFORE CONCEPTION

The first trimester of pregnancy is a crucial one for embryonic and fetal organ development. A healthful diet before conception is the best way to ensure that adequate nutrients are available for the developing fetus. Folate or folic acid intake is of particular concern in the periconceptual period. *Folate* is the form in which this vitamin is found naturally in foods, and *folic acid* is the form used in fortification of grain products and other foods and in vitamin supplements. Neural tube defects, or failure in closure of the neural tube, are more common in infants of women with poor folic acid intake. Researchers estimate that the incidence of neural tube defects can be decreased by as much as 70% if all women had an adequate folic acid intake during the periconceptual period (Cornel, Smit, & de Jong-van den Berg, 2005). All women capable of becoming pregnant are advised to consume 400 mcg of folic acid daily in fortified foods (e.g., ready-to-eat cereals, enriched grain products) or supplements, in addition to a diet rich in folate-containing foods such as green leafy vegetables, whole grains, and fruits (see Box 8-5 later in this chapter).

Both maternal and fetal risks in pregnancy are increased when the mother is significantly underweight or overweight when pregnancy begins. Ideally, all women achieve a desirable body weight before conception.

NUTRIENT NEEDS DURING PREGNANCY

Critical Thinking Exercise: Nutrition Education

Nutrient needs are determined, at least in part, by the stage of gestation. The amount of fetal growth varies during the different stages of pregnancy. During the first trimester, the synthesis of fetal tissues places relatively few demands on maternal nutrition. Therefore during the first trimester, when the embryo or fetus is very small, the needs are only slightly increased over those before pregnancy. In contrast, the last trimester is a period of noticeable fetal growth when most of the fetal stores of energy sources and minerals are deposited. Basal metabolic rates (BMRs), when expressed as kilocalories (kcal) per minute, are approximately 20% higher in pregnant women than in nonpregnant women. This increase includes the energy cost for tissue synthesis.

The Food and Nutrition Board of the National Academy of Sciences publishes recommendations for the people of the United States, the **Dietary Reference Intakes (DRIs)** (www.iom.edu). The DRIs consist of **Recommended Dietary Allowances (RDAs)** and **Adequate Intakes (AIs)**, as well as Upper Limits (ULs), guidelines for avoiding excessive intakes of nutrients that may be toxic if consumed in excess. RDAs for some nutrients have been available for many years, and they have been revised periodically. RDAs are recommendations for daily nutritional intakes that meet the needs of almost all (97%-98%) of the healthy members of the population. AIs are similar to the RDAs and are believed to cover the needs of virtually all healthy individuals in a group, except that they deal with nutrients for which the data are insufficient to be certain of their requirements. The RDAs and AIs include a wide variety of nutrients and food components, and they are divided into age, sex, and life-stage categories (e.g., infancy, pregnancy, lactation). They can be used as goals in planning the diets of individuals (Table 8-1).

Energy Needs

Energy (kilocalories or kcal) needs are met by carbohydrate, fat, and protein in the diet. No specific recommendations exist for the amount of carbohydrate and fat in the diet of the pregnant woman. However, intake of these nutrients should be adequate to support the recommended weight gain. Although protein can be used to supply energy, its primary role is to provide amino acids for the synthesis of new tissues (see the discussion later in this chapter). The estimated energy expenditure for the first trimester is the same as in the prepregnant state; during the second trimester of pregnancy the RDA is 340 kcal greater than the prepregnancy needs, and during the third trimester the amount is 462 kcal more than the prepregnant need (Institute of Medicine, 2003). Longitudinal assessment of weight gain during pregnancy is the best way to determine whether the kcal intake is adequate. Very underweight or active women or those with multifetal gestations will require more than the recommended increase in kcal to sustain the desired rate of weight gain.

Weight gain

The optimal weight gain during pregnancy is not known precisely. However, the amount of weight gained by the mother during pregnancy has an important bearing on the course and outcome of pregnancy. Adequate weight gain does not necessarily indicate that the diet is nutritionally adequate, but it is associated with a reduced risk of giving birth to a small-for-gestational-age (SGA) or preterm infant.

The desirable weight gain during pregnancy varies among women. The primary factor to consider in making a weight gain recommendation is the appropriateness of the prepregnancy weight for the woman's height. Maternal and fetal risks in pregnancy are increased when the mother is either significantly underweight or overweight before pregnancy and when weight gain during pregnancy is either too low or too high. Severely underweight women are more likely to have preterm labor and to give birth to LBW infants. Women with inadequate weight gain have an increased risk of giving birth to an infant with **intrauterine growth restriction (IUGR)**. Greater-than-expected weight gain during pregnancy may occur for many reasons, including multiple gestation, edema, preeclampsia, and overeating. Obesity (either preexisting or developed during pregnancy) increases the likelihood of macrosomia and fetopelvic disproportion; operative birth; emergency

TABLE 8-1

Recommendations for Daily Intakes of Selected Nutrients During Pregnancy and Lactation

NUTRIENT (UNITS)	RECOMMENDATION FOR NONPREGNANT WOMAN	RECOMMENDATION FOR PREGNANCY*	RECOMMENDATION FOR LACTATION*	ROLE IN RELATION TO PREGNANCY AND LACTATION	FOOD SOURCES
Energy (kilocalories [kcal] or kilojoules [kJ]†)	Variable	1st trimester, same as nonpregnant; second trimester, nonpregnant needs + 81 kcal (340 kJ); 3rd trimester, nonpregnant needs + 108 kcal (452 kJ)	1st 6 months, nonpregnant needs + 79 kcal (330 kJ); 2nd 6 months, nonpregnant needs + 55 kcal (230 kJ)	Growth of fetal and maternal tissues; milk production	Carbohydrate, fat, and protein
Protein (g)	46	1st trimester, same as nonpregnant; 2nd and 3rd trimesters, nonpregnant needs + 25 g‡	Nonpregnant needs + 25 g	Synthesis of the products of conception; growth of maternal tissue and expansion of blood volume; secretion of milk protein during lactation	Meats, eggs, cheese, yogurt, legumes (dry beans and peas, peanuts), nuts, grains
Water (L)	2.7 total (2.2 in beverages)	3 total (2.3 in beverages)	3.8 total (3.1 in beverages)	Expansion of blood volume, excretion of wastes; milk secretion	Water and beverages made with water, milk, juices; all foods, especially frozen desserts, fruits, lettuce and other fresh vegetables
Fiber (g)	25	28	29	Promote regular bowel elimination; reduce long-term risk of heart disease, diverticulosis, and diabetes	Whole grains, bran, vegetables, fruits, nuts and seeds
MINERALS					
Calcium (mg)	1300/1000	1300/1000	1300/1000	Fetal and infant skeleton and tooth formation; maintenance of maternal bone and tooth mineralization	Milk, cheese, yogurt, sardines or other fish eaten with bones left in, deep green leafy vegetables except spinach or Swiss chard, calcium-set tofu, baked beans, tortillas
Iron (mg)	15/18	30	10/9	Maternal hemoglobin formation, fetal liver iron storage	Liver, meats, whole grain or enriched breads and cereals, deep green leafy vegetables, legumes, dried fruits
Zinc (mg)	9/8	12/11	13/12	Component of numerous enzyme systems, possibly important in preventing congenital malformations	Liver, shellfish, meats, whole grains, milk
Iodine (mcg)	150	220	290	Increased maternal metabolic rate	Iodized salt, seafood, milk and milk products, commercial yeast breads, rolls, and donuts

Continued

TABLE 8-1

Recommendations for Daily Intakes of Selected Nutrients During Pregnancy and Lactation—cont'd

NUTRIENT (UNITS)	RECOMMENDATION FOR NONPREGNANT WOMAN	RECOMMENDATION FOR PREGNANCY*	RECOMMENDATION FOR LACTATION*	ROLE IN RELATION TO PREGNANCY AND LACTATION	FOOD SOURCES
Magnesium (mg)	360/310-320	400/350-360	360/310-320	Involved in energy and protein metabolism, tissue growth, muscle action	Nuts, legumes, cocoa, meats, whole grains
FAT-SOLUBLE VITAMINS					
A (mcg)	700	750/770	1200/1300	Essential for cell development, tooth bud formation, bone growth	Deep green leafy vegetables; dark yellow vegetables; and fruits, chili peppers, liver, fortified margarine and butter
D (mcg)	5	5	5	Involved in absorption of calcium and phosphorus, improves mineralization	Fortified milk and margarine, egg yolk, butter, liver, seafood
E (mg)	15	15	19	Antioxidant (protects cell membranes from damage), especially important for preventing breakdown of RBCs	Vegetable oils, green leafy vegetables, whole grains, liver, nuts and seeds, cheese, fish
WATER SOLUBLE VITAMINS					
C (mg)	65/75	80/85	115/120	Tissue formation and integrity, formation of connective tissue, enhancement of iron absorption	Citrus fruits, strawberries, melons, broccoli, tomatoes, peppers, raw deep green leafy vegetables
Folate (mcg)	400	600	500	Prevention of neural tube defects, support for increased maternal RBC formation	Fortified ready-to-eat cereals and other grain products, green leafy vegetables, oranges, broccoli, asparagus, artichokes, liver
B_6 or pyridoxine (mg)	1.2/1.3	1.9	2	Involved in protein metabolism	Meats, liver, deep green vegetables, whole grains
B_{12} (mcg)	2.4	2.6	2.8	Production of nucleic acids and proteins, especially important in formation of RBC and neural functioning	Milk and milk products, eggs, meats, liver, fortified soy milk

Sources: Institute of Medicine. (2002). *Dietary reference intakes for energy, carbohydrate, fiber, fat, fatty acids, cholesterol, protein, and amino acids.* Washington, DC: National Academies Press; Institute of Medicine. (2003). *Dietary reference intakes: Applications in dietary planning.* Washington, DC: National Academies Press; Institute of Medicine. (2004). *Dietary reference intakes for water, potassium, sodium, chloride, and sulfate.* Washington, DC: National Academies Press.

RBCs, Red blood cells.

*When two values appear, separated by a diagonal slash, the first is for females younger than 19 years, and the second is for those 19 to 50 years of age.

†The international metric unit of energy measurement is the joule (J). 1 kcal = 4.184 kJ.

‡Add an additional 25 g in twin pregnancies.

cesarean birth; postpartum hemorrhage; wound, genital tract, or urinary tract infection; birth trauma; and late fetal death. Obese women are more likely than normal-weight women to have gestational hypertension and gestational diabetes; their risk of giving birth to a child with a major congenital defect is double that of normal-weight women.

A commonly used method of evaluating the appropriateness of weight for height is the **body mass index (BMI)**, which is calculated by the following formula:

$$\text{BMI} = \text{weight}/\text{height}^2$$

where the weight is in kilograms and height is in meters. Therefore for a woman who weighed 51 kg before pregnancy and is 1.57 m tall:

$$\text{BMI} = 51/(1.57)^2, \text{ or } 20.7$$

Prepregnant BMI can be classified into the following categories: less than 18.5, underweight or low; 18.5 to 24.9, normal; 25 to 29.9, overweight or high; and greater than 30, obese (www.nhlbisupport.com/bmi/).

For women with single fetuses, current recommendations are that women with a normal BMI should gain 11.3-15.9 kg during pregnancy, underweight women should gain 12.7-18.1 kg, overweight women should gain 6.8-11.3 kg, and obese women should gain 5.0-9.1 kg (Institute of Medicine, 2009). Adolescents are encouraged to strive for weight gains at the upper end of the recommended range for their BMI because the fetus and the still-growing mother apparently compete for nutrients. The risk of mechanical complications at birth is reduced if the weight gain of short adult women (shorter than 157 cm) is near the lower end of their recommended range.

Pattern of weight gain

Weight gain should take place throughout pregnancy. The risk of giving birth to an SGA infant is greater when the weight gain early in pregnancy has been poor. The likelihood of preterm birth increases when the gains during the last half of pregnancy have been inadequate. These risks exist even when the total gain for the pregnancy is in the recommended range.

The optimal rate of weight gain depends on the stage of pregnancy. During the first and second trimesters, growth takes place primarily in maternal tissue; during the third trimester, growth occurs primarily in fetal tissues. During the first trimester the average total weight gain is only 1 to 2.5 kg. Thereafter the recommended weight gain increases to approximately 0.4 kg per week for a woman of normal weight. The recommended weekly weight gain for overweight women during the second and third trimesters is 0.3 kg and for underweight women is 0.5 kg.

In twin gestations the recommended weight gain for women in the normal BMI category is 16.8 to 24.5 kg, for women who are overweight, 14.1 to 22.7 kg, and for obese women 11.3 to 19.1 kg (Institute of Medicine, 2009). The ideal weight gain for higher multiples is likely to be greater, but no specific recommendations have been issued (Malone & D'Alton, 2009).

The recommended caloric intake corresponds to this pattern of gain. For the first trimester, no increment is necessary; during the second and third trimesters an additional 340 kcal per day and 462 kcal per day, respectively, over the prepregnant intake is recommended. The amount of food that provides the needed increase is not great. The 340 additional kcal needed during the second trimester can be provided by one additional serving from any one of the following groups: milk, yogurt, or cheese (all skim milk products); fruits; vegetables; and bread, cereal, rice, or pasta.

The reasons for an inadequate weight gain (less than 1 kg per month for normal-weight women or less than 0.5 kg/month for obese women during the last two trimesters) or excessive weight gain (more than 3 kg per month) should be evaluated thoroughly. Possible reasons for deviations from the expected rate of weight gain, besides inadequate or excessive dietary intake, include measurement or recording errors, differences in weight of clothing, time of day, and accumulation of fluids. An exceptionally high gain is likely to be caused by an accumulation of fluids, and a gain of more than 3 kg in a month, especially after the twentieth week of gestation, often indicates the development of gestational hypertension.

Hazards of restricting adequate weight gain

Figure-conscious women can have difficulty making the transition from guarding against weight gain before pregnancy to valuing weight gain during pregnancy. In counseling these women the nurse can emphasize the positive effects of good nutrition, as well as the adverse effects of maternal malnutrition (demonstrated by poor weight gain) on infant growth and development. This counseling includes information on the components of weight gain during pregnancy (Table 8-2) and the amount of this weight that will be lost at birth. Because lactation can help to reduce maternal energy stores gradually, this discussion provides an opportunity to promote breastfeeding.

In the United States, 20% of women who give birth are obese (Paul, 2008). However, pregnancy is not a time for weight-reduction. Even overweight or obese pregnant women need to gain at least enough weight to equal the weight of the products of conception (fetus, placenta, and amniotic fluid). If overweight women limit their caloric intake to prevent weight gain, they may also excessively limit their intake of important nutrients. Moreover, dietary restriction results in catabolism of fat stores, which, in turn, augments the production of ketones. The long-term effects of mild ketonemia during pregnancy are not known, but ketonuria has been found to be correlated with the occurrence of preterm labor. The idea that the quality of the weight gain is important should be stressed to obese

TABLE 8-2

Tissues Contributing to Maternal Weight Gain at 40 Weeks of Gestation

TISSUE	KILOGRAMS	POUNDS
Fetus	3.0-3.9	7.0-8.5
Placenta	0.9-1.1	2.0-2.5
Amniotic fluid	0.9	2
Increase in uterine tissue	0.9	2
Breast tissue	0.5-1.8	1-4
Increased blood volume	1.8-2.3	4-5
Increased tissue fluid	1.4-2.3	3-5
Increased stores (fat)	1.8-2.7	4-6

BOX 8-1

Bariatric Obstetric Care

Obstetricians today are seeing more morbidly obese pregnant women, those who weigh 400, 500, and even 600 pounds. Obesity creates many risks for pregnant women, including hypertension, diabetes, and prematurity. To manage their conditions and to meet their logistical needs, a new medical subspecialty, bariatric obstetrics, has arisen. Extra-wide blood pressure cuffs, scales that can accommodate up to 880 pounds, and extra-wide surgical tables designed to hold the weight of these women are used. Special techniques for ultrasound examination and longer surgical instruments for cesarean birth are required. In the St. Louis University, MO, bariatric obstetric clinic, women are counseled to avoid gaining weight and even to lose weight during pregnancy. New evidence indicates that when obese women maintain or lose weight during pregnancy, they have fewer complications and give birth to healthier babies (Paul, 2008).

women (and to all pregnant women), with emphasis placed on the consumption of nutrient-dense foods and the avoidance of empty-calorie foods.

Weight gain is important, but pregnancy is not an excuse for uncontrolled dietary indulgence. Excessive weight gained during pregnancy may be difficult to lose after pregnancy, thus contributing to chronic overweight or obesity, an etiologic factor in a host of chronic diseases, including hypertension, diabetes mellitus, and arteriosclerotic heart disease. The woman who gains 18 kg or more during pregnancy is especially at risk (Box 8-1 and the Critical Thinking/Clinical Decision Making Box).

Protein

Protein, with its essential constituent nitrogen, is the nutritional element basic to growth. Adequate protein intake is essential to meet increasing demands in pregnancy. These demands arise from the rapid growth of the fetus; the enlargement of the uterus and its supporting structures, mammary glands, and placenta; an increase in maternal circulating blood volume and subsequent demand for increased amounts of plasma protein to maintain colloidal osmotic pressure; and the formation of amniotic fluid.

Milk, meat, eggs, and cheese are complete-protein foods with a high biologic value. Legumes (dried beans and peas), whole grains, and nuts are also valuable sources of protein. In addition, these protein-rich foods are a source of other nutrients such as calcium, iron, and B vitamins; plant sources of protein often provide needed dietary fiber. The recommended daily food plan (Table 8-3) is a guide to the amounts of these foods that would supply the quantities of protein needed. The recommendations provide for only a modest increase in protein intake over the prepregnant levels in adult women.

Protein intake in many people in the United States is relatively high, thus many women may not need to increase their protein intake at all during pregnancy. Three servings of milk, yogurt, or cheese (four for adolescents) and 5 to 6 oz (140 to 168 g) (two servings) of meat, poultry, or fish supply the recommended protein for the pregnant woman. Additional protein is provided by vegetables and breads, cereals, rice, and pasta. Pregnant adolescents, women from

Critical Thinking/Clinical Decision Making

Nutrition and the Overweight Pregnant Woman

Tamara, of African-American and Asian heritage, is 3 months pregnant and comes to her initial appointment for diagnosis and care. She appears to be overweight for her height. To provide optimal care for her, you plan to calculate her prepregnancy body mass index. When her pregnancy is confirmed, you are asked to plan a diet with Tamara that meets the minimum daily requirements and allows for growth of the pregnancy. You know the importance of including consideration of personal preferences and cultural factors in your plan. With Tamara, identify barriers to implementing the plan.

1. Evidence—Is evidence sufficient to draw conclusions about an appropriate nutrition plan, taking into consideration personal preferences and cultural factors?
2. Assumptions—Describe the underlying assumptions about each of the following issues:
   a. Dietary reference intakes for pregnancy and lactation
   b. Indicators of nutritional risk in pregnancy
   c. Daily food guide for pregnancy and lactation
   d. Sources of calcium for women who do not drink milk
3. What implications and priorities for nursing care can be drawn at this time?
4. Does the evidence objectively support your conclusion?
5. Do alternative perspectives to your conclusion exist?

impoverished backgrounds, and women adhering to unusual diets, such as a macrobiotic (highly restricted vegetarian) diet, are those most likely to have inadequate protein intake. The use of high-protein supplements is not recommended because they have been associated with an increased incidence of preterm births. When choosing fish, pregnant and nursing women should be especially careful to select those that are low in mercury.

NURSING ALERT High levels of mercury can harm the developing nervous system of the fetus or young child, and certain fish are especially high in mercury. Women who may become pregnant, women who are pregnant or nursing, and young children need to follow some precautions: (1) Avoid eating shark, swordfish, king mackerel, and tilefish; (2) check local advisories about the safety of fish caught by family and friends in local bodies of water, but if no advisory is available, limit intake of these fish to 6 ounces, and eat no other fish that week; and (3) eat as much as 12 ounces a week of a variety of commercially caught fish and shellfish low in mercury, such as shrimp, salmon, pollock, catfish, and canned light tuna (but limit intake of albacore or "white" tuna and tuna steaks, which contain more mercury, to 6 ounces per week).

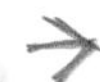

Fluids

Essential during the exchange of nutrients and waste products across cell membranes, water is the main substance of cells, blood, lymph, amniotic fluid, and other vital body fluids. It also aids in maintaining body temperature. A healthy fluid intake promotes good bowel function; constipation is sometimes a problem during pregnancy. The recommended daily intake of fluid is approximately six to eight glasses (1500-2000 ml). Water, milk, and juices are

TABLE 8-3

Daily Food Guide for Pregnancy and Lactation

		SUGGESTED NUMBER OF SERVINGS		
FOOD GROUP	SERVING SIZE	NONPREGNANT, NONLACTATING WOMAN	PREGNANT WOMAN	LACTATING WOMAN
GRAIN PRODUCTS				
Include whole-grain and enriched breads, cereals, pasta, and rice.	1 slice bread; ½ bun, bagel, or English muffin; 1 oz ready-to-eat cereal; ½ c cooked grains	6-11	6-11	6-11
VEGETABLES				
Eat dark-green leafy and deep-yellow vegetables often. Eat dried beans and peas often; count ½ c cooked dried beans or peas as a serving of vegetables or 1 oz from meat group.	1 c raw leafy greens; ½ c of others	3-5	3-5	3-5
FRUITS				
Include citrus fruits, strawberries, or melons frequently.	1 medium apple, orange, banana, peach, etc.; ½ c diced fruit; ¾ c juice	2-4	2-4	2-4
MILK AND MILK PRODUCTS				
	1 c milk or yogurt; 1½ oz cheese	2-3	3 or more	4 or more oz of meat
MEAT, POULTRY, FISH, DRY BEANS, NUTS, AND EGGS				
Eat peanut butter or nuts rarely to avoid excessive fat intake. Limit egg intake to reduce cholesterol intake; trim fat from meat, and remove skin from poultry.	½ c cooked dried beans, 1 egg, or 1½ T peanut butter is equivalent to 1 oz of meat	Up to 6 oz total	Up to 6 oz total	Up to 6 oz total

c, Cup; *T*, tablespoon.

good fluid sources. Dehydration may increase the risk of cramping, contractions, and preterm labor.

Caffeine in moderate amounts has not been proved to cause adverse effects during pregnancy. However, women who consume more than 300 mg of caffeine daily (equivalent to approximately 3 cups of coffee) may be at increased risk of miscarriage and of giving birth to infants with IUGR. The ill effects of caffeine have been proposed to result from vasoconstriction of the blood vessels supplying the uterus or from interference with cell division in the developing fetus. Consequently, caffeine-containing products such as caffeinated coffee, tea, soft drinks, and cocoa beverages should be avoided or consumed only in limited quantities.

No adverse effects on the normal mother or fetus have been found with the use of aspartame (NutraSweet, Equal), acesulfame potassium (Sunett), and sucralose (Splenda), artificial sweeteners commonly used in low- or no-calorie beverages and low-calorie food products. Aspartame, which contains phenylalanine, should be avoided by the woman with PKU (Box 8-2). Stevia (stevioside) is a food additive used as a sweetener but it has not been approved

BOX 8-2

Use of Artificial Sweeteners during Pregnancy

All of the following sweeteners are approved for use in all age groups, including pregnant women, in the United States:

Acesulfame K
- Brand names: Sunett, Sweet One
- Primary uses: baked goods, frozen desserts, candies, beverages
- Sweetness: 200 times sweeter than sugar
- Shelf life: long
- Suitability for cooking: good; does not break down when heated
- Health concerns: none known

Aspartame
- Brand names: Equal, NutraSweet, NatraTaste
- Primary uses: beverages, frozen desserts, dairy products, chewing gum, breakfast cereals, table-top sweetener
- Sweetness: 180 times sweeter than sugar
- Shelf life: relatively short (approximately 5 months in a soft drink)
- Suitability for cooking: breaks down and loses sweetness if cooked at high temperatures or for long periods
- Health concerns: contains phenylalanine, a consideration in the diets of people with phenylketonuria

Neotame
- Brand names: none (currently unavailable)
- Primary uses: approved in the United States but not currently marketed; proposed for use in beverages, frozen desserts, yogurt, chewing gum, toppings, fillings, fruit spreads, tabletop sweetener
- Sweetness: 8000 times sweeter than sugar
- Shelf life: similar to aspartame (approximately 5 months in a soft drink)
- Suitability for cooking: good, but loses sweetness if cooked at high temperatures or for prolonged periods
- Health concerns: none known; contains phenylalanine but not in a form that can be metabolized

Saccharin
- Brand name: Sweet 'n Low
- Primary uses: fountain drinks, chewable vitamins and medications, table-top sweetener
- Sweetness: 300 times sweeter than sugar
- Shelf life: long
- Suitability for cooking: good; does not lose sweetness during cooking
- Health concerns: linked to bladder cancer in rats

Sucralose
- Brand name: Splenda
- Primary uses: baked goods, beverages, frozen desserts, gelatins, table-top sweetener
- Sweetness: 600 times sweeter than sugar
- Shelf life: long
- Suitability for cooking: very good; does not break down during cooking (maltodextrin is added to give products better bulk and texture)
- Health concerns: none known

Sugar alcohols (not technically artificial sweeteners; contain almost as many calories as sugar) Types: sorbitol, xylitol, lactitol, mannitol, and maltitol
- Primary uses: sugar-free candy, cookies, and chewing gum
- Sweetness: most are approximately 70% as sweet as sugar; xylitol equals sugar in sweetness
- Shelf life: long
- Suitability for cooking: good
- Advantages over sugar: Sugar alcohols do not promote tooth decay and are more slowly metabolized, thus they do not create a rapid peak in blood glucose.
- Health concerns: Diarrhea can occur with large intakes.

Sugar is important for the volume and moisture of baked goods. Artificial sweeteners may produce a good-tasting product, but some sugar is necessary in many recipes to yield normal volume and texture.

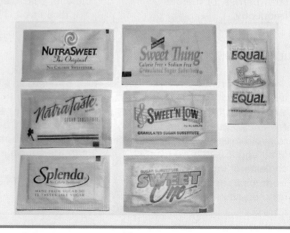

by the U.S. Food and Drug Administration (FDA) for that purpose.

Minerals and Vitamins

In general, the nutrient needs of pregnant women, except perhaps the need for folate and iron, can be met through dietary sources. Counseling about the need for a varied diet rich in vitamins and minerals should be a part of every pregnant woman's early prenatal care and should be reinforced throughout pregnancy. Supplements of certain nutrients (listed in the following discussion) are recommended whenever the woman's diet is very poor or whenever significant nutritional risk factors are present. Nutritional risk factors in pregnancy are listed in Box 8-3.

Iron

Iron is needed both to allow transfer of adequate iron to the fetus and to permit expansion of the maternal red blood cell (RBC) mass. The RDA of iron during pregnancy is 27 mg per day (National Institutes of Health, 2007). Pregnant women should receive a supplement of 30 mg of ferrous iron daily, starting by 12 weeks of gestation. (Iron supplements may be poorly tolerated during the nausea that is prevalent in the first trimester.) Iron supplementation of women with iron deficiency can improve maternal hematologic indices and appears to reduce LBW births. If maternal iron-deficiency anemia is present (preferably diagnosed by measurement of serum ferritin, a storage form of iron), increased doses (60-120 mg daily) are recommended. Certain foods taken with an iron supplement can promote or inhibit absorption of iron from the supplement. See the Patient Instructions for Self-Management box regarding iron supplementation. Even when a woman is taking an iron supplement, she should include good food sources of iron in her daily diet (see Table 8-1).

BOX 8-3

Indicators of Nutritional Risk in Pregnancy

- Adolescence
- Frequent pregnancies: three within 2 years
- Poor fetal outcome in a previous pregnancy
- Poverty
- Poor diet habits with resistance to change
- Use of tobacco, alcohol, or drugs
- Weight at conception under or over normal weight
- Problems with weight gain
- Any weight loss
- Weight gain of less than 1 kg/mo after the first trimester
- Weight gain of more than 1 kg/wk after the first trimester
- Multifetal pregnancy
- Low hemoglobin or hematocrit values (or both)

Calcium

The DRI shows no increase of calcium during pregnancy and lactation, in comparison with the recommendation for the nonpregnant woman (see Table 8-1). The DRI appears to provide sufficient calcium for fetal bone and tooth development to proceed while maintaining maternal bone mass.

Milk and yogurt are especially rich sources of calcium, providing approximately 300 mg per cup (240 ml). Nevertheless, many women do not consume these foods or do not consume adequate amounts to provide the recommended intakes of calcium. One problem that can interfere with milk consumption is **lactose intolerance**, the inability to digest milk sugar (lactose) caused by the absence of the lactase enzyme in the small intestine. Lactose intolerance is relatively common in adults, particularly African-Americans, Asians, Native Americans, and Inuits. Milk consumption may cause abdominal cramping, bloating, and diarrhea in such people, although many lactose-intolerant individuals can tolerate small amounts of milk without symptoms. Yogurt, sweet acidophilus milk, buttermilk, cheese, chocolate milk, and cocoa may be tolerated even when fresh fluid milk is not. Commercial lactase supplements (e.g., Lactaid) are widely

PATIENT INSTRUCTIONS FOR SELF-MANAGEMENT

Iron Supplementation

- Iron absorption is promoted by a diet rich in vitamin C (e.g., citrus fruits, melons) or "heme iron" (found in red meats, fish, and poultry).
- Iron supplements are best absorbed on an empty stomach; to this end, they can be taken between meals with beverages other than milk, tea, or coffee.
- Bran, milk, egg yolks, coffee, tea, or oxalate-containing vegetables such as spinach and Swiss chard will inhibit iron absorption if consumed at the same time as iron.
- Some women have gastrointestinal discomfort when they take the supplement on an empty stomach; therefore a good time for them to take the supplement is just before bedtime.
- Constipation is common with iron supplementation.
- Iron supplements should be kept away from any children in the household because ingestion of these supplements could result in acute iron poisoning and even death.
- Iron may cause black, tarry stools.

available to consume with milk. Many supermarkets stock lactase-treated milk. The lactase in these products hydrolyzes, or digests, the lactose in milk, thus enabling lactose-intolerant people to drink milk.

In some cultures, adults rarely drink milk. For example, Puerto Ricans and other Hispanic people may use milk only as an additive in coffee. Pregnant women from these cultures may need to consume nondairy sources of calcium. Vegetarian diets may also be deficient in calcium (Box 8-4). If calcium intake appears low and the woman does not change her dietary habits despite counseling, a daily supplement containing 600 mg of elemental calcium may be needed. Calcium supplements may also be recommended when a pregnant woman experiences leg cramps caused by an imbalance in the calcium/phosphorus ratio. Bone meal supplements are often contaminated with lead and should not be used in pregnancy.

Other Minerals and Electrolytes

Magnesium

Diets of women in the childbearing years are likely to be low in magnesium, and as many as one half of pregnant and lactating women may have inadequate intakes (Institute of Medicine, 2004). Adolescents and low-income women are especially at risk. Dairy products, nuts, whole grains, and green leafy vegetables are good sources of magnesium.

BOX 8-4

Calcium Sources for Women Who Do Not Drink Milk

Each of the following food items provides approximately the same amount of calcium as 1 cup of milk.

FISH
3-oz can of sardines
4½-oz can of salmon (if bones are eaten)

BEANS AND LEGUMES
3 cups cooked dried beans
2½ cups refried beans
2 cups baked beans with molasses
1 cup tofu (calcium is added in processing)

GREENS
1 cup collards
1½ cups kale or turnip greens

BAKED PRODUCTS
3 pieces cornbread
3 English muffins
4 slices French toast
2 waffles (7 inches in diameter)

FRUITS
11 dried figs
1⅛ cups orange juice with calcium added

SAUCES
3 oz pesto sauce
5 oz cheese sauce

Sodium

During pregnancy the need for sodium increases slightly, primarily because the body water is expanding (e.g., the expanding blood volume). Sodium is essential for maintaining body water balance. In the past, dietary sodium was routinely restricted in an effort to control the peripheral edema that commonly occurs during pregnancy. Moderate peripheral edema is now recognized as normal in pregnancy, occurring as a response to the fluid-retaining effects of elevated levels of estrogen. Severe sodium restriction may make achieving an adequate diet difficult for pregnant women. Grain, milk, and meat products, which are good sources of other nutrients needed during pregnancy, are significant sources of sodium. In addition, sodium restriction may stress the adrenal glands and the kidneys as they attempt to retain adequate sodium. In general, sodium restriction is necessary only if the woman has a medical condition such as renal or liver failure or hypertension that warrants such a restriction.

Excessive intake of sodium is discouraged during pregnancy just as it is in nonpregnant women, because it may contribute to development of hypertension in salt-sensitive individuals. An adequate sodium intake for pregnant and lactating women, as well as nonpregnant women in the childbearing years, is estimated to be 1.5 g/day, with a recommended upper limit of intake of 2.3 g/day (Institute of Medicine, 2003). Table salt (sodium chloride) is the richest source of sodium, with approximately 2.3 g of sodium contained in 1 teaspoon (6 g) of salt. Most canned foods contain added salt unless the label states otherwise. Large amounts of sodium are also found in many processed foods, including meats (e.g., smoked or cured meats, cold cuts, corned beef), frozen entrees and meals, baked goods, mixes for casseroles or grain products, soups, and condiments. Products low in nutritive value and excessively high in sodium include pretzels, potato and other chips, pickles, catsup, prepared mustard, steak and Worcestershire sauces, some soft drinks, and bouillon. A moderate sodium intake can usually be achieved by salting food lightly in cooking, adding no additional salt at the table, and avoiding low-nutrient, high-sodium foods.

Potassium

Diets that include AIs of potassium are associated with reduced risk of hypertension. Potassium has been identified as one of the nutrients most likely to be lacking in the diets of women of childbearing years (Institute of Medicine, 2004). A diet that includes 8 to 10 servings of unprocessed fruits and vegetables daily, along with moderate amounts of low-fat meats and dairy products, provides adequate amounts of potassium.

Zinc

Zinc is a constituent of numerous enzymes involved in major metabolic pathways. Zinc deficiency is associated with malformations of the central nervous system in infants. When large amounts of iron and folic acid are consumed the absorption of zinc is inhibited, and serum zinc levels are reduced as a result. Because iron and folic acid supplements are commonly prescribed during pregnancy, pregnant women should be encouraged to consume good sources of zinc daily (see Table 8-1). Women with anemia who receive high-dose iron supplements also need supplements of zinc and copper.

Fluoride

There is no evidence that prenatal fluoride supplementation reduces the child's likelihood of tooth decay during the preschool years. No increase in fluoride intake over the nonpregnant DRI is currently recommended during pregnancy (Institute of Medicine, 2003).

Fat-soluble vitamins

Fat-soluble vitamins–A, D, E, and K–are stored in the body tissues. These vitamins are of special concern during pregnancy because vitamin E intake is among the nutrients most likely to be lacking in the diets of women of childbearing age, and intake of vitamins A and D is also low in the diets of some women (Institute of Medicine, 2004). With chronic overdoses, these vitamins can reach toxic levels. Because of the high potential for toxicity, pregnant women are advised to take fat-soluble vitamin supplements only as prescribed.

Adequate intake of vitamin A is needed so that sufficient amounts of the vitamin can be stored in the fetus. A well-chosen diet that includes adequate amounts of deep-yellow and deep-green vegetables and fruits such as leafy greens, broccoli, carrots, cantaloupe, and apricots provides sufficient amounts of carotenes that can be converted in the body to vitamin A. Congenital malformations have occurred in infants of mothers who took excessive amounts of preformed vitamin A (from supplements) during pregnancy, and thus supplements are not recommended for pregnant women. Vitamin A analogs such as isotretinoin (Accutane), which are prescribed for the treatment of cystic acne, are a special concern. Isotretinoin use during early pregnancy has been associated with an increased incidence of heart malformations, facial abnormalities, cleft palate, hydrocephalus, and deafness and blindness in the infant, as well as an increased risk of miscarriage. Topical agents such as tretinoin (Retin-A) do not appear to enter the circulation in any substantial amounts, but their safety in pregnancy has not been confirmed.

Vitamin D plays an important role in absorption and metabolism of calcium. The main food sources of this vitamin are enriched or fortified foods such as milk and ready-to-eat cereals. Vitamin D is also produced in the skin by the action of ultraviolet light (in sunlight). Severe deficiency may lead to neonatal hypocalcemia and tetany, as well as hypoplasia of the tooth enamel. Women with lactose intolerance and those who do not include milk in their diet for any reason are at risk for vitamin D deficiency. Other risk factors are having dark skin, habitually using clothing that covers most of the skin (e.g., Muslim women with extensive body covering), and living in northern latitudes where sunlight exposure is limited, especially during the winter. Use of recommended amounts of sunscreen with a sun protection factor (SPF) rating of 15 or greater reduces skin vitamin D production by as much as 99%, reinforcing the need for regular intake of fortified foods or a supplement.

Vitamin E is needed for protection against oxidative stress, and pregnancy is associated with increased oxidative stress. Indeed, oxidative stress has been proposed as an explanation for the etiology of preeclampsia (Allen, 2005). Vegetable oils and nuts are especially good sources of vitamin E, and whole grains and leafy green vegetables are moderate sources.

Water-soluble vitamins

Body stores of water-soluble vitamins are much smaller than those of fat-soluble vitamins. Water-soluble vitamins, in contrast to fat-soluble vitamins, are readily excreted in the urine. Therefore good sources of these vitamins must be consumed frequently. Toxicity with overdose is less likely than with fat-soluble vitamins.

Folate and folic acid

Because of the increase in RBC production during pregnancy, as well as the nutritional requirements of the rapidly growing cells in the fetus and placenta, pregnant women should consume approximately 50% more folic acid than nonpregnant women, or approximately 0.6 mg (600 mcg) daily. In the United States, all enriched grain products, which includes most white breads, flour, and pasta, must contain folic acid at a level of 1.4 mg/kg of flour (Box 8-5). This level of fortification is designed to supply approximately 0.1 mg of folic acid daily in the average American diet and has significantly increased folic acid consumption in the population as a whole. Supplemental folic acid is usually prescribed to ensure that intake is adequate. Women who have borne a child with a neural tube defect are advised to consume 4 mg of folic acid daily, and a supplement is required for them to achieve this level of intake.

Pyridoxine

Pyridoxine, or vitamin B_6, is involved in protein metabolism. Although levels of a pyridoxine-containing enzyme have been reported to be low in women with preeclampsia, there is no evidence that supplementation prevents or cor-

EVIDENCE-BASED PRACTICE

What Nutritional Supplements, Besides Folic Acid, Promote Optimal Health during Pregnancy?

Pat Gingrich

ASK THE QUESTION

In addition to folic acid, what nutritional supplements should be recommended to pregnant women?

SEARCH FOR EVIDENCE

Search Strategies: Professional organization guidelines, meta-analyses, systematic reviews, randomized controlled trials, nonrandomized prospective studies, and retrospective studies since 2006.

Databases Searched: CINAHL, Cochrane, Medline, National Guideline Clearinghouse, and the websites for Association of Women's Health, Obstetric, and Neonatal Nurses; Centers for Disease Control and Prevention; and National Institute for Health and Clinical Excellence.

CRITICALLY ANALYZE THE EVIDENCE

The National Institute of Health and Clinical Evidence clinical guidelines for prenatal care included the recommendation that all women be informed about the importance of vitamin D supplementation, especially for women with darker skin, low vitamin D diets, obesity, or low sun exposure (National Institute for Health and Clinical Excellence [NICE], 2008). By facilitating the absorption of calcium, vitamin D prevents rickets and may protect against preeclampsia. Calcium is known to decrease the risk of preeclampsia by one half, especially for women with risk factors of low dietary calcium (Hofmeyr, Duley, & Atallah, 2007).

Norwegian women who were given vitamin A lowered their risk for giving birth to babies with cleft palate (Johansen, Lie, Wilcox, Andersen, & Drevon, 2008).

Because preeclampsia may be a result of oxidative stress, researchers have suggested that antioxidants may be protective. However, a Cochrane systematic review of 10 trials involving 6533 women found that vitamins C, E, selenium and lycopene supplements caused no improvement in preeclampsia, preterm birth, small-for-gestational age status, or perinatal death (Rumbold, Duley, Crowther, & Haslam, 2008).

Another Cochrane review of 17 trials involving more than 9000 women revealed that zinc supplementation in pregnancy may reduce preterm births in areas of high perinatal mortality but showed no evidence of benefit in other settings (Mahomed, Bhutta, & Middleton, 2007). The reviewers recommend a more comprehensive approach to dietary nutrition in pregnancy rather than focusing on specific micronutrients.

IMPLICATIONS FOR PRACTICE

Good nutrition is essential to good health, especially in pregnancy. Even though certain micronutrients may go in and out of scientific favor, women from low-resource areas will most benefit themselves and their fetuses with comprehensive vitamin and mineral supplementation, as well as dietary adequacy and variety. Women at risk for certain conditions can benefit from additional protective micronutrients such as vitamin D and calcium to decrease the risk of preeclampsia.

References:

Hofmeyr, G. J., Duley, L., & Atallah, A. (2007). Dietary calcium supplementation for prevention of pre-eclampsia and related problems: A systematic review and commentary. *British Journal of Obstetrics and Gynaecology, 1114*, 933-943.

Johansen, A. M., Lie, R. T., Wilcox, A. J., Andersen, L. F., & Drevon, C. A. (2008). Maternal dietary intake of vitamin A and risk of orofacial clefts: A population-based case-control study in Norway. *American Journal of Epidemiology, 167*(10), 1164-1170.

Mahomed, K., Bhutta, Z., & Middleton, P. (2007. Zinc supplementation for improving pregnancy and infant outcome. In *The Cochrane Database of Systematic Reviews 2007*, Issue 1, CD 000230.

National Institute for Health and Clinical Excellence (NICE). (2008). *Antenatal care: Routine care for the healthy pregnant woman.* NICE Clinical Guideline 62, London: NICE. Internet document available at http://www.nice.org.uk/nicemedia/pdf/CG062NICEguideline.pdf (accessed May 22, 2009).

Rumbold, A., Duley, L., Crowther, C. A., & Haslam R. R. (2008). Antioxidants for preventing pre-eclampsia. In *The Cochrane Database of Systematic Reviews 2008*, Issue 1, CD 004227.

rects the condition. No supplement is recommended routinely, but women with poor diets and those at nutritional risk (see Box 8-3) may need a supplement that provides 2 mg/day. In some trials, pyridoxine has been effective in reducing the nausea and vomiting of early pregnancy.

Vitamin C

Vitamin C, or ascorbic acid, plays an important role in tissue formation and enhances the absorption of iron. The vitamin C needs of most women are readily met by a diet that includes at least one daily serving of citrus fruit or juice or another good source of the vitamin (see Table 8-1), but women who smoke need more. For women at nutritional risk, a supplement of 50 mg/day is recommended. However, if the mother takes excessive doses of this vitamin during pregnancy, a vitamin C deficiency may develop in the infant after birth.

Multivitamin and multimineral supplements during pregnancy

Food can and should be the normal vehicle to meet the additional needs imposed by pregnancy, except for iron. In addition, the recommended folate or folic acid intake may be difficult for some women to achieve. Some women habitually consume diets that are deficient in necessary nutrients and, for whatever reason, may be unable to

BOX 8-5

Food Sources of Folate

FOODS PROVIDING 500 MCG OR MORE PER SERVING
- Liver: chicken, turkey, goose (3½ oz)

FOODS PROVIDING 200 MCG OR MORE PER SERVING
- Liver: lamb, beef, veal (3½ oz)

FOODS PROVIDING 100 MCG OR MORE PER SERVING
- Legumes, cooked (½ cup)
  - Peas: black-eyed peas, chickpeas (garbanzos)
  - Beans: black, kidney, pinto, red, navy
  - Lentils
- Vegetables (½ cup)
  - Asparagus
  - Spinach, cooked
- Papaya (1 medium)
- Breakfast cereal, ready-to-eat (½-1 cup)
- Wheat germ (½ cup)

FOODS PROVIDING 50 MCG OR MORE PER SERVING
- Vegetables (½ cup)
  - Broccoli
  - Beans: lima, baked, or pork and beans
  - Greens: collards or mustard, cooked
  - Spinach, raw
- Fruits (½ cup)
  - Avocado
  - Orange or orange juice
- Pasta, cooked (1 cup)
- Rice, cooked (1 cup)

FOODS PROVIDING 20 MCG OR MORE PER SERVING
- Bread (1 slice)
- Egg (1 large)
- Corn (½ cup)

change this intake. For these women, a multivitamin-multimineral supplement should be considered to ensure that they consume the RDA for most known vitamins and minerals. The pregnant woman needs to understand that the use of a vitamin-mineral supplement does not lessen the need to consume a nutritious, well-balanced diet.

Other Nutritional Issues during Pregnancy

Pica and food cravings

Pica, the practice of consuming nonfood substances (e.g., clay, dirt, laundry starch) or excessive amounts of foodstuffs low in nutritional value (e.g., cornstarch, ice, baking powder, baking soda), is often influenced by the woman's cultural background (Fig. 8-2). In the United

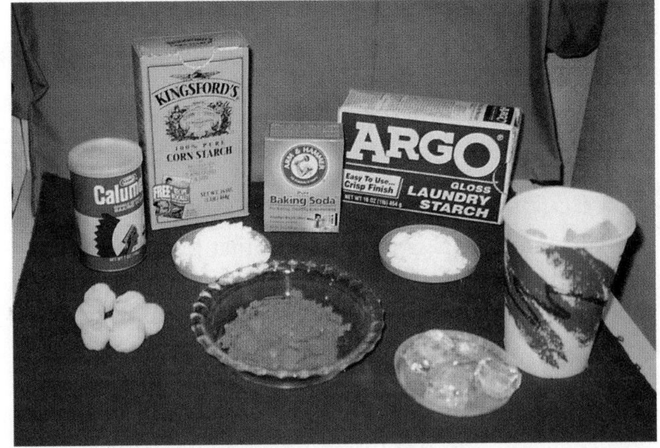

Fig. 8-2 Nonfood substances consumed in pica: (*center*) red clay from Georgia (*left to right*); *Nzu* from Eastern Nigeria, baking powder, corn starch, baking soda, laundry starch, and ice. Some individuals practice poly-pica (consuming more than one of these substances). (Courtesy Shannon Perry, Phoenix, AZ.)

States, pica appears to be most common among African-American women, women from rural areas, and women with a family history of pica. Regular and heavy consumption of low-nutrient products may cause more nutritious foods to be displaced from the diet, and the items consumed may interfere with the absorption of nutrients, especially minerals. As an example, cornstarch ingestion is popular among African-American women. It is a source of "empty" calories; one half cup (64 g) provides 240 kcal (57 kJ) but almost no vitamins, minerals, or protein. Grotegut, Dandolu, Katari, Whiteman, Geifman-Holtzman, and Teitelman (2006) reported a case of a 31-week gestation multigravida ingesting a box of baking soda (454 g of sodium bicarbonate) each day, which resulted in severe hypokalemic metabolic alkalosis and rhabdomyolysis. More than one substance may be ingested (Ngozi, 2008). Women with pica have lower hemoglobin levels than those without pica.

Moreover, a risk exists that nonfood items are contaminated with heavy metals or other toxic substances. Among Mexican-American women, consumption of "tierra" includes both soil and pulverized Mexican pottery (Klitzman, Sharma, Nicaj, Vitkevich, & Leighton, 2002; Shannon, 2003). Lead contamination of soils and soil-based products has caused high levels of lead in both pregnant women and their newborns. Regular household use of Mexican pottery in cooking or serving food or ingestion of ground pottery must be included in interviews or questionnaires regarding nutritional intake of pregnant women. The possibility of pica must be considered when pregnant women are found to be anemic, and the nurse should provide counseling about the health risks associated with pica (Corbett, Ryan, & Weinrich, 2003).

One hypothesis proposes that pica and food cravings (e.g., the urge to consume ice cream, pickles, or pizza) during pregnancy are caused by an innate drive to consume nutrients missing from the diet. However, research has not supported this hypothesis.

Adolescent pregnancy needs

Many adolescent girls have diets that provide less than the recommended intakes of key nutrients, including energy, calcium, and iron. Pregnant adolescents and their infants are at increased risk of complications during pregnancy and parturition. Growth of the pelvis is delayed in comparison with growth in stature, which helps to explain why cephalopelvic disproportion and other mechanical problems associated with labor are common among young adolescents. Competition for nutrients between the growing adolescent and the fetus may also contribute to some of the poor outcomes apparent in teen pregnancies. Pregnant adolescents are encouraged to choose a weight gain goal at the upper end of the range for their BMI.

Efforts to improve the nutritional health of pregnant adolescents focus on improving the nutrition knowledge, meal planning, and food preparation and selection skills of young women; promoting access to prenatal care; developing nutrition interventions and educational programs that are effective with adolescents; and striving to understand the factors that create barriers to change in the adolescent population.

Nutrition needs related to physical activity during pregnancy

Moderate exercise during pregnancy yields numerous benefits, including improving muscle tone, potentially shortening the course of labor, and promoting a sense of well-being. If no medical or obstetric problems contraindicate physical activity, pregnant women should perform 30 minutes of moderate physical exercise on most, if not all, days of the week. Two nutritional concepts are especially important for women who choose to exercise during pregnancy. First, a liberal amount of fluid should be consumed before, during, and after exercise because dehydration can trigger premature labor. Second, the calorie intake should be sufficient to meet the increased needs of pregnancy and the demands of exercise.

NUTRIENT NEEDS DURING LACTATION

Nutritional needs during lactation are similar in many ways to those during pregnancy (see Table 8-1). Needs for energy (calories), protein, calcium, iodine, zinc, the B vitamins (thiamine, riboflavin, niacin, pyridoxine, and vitamin B_{12}), and vitamin C remain greater than nonpregnant needs. The recommendations for some of these (e.g., vitamin C, zinc, protein) are slightly to moderately higher than during pregnancy (see Table 8-1). This allowance covers the amount of the nutrients released in the milk, as well as the needs of the mother for tissue maintenance. In the case of iron and folic acid, the recommendation during lactation is lower than during pregnancy. With the decrease in maternal blood volume to nonpregnant levels after birth, maternal iron and folic acid needs also decrease. Many lactating women have a delay in the return of menses; this delay conserves blood cells and reduces iron and folic acid needs. The calcium intake must be adequate; if it is not and the women does not respond to diet counseling, a supplement of 600 mg of calcium per day may be needed.

Fluid intake must be adequate to maintain milk production, but the mother's level of thirst is the best guide to the right amount. Consuming more fluids than those needed to satisfy thirst is unnecessary.

Alcohol intake and excessive caffeine intake should be avoided during lactation. Researchers have speculated that the infant's psychomotor development may be affected by maternal alcohol use, and alcoholic beverages (two drinks per day) may impair the milk ejection reflex. Caffeine intake may lead to a reduced iron concentration in milk and consequently contribute to the development of anemia in the infant. The caffeine concentration in milk is only approximately 1% of the mother's plasma level, but caffeine tends to accumulate in the infant. Breastfed infants of mothers who drink large amounts of coffee or caffeine-containing soft drinks may be unusually active and wakeful.

CARE MANAGEMENT

During pregnancy, nutrition plays a key role in achieving an optimal outcome for the mother and her unborn baby. Motivation to learn about nutrition is usually higher during pregnancy as parents strive to "do what's right for the baby." Optimal nutrition cannot eliminate all problems that can arise during pregnancy, but it does establish a good foundation for supporting the needs of the mother and her unborn baby (see Nursing Process and Community Activity boxes).

Diet History

A diet history is a description of the woman's usual food and beverage intake and factors affecting her nutritional status. Such factors include medications being taken and adequacy of income to allow her to purchase the necessary foods.

Obstetric and gynecologic effects on nutrition

Nutritional reserves may be depleted in the multiparous woman or one who has had frequent pregnancies (especially three pregnancies within 2 years). A history of preterm birth or the birth of an LBW or SGA infant may indicate inadequate dietary intake. Preeclampsia may also

NURSING PROCESS *Nutrition*

ASSESSMENT

- Take a thorough diet history using interview and review of the woman's health records.
- Perform a physical examination with attention to blood pressure, weight, and condition of teeth and skin.
- Review laboratory results for evidence of anemia or iron deficiency.

Ideally, a nutritional assessment is performed before conception so that any recommended changes in diet, lifestyle, and weight can be undertaken before the woman becomes pregnant.

NURSING DIAGNOSES

Nursing diagnoses include:

- *Imbalanced nutrition: less than body requirements* related to:
  - Inadequate information about nutritional needs and weight gain during pregnancy
  - Misperceptions regarding normal body changes during pregnancy and inappropriate fear of becoming fat
  - Inadequate income or skills in meal planning and preparation
- *Imbalanced nutrition: more than body requirements* related to:
  - Excessive intake of energy (calories) or decrease in activity during pregnancy
  - Use of unnecessary dietary supplements
- *Constipation* related to:
  - Decrease in gastrointestinal motility because of elevated progesterone levels
  - Compression of intestines by the enlarging uterus
  - Oral iron supplementation

EXPECTED OUTCOMES OF CARE

Nutrition-related outcomes are that the woman will take the following actions:

- Achieve an appropriate weight gain during pregnancy that takes into account such factors as prepregnancy weight, whether she is overweight, obese, or underweight, and whether the pregnancy is single or multifetal.
- Consume adequate nutrients from the diet and supplements to meet estimated needs.
- Cope successfully with nutrition-related discomforts associated with pregnancy, such as morning sickness, pyrosis (heartburn), and constipation.
- Avoid or reduce potentially harmful practices such as smoking, alcohol consumption, and caffeine intake.
- Return to prepregnancy weight (or an appropriate weight for height) within 6 months of giving birth.

PLAN OF CARE AND INTERVENTIONS

- Acquaint the woman with nutritional needs during pregnancy and, if necessary, the characteristics of an adequate diet.
- Help the woman individualize her diet so that she achieves an adequate intake while conforming to her personal, cultural, financial, and health circumstances.
- Acquaint the woman with strategies for coping with the nutrition-related discomforts of pregnancy.
- Help the woman use nutrition supplements appropriately.
- Consult with and make referrals to other professionals or services as indicated.
- Compare the woman's weight gain with standardized grids showing recommended patterns.
- Compare the woman's diet with the plan in Table 8-2. Individual factors affecting nutritional needs and dietary intake must be considered.

EVALUATION

Care has been effective when the woman's nutritional intake meets recommendations, she copes with nutrition-related discomforts of pregnancy, and her weight gain is appropriate for gestational age.

COMMUNITY ACTIVITY

Visit a prenatal clinic. Identify sources of nutrition education that are evident in the waiting room. Is education and assistance from the WIC program available? Does the clinic employ a nutritionist or dietitian? Who provides nutrition counseling in the clinic? Are materials promoting breastfeeding prominently displayed? Are print materials available in multiple languages? Are interpreters available? Are sources of free materials on nutrition available that can be placed in the clinic? Are the nutrition education materials culturally relevant? Identify strengths and weaknesses of nutrition education in this setting. Develop a feasible plan for improving nutrition education in the clinic.

WIC, Special Supplemental Nutrition Program for Women, Infants, and Children.

be a factor in poor maternal nutrition. Birth of a large-for-gestational-age (LGA) infant may indicate the existence of maternal diabetes mellitus. Previous contraceptive methods also may affect reproductive health. Increased menstrual blood loss often occurs during the first 3 to 6 months after placement of an intrauterine contraceptive device. Consequently the user may have low iron stores or even iron deficiency anemia. Oral contraceptive agents, on the other hand, are associated with decreased menstrual losses and increased iron stores. Oral contraceptives, however, may interfere with folic acid metabolism.

Medical history

Chronic maternal illnesses such as diabetes mellitus, renal disease, liver disease, cystic fibrosis or other malabsorptive disorders, seizure disorders and the use of anticonvulsant agents, hypertension, and PKU may affect a woman's nutritional status and dietary needs. In women with illnesses that have resulted in nutritional deficits or that require dietary treatment (e.g., diabetes mellitus, PKU), nutritional care must be started and the condition must be optimally controlled before conception. A registered dietitian can provide in-depth counseling for the woman who requires a therapeutic diet during pregnancy and lactation.

Usual maternal diet

The woman's usual food and beverage intake, adequacy of income and other resources to meet her nutritional needs, any dietary modifications, food allergies and intolerances, and all medications and nutrition supplements being taken, as well as pica and cultural dietary requirements, should be ascertained. In addition, the presence and severity of nutrition-related discomforts of pregnancy, such as morning sickness, constipation, and pyrosis (heartburn), should be determined. The nurse should be alert to any evidence of eating disorders such as anorexia nervosa, bulimia, or frequent and rigorous dieting before or during pregnancy.

The impact of food allergies and intolerances on nutritional status ranges from very important to almost none. Lactose intolerance is of special concern in pregnant and lactating women because no other food group equals milk and milk products in terms of calcium content. If a woman has lactose intolerance, then the interviewer should explore her intake of other calcium sources (see Box 8-4).

The assessment must include an evaluation of the woman's financial status and her knowledge of sound dietary practices. The quality of the diet improves with increasing socioeconomic status and educational level. Poor women may not have access to adequate refrigeration and cooking facilities and can have difficulty obtaining adequate nutritious food. The pregnancy rates are high among homeless women, and many such women cannot or do not take advantage of services such as food stamps.

Box 8-6 provides a simple tool for obtaining diet history information. When potential problems are identified, they should be followed up with a thorough interview.

Physical Examination

Anthropometric (body) **measurements** provide short- and long-term information about a woman's nutritional status and are therefore essential to the assessment. At a minimum, the woman's height and weight must be determined at the time of her first prenatal visit, and her weight should be measured at each subsequent visit (see earlier discussion of BMI).

A thorough physical examination can reveal objective signs of malnutrition (Table 8-4). An important point to note, however, is that some of these signs are nonspecific and that the physiologic changes of pregnancy may complicate the interpretation of physical findings. For example, lower-extremity edema often occurs in calorie and protein deficiency, but it may also be a normal finding in the third trimester of pregnancy. Interpretation of physical findings is made relatively easy by a thorough health history and by laboratory testing, if indicated.

Laboratory Testing

The only nutrition-related laboratory testing needed by most pregnant women is a hematocrit or hemoglobin measurement to screen for the presence of anemia. Because of the physiologic anemia of pregnancy, the reference values for hemoglobin and hematocrit must be adjusted during pregnancy. The lower limit of the normal range for hemoglobin during pregnancy is 11 g/dl in the first and third trimesters and 10.5 g/dl in the second trimester (compared with 12 g/dl in the nonpregnant state). The lower limit of the normal range for hematocrit is 33% during the first and third trimesters and 32% in the second trimester (compared with 37% in the nonpregnant state). Cutoff values for anemia are higher in women who smoke or who live at high altitudes because the decreased oxygen-carrying capacity of their RBCs causes them to produce more RBCs than other women.

A woman's history or physical findings may indicate the need for additional testing. These tests can include a complete blood cell count with differential to identify megaloblastic or macrocytic anemia, and measurement of levels of specific vitamins or minerals believed to be lacking in the diet.

For many women with uncomplicated pregnancies, the nurse can serve as the primary source of nutrition education during pregnancy. The registered dietitian, who has specialized training in diet evaluation and planning, nutritional needs during illness, and ethnic and cultural food patterns, as well as translating nutrient needs into food patterns, often serves as a consultant. Pregnant women with serious nutritional problems, those with intervening illnesses such as diabetes (either preexisting or gestational), and any others requiring in-depth dietary counseling should be referred to the dietitian.

Two programs that provide nutrition services are the food stamp program and the Special Supplemental Program for Women, Infants, and Children (WIC). These programs provide vouchers for selected foods to pregnant and lactating women, as well as infants and children at nutritional risk. WIC foods include items such as eggs, cheese, milk, juice, and fortified cereals–foods chosen because they provide iron, protein, vitamin C, and other vitamins.

Spanish Guidelines: Diet and Nutrition

Adequate Dietary Intake

Nutrition teaching can take place in a one-on-one interview or in a group setting. In either case, teaching should emphasize the importance of choosing a varied diet composed of readily available foods, rather than specialized diet supplements. The importance of consuming adequate amounts from the milk, yogurt, and cheese group must be emphasized, especially for adolescents and women younger

BOX 8-6

Food Intake Questionnaire

Which of the following did you eat or drink yesterday? If the way you ate yesterday was not the way you usually eat, choose a recent day that was typical for you.

FOOD OR DRINK	NUMBER OF SERVINGS	FOOD OR DRINK	NUMBER OF SERVINGS
Beer, wine, other alcoholic drinks	_____	Orange or grapefruit juice	_____
Tea	_____	Fruit juice other than orange or grapefruit	_____
Coffee		Soft drinks	_____
Caffeinated	_____	Milk	_____
Decaffeinated	_____	Cereal with milk	_____
Fruit drink	_____	Yogurt	_____
Water	_____	Pizza	_____
Cheese	_____	Melon (e.g., watermelon, cantaloupe)	_____
Macaroni and cheese	_____	Berries (e.g., raspberries, strawberries)	_____
Other foods with cheese (e.g., lasagna, enchiladas, cheeseburgers)	_____	Apples	_____
Orange or grapefruit	_____	Other fruit	_____
Bananas	_____	Broccoli	_____
Peaches or apricots	_____	Green beans	_____
Green salad	_____	Potatoes (other than fried)	_____
Spinach or greens	_____	Corn	_____
Green peas	_____	Other vegetables	_____
Sweet potatoes	_____	Chicken or turkey	_____
Carrots	_____	Egg	_____
Meat	_____	Nuts	_____
Fish	_____	Hot dog	_____
Peanut butter	_____	Cold cuts (e.g., bologna)	_____
Dried beans or peas	_____	Roll/bagel	_____
Bacon or sausage	_____	Noodles	_____
Bread	_____	Chips	_____
Rice	_____	Cake	_____
Spaghetti or other pasta	_____	Donut or pastry	_____
Tortillas	_____	Cookie	_____
French fries	_____	Pie	_____

Are you often bothered by any of the following? (Circle all that apply.)

Nausea Vomiting Heartburn Constipation

Are you on a special diet? No _____ Yes _____ If yes, what kind? _____________________

Do you try to limit the amount or kind of food you eat to control your weight? No _____ Yes _____

Do you avoid any foods for health or religious reasons? No _____ Yes _____ If yes, what foods? _____________

Do you take any prescribed drugs or medications? No_____ Yes _____ If yes, what are they? _________________

____

Do you take any over-the-counter medications (e.g., aspirin, cold medicines, acetaminophen [Tylenol])?

No _____ Yes _____ If yes, what are they? _____________________________

Do you take any herbal supplements? No _____ Yes _____ If yes, what are they? ______________________

____

Do you ever have trouble affording the food you need? No _____ Yes _____

Do you have any help getting the food you need? No _____ Yes _____

Food stamps? _____ WIC? _____ School lunch or breakfast? _____

Food from a food pantry, soup kitchen, or food bank? _____________

WIC, Special Supplemental Nutrition Program for Women, Infants, and Children.

TABLE 8-4

Physical Assessment of Nutritional Status

SIGNS OF GOOD NUTRITION	SIGNS OF POOR NUTRITION
GENERAL APPEARANCE	
Alert, responsive, energetic, good endurance	Listless, apathetic, cachectic, easily fatigued, looks tired
MUSCLES	
Well developed, firm, good tone, some fat under skin	Flaccid, poor tone, undeveloped, tender, "wasted" appearance
CENTRAL NERVOUS SYSTEM CONTROL	
Good attention span, not irritable or restless, normal reflexes, psychologic stability	Inattentive, irritable, confused, burning and tingling of hands and feet, loss of position and vibratory sense, weakness and tenderness of muscles, decrease or loss of ankle and knee reflexes
GASTROINTESTINAL FUNCTION	
Good appetite and digestion, normal regular elimination, no palpable organs or masses	Anorexia, indigestion, constipation or diarrhea, liver or spleen enlargement
CARDIOVASCULAR FUNCTION	
Normal heart rate and rhythm, no murmurs, normal blood pressure for age	Rapid heart rate, enlarged heart, abnormal rhythm, elevated blood pressure
HAIR	
Shiny, lustrous, firm, not easily plucked, healthy scalp	Stringy, dull, brittle, dry, thin and sparse, depigmented, can be easily plucked
SKIN (GENERAL)	
Smooth, slightly moist, good color	Rough, dry, scaly, pale, pigmented, irritated, easily bruised, petechiae
FACE AND NECK	
Skin color uniform, smooth, pink, healthy appearance; no enlargement of thyroid gland; lips not chapped or swollen	Scaly, swollen, skin dark over cheeks and under eyes, lumpiness or flakiness of skin around nose and mouth; thyroid enlarged; lips swollen, angular lesions or fissures at corners of mouth
ORAL CAVITY	
Reddish pink mucous membranes and gums; no swelling or bleeding of gums; tongue healthy pink or deep reddish in appearance, not swollen or smooth, surface papillae present; teeth bright and clean, no cavities, no pain, no discoloration	Gums spongy, bleed easily, inflamed or receding; tongue swollen, scarlet and raw, magenta color, beefy, hyperemic and hypertrophic papillae, atrophic papillae; teeth with unfilled caries, absent teeth, worn surfaces, mottled
EYES	
Bright, clear, shiny, no sores at corners of eyelids, membranes moist and healthy pink color, no prominent blood vessels or mound of tissue (Bitot spots) on sclera, no fatigue circles beneath	Eye membranes pale, redness of membrane, dryness, signs of infection, Bitot's spots, redness and fissuring of eyelid corners, dryness of eye membrane, dull appearance of cornea, soft cornea, blue sclerae
EXTREMITIES	
No tenderness, weakness, or swelling; nails firm and pink	Edema, tender calves, tingling, weakness; nails spoon-shaped, brittle
SKELETON	
No malformations	Bowlegs, knock-knees, chest deformity at diaphragm, beaded ribs, prominent scapulas

than 25 years who are still actively adding calcium to their skeletons; adolescents need at least 3 to 4 servings from the milk group daily. Good nutrition practices (and avoidance of poor practices such as smoking and alcohol or drug use) are essential content for prenatal classes designed for women in early pregnancy.

MyPyramid provides a plan for guiding nutrition choices (Fig. 8-3). Additional individualized information and resources are available from the website www.mypyramid.gov. For example, MyPyramid for Moms can be used as a guide for making daily good choices during pregnancy and lactation. On the website, select the option for MyPyramid for Moms. By selecting pregnancy or breastfeeding as appropriate a women can fill in the requested information (age, due date, height, prepregnancy weight, amount of exercise), and the program will calculate a plan for calories and amounts of food to be consumed daily to promote an appropriate weight gain. MyPyramid is also available in Spanish (MiPirámide).

Pregnancy

The pregnant woman must understand what adequate weight gain during pregnancy means, recognize the reasons for its importance, and be able to evaluate her own gain in terms of the desirable pattern. Many women, particularly those who have worked hard to control their weight before pregnancy, may have difficulty understanding why the weight gain goal is so high when a newborn infant is so small. The nurse can explain that maternal weight gain consists of increments in the weight of many tissues, not just the growing fetus (see Table 8-2).

Dietary overindulgence, which may result in excessive fat stores that persist after giving birth, should be discouraged. Nevertheless, the nurse should not focus unduly on weight gain because doing so could result in feelings of stress and guilt in the woman who does not follow the preferred pattern of gain.

Postpartum nutrition needs

The need for a varied diet with portions of food from all food groups continues throughout lactation. As mentioned previously, the lactating woman should be advised to consume at least 1800 kcal daily, and she should receive counseling if her diet appears to be inadequate in any nutrients.

The recommended energy intake for the first 6 months is an increase of 330 kcal more than the woman's nonpregnant intake. Obtaining adequate nutrients for maintenance of lactation is difficult if total caloric intake is less than 1800 kcal. Because of the deposition of energy stores, the woman who has gained the optimal amount of weight during pregnancy is heavier after birth than at the beginning of pregnancy. As a result of the caloric demands of lactation, however, the lactating mother usually experiences a gradual but steady weight loss. Most women rapidly lose several pounds during the first month after birth whether or not they breastfeed. After the first month the average loss during lactation is 0.5 to 1 kg a month.

The woman who does not breastfeed loses weight gradually if she consumes a balanced diet that provides slightly less than her daily energy expenditure. A reasonable weight loss goal for nonlactating women is 0.5 to 1 kg per week; a loss of 1 kg per month is recommended for most lactating women who need to lose weight. On average, at 6 weeks postpartum, women retain 3 to 7 kg of the weight gained during pregnancy, and two thirds of them weigh more than they did before pregnancy (Walker, Sterling, & Timmerman, 2005). Those at risk for obesity and overweight need follow-up to ensure that they know how to make wise food choices, primarily from fruits, vegetables, whole grains, lean meats, and low-fat dairy products. An hour of moderately vigorous physical activity (walking, jogging, swimming, cycling, aerobic dance, etc.) most days of the week will improve the ability of the woman to lose weight gradually and maintain the weight loss.

Medical nutrition therapy. During pregnancy and lactation the food plan for women with special medical nutrition therapy may have to be modified. The registered dietitian can instruct these women about their diet and assist them in meal planning. However, the nurse should understand the basic principles of the diet and be able to reinforce the diet teaching.

The nurse should be especially aware of the dietary modifications necessary for women with diabetes mellitus (either gestational or preexisting). This disease is relatively common, and fetal morbidity and mortality occur more often in pregnancies complicated by hyperglycemia or hypoglycemia (see discussion of diabetes in Chapter 20). Every effort should be made to maintain blood glucose levels in the normal range throughout pregnancy. The food plan of the woman with diabetes usually includes four to six meals and snacks daily, with the daily carbohydrate intake distributed fairly evenly among the meals and snacks. The complex carbohydrates–fibers and starches–should be well represented in the diet. To maintain strict control of the blood glucose level, the pregnant woman with diabetes usually must monitor her own blood glucose daily.

Counseling about Iron Supplementation

As mentioned earlier, the nutritional supplement most commonly needed during pregnancy is iron. However, a variety of dietary factors can affect the completeness of absorption of an iron supplement. The Patient Instructions for Self-Management box on p. 247 summarizes important points regarding iron supplementation.

Coping with Nutrition-Related Discomforts of Pregnancy

The most common nutrition-related discomforts of pregnancy are nausea and vomiting (or "morning sickness"), constipation, and pyrosis.

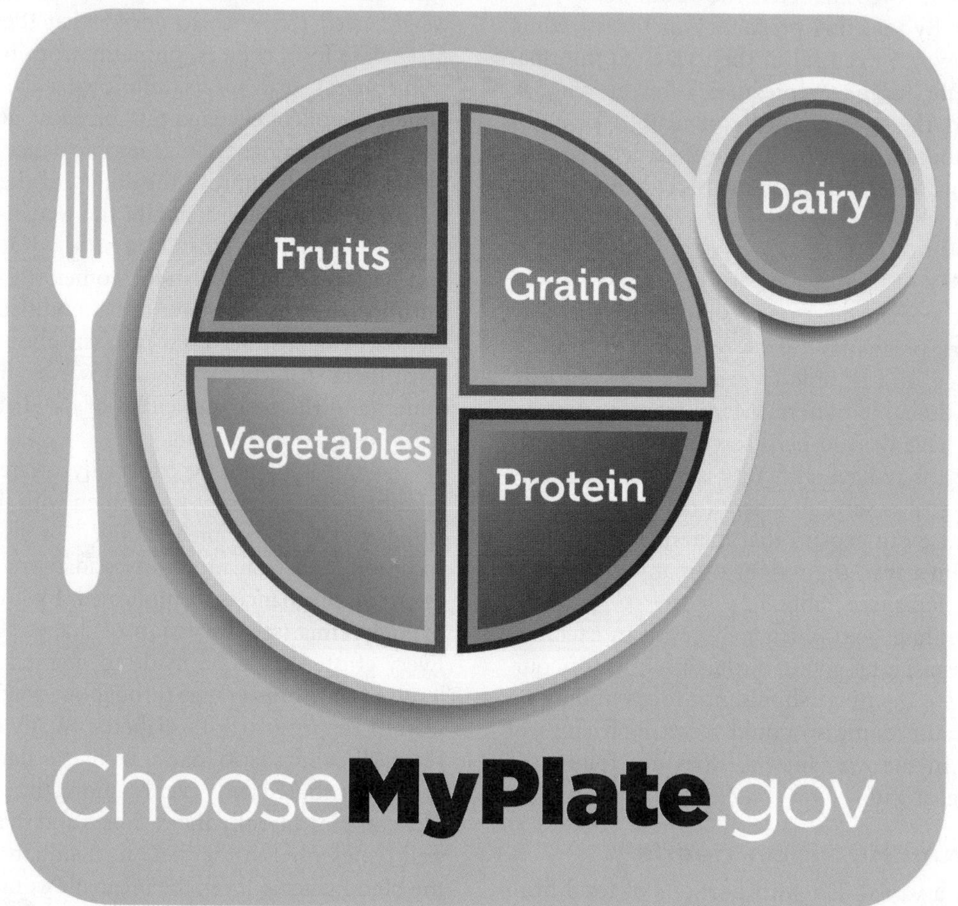

Fig. 8-3 Choose My Plate describes a healthy diet focusing on vegetables, fruits, fat-free or low-fat milk and milk products, as well as whole grains. MyPlate food guidelines suggest more lean meat consumption, nuts, eggs, beans, fish, and poultry; and a diet that is low in trans fats, saturated fats, cholesterol, and added sugars and salt. (Courtesy U.S. Department of Agriculture, Washington, DC; www.choosemyplate.gov.)

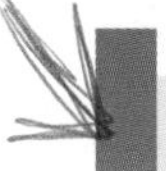

PATIENT INSTRUCTIONS FOR SELF-MANAGEMENT

Nausea and Vomiting

- Eat dry, starchy foods such as dry toast, Melba toast, or crackers on awakening in the morning and at other times when nausea occurs.
- Avoid consuming excessive amounts of fluids early in the day or when nauseated (but compensate by drinking fluids at other times).
- Eat small amounts frequently (every 2 to 3 hours), and avoid large meals that distend the stomach.
- Avoid skipping meals and thereby becoming extremely hungry, which may worsen nausea. Have a snack such as cereal with milk, a small sandwich, or yogurt before bedtime.
- Avoid sudden movements. Get out of bed slowly.
- Decrease intake of fried and other fatty foods. Starches such as pastas, rice, and breads and low-fat, high-protein foods such as skinless broiled or baked poultry, cooked dry beans or peas, lean meats, and broiled or canned fish are good choices.
- Tart foods or drinks (e.g., lemonade) or salty foods (e.g., potato chips) may be tolerated during periods of nausea.
- Fresh air may help relieve nausea. Keep the environment well ventilated (e.g., open a window), go for a walk outside, or decrease cooking odors by using an exhaust fan.
- During periods of nausea, eat foods served at cool temperatures and foods that give off little aroma.
- Try herbal teas such as those made with raspberry leaf or peppermint to decrease nausea.
- Ginger root may be effective in reducing nausea.
- Avoid brushing teeth immediately after eating.

Nausea and vomiting

Nausea and vomiting are most common during the first trimester. Usually, nausea and vomiting cause only mild to moderate problems nutritionally, although they may cause substantial discomfort. Antiemetic medications, vitamin B_6, and p6 acupressure (see Fig. 7-18, *A*) may be effective in reducing the severity of nausea (Jewell & Young, 2003). The Patient Instructions for Self-Management box summarizes important points regarding nausea and vomiting.

Hyperemesis gravidarum (severe and persistent vomiting causing weight loss, dehydration, and electrolyte abnormalities) occurs in up to 1% of pregnant women. Intravenous fluid and electrolyte replacement is usually necessary for women who lose 5% of their body weight. See Chapter 21 for a discussion of the condition.

Constipation

Improved bowel function generally results from increasing the intake of fiber (e.g., wheat bran and whole-wheat products, popcorn, and raw or lightly steamed vegetables) in the diet. Fiber helps retain water within the stool, creating a bulky stool that stimulates intestinal peristalsis. The recommendation for pregnant women for fiber is 28 g/day. An adequate fluid intake (at least 50 ml/kg/day) helps hydrate the fiber and increase the bulk of the stool. Making a habit of regular exercise that uses large muscle groups (walking, swimming, cycling) also helps stimulate bowel motility.

Pyrosis

Pyrosis, or heartburn, is usually caused by reflux of gastric contents into the esophagus. This condition can be minimized by eating small, frequent meals rather than two or three larger meals daily. Because fluids increase the distention of the stomach, they should not be consumed with foods. The woman needs to be sure to drink adequate amounts between meals. Avoiding spicy foods may help alleviate the problem. Reflux can be exacerbated by lying down immediately after eating and wearing clothing that is tight across the abdomen.

Cultural Influences

Consideration of a woman's cultural food preferences enhances communication and provides a greater opportunity for following the agreed-on pattern of intake. Women in most cultures are encouraged to eat a diet typical for them. The nurse needs to be aware of what constitutes a typical diet for each cultural or ethnic group that is present in her patient population. However, several variations may occur within one cultural group. Therefore a thorough exploration of individual preferences is needed. Although some ethnic and cultural food beliefs may seem, at first glance, to conflict with the dietary instruction provided by physicians, nurses, and dietitians, the empathic health care provider can often identify cultural beliefs that are congruent with the modern understanding of pregnancy and fetal development. Many cultural food practices have some merit; otherwise the culture would not have survived. Food cravings during pregnancy are considered normal by many cultures, but the kinds of cravings are often culturally specific. In most cultures, women crave acceptable foods, such as chicken, fish, and greens among African-Americans. Cultural influences on food intake usually lessen if the woman and her family become more integrated into the dominant culture. Nutrition beliefs and the practices of selected cultural groups are summarized in Table 8-5.

TABLE 8-5

Characteristic Food Patterns of Selected Cultures

MILK GROUP	PROTEIN GROUP	FRUITS AND VEGETABLES	BREADS AND CEREALS	POSSIBLE DIETARY PROBLEMS
NATIVE AMERICAN (MANY TRIBAL VARIATIONS; MANY "AMERICANIZED")				
Fresh milk Evaporated milk for cooking Ice cream Cream pie	Pork, beef, lamb, rabbit Fowl, fish, eggs Legumes Sunflower seeds Nuts: walnuts, acorn, pine, peanut butter Game meat	Green peas, beans Beets, turnips Leafy green and other vegetables Grapes, bananas, peaches, other fresh fruits Roots	Refined bread Whole wheat Cornmeal Rice Dry cereals "Fry" bread Tortillas	Obesity, diabetes, alcoholism, nutritional deficiencies expressed in dental problems and iron-deficiency anemia Inadequate amounts of all nutrients Excessive use of sugar
MIDDLE EASTERN* (ARMENIAN, GREEK, SYRIAN, TURKISH)				
Yogurt Little butter	Lamb Nuts Dried peas, beans, lentils Sesame seeds	Peppers, tomatoes, cabbage, grape leaves, cucumbers, squash Dried apricots, raisins, dates	Cracked wheat and dark bread	Fry many meats and vegetables Lack of fresh fruits Insufficient foods from milk group High consumption of sweeteners, lamb fat, and olive oil
AFRICAN-AMERICAN (PARTICULARLY SOUTHERN AND RURAL)				
Milk† Ice cream Cheese: longhorn, American	Pork: all cuts, plus organs, chitterlings Beef, lamb Chicken, giblets Eggs Nuts Legumes Fish, game	Leafy vegetables Green and yellow vegetables Potato: white, sweet Stewed fruit Bananas and other fresh fruit	Cornmeal and hominy grits Rice Biscuits, pancakes, white breads Puddings: bread, rice	Extensive use of frying, smothering in gravy, or simmering Fats: salt pork, bacon drippings, lard, and gravies High consumption of sweets Insufficient citrus Vegetables often boiled for long periods with pork fat and much salt Limited amounts from milk group†
CHINESE (CANTONESE MOST PREVALENT)				
Milk: water buffalo	Pork sausage‡ Eggs and pigeon eggs Fish Lamb, beef, goat Fowl: chicken, duck Nuts Legumes Soybean curd (tofu)	Many vegetables Radish leaves Bean, bamboo sprouts	Rice and rice-flour products Cereals, noodles Wheat, corn, millet seed	Tendency of some immigrants to use large amounts of grease in cooking Limited use of milk and milk products Often low in protein, calories, or both Soy sauce (high sodium)
FILIPINO (SPANISH-CHINESE INFLUENCE)				
Flavored milk Milk in coffee Cheese: gouda, cheddar	Pork, beef, goat, rabbit Chicken Fish Eggs, nuts, legumes	Many vegetables and fruits	Rice, cooked cereals Noodles: rice, wheat	Limited use of milk and milk products Tendency to prewash rice Tendency to have only small portions of protein foods

TABLE 8-5

Characteristic Food Patterns of Selected Cultures—cont'd

MILK GROUP	PROTEIN GROUP	FRUITS AND VEGETABLES	BREADS AND CEREALS	POSSIBLE DIETARY PROBLEMS
ITALIAN				
Cheese Some ice cream	Meat Eggs Dried beans	Leafy vegetables Potatoes Eggplant, tomatoes, peppers Fruits	Pasta White breads, some whole wheat Farina Cereals	Prefer expensive imported cheeses; reluctant to substitute less expensive domestic varieties Tendency to overcook vegetables Limited use of whole grains High consumption of sweets Extensive use of olive oil Insufficient servings from milk group
JAPANESE (ISEI, MORE JAPANESE INFLUENCE; NISEI, MORE WESTERNIZED)				
Increasing amounts being used by younger generations	Pork, beef, chicken Fish Eggs Legumes: soys, red, lima beans Tofu Nuts	Many vegetables and fruits Seaweed	Rice, rice cakes Wheat noodles Refined bread, noodles	Excessive sodium: pickles, salty crisp seaweed, MSG, and soy sauce Insufficient servings from milk group May use prewashed rice
HISPANIC, MEXICAN-AMERICAN				
Milk Cheese Flan, ice cream	Beef, pork, lamb, chicken, tripe, hot sausage, beef intestines Fish Eggs Nuts Dry beans: pinto, chickpeas (often eaten more than once daily)	Spinach, wild greens, tomatoes, chilies, corn, cactus leaves, cabbage, avocado, potatoes Pumpkin, zapote, peaches, guava, papaya, citrus	Rice, cornmeal Sweet bread, pastries Tortilla: corn, flour Vermicelli (fideo)	Limited meats primarily because of cost Limited use of milk and milk products Large amounts of lard Abundant use of sugar Tendency to boil vegetables for long periods
PUERTO RICAN				
Limited use of milk products Coffee with milk (café con leche)	Pork Poultry Eggs (Fridays) Dried codfish Beans (habichuelas)	Avocado, okra Eggplant Sweet yams Starchy vegetables and fruits (viandas)	Rice Cornmeal	Small amounts of pork and poultry Extensive use of fat, lard, salt pork, and olive oil Lack of milk products
SCANDINAVIAN (DANISH, FINNISH, NORWEGIAN, SWEDISH)				
Cream Butter Cheeses	Wild game Reindeer Fish (fresh or dried) Eggs	Berries Dried fruit Vegetables: cole slaw, roots	Whole wheat, rye, barley, sweets (cookies and sweet breads)	Insufficient fresh fruits and vegetables High consumption of sweets, pickled or salted meats, and fish

Continued

TABLE 8-5

Characteristic Food Patterns of Selected Cultures—cont'd

MILK GROUP	PROTEIN GROUP	FRUITS AND VEGETABLES	BREADS AND CEREALS	POSSIBLE DIETARY PROBLEMS
SOUTHEAST ASIAN (VIETNAMESE, CAMBODIAN)				
Generally not taken Coffee with condensed cow's milk Plain yogurt Ice cream (rare) Soybean milk	Fish (daily): fresh, dried, salted Poultry and eggs: duck, chicken Pork Beef (seldom) Dry beans Tofu	Seasonal variety: fresh or preserved Green, leafy vegetables Yams Corn	Rice: grains, flour, noodles French bread "Cellophane" (bean starch) noodles	Fresh milk products generally not consumed Poultry/eggs may be limited Meat considered "unclean" is avoided Preference for a diet high in salt and pepper, as well as rice and pork High intake of MSG and soy sauce
JEWISH: ORTHODOX*				
Milk† Cheese†	Meat (bloodless; Kosher prepared): beef, lamb, goat, deer, poultry (all types), no pork Fish with fins and scales only No crustaceans	Wide variety	Wide variety	High intake of sodium in meat products

MSG, monosodium L-glutamate.
*Religious holidays may involve fasting, which is believed to increase the likelihood of preterm labor. Fasting requirement may be waived during pregnancy.
†Lactose intolerance relatively common in adults.
‡Lower in fat content than Western sausage.

Vegetarian diets

Vegetarian diets represent another cultural effect on nutritional status. Foods basic to almost all vegetarian diets are vegetables, fruits, legumes, nuts, seeds, and grains, but with many variations. Semivegetarians, who are not truly vegetarians, include fish, poultry, eggs, and dairy products in their diets but do not eat beef or pork. Such a diet can be completely adequate for pregnant women. Another type of vegetarian, lacto-ovovegetarian, consumes dairy products and eggs in addition to plant products. Iron and zinc intake may not be adequate in these women, but such diets can be otherwise nutritionally sound. Strict vegetarians, or vegans, consume only plant products. Because vitamin B_{12} is found only in foods of animal origin, this diet is therefore deficient in vitamin B_{12}. As a result, strict vegetarians should take a supplement or regularly consume vitamin B_{12}–fortified foods (e.g., soy milk). Vitamin B_{12} deficiency can result in megaloblastic anemia, glossitis (inflamed red tongue), and neurologic deficits in the mother. Infants born to affected mothers are likely to have megaloblastic anemia and exhibit neurodevelopmental delays. Iron, calcium, zinc, and vitamin B_6 intake may also be low in women on this diet, and some strict vegetarians have excessively low caloric intakes. The protein intake should be assessed especially carefully because plant proteins tend to be incomplete in that they lack one or more amino acids required for growth and maintenance of body tissues. The daily consumption of a variety of different plant proteins–grains, dried beans and peas, nuts, and seeds–helps to provide all of the essential amino acids.

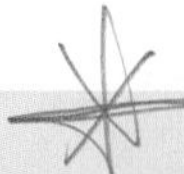

NURSING CARE PLAN *Nutrition during Pregnancy*

NURSING DIAGNOSIS Deficient knowledge related to nutritional requirements during pregnancy

Expected Outcome *The patient will delineate nutritional requirements and exhibit evidence of incorporating requirements into diet.*

Nursing Interventions/*Rationales*

- Review basic nutritional requirements for a healthy diet using recommended dietary guidelines and MyPyramid *to provide knowledge baseline for discussion.*
- Discuss increased nutrient needs (calories, protein, minerals, vitamins) that occur as a result of being pregnant *to increase knowledge needed for altered dietary requirements.*
- Discuss the relationship between weight gain and fetal growth *to reinforce interdependence of fetus and mother.*
- Calculate the appropriate total weight gain range during pregnancy using the woman's body mass index (BMI) as a guide and discuss recommended rates of weight gain during the various trimesters of pregnancy *to provide concrete measures of dietary success.*
- Review food preferences, cultural eating patterns or beliefs, and prepregnancy eating patterns *to enhance integration of new dietary needs.*
- Discuss how to fit nutritional needs into usual dietary patterns and how to alter any identified nutritional deficits or excesses *to increase chances of success with dietary alterations.*
- Discuss food aversions or cravings that may occur during pregnancy and strategies to deal with them if they are detrimental to fetus (e.g., pica) *to ensure the well-being of the fetus.*
- Have the woman keep a food diary delineating eating habits, dietary alterations, aversions, and cravings *to track eating habits and potential problem areas.*

NURSING DIAGNOSIS Imbalanced nutrition: more than body requirements related to excessive intake or inadequate activity levels (or both)

Expected Outcome *The woman's weekly weight gain will be reduced to the appropriate rate using her BMI and recommended weight gain ranges as guidelines.*

Nursing Interventions/*Rationales*

- Review recent diet history (including food cravings) using a food diary, 24-hour recall, or food frequency approach *to ascertain food excesses contributing to excess weight gain.*
- Review normal activity and exercise routines *to determine the level of energy expenditure;* discuss eating patterns and reasons that lead to increased food intake (e.g., cultural beliefs or myths, increased stress, boredom) *to identify habits that contribute to excess weight gain.*
- Review optimal weight gain guidelines and their rationale *to ensure that the woman is knowledgeable about healthful weight gain rates.*
- Set target weight gains for the remaining weeks of the pregnancy *to establish goals.*
- Discuss with the woman what changes can be made in diet, activity, and lifestyle *to enhance chances of meeting weight gain goals and dietary needs.* Weight-reduction diets should be avoided *because they may deprive the mother and fetus of needed nutrients and lead to ketonemia.*

NURSING DIAGNOSIS Imbalanced nutrition: less than body requirements related to inadequate intake of needed nutrients

Expected Outcome *The woman's weekly weight gain will be increased to the appropriate rate using her BMI and recommended weight gain ranges as guidelines.*

Nursing Interventions/*Rationales*

- Review recent diet history (including food aversions) using a food diary, 24-hour recall, or food frequency approach *to ascertain dietary inadequacies contributing to a lack of sufficient weight gain.*
- Review normal activity and exercise routines *to determine the level of energy expenditure;* discuss eating patterns and reasons that lead to decreased food intake (e.g., morning sickness, pica, fear of becoming fat, stress, boredom) *to identify habits that contribute to inadequate weight gain.*
- Review optimal weight gain guidelines and their rationale *to ensure that the woman is knowledgeable about healthful weight gain rates.*
- Set target weight gains for the remaining weeks of the pregnancy *to establish goals.*
- Review increased nutrient needs (calories, protein, minerals, vitamins) that occur as a result of being pregnant *to ensure that the woman is knowledgeable about altered dietary requirements.*
- Review the relationship between weight gain and fetal growth *to reinforce that adequate weight gain is needed to promote fetal well-being.*
- Discuss with the woman what changes can be made in diet, activity, and lifestyle *to enhance chances of meeting the set weight gain goals and nutrient needs of the mother and fetus.*
- If woman has fear of being fat, if symptoms of an eating disorder are evident, or if problems in adjusting to a changing body image surface, refer the woman to the appropriate mental health professional for evaluation *because intensive treatment and follow-up may be required to ensure fetal health.*

KEY POINTS

- A woman's nutritional status before, during, and after pregnancy contributes significantly to her well-being and that of her infant.
- Many physiologic changes occurring during pregnancy influence the need for additional nutrients and the efficiency with which the body uses them.
- Both the total maternal weight gain and the pattern of weight gain are important determinants of the outcome of pregnancy.
- The appropriateness of the mother's prepregnancy weight for height (BMI) is a major determinant of her recommended weight gain during pregnancy.
- Nutritional risk factors include adolescent pregnancy, nicotine use, alcohol or drug use, bizarre or faddish food habits, a low weight for height, and frequent pregnancies.
- Iron supplementation is usually routinely recommended during pregnancy. Other supplements can be warranted when nutritional risk factors are present.
- The nurse and the woman are influenced by cultural and personal values and beliefs during nutrition counseling.
- Pregnancy complications that may be nutrition related include anemia, gestational hypertension, gestational diabetes, and IUGR.
- Dietary adaptation can be an effective intervention for some of the common discomforts of pregnancy, including nausea and vomiting, constipation, and heartburn.

Audio Chapter Summaries Access an audio summary of these Key Points on evolve

References

Allen, L. (2005). Multiple micronutrients in pregnancy and lactation: An overview. *American Journal of Clinical Nutrition, 81*(5), 1206S-1212S.

Corbett, R., Ryan, C., & Weinrich, S. (2003). Pica in pregnancy: Does it affect pregnancy outcomes? *MCN American Journal of Maternal/Child Nursing, 28*(3), 183-189.

Cornel, M., Smit, D., & de Jong-van den Berg, L. (2005). Folic acid–the scientific debate as a base for public health policy. *Reproductive Toxicology, 20*(3), 411-415.

Gardiner, P. M., Nelson, L., Shellhaas, C. S., Dunlop, A. L., Long, R., Andrist, S., et al. (2008). The clinical content of preconception care: Nutrition and dietary supplements. *American Journal of Obstetrics & Gynecology, 199* (6 Suppl), S345-S356.

Grotegut, C. A., Dandolu, V., Katari, S., Whiteman, V. E., Geifman-Holtzman, O., & Teitelman, M. (2006). Baking soda pica: A case of hypokalemic metabolic alkalosis and rhabdomyolysis in pregnancy. *Obstetrics & Gynecology, 107*(2 Pt 2), 484-486.

Institute of Medicine. (2003). *Dietary reference intakes: Applications in dietary planning.* Washington, DC: National Academies Press.

Institute of Medicine. (2004). *Dietary reference intakes for water, potassium, sodium, chloride, and sulfate.* Washington, DC: National Academies Press.

Institute of Medicine. (2009). *Weight gain during pregnancy: Reexamining the guidelines.* Internet document available at www.iom.edu/?ID=68004 (accessed June 23, 2009).

Jewell, D., & Young, G. (2003). Interventions for nausea and vomiting in early pregnancy. In *The Cochrane Database of Systematic Reviews*, 2003, Issue 4, CD 000125.

Klitzman, S., Sharma, A., Nicaj, L., Vitkevich, R., & Leighton, J. (2002). Lead poisoning among pregnant women in New York City: Risk factors and screening practices. *Journal of Urban Health, 79*(2), 225-237.

Malone, F. D., & D'Alton, M. E. (2009). Multiple gestation: Clinical characteristics and management. In R. Creasy, R. Resnik, J. Iams, C. J. Lockwood, & T. R. Moore (Eds.), *Creasy & Resnick's maternal-fetal medicine: Principles and practice* (6th ed.). Philadelphia: Saunders.

Mathews, T. J., & MacDorman, M.F. (2008). Infant mortality statistics from the 2005 period linked birth/infant death data set. *National Vital Statistics Report, 57*(2), 1-32.

National Institutes of Health, Office of Dietary Supplements. (2007). *Dietary supplement fact sheet: Iron.* Internet document available at http://dietary-supplements.info.nih.gov/factsheets/iron.asp (accessed January 23, 2009).

Ngozi, P. O. (2008). Pica practices of pregnant women in Nairobi, Kenya. *East Africa Medical Journal, 85*(2), 72-79.

Paul, A. M. (July 13, 2008). Too fat and pregnant. *New York Times.*

Shannon, M. (2003). Severe lead poisoning in pregnancy. *Ambulatory Pediatrics, 3*(1), 37-39.

Walker, L., Sterling, B., & Timmerman, G. (2005). Retention of pregnancy-related weight in the early postpartum period: Implications for women's health services. *Journal of Obstetric, Gynecologic, & Neonatal Nursing, 34*(4), 418-427.

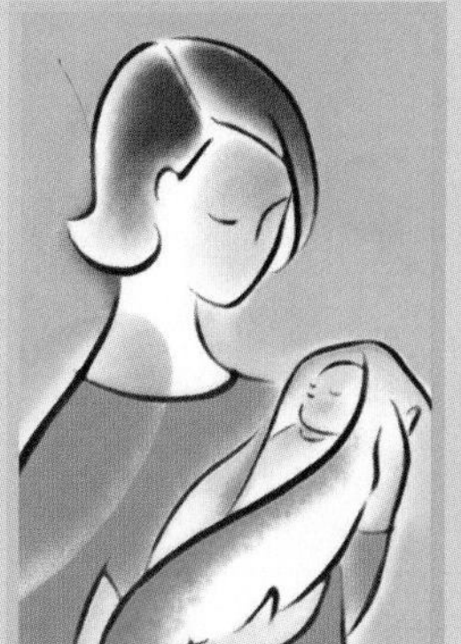

CHAPTER 9

Labor and Birth Processes

DEITRA LEONARD LOWDERMILK

LEARNING OBJECTIVES

- *Explain five factors that affect the labor process.*
- *Describe the anatomic structure of the bony pelvis.*
- *Recognize the normal measurements of the diameters of the pelvic inlet, cavity, and outlet.*
- *Explain the significance of the size and position of the fetal head during labor and birth.*
- *Summarize the cardinal movements of the mechanism of labor for a vertex presentation.*
- *Identify the maternal anatomic and physiologic adaptations to labor.*
- *Describe fetal adaptations to labor.*

KEY TERMS AND DEFINITIONS

asynclitism Oblique presentation of the fetal head at the superior strait of the pelvis; the pelvic planes and those of the fetal head are not parallel

attitude Relationship of fetal parts to each other in the uterus (e.g., all parts flexed or all parts flexed except neck extended)

biparietal diameter Largest transverse diameter of the fetal head; measured between the parietal bones

bloody show Vaginal discharge that originates in the cervix and consists of blood and mucus; increases as the cervix dilates during labor

dilation Stretching of the external os from an opening a few millimeters in size to an opening large enough to allow the passage of the fetus

effacement Thinning and shortening or obliteration of the cervix that occurs during late pregnancy or labor or both

engagement In obstetrics, the entrance of the fetal presenting part into the superior pelvic strait and the beginning of the descent through the pelvic canal; usually the lowest part of the presenting part is at or below the level of ischial spines

Ferguson reflex Reflex contractions (urge to push) of the uterus after stimulation of the cervix when the presenting part of the fetus reaches the perineal floor

fontanels Broad areas, or soft spots, consisting of a strong band of connective tissue contiguous with cranial bones and located at the junctions of the bones

lie Relationship existing between the long axis of the fetus and the long axis of the mother; in a longitudinal lie, the fetus is lying lengthwise or vertically, whereas in a transverse lie, the fetus is lying crosswise or horizontally in the uterus

lightening Sensation of decreased abdominal distention produced by uterine descent into the pelvic cavity as the fetal presenting part settles into the pelvis; usually occurs 2 weeks before the onset of labor in nulliparas

molding Overlapping of cranial bones or shaping of the fetal head to accommodate and conform to the bony and soft parts of the mother's birth canal during labor

position Relationship of a reference point on the presenting part of the fetus, such as the occiput, sacrum, chin, or scapula, to its location in the front, back, or sides of the maternal pelvis

presentation That part of the fetus that first enters the pelvis and lies over the inlet; may be the head, face, breech, or shoulder

presenting part That part of the fetus that lies closest to the internal os of the cervix

station Relationship of the presenting fetal part to an imaginary line drawn between the ischial spines of the pelvis

suboccipitobregmatic diameter Smallest anterior-posterior diameter of the fetal head; follows a line drawn from the middle of the anterior fontanel to the undersurface of the occipital bone

Valsalva maneuver Forced expiratory effort against a closed airway, such as holding one's breath and tightening the abdominal muscles (e.g., pushing during the second stage of labor)

vertex Crown, or top, of the head

WEB RESOURCES

Additional related content can be found on the companion website at evolve
http://evolve.elsevier.com/Lowdermilk/Maternity/

- NCLEX Review Questions
- Assessment Videos: Fetal Lie, Presentation, Position
- Critical Thinking Exercise: Fetal Presentation

During late pregnancy the woman and fetus prepare for the labor process. The fetus has grown and developed in preparation for extrauterine life. The woman has undergone various physiologic adaptations during pregnancy that prepare her for birth and motherhood. Labor and birth represent the end of pregnancy, the beginning of extrauterine life for the newborn, and a change in the lives of the family. This chapter discusses the factors affecting labor, the process involved, the normal progression of events, and the adaptations made by both the woman and the fetus.

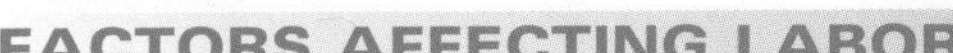

FACTORS AFFECTING LABOR

At least five factors affect the process of labor and birth. These factors are easily remembered as the five *P*s: passenger (fetus and placenta), passageway (birth canal), powers (contractions), position of the mother, and psychologic response. The first four factors are presented here as the basis of understanding the physiologic process of labor. The fifth factor is discussed in Chapter 12. Other factors that may be a part of the woman's labor experience may be important as well. VandeVusse (1999) identified external forces that include place of birth, preparation, type of provider (especially nurses), and procedures. Physiologic response (sensations) was identified as an internal force. These factors are discussed generally in Chapter 12 because they relate to nursing care during labor. Further research investigating essential forces of labor is recommended.

Passenger

Critical Thinking Exercise: Fetal Presentation

The way the passenger, or fetus, moves through the birth canal is determined by several interacting factors: the size of the fetal head, fetal presentation, fetal lie, fetal attitude, and fetal position. Because the placenta also must pass through the birth canal, it can be considered a passenger along with the fetus; however, the placenta rarely impedes the process of labor in a normal vaginal birth, except in cases of placenta previa.

Size of the fetal head

Because of its size and relative rigidity, the fetal head has a major effect on the birth process. The fetal skull is composed of two parietal bones, two temporal bones, the frontal bone, and the occipital bone (Fig. 9-1, *A*). These bones are united by membranous sutures: the sagittal, lambdoidal, coronal, and frontal (Fig. 9-1, *B*). Membrane-filled spaces called **fontanels** are located where the sutures intersect. During labor, after rupture of membranes, palpation of fontanels and sutures during vaginal examination reveals fetal presentation, position, and attitude.

The two most important fontanels are the anterior and posterior ones (see Fig. 9-1, *B*). The larger of these, the anterior fontanel, is diamond shaped, is approximately 3 cm by 2 cm, and lies at the junction of the sagittal, coronal, and frontal sutures. It closes by 18 months after birth. The posterior fontanel lies at the junction of the sutures of the two parietal bones and the occipital bone, is triangular, and is approximately 1 cm by 2 cm. It closes 6 to 8 weeks after birth.

Sutures and fontanels make the skull flexible to accommodate the infant brain, which continues to grow for some time after birth. Because the bones are not firmly united, however, slight overlapping of the bones, or **molding** of the shape of the head, occurs during labor. This capacity of the bones to slide over one another also permits adaptation to the various diameters of the maternal pelvis. Molding can be extensive, but the heads of most newborns assume their normal shape within 3 days after birth.

Although the size of the fetal shoulders may affect passage, their position can be altered relatively easily during labor; thus one shoulder may occupy a lower level than the other. This position creates a shoulder diameter that is smaller than the skull, facilitating passage through the birth canal. The circumference of the fetal hips is usually small enough not to create problems.

Fetal presentation

Presentation refers to the part of the fetus that enters the pelvic inlet first and leads through the birth canal during labor at term. The three main presentations are *cephalic* presentation (head first), occurring in 96% of births (Fig. 9-2); *breech* presentation (buttocks or feet first), occurring in 3% of births (Fig. 9-3, *A-C*); and *shoulder* presentation, seen in 1% of births (Fig. 9-3, *D*). The **presenting part** is that part of the fetal body first felt by the examining finger during a vaginal examination. In a cephalic presentation the presenting part is usually the occiput, in a breech presentation it is the sacrum, and in the shoulder

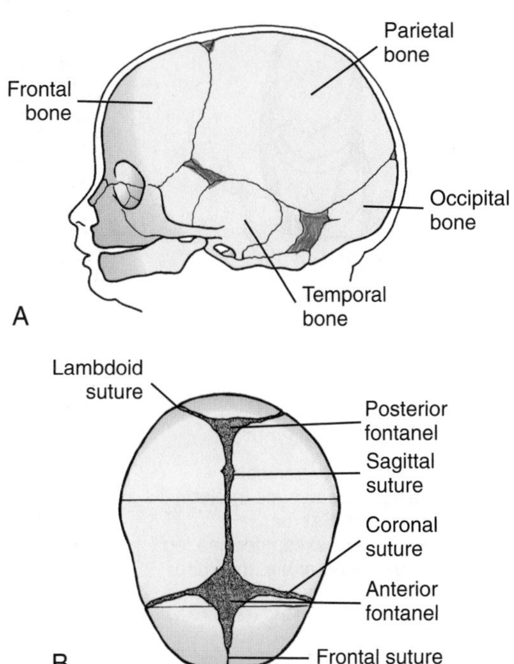

Fig. 9-1 Fetal head at term. **A,** Bones. **B,** Sutures and fontanels.

presentation it is the scapula. When the presenting part is the occiput, the presentation is noted as **vertex** (see Fig. 9-2). Factors that determine the presenting part include fetal lie, fetal attitude, and extension or flexion of the fetal head.

Assessment Video: Presentation

Fetal Lie

Lie is the relation of the long axis (spine) of the fetus to the long axis (spine) of the mother. The two primary lies are longitudinal, or vertical, in which the long axis of the fetus is parallel with the long axis of the mother (see Fig. 9-2); and transverse, horizontal, or oblique, in which the long axis of the fetus is at a right angle diagonal to the long axis of the mother (see Fig. 9-3, *D*). Longitudinal lies are either cephalic or breech presentations, depending on the fetal structure that first enters the mother's pelvis. Vaginal birth cannot occur when the fetus stays in a transverse lie. An oblique lie, one in which the long axis of the fetus is lying at an angle to the long axis of the mother, is uncommon and usually converts to a longitudinal or transverse lie during labor (Cunningham, Bloom, Gilstrap, Leveno, Hauth, & Wenstrom, 2005).

Assessment Video: Fetal Lie

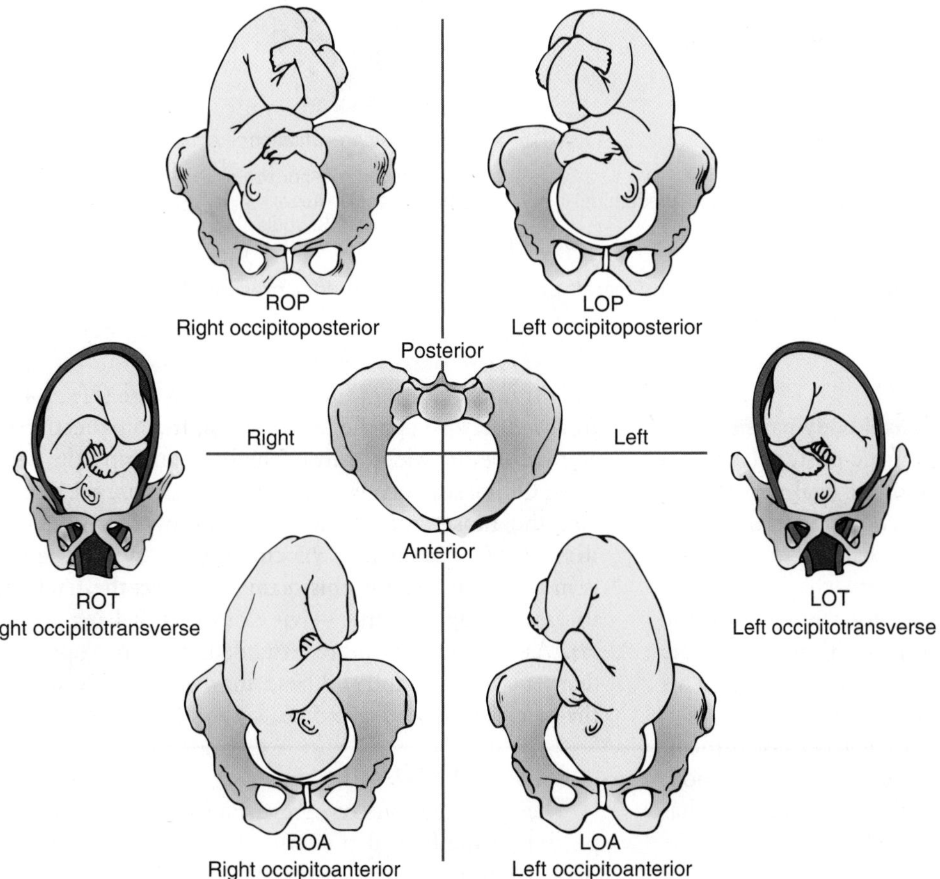

Fig. 9-2 Examples of fetal vertex (occiput) presentations in relation to front, back, or side of maternal pelvis.

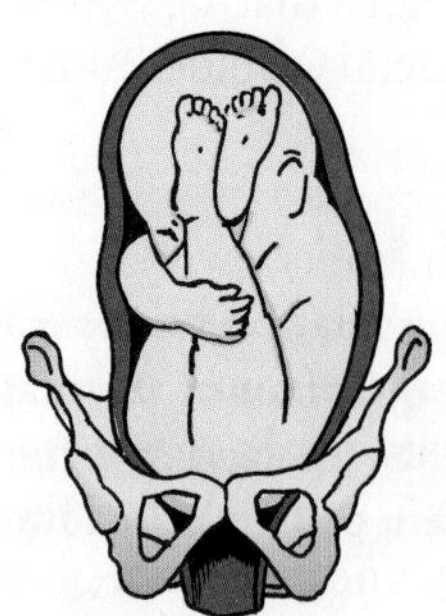

Frank breech

Lie: Longitudinal or vertical
Presentation: Breech (incomplete)
Presenting part: Sacrum
A Attitude: Flexion, except for legs at knees

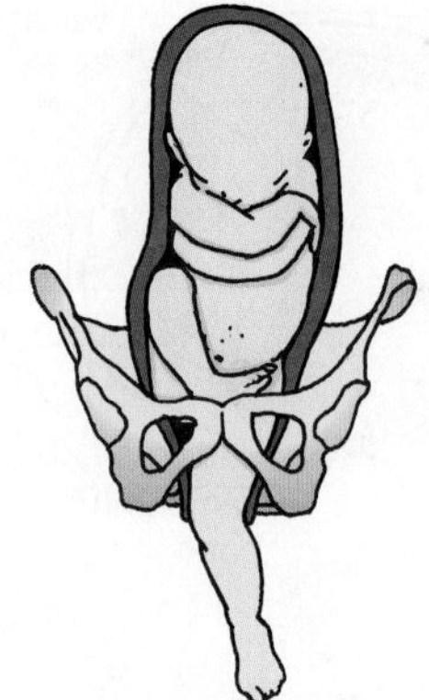

Single footling breech

Lie: Longitudinal or vertical
Presentation: Breech (incomplete)
Presenting part: Sacrum
Attitude: Flexion, except for one leg extended at hip and knee
B

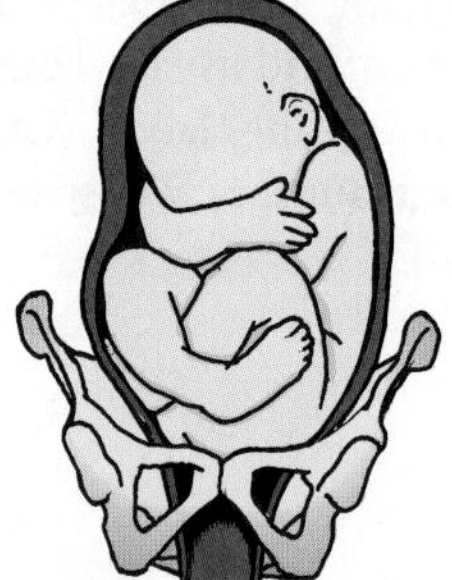

Complete breech

Lie: Longitudinal or vertical
Presentation: Breech (sacrum and feet presenting)
Presenting part: Sacrum (with feet)
C Attitude: General flexion

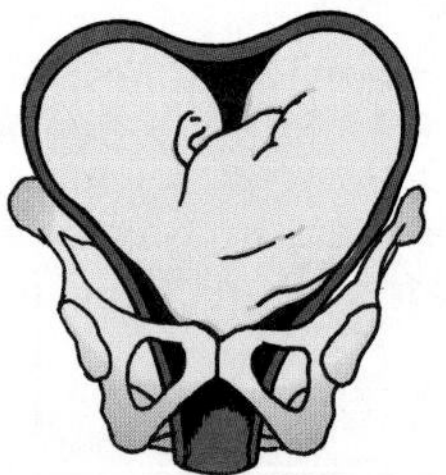

Shoulder presentation

Lie: Transverse or horizontal
Presentation: Shoulder
Presenting part: Scapula
D Attitude: Flexion

Fig. 9-3 Fetal presentations. **A-C,** Breech (sacral) presentation. **D,** Shoulder presentation.

Fetal Attitude

Attitude is the relationship of the fetal body parts to each other. The fetus assumes a characteristic posture (attitude) in utero partly because of the mode of fetal growth and partly because of the way the fetus conforms to the shape of the uterine cavity. Normally the back of the fetus is rounded so that the chin is flexed on the chest, the thighs are flexed on the abdomen, and the legs are flexed at the knees. The arms are crossed over the thorax, and the umbilical cord lies between the arms and the legs. This attitude is termed *general flexion* (see Fig. 9-2).

Assessment Video: Position

Deviations from the normal attitude may cause difficulties in childbirth. For example, in a cephalic presentation, the fetal head may be extended or flexed in a manner that presents a head diameter that exceeds the limits of the maternal pelvis, leading to prolonged labor, forceps- or vacuum-assisted birth, or cesarean birth.

Certain critical diameters of the fetal head are usually measured. The **biparietal diameter,** which is approximately 9.25 cm at term, is the largest transverse diameter and an important indicator of fetal head size (Fig. 9-4, *B*). In a well-flexed cephalic presentation, the biparietal diameter will be the widest part of the head entering the pelvic inlet. Of the several anteroposterior diameters, the smallest and the most critical one is the **suboccipitobregmatic diameter** (approximately 9.5 cm at term). When the head is in complete flexion, this diameter allows the fetal head to pass through the true pelvis easily (Fig. 9-4, *A*; Fig. 9-5, *A*). As the head is more extended, the anteroposterior diameter widens, and the head may not be able to enter the true pelvis (see Fig. 9-5, *B, C*).

Fetal position

The presentation or presenting part indicates the portion of the fetus that overlies the pelvic inlet. **Position** is the relationship of the presenting part (occiput, sacrum, mentum [chin], or sinciput [deflexed vertex]) to the four quadrants of the mother's pelvis (see Fig. 9-2). Position is denoted by a three-letter abbreviation. The first letter of the abbreviation denotes the location of the presenting

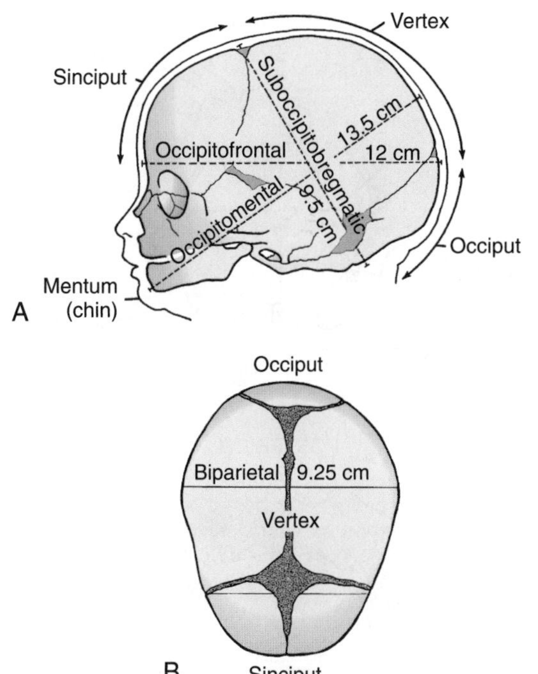

Fig. 9-4 Diameters of the fetal head at term. **A,** Cephalic presentations: occiput, vertex, and sinciput; and cephalic diameters: suboccipitobregmatic, occipitofrontal, and occipitomental. **B,** Biparietal diameter.

part in the right (R) or left (L) side of the mother's pelvis. The middle letter stands for the specific presenting part of the fetus (O for occiput, S for sacrum, M for mentum [chin], and Sc for scapula [shoulder]). The third letter stands for the location of the presenting part in relation to the anterior (A), posterior (P), or transverse (T) portion of the maternal pelvis. For example, ROA means that the occiput is the presenting part and is located in the right anterior quadrant of the maternal pelvis (see Fig. 9-2). LSP means that the sacrum is the presenting part and is located in the left posterior quadrant of the maternal pelvis (see Fig. 9-3).

Station is the relationship of the presenting part of the fetus to an imaginary line drawn between the maternal ischial spines and is a measure of the degree of descent of the presenting part of the fetus through the birth canal. The placement of the presenting part is measured in centimeters above or below the ischial spines (Fig. 9-6). For example, when the lowermost portion of the presenting part is 1 cm above the spines, it is noted as being minus (–) 1. At the level of the spines, the station is said to be 0 (zero). When the presenting part is 1 cm below the spines, the station is said to be plus (+) 1. Birth is imminent when the presenting part is at +4 to +5 cm. The station of the presenting part should be determined when labor begins so that the rate of descent of the fetus during labor can be accurately determined.

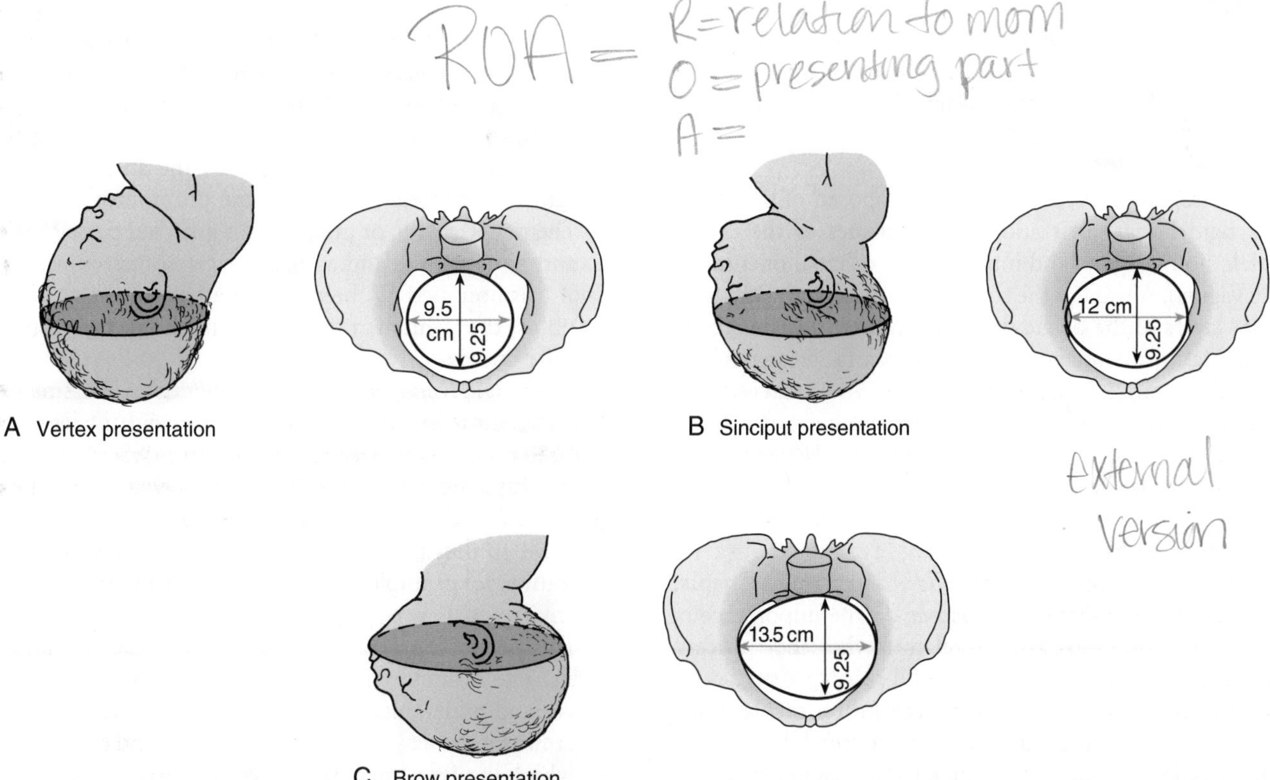

Fig. 9-5 Head entering pelvis. Biparietal diameter is indicated with shading (9.25 cm). **A,** Suboccipitobregmatic diameter: complete flexion of head on chest so that smallest diameter enters. **B,** Occipitofrontal diameter: moderate extension (military attitude) so that large diameter enters. **C,** Occipitomental diameter: marked extension (deflection) so that the largest diameter, which is too large to permit head to enter pelvis, is presenting.

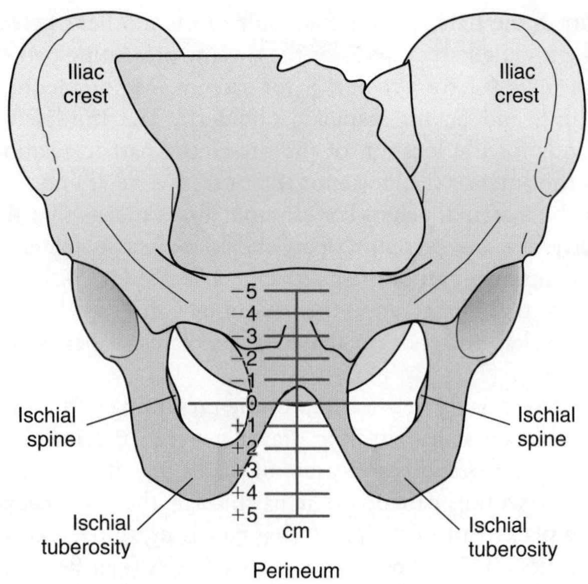

Fig. 9-6 Stations of presenting part, or degree of descent. The lowermost portion of the presenting part is at the level of the ischial spines, station 0.

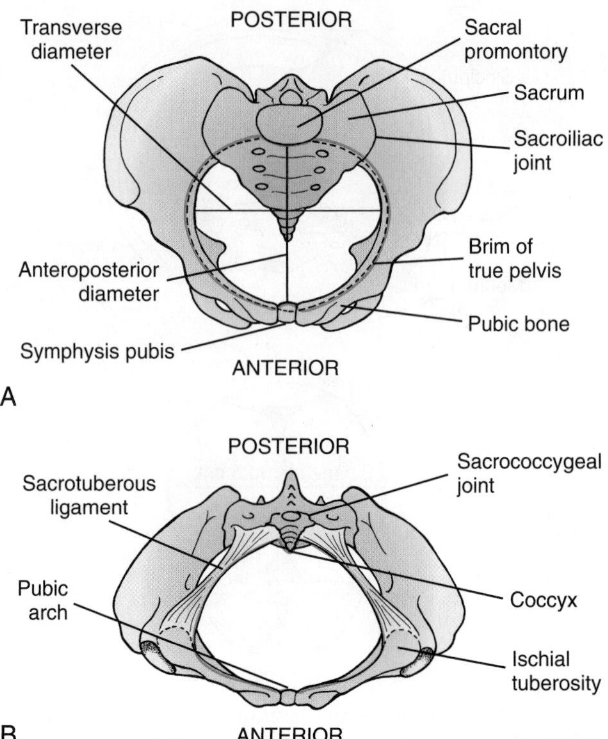

Fig. 9-7 Female pelvis. **A,** Pelvic brim above. **B,** Pelvic outlet from below.

Engagement is the term used to indicate that the largest transverse diameter of the presenting part (usually the biparietal diameter) has passed through the maternal pelvic brim or inlet into the true pelvis and usually corresponds to station 0. Engagement often occurs in the weeks just before labor begins in nulliparas and may occur before labor or during labor in multiparas. Engagement can be determined by abdominal or vaginal examination.

Passageway

The passageway, or birth canal, is composed of the mother's rigid bony pelvis and the soft tissues of the cervix, pelvic floor, vagina, and introitus (the external opening to the vagina). Although the soft tissues, particularly the muscular layers of the pelvic floor, contribute to vaginal birth of the fetus, the maternal pelvis plays a far greater role in the labor process because the fetus must successfully accommodate itself to this relatively rigid passageway. Therefore the size and shape of the pelvis need to be determined before labor begins.

Bony pelvis

The anatomy of the bony pelvis is described in Chapter 2. The following discussion focuses on the importance of pelvic configurations as they relate to the labor process. (Referring to Fig. 2-4 may be helpful.)

The bony pelvis is formed by the fusion of the ilium, ischium, pubis, and sacral bones. The four pelvic joints are the symphysis pubis, the right and left sacroiliac joints, and the sacrococcygeal joint (Fig. 9-7, *A*). The bony pelvis is separated by the brim, or inlet, into two parts: the false pelvis and the true pelvis. The false pelvis is the part above the brim and plays no part in childbearing. The true pelvis, the part involved in birth, is divided into three planes: the inlet, or brim; the midpelvis, or cavity; and the outlet.

The pelvic inlet, which is the upper border of the true pelvis, is formed anteriorly by the upper margins of the pubic bone, laterally by the iliopectineal lines along the innominate bones, and posteriorly by the anterior, upper margin of the sacrum and the sacral promontory.

The pelvic cavity, or midpelvis, is a curved passage with a short anterior wall and a much longer concave posterior wall. It is bounded by the posterior aspect of the symphysis pubis, the ischium, a portion of the ilium, the sacrum, and the coccyx.

The pelvic outlet is the lower border of the true pelvis. Viewed from below, it is ovoid, somewhat diamond shaped, bounded by the pubic arch anteriorly, the ischial tuberosities laterally, and the tip of the coccyx posteriorly (Fig. 9-7, *B*). In the latter part of pregnancy, the coccyx is movable (unless it has been broken in a fall during skiing or skating, for example, and has fused to the sacrum during healing).

The pelvic canal varies in size and shape at various levels. The diameters at the plane of the pelvic inlet, midpelvis, and outlet, plus the axis of the birth canal (Fig. 9-8), determine whether vaginal birth is possible and the manner by which the fetus may pass down the birth canal.

The subpubic angle, which determines the type of pubic arch, together with the length of the pubic rami and the intertuberous diameter, is of great importance. Because the fetus must first pass beneath the pubic arch, a narrow

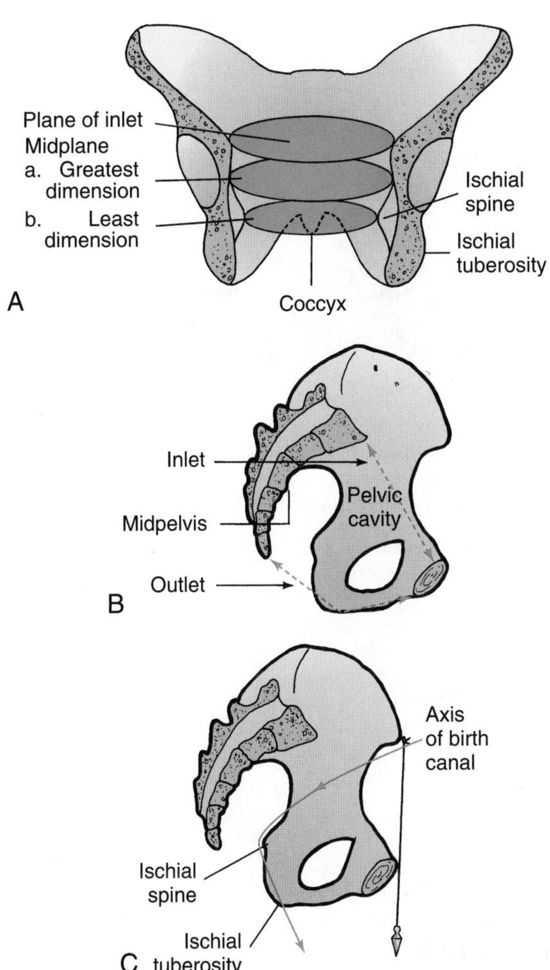

Fig. 9-8 Pelvic cavity. **A,** Inlet and midplane. Outlet not shown. **B,** Cavity of true pelvis. **C,** Note curve of sacrum and axis of birth canal.

subpubic angle will be less accommodating than a rounded wide arch. The method of measurement of the subpubic arch is shown in Fig. 9-9. A summary of obstetric measurements is given in Table 9-1.

The four basic types of pelves are classified as follows:

1. Gynecoid (the classic female type)
2. Android (resembling the male pelvis)
3. Anthropoid (resembling the pelvis of anthropoid apes)
4. Platypelloid (the flat pelvis)

The gynecoid pelvis is the most common, with major gynecoid pelvic features present in 50% of all women. Anthropoid and android features are less common than the gynecoid pelvis, and platypelloid pelvic features are the least common. Mixed types of pelves are more common than are pure types (Cunningham et al., 2005). Examples of pelvic variations and their effects on mode of birth are given in Table 9-2.

Assessment of the bony pelvis can be performed during the first prenatal evaluation and need not be repeated if the pelvis is of adequate size and suitable shape. In the third trimester of pregnancy, the examination of the bony

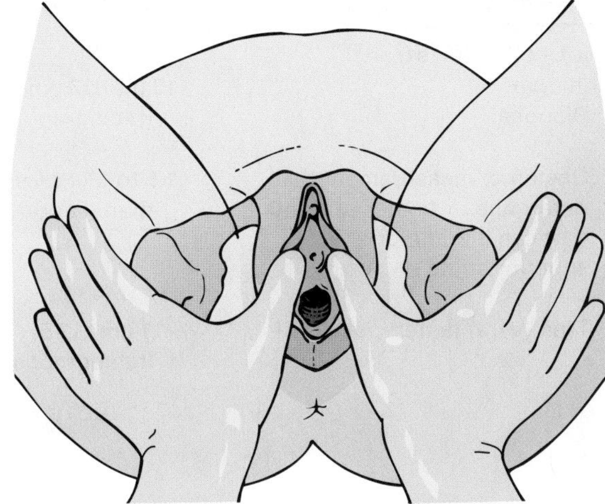

Fig. 9-9 Estimation of angle of subpubic arch. With both thumbs, examiner externally traces descending rami down to tuberosities. (From Barkauskas, V., Baumann, L., & Darling-Fisher, C. [2002]. *Health and physical assessment* [3rd ed.]. St. Louis: Mosby.)

pelvis may be more thorough and the results more accurate because of the relaxation and increased mobility of the pelvic joints and ligaments owing to hormonal influences. Widening of the joint of the symphysis pubis and the resulting instability may cause pain in any or all of the pelvic joints.

Because the examiner does not have direct access to the bony structures and because the bones are covered with varying amounts of soft tissue, estimates of size and shape are approximate. Precise bony pelvis measurements can be determined by use of computed tomography, ultrasound, or x-ray films. However, radiographic examination is rarely performed during pregnancy because the x-rays may damage the developing fetus.

Soft tissues

The soft tissues of the passageway include the distensible lower uterine segment, cervix, pelvic floor muscles, vagina, and introitus. Before labor begins, the uterus is composed of the uterine body (corpus) and cervix (neck). After labor has begun, uterine contractions cause the uterine body to have a thick and muscular upper segment and a thin-walled, passive, muscular lower segment. A *physiologic retraction ring* separates the two segments (Fig. 9-10). The lower uterine segment gradually distends to accommodate the intrauterine contents as the wall of the upper segment thickens, and its accommodating capacity is reduced. The contractions of the uterine body thus exert downward pressure on the fetus, pushing it against the cervix.

The cervix effaces (thins) and dilates (opens) sufficiently to allow the first fetal portion to descend into the vagina. As the fetus descends, the cervix is actually drawn upward and over this first portion.

The pelvic floor is a muscular layer that separates the pelvic cavity above from the perineal space below. This

TABLE 9-1

Obstetric Measurements

PLANE	DIAMETER	MEASUREMENTS
Inlet (superior strait)		
Conjugate Diagonal	12.5 to 13 cm (radiographic)	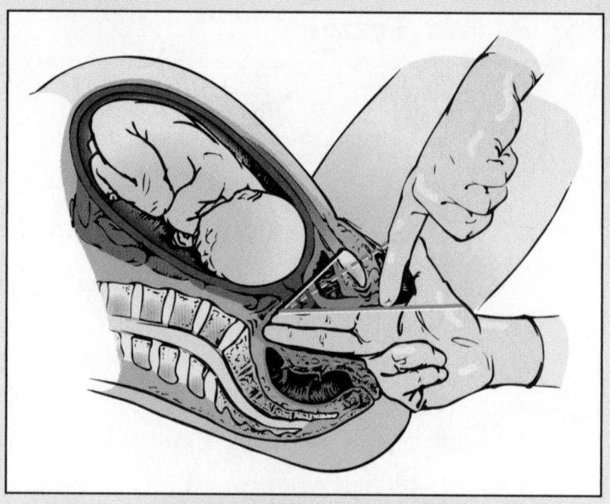
Obstetric: measurement that determines whether presenting part can engage or enter superior strait	1.5 to 2 cm less than diagonal	
True (vera) (anteroposterior)	≥11 cm (12.5) (radiographic)	Length of diagonal conjugate (blue line), obstetric conjugate (broken blue line), and true conjugate (white line)*
Midplane		
Transverse diameter (interspinous diameter)	10.5 cm	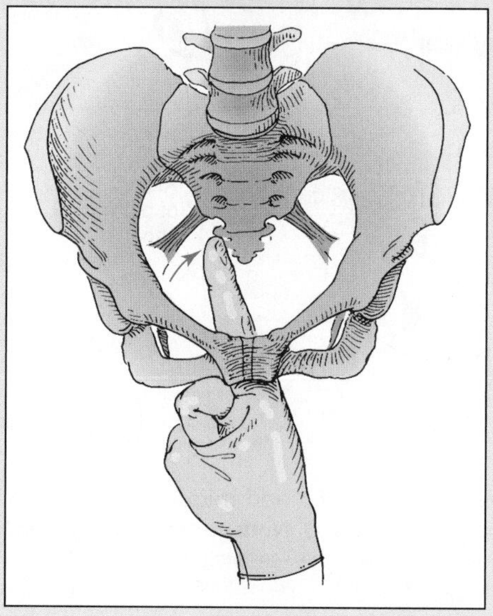
The midplane of the pelvis normally is its largest plane and the one of greatest diameter		Measurement of interspinous diameter*
Outlet		
Transverse diameter (intertuberous diameter) (biischial)	≥8 cm	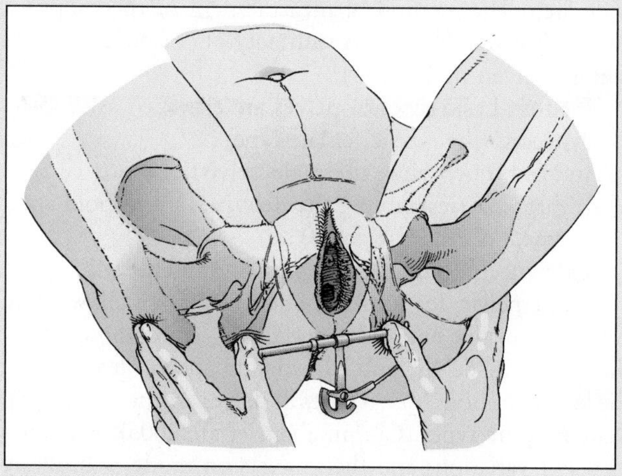
The outlet presents the smallest plane of the pelvic canal		Use of Thom's pelvimeter to measure intertuberous diameter*

*From Seidel, H., Ball, J., Dains, J., & Benedict, G. (2006). *Mosby's guide to physical examination* (6th ed.). St. Louis: Mosby.

TABLE 9-2

Comparison of Pelvic Types

CHARACTERISTICS OF PELVIS TYPE	GYNECOID (50% OF WOMEN)	ANDROID (23% OF WOMEN)	ANTHROPOID (24% OF WOMEN)	PLATYPELLOID (3% OF WOMEN)
Brim	Slightly ovoid or transversely rounded	Heart shaped, angulated	Oval, wider anteroposteriorly	Flattened anteroposteriorly, wide transversely
Shape	◯ Round	♡ Heart	0 Oval	⬭ Flat
Depth	Moderate	Deep	Deep	Shallow
Sidewalls	Straight	Convergent	Straight	Straight
Ischial spines	Blunt, somewhat widely separated	Prominent, narrow interspinous diameter	Prominent, often with narrow interspinous diameter	Blunted, widely separated
Sacrum	Deep, curved	Slightly curved, terminal portion often beaked	Slightly curved	Slightly curved
Subpubic arch	Wide	Narrow	Narrow	Wide
Usual mode of birth	Vaginal Spontaneous Occipitoanterior position	Cesarean Vaginal Difficult with forceps	Vaginal Forceps Spontaneous Occipitoposterior or occipitoanterior position	Vaginal Cesarean

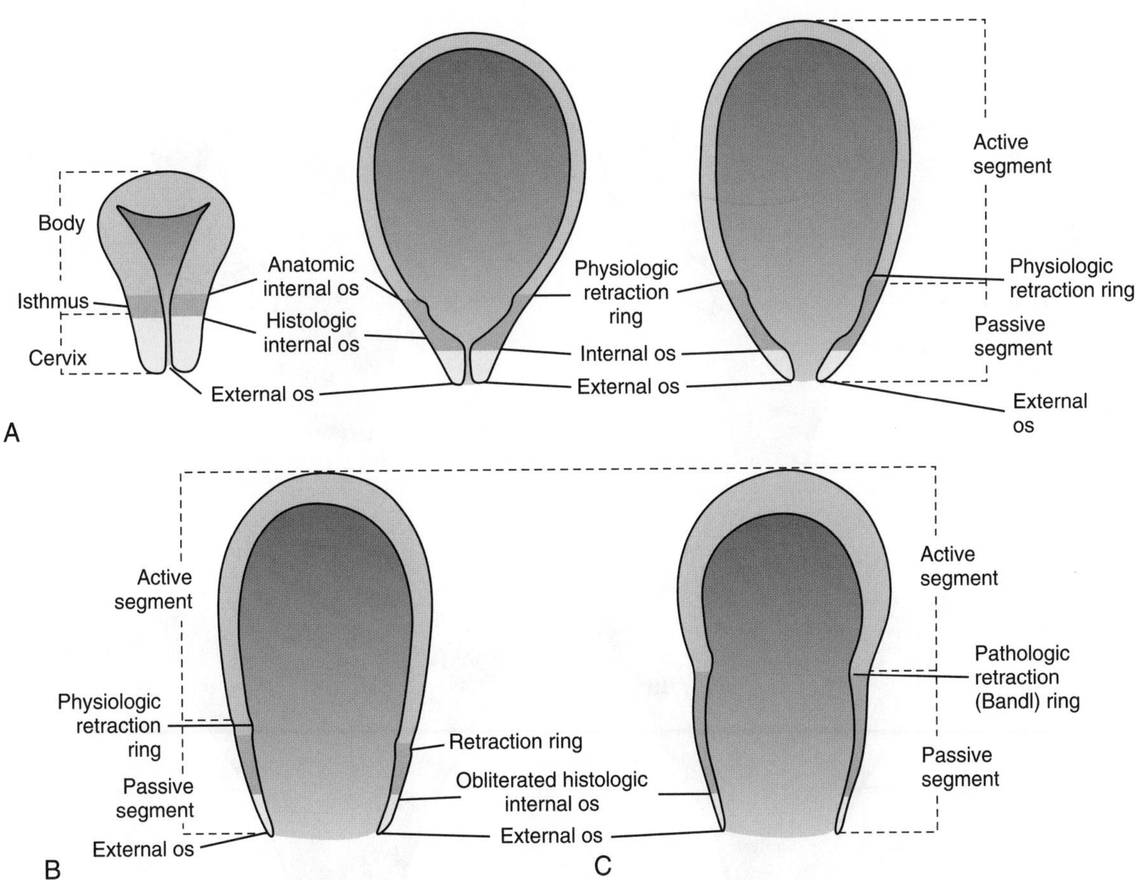

Fig. 9-10 **A,** Uterus in normal labor in early first stage, and **B,** in second stage. Passive segment is derived from lower uterine segment (isthmus) and cervix, and physiologic retraction ring is derived from anatomic internal os. **C,** Uterus in abnormal labor in second-stage dystocia. Pathologic retraction (Bandl) ring that forms under abnormal conditions develops from the physiologic ring.

structure helps the fetus rotate anteriorly as it passes through the birth canal. As noted earlier, the soft tissues of the vagina develop throughout pregnancy until at term the vagina can dilate to accommodate the fetus and permit passage of the fetus to the external world.

Powers

Involuntary and voluntary powers combine to expel the fetus and the placenta from the uterus. Involuntary uterine contractions, called the *primary powers,* signal the beginning of labor. Once the cervix has dilated, voluntary bearing-down efforts by the woman, called the *secondary powers,* augment the force of the involuntary contractions.

Primary powers

The involuntary contractions originate at certain pacemaker points in the thickened muscle layers of the upper uterine segment. From the pacemaker points, contractions move downward over the uterus in waves, separated by short rest periods. Terms used to describe these involuntary contractions include *frequency* (the time from the beginning of one contraction to the beginning of the next), *duration* (length of contraction from the beginning to the end), and *intensity* (strength of contraction).

The primary powers are responsible for the effacement and dilation of the cervix and descent of the fetus. **Effacement** of the cervix means the shortening and thinning of the cervix during the first stage of labor. The cervix, normally 2 to 3 cm long and approximately 1 cm thick, is obliterated or "taken up" by a shortening of the uterine muscle bundles during the thinning of the lower uterine segment that occurs in advancing labor. Only a thin edge of the cervix can be palpated when effacement is complete. Effacement is generally advanced in first-time term pregnancy before more than slight dilation occurs. In subsequent pregnancies, effacement and dilation of the cervix tend to progress together. Degree of effacement is expressed in percentages from 0% to 100% (e.g., a cervix is 50% effaced) (see Fig. 9-9, *A-C*).

Dilation of the cervix is the enlargement or widening of the cervical opening and the cervical canal that occurs once labor has begun. The diameter of the cervix increases from less than 1 cm to full dilation (approximately 10 cm) to allow birth of a term fetus. When the cervix is fully dilated (and completely retracted), it can no longer be palpated (Fig. 9-11, *D*). Full cervical dilation marks the end of the first stage of labor.

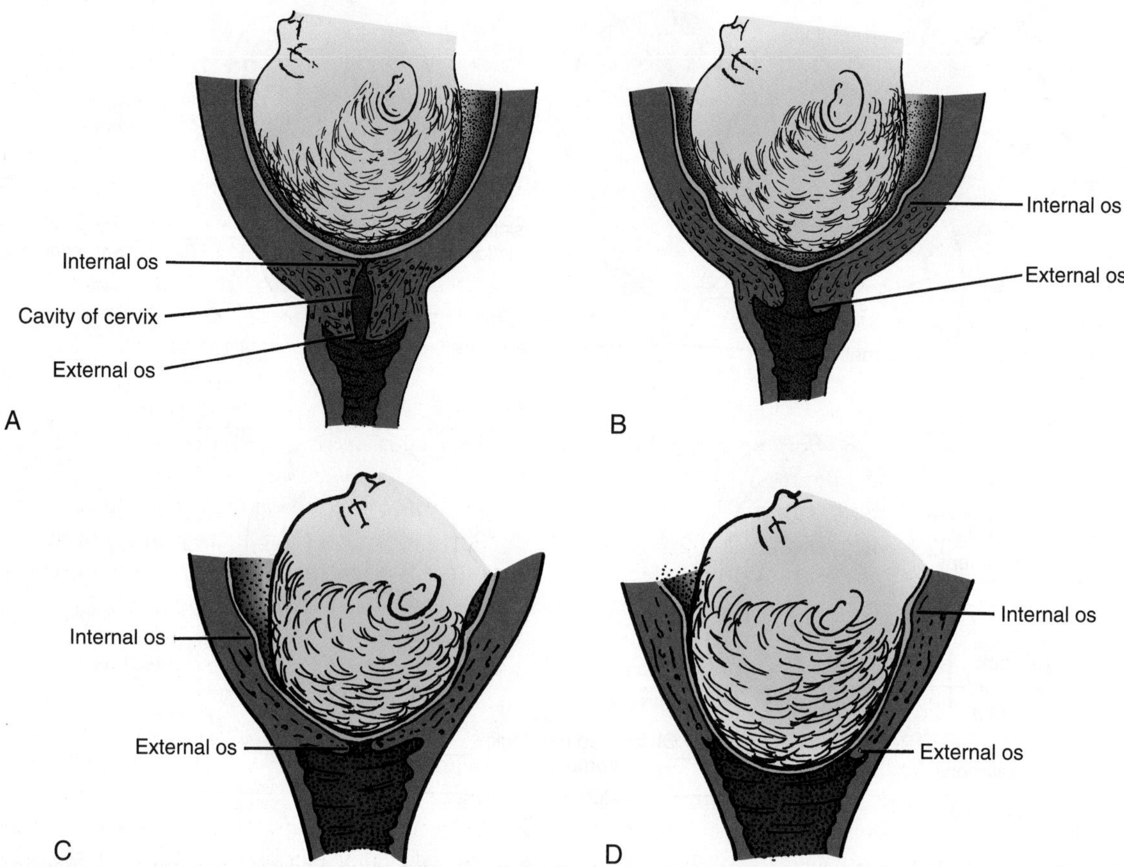

Fig. 9-11 Cervical effacement and dilation. Note how cervix is drawn up around presenting part (internal os). Membranes are intact, and head is not well applied to cervix. **A,** Before labor. **B,** Early effacement. **C,** Complete effacement (100%). Head is well applied to cervix. **D,** Complete dilation (10 cm). Cranial bones overlap somewhat, and membranes are still intact.

Dilation of the cervix occurs by the drawing upward of the musculofibrous components of the cervix, caused by strong uterine contractions. Pressure exerted by the amniotic fluid while the membranes are intact or by the force applied by the presenting part also can promote cervical dilation. Scarring of the cervix as a result of prior infection or surgery may slow cervical dilation.

In the first and second stages of labor, increased intrauterine pressure caused by contractions exerts pressure on the descending fetus and the cervix. When the presenting part of the fetus reaches the perineal floor, mechanical stretching of the cervix occurs. Stretch receptors in the posterior vagina cause release of endogenous oxytocin that triggers the maternal urge to bear down, or the **Ferguson reflex.**

Uterine contractions are usually independent of external forces. For example, laboring women who are paralyzed because of spinal cord lesions above the twelfth thoracic vertebra will have normal but painless uterine contractions (Cunningham et al., 2005). However, uterine contractions may decrease temporarily in frequency and intensity if narcotic analgesic medication is given early in labor. Studies of the effects of epidural analgesia have demonstrated prolonged length of labor for nulliparas both in the active phase of first-stage labor and in the second stage (Salim, Nachum, Moscovici, Lavee, & Shalev, 2005; Schiessl, Janni, Jundt, Rammel, Peschers, & Kainer, 2005).

Secondary powers

As soon as the presenting part reaches the pelvic floor, the contractions change in character and become expulsive. The laboring woman experiences an involuntary urge to push. She uses secondary powers (bearing-down efforts) to aid in expulsion of the fetus as she contracts her diaphragm and abdominal muscles and pushes. These bearing-down efforts result in increased intraabdominal pressure that compresses the uterus on all sides and adds to the power of the expulsive forces.

The secondary powers have no effect on cervical dilation, but they are of considerable importance in the expulsion of the infant from the uterus and vagina after the cervix is fully dilated. Studies have shown that pushing in the second stage is more effective and the woman is less fatigued when she begins to push only after she has the urge to do so rather than beginning to push when she is fully dilated without an urge to do so (Jacobson & Turner, 2008; Simpson & James, 2005; Yildirim & Beji, 2008).

When and how a woman pushes in the second stage is a much-debated topic. Studies have investigated the effects of spontaneous bearing-down efforts, directed pushing, delayed pushing, **Valsalva maneuver** (closed glottis and prolonged bearing down), and open-glottis pushing both with and without epidural analgesia (Brancato, Church, & Stone, 2008; Gupta, Hofmeyr, & Smyth, 2004; Simpson & James, 2005). The benefits of delayed pushing include an increased chance of spontaneous vaginal birth and decreased pushing time. Adverse effects associated with prolonged breath holding and forceful pushing efforts include increased fetal hypoxia and subsequent acidosis (Simpson & James). Pelvic floor problems also have been associated with directed pushing (Schaffer, Bloom, Casey, McIntire, Nihira, & Leveno, 2005). Continued study is needed to determine the effectiveness and appropriateness of strategies used by nurses to teach pushing techniques, the suitability and effectiveness of various pushing techniques related to nonreassuring fetal heart patterns, and the standards for length of duration of pushing in terms of maternal and fetal outcomes (Gennero, Mayberry, & Kafulafula, 2007) (See Chapter 12 for further discussion).

Position of the Laboring Woman

Position affects the woman's anatomic and physiologic adaptations to labor. Frequent changes in position relieve fatigue, increase comfort, and improve circulation. Therefore a laboring woman should be encouraged to find positions that are most comfortable for her (Fig. 9-12, *A*).

An upright position (walking, sitting, kneeling, or squatting) offers several advantages. Gravity can promote the descent of the fetus. Uterine contractions are generally stronger and more efficient in effacing and dilating the cervix, resulting in shorter labor (Gupta et al., 2004).

An upright position also is beneficial to the mother's cardiac output, which normally increases during labor as uterine contractions return blood to the vascular bed. The increased cardiac output improves blood flow to the uteroplacental unit and the maternal kidneys. Cardiac output is compromised if the descending aorta and ascending vena cava are compressed during labor. Compression of these major vessels may result in supine hypotension that decreases placental perfusion. With the woman in an upright position, pressure on the maternal vessels is reduced, and compression is prevented. If the woman wishes to lie down, a lateral position is suggested (Blackburn, 2007). Upright positions for women who have epidural analgesia are associated with a reduced labor duration (Roberts, Algert, Cameron, & Torvaldsen, 2005).

The "all fours" position (hands and knees) may be used to relieve backache if the fetus is in an occipitoposterior position and may assist in anterior rotation of the fetus and in cases of shoulder dystocia (Hunter, Hofmeyr & Kulier, 2007).

Positioning for second-stage labor (Fig. 9-12, *B*) may be determined by the woman's preference, but it is constrained by the condition of the woman and fetus, the environment, and the health care provider's confidence in assisting with a birth in a specific position. No evidence has been found that any of these positions suggested for second-stage labor increases the need for use of operative techniques (e.g., forceps or vacuum-assisted birth, cesarean birth, episiotomy) or causes perineal trauma. No evidence has been found that use of any of these positions adversely

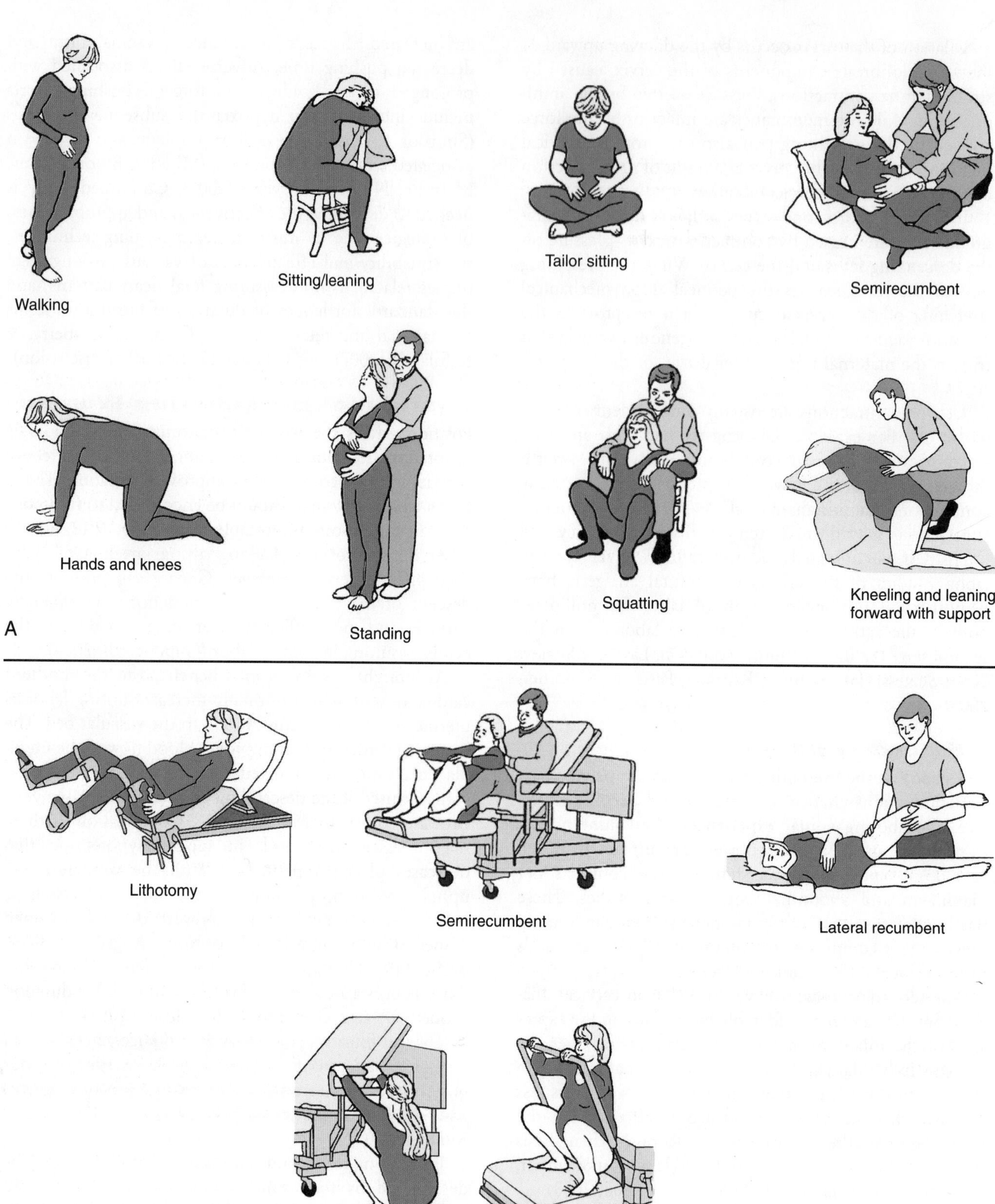

Fig. 9-12 Positions for labor and birth. **A,** Positions for labor. **B,** Positions for birth.

affects the newborn (Gupta et al., 2004; Roberts et al., 2005).

PROCESS OF LABOR

The term *labor* refers to the process of moving the fetus, placenta, and membranes out of the uterus and through the birth canal. Various changes take place in the woman's reproductive system in the days and weeks before labor begins. Labor itself can be discussed in terms of the mechanisms involved in the process and the stages through which the woman moves.

Signs Preceding Labor

In first-time pregnancies the uterus sinks downward and forward approximately 2 weeks before term, when the fetus's presenting part (usually the fetal head) descends into the true pelvis. This settling is called **lightening**, or "dropping," and usually happens gradually. After lightening, women feel less congested and breathe more easily, but usually more bladder pressure results from this shift, and consequently a return of urinary frequency occurs. In a multiparous pregnancy, lightening may not take place until after uterine contractions are established and true labor is in progress.

The woman may complain of persistent low backache and sacroiliac distress as a result of relaxation of the pelvic joints. She may identify strong and frequent but irregular uterine (Braxton Hicks) contractions.

The vaginal mucus becomes more profuse in response to the extreme congestion of the vaginal mucous membranes. The thick mucus that has obstructed the cervical canal since conception (commonly referred to as the mucus plug) is passed. Brownish or blood-tinged cervical mucus may be passed (**bloody show**). The cervix becomes soft (ripens) and partially effaced and may begin to dilate. The membranes may rupture spontaneously.

Other phenomena are common in the days preceding labor: (1) loss of 0.5 to 1.5 kg in weight, caused by water loss resulting from electrolyte shifts that in turn are produced by changes in estrogen and progesterone levels, and (2) a surge of energy. Women speak of having a burst of energy that they often use to clean the house and put everything in order. Less commonly, some women have diarrhea, nausea, vomiting, and indigestion. Box 9-1 lists signs that may precede labor.

BOX 9-1

Signs Preceding Labor

- Lightening
- Return of urinary frequency
- Backache
- Stronger Braxton Hicks contractions
- Weight loss: 0.5-1.5 kg
- Surge of energy
- Increased vaginal discharge; bloody show
- Cervical ripening
- Possible rupture of membranes

Onset of Labor

The onset of true labor cannot be ascribed to a single cause. Many factors, including changes in the maternal uterus, cervix, and pituitary gland, are involved. Hormones produced by the normal fetal hypothalamus, pituitary, and adrenal cortex probably contribute to the onset of labor. Progressive uterine distention, increasing intrauterine pressure, and aging of the placenta seem to be associated with increasing myometrial irritability. These factors are a result of increased concentrations of estrogen and prostaglandins, as well as decreasing progesterone levels. The mutually coordinated effects of these factors result in the occurrence of strong, regular, rhythmic uterine contractions. The outcome of these factors working together is normally the birth of the fetus and the expulsion of the placenta; however, how certain alterations trigger others and how proper checks and balances are maintained is not known.

Stages of Labor

Labor is considered "normal" when the woman is at or near term, no complications exist, a single fetus presents by vertex, and labor is completed within 18 hours. The course of normal labor, which is remarkably constant, consists of (1) regular progression of uterine contractions, (2) effacement and progressive dilation of the cervix, and (3) progress in descent of the presenting part. Four stages of labor are recognized. An overview of these stages is discussed here. These stages are discussed in greater detail, along with nursing care for the laboring woman and family, in Chapter 12.

The *first stage of labor* is considered to last from the onset of regular uterine contractions to full dilation of the cervix. Commonly the onset of labor is difficult to establish because the woman may be admitted to the labor unit just before birth, and the beginning of labor may be only an estimate. The first stage is much longer than the second and third combined. Great variability is the rule, however, depending on the factors discussed previously in this chapter. Parity has a strong effect on the duration of first-stage labor (Gross, Drobnic, & Keirse, 2005). Full dilation may occur in less than 1 hour in some multiparous pregnancies. In first-time pregnancy, complete dilation of the cervix can take 20 hours or longer. Variations may reflect differences in the patient population (e.g., risk status, age) or in clinical management of the labor and birth.

The first stage of labor has been divided into three phases: a latent phase, an active phase, and a transition phase. The latent phase heralds more progress in effacement of the cervix and little increase in descent. During the active phase and the transition phase, more rapid dilation of the cervix and increased rate of descent of the presenting part occur. Maternal prepregnancy overweight and obesity can cause the active phase of labor to be longer than for women of normal weight (Liao, Buhimschi, & Norwitz, 2005).

The *second stage of labor* lasts from the time the cervix is fully dilated to the birth of the fetus. The second stage takes an average of 20 minutes for a multiparous woman and 50 minutes for a nulliparous woman. Ethnicity may play a role in length of second-stage labor. Greenberg, Cheng, Hopkins, Stotland, Bryant, and Caughey (2006) found that nulliparous Asian women had a longer second stage and African-American and Latina women had shorter second stages of labor than Caucasian women.

Roberts (2002) described three phases of second-stage labor. The first phase is a period that begins approximately the time of complete dilation of the uterus, when the contractions are weak or not noticeable and the woman is not feeling the urge to push, is resting, or is exerting only small bearing-down efforts with contractions. The second phase is a period when contractions resume, the woman is making strong bearing-down efforts, and the fetal station is advancing. The third phase is a period lasting from crowning until the birth.

The *third stage of labor* lasts from the birth of the fetus until the placenta is delivered. The placenta normally separates with the third or fourth strong uterine contraction after the infant has been born. After it has separated, the placenta can be delivered with the next uterine contraction. The duration of the third stage may be as short as 3 to 5 minutes, although up to 30 minutes is considered within normal limits. The risk of hemorrhage increases as the length of the third stage increases (Battista & Wing, 2007).

The fourth stage of labor arbitrarily lasts approximately 2 hours after delivery of the placenta. It is the period of immediate recovery, when homeostasis is reestablished. The fourth stage is an important period of observation for complications, such as abnormal bleeding (see Chapter 12).

Mechanism of Labor

As already discussed, the female pelvis has varied contours and diameters at different levels, and the presenting part of the passenger is large in proportion to the passage. Therefore for vaginal birth to occur, the fetus must adapt to the birth canal during the descent. The turns and other adjustments necessary in the human birth process are termed the *mechanism of labor* (Fig. 9-13). The seven cardinal movements of the mechanism of labor that occur in a vertex presentation are engagement, descent, flexion, internal rotation, extension, external rotation (restitution), and finally birth by expulsion. Although these movements are discussed separately, in actuality a combination of movements occurs simultaneously. For example, engagement involves both descent and flexion.

Engagement

When the biparietal diameter of the head passes the pelvic inlet, the head is said to be engaged in the pelvic inlet (Fig. 9-13, *A*). In most nulliparous pregnancies, this event occurs before the onset of active labor because the firmer abdominal muscles direct the presenting part into the pelvis. In multiparous pregnancies, in which the abdominal musculature is more relaxed, the head often remains freely movable above the pelvic brim until labor is established.

Asynclitism. The head usually engages in the pelvis in a synclitic position–one that is parallel to the anteroposterior plane of the pelvis. Frequently, **asynclitism** occurs (the head is deflected anteriorly or posteriorly in the pelvis), which can facilitate descent because the head is being positioned to accommodate to the pelvic cavity (Fig. 9-14). Extreme asynclitism can cause cephalopelvic disproportion, even in a normal-size pelvis, because the head is positioned so that it cannot descend.

Descent

Descent refers to the progress of the presenting part through the pelvis. Descent depends on at least four forces: (1) pressure exerted by the amniotic fluid, (2) direct pressure exerted by the contracting fundus on the fetus, (3) force of the contraction of the maternal diaphragm and abdominal muscles in the second stage of labor, and (4) extension and straightening of the fetal body. The effects of these forces are modified by the size and shape of the maternal pelvic planes and the size of the fetal head and its capacity to mold.

Critical Thinking/Clinical Decision Making

Second Stage Labor

You are assigned to a woman in the labor unit who is having her first baby. Her cervix is completely dilated and effaced, and the fetus is at −1 station. She is lying in a semirecumbent position and is holding her breath and pushing with each contraction. She is complaining of a lot of back pain. She does not have an epidural but she had Stadol 1 mg intravenously an hour ago. What interventions would be appropriate?

1. Evidence—Is evidence sufficient to draw conclusions about what intervention is needed?
2. Assumptions—Describe underlying assumptions about the following issues:
   a. Positions for second stage labor
   b. Immediate versus delayed pushing
   c. Comfort measures for back pain
3. What implications and priorities for nursing care can be drawn at this time?
4. Does the evidence objectively support your conclusion?
5. Do alternative perspectives to your conclusion exist?

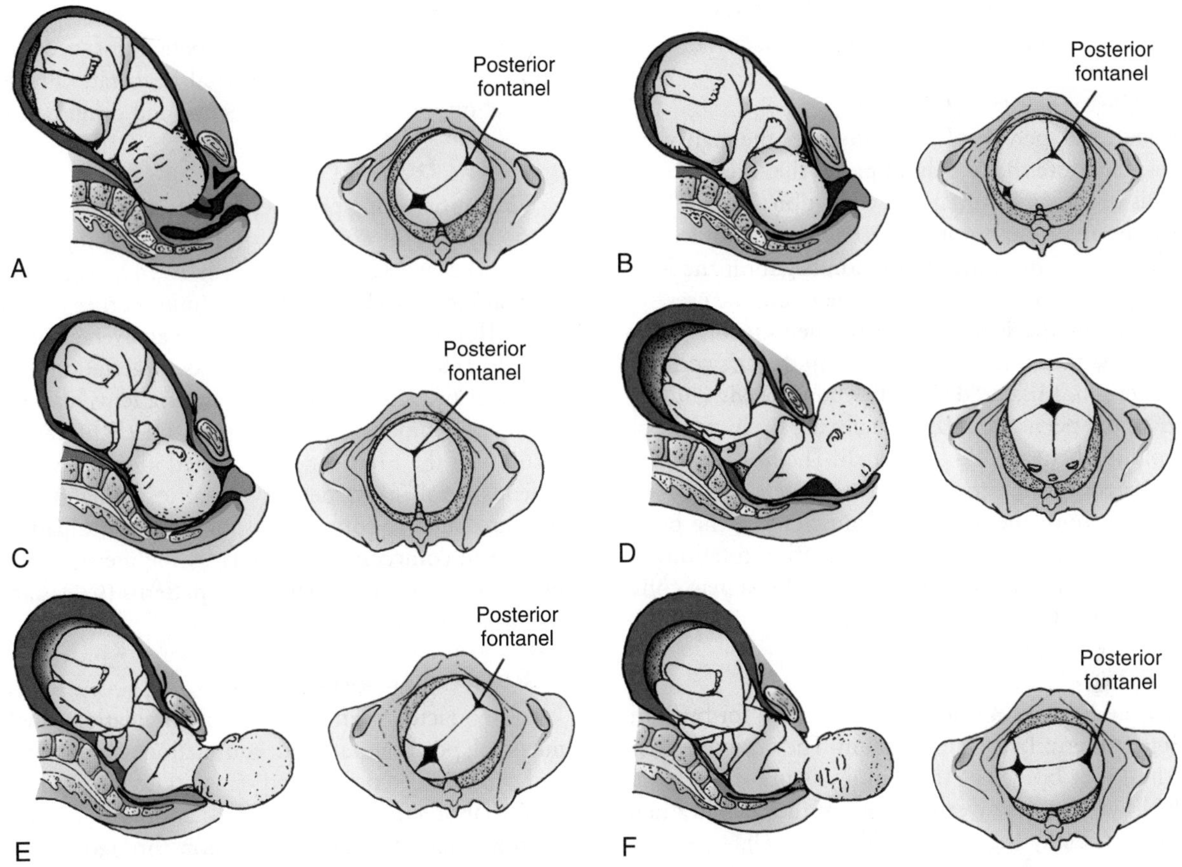

Fig. 9-13 Cardinal movements of the mechanism of labor. Left occipitoanterior (LOA) position. Woman is lying on her back. Pelvic view is from the perineum. **A,** Engagement and descent. **B,** Flexion. **C,** Internal rotation to occipitoanterior position (OA). **D,** Extension. **E,** External rotation beginning (restitution). **F,** External rotation.

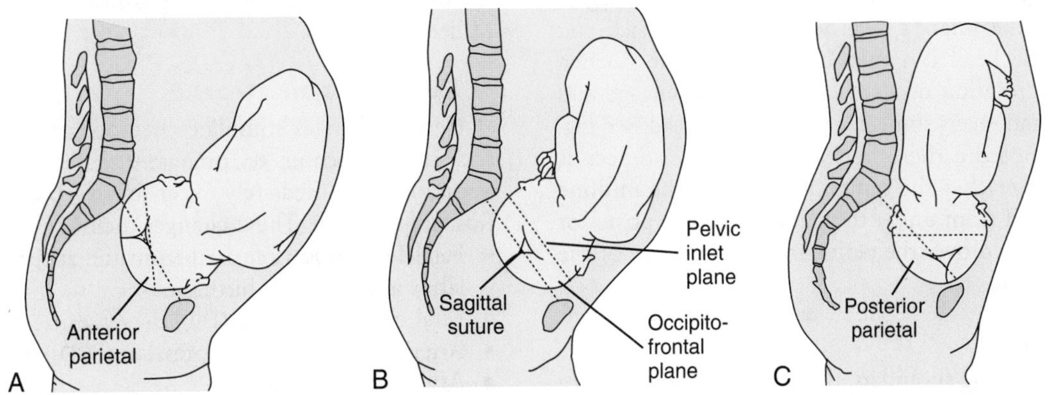

Fig. 9-14 Synclitism and asynclitism. **A,** Anterior asynclitism. **B,** Normal synclitism. **C,** Posterior asynclitism.

The degree of descent is measured by the station of the presenting part (see Fig. 9-6). As mentioned, little descent occurs during the latent phase of the first stage of labor. Descent accelerates in the active phase when the cervix has dilated to 5 to 7 cm. It is especially apparent when the membranes have ruptured.

In a first-time pregnancy, descent is usually slow but steady; in subsequent pregnancies, descent may be rapid. Progress in descent of the presenting part is determined by abdominal palpation (Leopold maneuvers) [see Chapter 12)] and vaginal examination until the presenting part can be seen at the introitus.

Flexion

As soon as the descending head meets resistance from the cervix, pelvic wall, or pelvic floor, it normally flexes, and the chin is brought into closer contact with the fetal chest (see Fig. 9-13, *B*). Flexion permits the smaller suboccipitobregmatic diameter (9.5 cm) rather than the larger diameters to present to the outlet.

Internal rotation

The maternal pelvic inlet is widest in the transverse diameter; therefore the fetal head passes the inlet into the true pelvis in the occipitotransverse position. The outlet is widest in the anteroposterior diameter; for the fetus to exit, the head must rotate. Internal rotation begins at the level of the ischial spines but is not completed until the presenting part reaches the lower pelvis. As the occiput rotates anteriorly, the face rotates posteriorly. With each contraction the fetal head is guided by the bony pelvis and the muscles of the pelvic floor. Eventually the occiput will be in the midline beneath the pubic arch. The head is almost always rotated by the time it reaches the pelvic floor (see Fig. 9-13, *C*). Both the levator ani muscles and the bony pelvis are important for achieving anterior rotation. A previous childbirth injury or regional anesthesia may compromise the function of the levator sling.

Extension

When the fetal head reaches the perineum for birth, it is deflected anteriorly by the perineum. The occiput passes under the lower border of the symphysis pubis first, and then the head emerges by extension: first the occiput, then the face, and finally the chin (see Fig. 9-13, *D*).

Restitution and external rotation

After the head is born, it rotates briefly to the position it occupied when it was engaged in the inlet. This movement is called *restitution* (see Fig. 9-13, *E*). The 45-degree turn realigns the infant's head with her or his back and shoulders. The head can then be seen to rotate further. This external rotation occurs as the shoulders engage and descend in maneuvers similar to those of the head (see Fig. 9-13, *F*). As noted earlier, the anterior shoulder descends first. When it reaches the outlet, it rotates to the midline and is delivered from under the pubic arch. The posterior shoulder is guided over the perineum until it is free of the vaginal introitus.

Expulsion

After birth of the shoulders, the head and shoulders are lifted up toward the mother's pubic bone and the trunk of the baby is born by flexing it laterally in the direction of the symphysis pubis. When the baby has completely emerged, birth is complete, and the second stage of labor ends.

PHYSIOLOGIC ADAPTATIONS TO LABOR

In addition to the maternal and fetal anatomic adaptations that occur during birth, physiologic adaptations must occur. Accurate assessment of the laboring woman and fetus requires knowledge of these expected adaptations.

Fetal Adaptation

Several important physiologic adaptations occur in the fetus. These changes occur in fetal heart rate (FHR), fetal circulation, respiratory movements, and other behaviors.

Fetal heart rate

FHR monitoring provides reliable and predictive information about the condition of the fetus related to oxygenation. The average FHR at term is 140 beats/min. The normal range is 110 to 160 beats/min. Earlier in gestation the FHR is higher than normal, with an average of approximately 160 beats/min at 20 weeks of gestation. The rate decreases progressively as the maturing fetus reaches term. However, temporary accelerations and slight early decelerations of the FHR can be expected in response to spontaneous fetal movement, vaginal examination, fundal pressure, uterine contractions, abdominal palpation, and fetal head compression. Stresses to the uterofetoplacental unit result in characteristic FHR patterns (see Chapter 11 for further discussion).

Fetal circulation

Many factors can affect fetal circulation, including maternal position, uterine contractions, blood pressure, and umbilical cord blood flow. Uterine contractions during labor tend to decrease circulation through the spiral arterioles and subsequent perfusion through the intervillous space. Most healthy fetuses are well able to compensate for this stress and exposure to increased pressure while moving passively through the birth canal during labor. Usually, umbilical cord blood flow is undisturbed by uterine contractions or fetal position (Tucker, Miller, & Miller, 2009).

Fetal respiration

Certain changes stimulate chemoreceptors in the aorta and carotid bodies to prepare the fetus for initiating respirations immediately after birth (Blackburn, 2007; Rosenberg, 2007). These changes include the following:

- Fetal lung fluid is cleared from the air passages during labor and (vaginal) birth.
- Fetal oxygen pressure (PO_2) decreases.
- Arterial carbon dioxide pressure (PCO_2) increases.
- Arterial pH decreases.
- Bicarbonate level decreases.
- Fetal respiratory movements decrease during labor.

Maternal Adaptation

As the woman progresses through the stages of labor, various body system adaptations cause the woman to exhibit both objective and subjective symptoms (Box 9-2).

Cardiovascular changes

During each contraction, an average of 400 ml of blood is emptied from the uterus into the maternal vascular system. This event increases cardiac output by

BOX 9-2

Maternal Physiologic Changes during Labor

- Cardiac output increases 10%-15% in the first stage, 30%-50% in the second stage.
- Heart rate increases slightly in the first and second stages.
- Systolic blood pressure increases during uterine contractions in the first stage; systolic and diastolic pressures increase during uterine contractions in the second stage.
- White blood cell count increases.
- Respiratory rate increases.
- Temperature may be slightly elevated.
- Proteinuria may occur.
- Gastric motility and absorption of solid food is decreased; nausea and vomiting may occur during the transition to second-stage labor.
- Blood glucose level decreases.

approximately 12% to 31% in the first stage and by approximately 50% in the second stage. The heart rate increases slightly (Gordon, 2007).

Changes in the woman's blood pressure also occur. Blood flow, which is reduced in the uterine artery by contractions, is redirected to peripheral vessels. As a result, peripheral resistance increases, and blood pressure increases (Gordon, 2007). During the first stage of labor, uterine contractions cause systolic readings to increase by approximately 10 mm Hg; assessing blood pressure between contractions therefore provides more accurate readings. During the second stage, contractions may cause systolic pressures to increase by 30 mm Hg and diastolic readings to increase by 25 mm Hg, with both systolic and diastolic pressures remaining somewhat elevated even between contractions (Gordon). Therefore the woman already at risk for hypertension is at increased risk for complications such as cerebral hemorrhage.

Supine hypotension (see Fig. 12-5) occurs when the ascending vena cava and descending aorta are compressed. The laboring woman is at greater risk for supine hypotension if the uterus is particularly large because of multifetal pregnancy, hydramnios, or obesity or if the woman is dehydrated or hypovolemic. In addition, anxiety and pain, as well as some medications, can cause hypotension.

The woman should be discouraged from using the Valsalva maneuver (holding one's breath and tightening abdominal muscles) for pushing during the second stage. This activity increases intrathoracic pressure, reduces venous return, and increases venous pressure. The cardiac output and blood pressure increase, and the pulse slows temporarily. During the Valsalva maneuver, fetal hypoxia may occur. The process is reversed when the woman takes a breath.

The white blood cell (WBC) count can increase (Blackburn, 2007). Although the mechanism leading to this increase in WBCs is unknown, it may be secondary to physical or emotional stress or to tissue trauma. Labor is strenuous, and physical exercise alone can increase the WBC count.

Some peripheral vascular changes occur, perhaps in response to cervical dilation or to compression of maternal vessels by the fetus passing through the birth canal. Flushed cheeks, hot or cold feet, and eversion of hemorrhoids may result.

Respiratory changes

Increased physical activity with greater oxygen consumption is reflected in an increase in the respiratory rate. Hyperventilation may cause respiratory alkalosis (an increase in pH), hypoxia, and hypocapnia (decrease in carbon dioxide). In the unmedicated woman in the second stage, oxygen consumption almost doubles. Anxiety also increases oxygen consumption.

Renal changes

During labor, spontaneous voiding may be difficult for various reasons: tissue edema caused by pressure from the presenting part, discomfort, analgesia, and embarrassment. Proteinuria up to +1 is a normal finding because it can occur in response to the breakdown of muscle tissue from the physical work of labor.

Integumentary changes

The integumentary system changes are evident, especially in the great distensibility (stretching) in the area of the vaginal introitus. The degree of distensibility varies with the individual. Despite this ability to stretch, even in the absence of episiotomy or lacerations, minute tears in the skin around the vaginal introitus do occur.

Musculoskeletal changes

The musculoskeletal system is stressed during labor. Diaphoresis, fatigue, proteinuria (+1), and possibly an increased temperature accompany the marked increase in muscle activity. Backache and joint ache (unrelated to fetal position) occur as a result of increased joint laxity at term. The labor process itself and the woman's pointing her toes can cause leg cramps.

Neurologic changes

Sensorial changes occur as the woman moves through the phases of the first stage of labor and as she moves from one stage to the next. Initially, she may be euphoric. Euphoria gives way to increased seriousness, then to amnesia between contractions during the second stage, and finally to elation or fatigue after giving birth. Endogenous endorphins (morphine-like chemicals produced naturally by the body) raise the pain threshold and produce sedation. In addition, physiologic anesthesia of perineal tissues, caused by pressure of the presenting part, decreases perception of pain.

Gastrointestinal changes

During labor, gastrointestinal motility and absorption of solid foods are decreased, and stomach-emptying time is slowed. Nausea and vomiting of undigested food eaten after the onset of labor are common. Nausea and belching also occur as a reflex response to full cervical dilation. The woman may state that diarrhea accompanied the onset of labor, or the nurse may palpate the presence of hard or impacted stool in the rectum.

Endocrine changes

The onset of labor may be triggered by decreasing levels of progesterone and increasing levels of estrogen, prostaglandins, and oxytocin. Metabolism increases, and blood glucose levels may decrease with the work of labor.

KEY POINTS

- Labor and birth are affected by at least five *Ps*: passenger, passageway, powers, position of the woman, and psychologic responses.
- Because of its size and relative rigidity, the fetal head is a major factor in determining the course of birth.
- The diameters at the plane of the pelvic inlet, midpelvis, and outlet, plus the axis of the birth canal, determine whether vaginal birth is possible and the manner in which the fetus passes down the birth canal.
- Involuntary uterine contractions act to expel the fetus and placenta during the first stage of labor; these contractions are augmented by voluntary bearing-down efforts during the second stage.
- The first stage of labor lasts from the time dilation begins to the time when the cervix is fully dilated. The second stage of labor lasts from the time of full dilation to the birth of the infant. The third stage of labor lasts from the infant's birth to the expulsion of the placenta. The fourth stage is the first 2 hours after birth.
- The cardinal movements of the mechanism of labor are engagement, descent, flexion, internal rotation, extension, restitution and external rotation, and expulsion of the infant.
- Although the events precipitating the onset of labor are unknown, many factors, including changes in the maternal uterus, cervix, and pituitary gland, are thought to be involved.
- A healthy fetus with an adequate uterofetoplacental circulation will be able to compensate for the stress of uterine contractions.
- As the woman progresses through labor, various body systems adapt to the birth process.

Audio Chapter Summaries: Access an audio summary of these Key Points on evolve

References

Battista, L., & Wing, D. (2007). Abnormal labor and induction of labor. In S. Gabbe, J. Niebyl, & J. Simpson (Eds.), *Obstetrics: Normal and problem pregnancies* (5th ed.). Philadelphia: Churchill Livingstone.

Blackburn, S. (2007). *Maternal, fetal, and neonatal physiology: A clinical perspective* (3rd ed.). St. Louis: Saunders.

Brancato, R., Church, S., & Stone, P. (2008). A meta-analysis of passive descent versus immediate pushing in nulliparous women with epidural analgesia in the second stage of labor. *Journal of Obstetric, Gynecologic, and Neonatal Nursing, 37*(1), 4-12.

Cunningham, F., Bloom, S., Gilstrap, L., Leveno, K., Hauth, J., & Wenstrom, K. (2005). *Williams obstetrics* (22nd ed.). New York: McGraw-Hill.

Gennero, S., Mayberry, L., & Kafulafula, U. (2007). The evidence supporting nursing management of labor. *Journal of Obstetric, Gynecologic, and Neonatal Nursing, 36*(6), 598-604.

Gordon, M. (2007). Maternal physiology. In S. Gabbe, J. Niebyl, & J. Simpson (Eds.), *Obstetrics: Normal and problem pregnancies* (5th ed.). New York: Churchill Livingstone.

Greenberg, M., Cheng, Y., Hopkins, L., Stotland, N., Bryant, A., & Caughey, A. (2006). Are there ethnic differences in the length of labor? *American Journal of Obstetrics and Gynecology, 195*(3), 743-748.

Gross, M., Drobnic, S., & Keirse, M. (2005). Influence of fixed and time-dependent factors on duration of normal first stage labor. *Birth, 32*(1), 27-33.

Gupta, J., Hofmeyr, G., & Smyth, R. (2004). Position in the second stage of labor of women with epidural analgesia. In *The Cochrane Database of Systematic Reviews*, 2004, Issue 1, CD002006.

Hunter, S., Hofmeyr, G., & Kulier, R. (2007). Hands and knees posture in late pregnancy or labour for fetal malposition (lateral or posterior). In *The Cochrane Database of Systematic Reviews*, 2007, Issue 4, CD 001063.

Jacobson, P., & Turner, L. (2008). Management of the second stage of labor in women with epidural analgesia. *Journal of Midwifery and Women's Health, 53*(10), 82-85.

Liao, J., Buhimschi, D., & Norwitz, E. (2005). Normal labor: Mechanism and duration. *Obstetric and Gynecologic Clinics of North America, 32*(2), 145-164.

Roberts, C., Algert, C., Cameron, C., & Torvaldsen, S. (2005). A meta-analysis of upright positions in the second stage to reduce instrumental deliveries in women with epidural analgesia. *Acta Obstetricia et Gynecologogica Scandinavica, 84*(8), 794-798.

Roberts, J. (2002). The "push" for evidence: Management of the second stage. *Journal of Midwifery & Women's Health, 47*(1), 2-15.

Rosenberg, A. (2007). The neonate. In S. Gabbe, J. Niebyl, & J. Simpson (Eds.), *Obstetrics: Normal and problem pregnancies* (5th ed.). New York: Churchill Livingstone.

Salim, R., Nachum, Z., Moscovici R., Lavee, M., & Shalev, E. (2005). Continuous compared with intermittent epidural infusion on progress of labor and patient satisfaction. *Obstetrics and Gynecology, 106*(2), 301-306.

Schaffer, J., Bloom, S., Casey, B., McIntire, D., Nihira, M., & Leveno, K. (2005). A randomized trial of the effects of coached vs. uncoached maternal pushing during the second stage of labor on postpartum pelvic floor structure and function. *American Journal of Obstetrics and Gynecology, 192*(5), 1692-1696.

Schiessl, B., Janni, W., Jundt, K., Rammel, G., Peschers, U., & Kainer, F. (2005). Obstetrical parameters influencing the duration of second stage labor. *European Journal of Obstetric and Gynecologic Reproductive Biology, 118*(1), 17-20.

Simpson, K., & James, D. (2005). Effects of immediate versus delayed pushing during second-stage labor on fetal well-being: A randomized clinical trial. *Nursing Research, 54*(3), 149-157.

Tucker, S., Miller, L., & Miller, D. (2009). *Mosby's pocket guide to fetal monitoring: A multidisciplinary approach.* (6th ed.). St. Louis: Mosby.

VandeVusse, L. (1999). The essential forces of labor revisited: 13 *P*s reported in women's birth stories. *MCN American Journal of Maternal Child Nursing, 24*(4), 176-184.

Yildirim, G., & Beji, N. (2008). Effects of pushing techniques in birth on mother and fetus: A randomized study. *Birth, 35*(10), 25-30.

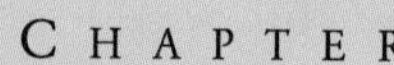
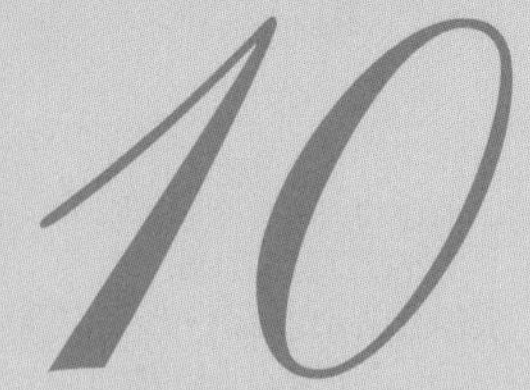
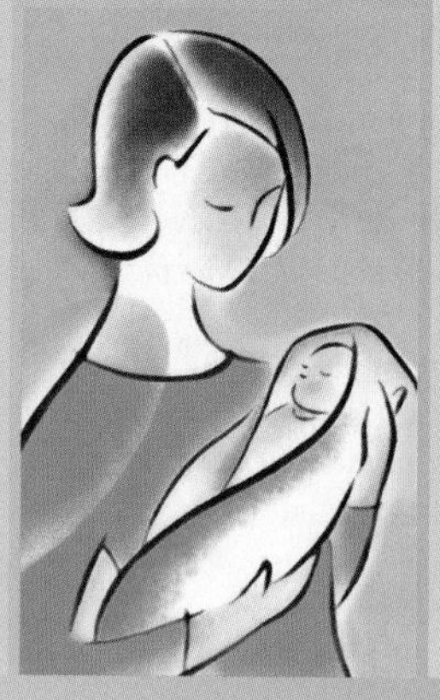

CHAPTER 10

Management of Discomfort

KITTY CASHION

LEARNING OBJECTIVES

- *Describe breathing and relaxation techniques used for each stage of labor.*
- *Identify nonpharmacologic strategies to enhance relaxation and decrease discomfort during labor.*
- *Compare pharmacologic methods used to relieve discomfort in different stages of labor and for vaginal or cesarean births.*
- *Discuss the use of naloxone (Narcan).*
- *Apply the nursing process to the management of the discomfort of a woman in labor.*
- *Summarize the nursing responsibilities appropriate for a woman receiving analgesia or anesthesia during labor.*

KEY TERMS AND DEFINITIONS

analgesia Absence of pain without loss of consciousness

anesthesia Partial or complete absence of sensation with or without loss of consciousness

counterpressure Pressure applied to the sacral area of the back during uterine contractions

effleurage Gentle stroking used in massage, usually on the abdomen

epidural block Type of regional anesthesia produced by injection of a local anesthetic alone or in combination with a narcotic analgesic into the epidural (peridural) space

epidural blood patch A patch formed by a few milliliters of the mother's blood occluding a tear in the dura mater around the spinal cord that occurs during induction of spinal or epidural block; its purpose is to relieve headache associated with leakage of spinal fluid

gate-control theory of pain Pain theory used to explain the neurophysiologic mechanism underlying the perception of pain: the capacity of nerve pathways to transmit pain is reduced or completely blocked by using distraction techniques

local perineal infiltration anesthesia Process by which a local anesthetic medication is deposited within the tissue to anesthetize a limited region of the body

neonatal narcosis Central nervous system depression in the newborn caused by an opioid (narcotic); may be signaled by respiratory depression, hypotonia, lethargy, and delay in temperature regulation

opioid (narcotic) agonist analgesics Medications that relieve pain by activating opioid receptors

opioid (narcotic) agonist-antagonist analgesics Medications that combine agonist activity (activates or stimulates a receptor to perform a function) and antagonist activity (blocks a receptor or medication designed to activate a receptor) to relieve pain without causing significant maternal or fetal or newborn respiratory depression

opioid (narcotic) antagonists Medications used to reverse the central nervous system depressant effects of an opioid, especially respiratory depression

pudendal nerve block Injection of a local anesthetic at the pudendal nerve root to produce numbness of the genital and perianal region

spinal anesthesia (block) Regional anesthesia induced by injection of a local anesthetic agent into the subarachnoid space at the level of the third, fourth, or fifth lumbar interspace

systemic analgesia Pain relief induced when an analgesic is administered parenterally (e.g., subcutaneous [SC], intramuscular [IM], or intravenous [IV] route) and crosses the blood-brain barrier to provide central analgesic effects

WEB RESOURCES

Additional related content can be found on the companion website at evolve

http://evolve.elsevier.com/Lowdermilk/Maternity/

- NCLEX Review Questions
- Critical Thinking Exercise: Patient Receiving Epidural Block
- Nursing Care Plan: Epidural Block during Labor
- Nursing Care Plan: Nonpharmacologic Management of Discomfort
- Spanish Guidelines: Pain Management

Pain is an unpleasant, complex, highly individualized phenomenon with both sensory and emotional components. Pregnant women commonly worry about the pain they will experience during labor and birth and how they will react to and deal with that pain. Many physiologic, emotional, psychosocial, and environmental factors influence the nature and degree of pain experienced by the laboring woman and how she will respond to and cope with the pain (Zwelling, Johnson, & Allen, 2006). A variety of nonpharmacologic and pharmacologic methods can help the woman or the couple cope with the discomfort of labor. The methods selected depend on the situation, availability, and the preferences of the woman and her health care provider.

DISCOMFORT DURING LABOR AND BIRTH

Neurologic Origins

The pain and discomfort of labor have two origins, visceral and somatic. During the first stage of labor, uterine contractions cause cervical dilation and effacement. Uterine ischemia (decreased blood flow and therefore local oxygen deficit) results from compression of the arteries supplying the myometrium during uterine contractions. Pain impulses during the first stage of labor are transmitted via the T-1 to T-12 spinal nerve segment and accessory lower thoracic and upper lumbar sympathetic nerves. These nerves originate in the uterine body and cervix (Blackburn, 2007).

The pain from cervical changes, distention of the lower uterine segment, stretching of cervical tissue as it dilates, and pressure on adjacent structures and nerves during the first stage of labor is visceral pain. It is located over the lower portion of the abdomen. Referred pain occurs when the pain that originates in the uterus radiates to the abdominal wall, lumbosacral area of the back, iliac crests, gluteal area, thighs, and lower back (Blackburn, 2007; Zwelling et al., 2006).

During the second stage of labor the woman has somatic pain, which is often described as intense, sharp, burning, and well localized. Pain results from stretching and distention of perineal tissues and the pelvic floor to allow passage of the fetus, from distention and traction on the peritoneum and uterocervical supports during contractions, and from lacerations of soft tissue (e.g., cervix, vagina, perineum). Other physical factors related to pain during second stage labor include fetal position, rapidity of fetal descent, maternal position, interval and duration of contractions, and fatigue (Zwelling et al., 2006). Pain impulses during the second stage of labor are transmitted via the pudendal nerve through S2 to S4 spinal nerve segments and the parasympathetic system (Blackburn, 2007).

Pain experienced during the third stage of labor and the afterpains of the early postpartum period are uterine, similar to the pain experienced early in the first stage of labor. Areas of discomfort during labor are shown in Fig. 10-1.

Perception of Pain

Although the pain threshold is remarkably similar in all persons regardless of gender, social, ethnic, or cultural differences, these differences play a definite role in the person's perception of and behavioral responses to pain. The effects of factors such as culture, counterstimuli, and distraction in coping with pain are not fully understood. The meaning of pain and the verbal and nonverbal expressions given to pain are apparently learned from interactions within the primary social group. Cultural influences impose certain behavioral expectations regarding acceptable and unacceptable behavior when experiencing pain.

Expression of Pain

Pain results in physiologic effects and sensory and emotional (affective) responses. During childbirth, pain gives rise to identifiable physiologic effects. Sympathetic nervous system activity is stimulated in response to intensifying pain, resulting in increased catecholamine levels. Blood pressure and heart rate increase. Maternal respiratory patterns change in response to an increase in oxygen consumption. Hyperventilation, sometimes accompanied by respiratory alkalosis, can occur as pain intensifies. Pallor and diaphoresis may be seen. Gastric acidity increases, and nausea and vomiting are common in the active phase of labor. Placental perfusion may decrease, and uterine

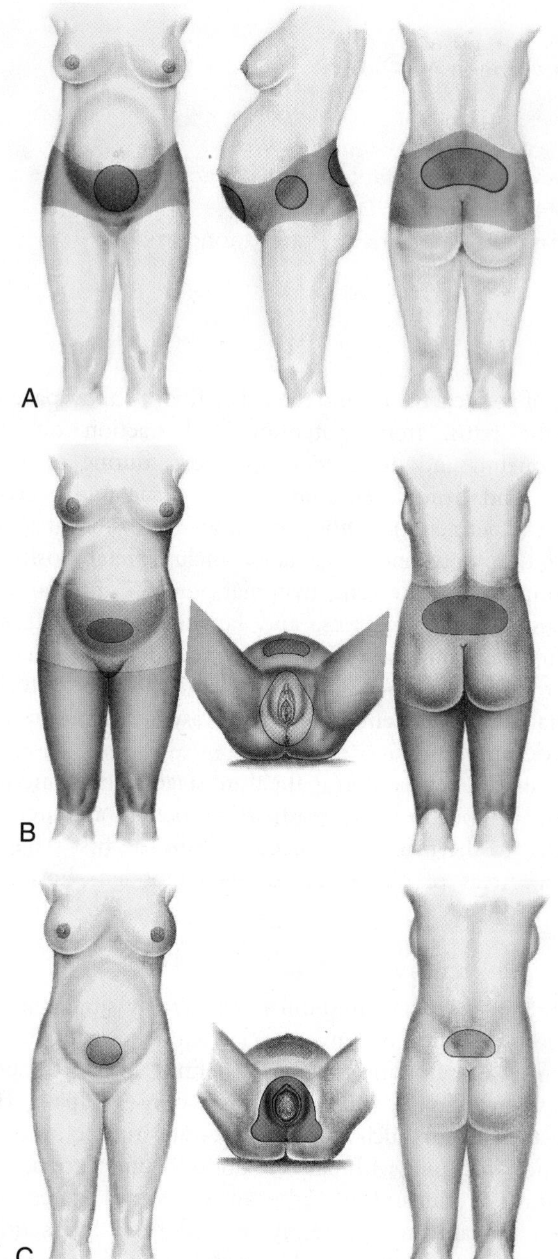

Fig. 10-1 Discomfort during labor. **A,** Distribution of labor pain during first stage. **B,** Distribution of labor pain during transition and early phase of second stage. **C,** Distribution of pain during late second stage and actual birth. (Gray areas indicate mild discomfort; light-colored areas indicate moderate discomfort; dark-colored areas indicate intense discomfort.)

activity may diminish, potentially prolonging labor and affecting fetal well-being.

Certain emotional (affective) expressions of pain are often seen. Such changes include increasing anxiety with lessened perceptual field, writhing, crying, groaning, gesturing (hand clenching and wringing), and excessive muscular excitability throughout the body.

Factors Influencing Pain Response

Pain during childbirth is unique to each woman. How she perceives or interprets that pain is influenced by a variety of physical, emotional, psychosocial, cultural, and environmental factors (Zwelling et al., 2006).

Physiologic factors

A variety of physiologic factors can affect the intensity of pain that women experience during childbirth. Women with a history of dysmenorrhea may experience increased pain during childbirth as a result of higher prostaglandin levels. Back pain associated with menstruation also may increase the likelihood of contraction-related low back pain. Other physical factors include fatigue, the interval and duration of contractions, fetal position, rapidity of fetal descent, and maternal position (Zwelling et al., 2006).

Endorphins are endogenous opioids secreted by the pituitary gland that act on the central and peripheral nervous systems to reduce pain. Beta-endorphin is the most potent of the endorphins. Endorphin levels increase during pregnancy and birth in humans. Endorphins are associated with feelings of euphoria and analgesia. Increased endorphin levels may increase the pain threshold and enable women in labor to tolerate acute pain (Blackburn, 2007).

Culture

The obstetric population reflects the increasingly multicultural nature of U.S. society. As nurses care for women and families from a variety of cultural backgrounds, they must have knowledge and understanding of how culture mediates pain. Although all women expect to experience at least some pain and discomfort during childbirth, their culture and religious belief system determines how they will perceive, interpret, and respond to and manage the pain. For example, women with strong religious beliefs often accept pain as a necessary and inevitable part of bringing a new life into the world (Callister, Khalaf, Semenic, Kartchner, & Vehvilainen-Julkunen, 2003). An understanding of the beliefs, values, and practices of various cultures will narrow the cultural gap and help the nurse to assess the woman's pain experience more accurately. The nurse can then provide appropriate culturally sensitive care by using pain-relief measures that preserve the woman's sense of control and self-confidence (see Cultural Considerations box). Recognize that although a woman's behavior in response to pain may vary according to her cultural background, it may not accurately reflect the intensity of the pain she is experiencing. Assess the woman for the physiologic effects of pain and listen to the words she uses to describe the sensory and affective qualities of her pain.

Anxiety

Anxiety is commonly associated with increased pain during labor. Mild anxiety is considered normal for a woman during labor and birth. However, excessive anxiety

Cultural Considerations

Some Cultural Beliefs about Pain

The following examples demonstrate how women of different cultural backgrounds may react to pain. Because they are generalizations the nurse must assess each woman experiencing pain related to childbirth.

- Chinese women may not exhibit reactions to pain, although exhibiting pain during childbirth is acceptable. They consider accepting something when it is first offered as impolite; therefore pain interventions must be offered more than once. Acupuncture may be used for pain relief.
- Arab or Middle Eastern women may be vocal in response to labor pain. They may prefer medication for pain relief.
- Japanese women may be stoic in response to labor pain, but they may request medication when pain becomes severe.
- Southeast Asian women may endure severe pain before requesting relief.
- Hispanic women may be stoic until late in labor, when they may become vocal and request pain relief.
- Native American women may use medications or remedies made from indigenous plants. They are often stoic in response to labor pain.
- African-American women may express pain openly. Use of medication for pain relief varies.

COMMUNITY ACTIVITY

Talk to a man and a woman from a culture different from your own who have experienced childbirth. Ask her to describe her reactions to pain, how she sought relief of pain, the atmosphere of the childbirth setting, and the attitudes of the health care providers. Ask him if he was present for the birth and what his role in the birth was. How did his culture influence his role and reaction to childbirth? How did her culture influence her response to labor and the associated pain? What expressions of pain are "acceptable" in her culture? If he was present, how did he help her deal with the pain? What is the role of support persons in the labor process? Are the responses of the couple different from your responses to those same questions?

and fear cause additional catecholamine secretion, which increases the stimuli to the brain from the pelvis because of decreased blood flow and increased muscle tension; this action, in turn, magnifies pain perception (Zwelling et al., 2006). Thus, as fear and anxiety heighten, muscle tension increases, the effectiveness of uterine contractions decreases, the experience of discomfort increases, and a cycle of increased fear and anxiety begins. Ultimately this cycle will slow the progress of labor. The woman's confidence in her ability to cope with pain will be diminished, potentially resulting in reduced effectiveness of pain-relief measures being used.

Previous experience

Previous experience with pain and childbirth may affect a woman's description of her pain and her ability to cope with the pain. Childbirth, for a healthy young woman, may be her first experience with significant pain, and as a result, she may not have developed effective pain-coping strategies. She may describe the intensity of even early labor pain as a "10" on a 10-point scale. The nature of previous childbirth experiences also may affect a woman's responses to pain. For women who have had a difficult and painful previous birth experience, anxiety and fear from this past experience may lead to increased pain perception.

Sensory pain for nulliparous women is often greater than that for multiparous women during early labor (dilation less than 5 cm) because their reproductive tract structures are less supple. During the transition phase of the first stage of labor and during the second stage of labor, multiparous women may experience greater sensory pain than nulliparous women because their more supple tissue increases the speed of fetal descent and thereby intensifies pain. The firmer tissue of nulliparous women results in a slower, more gradual descent. Affective pain is usually increased for nulliparous women throughout the first stage of labor but decreases for both nulliparous and multiparous women during the second stage of labor (Lowe, 2002).

Parity may affect perception of labor pain because nulliparous women often have longer labors and therefore greater fatigue. Because fatigue magnifies pain, the combination of increased pain, fatigue, and reduced ability to cope may lead to more use of pharmacologic support.

Gate-control theory of pain

Even particularly intense pain stimuli can, at times, be ignored. This phenomenon is possible because certain nerve cell groupings within the spinal cord, brainstem, and cerebral cortex have the ability to modulate the pain impulse through a blocking mechanism. This **gate-control theory of pain** helps explain the way hypnosis and the pain-relief techniques taught in childbirth preparation classes work to relieve the pain of labor. According to this theory, pain sensations travel along sensory nerve pathways to the brain, but only a limited number of sensations, or messages, can travel through these nerve pathways at one time. Using distraction techniques such as massage or stroking, music, focal points, and imagery reduces or completely blocks the capacity of nerve pathways to transmit pain. These distractions are thought to work by closing down a hypothetic gate in the spinal cord, thus preventing pain signals from reaching the brain. The perception of pain is thereby diminished.

In addition, when the laboring woman engages in neuromuscular and motor activity, activity within the spinal cord itself further modifies the transmission of pain. Cognitive work involving concentration on breathing and relaxation requires selective and directed cortical activity that activates and closes the gating mechanism as well. As

Spanish Guidelines: Pain Management

labor intensifies, more complex cognitive techniques are required to maintain effectiveness. The gate-control theory underscores the need for a supportive birth setting that allows the laboring woman to relax and use various higher mental activities.

Comfort

Although the predominant medical approach to labor is that it is painful, and the pain must be removed, an alternative view is that labor is a natural process, and women can experience comfort and transcend the discomfort or pain to reach the joyful outcome of birth. Having needs and desires met promotes a feeling of comfort. The most helpful interventions in enhancing comfort are a caring nursing approach and a supportive presence.

Support. Current evidence indicates that a woman's satisfaction with her labor and birth experience is determined by how well her personal expectations of childbirth were met and the quality of support and interaction she receives from her caregivers. In addition, satisfaction is influenced by the degree to which the woman was able to stay in control of her labor and to participate in decision making regarding her labor, including the pain-relief measures to be used (Albers, 2007; Zwelling et al., 2006).

The value of the continuous supportive presence of a person (e.g., doula, childbirth educator, family member, friend, nurse, partner) during labor has long been known. Women who have continuous support beginning early in labor are less likely to use pain medication or epidurals, more likely to have a spontaneous vaginal birth, and less likely to report dissatisfaction with their birth experience. No harmful effects from continuous labor support have been identified. To the contrary, good evidence exists that labor support improves important health outcomes. Interestingly, a more positive effect was achieved when the continuous support was provided by people who were not hospital staff members (Albers, 2007; Berghella, Baxter, & Chauhan, 2008; Hodnett, Gates, Hofmeyr, & Sakala, 2007).

Environment. The quality of the environment can influence pain perception. Environment includes both the persons present (e.g., how they communicate, their philosophy of care, practice policies, and quality of support) and the physical space in which the labor occurs (Zwelling et al., 2006). Women usually prefer to be cared for by familiar caregivers in a comfortable, homelike setting. The environment should be safe and private, allowing a woman to feel free to be herself as she tries out different comfort measures. Stimuli that includes light, noise, and temperature should be adjusted according to the woman's preferences. The environment should have space for movement, and equipment such as birth balls, comfortable chairs, tubs, and showers should be readily available to facilitate a variety of nonpharmacologic pain-relief measures. The familiarity of the environment can be enhanced by bringing items from home such as pillows, objects for a focal point, music, and DVDs.

NONPHARMACOLOGIC MANAGEMENT OF DISCOMFORT

Pain management is important. Commonly, it is not the amount of pain the woman experiences, but whether she meets her goals for herself in coping with the pain that influences her perception of the birth experience as "good" or "bad." The observant nurse looks for clues to the woman's desired level of control in the management of pain and its relief. Nonpharmacologic measures are often simple, safe, and relatively inexpensive and provide the woman with a sense of control over her childbirth as she makes choices about the measures that are best for her. During the prenatal period the woman should explore a variety of nonpharmacologic measures. Techniques she finds helpful in relieving stress and enhancing relaxation (e.g., music, meditation, massage, warm baths) also may be very effective as components of a plan for managing labor pain. The woman should be encouraged to communicate to her health care providers her preferences for relaxation and pain-relief measures and to actively participate in their implementation.

Many of the nonpharmacologic methods for relief of discomfort are taught in different types of prenatal preparation classes, or the woman or couple may have read various books and magazine articles on the subject in advance. Many of these methods require practice for best results (e.g., hypnosis, patterned breathing and controlled relaxation techniques, biofeedback), although the nurse may use some of them successfully without the woman or couple having prior knowledge (e.g., slow paced breathing, massage and touch, effleurage, counterpressure). Women should be encouraged to try a variety of methods and to seek alternatives, including pharmacologic methods, if the measure being used is no longer effective (Box 10-1).

Childbirth Preparation Methods

The childbirth education movement began in the 1950s and grew. Prepared childbirth classes are now recommended for expectant parents by most caregivers. Historically, popular childbirth methods taught in the United States included the Dick-Read method; the Lamaze (psychoprophylaxis) method, and the Bradley (husband-coached childbirth) method.

An English physician, Grantly Dick-Read, published two books in which he theorized that pain in childbirth is socially conditioned and caused by a *fear-tension-pain syndrome.* His first book, *Natural Childbirth,* was published in 1933. Dick-Read's second book, *Childbirth without Fear,* was published in the United States in 1944. The work of Dick-Read became the foundation for organized programs of preparation for childbirth and teacher training throughout the United States, Canada, Great Britain, and South Africa. In 1960, persons prepared through such programs established the International Childbirth Education Association (ICEA). The *Grantly Dick-Read method,* known as

BOX 10-1

Nonpharmacologic Strategies to Encourage Relaxation and Relieve Pain

CUTANEOUS STIMULATION STRATEGIES
- Counterpressure
- Effleurage (light massage)
- Therapeutic touch and massage
- Walking
- Rocking
- Changing positions
- Application of heat or cold
- Transcutaneous electrical nerve stimulation (TENS)
- Acupressure
- Water therapy (showers, baths)
- Intradermal water block

SENSORY STIMULATION STRATEGIES
- Aromatherapy
- Breathing techniques
- Music
- Imagery
- Use of focal points

COGNITIVE STRATEGIES
- Childbirth education
- Hypnosis
- Biofeedback

Childbirth without Fear, initially recommended deep abdominal breathing during early first-stage contractions, shallow breathing for later first stage, and sustained pushing with breath holding (Dick-Read, 1987). Women were taught to relax different muscle groups through the entire body, consciously and progressively, until a high degree of skill at relaxation was achieved. Consequently, a woman was taught to relax completely between contractions and keep all muscles except the uterus relaxed during contractions.

During the 1960s the *Lamaze method,* originally known as the *psychoprophylactic method* (PPM), gained popularity in the United States. PPM offered new perspectives on preparation for childbirth by emphasizing control by using the mind. Marjorie Karmel introduced PPM to the United States in her book *Thank You, Dr. Lamaze,* which was published in the United States in 1959. PPM combined controlled muscular relaxation and breathing techniques. Active relaxation was an integral part of the Lamaze method. The woman was taught to contract specific muscle groups (neuromuscular control) while relaxing the remainder of her body. The goal was to be able to relax the uninvolved muscles in her body while her uterine muscle contracted. Rather than tensing during uterine contractions, women were conditioned to respond with relaxation and breathing patterns.

In 1960 the American Society for Psychoprophylaxis in Obstetrics (ASPO) was formed in New York and became a national organization to promote use of the Lamaze method and prepare teachers of the method. It continues to be an active organization, known since 1998 as Lamaze International and dedicated to advancing normal birth. Lamaze's Institute of Normal Birth publishes reviews of research related to normal birth. In the official *Lamaze Guide to Giving Birth with Confidence,* the authors state that "Mothers do know how to give birth, simply. And doctors, hospitals and technology have not made normal birth safer" (Lothian & Devries, 2005). They further state that women need to rediscover birth as a natural part of life based on research that confirms that interfering in the normal birth process is harmful unless clear evidence exists that interference provides benefits.

A third early advocate of prepared childbirth was the Denver obstetrician, Robert Bradley, who published *Husband-Coached Childbirth* in 1965. He advocated what he called true "natural" childbirth, without any form of anesthesia or analgesia and with a husband-coach and breathing techniques for labor. The American Academy of Husband-Coached Childbirth (AAHCC) was founded to make the *Bradley method* available and to prepare teachers (www.bradleybirth.com). This method of partner-coached childbirth used breath control, abdominal breathing, and general body relaxation. Working in harmony with the body was emphasized (Bradley, 1965). Bradley's technique emphasized environmental variables such as darkness, solitude, and quiet to make childbirth a more natural experience. Women using the Bradley method may appear to be sleeping during labor because they are in such a deep state of mental relaxation.

Even though these three organizations continue to exist, they are now less focused on a "method" approach. Rather, women are assisted to develop their birth philosophy and inner knowledge and then offered many skills from which to choose. Many childbirth educators teach a variety of techniques that originated in several different organizations or publications. Women are encouraged to choose the techniques that work for them.

Currently gaining popularity are methods developed and promoted by Birthing From Within, Birth Works, Association of Childbirth Educators and Labor Assistants (ALACE), Childbirth and Postpartum Professional Association (CAPPA), and HypnoBirthing, to name a few. These methods offer classes and other services that focus on fostering a woman's confidence in her innate ability to give birth. The woman or couple is helped to recognize the uniqueness of their pregnancy and childbirth experience (see Resources online for contact information).

Relaxing and Breathing Techniques

Focusing and relaxation

By reducing tension and stress, focusing and relaxation techniques allow a woman in labor to rest and to conserve energy for the task of giving birth. Attention-focusing and

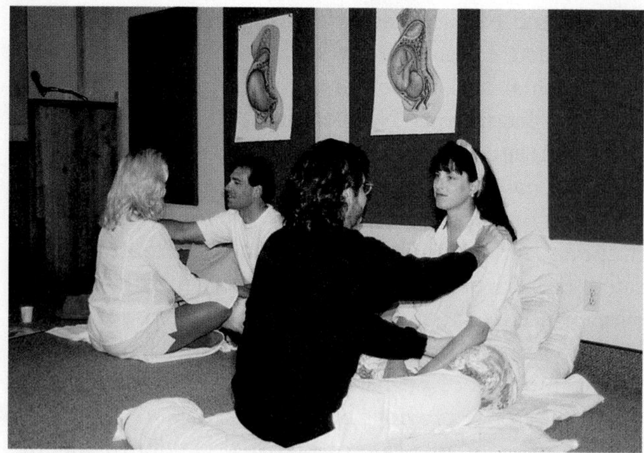

Fig. 10-2 Expectant parents learning relaxation techniques. (Courtesy Marjorie Pyle, RNC, Lifecircle, Costa Mesa, CA.)

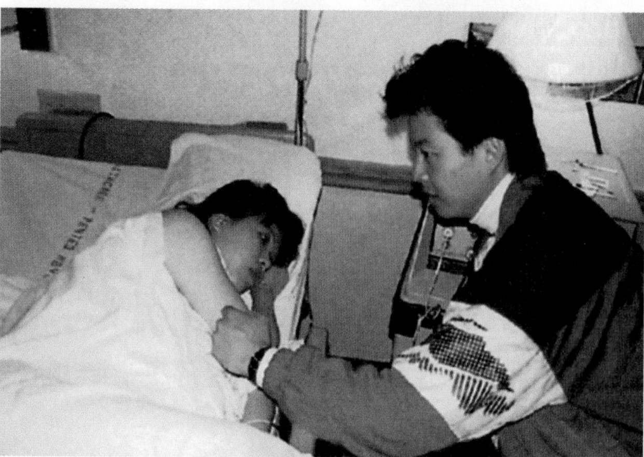

Fig. 10-3 Laboring woman using focusing and breathing techniques during a uterine contraction with coaching from her partner. (Courtesy Marjorie Pyle, RNC, Lifecircle, Costa Mesa, CA.)

distraction techniques are forms of care that are effective to some degree in relieving labor pain (Albers, 2007). Some women bring a favorite object such as a photograph or stuffed animal to the labor room and focus their attention on this object during contractions. Others choose to fix their attention on some object in the labor room. As the contraction begins, they focus on their chosen object and perform a breathing technique to reduce their perception of pain.

With imagery the woman focuses her attention on a pleasant scene, a place where she feels relaxed, or an activity she enjoys. She can imagine walking through a restful garden or breathing in light, energy, and healing color and breathing out worries and tension. Choosing the subject for the imagery and practicing the technique during pregnancy will enhance effectiveness during labor.

These techniques, coupled with feedback relaxation, help the woman work with her contractions rather than against them. The support person monitors this process, telling the woman when to begin the breathing techniques (Fig. 10-2).

During childbirth preparation classes the coach can learn how to palpate a woman's body to detect tense and contracted muscles. The woman then learns how to relax the tense muscle in response to the gentle stroking of the muscle by the coach (Fig. 10-3). In a common feedback mechanism the woman and her coach say the word "relax" at the onset of each contraction and throughout it as needed. With practice the coach can effectively use support, feedback, and touch to facilitate the woman's relaxation and thereby reduce tension and stress and enhance the progress of labor (Humenick, Schrock, & Libresco, 2000). The nurse can assist the woman by providing a quiet environment and offering cues as needed.

Breathing techniques

Different approaches to childbirth preparation stress varying breathing techniques to provide distraction, thereby reducing the perception of pain and helping the woman maintain control throughout contractions. In the first stage of labor, such breathing techniques can promote relaxation of the abdominal muscles and thereby increase the size of the abdominal cavity. This approach lessens discomfort generated by friction between the uterus and abdominal wall during contractions. Because the muscles of the genital area also become more relaxed, they do not interfere with fetal descent. In the second stage, breathing is used to increase abdominal pressure and thereby assist in expelling the fetus. Breathing also can be used to relax the pudendal muscles to prevent precipitate expulsion of the fetal head.

For couples who have prepared for labor by practicing relaxing and breathing techniques, occasional reminders may be all that are necessary to help them along. For those who have had no preparation, instruction in simple breathing and relaxation can be given early in labor and is often surprisingly successful. Motivation is high, and readiness to learn is enhanced by the reality of labor.

Various breathing techniques can be used for controlling pain during contractions (Box 10-2). The nurse needs to determine what, if any, techniques the laboring couple knows before giving them instruction. Simple patterns are more easily learned. Paced breathing is the technique most associated with prepared childbirth and includes slow-paced, modified-paced, and pant-blow breathing techniques. Each labor is different, and nursing support includes assisting couples to adapt breathing techniques to their individual labor experience.

All patterns begin with a deep relaxing cleansing breath to "greet the contraction" and end with another deep breath exhaled to "gently blow the contraction away." In general, *slow-paced breathing* is performed at approximately one half the woman's normal breathing rate. The woman should take no fewer than three to four breaths per minute. Slow-paced breathing aids in relaxation and provides

BOX 10-2

Paced Breathing Techniques

CLEANSING BREATH

- Relaxed breath in through nose and out mouth. Used at the beginning and end of each contraction

SLOW-PACED BREATHING (APPROXIMATELY 6 TO 8 BREATHS PER MINUTE)

- Performed at approximately one half the normal breathing rate (number of breaths per minute divided by 2):

IN-2-3-4/OUT-2-3-4/IN-2-3-4/OUT-2-3-4 ...

MODIFIED-PACED BREATHING (APPROXIMATELY 32 TO 40 BREATHS PER MINUTE)

- Not more than twice normal breathing rate (number of breaths per minute multiplied by 2)
- IN-OUT/IN-OUT/IN-OUT/IN-OUT ...
- For more flexibility and variety the woman may combine the slow and modified breathing by using the slow breathing for beginnings and ends of contractions and modified breathing for more intense peaks. This technique conserves energy, lessens fatigue, and reduces risk for hyperventilation.

PATTERNED-PACED OR PANT-BLOW BREATHING (SAME RATE AS MODIFIED)

- Enhances concentration
  3:1 Patterned breathing IN-OUT/IN-OUT/IN-OUT/IN-BLOW (repeat through contraction)
  4:1 Patterned breathing IN-OUT/IN-OUT/IN-OUT/IN-OUT/IN-BLOW (repeat through contraction)

Sources: Nichols, F. (2000). Paced breathing techniques. In F. Nichols & S. Humenick (Eds.), *Childbirth education: Practice, research, and theory* (2nd ed.). Philadelphia: Saunders; Perinatal Education Associates. (2008). *Breathing.* Internet document available at http://www.birthsource.com/scripts/article.asp?articleid=211 (accessed May 26, 2009).

optimal oxygenation. As contractions increase in frequency and intensity the woman often needs to change to a more complex breathing technique, which is shallower and faster than the woman's normal rate of breathing, but should not exceed twice her resting respiratory rate. This *modified-paced breathing* pattern allows the woman to be more focused and alert (Perinatal Education Associates, 2008 [www.birthsource.com]).

The most difficult time to maintain control during contractions comes during the transition phase of the first stage of labor, when the cervix dilates from 8 cm to 10 cm. Even for the woman who has prepared for labor, concentration on breathing techniques is difficult to maintain. The *pant-blow breathing* technique is suggested for use during this phase. It is performed at the same rate as modified-paced breathing and consists of panting breaths combined with soft blowing breaths at regular intervals. The patterns may vary (i.e., *pant, pant, pant, pant, blow* or *pant, pant, pant, blow*) (Perinatal Education Associates, 2008). An undesirable side effect of this type of breathing is hyperventilation. The woman and her support person must be aware of and watch for symptoms of the resultant respiratory alkalosis: light-headedness, dizziness, tingling of the fingers, or circumoral numbness. Respiratory alkalosis may be eliminated by having the woman breathe into a paper bag held tightly around her mouth and nose, which enables her to rebreathe carbon dioxide and replace the bicarbonate ion. The woman also can breathe into her cupped hands if no bag is available. Maintaining a breathing rate that is no more than twice the normal rate will lessen chances of hyperventilation. The partner can help the woman maintain her breathing rate with visual, tactile, or auditory cues.

As the fetal head reaches the pelvic floor the woman may feel the urge to push and may automatically begin to exert downward pressure by contracting her abdominal muscles. During second stage pushing the woman should find a breathing pattern that is relaxing and feels good for her and her baby. Any regular or rhythmic breathing that avoids prolonged breath holding during pushing should maintain a good oxygen flow to the fetus (Perinatal Education Associates, 2008).

The woman can control the urge to push by taking panting breaths (as though blowing out a candle) or by slowly exhaling through pursed lips. This type of breathing can be used to overcome the urge to push when the cervix is not fully prepared (e.g., less than 8 cm dilated, not retracting) and to facilitate a slow birth of the fetal head.

Effleurage and Counterpressure

Effleurage (light massage) and counterpressure have brought relief to many women during the first stage of labor. The gate-control theory may supply the reason for the effectiveness of these measures. **Effleurage** is light stroking, usually of the abdomen, in rhythm with breathing during contractions. It is used to distract the woman from contraction pain. The presence of monitor belts often makes performing effleurage on the abdomen difficult; therefore a thigh or the chest may be used. As labor progresses, hyperesthesia may make effleurage uncomfortable and thus less effective.

Counterpressure is steady pressure applied by a support person to the sacral area with the fist or heel of the hand. This technique helps the woman cope with the sensations of internal pressure and pain in the lower back. It is especially helpful when back pain is caused by pressure of the occiput against spinal nerves when the fetal head is in a posterior position. Counterpressure lifts the occiput off these nerves, thereby providing pain relief. The support person will need to be relieved occasionally because application of counterpressure is hard work.

Music

Music, recorded or live, can enhance relaxation and lift spirits during labor, thereby reducing the woman's level of stress, anxiety, and perception of pain. It can be used to promote relaxation in early labor and to stimulate movement as labor progresses (Zwelling et al., 2006). Women should be encouraged to prepare their musical preferences in advance and bring a compact disk player or iPod to the hospital or birthing center. Use of a headset or earphones may increase the effectiveness of the music because other sounds will be shut out. Live music provided at the bedside by a support person may also be very helpful in transmitting energy that decreases tension and elevates mood. Although promising, evidence at the present time is insufficient to support the effectiveness of music as a method of pain relief during labor. Further research is recommended (Smith, Collins, Cyna, & Crowther, 2006).

Water Therapy (Hydrotherapy)

Bathing, showering, and jet hydrotherapy (whirlpool baths) with warm water (e.g., at or below body temperature) are nonpharmacologic measures that can be used to promote comfort and relaxation during labor (Fig. 10-4). The warm water stimulates the release of endorphins, relaxes fibers to close the gate on pain, and promotes better circulation and oxygenation. Most women find immersion in water to be soothing, relaxing, and comforting. While immersed, they may find it easier to let go and allow labor to take its course (Gilbert, 2007). Immersion in water has been reported to be effective in relieving pain by women who used this technique during labor (Albers, 2007).

In addition to pain relief, hydrotherapy offers other benefits. If the woman is having "back labor" as the result of an occiput posterior or transverse position, hydrotherapy can enhance fetal rotation to the occiput anterior position as a result of increased buoyancy. Hydrotherapy may also encourage a greater use of the upright position and more movements that facilitate labor progress and coping (Stark, Rudell, & Haus, 2008). In addition, it promotes faster labor, less use of intramuscular and intravenous pain medications, less use of epidural anesthesia, fewer forceps- or vacuum-assisted births, fewer episiotomies, less perineal trauma, and increased satisfaction with the birth experience (Zwelling et al., 2006).

When hydrotherapy is in use the fetal heart rate (FHR) is monitored by Doppler device, fetoscope, or wireless external monitor device (Fig. 10-4, *C*). Placement of internal electrodes is contraindicated for jet hydrotherapy. Several studies have investigated the risks of using hydrotherapy with ruptured membranes. Findings have shown no increases in chorioamnionitis, postpartum endometritis, neonatal infections, or antibiotic use. However, care must be taken to use tubs that can easily be thoroughly cleaned and a unit policy should be developed for cleaning the tubs (Tournaire & Theau-Yonneau, 2007; Zwelling et al., 2006).

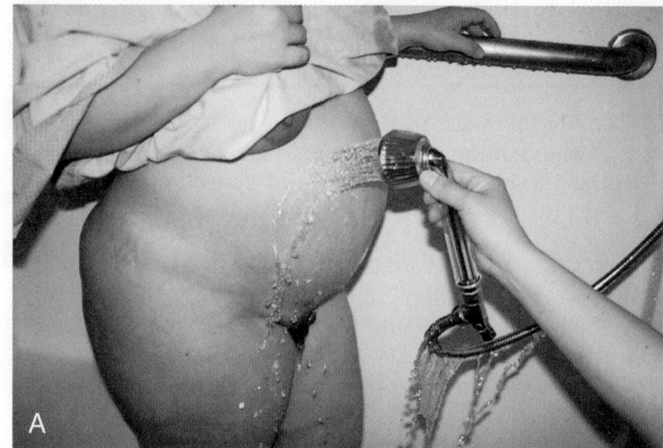
A

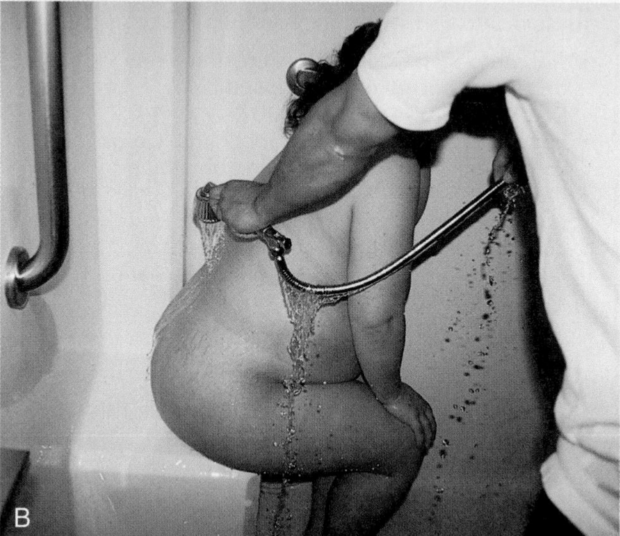
B

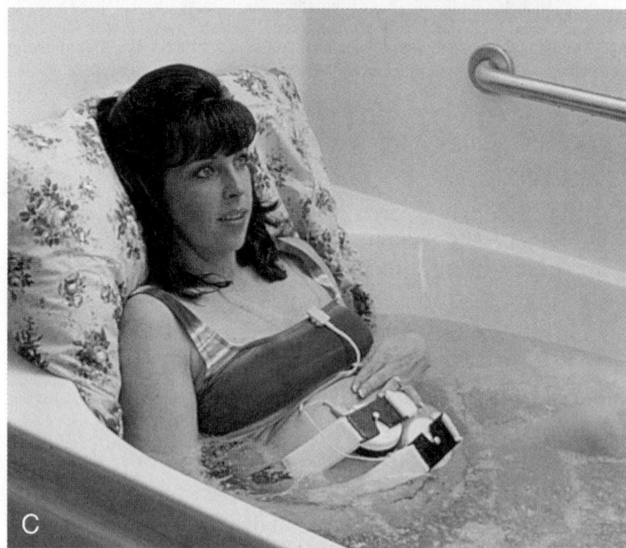
C

Fig. 10-4 Water therapy during labor. **A,** Use of shower during labor. **B,** Woman experiencing back labor relaxes as partner sprays warm water on her back. **C,** Laboring woman relaxes in Jacuzzi. Note that fetal monitoring can continue during time in the Jacuzzi. (**A** and **B,** Courtesy Marjorie Pyle, RNC, Lifecircle, Costa Mesa, CA; **C,** Courtesy Spacelabs Medical, Redmond, WA.)

Transcutaneous Electrical Nerve Stimulation

Transcutaneous electrical nerve stimulation (TENS) involves the placing of two pairs of flat electrodes on either side of the woman's thoracic and sacral spine (Fig. 10-5). These electrodes provide continuous low-intensity electrical impulses or stimuli from a battery-operated device. Women describe the resulting sensation as a tingling or buzzing. TENS is most useful for lower back pain during the early first stage of labor. Patients tend to rate the device as helpful, although its use does not decrease pain scores or the use of additional analgesics. Although TENS units do not change the degree of pain, apparently they somehow may make the pain less disturbing. No serious safety concerns associated with the use of TENS have been found (Hawkins, Goetzl, & Chestnut, 2007).

Acupressure and Acupuncture

Acupressure and acupuncture techniques can be used in pregnancy, in labor, and postpartum to relieve pain and other discomforts. Pressure, heat, or cold is applied to acupuncture points called *tsubos.* These points have an increased density of neuroreceptors and increased electrical conductivity. Acupressure is said to promote circulation of blood, the harmony of yin and yang and the secretion of neurotransmitters, thus maintaining normal body functions and enhancing well-being (Tournaire & Theau-Yonneau, 2007). Acupressure is best applied over the skin without using lubricants. Pressure is usually applied with the heel of the hand, fist, or pads of the thumbs and fingers (Fig. 10-6). Tennis balls or other devices also may be used to apply pressure. Pressure is applied with contractions initially and then continuously as labor progresses to the transition phase at the end of the first stage of labor (Tournaire & Theau-Yonneau). Synchronized breathing by the caregiver and the woman is suggested for greater effectiveness. Acupressure points are found on the neck, the shoulders, the wrists, the lower back, including sacral points, the hips, the area below the kneecaps, the ankles, the nails on the small toes, and the soles of the feet.

Acupuncture is the insertion of fine needles into specific areas of the body to restore the flow of *qi* (energy) and to decrease pain, which is thought to be obstructing the flow of energy. Acupuncture may work by altering the level of chemical neurotransmitters in the body or by releasing endorphins as a result of activation of the hypothalamus. It should be performed by a trained certified therapist. Current evidence indicates that acupuncture may be beneficial for relief of labor pain; however, further study is indicated (Hawkins et al., 2007; Smith et al., 2006; Tournaire & Theau-Yonneau, 2007).

Application of Heat and Cold

Warmed blankets, warm compresses, heated rice bags, a warm bath or shower, or a moist heating pad can enhance relaxation and reduce pain during labor. Heat relieves muscle ischemia and increases blood flow to the area of discomfort. Heat application is effective for back pain caused by a posterior presentation or general backache from fatigue.

Cold application such as cool cloths or ice packs applied to the back, the chest, or the face during labor may be effective in increasing comfort when the woman feels warm. They may also be applied to areas of pain. Cooling relieves pain by reducing the muscle temperature and relieving muscle spasms. A woman's culture may make the use of cold during labor unacceptable, however.

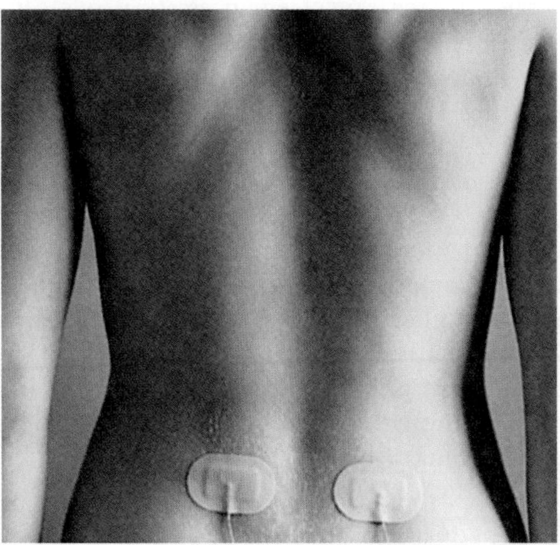

Fig. 10-5 Placement of transcutaneous electrical nerve stimulation (TENS) electrodes on back for relief of labor pain.

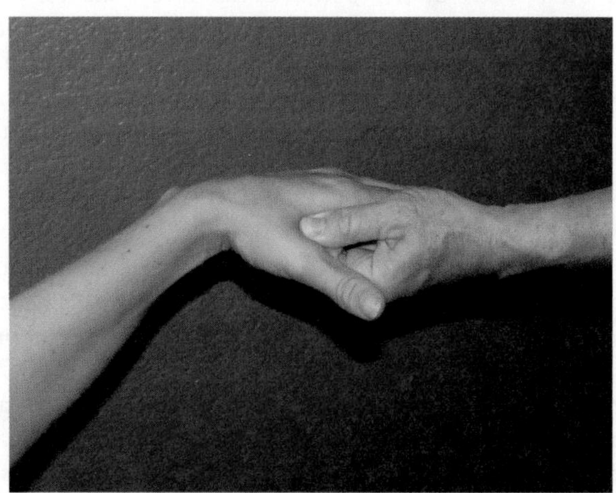

Fig. 10-6 Ho-Ku acupressure point (back of hand where thumb and index finger come together) used to enhance uterine contractions without increasing pain. (Courtesy Julie Perry Nelson, Loveland, CO.)

Heat and cold may be used alternately for a greater effect. Neither heat nor cold should be applied over ischemic or anesthetized areas because tissues can be damaged. One or two layers of cloth should be placed between the skin and a hot or cold pack to prevent damage to the underlying integument.

Touch and Massage

Touch and massage have been an integral part of the traditional care process for women in labor. A variety of massage techniques have been shown to be safe and effective during labor (Gilbert, 2007; Zwelling et al., 2006).

Touch can be as simple as holding the woman's hand, stroking her body, and embracing her. When using touch to communicate caring, reassurance, and concern, the woman's preferences for touch (e.g., who can touch her, where they can touch her, and how they can touch her) and responses to touch should be determined. Women who perceive touch during labor as positive have less pain, anxiety, and need for pain medication (Tournaire & Theau-Yonneau, 2007). Touch also can involve very specialized techniques that require manipulation of the human energy field. Therapeutic touch (TT) uses the concept of energy fields within the body called *prana.* Prana are thought to be deficient in some people who are in pain. TT uses laying-on of hands by a specially trained person to redirect energy fields associated with pain (Aghabati, Mohammadi, & Pour Esmaiel, 2008). Research has demonstrated the effectiveness of TT to enhance relaxation, reduce anxiety, and relieve pain (Aghabati et al.); however, little is known about the use or effectiveness of TT for relieving labor pain.

Head, arm, hand, leg, foot, or back massage may be very effective in reducing tension and enhancing comfort and it can easily be taught to support persons. Hand and foot massage may be especially relaxing in advanced labor when hyperesthesia limits a woman's tolerance for touch on other parts of her body. Combining massage with aromatherapy oil or lotion enhances relaxation both during and between contractions. The woman and her partner should be encouraged to experiment with different types of massage during pregnancy to determine what might feel best and be most relaxing during labor.

Hypnosis

Hypnosis is a form of deep relaxation, similar to daydreaming or meditation. While under hypnosis, women are in a state of focused concentration, and the subconscious mind can be more easily accessed (Gilbert, 2007). Hypnosis techniques used for labor and birth place an emphasis on enhancing relaxation and diminishing fear, anxiety, and perception of pain. Current evidence suggests that hypnosis seems to reduce fear, tension, and pain during labor and to raise the pain threshold. Women using this technique report a greater sense of control over painful contractions. Because it reduces the need for pain medication, hypnosis can be helpful when used with other interventions during labor. A few negative effects of hypnosis have been reported, including mild dizziness, nausea, and headache. These effects seem to be associated with failure to dehypnotize the patient properly (Tournaire & Theau-Yonneau, 2007).

Biofeedback

Biofeedback may provide another relaxation technique that can be used for labor. Biofeedback is based on the theory that if a person can recognize physical signals, certain internal physiologic events can be changed (i.e., whatever signs the woman has that are associated with her pain). For biofeedback to be effective the woman must be educated during the prenatal period to become aware of her body and its responses and how to relax. The woman must learn how to use thinking and mental processes (e.g., focusing) to control body responses and functions. Informational biofeedback helps couples develop awareness of their bodies and use strategies to change their responses to stress. If the woman responds to pain during a contraction with tightening of muscles, frowning, moaning, and breath holding, her partner uses verbal and touch feedback to help her relax. Formal biofeedback, which uses machines to detect skin temperature, blood flow, or muscle tension, can also prepare women to intensify their relaxation responses. Biofeedback-assisted relaxation techniques are not always successful in reducing labor pain. Using these techniques effectively requires the strong support of caregivers (Tournaire & Theau-Yonneau, 2007).

Aromatherapy

Aromatherapy uses oils distilled from plants, flowers, herbs, and trees to treat and balance the mind, body, and spirit. These essential oils are highly concentrated, complex essences, and are mixed with lotions or creams before they are applied to the skin. Certain essential oils can tone the uterus, encourage contractions, reduce pain, relieve tension, diminish fear and anxiety, and enhance the feeling of well-being. Lavender or jasmine oils can promote relaxation and reduce pain, for example, and rose oil acts as an antidepressant, sedative, and uterine tonic (Gilbert, 2007; Tournaire & Theau-Yonneau, 2007). Oils may also be used by adding a few drops to a warm bath, to warm water used for soaking compresses that can be applied to the body, or to an aromatherapy lamp to vaporize a room (Zwelling et al., 2006). Currently, evidence is insufficient to support the effectiveness of aromatherapy for pain relief in labor although its use has elicited promising results (Berghella et al., 2008; Smith et al., 2006; Zwelling et al.).

NURSING ALERT Caution: Only a trained aromatherapist should administer aromatherapy. Essential oils vary in terms of safe use during pregnancy (Gilbert, 2007).

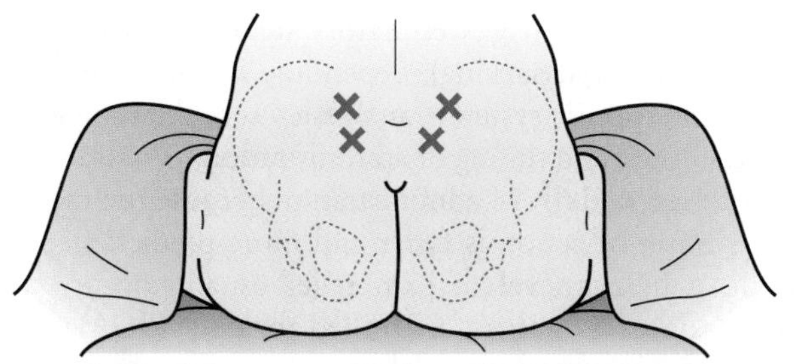

Fig. 10-7 Intradermal injection of 0.1 ml of sterile water in the treatment of women with back pain during labor. Sterile water is injected into four locations on the lower back, two over each posterior superior iliac spine (PSIS) and two 3 cm below and 1 cm medial to the PSIS. The injections should raise a bleb on the skin. Simultaneous injections administered by two clinicians will decrease the pain of the injections. (From Leeman, L., Fontaine, P., King, V., Klein, M., & Ratcliffe, S. [2003]. The nature and management of labor pain: part 1: Nonpharmacologic pain relief. *American Family Physician, 68*[6], 1109-1112.)

Intradermal Water Block

An intradermal water block involves the injection of small amounts of sterile water (e.g., 0.05 to 0.1 ml) by using a fine needle (e.g., 25 gauge) into four locations on the lower back to relieve back pain (Fig. 10-7). It is simple to perform and is effective in early labor and in an effort to delay the initiation of pharmacologic pain-relief measures (Hawkins et al., 2007). Stinging will occur for approximately 20 to 30 seconds after injection, but relief of back pain for up to 2 hours has been reported. Effectiveness of this method is probably related to the mechanism of counterirritation (i.e., reducing localized pain in one area by irritating the skin in an area nearby). When the effect wears off, the treatment can be repeated, or another method of pain relief can be used (Fogarty, 2008; Tournaire & Theau-Yonneau, 2007).

PHARMACOLOGIC MANAGEMENT OF DISCOMFORT

Pharmacologic measures for pain management should be implemented before pain becomes so severe that catecholamines increase and labor is prolonged. Pharmacologic and nonpharmacologic measures, when used together, increase the level of pain relief and create a more positive labor experience for the woman and her family. Nonpharmacologic measures can be used for relaxation and for pain relief, especially in early labor. Pharmacologic measures can be implemented as labor becomes more active and discomfort and pain intensify. Less pharmacologic intervention is often required because nonpharmacologic measures enhance relaxation and potentiate the analgesic's effect. However, from 1981 to 2001, more women took advantage of pharmacologic measures to relieve their pain during labor and birth and fewer opted for no pharmacologic support. The largest increase was noted in the use of epidural forms of analgesia (Bucklin, Hawkins, Anderson, & Ullrich, 2005).

Sedatives

Sedatives relieve anxiety and induce sleep. They may be given to a woman experiencing a prolonged latent phase of labor when a need exists to decrease anxiety or promote sleep. They may also be given to augment analgesics and reduce nausea when an opioid is used. Barbiturates such as secobarbital sodium (Seconal) can cause undesirable side effects, including respiratory and vasomotor depression affecting the woman and newborn. These effects are increased if a barbiturate is administered with another central nervous system (CNS) depressant such as an opioid analgesic. However, pain will be magnified if a barbiturate is given without an analgesic to a woman experiencing pain because her normal coping mechanisms may be blunted. Because of these disadvantages, barbiturates are seldom used during labor (Hawkins et al., 2007).

Phenothiazines (e.g., promethazine [Phenergan], hydroxyzine [Vistaril]) do not relieve pain but are often given to decrease anxiety and apprehension, increase sedation, and potentiate opioid analgesic effects. Promethazine is probably the most widely used drug in this class. It causes significant sedation and has been shown to actually impair the analgesic efficacy of opioids. Using opioids with less potential to cause nausea and vomiting should make routine use of promethazine unnecessary (Hawkins et al., 2007). Metoclopramide (Reglan) is an antiemetic that causes little sedation and may potentiate the effects of analgesics (Hawkins et al.).

Benzodiazepines (e.g., diazepam [Valium], lorazepam [Ativan]), when given with an opioid analgesic, seem to enhance pain relief and reduce nausea and vomiting. Because all of the benzodiazepines cause significant maternal amnesia, however, their use should be avoided in labor. A major disadvantage of diazepam is that it disrupts thermoregulation in newborns, making them less able to maintain body temperature (Hawkins et al., 2007).

Analgesia and Anesthesia

The use of analgesia and anesthesia was not generally accepted as part of obstetric management until Queen Victoria used chloroform during the birth of her son in 1853. Since then, much study has gone into the development of pharmacologic measures for controlling discomfort during the birth period. The goal of researchers is to develop methods that will provide adequate pain relief to women without increasing maternal or fetal risk or affecting the progress of labor.

Nursing management of obstetric analgesia and anesthesia combines the nurse's expertise in maternity care with a knowledge and understanding of anatomy and physiology and of medications and their therapeutic effects, adverse reactions, and methods of administration.

BOX 10-3

Pharmacologic Control of Discomfort by Stage of Labor and Method of Birth

FIRST STAGE
- Systemic analgesia
- Opioid agonist analgesics
- Opioid agonist-antagonist analgesics
- Epidural (block) analgesia
- Combined spinal-epidural (CSE) analgesia
- Nitrous oxide

SECOND STAGE
- Nerve block analgesia and anesthesia
- Local infiltration anesthesia
- Pudendal block
- Spinal (block) anesthesia
- Epidural (block) analgesia
- CSE analgesia
- Nitrous oxide

VAGINAL BIRTH
- Local infiltration anesthesia
- Pudendal block
- Epidural (block) analgesia and anesthesia
- Spinal (block) anesthesia
- CSE analgesia and anesthesia
- Nitrous oxide

CESAREAN BIRTH
- Spinal (block) anesthesia
- Epidural (block) anesthesia
- General anesthesia

Anesthesia encompasses analgesia, amnesia, relaxation, and reflex activity. Anesthesia abolishes pain perception by interrupting the nerve impulses to the brain. The loss of sensation may be partial or complete, sometimes with the loss of consciousness.

The term *analgesia* refers to the alleviation of the sensation of pain or the raising of the threshold for pain perception without loss of consciousness.

The type of analgesic or anesthetic chosen is determined in part by the stage of labor of the woman and by the method of birth planned (Box 10-3).

Systemic analgesia

Use of systemic analgesia for relieving the pain of labor has been declining, although it still remains the major pharmacologic method used when personnel trained in regional analgesia (e.g., epidural analgesia) are not available (Bucklin et al., 2005). Systemic analgesics cross the maternal blood-brain barrier to provide central analgesic effects. They also cross the placenta. Once transferred to the fetus, analgesics cross the fetal blood-brain barrier more readily than the maternal blood-brain barrier. The duration of action also will be longer because the systemic analgesics used during labor have a significantly longer half-life in the fetus and newborn. Effects on the fetus and newborn can be profound (e.g., respiratory depression, decreased alertness, delayed sucking), depending on the characteristics of the specific systemic analgesic used, the dose given, and the route and timing of administration. IV administration is preferred to IM administration because the medication's onset of action is faster and more predictable; as a result, a higher level of pain relief usually occurs with smaller doses. IV patient-controlled analgesia (PCA) is now available for use during labor. With this method the woman self-administers small doses of an opioid analgesic by using a pump programmed for dose and frequency. Overall, a lower total amount of analgesic is used and women appreciate the sense of autonomy provided by this method of pain relief (Hawkins et al., 2007).

Classifications of analgesic drugs used to relieve the pain of childbirth include opioid (narcotic) agonists and opioid (narcotic) agonist-antagonists. Choice of which medication to use is often dependent on preferences of the primary health care provider and characteristics of the laboring woman. Type of systemic analgesics used, therefore, often varies among obstetric units.

Opioid agonist analgesics. Opioid (narcotic) agonist analgesics such as hydromorphone hydrochloride (Dilaudid), meperidine (Demerol), fentanyl (Sublimaze), and sufentanil citrate (Sufenta) are effective for relieving severe, persistent, or recurrent pain. As pure opioid agonists, they stimulate both major opioid receptors, mu and kappa. They have no amnesic effect but create a feeling of well-being or euphoria. These analgesics decrease gastric emptying and increase nausea and vomiting. Bladder and bowel elimination can be inhibited. Because heart rate (e.g., bradycardia, tachycardia), blood pressure (e.g., hypotension), and respiratory effort (e.g., depression) can be adversely affected, opioid analgesics should be used cautiously in women with respiratory and cardiovascular disorders. Safety precautions should be taken because sedation and dizziness can occur after administration, increasing the risk for injury.

Hydromorphone hydrochloride (Dilaudid) is a potent opioid agonist analgesic that can be administered by IV or IM route during labor. After IV administration the onset of action occurs within 10 to 15 minutes, the peak effect is reached in 15 to 30 minutes, and the duration of action is approximately 2 to 3 hours. IM administration has an onset of action in 15 minutes, with a peak in 30 to 60 minutes and a duration of action approximately 4 to 5 hours.

Meperidine (Demerol) used to be the most commonly used opioid agonist analgesic for women in labor but is no longer the preferred choice because other medications have fewer side effects. In particular, the accumulation of normeperidine, a toxic metabolite of meperidine, causes prolonged neonatal sedation and neurobehavioral changes that are evident for the first 2 to 3 days of life (Hawkins et al., 2007). After IV administration the onset of action is almost immediate, and the duration of action is approxi-

EVIDENCE-BASED PRACTICE

Regional Pain Relief for Laboring Women

Pat Gingrich

ASK THE QUESTION

When in labor, should a woman be offered neuraxial (regional) analgesia? Does a difference in outcomes exist between epidurals and combined spinal-epidurals? When should women receiving neuraxial analgesia begin pushing?

SEARCH FOR EVIDENCE

Search Strategies: Professional organization guidelines, meta-analyses, systematic reviews, randomized controlled trials, nonrandomized prospective studies, and retrospective studies since 2006.

Databases Searched: CINAHL, Cochrane, Medline, National Guideline Clearinghouse, National Institute for Health and Clinical Excellence, TRIP Database and websites for Association of Women's Health, Obstetric, and Neonatal Nurses and the Royal College of Obstetrics & Gynaecology.

CRITICALLY ANALYZE THE DATA

Severe pain in labor can prolong labor and stress the fetus. The ideal pain-control measure would relieve the pain without maternal or fetal side effects. It would be easy to administer, compatible with other obstetric medications, allow maternal freedom of movement, and be readily available as soon as women request it.

The National Institute for Health and Clinical Excellence (NICE, 2007) recommends counseling women interested in neuraxial (regional) anesthesia that epidurals give better pain relief than intravenous opioids or inhaled analgesia, but they may prolong second stage and increase the risk of instrumental birth. The NICE guidelines recommend neuraxial analgesia be offered to any woman in severe pain, even in early (less than 4 cm dilation) labor.

A Cochrane meta-analysis of 19 trials, involving 2658 women, compared epidural with combined spinal-epidural (CSE) analgesia and found that CSE relieved pain faster and with less urinary retention but with increased risk of pruritus (Simmons, Cyna, Dennis, & Hughes, 2007). No differences between the two methods were found for maternal satisfaction, headaches, maternal hypotension, cesarean birth, need for blood patch, or adverse fetal effects. According to the American Society of Anesthesiologists (ASA) (2007) the use of low-dose local anesthesia allows for increased patient mobility and decreased pruritus, and patient-controlled analgesia results in lower overall dose. NICE (2007) recommends initiating CSE with bupivacaine and fentanyl.

In settings that offer neuraxial analgesia, the ASA guidelines (2007) recommend appropriate resources for possible complications such as malplacement, toxicity, hypotension, pruritus, nausea, and respiratory depression. IV access is essential, but a bolus of fluid is not required.

Finally, a meta-analysis of seven studies involving 2827 nulliparous women receiving epidural analgesia compared the practice of instructing women to push as soon as dilation is complete with passive descent or allowing a woman to "labor down" until she feels the urge to push. When compared with immediate pushing, passive descent is associated with an increased chance of vaginal birth, shortened pushing time, and decreased risk for instrumental (forceps or vacuum) birth (Brancato, Church, & Stone, 2008).

IMPLICATIONS FOR PRACTICE

Women should not have to suffer severe pain during labor. Nurses need to assess their patients' pain frequently and advocate for appropriate pain-relief measures. In settings in which neuraxial analgesia is offered, the CSE and low-dose medications are currently the first choice for women who request it, even in early labor. The medical team needs to be ready for complications. Respiratory monitoring, oxygen, and suction may be necessary for respiratory depression resulting from opioid use or high spinal anesthesia. Intravenous access is required for epidurals or CSE, but the bolus of fluid is no longer required. Nurses need to monitor maternal urinary output and blood pressure. Medications should be readily available for the reversal of opioid effects, as well as for relief of itching or nausea. Electronic fetal monitoring is important, as is availability of cesarean birth, in the event of fetal compromise.

References:

American Society of Anesthesiologists Task Force on Obstetric Anesthesia. (2007). Practice guidelines for obstetric anesthesia: an updated report. *Anesthesiology, 106*(4), 843-863.

Brancato, R. M., Church, S., & Stone, P. W. (2008). A meta-analysis of passive descent versus immediate pushing in nulliparous women with epidural analgesia in the second stage of labor. *Journal of Obstetric, Gynecologic, and Neonatal Nursing, 37*(1), 4-12.

National Institute for Health and Clinical Excellence. (2007). *Intrapartum care. NICE clinical guideline 55.* London: NICE.

Simmons, S. W., Cyba, A. M., Dennis, A. T., & Hughes, D. (2007). Combines spinal-epidural versus epidural analgesia in labour. In *The Cochrane Database of Systematic Reviews*, 2007, Issue 3, CD 003401.

mately 1½ to 2 hours. The onset of action begins in 10 to 20 minutes after an IM injection of meperidine and the duration is 2 to 3 hours (Hawkins et al.).

Fentanyl citrate (Sublimaze) and sufentanil citrate (Sufenta) are potent, short-acting opioid agonist analgesics. Sufentanil use is increasing because it has a more potent analgesic action than fentanyl when given through an epidural catheter. Also, less sufentanil will cross the placenta resulting in reduced fetal exposure. Onset of action after IV injection occurs within 2 to 5 minutes, the action peaks in 3 to 5 minutes, and the duration of action is approximately 30 to 60 minutes. Onset of the medication action occurs in 7 to 8 minutes after IM injection, reaches its peak effect in 20 to 30 minutes, and lasts for 1 to 2 hours. More frequent dosing is required with fentanyl and sufentanil because of their relatively short duration of action (Hawkins et al., 2007). As a result, these opioids are most commonly administered intrathecally or epidurally, alone or in combination with a local anesthetic agent (e.g., bupivacaine [Marcaine]) (see Medication Guide: Opioid Agonist Analgesics).

Ideally, birth should occur less than 1 hour or more than 4 hours after administration of an opioid agonist analgesic so that neonatal CNS depression resulting from the opioid is minimized.

Opioid agonist-antagonist analgesics. An agonist is an agent that activates or stimulates a receptor to act; an antagonist is an agent that blocks a receptor or a medication designed to activate a receptor. **Opioid (narcotic) agonist-antagonist analgesics** such as butorphanol (Stadol) and nalbuphine (Nubain) are agonists at kappa opioid receptors and are either antagonists or weak agonists at mu opioid receptors. In the doses used during labor, these mixed opioids provide adequate analgesia without causing significant respiratory depression in the mother or neonate. They are less likely to cause nausea and vomiting, but sedation may be as great or greater when compared with pure opioid agonists. As a result of these effects, parenteral opioid agonist-antagonist analgesics are used more commonly during labor than the opioid agonist analgesics. Both IM and IV routes of administration are used, but the IV route is preferred. This classification of opioid analgesics, especially nalbuphine hydrochloride is not suitable for women with an opioid dependence because the antagonist activity could precipitate withdrawal symptoms (abstinence syndrome) in both the mother and her newborn (Hawkins et al., 2007) (see Medication Guide: Opioid Agonist-Antagonist Analgesics and Signs of Potential Complications box).

Medication Guide

Opioid Agonist Analgesics

FENTANYL CITRATE (SUBLIMAZE)
SUFENTANIL CITRATE (SUFENTA)

Action

Opioid agonist analgesics that stimulate both mu and kappa opioid receptors to decrease the transmission of pain impulses, rapid action with short duration (0.5-1 hr IV; 1-2 hr epidural); sufentanil citrate has a more potent analgesic action than fentanyl citrate with less passage across the placenta to the fetus.

Indication

Because of their short duration of action when given intravenously, they are most commonly administered epidurally or intrathecally, alone or in combination with a local anesthetic agent, to relieve moderate to severe labor pain and postoperative pain after cesarean birth.

Dosage and route

Fentanyl citrate: 25 to 50 mcg IV; 1 to 2 mcg with 0.125% bupivacaine at rate of 8 to 10 ml/hr epidurally
Sufentanil citrate: 10 to 15 mcg with 0.125% bupivacaine at rate of 10 ml/hr epidurally

Adverse effects

Dizziness, drowsiness, allergic reactions, rash, pruritus, maternal and fetal or neonatal respiratory depression, nausea and vomiting, urinary retention

Nursing considerations

Assess for respiratory depression; naloxone should be available as an antidote.

IV, Intravenous.

Medication Guide

Opioid Agonist-Antagonist Analgesics

BUTORPHANOL TARTRATE (STADOL)
NALBUPHINE HYDROCHLORIDE (NUBAIN)

Action

Mixed agonist-antagonist analgesics that stimulate kappa opioid receptors and block or weakly stimulate mu opioid receptors, resulting in good analgesia but with less respiratory depression and nausea and vomiting when compared with opioid agonist analgesics

Indication

Moderate to severe labor pain and postoperative pain after cesarean birth

Dosage and route

Butorphanol tartrate: 1 mg (range 0.5 to 2 mg) IV every 3-4 hr as needed; 2 mg (range 1 to 4 mg) IM every 3-4 hr as needed
Nalbuphine hydrochloride: 10 mg IV; 10 to 20 mg IM every 3-4 hours as needed

Adverse effects

Confusion, sedation, hallucinations, "floating" feeling, drowsiness, headache, dizziness, nervousness, sweating; maternal palpitations and tachycardia or bradycardia; transient nonpathologic sinusoidal-like fetal heart rate rhythm; respiratory depression; nausea and vomiting; difficulty with urination (retention, urgency)

Nursing considerations

May precipitate withdrawal symptoms in opioid-dependent women and their newborns. Assess maternal vital signs, degree of pain, FHR, and uterine activity before and after administration; observe for maternal respiratory depression, notifying primary health care provider if maternal respirations are ≤12 breaths/min; encourage voiding every 2 hours and palpate for bladder distention; if birth occurs within 1 to 4 hours of dose administration, observe newborn for respiratory depression; implement safety measures as appropriate, including use of side rails and assistance with ambulation; continue use of nonpharmacologic pain-relief measures.

IM, Intramuscular; *IV,* intravenous.

signs of POTENTIAL COMPLICATIONS

Maternal Opioid Abstinence Syndrome (Opioid/Narcotic Withdrawal)

- Yawning, rhinorrhea (runny nose), sweating, lacrimation (tearing), mydriasis (dilation of pupils)
- Anorexia
- Irritability, restlessness, generalized anxiety
- Tremor
- Chills and hot flashes
- Piloerection ("gooseflesh" or "chill bumps")
- Violent sneezing
- Weakness, fatigue, and drowsiness
- Nausea and vomiting
- Diarrhea, abdominal cramps
- Bone and muscle pain, muscle spasm, kicking movements

Opioid (narcotic) antagonists. Opioids such as hydromorphone, meperidine, and fentanyl can cause excessive CNS depression in the mother, the newborn, or both, although the current practice of giving lower doses of opioids intravenously has reduced the incidence and severity of opioid-induced CNS depression. Opioid antagonists such as naloxone (Narcan) can promptly reverse the CNS depressant effects, especially respiratory depression. In addition, the antagonist counters the effect of the stress-induced levels of endorphins. An opioid antagonist is especially valuable if labor is more rapid than expected and birth is anticipated when the opioid is at its peak effect. The antagonist may be given through the woman's IV line, or it can be administered intramuscularly (see Medication Guide: Opioid Antagonist).

NURSING ALERT An opioid antagonist (e.g., naloxone [Narcan]) is contraindicated for opioid-dependent women because it may precipitate abstinence syndrome (withdrawal symptoms). For the same reason, opioid agonist-antagonist analgesics such as butorphanol (Stadol) and nalbuphine (Nubain) should not be given to opioid–dependent women (see Signs of Potential Complications box).

An opioid antagonist can be given to the newborn as one part of the treatment for **neonatal narcosis**, which is a state of CNS depression in the newborn produced by an opioid. Prophylactic administration of naloxone is controversial. Affected infants may exhibit respiratory depression, hypotonia, lethargy, and a delay in temperature regulation. Risk for hypoxia, hypercarbia, and acidosis increases if neonatal narcosis is not treated promptly. Treatment involves ventilation, administration of oxygen, and gentle stimulation. Naloxone is administered, if still required, to reverse CNS depression. More than one dose of naloxone may be required because its half-life is shorter than the half-life of opioids. Alterations in neurologic and behavioral responses may be evident in the newborn for as long as 2 to 4 days after birth. The significance of these neurobehavioral changes is unknown (Hawkins et al., 2007).

Medication Guide

Opioid Antagonist

NALOXONE HYDROCHLORIDE (NARCAN)

Action

Opioid antagonist that blocks both mu and kappa opioid receptors from the effects of opioid agonists

Indication

Reverses opioid-induced respiratory depression in woman or newborn; may be used to reverse pruritus from epidural opioids

Dosage and route

Adult

Opioid overdose: 0.4 to 2 mg IV, may repeat IV at 2- to 3-minute intervals until a maximum of 10 mg has been given; if IV route unavailable, IM or SC administration may be used.

Newborn

Opioid-induced depression: Initial dose is 0.1 mg/kg; preferred route is IV but may be administered IM.

Adverse effects

Maternal hypotension and hypertension, tachycardia, hyperventilation, nausea or vomiting, sweating, tremulousness

Nursing considerations

Woman should delay breastfeeding until medication is out of her system; do not give to mother or newborn if woman is opioid dependent—may cause abrupt withdrawal in woman and newborn; if given to woman for reversal of respiratory depression caused by opioid analgesic, pain will return suddenly.

The duration of action of naloxone is shorter than that of most opioids. Therefore the patient must be monitored closely for the return of opioid depression when the effects of naloxone are gone. Additional doses of naloxone may be necessary to maintain reversal.

IM, Intramuscular; *IV*, intravenous; *SC*, subcutaneous.

Nerve block analgesia and anesthesia

A variety of local anesthetic agents are used in obstetrics to produce regional analgesia (some pain relief and motor block) and anesthesia (complete pain relief and motor block). Most of these agents are related chemically to cocaine and end with the suffix *-caine,* which helps to identify a local anesthetic.

The principal pharmacologic effect of local anesthetics is the temporary interruption of the conduction of nerve impulses, notably pain. Examples of common agents given are bupivacaine (Marcaine), chloroprocaine (Nesacaine) lidocaine (Xylocaine), ropivacaine (Naropin or Naropeine), and mepivacaine (Carbocaine). Rarely, people are sensitive (allergic) to one or more local anesthetics. Such a reaction may include respiratory depression, hypotension, and other serious adverse effects. Epinephrine, antihistamines, oxygen, and supportive measures should reverse these effects. Sensitivity may be identified by administering minute amounts of the drug to test for an allergic reaction.

Local perineal infiltration anesthesia. Local perineal infiltration anesthesia may be used when an episiotomy is to be performed or when lacerations must be sutured after birth in a woman who does not have regional anesthesia. Rapid anesthesia is produced by injecting approximately 10 to 20 ml of 1% lidocaine or 2% chloroprocaine into the skin and then subcutaneously into the region to be anesthetized. Epinephrine is often added to the solution to prolong the effects of the anesthetic (Cunningham, Leveno, Bloom, Hauth, Gilstrap, & Wenstrom, 2005). Injections can be repeated as needed to keep the woman comfortable while postbirth repairs are completed.

Pudendal nerve block. A pudendal nerve block, administered late in the second stage of labor, is useful if an episiotomy is to be performed or if forceps or a vacuum extractor are to be used to facilitate birth. It can also be administered during the third stage of labor if an episiotomy or lacerations must be repaired (American Academy of Pediatrics [AAP] & American College of Obstetricians and Gynecologists [ACOG], 2007). A pudendal nerve block is considered to be reasonably effective for pain relief and very safe (Hawkins et al., 2007). Although a pudendal nerve block does not relieve the pain from uterine contractions, it does relieve pain in the lower vagina, vulva, and perineum (Fig. 10-8, *A* and *B*). A pudendal nerve block should be administered 10 to 20 minutes before perineal anesthesia is needed.

The pudendal nerve traverses the sacrosciatic notch just medial to the tip of the ischial spine on each side. Injection of an anesthetic solution at or near these points anesthetizes the pudendal nerves peripherally (Fig. 10-9). A pudendal block does not change maternal hemodynamic or respiratory functions, vital signs, or the FHR. However, the bearing-down reflex is lessened or lost completely.

Spinal anesthesia. In spinal anesthesia (block) an anesthetic solution containing a local anesthetic alone or in combination with an opioid analgesic is injected through the third, fourth, or fifth lumbar interspace into the subarachnoid space (Fig. 10-10, *A* and *B*), where the anesthetic solution mixes with cerebrospinal fluid (CSF). The use of this technique has increased for both elective and emergent cesarean births and is more common than epidural anesthesia for these types of births (Bucklin et al., 2005). Low spinal anesthesia (block) may be used for vaginal birth, but it is not suitable for labor. Spinal anesthesia (block) used for cesarean birth provides anesthesia from the nipple (T6) to the feet. If it is used for vaginal birth, the anesthesia level is from the hips (T10) to the feet (Fig. 10-10, *C*).

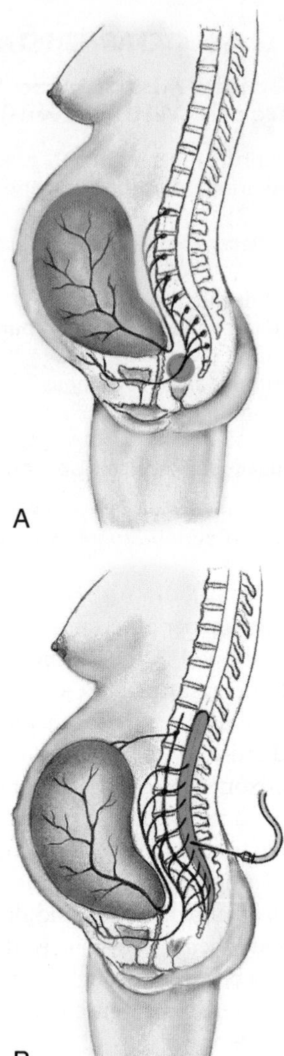

Fig. 10-8 Pain pathways and sites of pharmacologic nerve blocks. **A,** Pudendal block: suitable during second and third stages of labor and for repair of episiotomy or lacerations. **B,** Epidural block: suitable for all stages of labor and for repair of episiotomy and lacerations.

For spinal anesthesia (block) the woman sits or lies on her side (e.g., modified Sims position) with the back curved to widen the intervertebral space to facilitate insertion of a small-gauge spinal needle and injection of the anesthetic solution into the spinal canal. The nurse supports the woman because she must remain still during the placement of the spinal needle. The needle is inserted and the anesthetic injected between contractions. After the anesthetic solution has been injected the woman is positioned upright to allow the heavier (hyperbaric) anesthetic solution to flow downward to obtain the lower level of anesthesia suitable for a vaginal birth. To obtain the higher level of anesthesia desired for cesarean birth, she will be positioned supine with head and shoulders slightly elevated and the

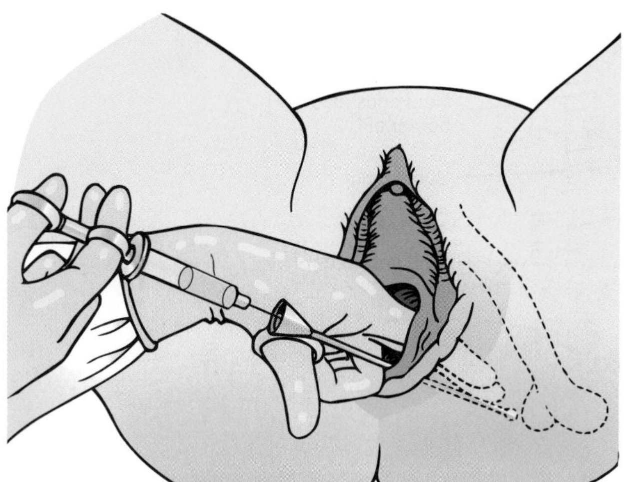

Fig. 10-9 Pudendal block. Use of needle guide (Iowa trumpet) and Luer-Lok syringe to inject medication.

uterus displaced by tilting the operating table or placing a wedge under one of her hips. Usually the level of the block will be complete and fixed within 5 to 10 minutes after the anesthetic is injected, but it can continue to creep upward for 20 minutes or longer (Hawkins et al., 2007) (Fig. 10-11, *A* and *B*).

Marked hypotension, impaired placental perfusion, and an ineffective breathing pattern may occur during spinal anesthesia. Before induction of the spinal anesthetic, the woman may be preloaded with IV fluid (usually 500 to 1,000 ml) to decrease the potential for hypotension caused by sympathetic blockade (vasodilation with pooling of blood in the lower extremities decreases cardiac output). Although the practice guidelines for obstetric anesthesia published by the American Society of Anesthesiologists (2007) state that this pre-anesthetic fluid bolus is not required, it is still usually administered in most clinical settings.

After induction of the anesthetic, maternal blood pressure, pulse, and respirations and fetal heart rate must be checked and documented every 5 to 10 minutes. If signs of serious maternal hypotension (e.g., a drop in the baseline blood pressure of more than 20%) or fetal distress (e.g., bradycardia, minimal or absent variability, late decelerations) develop, emergency care must be given (see Emergency box).

Because the woman is unable to sense her contractions, she must be instructed when to bear down during a vaginal birth. Use of a combination of local anesthetic agent and an opioid reduces the degree of motor function loss, thereby enhancing a woman's ability to push effectively. If the birth occurs in a delivery room (rather than a labor-delivery-recovery room), then the woman will need assistance in the transfer to a recovery bed after expulsion of the placenta.

Advantages of spinal anesthesia include ease of administration and absence of fetal hypoxia with maintenance of normal maternal blood pressure. Maternal consciousness is maintained, excellent muscular relaxation is achieved, and blood loss is not excessive.

Disadvantages of spinal anesthesia include possible medication reactions (e.g., allergy), hypotension, and an ineffective breathing pattern; cardiopulmonary resuscitation may be needed. When a spinal anesthetic is given, the need for operative birth (e.g., episiotomy, forceps-assisted birth, vacuum-assisted birth) tends to increase because voluntary expulsive efforts are reduced or eliminated. After birth the incidence of bladder and uterine atony, as well as postspinal headache, is higher.

Leakage of CSF from the site of puncture of the dura mater (membranous covering of the spinal cord) is thought to be the major causative factor in *postdural puncture headache* (PDPH), commonly called a spinal headache. Spinal headache is much more likely to occur when the dura is punctured during the process of administering an epidural block. The needle used for an epidural block has a much larger gauge than the one used for spinal anesthesia and thus creates a bigger opening in the dura, resulting in greater loss of CSF. Presumably, postural changes cause the diminished volume of CSF to exert traction on pain-sensitive CNS structures. Characteristically, assuming an upright position triggers or intensifies the headache, whereas assuming a supine position achieves relief (Hawkins et al., 2007).

The likelihood of headache after dural puncture can be reduced if the anesthesia care provider uses a small-gauge

EMERGENCY

Maternal Hypotension with Decreased Placental Perfusion

SIGNS AND SYMPTOMS

- Maternal hypotension (20% decrease from preblock baseline level or <100 mm Hg systolic)
- Fetal bradycardia
- Absent or minimal FHR variability

INTERVENTIONS

- Turn the woman to lateral position or place pillow or wedge under hip to deflect uterus.
- Maintain IV infusion at rate specified, or increase *as-needed* administration per hospital protocol.
- Administer oxygen by facemask at 10-12 L/min or per protocol.
- Elevate the woman's legs.
- Notify the primary health care provider, anesthesiologist, or nurse anesthetist.
- Administer IV vasopressor (e.g., ephedrine 5-10 mg or phenylephrine 50-100 mcg) per protocol if previous measures are ineffective.
- Remain with the woman and continue to monitor maternal blood pressure and FHR every 5 minutes until her condition is stable or per primary health care provider's order.

FHR, Fetal heart rate; *IV,* intravenous.

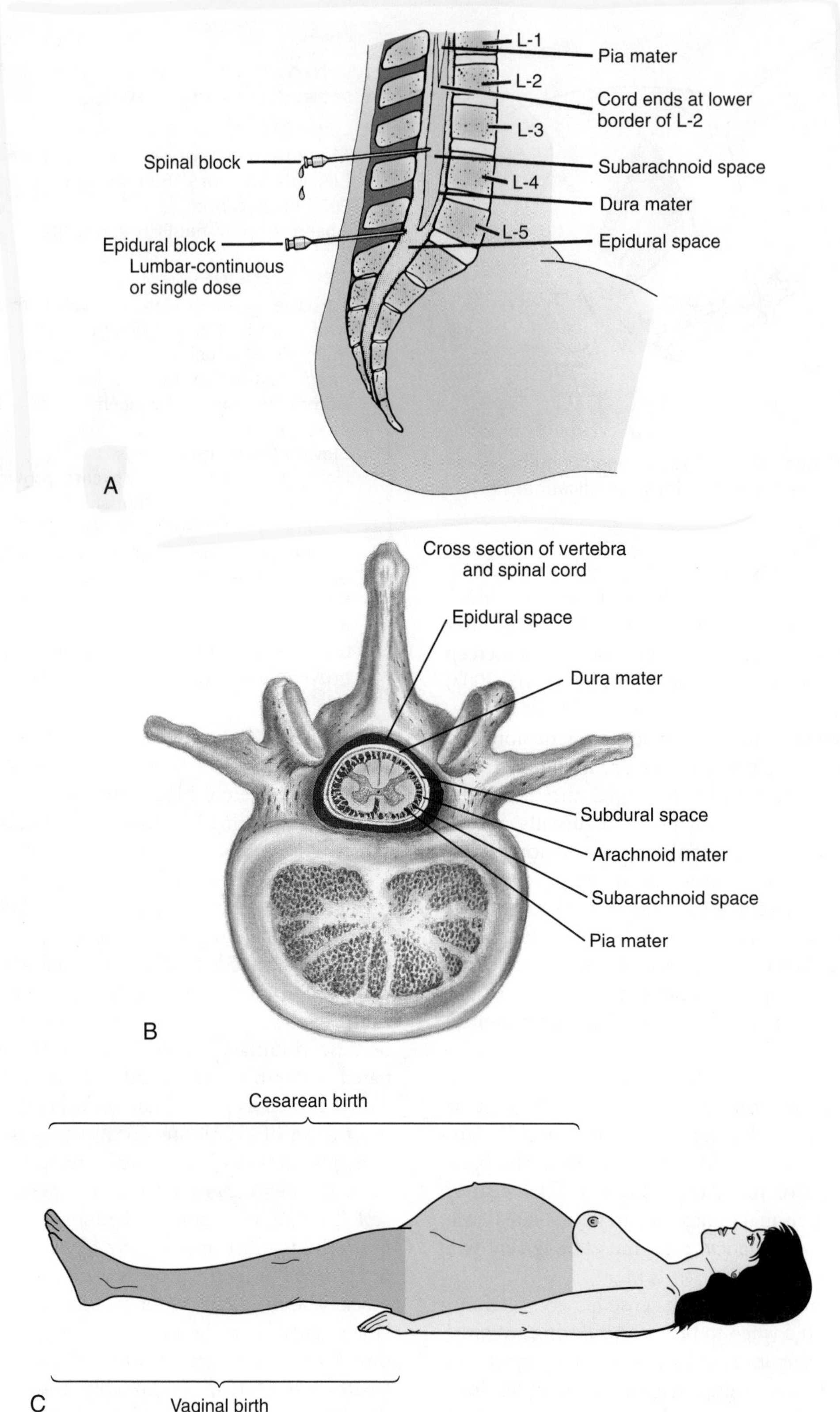

Fig. 10-10 **A,** Membranes and spaces of spinal cord and levels of sacral, lumbar, and thoracic nerves. **B,** Cross-section of vertebra and spinal cord. **C,** Level of anesthesia necessary for cesarean birth and for vaginal births.

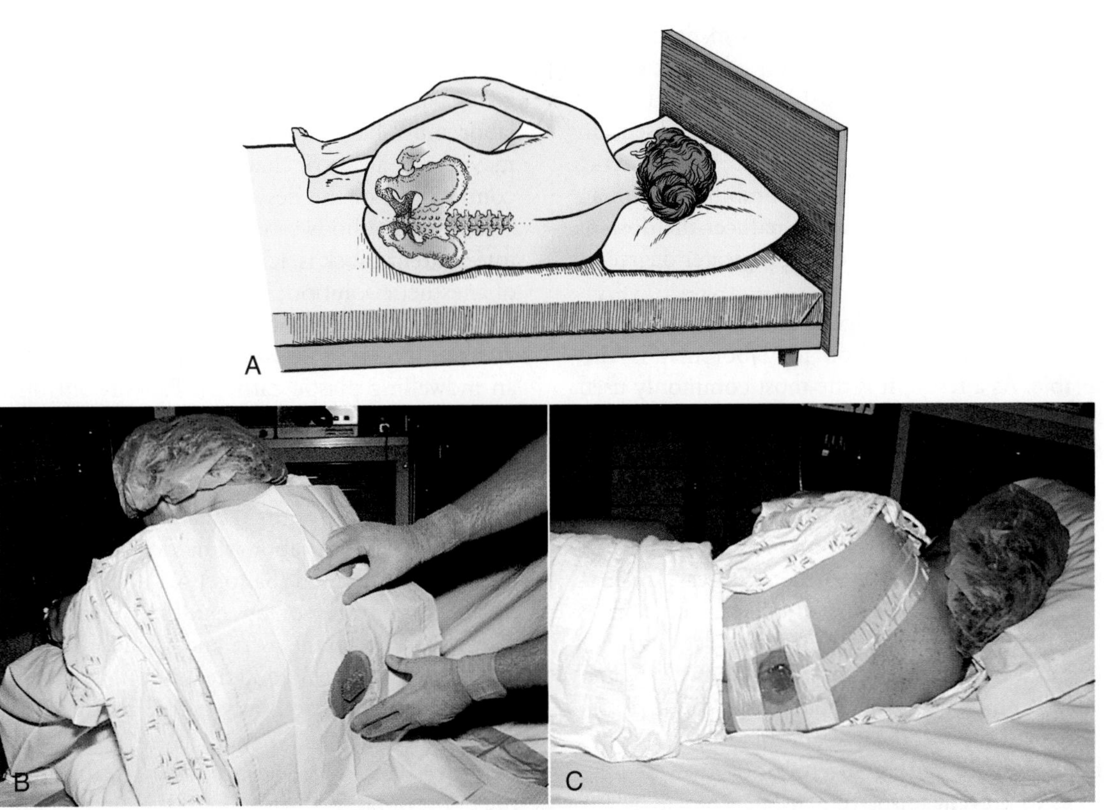

Fig. 10-11 Positioning for spinal and epidural blocks. **A,** Lateral position. **B,** Upright position. **C,** Catheter for epidural taped to woman's back with port segment located near shoulder. (**B** and **C,** Courtesy Michael S. Clement, MD, Mesa, AZ.)

spinal needle and avoids making multiple punctures of the meninges. Passing an epidural catheter through the dural opening at the time of puncture to provide continuous spinal anesthesia, with removal of the catheter 24 hours later, may help to prevent spinal headache. Injecting preservative-free saline through the spinal catheter before removing it may also decrease the incidence of headache. Hydration and bedrest in the prone position have been recommended in the past as preventive measures, but they have not been proven to be of much value (Hawkins et al., 2007).

Conservative treatment for a PDPH consists of oral analgesics and caffeine or theophylline. Caffeine and theophylline cause constriction of cerebral blood vessels, and may provide symptomatic relief. An autologous **epidural blood patch** is the most rapid, reliable, and beneficial relief measure for PDPH. The woman's blood (i.e., 20 ml) is injected slowly into the lumbar epidural space, creating a clot that patches the tear or hole in the dura mater around the spinal cord. Treatment with a blood patch is considered if the headache is severe and debilitating or does not resolve after conservative management (Fig. 10-12). The blood patch is remarkably effective and is nearly complication free (Hawkins et al., 2007).

The woman should be observed for alteration in vital signs, pallor, clammy skin, and leakage of CSF for 1 to 2 hours after the blood patch is performed. If no complications occur, she can resume normal activity after that time. She should, however, be instructed to avoid coughing or straining for several days (Hawkins et al., 2007).

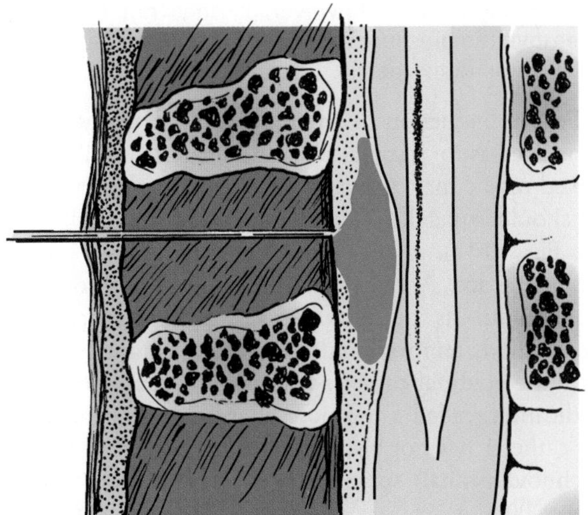

Fig. 10-12 Blood-patch therapy for spinal headache.

Epidural anesthesia or analgesia (block). Relief from the pain of uterine contractions and birth (vaginal and cesarean) can be relieved by injecting a suitable local anesthetic agent (e.g., bupivacaine, ropivacaine), an opioid analgesic (e.g., fentanyl, sufentanil), or both into

Critical Thinking/Clinical Decision Making: Patient Receiving Epidural Block
Nursing Care Plan: Epidural Block during Labor

the epidural (peridural) space. Injection is made between the fourth and fifth lumbar vertebrae for a lumbar **epidural block** (see Figs. 10-8, *B*, and 10-10, *A*). Depending on the type, amount, and number of medications used, an anesthetic or analgesic effect will occur with varying degrees of motor impairment. The combination of an opioid with the local anesthetic agent reduces the dose of anesthetic required, thereby preserving a greater degree of motor function.

Epidural anesthesia and analgesia is the most effective pharmacologic pain-relief method for labor that is currently available. As a result, it is the most commonly used method for relieving pain during labor in the United States and its use has been increasing. Nearly two thirds of American women giving birth choose epidural analgesia (AAP & ACOG, 2007; Bucklin et al., 2005; Hawkins et al., 2007). For relieving the discomfort of labor and vaginal birth, a block from T10 to S5 is required. For cesarean birth, a block from at least T8 to S1 is essential. The diffusion of epidural anesthesia depends on the location of the catheter tip, the dose and volume of the anesthetic agent used, and the woman's position (e.g., horizontal or head-up position). The woman must cooperate and maintain her position without moving during insertion of the epidural catheter so as to prevent misplacement, neurologic injury, or hematoma formation (Cunningham et al., 2005).

NURSING ALERT Epidural anesthesia effectively relieves the pain caused by uterine contractions. For most women, however, it does not completely remove the pressure sensations that occur as the fetus descends in the pelvis.

For the induction of an epidural block, the woman is positioned as for a spinal block. She may sit with her back curved or she may assume a modified Sims position with her shoulders parallel, legs slightly flexed, and back arched (see Fig. 10-11). A large-bore needle is inserted into the epidural space. A catheter is then threaded through the needle until its tip rests in the epidural space. Then the needle is removed and the catheter is taped in place. After the epidural catheter is inserted, a small amount of medication, called a test dose, is injected to be sure that the catheter has not been accidentally placed in the subarachnoid (spinal) space or in a blood vessel (Hawkins et al., 2007).

After the epidural has been initiated the woman is positioned preferably on her side so that the uterus does not compress the ascending vena cava and descending aorta, which can impair venous return, reduce cardiac output and blood pressure, and decrease placental perfusion. Her position should be alternated from side to side every hour. Upright positions and ambulation may be possible, depending on the degree of motor impairment. Oxygen should be available if hypotension occurs despite maintenance of hydration with IV fluid and displacement of the uterus to the side. Ephedrine or phenylephrine (vasopressors used to increase maternal blood pressure) and increased IV fluid infusion may be needed (see Emergency box). The FHR, contraction pattern, and progress in labor must be monitored carefully because the woman may not be aware of changes in the strength of the uterine contractions or the descent of the presenting part.

Several methods can be used for an epidural block. An intermittent block is achieved by using repeated injections of anesthetic solution; it is the least common method. The most common method is the continuous block, achieved by using a pump to infuse the anesthetic solution through an indwelling plastic catheter. Patient-controlled epidural analgesia (PCEA) is the newest method; it uses an indwelling catheter and a programmed pump that allows the woman to control the dosing. This method has been found to provide optimal analgesia with better maternal satisfaction during labor while decreasing the amount of local anesthetic used (Saito et al., 2005).

The advantages of an epidural block are numerous: The woman remains alert and is more comfortable and able to participate, good relaxation is achieved, airway reflexes remain intact, only partial motor paralysis develops, gastric emptying is not delayed, and blood loss is not excessive. Fetal complications are rare but may occur in the event of rapid absorption of the medication or marked maternal hypotension. The dose, volume, type, and number of medications used can be modified to allow the woman to push and to assume upright positions and even to walk, to produce perineal anesthesia, and to permit forceps-assisted, vacuum-assisted, or cesarean birth if required (Cunningham et al., 2005).

The disadvantages of epidural block also are numerous. The woman's ability to move freely and to maintain control of her labor is limited, related to the use of numerous medical interventions (e.g., an IV infusion and electronic monitoring) and the occurrence of orthostatic hypotension and dizziness, sedation, and weakness of the legs. CNS effects (Box 10-4) can occur if a solution containing a local anesthetic agent is accidentally injected into a blood vessel or if excessive amounts of local anesthetic are given. High spinal or "total spinal" anesthesia, resulting in respiratory arrest, can occur if the relatively high dose of local anesthetic used with an epidural block is accidentally injected into the subarachnoid space. Women who receive an epidural have a higher rate of fever (i.e., intrapartum temperature of 38° C or higher), especially when labor lasts longer that 12 hours; the temperature elevation most likely is related to thermoregulatory changes, although infection cannot be ruled out. The elevation in temperature can result in fetal tachycardia and neonatal workup for sepsis, whether or not signs of infection are present (see Box 10-4).

Severe hypotension (more than a 20% decrease in baseline blood pressure) as a result of sympathetic blockade can be an outcome of an epidural block (Anim-Somuah, Smyth, & Howell, 2005) (see Emergency box). It can result

BOX 10-4

Side Effects of Epidural and Spinal Anesthesia

- Hypotension
- Local anesthetic toxicity
  - Light-headedness
  - Dizziness
  - Tinnitus (ringing in the ears)
  - Metallic taste
  - Numbness of the tongue and mouth
  - Bizarre behavior
  - Slurred speech
  - Convulsions
  - Loss of consciousness
- High or total spinal anesthesia
- Fever
- Urinary retention
- Pruritus (itching)
- Limited movement
- Longer second stage labor
- Increased use of oxytocin
- Increased likelihood of forceps- or vacuum-assisted birth

in a significant decrease in uteroplacental perfusion and oxygen delivery to the fetus. Urinary retention and stress incontinence can occur in the immediate postpartum period. Pruritus (itching) is a side effect that often occurs with the use of an opioid, especially fentanyl. A relationship between epidural analgesia and longer second-stage labor, use of oxytocin, and forceps-assisted or vacuum-assisted birth has been documented. Research findings have been unable to demonstrate a significant increase in cesarean birth associated with epidural analgesia (Anim-Somuah et al.). For some women, the epidural block is not effective, and a second form of analgesia is required to establish effective pain relief. When women progress rapidly in labor, pain relief may not be obtained before birth occurs.

Combined spinal-epidural analgesia. In the combined spinal-epidural (CSE) analgesia technique, sometimes called a "walking epidural," an epidural needle is inserted into the epidural space. Before the epidural catheter is placed, a smaller-gauge spinal needle is inserted through the bore of the epidural needle into the subarachnoid space. A small amount of opioid or combination of opioid and local anesthetic is then injected intrathecally to provide analgesia rapidly. Afterward the epidural catheter is inserted as usual. The CSE technique is an increasingly popular approach that can be used to block pain transmission without compromising motor ability. The concentration of opioid receptors is high along the pain pathway in the spinal cord, in the brainstem, and in the thalamus. Because these receptors are highly sensitive to opioids, a small quantity of an opioid-agonist analgesic produces marked pain relief lasting for several hours. If additional pain relief is needed, medication can be injected through the epidural catheter (see Fig. 10-10, *A*). The most common side effects of CSE are pruritus and nausea (Hawkins et al., 2007). CSE analgesia may also be associated with fetal bradycardia, necessitating close assessment of fetal heart rate (Cunningham et al., 2005).

Although women can walk, they often choose not to do so because of sedation and fatigue, abnormal sensations perceived in their legs, weakness of the legs, and a feeling of insecurity. Health care providers are often reluctant to encourage or assist women to ambulate for fear of injury. However, women can be assisted to change positions and use upright positions during labor and birth. Upright positioning is associated with less pain, more efficient labor progress, and a lower incidence of forceps- or vacuum-assisted birth (Albers, 2007; Berghella et al., 2008). Laboring upright also conveys a sense of normalcy, autonomy, and personal control (Albers).

Epidural and intrathecal (spinal) opioids. Opioids also can be used alone, eliminating the effect of a local anesthetic altogether. The use of epidural or intrathecal opioids without the addition of a local anesthetic agent during labor has several advantages. Opioids administered in this manner do not cause maternal hypotension or affect vital signs. The woman feels contractions but not pain. Her ability to bear down during the second stage of labor is preserved because the pushing reflex is not lost, and her motor power remains intact.

Fentanyl, sufentanil, or preservative-free morphine may be used. Fentanyl and sufentanil produce short-acting analgesia (i.e., 1.5 to 3.5 hours), and morphine may provide pain relief for 4 to 7 hours. Morphine may be combined with fentanyl or sufentanil. Using short-acting opioids with multiparous women and morphine with nulliparous women or women with a history of long labor would be appropriate. For most women, intrathecal opioids do not provide adequate analgesia for second-stage labor pain, episiotomy, or birth (Cunningham et al., 2005). Pudendal nerve blocks or local perineal infiltration anesthesia may be necessary.

A more common indication for the administration of epidural or intrathecal analgesics is the relief of postoperative pain. For example, women who give birth by cesarean can receive fentanyl or morphine through a catheter. The catheter may then be removed, and the women are usually free of pain for 24 hours. The catheter is occasionally left in place in the epidural space in case another dose is needed.

Women receiving epidurally administered morphine after a cesarean birth may ambulate sooner than women who do not. The early ambulation and freedom from pain also facilitate bladder emptying, enhance peristalsis, and prevent clot formation in the lower extremities (e.g., thrombophlebitis). Women may require additional medication for pain during the first 24 hours after surgery. If so, they will usually be given oral analgesics (e.g., oxycodone/acetaminophen [Percocet]), rather than IV or IM narcotics.

Side effects of opioids administered by the epidural and intrathecal routes include nausea, vomiting, pruritus, urinary retention, and delayed respiratory depression. These side effects are more common when morphine is administered. Antiemetics, antipruritics, and opioid antagonists are used to relieve these symptoms. For example, naloxone (Narcan), nalbuphine (Nubain), or metoclopramide (Reglan) may be administered. Hospital protocols or detailed physician orders should provide specific instructions for the treatment of these side effects. Use of epidural opioids is not without risk. Respiratory depression is a serious concern; for this reason the woman's respiratory rate should be assessed and documented every hour for 24 hours, or as designated by hospital protocol. Naloxone should be readily available for use if the respiratory rate decreases to less than 10 breaths per minute or if the oxygen saturation rate decreases to less than 89%. Administration of oxygen by facemask also may be initiated, and the anesthesia care provider should be notified.

Contraindications to epidural blocks. Some contraindications to epidural analgesia include the following (Cunningham et al., 2005; Hawkins et al., 2007):

- Active or anticipated serious maternal hemorrhage (Acute hypovolemia leads to increased sympathetic tone to maintain the blood pressure. Any anesthetic technique that blocks the sympathetic fibers can produce significant hypotension that can endanger the mother and baby.)
- Coagulopathy (If a woman is receiving anticoagulant therapy or has a bleeding disorder, injury to a blood vessel may cause the formation of a hematoma that may compress the cauda equina or the spinal cord and lead to serious CNS complications.)
- Infection at the injection site (Infection can be spread through the peridural or subarachnoid spaces if the needle traverses an infected area.)
- Increased intracranial pressure caused by a mass lesion.
- Maternal refusal.
- Some types of maternal cardiac conditions.

Epidural block effects on the neonate. Analgesia or anesthesia during labor and birth has little or no lasting effect on the physiologic status of the neonate. Currently, no evidence has been found that the administration of analgesia or anesthesia during labor and birth has a significant effect on the child's later mental and neurologic development (AAP & ACOG, 2007).

Nitrous oxide for analgesia

Nitrous oxide mixed with oxygen can be inhaled in a low concentration (50% or less) to reduce but not eliminate pain during the first and second stages of labor. At the lower doses used for analgesia the woman remains awake, and the danger of aspiration is avoided because the laryngeal reflexes are unaffected. Nitrous oxide can be used in combination with other nonpharmacologic and pharmacologic measures for pain relief. Many women report significant analgesia with nitrous oxide use and would choose to use it again for a subsequent labor (Tournaire & Theau-Yonneau, 2007).

A facemask or mouthpiece is used to self-administer the gas. The woman places the mask over her mouth and nose or inserts the mouthpiece 30 seconds before the onset of a contraction (if regular) or as soon as a contraction begins (if irregular). When she inhales, a valve opens, and the gas is released. She should continue to inhale the gas slowly and deeply until the contraction starts to subside. When inhalation stops, the valve closes. Between contractions the woman should remove the device and breathe normally. The nurse should observe the woman for nausea and vomiting, drowsiness, dizziness, hazy memory, and loss of consciousness. Loss of consciousness is more likely to occur if opioids are used with the nitrous oxide (Cunningham et al., 2005).

General anesthesia

General anesthesia is rarely used for uncomplicated vaginal birth and is infrequently used for elective cesarean birth. It may be necessary if a contraindication to a spinal or epidural block exists, if regional anesthesia (e.g., epidural or spinal block) is ineffective, or if indications necessitate rapid birth (vaginal or emergent cesarean) without sufficient time or available personnel to perform a block (Bucklin et al., 2005). In addition, being awake and aware during major surgery may be unacceptable for some

Critical Thinking/Clinical Decision Making

Laboring Without an Epidural

Jamie is a 16-year-old G1 P0 who has been admitted with severe preeclampsia (HELLP syndrome) at 34 weeks of gestation. Jamie's physician plans to induce labor and anticipates a vaginal birth. Jamie has not attended any childbirth preparation classes and has been planning to have an epidural for labor and birth. Unfortunately, because her platelet count is very low (28,000), the anesthesia care provider refuses to place an epidural block. Jamie bursts into tears and says, "I can't make it through labor without an epidural! It's going to hurt too much! Help me!!"

1. Evidence—Is evidence sufficient to support the anesthesia care provider's decision to avoid epidural anesthesia for Jamie?
2. Assumptions—What assumptions can be made about the following methods for relieving pain during labor that would likely be available to Jamie?
   a. Breathing and relaxation techniques
   b. Application of heat and cold
   c. Intradermal water block
   d. Systemic analgesia
3. What implications and priorities for nursing care can be drawn at this time?
4. Does the evidence objectively support your conclusion?
5. Do alternative perspectives to your conclusion exist?

women having a cesarean birth. The major risks associated with general anesthesia are difficulty with or inability to intubate and aspiration of gastric contents (Cunningham et al., 2005; Hawkins et al., 2007).

If general anesthesia is being considered, give the woman nothing by mouth and ensure that an IV infusion is in place. If time allows, premedicate the woman with a nonparticulate (clear) oral antacid (e.g., sodium citrate [Bicitra], Alka-Seltzer) to neutralize the acidic contents of the stomach. Aspiration of highly acidic gastric contents will damage lung tissue. Some anesthesia care providers also order the administration of a histamine (H_2)-receptor blocker such as cimetidine (Tagamet) to decrease the production of gastric acid and metoclopramide (Reglan) to accelerate gastric emptying (Hawkins et al., 2007). Before the anesthesia is given, a wedge should be placed under one of the woman's hips to displace the uterus. Uterine displacement prevents aortocaval compression, which interferes with placental perfusion.

Before the induction of anesthesia the woman will be preoxygentated with 100% oxygen by facemask for 2 to 3 minutes. This step is especially important in pregnant women, who are more likely than other adults to become hypoxemic rapidly if a delay occurs in successful intubation. Thiopental, a short-acting barbiturate, or ketamine is then administered intravenously to render the woman unconscious. Next, succinylcholine, a muscle relaxer, is administered to facilitate passage of an endotracheal tube (Hawkins et al., 2007). The nurse is sometimes asked to assist with applying cricoid pressure before intubation as the woman begins to lose consciousness. This maneuver blocks the esophagus and prevents aspiration should the woman vomit or regurgitate (Fig. 10-13). Pressure is released once the endotracheal tube is securely in place.

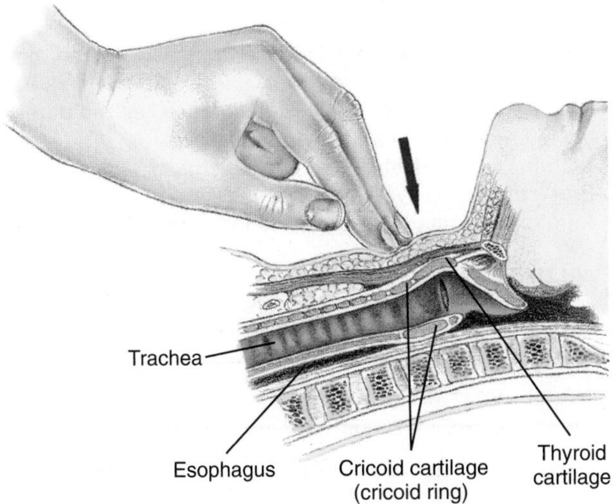

Fig. 10-13 Technique for applying pressure on cricoid cartilage to occlude esophagus to prevent pulmonary aspiration of gastric contents during induction of general anesthesia.

After the woman is intubated, nitrous oxide and oxygen in a 50:50 mixture are administered. A low concentration of a volatile halogenated agent (e.g., isoflurane) also may be administered to increase pain relief and to reduce maternal awareness and recall (Hawkins et al., 2007). In higher concentrations, isoflurane or methoxyflurane relaxes the uterus quickly and facilitates intrauterine manipulation, version, and extraction. However, at higher concentrations, these agents cross the placenta readily and can produce narcosis in the fetus and could reduce uterine tone after birth, increasing the risk for hemorrhage.

Priorities for recovery room care are to maintain an open airway and cardiopulmonary function and to prevent postpartum hemorrhage. Women who had surgery under general anesthesia will require pain medication soon after regaining consciousness. Routine postpartum care is organized to facilitate parent-infant attachment as soon as possible and to answer the mother's questions. When appropriate, the nurse assesses the mother's readiness to see the baby, as well as her response to the anesthesia and to the event that necessitated general anesthesia (e.g., emergency cesarean birth when vaginal birth was anticipated).

CARE MANAGEMENT

The choice of pain relief interventions depends on a combination of factors, including the woman's special needs and wishes, the availability of the desired method or methods, the knowledge and expertise in nonpharmacologic and pharmacologic methods of the health care providers involved in the woman's care, and the phase and stage of labor. The nurse is responsible for assessing maternal and fetal status, establishing mutual goals with the woman (and her family), formulating nursing diagnoses, planning and implementing nursing care, and evaluating the effects of care (see Nursing Process box).

Nonpharmacologic Interventions

The nurse supports and assists the woman as she uses nonpharmacologic interventions for pain relief and relaxation. During labor, ask the woman how she feels so as to evaluate the effectiveness of the specific pain-management techniques used. Appropriate interventions can then be planned or continued for effective care, such as trying other nonpharmacologic methods or combining nonpharmacologic methods with medications (see Nursing Care Plan).

The woman's perception of her behavior during labor is of utmost importance. If she planned a nonmedicated birth but then needs and accepts medication, her self-esteem may falter. Verbal and nonverbal acceptance of her behavior is given as necessary by the nurse and reinforced by discussion and reassurance after birth. Providing explanations about the fetal response to maternal discomfort, the effects of maternal stress and fatigue on the progress of labor, and the medication itself is a supportive measure. The woman may also experience anxiety and stress related

NURSING PROCESS *Management of Discomfort*

ASSESSMENT

History

- Review of prenatal record (parity, estimated date of birth, complications, medications)
- History of smoking; neurologic or spinal disorders

Interview

- Time of woman's last meal: type of food and fluid consumed
- Nature of existing respiratory condition (cold, allergy)
- Allergies to medications, cleansing agents, latex, or tape
- Childbirth preparation, knowledge and preferences for management of discomfort
- Type of analgesia or anesthesia chosen (see Box 10-3)
- If evidence of substance abuse, identify type of drug, last time drug taken, and method of administration. A urine drug screen may be ordered.
- Determine if woman wears contact lenses or dentures.

Physical Examination

- Character and status of labor and fetal response
- Hydration status
- Bladder distention
- Signs of apprehension (fist clenching; restlessness)

Review of results of laboratory tests

- Hemoglobin and hematocrit (anemia)
- Prothrombin time and platelet count (coagulopathy or bleeding disorder)*
- White blood cell count and differential (infection)*

Anesthesia Interview†

- Time of woman's last meal; type of food and fluid consumed
- Nature of existing respiratory conditions (cold, allergy)
- Allergies to medications, cleansing agents, latex, or tape
- Personal or family history of problems with anesthesia (e.g., history of malignant hypertension)
- Past or current neurologic or spinal disorders
- Current medical problems that might affect her choice of anesthesia for labor and birth (e.g., thrombocytopenia, low hematocrit [e.g., <25], vaginal bleeding, rash or infection on lower back, fever of unknown origin)
- Type of analgesia or anesthesia chosen (see Box 10-3)
- Brief physical examination, focusing especially on the woman's airway

NURSING DIAGNOSES

Possible nursing diagnoses include:

- *Acute pain* related to:
  - Processes of labor and birth
- *Risk for ineffective tissue perfusion* related to:
  - Effects of analgesia or anesthesia
  - Maternal position
- *Situational low self-esteem* related to:
  - Negative perception of the woman's (or her family's) behavior
- *Anxiety* or *fear* related to *deficient knowledge of*:
  - Procedure for nerve block analgesia
  - Expected sensations during nerve block analgesia
- *Risk for injury to fetus* related to:
  - Maternal hypotension
  - Maternal position (aortocaval compression)
- *Risk for maternal injury* related to:
  - Effects of analgesia and anesthesia on sensation and motor control

EXPECTED OUTCOMES OF CARE

The woman will do the following:

- Promptly report the characteristics of her pain and discomfort.
- Verbalize understanding of her needs and rights with regard to pain-relief management that uses a variety of nonpharmacologic and pharmacologic methods reflecting her preferences.
- Experience adequate pain relief without adding to maternal risk (e.g., through the use of appropriate nonpharmacologic methods and appropriate medication, including the appropriate dose, timing, and route of administration).
- Give birth to a neonate who adjusts to extrauterine life without problems related to the management of maternal pain.

PLAN OF CARE AND INTERVENTIONS

- Assist woman in use of nonpharmacologic interventions.
- Provide explanations of fetal response to maternal discomfort and effects of maternal stress and fatigue on the progress of labor.
- Ensure informed consent to procedures and anesthesia.
- Administer pharmacologic measures as ordered or desired.
- Prepare woman for procedures, such as epidural catheter insertion, as ordered or desired.
- Monitor for signs of potential problems.
- Protect from injury.
- Monitor and record response to interventions.

EVALUATION

The expected outcomes of care are used to evaluate the care related to management of discomfort.

*Only if ordered.
†The anesthesia interview should be completed by a member of the anesthesia care team as soon as possible after the woman's admission to the labor and birth unit.

NURSING CARE PLAN Nonpharmacologic Management of Discomfort

NURSING DIAGNOSIS Anxiety related to lack of confidence in ability to cope effectively with pain during labor

Expected Outcomes *Woman will express decrease in anxiety and experience satisfaction with her labor and birth performance.*

Nursing Interventions/*Rationales*

- Assess whether the woman and significant other have attended childbirth classes, their knowledge of the labor process, and their current level of anxiety *to plan supportive strategies that address this couple's specific needs.*
- Encourage support person to remain with woman in labor *to provide support and increase probability of response to comfort measures.*
- Teach or review nonpharmacologic techniques available to decrease anxiety and pain during labor (e.g., focusing, relaxation and breathing techniques, effleurage, sacral pressure) *to enhance the chances of success in using the techniques.*
- Explore other techniques that the woman or significant other may have learned in childbirth classes (e.g., hypnosis, water immersion, acupressure, biofeedback, therapeutic touch, aromatherapy, imaging, music) *to provide more options for coping strategies.*
- Explore the use of transcutaneous nerve stimulation if ordered by the primary health care provider *to provide an increased perception of control over pain and an increase in release of endogenous opiates.*
- Assist the woman to change positions and to use pillows *to reduce stiffness, aid circulation, and promote comfort.*
- Assess the bladder for distention and encourage voiding often *to prevent bladder distention and subsequent discomfort.*
- Encourage rest between contractions *to minimize fatigue.*
- Keep woman and significant other informed about progress *to allay anxiety.*
- Guide the couple through the labor stages and phases, helping them use and modify comfort techniques that are appropriate to each phase, *to ensure the greatest effectiveness of the techniques employed.*
- Support the couple if pharmacologic measures are required to increase pain relief, explaining safety and effectiveness, *to reduce anxiety and maintain self-esteem and sense of control over the labor process.*

NURSING DIAGNOSIS Health-seeking behavior (labor) related to desire for a healthy outcome of labor and birth

Expected Outcome *Woman will participate in planning care for labor.*

Nursing Interventions/*Rationales*

- Discuss the woman's birth plan and knowledge about the birth process *to collect data for the nursing care plan.*
- Provide information about the labor process *to correct any misconceptions.*
- Inform the woman about her labor status and the fetus's well-being *to promote comfort and confidence.*
- Discuss rationales for all interventions *to incorporate woman into the plan of care.*
- Incorporate nonpharmacologic interventions into nursing care plan *to increase the woman's sense of control during labor.*
- Provide emotional support and ongoing positive feedback *to enhance positive coping mechanisms.*

to anticipated or actual pain. Stress can cause increased maternal catecholamine production. Increased levels of catecholamines have been linked to dysfunctional labor and fetal and neonatal distress and illness. Nurses must be able to implement strategies aimed at reducing this stress.

Pharmacologic Interventions

Informed consent

Pregnant women have the right to be active participants in determining the best pain care approach to use during labor and birth. The primary health care provider and anesthesia care provider are responsible for fully informing women of the alternative methods of pharmacologic pain relief available in the hospital. A description of the various anesthetic techniques and what they entail is essential to informed consent, even if the woman received information about analgesia and anesthesia earlier in her pregnancy. The initial discussion of pain management options should ideally take place in the third trimester so the woman has time to consider alternatives. Nurses play a part in the informed consent by clarifying and describing procedures or by acting as the woman's advocate and asking the primary health care provider for further explanations. Informed consent consists of three essential components. First, the procedure and its advantages and disadvantages must be thoroughly explained. Second, the woman must agree with the plan of labor pain care as explained to her. Third, her consent must be given freely without coercion or manipulation from her health care provider.

LEGAL TIP Informed Consent for Anesthesia

The woman receives (in an understandable manner) the following:

- Explanation of alternative methods of anesthesia and analgesia available
- Description of the anesthetic, including its effects and the procedure for its administration
- Description of the benefits, discomforts, risks, and consequences for the mother and the fetus
- Explanation of how complications can be treated
- Information that the anesthetic is not always effective
- Indication that the woman may withdraw consent at any time

- Opportunity to have any question answered
- Opportunity to have components of the consent explained in the woman's own words

The consent form will:

- Be written or explained in the woman's primary language
- Have the woman's signature
- Have the date of consent
- Carry the signature of the anesthetic care provider, certifying that the woman has received and appears to understand the explanation

Timing of administration

The nurse is often the person who notifies the primary health care provider that the woman is in need of pharmacologic measures to relieve her discomfort. Orders are often written for the administration of pain medication as needed by the woman and based on the nurse's clinical judgment. In the past, pharmacologic measures for pain relief were usually not implemented until labor had advanced to the active phase of the first stage of labor and the cervix had dilated approximately 4 to 5 cm to prevent suppressing the progress of labor. However, research has shown that epidural anesthesia in early labor does not increase the rate of cesarean birth and may shorten the duration of labor. Consequently, women in labor must no longer reach a certain level of cervical dilation or fetal station before receiving epidural anesthesia (AAP & ACOG, 2007; Cunningham et al., 2005). Nonpharmacologic measures can be used to relieve pain at any time in labor.

Preparation for procedures

The methods of pain relief available to the woman are reviewed, and information is clarified as necessary. The procedure and what will be asked of the woman (e.g., to maintain a flexed position during insertion of the epidural needle) must be explained. The woman also can benefit from knowing the way that the medication is to be given, the interval before the medication takes effect, and the expected pain relief from the medication. Skin-preparation measures are described, and an explanation is given for the need to empty the bladder before the analgesic or anesthetic is administered and the reason for keeping the bladder empty. When an indwelling catheter is to be threaded into the epidural space, the woman should be told that she may have a momentary twinge down her leg, hip, or back, and that this feeling is not a sign of injury (Box 10-5).

Administration of medication

Accurate monitoring of the progress of labor forms the basis for the nurse's judgment that a woman needs pharmacologic control of discomfort. Knowledge of the medications used during childbirth is essential. The most effective route of administration is selected for each woman; then the medication is prepared and administered correctly.

Any medication can cause a minor or severe allergic reaction. As part of the assessment for such allergic reactions the nurse should monitor the woman's vital signs, respiratory status, cardiovascular status, integument, and platelet and white blood cell count. The woman is observed for side effects of drug therapy, especially drowsiness. Minor reactions can consist of a rash, rhinitis, fever, asthma, or pruritus. Management of the less acute allergic response is not an emergency.

Severe allergic reactions (anaphylaxis) may occur suddenly and lead to shock or death. The most dramatic form of anaphylaxis is sudden severe bronchospasm, upper airway obstruction, and hypotension (Brown, Mullins, & Gold, 2006). Signs of anaphylaxis are largely caused by contraction of smooth muscles and may begin with irritability, extreme weakness, nausea, and vomiting. This situation may lead to dyspnea, cyanosis, convulsions, and cardiac arrest. Anaphylaxis must be diagnosed and treated immediately. Initial treatment usually consists of placing the patient in the supine position, injecting epinephrine intramuscularly, administering fluid intravenously, supporting the airway with ventilation if necessary, and giving oxygen. If response to these measures is inadequate, intravenous epinephrine should be given (Brown et al.). Cardiopulmonary resuscitation may be necessary.

Intravenous route. The preferred route of administration of medications such as hydromorphone, butorphanol, fentanyl, or nalbuphine is through IV tubing, administered into the port nearest the woman (proximal port). The medication is given slowly in small doses during a contraction. It may be given over a period of three to five consecutive contractions if needed to complete the dose. It is given during contractions to decrease fetal exposure to the medication because uterine blood vessels are constricted during contractions, and the medication stays within the maternal vascular system for several seconds before the uterine blood vessels reopen. With this method of injection, along with smaller but more frequent dosing, the amount of medication crossing the placenta to the fetus is reduced while the woman's degree of pain relief is maximized. The IV route is associated with the following advantages:

- The onset of pain relief is more predictable.
- Pain relief is obtained with small doses of the drug.
- The duration of effect is more predictable.

Intramuscular route. IM injection of analgesics, although still used, is not the preferred route for administration for women in labor. Disadvantages of the IM route include the following:

- The onset of pain relief is delayed.
- Higher doses of medication are required.
- Medication from muscle tissue is released at an unpredictable rate and is available for transfer across the placenta to the fetus.

BOX 10-5

Nursing Interventions for the Woman Receiving Regional Anesthesia or Analgesia

BEFORE THE BLOCK

- Assist primary health care provider or anesthesia care provider with explaining the procedure and obtaining the woman's informed consent.
- Start an intravenous line and infuse a bolus of fluid if ordered.
- Obtain laboratory results (hematocrit or hemoglobin level, other tests as necessary).
- Assess the woman's level of pain using a pain scale (from 0 [no pain] to 10 [pain as bad as it could possibly be]).
- Encourage the woman to void.

DURING INITIATION OF THE BLOCK

- Assist the woman with assuming and maintaining proper positioning.
- Verbally guide the woman through the procedure, explaining sounds and sensations as she experiences them.
- Assist the anesthesia care provider with documentation of vital signs, time and amount of medications given, etc.
- Monitor maternal vital signs (especially blood pressure) and fetal heart rate as ordered.
- Have oxygen and suction readily available.
- Monitor for signs of local anesthetic toxicity (see Box 10-4) as the test dose of medication is administered.

WHILE THE BLOCK IS IN EFFECT

- Continue to monitor maternal vital signs and fetal heart rate as ordered.
- Continue to assess the woman's level of pain using a pain scale (from 0 [no pain] to 10 [pain as bad as it could possibly be]).
- Monitor for bladder distention.
  - Assist with spontaneous voiding on bedpan or toilet.
  - Place urinary catheter if necessary.
- Encourage or assist the woman to change positions often.
- Promote safety.
  - Keep side rails up on the bed.
  - Place telephone and call light within easy reach.
  - Instruct woman not to get out of bed without help.
  - Make sure no prolonged pressure occurs on anesthetized body parts.
- Keep the catheter insertion site clean and dry.
- Continue to monitor for anesthetic side effects (see Box 10-4).

WHILE THE BLOCK IS WEARING OFF AFTER BIRTH

- Assess regularly for the return of sensory and motor function
- Continue to monitor maternal vital signs as ordered.
- Monitor for bladder distension.
  - Assist with spontaneous voiding on bedpan or toilet.
  - Place urinary catheter if necessary.
- Promote safety.
  - Keep side rails up on the bed.
  - Place telephone and call light within easy reach.
  - Instruct woman not to get out of bed without help.
  - Make sure no prolonged pressure occurs on anesthetized body parts.
- Keep the catheter insertion site clean and dry.
- Continue to monitor for anesthetic side effects (see Box 10-4).

The maternal plasma level of the medication necessary to bring pain relief is usually reached 45 minutes after IM injection, followed by a decline in plasma levels. The maternal medication levels (after IM injections) also are unequal because of uneven distribution (maternal uptake) and metabolism. The advantage of using the IM route is quick administration by the health care provider. IM injections given in the upper arm (deltoid muscle) seem to result in more rapid absorption and higher blood levels of the medication (Bricker & Lavender, 2002). If regional anesthesia is planned later in labor, the autonomic blockade from the regional (e.g., epidural) anesthesia increases blood flow to the gluteal region and accelerates absorption of medication that may be sequestered there.

Regional (epidural or spinal) anesthesia. An IV infusion is established before the induction of regional anesthesia (epidural or spinal). Anesthesia protocols may include the prophylactic administration of IV fluid before epidural and spinal anesthesia for blood volume expansion to prevent maternal hypotension. Hypotension is one of the most common complications of regional anesthesia (see Box 10-4) (AAP & ACOG, 2007; Cunningham et al., 2005).

Lactated Ringer's or normal saline solutions are commonly used infusion solutions. Infusion solutions without dextrose are preferred, especially when the solution must be infused rapidly (e.g., to treat dehydration or to maintain blood pressure) because solutions containing dextrose rapidly increase maternal blood glucose levels. The fetus responds to high blood glucose levels by increasing insulin production; neonatal hypoglycemia may result. In addition, dextrose changes the osmotic pressure so that fluid is excreted from the kidneys more rapidly.

According to professional standards (Association of Women's Health, Obstetric and Neonatal Nurses [AWHONN], 2007) the nonanesthetist registered nurse is permitted to monitor the status of the woman, the fetus, and the progress of labor; replace empty infusion syringes or bags with the same medication and concentration; stop the infusion and initiate emergency measures if the need arises; and remove the catheter if properly educated to do so. Only qualified, licensed anesthesia care providers are permitted to insert a catheter and initiate epidural anesthesia, verify catheter placement, inject the medication through the catheter, and alter the medication or medications, including the type, the amount, and the rate of infusion.

NURSING ALERT Complications may occur with epidural analgesia, including injection-related emergencies and compression problems. These complications can require immediate interventions. Nurses must be prepared to provide safe and effective care during the emergency situation. Clear procedures or protocols should be in place in labor and birth units delineating responsibilities and actions needed (Mahlmeister, 2003).

Because spinal nerve blocks can reduce bladder sensation, resulting in difficulty voiding, the woman should empty her bladder before the induction of the block and should be encouraged to void at least every 2 hours thereafter. The nurse should palpate for bladder distention and measure urinary output to ensure that the bladder is being completely emptied. A distended bladder can inhibit uterine contractions and fetal descent, resulting in a slowing of the progress of labor. For this reason an indwelling urinary catheter is often routinely inserted immediately after epidural or spinal anesthesia is initiated and left in place for the remainder of the first stage of labor.

The status of the maternal-fetal unit and the progress of labor must be established before the block is performed. The nurse must assist the woman to assume and maintain the correct position for induction of epidural and spinal anesthesia (see Fig. 10-11, *A* and *B*) Depending on the level of motor blockade the woman should be assisted to remain as mobile as possible. When in bed, her position should be alternated from side to side every hour to ensure adequate distribution of the anesthetic solution and to maintain circulation to the uterus and placenta. Assisting the woman to assume upright positions such as sitting (e.g., modified throne position in which the woman sits on the bed with the bottom part lowered to place her feet below her body) (Fig. 10-14), tug-of-war position (woman tugs on towel or sheet that is tied to the bar on the bed or held by the nurse), and squatting by using the head of the bed for support will facilitate fetal descent and enhance bearing-down efforts (Gilder, Mayberry, Gennaro, & Clemmons, 2002).

Health care providers should recognize that the second stage of labor may be prolonged in women who use epidural analgesia for pain management. Research evidence indicates that as long as the well-being of the maternal-fetal unit is established, a period of passive descent or "laboring down" can be implemented to allow the fetus to passively descend and rotate with uterine contractions until the woman perceives the urge to bear down (Brancato, Church, & Stone, 2008; Simpson & James, 2005). Fetal well-being along with less maternal fatigue, fever, and perineal trauma and fewer operative vaginal births are beneficial outcomes

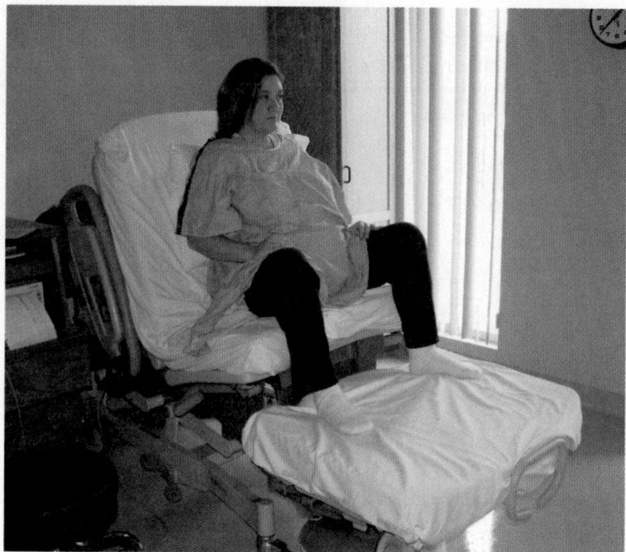

Fig. 10-14 Modified throne position for labor. (Courtesy Julie Perry Nelson, Loveland, CO.)

of this approach for the management of the second stage of labor for women with epidural analgesia. Evidence is insufficient to support the practice of discontinuing epidural analgesia during the second stage to help enhance the effectiveness of bearing-down efforts and decrease the risk for forceps- or vacuum-assisted birth. This practice does result in an increase in the woman's level of pain (Torvaldsen, Roberts, Bell, & Raynes-Greenow, 2004). (See Chapter 12 for a full discussion of second stage labor management.)

Safety and general care

The nurse monitors and records the woman's response to nonpharmacologic pain-relief methods and to the medication or medications. This assessment includes the degree of pain relief, the level of apprehension, the return of sensations and perception of pain, and allergic or adverse reactions (e.g., hypotension, respiratory depression, fever, pruritus, nausea, vomiting). The nurse continues to monitor maternal vital signs and FHR at frequent intervals, the strength and frequency of uterine contractions, changes in the cervix and station of the presenting part, the presence and quality of the bearing-down reflex, bladder filling, and state of hydration. Determining the fetal response after administration of analgesia or anesthesia is vital. The woman is asked if she (or the family) has any questions. The nurse also assesses the woman's and her family's understanding of the need for ensuring her safety (e.g., keeping side rails up, calling for assistance as needed).

After birth the woman who has had spinal, epidural, or general anesthesia is assessed for return of sensory and motor function in addition to the usual postpartum assessments. Both the nurse and the anesthesia provider are responsible for documenting assessments and care in relation to the epidural (Mahlmeister, 2003).

KEY POINTS

- Nonpharmacologic pain and stress-management strategies are valuable for managing labor discomfort alone or in combination with pharmacologic methods.
- The gate-control theory of pain and the stress response are the bases for many of the nonpharmacologic methods of pain relief.
- The type of analgesic or anesthetic to be used is determined in part by the stage of labor and the method of birth.
- Sedatives may be appropriate for women in prolonged early labor when a need exists to decrease anxiety or promote sleep or therapeutic rest.
- Naloxone (Narcan) is an opioid antagonist that can reverse opioid effects, especially respiratory depression.
- Pharmacologic control of discomfort during labor requires collaboration among the health care providers and the laboring woman.
- The nurse must understand medications, their expected effects, their potential adverse reactions, and their methods of administration.
- Maintenance of maternal fluid balance is essential during spinal and epidural nerve blocks.
- Maternal analgesia or anesthesia potentially affects initial neonatal neurobehavioral response.
- The use of opioid agonist-antagonist analgesics in women with preexisting opioid dependence may cause symptoms of abstinence syndrome (opioid withdrawal).
- Epidural anesthesia and analgesia is the most effective pharmacologic pain-relief method for labor that is currently available. As a result, it is the most commonly used method for relieving pain during labor in the United States.
- General anesthesia is rarely used for vaginal birth but may be used for cesarean birth or whenever rapid anesthesia is needed in an emergency.

Audio Chapter Summaries: Access an audio summary of these Key Points on evolve

References

Aghabati, N., Mohammadi, E., & Pour Esmaiel, Z. (2008). The effect of therapeutic touch on pain and fatigue of cancer patients undergoing chemotherapy. *Evidence-based complementary and alternative medicine.* Internet document available at http://ecam.oxfordjournals.org/cgi/content/abstract/nen006 (accessed May 24, 2009).

Albers, L. L. (2007). The evidence for physiologic management of the active phase of the first stage of labor. *Journal of Midwifery & Women's Health, 52*(3), 207-215.

American Academy of Pediatrics (AAP) & American College of Obstetricians and Gynecologists (ACOG). (2007). *Guidelines for perinatal care* (6th ed.). Washington, DC: ACOG.

American Society of Anesthesiologists Task Force on Obstetric Anesthesia. (2007). Practice guidelines for obstetric anesthesia: an updated report. *Anesthesiology, 106*(4), 843-863.

Anim-Somuah M., Smyth R., & Howell, C. Epidural versus non-epidural or no analgesia in labour. In *The Cochrane Database of Systematic Reviews,* 2005, Issue 4, CD 000331.

Association of Women's Health, Obstetric and Neonatal Nurses (AWHONN). (2007). *The role of the registered nurse (RN) in the care of pregnant women receiving analgesia/anesthesia by catheter techniques (epidural, intrathecal, spinal, PCEA catheters).* Clinical Position Statement. Internet document available at www.awhonn.org (accessed July 8, 2009).

Berghella,V., Baxter, J. K., & Chauhan, S. P. (2008). Evidence-based labor and delivery management. *American Journal of Obstetrics & Gynecology, 199*(5), 445-454.

Blackburn, S. T. (2007). *Maternal, fetal, and neonatal physiology: A clinical perspective* (3rd ed.). St. Louis: Saunders.

Bradley, R. (1965). *Husband-coached childbirth.* New York: HarperCollins.

Brancato, R. M., Church, S., & Stone, P. W. (2008). A meta-analysis of passive descent versus immediate pushing in nulliparous women with epidural analgesia in the second stage of labor. *Journal of Obstetric, Gynecologic, and Neonatal Nursing, 37*(1), 4-12.

Bricker, L., & Lavender, T. (2002). Parenteral opioids for labor pain relief: A systematic review. *American Journal of Obstetrics and Gynecology, 186*(5), S94-S109.

Brown, S. G., Mullins, R. J., & Gold, M. S. (2006). Anaphylaxis: Diagnosis and management. *Medical Journal of Australia, 185*(5), 283-289.

Bucklin, B., Hawkins, J., Anderson, J., & Ullrich, F. (2005). Obstetric anesthesia workforce survey. *Anesthesiology, 103*(3), 645-653.

Callister, L., Khalaf, I., Semenic, S., Kartchner, R., & Vehvilainen-Julkunen, K. (2003). The pain of childbirth: Perceptions of culturally diverse women. *Pain Management Nursing, 4*(4), 145-154.

Cunningham, F., Leveno, K., Bloom, S., Hauth, J., Gilstrap, L., & Wenstrom, K. (2005). *Williams obstetrics* (22nd ed.). New York: McGraw-Hill.

Dick-Read, G. (1987). *Childbirth without fear* (5th ed.). New York: Harper & Collins.

Fogarty, V. (2008). Intradermal sterile water injections for the relief of low back pain in labour: A systematic review of the literature. *Women and Birth, 21,* 157-163. Internet document available at www.sciencedirect.com (accessed Sept 25, 2009).

Gilbert, E. S. (2007). *Manual of high risk pregnancy and delivery* (4th ed.). St. Louis: Mosby.

Gilder, K., Mayberry, L., Gennaro, S., & Clemmons, D. (2002). Maternal positions in labor with epidural analgesia: Results from a multi-site survey. *AWHONN Lifelines, 6*(1), 40-45.

Hawkins, J. L., Goetzl, L., & Chestnut, D. H. (2007). Obstetric anesthesia. In S. Gabbe, J. Niebyl, & J. Simpson (Eds.), *Obstetrics: Normal and problem pregnancies* (5th ed.). Philadelphia: Churchill Livingstone.

Hodnett, E. D., Gates, S., Hofmeyr, G. J., & Sakala, C. (2007). Continuous support for women during childbirth. In *The Cochrane Database of Systematic Reviews,* 2007, Issue 3, CD 003766.

Humenick, S., Schrock, P., & Libresco, M. (2000). Relaxation. In F. Nichols & S. Humenick (Eds.), *Childbirth education: Practice, research, and theory* (2nd ed.). Philadelphia: Saunders.

Lothian, J., & Devries, C. (2005). *The official Lamaze guide: Giving birth with confidence.* New York: Meadowbrook Press.

Lowe, N. (2002). The nature of labor pain. *American Journal of Obstetrics and Gynecology, 186*(5), S16-S24.

Mahlmeister, L. (2003). Nursing responsibilities in preventing, preparing for, and managing epidural emergencies. *Journal of Perinatal and Neonatal Nursing, 17*(1), 19-32.

Perinatal Education Associates. (2009). *Breathing.* Internet document available at www.birthsource.com (accessed Sept 25, 2009).

Saito, M., Okutomi, T., Kanai, Y., Mochizuki, J., Tani, A., Amano, K., et al. (2005). Patient-controlled epidural analgesia during labor using ropivacaine and fentanyl provides better maternal satisfaction with less local anesthetic requirement. *Journal of Anesthesia, 19*(3), 208-212.

Simpson, K., & James, D. (2005). Effects of immediate versus delayed pushing during second-stage labor on fetal well-being: A randomized clinical trial. *Nursing Research, 54*(3), 149-157.

Smith, C. A., Collins, C. T., Cyna, A. M., & Crowther, C. A. (2006). Complementary and alternative therapies for pain management in labour. In *The Cochrane Database of Systematic Reviews*, 2006, Issue 4, CD 003521.

Stark, M. A., Rudell, B., & Haus, G. (2008). Observing position and movements in hydrotherapy: A pilot study. *Journal of Obstetric, Gynecologic, and Neonatal Nursing, 37*(1), 116-122.

Torvaldsen, S., Roberts, C., Bell, J., & Raynes-Greenow, C. (2004). Discontinuation of epidural analgesia late in labour for reducing the adverse delivery outcomes associated with epidural analgesia. In *The Cochrane Database of Systematic Reviews*, 2004, Issue 4, CD 004457.

Tournaire, M., & Theau-Yonneau, A. (2007). Complementary and alternative approaches to pain relief during labor. *Evidence-based Complementary and Alternative Medicine, 4*(4), 409-417. Internet document available at http://ecam.oxfordjournals.org/cgi/content/full/nem012v1 (accessed May 25, 2009).

Zwelling, E., Johnson, K., & Allen, J. (2006). How to implement complementary therapies for laboring women. *MCN American Journal of Maternal Child Nursing, 30*(6), 364-372.

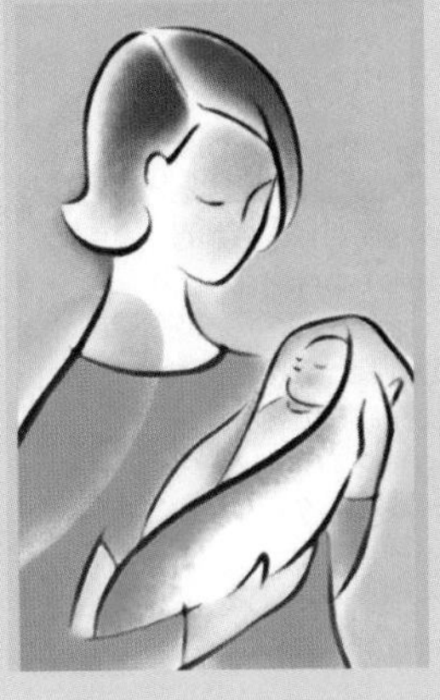

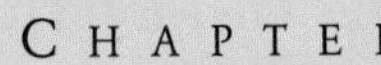

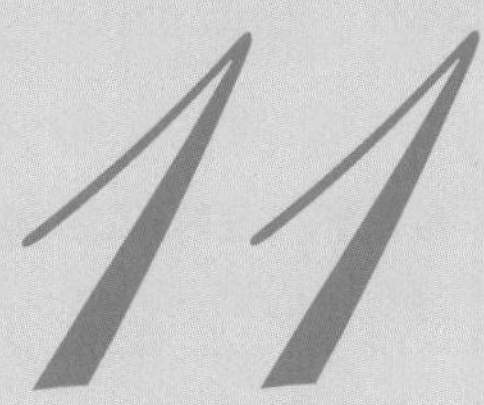

CHAPTER 11

Fetal Assessment during Labor

KITTY CASHION

LEARNING OBJECTIVES

- *Identify typical signs of normal (reassuring) and abnormal (nonreassuring) fetal heart rate (FHR) patterns.*
- *Compare FHR monitoring performed by intermittent auscultation with external and internal electronic methods.*
- *Explain the baseline FHR and evaluate periodic changes.*
- *Describe nursing measures that can be used to maintain FHR patterns within normal limits.*
- *Differentiate among the nursing interventions used for managing specific FHR patterns, including tachycardia and bradycardia, absent or minimal variability, and late and variable decelerations.*
- *Review the documentation of the monitoring process necessary during labor.*

KEY TERMS AND DEFINITIONS

acceleration Increase in fetal heart rate (FHR); usually interpreted as a reassuring sign

amnioinfusion Infusion of normal saline or lactated Ringer's solution through an intrauterine catheter into the uterine cavity in an attempt to increase the fluid around the umbilical cord and prevent compression during uterine contractions

baseline fetal heart rate Average FHR during a 10-minute period that excludes periodic and episodic changes and periods of marked variability; normal FHR baseline is 110-160 beats/min

bradycardia Baseline FHR below 110 beats/min and lasting for 10 minutes or longer

deceleration Slowing of FHR attributed to a parasympathetic response and described in relation to uterine contractions. Types of decelerations include:

- **early deceleration** A visually apparent gradual decrease of FHR before the peak of a contraction and return to baseline as the contraction ends; caused by fetal head compression
- **late deceleration** A visually apparent gradual decrease of FHR, with the lowest point of the deceleration occurring after the peak of the contraction and returning to baseline after the contraction ends; caused by uteroplacental insufficiency
- **prolonged deceleration** A visually apparent decrease (may be either gradual or abrupt) in FHR of at least 15 beats/min below the baseline and lasting more than 2 minutes but less than 10 minutes
- **variable deceleration** A visually apparent abrupt decrease in FHR below the baseline occurring any time during the uterine contracting phase; caused by compression of the umbilical cord

electronic fetal monitoring (EFM) Electronic surveillance of FHR by external and internal methods

episodic changes Changes from baseline patterns in the FHR that are not associated with uterine contractions

hypoxemia Reduction in arterial oxygen pressure resulting in metabolic acidosis by forcing anaerobic glycolysis, pulmonary vasoconstriction, and direct cellular damage

hypoxia Insufficient availability of oxygen to meet the metabolic needs of body tissue

intermittent auscultation Listening to fetal heart sounds at periodic intervals using nonelectronic or ultrasound devices placed on the maternal abdomen

periodic changes Changes from baseline of the FHR that occur with uterine contractions

tachycardia Baseline FHR above 160 beats/min and lasting for 10 minutes or longer

KEY TERMS AND DEFINITIONS—cont'd

tachysystole More than five uterine contractions in 10 minutes, averaged over a 30-minute window

tocolysis Inhibition of uterine contractions through administration of medications; used as an adjunct to other interventions in the management of fetal compromise related to increased uterine activity

uteroplacental insufficiency Decline in placental function (exchange of gases, nutrients, and wastes) leading to fetal hypoxia and acidosis; evidenced by late FHR decelerations in response to uterine contractions

variability Normal irregularity of fetal cardiac rhythm or fluctuations from the baseline FHR of two cycles or more

WEB RESOURCES

Additional related content can be found on the companion website at evolve

http://evolve.elsevier.com/Lowdermilk/Maternity/

- NCLEX Review Questions
- Critical Thinking Exercise: Fetal Monitoring
- Nursing Care Plan: Electronic Fetal Monitoring during Labor
- Spanish Guidelines: Fetal Monitoring

Spanish Guidelines: Fetal Monitoring

The ability to assess the fetus by auscultation of the fetal heart was initially described more than 300 years ago. With the advent of the fetoscope and stethoscope after the turn of the twentieth century the listener could hear clearly enough to count the fetal heart rate (FHR). When electronic FHR monitoring made its debut for clinical use in the early 1970s, the anticipation was that its use would result in fewer cases of cerebral palsy and be more sensitive than stethoscopic auscultation in predicting and preventing fetal compromise (Garite, 2007). Consequently, the use of electronic fetal monitoring rapidly expanded. However, the rate of cerebral palsy has risen slightly since that time and is not likely to improve (Gilbert, 2007). Moreover, in 2006 the cesarean birth rate in the United States reached an all-time high of 31.1% (Collard, Diallo, Habinsky, Hentschell, & Vezeau, 2008/2009).

Still, **electronic fetal monitoring (EFM)** is a useful tool for visualizing FHR patterns on a monitor screen or printed tracing and continues to be the primary mode of intrapartum fetal assessment. Currently in the United States, approximately 85% of women giving birth have continuous EFM during labor, making it the most commonly performed obstetric procedure (American College of Obstetricians and Gynecologists [ACOG], 2009; Tucker, Miller, & Miller, 2009). Pregnant women should be informed about the equipment and procedures used and the risks, benefits, and limitations of intermittent auscultation (IA) and EFM. This chapter discusses the basis for intrapartum fetal monitoring, the types of monitoring, and nursing assessment and management of abnormal fetal status.

BASIS FOR MONITORING

Fetal Response

Because labor is a period of physiologic stress for the fetus, frequent monitoring of fetal status is part of the nursing care during labor. The fetal oxygen supply must be maintained during labor to prevent fetal compromise and to promote newborn health after birth. The fetal oxygen supply can decrease in several ways:

- Reduction of blood flow through the maternal vessels as a result of maternal hypertension (chronic hypertension, preeclampsia, or gestational hypertension), hypotension (caused by supine maternal position, hemorrhage, or epidural analgesia or anesthesia), or hypovolemia (caused by hemorrhage)
- Reduction of the oxygen content in the maternal blood as a result of hemorrhage or severe anemia
- Alterations in fetal circulation, occurring with compression of the umbilical cord (transient, during uterine contractions [UCs], or prolonged, resulting from cord prolapse), placental separation or complete abruption, or head compression (head compression causes increased intracranial pressure and vagal nerve stimulation with an accompanying decrease in the FHR)
- Reduction in blood flow to the intervillous space in the placenta secondary to uterine hypertonus (generally caused by excessive exogenous oxytocin) or secondary to deterioration of the placental vasculature associated with maternal disorders such as hypertension or diabetes mellitus

Fetal well-being during labor can be measured by the response of the FHR to UCs. A group of fetal monitoring

EVIDENCE-BASED PRACTICE

Fetal Monitoring and the Machine that Goes "Beep"

Pat Gingrich

ASK THE QUESTION

What are the optimal methods of assessing fetal well-being during labor?

SEARCH FOR EVIDENCE

Search Strategies: Professional organization guidelines, meta-analyses, systematic reviews, randomized controlled trials, nonrandomized prospective studies, and retrospective studies since 2006.

Databases Searched: CINAHL, Cochrane, Medline, National Guideline Clearinghouse, TRIP Database Plus, and the websites for American College of Obstetricians and Gynecologists; Association of Women's Health, Obstetric, and Neonatal Nurses; and National Institute for Health and Clinical Excellence.

CRITICALLY ANALYZE THE EVIDENCE

Electronic fetal heart monitoring (EFM; also known as cardiotocography [CTG]) has become standard procedure in the labor and birth setting for many decades, especially in the United States. The suggestion has been made that such monitoring is not necessary for the low-risk labor patient and may even present a risk of false abnormal readings that lead to high rates of cesarean births.

A meta-analysis of trials measuring fetal outcomes and use of EFM revealed no significant change in Apgar scores for women who had EFM on admission for labor when compared with women who were not monitored on admission. However, a statistically increased risk was noted for cesarean birth in the monitored women (Gourounti & Sandall, 2007).

The National Institute for Health and Clinical Excellence (NICE) issued professional guidelines for intrapartum care that do not recommend EFM for the low-risk laboring patient (NICE, 2007). Instead, the guidelines recommend intermittent auscultation on admission and during labor, using a stethoscope or Doppler. Use of continuous EFM should begin in the presence of meconium, bleeding, abnormal fetal heart rate (<110 bpm or >160 bpm), oxytocin use, or patient request. Similar clinical practice guidelines from the Society of Obstetricians and Gynaecologists of Canada (2007) also recommend intermittent auscultation in the absence of risk factors. EFM should be used for high-risk women, with fetal scalp blood pH testing if abnormal patterns arise. The guidelines do not recommend the routine use of fetal pulse oximetry.

Some question remains about the use of fetal pulse oximetry as an adjunct assessment that might be more reassuring and thus decrease cesarean rates. A Cochrane systematic analysis examined five trials, involving 7424 women, and showed no difference in cesarean rates between women with EFM alone versus women being monitored with EFM and fetal pulse oximetry together (East, Chan, Colditz, & Begg, 2007). However, the reviewers believed that the use of the fetal pulse oximeters may have provided some reassurance, thus buying some additional time for providers to adequately prepare for cesarean birth.

IMPLICATIONS FOR PRACTICE

EFM is here to stay, but it is only a tool. Women and providers have come to expect the constant feedback, and busy nurses have come to rely on the remote screens as they move from room to room. However, the risks of false alarms, as well as the legal vulnerability of ambiguous patterns, may be contributing to the soaring cesarean rate, which carries its own risks. Continuous monitoring of low risk women restricts patient mobility, which may prolong labor and increase discomfort. In high risk situations, EFM can be valuable for picking up some fetal stress early, but it may also be inaccurate, ambiguous, and cause needless anxiety. Women who expect routine monitoring need explanations about the risks and benefits of continuous monitoring versus intermittent auscultation, and to be given informed choices. The health care team may also need to become more proficient and familiar with auscultation as an assessment tool.

References:

East, C. E., Chan, F. Y., Colditz, P. B., & Begg, L. (2007). Fetal pulse oximetry for fetal assessment in labor. In *The Cochrane Database of Systematic Reviews,* 2007, Issue 2, CD 004075.

Gourounti, K., & Sandall, J. (2007). Admission cardiotocography versus intermittent auscultation of fetal heart rate: Effects on neonatal Apgar score, on the rate of caesarean sections and on the rate of instrumental delivery: A systematic review. *International Journal of Nursing Studies, 44*(6), 1029-1035.

National Institute for Health and Clinical Excellence (NICE). (2007). *Intrapartal care: Care for healthy women and their babies during childbirth. NICE Clinical Guideline No. 55.* London: NICE. Internet document available at www.nice.org.uk/nicemedia/pdf/IPCNICEGuidance.pdf (accessed May 27, 2009).

Society of Obstetricians and Gynaecologists of Canada (SOGC). (2007). *Fetal health surveillance: Antepartum and intrapartum consensus guideline. Clinical Practice Guideline No. 197.* Ottawa, Ontario, Canada: SOGC. Internet document available at www.sogc.org/guidelines/documents/gui197CPG0709.pdf (accessed May 27, 2009).

experts have recently recommended that FHR tracings that demonstrate the following characteristics be described as *normal* (Macones, Hankins, Spong, Hauth, & Moore, 2008):

- A baseline FHR rate of 110 to 160 beats/min
- Moderate baseline FHR variability
- Late or variable decelerations absent
- Early decelerations present or absent
- Accelerations present or absent

Uterine Activity

Table 11-1 describes normal uterine activity (UA) during labor.

Fetal Compromise

The goals of intrapartum FHR monitoring are to identify and differentiate the normal (reassuring) patterns from the abnormal (nonreassuring) patterns, which can be indicative of fetal compromise. Although the 2008 National

TABLE 11-1

Normal Uterine Activity during Labor

CHARACTERISTIC	DESCRIPTION
Frequency	Contraction frequency overall generally ranges from two to five per 10 minutes during labor, with lower frequencies seen in the first stage of labor and higher frequencies (up to five contractions in 10 minutes) seen during the second stage of labor.
Duration	Contraction duration remains fairly stable throughout the first and second stages, ranging from 45-80 seconds, not generally exceeding 90 seconds.
Intensity (peak less resting tone)	Intensity of uterine contractions generally range from 25-50 mm Hg in the first stage of labor and may rise to over 80 mm Hg in second stage. Contractions palpated as "mild" would likely peak at less than 50 mm Hg if measured internally, whereas contractions palpated as "moderate" or greater would likely peak at 50 mm Hg or greater if measured internally.
Resting tone	Average resting tone during labor is 10 mm Hg; if using palpation, should palpate as "soft" (i.e., easily indented, no palpable resistance).
Montevideo units (MVUs)	Ranges from 100-250 MVUs in the first stage, may rise to 300-400 in the second stage. Contraction intensities of 40 mm Hg or more and MVUs of 80-120 are generally sufficient to initiate spontaneous labor.

Source: Tucker, S. M., Miller, L. A, & Miller, D. A. (2009). *Mosby's pocket guide to fetal monitoring: A multidisciplinary approach* (6th ed.). St. Louis: Mosby.

Institute of Child Health and Human Development workshop (Macones et al., 2008) and a recent ACOG Practice Bulletin (2009) both recommend use of the terms *normal* and *abnormal* to describe FHR tracings, the terms *reassuring* and *nonreassuring* are still frequently used clinically.

Abnormal FHR patterns are those associated with fetal **hypoxemia,** which is a deficiency of oxygen in the arterial blood. If uncorrected, hypoxemia can deteriorate to severe fetal **hypoxia,** which is an inadequate supply of oxygen at the cellular level. Examples of abnormal FHR patterns include the following (Macones et al., 2008).

Absent baseline FHR variability and any of the following:

- Recurrent late decelerations
- Recurrent variable decelerations
- Bradycardia
- Sinusoidal FHR pattern

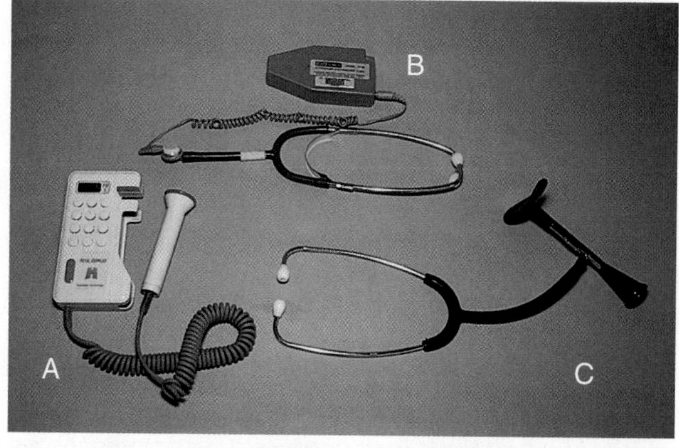

Fig. 11-1 **A,** Ultrasound fetoscope; **B,** Ultrasound stethoscope; **C,** DeLee-Hillis fetoscope. (Courtesy Michael S. Clement, MD, Mesa, AZ.)

MONITORING TECHNIQUES

The ideal method of fetal assessment during labor continues to be debated. When performed at prescribed intervals, especially during and immediately after contractions, IA has been shown to be as valuable as EFM at predicting fetal outcomes (Gilbert, 2007).

Intermittent Auscultation

Intermittent auscultation (IA) involves listening to fetal heart sounds at periodic intervals to assess the FHR. IA of the fetal heart can be performed with a Pinard stethoscope, a Doppler ultrasound device (Fig.11-1, *A*) an ultrasound stethoscope (Fig. 11-1, *B*) or a DeLee-Hillis fetoscope (Fig. 11-1, *C*). The fetoscope is applied to the listener's forehead because bone conduction amplifies the fetal heart sounds for counting. The Doppler ultrasound device and ultrasound stethoscope transmit ultrahigh-frequency sound waves reflecting movement of the fetal heart and convert these sounds into an electronic signal that can be counted. Box 11-1 describes how to perform IA.

IA is easy to use, inexpensive, and less invasive than EFM. It is often more comfortable for the woman and gives her more freedom of movement. Other care measures, such as ambulation and the use of baths or showers, are easier to carry out when IA is used. On the other hand, IA may be difficult to perform in women who are obese. Because IA is intermittent, significant events may occur during a time when the FHR is not auscultated. Also, IA

BOX 11-1

Procedure for Intermittent Auscultation of the Fetal Heart Rate

1. Palpate the maternal abdomen to identify fetal presentation and position.
2. Apply ultrasonic gel to the device if using a Doppler ultrasound. Place the listening device over the area of maximal intensity (see Fig. 11-1) and clarity of the fetal heart sounds to obtain the clearest and loudest sound, which is easiest to count. This location will usually be over the fetal back. If using the fetoscope, firm pressure may be needed.
3. Count the maternal radial pulse while listening to the FHR to differentiate it from the fetal rate.
4. Palpate the abdomen for the presence or absence of UA so as to count the FHR between contractions.
5. Count the FHR for 30 to 60 seconds between contractions to identify the auscultated rate, best assessed in the absence of UA.
6. Auscultate the FHR before, during, and after a contraction to identify the FHR during the contraction, as a response to the contraction, and to assess for the absence or presence of increases or decreases in FHR.
7. When distinct discrepancies in the FHR are noted during listening periods, auscultate for a longer period during, after, and between contractions to identify significant changes that may indicate the need for another mode of FHR monitoring

Source: Tucker, S. M., Miller, L. A, & Miller, D. A. (2009). *Mosby's pocket guide to fetal monitoring: A multidisciplinary approach* (6th ed.). St. Louis: Mosby.
FHR, Fetal heart rate; *UA*, uterine activity.

does not provide a permanent documented visual record of the FHR and cannot be used to assess visual patterns of the FHR variability or periodic changes (Albers, 2007; Tucker et al., 2009). By using IA the nurse can assess the baseline FHR, rhythm, and increases and decreases from baseline. The recommended optimal frequency for IA in low risk women during labor has not been determined (Nageotte & Gilstrap, 2009).

NURSING ALERT When the FHR is auscultated and documented, using the descriptive terms associated with EFM (e.g., moderate variability, variable deceleration) is inappropriate because most of the terms are visual descriptions of the patterns produced on the monitor tracing. Terms that are numerically defined, however, such as bradycardia and tachycardia, can be used.

Every effort should be made to use the method of fetal assessment the woman desires, if possible. However, adherence to the frequency guides can make using IA difficult in today's busy labor and birth units because when used as the primary method of fetal assessment, auscultation requires a 1:1 nurse-to-patient staffing ratio. If acuity and census change such that auscultation standards are no longer met, then the nurse must inform the physician or nurse-midwife that continuous EFM will be used until staffing can be arranged to meet the standards.

The woman can become anxious if the examiner cannot readily count the fetal heartbeats. The inexperienced listener often needs time to locate the heartbeat and find the area of maximal intensity. To allay the mother's concerns, she can be told that the nurse is "finding the spot where the sounds are loudest." If the examiner cannot locate the fetal heartbeat, assistance should be requested. In some cases, ultrasound can be used to help locate the fetal heartbeat. Seeing the FHR on the ultrasound screen will be reassuring to the mother if locating the best area for auscultation was initially difficult.

When using IA, UA is assessed by palpation. The examiner should keep his or her hand placed over the fundus before, during, and after contractions. The contraction intensity is usually described as mild, moderate, or strong. The contraction duration is measured in seconds, from the beginning to the end of the contraction. The frequency of contractions is measured in minutes, from the beginning of one contraction to the beginning of the next. The examiner should keep his or her hand on the fundus after the contraction is over to evaluate uterine resting tone or relaxation between contractions. Resting tone between contractions is usually described as soft or relaxed.

Accurate and complete documentation of fetal status and UA is especially important when IA and palpation are being used because no paper tracing record or computer storage of these assessments is provided, as is the case with continuous EFM. Labor flow records or computer charting systems that prompt notations of all assessments are useful for ensuring such comprehensive documentation.

Electronic Fetal Monitoring

Critical Thinking Exercise: Fetal Monitoring

The purpose of electronic FHR monitoring is the ongoing assessment of fetal oxygenation. The goal is to detect fetal hypoxia and metabolic acidosis during labor so that interventions to resolve the problem can be implemented in a timely manner before permanent damage or death occur (Garite, 2007).

The two modes of EFM include the external mode, which uses external transducers placed on the maternal abdomen to assess FHR and UA, and the internal mode, which uses a spiral electrode applied to the fetal presenting part to assess the FHR and an intrauterine pressure catheter (IUPC) to assess UA and pressure. The differences between the external and internal modes of EFM are summarized in Table 11-2.

External monitoring

Separate transducers are used to monitor the FHR and UCs (Fig. 11-2). The ultrasound transducer works by reflecting high-frequency sound waves off a moving interface: in this case the fetal heart and valves. Reproducing a

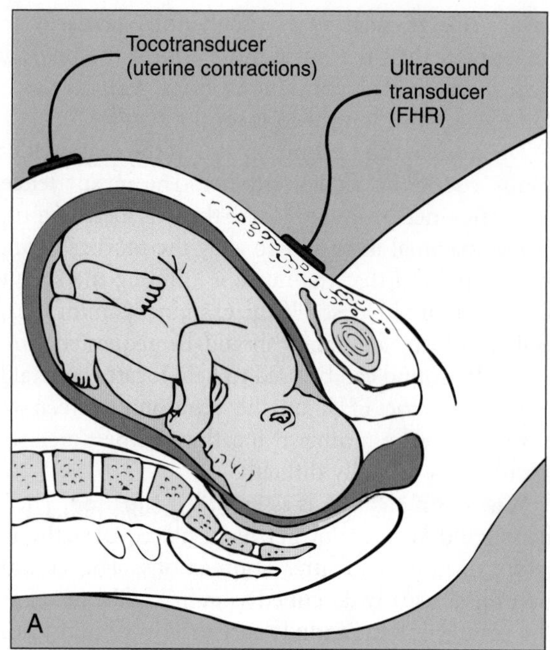

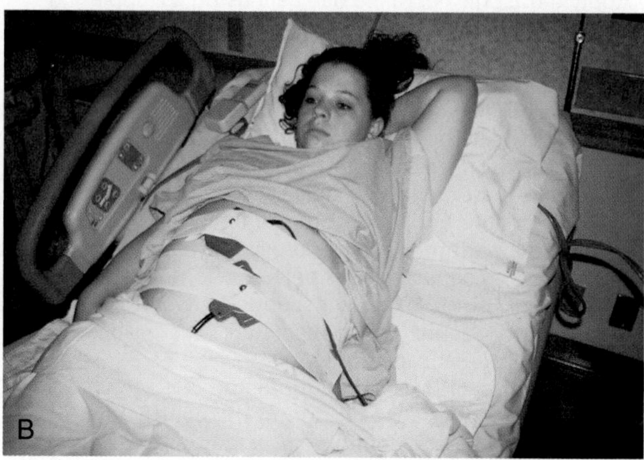

Fig. 11-2 **A,** External noninvasive fetal monitoring with tocotransducer and ultrasound transducer. **B,** Ultrasound transducer is placed below umbilicus, over the area where fetal heart rate is best heard, and tocotransducer is placed on uterine fundus. (**B,** Courtesy Marjorie Pyle, RNC, Lifecircle, Costa Mesa, CA.)

TABLE 11-2

External and Internal Modes of Monitoring

EXTERNAL MODE	INTERNAL MODE
FETAL HEART RATE	
Ultrasound transducer: High-frequency sound waves reflect mechanical action of the fetal heart. Noninvasive. Does not require rupture of membranes or cervical dilation. Used during both the antepartum and intrapartum periods.	*Spiral electrode:* Converts the fetal ECG as obtained from the presenting part to the FHR via a cardiotachometer. Can be used only when membranes are ruptured and the cervix is sufficiently dilated during the intrapartum period. Electrode penetrates into fetal presenting part by 1.5 mm and must be attached securely to ensure a good signal.
UTERINE ACTIVITY	
Tocotransducer: Monitors frequency and duration of contractions by means of pressure-sensing device applied to the maternal abdomen. Used during both the antepartum and intrapartum periods.	*Intrauterine pressure catheter* (IUPC): Monitors the frequency, duration, and intensity of contractions. The two types of IUPCs are a fluid-filled system and a solid catheter. Both measure intrauterine pressure at the catheter tip and convert the pressure into millimeters of mercury on the uterine activity panel of the strip chart. Both can be used only when membranes are ruptured and the cervix is sufficiently dilated during the intrapartum period.

ECG, Electrocardiogram; *FHR,* fetal heart rate.

continuous and precise record of the FHR is sometimes difficult because of artifacts introduced by fetal and maternal movement. The FHR is printed on specially formatted monitor paper. The standard paper speed used in the United States is 3 cm/min. Once the area of maximal intensity of the FHR has been located, conductive gel is applied to the surface of the ultrasound transducer, and the transducer is then positioned over this area and held securely in place using an elastic belt.

The tocotransducer (tocodynamometer) measures UA transabdominally. The device is placed over the uterine fundus and held securely in place using an elastic belt (see Fig. 11-2). UCs or fetal movements depress a pressure-sensitive surface on the side next to the abdomen. The tocotransducer can measure and record the frequency and approximate duration of UCs but not their intensity. This method is especially valuable for measuring UA during the first stage of labor in women with intact membranes or for

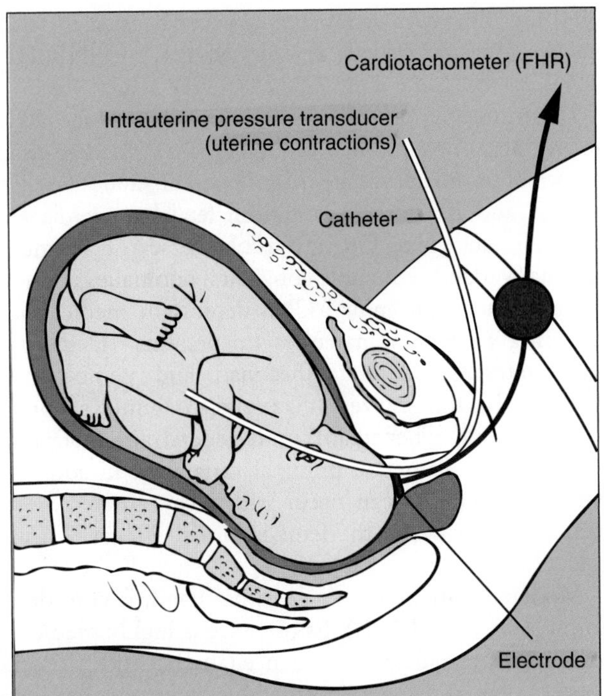

Fig. 11-3 Diagrammatic representation of internal invasive fetal monitoring with intrauterine pressure catheter and spiral electrode in place (membranes ruptured and cervix dilated).

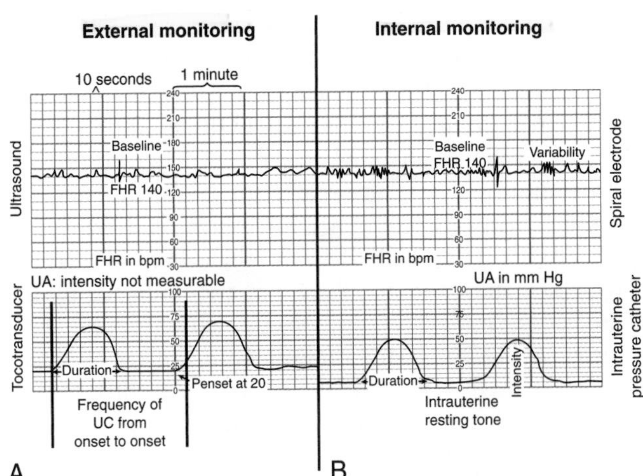

Fig. 11-4 Display of fetal heart rate and uterine activity on monitor paper. **A,** External mode with ultrasound and tocotransducer as signal source. **B,** Internal mode with spiral electrode and intrauterine catheter as signal source. Frequency of contractions is measured from the beginning of one contraction to the beginning of the next. (From Tucker, S. M., Miller, L. A., & Miller, D. A. [2009]. *Mosby's pocket guide to fetal monitoring: A multidisciplinary approach* [6th ed.]. St. Louis: Mosby.

antepartum testing. Because the tocotransducer of most electronic fetal monitors is designed for assessing UA in the term pregnancy, it may not be sensitive enough to detect preterm UA. When monitoring the woman in preterm labor, remember that the fundus may be located below the level of the umbilicus. The nurse may need to rely on the woman to indicate when UA is occurring and to use palpation as an additional way of assessing contraction frequency and validating the monitor tracing.

The external transducer is easily applied by the nurse, but it must be repositioned as the woman or fetus changes position (see Fig. 11-2, *B*). The woman is asked to assume a semi-sitting or a lateral position. Use of an external transducer confines the woman to bed. Portable telemetry monitors allow observation of the FHR and UC patterns by means of centrally located electronic display stations. These portable units permit the woman to walk around during electronic monitoring.

Internal monitoring

The technique of continuous internal FHR or UA monitoring allows a more accurate appraisal of fetal well-being during labor than external monitoring because it is not interrupted by fetal or maternal movement or affected by maternal size (Fig. 11-3). For this type of monitoring the membranes must be ruptured and the cervix sufficiently dilated (at least 2-3 cm) to allow placement of the spiral electrode or IUPC or both. Internal and external modes of monitoring may be combined (i.e., internal FHR with external UA or external FHR with internal UA) without difficulty.

Internal monitoring of the FHR is accomplished by attaching a small spiral electrode to the presenting part. For UA to be monitored internally, a solid IUPC is introduced into the uterine cavity. The catheter has a pressure-sensitive tip that measures changes in intrauterine pressure. As the catheter is compressed during a contraction, pressure is placed on the pressure transducer. This pressure is then converted into a pressure reading in millimeters of mercury. The average pressure during a contraction ranges from 50 to 85 mm Hg. The IUPC can measure the frequency, duration, and intensity of UC, as well as uterine resting tone.

The FHR and UA are displayed on the monitor paper, with the FHR in the upper section and UA in the lower section. Fig. 11-4 contrasts the internal and external modes of electronic monitoring. Note that each small square on the monitor paper or screen represents 10 seconds; each larger box of six squares equals 1 minute (when paper is moving through the monitor at the rate of 3 cm/min).

FETAL HEART RATE PATTERNS

Characteristic FHR patterns are associated with fetal and maternal physiologic processes and have been identified for many years. Because EFM was introduced into clinical practice before consensus was reached in regard to standardized terminology, however, variations in the description and interpretation of common fetal heart rate patterns were often great. In 1997 the National Institute of Child Health and Human Development (NICHD) published a proposed nomenclature system for EFM interpretation with standardized definitions for FHR monitoring. The NICHD recommendations were not widely incorporated into clinical practice, however, until they were endorsed by the American College of Obstetricians and Gynecologists (ACOG) in 2005. Shortly thereafter, use of the NICHD standard terminology was also endorsed by the Association of Women's Health, Obstetric, and Neonatal Nurses (AWHONN), and the American College of Nurse-Midwives (ACNM) (Tucker et al., 2009). All three organizations cited concerns regarding patient safety and the need for improved communication among caregivers as reasons for using standard EFM definitions in clinical practice.

In April 2008 the NICHD, ACOG, and the Society for Maternal-Fetal Medicine partnered to sponsor another workshop to revisit the FHR definitions recommended by the NICHD in 1997. The 1997 FHR definitions were reaffirmed at this workshop. In addition, new definitions related to UA were recommended, as well as a three-tier system of FHR pattern interpretation and categorization (Macones et al., 2008). ACOG (2009) has recently published a practice bulletin which supports use of the 2008 NICHD workshop recommendations.

Baseline Fetal Heart Rate

The intrinsic rhythmicity of the fetal heart, the central nervous system (CNS), and the fetal autonomic nervous system control the FHR. An increase in sympathetic response results in acceleration of the FHR, whereas an increase in parasympathetic response produces a slowing of the FHR. A balanced increase of sympathetic and parasympathetic response usually occurs during contractions, with no observable change in the baseline FHR.

The **baseline fetal heart rate** is the average rate during a 10-minute segment that excludes periodic or episodic changes, periods of marked variability, and segments of the baseline that differ by more than 25 beats/min (Macones et al., 2008). The normal range at term is 110 to 160 beats/min. The baseline rate is documented as a single number, rather than a range (Tucker et al., 2009).

Variability

Variability of the FHR can be described as irregular waves or fluctuations in the baseline FHR of two cycles per minute or greater (Macones, et al., 2008). It is a characteristic of the baseline FHR and does not include accelerations or decelerations of the FHR. Variability is quantified in beats per minute and is measured from the peak to the trough of a single cycle. Four possible categories of variability have been identified: absent, minimal, moderate, and marked (Fig. 11-5). In the past, variability was described as either long term or short term (beat to beat). The NICHD definitions do not distinguish between long- and short-term variability, however, because in actual practice, they are visually determined as a unit (NICHD, 1997).

Depending upon other characteristics of the FHR tracing, absent or minimal variability is classified as either abnormal or indeterminate (Macones et al., 2008) (see Fig. 11-5, *A* and *B*). It can result from fetal hypoxemia and metabolic acidemia. Other possible causes of absent or minimal variability include congenital anomalies and preexisting neurologic injury. CNS depressant medications, including analgesics, narcotics (meperidine [Demerol]), barbiturates (secobarbital [Seconal] and pentobarbital [Nembutal]), tranquilizers (diazepam [Valium]), ataractics (promethazine [Phenergan]), and general anesthetics are other possible causes of minimal variability. In addition, minimal variability can occur with tachycardia, extreme prematurity, or when the fetus is in a sleep state (Tucker et al., 2009).

Moderate variability, on the other hand, is considered normal (see Fig. 11-5, *C*). Its presence is highly predictive of a normal fetal acid-base balance (absence of fetal metabolic acidemia). Moderate variability indicates that FHR regulation is not significantly affected by fetal sleep cycles, tachycardia, prematurity, congenital anomalies, preexisting neurologic injury, or CNS depressant medications (Macones et al., 2008; Tucker et al., 2009).

The significance of marked variability (see Fig. 11-5, *D*) is unclear (Macones et al., 2008).

A sinusoidal pattern–a regular smooth, undulating wavelike pattern–is not included in the definition of FHR variability. This uncommon pattern classically occurs with severe fetal anemia (Fig. 11-6) (Tucker et al., 2009).

Tachycardia

Tachycardia is a baseline FHR greater than 160 beats/min for a duration of 10 minutes or longer (Fig. 11-7). It can be considered an early sign of fetal hypoxemia, especially when associated with late decelerations and minimal or absent variability. Fetal tachycardia can result from maternal or fetal infection (e.g., prolonged rupture of membranes with amnionitis), from maternal hyperthyroidism or fetal anemia, or in response to medications such as atropine, hydroxyzine (Vistaril), terbutaline (Brethine), or illicit drugs such as cocaine or methamphetamines. Table 11-3 lists causes, clinical significance, and nursing interventions for tachycardia.

Bradycardia

Bradycardia is a baseline FHR less than 110 beats/min for a duration of 10 minutes or longer (Fig. 11-8). True bradycardia occurs rarely and is not specifically related to fetal oxygenation. True bradycardia must be distinguished from a prolonged deceleration because the causes and management of these two conditions are very different. Bradycardia is often caused by some type of fetal cardiac problem such as structural defects involving the pacemak-

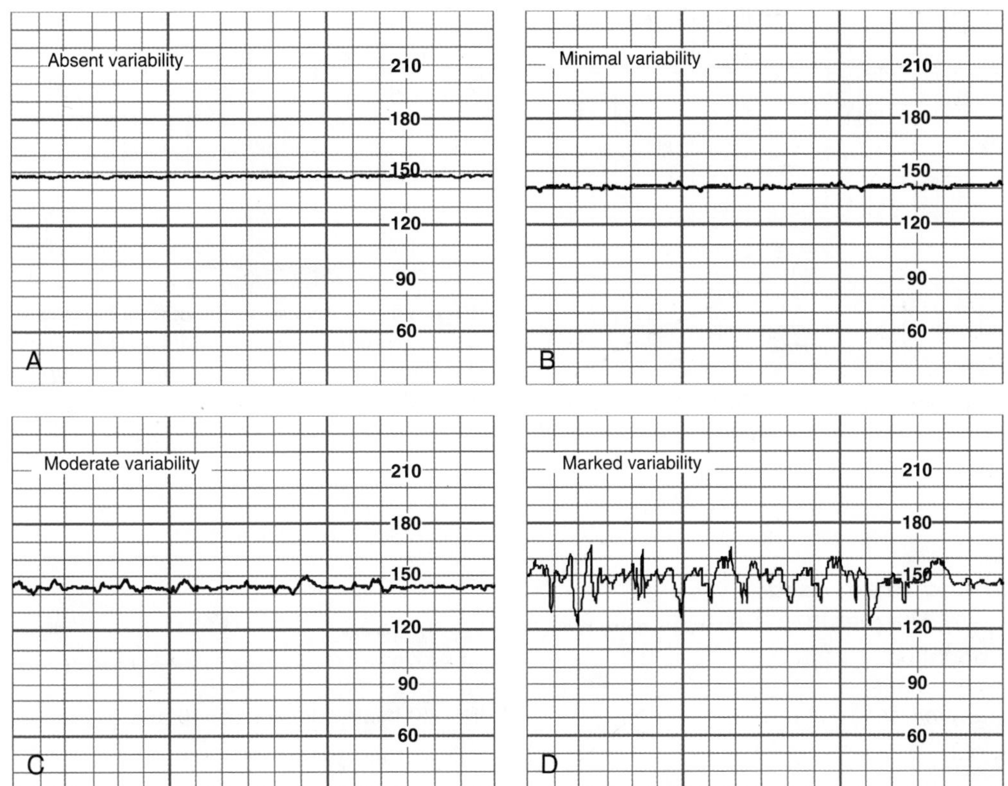

Fig. 11-5 Fetal heart rate variability. **A,** Absent variability; amplitude range undetectable. **B,** Minimal variability; amplitude range detectable up to and including 5 beats/min. **C,** Moderate variability; amplitude range 6-25 beats/min. **D,** Marked variability; amplitude range >25 beats/min. (From Tucker, S. M., Miller, L. A., & Miller, D. A. [2009]. *Mosby's pocket guide to fetal monitoring: A multidisciplinary approach* [6th ed.]. St. Louis: Mosby.

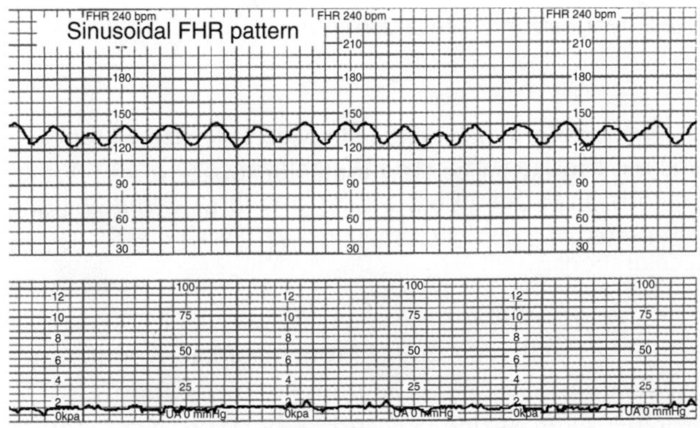

Fig. 11-6 Sinusoidal pattern. (From Tucker, S. M., Miller, L. A., & Miller, D. A. [2009]. *Mosby's pocket guide to fetal monitoring: A multidisciplinary approach* [6th ed.]. St. Louis: Mosby.

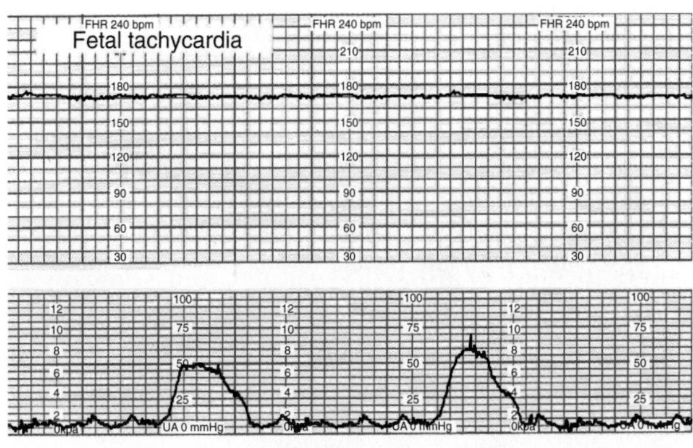

Fig. 11-7 Fetal tachycardia. (From Tucker, S. M., Miller, L. A., & Miller, D. A. [2009]. *Mosby's pocket guide to fetal monitoring: A multidisciplinary approach* [6th ed.]. St. Louis: Mosby.

ers or conduction system or fetal heart failure. Other causes of bradycardia include viral infections (e.g., cytomegalovirus), maternal hypoglycemia, and maternal hypothermia. The clinical significance of the bradycardia depends on the underlying cause and accompanying FHR patterns, including variability and the presence of accelerations or decelerations (Tucker et al., 2009). (See Table 11-3 for a list of causes, clinical significance, and nursing interventions for bradycardia.)

Periodic and Episodic Changes in Fetal Heart Rate

Changes in FHR from the baseline are categorized as periodic or episodic. **Periodic changes** are those that occur

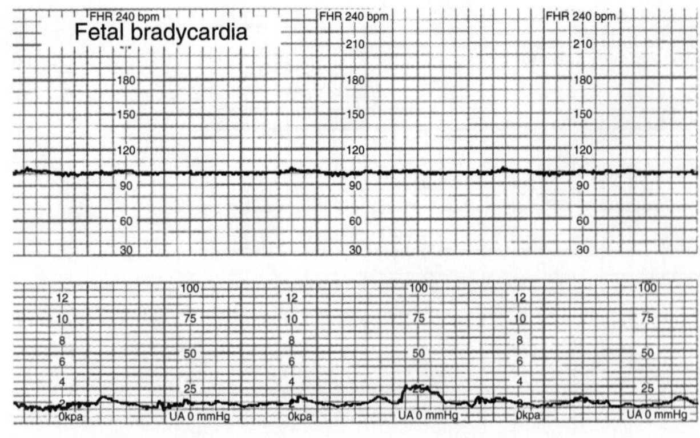

Fig. 11-8 Fetal bradycardia. (From Tucker, S. M., Miller, L. A., & Miller, D. A. [2009]. *Mosby's pocket guide to fetal monitoring: A multidisciplinary approach* [6th ed.]. St. Louis: Mosby.)

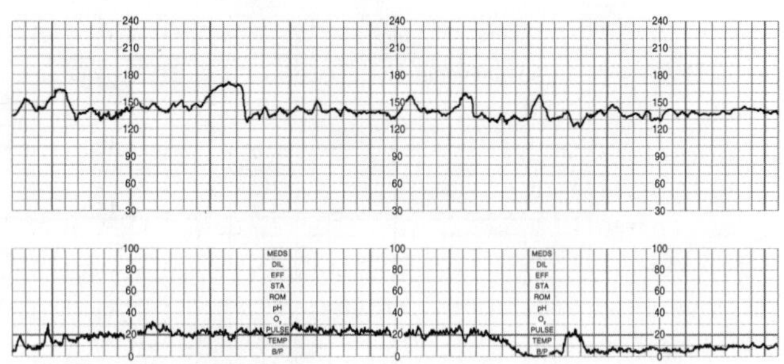

Fig. 11-9 Accelerations of fetal heart rate in a term pregnancy. (From Miller, L.A., Miller, D.A., Tucker, S.M. [2013]. *Mosby's pocket guide to fetal monitoring: A multidisciplinary approach* [7th ed.]. Mosby.)

TABLE 11-3

Tachycardia and Bradycardia

TACHYCARDIA	BRADYCARDIA
DEFINITION	
FHR >160 beats/min lasting >10 min	FHR <110 beats/min lasting >10 min
POSSIBLE CAUSES	
Early fetal hypoxemia	Atrioventricular dissociation (heart block)
Fetal cardiac arrhythmias	Structural defects
Maternal fever	Viral infections (e.g., cytomegalovirus)
Infection (including chorioamnionitis)	Medications
Parasympatholytic drugs (atropine, hydroxyzine)	Fetal heart failure
β-Sympathomimetic drugs (terbutaline)	Maternal hypoglycemia
Maternal hyperthyroidism	Maternal hypothermia
Fetal anemia	
Drugs (caffeine, cocaine, methamphetamines)	
CLINICAL SIGNIFICANCE	
Persistent tachycardia in absence of periodic changes does not appear serious in terms of neonatal outcome (especially true if tachycardia is associated with maternal fever); tachycardia is abnormal when associated with late decelerations, severe variable decelerations, or absent variability.	Baseline bradycardia alone is not specifically related to fetal oxygenation. The clinical significance of bradycardia depends on the underlying cause and the accompanying FHR patterns, including variability, accelerations, or decelerations.
NURSING INTERVENTIONS	
Dependent on cause; reduce maternal fever with antipyretics as ordered and cooling measures; oxygen at 10 L/min by rebreather facemask may be of some value; carry out health care provider's orders based on alleviating cause.	Dependent on cause

ECG; Electrocardiogram; *FHR,* fetal heart rate.

with UCs. **Episodic changes** are those that are not associated with UCs. These patterns include both accelerations and decelerations (NICHD, 1997).

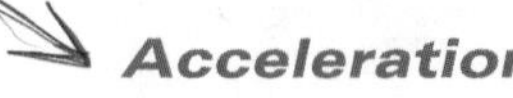

Accelerations

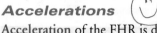

Acceleration of the FHR is defined as a visually apparent abrupt (onset to peak <30 seconds) increase in FHR above the baseline rate (Fig. 11-9). The peak is at least 15 beats/min above the baseline, and the acceleration lasts 15 seconds or more, with the return to baseline less than 2 minutes from the beginning of the acceleration. Before 32 weeks gestation the definition of an acceleration is a peak of 10 beats/min or more above the baseline and a duration of at least 10 seconds. Acceleration of the FHR for more than 10 minutes is considered a change in baseline rate (Tucker et al., 2009).

Accelerations can be periodic or episodic. They may occur in association with fetal movement or spontaneously. If accelerations do not occur spontaneously, they can be elicited by fetal scalp stimulation or vibroacoustic stimulation. Similar to moderate variability, accelerations are considered an indication of fetal well-being. Their presence is highly predictive of a normal fetal acid-base balance (absence of fetal metabolic acidemia) (Tucker et al., 2009). Box 11-2 lists causes, clinical significance, and nursing interventions for accelerations.

Decelerations

FHR **decelerations** are categorized as early, late, variable, or prolonged. FHR decelerations are defined according to their visual relationship to the onset and end of a contraction and by their shape.

BOX 11-2

Accelerations

CAUSES

- Spontaneous fetal movement
- Vaginal examination
- Electrode application
- Scalp stimulation
- Reaction to external sounds
- Breech presentation
- Occiput posterior position
- Uterine contractions
- Fundal pressure
- Abdominal palpation

CLINICAL SIGNIFICANCE

Normal pattern. Acceleration with fetal movement signifies fetal well-being representing fetal alertness or arousal states

NURSING INTERVENTIONS

None required

Early decelerations. Early deceleration of the FHR is a visually apparent gradual (onset to lowest point 30 seconds or more) decrease in and return to the baseline FHR associated with UCs (Macones et al., 2008). Generally the onset, nadir, and recovery of the deceleration correspond to the beginning, peak, and end of the contraction (Fig. 11-10). For this reason, early decelerations are sometimes called the "mirror image" of a contraction.

Early decelerations are thought to be caused by transient fetal head compression and are considered a benign finding (Tucker et al., 2009). Early decelerations may also occur during vaginal examinations, as a result of fundal pressure, and during placement of the internal mode of fetal monitoring. When present, they usually occur during the first stage of labor when the cervix is dilated 4 to 7 cm but can also be seen during the second stage when the woman is pushing.

Because early decelerations are considered to be benign, interventions are not necessary. Early decelerations should be identified, however, so that they can be distinguished from late or variable decelerations, for which interventions are appropriate. Box 11-3 lists cause, clinical significance, and nursing interventions for early decelerations.

Late decelerations. Late deceleration of the FHR is a visually apparent gradual (onset to lowest point 30 seconds or more) decrease in and return to baseline FHR associated with UCs (Macones et al., 2008). The deceleration begins after the contraction has started, and the lowest point of the deceleration occurs after the peak of the contraction. The deceleration usually does not return to baseline until after the contraction is over (Fig. 11-11).

Uteroplacental insufficiency causes late decelerations. Persistent and repetitive late decelerations indicate the presence of fetal hypoxemia stemming from insufficient placental perfusion during UCs. If recurrent or sustained, late decelerations can lead to metabolic acidemia (Tucker

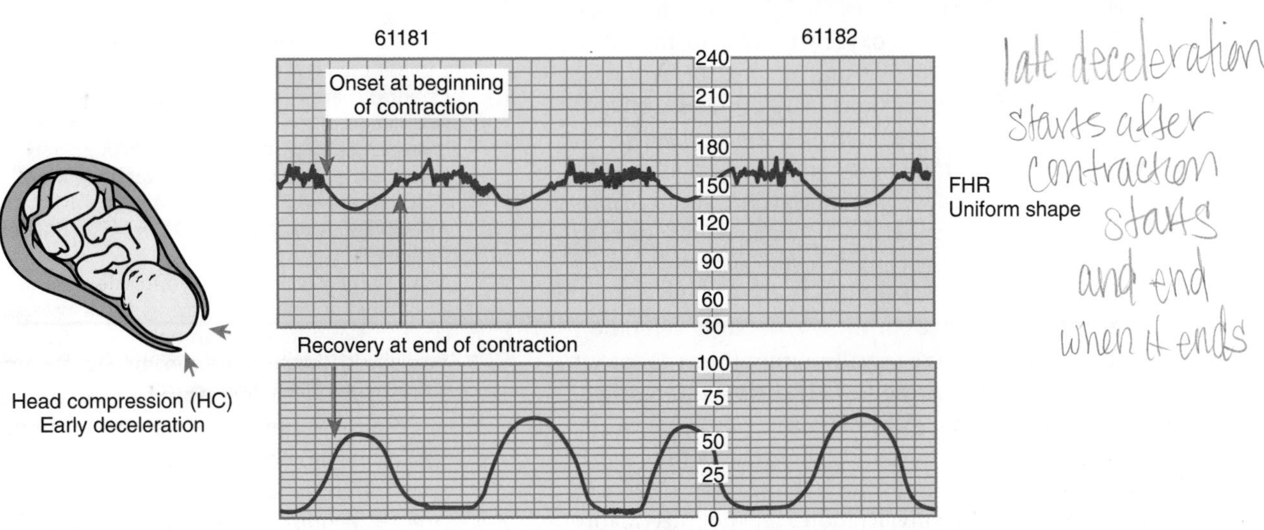

Fig. 11-10 Early decelerations. (From Tucker, S. [2004]. *Pocket guide to fetal monitoring and assessment* [5th ed.]. St. Louis: Mosby.)

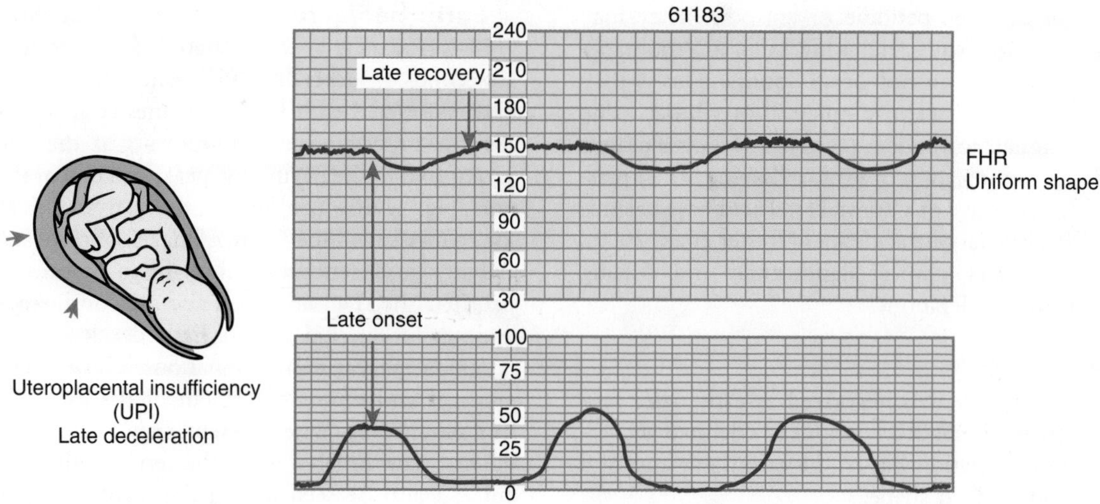

Fig. 11-11 Late decelerations. (From Tucker, S. [2004]. *Pocket guide to fetal monitoring and assessment* [5th ed.]. St. Louis: Mosby.)

BOX 11-3

Early Decelerations

CAUSE

Head compression resulting from the following:

- Uterine contractions
- Vaginal examination
- Fundal pressure
- Placement of internal mode of monitoring

CLINICAL SIGNIFICANCE

Normal pattern. Not associated with fetal hypoxemia, acidemia, or low Apgar scores

NURSING INTERVENTIONS

None required

et al., 2009). They should be considered an ominous sign when they are uncorrectable, especially if they are associated with absent or minimal variability and tachycardia. Several factors can disrupt oxygen transfer to the fetus, including maternal hypotension, uterine **tachysystole** (e.g., more than five contractions in 10 minutes, averaged over a 30-minute window), preeclampsia, postdate or postterm pregnancy, amnionitis, small-for-gestational-age fetuses, maternal diabetes, placenta previa, abruptio placentae, conduction anesthetics, maternal cardiac disease, and maternal anemia. The clinical significance and nursing interventions are described in Box 11-4.

Variable decelerations. Variable deceleration of the FHR is defined as a visually abrupt (onset to lowest point <30 seconds) decrease in FHR below the baseline. The decrease is at least 15 beats/min or more below the baseline, lasts at least 15 seconds, and returns to baseline in less than 2 minutes from the time of onset (Macones et al., 2008). Variable decelerations are not necessarily associated with UCs. Variable decelerations are caused by compression of the umbilical cord (Fig. 11-12).

BOX 11-4

Late Decelerations

CAUSE

Uteroplacental insufficiency caused by the following:

- Uterine tachysystole
- Maternal supine hypotension
- Epidural or spinal anesthesia
- Placenta previa
- Abruptio placentae
- Hypertensive disorders
- Postmaturity
- Intrauterine growth restriction
- Diabetes mellitus
- Intraamniotic infection

CLINICAL SIGNIFICANCE

Abnormal pattern associated with fetal hypoxemia, acidemia, and low Apgar scores; considered ominous if persistent and uncorrected, especially when associated with fetal tachycardia and loss of variability

NURSING INTERVENTIONS

The usual priority is as follows:

1. Change maternal position (lateral).
2. Correct maternal hypotension by elevating legs.
3. Increase rate of maintenance IV solution.
4. Palpate uterus to assess for tachysystole.
5. Discontinue oxytocin if infusing.
6. Administer oxygen at 8-10 L/min by nonrebreather facemask.
7. Notify physician or nurse-midwife.
8. Consider internal monitoring for a more accurate fetal and uterine assessment.
9. Assist with birth (cesarean or vaginal assisted) if pattern cannot be corrected.

IV, Intravenous.

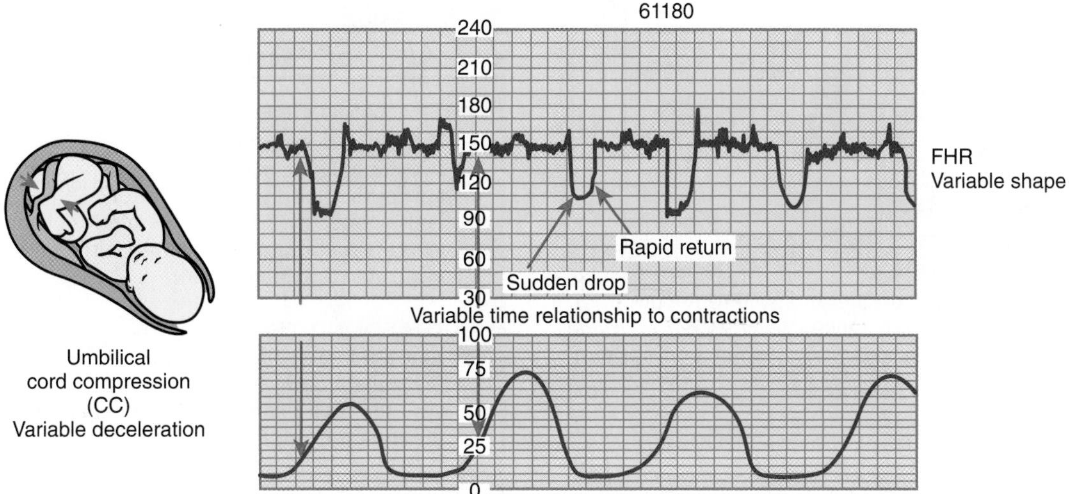

Fig. 11-12 Variable decelerations. (From Tucker, S. [2004]. *Pocket guide to fetal monitoring and assessment* [5th ed.]. St. Louis: Mosby.)

The appearance of variable decelerations differs from those of early and late decelerations, which closely approximate the shape of the corresponding UC. Instead, variable decelerations often have a U, V, or W shape characterized by a rapid descent to and ascent from the nadir (lowest point) of the deceleration (see Fig. 11-12). Some variable decelerations are preceded and followed by brief accelerations of the FHR, known as "shoulders," which is an appropriate compensatory response to compression of the umbilical cord.

Occasional variable decelerations have little clinical significance. Repetitive variable decelerations, on the other hand, indicate recurrent disruption in the fetus' oxygen supply. This disruption can result in hypoxemia and eventually metabolic acidemia (Tucker et al., 2009). Variable decelerations are most commonly found during the transition phase of first stage labor or the second stage of labor as a result of umbilical cord compression and stretching during fetal descent (Garite, 2007). Box 11-5 lists causes, clinical significance, and nursing interventions for variable decelerations.

Prolonged decelerations. A prolonged deceleration is a visually apparent decrease (may be either gradual or abrupt) in FHR of at least 15 beats/min below the baseline and lasting more than 2 minutes but less than 10 minutes. A deceleration lasting more than 10 minutes is considered a baseline change (Macones et al., 2008) (Fig. 11-13).

Prolonged decelerations are caused by a disruption in the fetal oxygen supply. They usually begin as a reflex response to hypoxia. If the disruption continues, however, the fetal cardiac tissue itself will become hypoxic, resulting in direct myocardial depression of the FHR (Tucker et al., 2009). Prolonged decelerations may be caused by prolonged cord compression, profound uteroplacental insufficiency, or perhaps sustained head compression. The presence and degree of hypoxia present are thought to correlate with the depth and duration of the deceleration, how abruptly it returns to the baseline, how much variability is lost during the deceleration, and whether rebound tachycardia and loss of variability occur after the deceleration (Garite, 2007).

Significant stimuli that may result in prolonged decelerations are a prolapsed umbilical cord or other forms of prolonged cord compression, prolonged uterine tachysystole, hypotension after spinal or epidural anesthesia or analgesia, abruptio placentae, eclamptic seizure, and rapid descent through the birth canal. Other more benign causes of prolonged decelerations include pelvic examination, application of a spiral electrode, and sustained maternal Valsalva maneuver (Garite, 2007).

Critical Thinking/Clinical Decision Making

Management of Variable Decelerations

You are the nurse assigned to care for Ashley, a G1 P0 at 39 weeks of gestation in active labor. At last check, approximately an hour ago, Ashley's cervix was dilated to 6 cm. Suddenly, you notice the appearance of repetitive abrupt decreases in the FHR below the baseline on her EFM tracing. The decelerations are V shaped, with a rapid descent to and ascent from the nadir of the deceleration.

1. Based on the above description, what type of FHR deceleration is Ashley's fetus experiencing?
2. What assumptions can be made about the following issues:
   a. The cause of this deceleration
   b. The goal of interventions for this deceleration
   c. Nursing interventions to correct this type of deceleration
3. Of the interventions listed in 2 c, which is the least important to implement initially? Why?
4. Does the evidence objectively support your conclusion?
5. Do alternative perspectives to your conclusion exist?

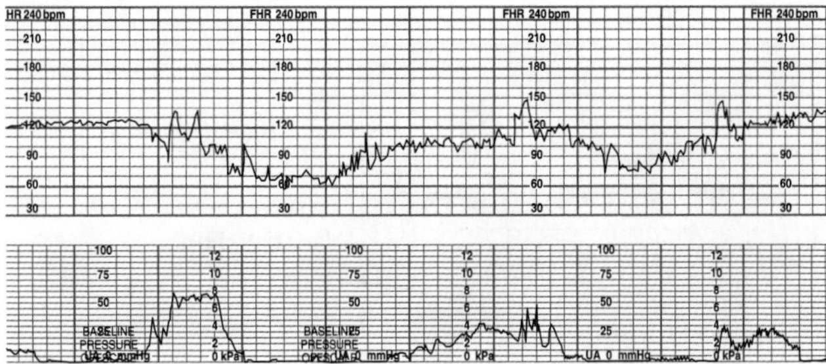

Fig. 11-13 Prolonged decelerations. (From Tucker, S. M., Miller, L. A., & Miller, D. A. [2009]. *Mosby's pocket guide to fetal monitoring: A multidisciplinary approach* [6th ed.]. St. Louis: Mosby.

BOX 11-5

Variable Decelerations

CAUSE

Umbilical cord compression caused by the following:
- Maternal position with cord between fetus and maternal pelvis
- Cord around fetal neck, arm, leg, or other body part
- Short cord
- Knot in cord
- Prolapsed cord

CLINICAL SIGNIFICANCE

Variable decelerations occur in approximately 50% of all labors and usually are transient and correctable

NURSING INTERVENTIONS

The usual priority is as follows:
1. Change maternal position (side to side, knee chest).
2. Discontinue oxytocin if infusing.
3. Administer oxygen at 8-10 L/min by nonrebreather facemask.
4. Notify physician or nurse-midwife.
5. Assist with vaginal or speculum examination to assess for cord prolapse.
6. Assist with amnioinfusion if ordered.
7. Assist with birth (vaginal assisted or cesarean) if pattern cannot be corrected.

NURSING ALERT Nurses should notify the physician or nurse-midwife immediately and initiate appropriate treatment when they see a prolonged deceleration.

CARE MANAGEMENT

Care of the woman receiving EFM in labor begins with evaluation of the EFM equipment. The nurse must ensure that the monitor is recording FHR and UA accurately and that the tracing is interpretable. If external monitoring is not adequate, changing to a fetal spiral electrode or IUPC may be necessary. A checklist for fetal monitoring equipment can be used to evaluate the equipment functions (Box 11-6).

BOX 11-6

Checklist for Fetal Monitoring Equipment

PREPARATION OF MONITOR

1. Is the paper inserted correctly?
2. Are transducer cables plugged securely into the appropriate port on the monitor?
3. Is the paper speed set to 3 cm/min?
4. Was the monitor date and time verified (when using electronic documentation)?

ULTRASOUND TRANSDUCER

1. Has ultrasound transmission gel been applied to the transducer?
2. Was the fetal heart rate (FHR) tested and noted on the monitor strip?
3. Was the FHR compared with the maternal pulse and noted?
3. Does a signal light flash or an audible beep occur with each heartbeat?
4. Is the belt secure and snug but comfortable for the laboring woman?

TOCOTRANSDUCER

1. Is the tocotransducer firmly positioned at the site of the least maternal tissue?
2. Has it been applied without gel or paste?
3. Was the uterine activity (UA) baseline adjusted between contractions to print at the 20 mm Hg line?
4. Is the belt secure and snug but comfortable for the laboring woman?

SPIRAL ELECTRODE

1. Is the connector attached firmly to the electrode pad (on the leg plate or abdomen)?
2. Is the spiral electrode attached to the presenting part of the fetus?
3. Is the inner surface of the electrode pad pre-gelled or covered with electrode gel?
4. Is the electrode pad properly secured to the woman's thigh or abdomen?

INTERNAL CATHETER OR STRAIN GAUGE

1. Is the length line on the catheter visible at the introitus?
2. Is it noted on the monitor paper that a UA test or calibration was performed?
3. Has the monitor been set to zero according to manufacturer's directions?
4. Is the intrauterine pressure catheter properly secured to the woman?
5. Is the baseline resting tone of the uterus documented?

Modified from Tucker, S. M., Miller, L. A., & Miller, D. A. (2009). *Mosby's pocket guide to fetal monitoring: A multidisciplinary approach* (6th ed.). St. Louis: Mosby.

After ensuring that the monitor is recording properly, the FHR and UA tracings are evaluated regularly throughout labor. *Guidelines for Perinatal Care* published jointly by the American Academy of Pediatrics (AAP) and ACOG (2007) recommends that the FHR tracing be evaluated at

Nursing Care Plan: Electronic Fetal Monitoring during Labor

NURSING PROCESS *Fetal Heart Rate Monitoring*

ASSESSMENT

Assessment should be performed at least every 30 minutes during the first stage of labor and every 15 minutes during the second stage of labor in low risk women. If risk factors are present, assessment should be performed every 15 minutes in the first stage of labor and every 5 minutes in the second stage of labor.

- Fetal heart rate (FHR) tracing
  - Baseline rate
  - Baseline variability (absent, minimal, moderate, or marked)
  - Presence of accelerations
  - Presence of early, late, variable, or prolonged decelerations
  - Changes in the FHR pattern over time
- Uterine activity (UA)
  - Contraction frequency
  - Contraction duration
  - Contraction intensity
  - Uterine resting tone
- Maternal vital signs (usually assessed at the same time as the FHR and UA)
  - Blood pressure
  - Pulse
  - Respirations

NURSING DIAGNOSES

Possible nursing diagnoses include the following:

- *Decreased maternal cardiac output* related to:
  - Supine hypotension secondary to maternal position or regional (epidural) anesthesia
- *Anxiety* related to:
  - Lack of knowledge concerning fetal monitoring during labor
  - Restriction of mobility or movement during EFM
- *Impaired fetal gas exchange* related to:
  - Umbilical cord compression
  - Placental insufficiency
- *Risk for fetal injury* related to:
  - Unrecognized hypoxemia or metabolic acidemia
  - Maternal hypotension
  - Maternal position (aortocaval compression)

EXPECTED OUTCOMES OF CARE

Expected outcomes for the pregnant woman, her family, and the fetus include the following:

- The pregnant woman and family will verbalize their understanding of the need for monitoring.
- The pregnant woman and family will recognize and avoid situations that compromise maternal and fetal circulation.
- The fetus will not develop hypoxemia or metabolic acidemia.
- Should fetal compromise occur, it will be identified promptly, and appropriate nursing interventions such as intrauterine resuscitation will be initiated and the physician or nurse-midwife notified.

PLAN OF CARE AND INTERVENTIONS

Implement basic corrective actions immediately whenever one of the essential components of the FHR tracing (see Assessment, above) is determined to be abnormal (see Boxes 11-4, 11-5, 11-8, and Table 11-3 for specific interventions).

EVALUATION

The expected outcomes of care are used to evaluate the care related to FHR and UA monitoring.

Source: American Academy of Pediatrics (AAP) & American College of Obstetricians and Gynecologists (ACOG). (2007). *Guidelines for perinatal care* (6th ed.). Washington, DC: AAP & AGOG.

least every 30 minutes during the first stage of labor and every 15 minutes during the second stage of labor in low risk women. If risk factors are present, then the FHR tracing should be evaluated more frequently, every 15 minutes in the first stage of labor and every 5 minutes in the second stage of labor.

Based on assessment findings the nurse identifies relevant nursing diagnoses and expected outcomes of care, implements appropriate interventions, and evaluates the care provided (see Nursing Process box). Assessing FHR and UA patterns, implementing independent nursing interventions, documenting observations and actions according to the established standard of care, and reporting abnormal patterns to the primary care provider (e.g., physician, certified nurse-midwife) are the responsibilities of the nurse providing care to women in labor.

Electronic Fetal Monitoring Pattern Recognition

Nurses must evaluate many factors to determine whether an FHR pattern is normal or abnormal (see Nursing Process box). Nurses evaluate these factors based on the presence of other obstetric complications, progress in labor, and use of analgesia or anesthesia. They must also consider the estimated time interval until birth. Interventions are therefore based on clinical judgment of a complex, integrated process (Simpson & James, 2005).

LEGAL TIP Fetal Monitoring Standards

Nurses who care for women during childbirth are legally responsible for correctly interpreting FHR patterns, initiating appropriate nursing interventions based on those patterns, and documenting the outcomes of those interventions. Perinatal nurses are responsible for the timely notification of the physician or nurse-midwife in the event of abnormal FHR patterns. Perinatal nurses are also responsible for initiating the institutional chain of command should differences in opinion arise among health care providers concerning the interpretation of the FHR pattern and the intervention required.

Nursing Management of Abnormal Patterns

The five essential components of the fetal heart rate tracing that must be evaluated regularly are baseline rate, baseline variability, accelerations, decelerations, and changes or trends over time (Tucker et al., 2009). Whenever one of these five essential components is assessed as abnormal, corrective measures must immediately be taken (see Nursing Process box). The purpose of these actions is to improve fetal oxygenation (Tucker et al.). The term *intrauterine resuscitation* is sometimes used to refer to specific interventions initiated when an abnormal FHR pattern is noted. Basic corrective measures include providing supplemental oxygen, instituting maternal position changes, and increasing intravenous fluid administration. The purpose of these interventions is to improve uterine and intervillous space blood flow and increase maternal oxygenation and cardiac output (Simpson & James, 2005). Box 11-7 lists basic interventions to improve maternal and fetal oxygenation status.

Depending on the underlying cause of the abnormal FHR pattern, other interventions, such as correcting maternal hypotension, reducing uterine activity, and altering second stage pushing techniques, may also be instituted (Tucker et al., 2009). Box 11-7 also lists interventions for these specific problems. Realize that some of the items listed are not independent nursing interventions. Any medications administered, for example, must be authorized either through inclusion in a specific unit protocol or by a specific order. Some interventions are specific to the FHR pattern. See Table 11-3 and Boxes 11-4 and 11-5 for nursing interventions for tachycardia, late decelerations, and variable decelerations. Based on the FHR response to these interventions the primary health care provider decides whether additional interventions should be instituted or whether immediate vaginal or cesarean birth should be performed.

Other Methods of Assessment and Intervention

A major shortcoming of EFM is its high rate of false-positive results. Even the most abnormal patterns are poorly predictive of neonatal morbidity. Therefore other methods of assessment have been developed to evaluate fetal status. Fetal scalp stimulation and vibroacoustic stimulation and umbilical cord acid-base determination are frequently performed assessments. On the other hand, fetal scalp blood sampling and fetal pulse oximetry are assessments that are rarely performed in the United States. Amnioinfusion and tocolytic therapy are two interventions often used in an attempt to improve abnormal FHR patterns.

BOX 11-7

Management of Abnormal Fetal Heart Rate (FHR) Patterns

BASIC INTERVENTIONS

- Administer oxygen by nonrebreather facemask at a rate of 10 L/min for approximately 15-30 minutes.
- Assist the woman to a side-lying (lateral) position.
- Increase maternal blood volume by increasing the rate of the primary IV infusion.

INTERVENTIONS FOR SPECIFIC PROBLEMS

- Maternal hypotension
  - Increase the rate of the primary IV infusion.
  - Change to lateral or Trendelenburg positioning.
  - Administer ephedrine or phenylephrine if other measures are unsuccessful in increasing blood pressure.
- Uterine tachysystole
  - Reduce or discontinue the dose of any uterine stimulants in use (e.g., oxytocin [Pitocin]).
  - Administer a uterine relaxant (tocolytic) (e.g., terbutaline [Brethine]).
- Abnormal FHR tracing during the second stage of labor
  - Use open glottis pushing.
  - Use fewer pushing efforts during each contraction.
  - Make individual pushing efforts shorter.
  - Push only with every other or every third contraction.
  - Push only with a perceived urge to push (in patients with regional anesthesia).

IV, Intravenous.

Assessment techniques

Fetal scalp stimulation and vibroacoustic stimulation. Several research studies undertaken in the 1980s found that a FHR acceleration in response to digital or vibroacoustic stimulation was highly predictive of a normal scalp blood pH. The two methods of fetal stimulation currently used most often in clinical practice are scalp stimulation (using digital pressure during a vaginal examination) and vibroacoustic stimulation (using an artificial larynx or fetal acoustic stimulation device on the maternal abdomen over the fetal head for 1 to 5 seconds). The desired result of both methods of stimulation is an acceleration in the FHR of at least 15 beats/min for at least 15 seconds (Tucker et al., 2009). A FHR acceleration indicates the absence of metabolic acidemia. If the fetus does not respond to stimulation with an acceleration, fetal compromise is not necessarily indicated; however, further evaluation of fetal well-being is needed. Fetal stimulation should be performed at times when the FHR is at baseline. Neither fetal scalp stimulation nor vibroacoustic stimulation should be instituted if FHR decelerations or bradycardia is present (Tucker et al.).

Umbilical cord acid-base determination. In assessing the immediate condition of the newborn after birth, a sample of cord blood is a useful adjunct to the Apgar score. The procedure is generally performed by withdrawing blood from both the umbilical artery and the umbilical vein. Both samples are then tested for pH, carbon dioxide pressure (PCO_2), oxygen pressure (PO_2), and base deficit or base excess (Garite, 2007; Tucker et al., 2009). Umbilical arterial values reflect fetal condition, whereas umbilical vein values indicate placental function (Tucker et al.).

ACOG (2006a) suggests obtaining cord blood values in the following clinical situations: cesarean birth for fetal compromise, low 5-minute Apgar score, severe intrauterine growth restriction, abnormal FHR tracing, maternal thyroid disease, intrapartum fever, and multifetal gestation. Normal umbilical artery and vein cord blood values are listed in Table 11-4. Normal findings preclude the presence of acidemia at, or immediately before, birth (Tucker et al., 2009). If acidemia is present (e.g., pH <7.20), then the type of acidemia is determined (respiratory, metabolic, or mixed) by analyzing the blood gas values (Table 11-5) (Tucker et al.).

Fetal scalp blood sampling. Sampling of the fetal scalp blood for pH determination was first described in the 1960s and performed extensively in the 1970s. The procedure is performed by obtaining a sample of fetal scalp blood through the dilated cervix after the membranes have ruptured. Its use is limited by many factors, including the requirement for cervical dilation and membrane rupture, technical difficulty of the procedure, need for repetitive pH determinations, and uncertainty regarding interpretation and application of results. This procedure is now seldom used in the United States but remains a common practice in other countries (Tucker et al., 2009).

Fetal pulse oximetry. Fetal pulse oximetry or continuous monitoring of fetal oxygen saturation levels is a method of fetal assessment that indirectly measures the oxygen saturation of hemoglobin in fetal blood. An intrauterine sensor placed in contact with the fetal cheek or temple area provides a continuous estimation of fetal oxygen saturation. Fetal pulse oximetry was approved for clinical use by the U.S. Food and Drug Administration in May 2000. The hope was that this technology would help to interpret nonreassuring FHR patterns more accurately and perhaps decrease the number of cesarean births performed for nonreassuring FHR tracings (Garite, 2007). Several studies, however, found that although fetal pulse oximetry did decrease the incidence of cesarean births for fetal indications, it had no consistent impact on overall cesarean birth rates or newborn outcomes. Therefore, fetal pulse oximetry has not been proven to be a clinically useful test for determining fetal status (ACOG, 2009). Because the manufacturer no longer distributes the sensors, the product has in effect been taken off the market (Tucker et al., 2009).

TABLE 11-4

Approximate Normal Values for Cord Blood

CORD BLOOD	pH	CARBON DIOXIDE PRESSURE (PCO_2) (mm Hg)	OXYGEN PRESSURE (PO_2) (mm Hg)	BASE DEFICIT (mmol/L)
Artery	7.2-7.3	45-55	15-25	<12
Vein	7.3-7.4	35-45	25-35	<12

From Tucker, S. M., Miller, L. A, & Miller, D. A. (2009). *Mosby's pocket guide to fetal monitoring: A multidisciplinary approach* (6th ed.). St. Louis: Mosby.

TABLE 11-5

Types of Acidemia

BLOOD GASES	RESPIRATORY	METABOLIC	MIXED
pH	<7.20	<7.20	<7.20
Carbon dioxide pressure (PCO_2)	Elevated	Normal	Elevated
Base deficit	<12 mmol/L	≥12 mmol/L	≥12 mmol/L

From Tucker, S. M., Miller, L. A, & Miller, D. A. (2009). *Mosby's pocket guide to fetal monitoring: A multidisciplinary approach* (6th ed.). St. Louis: Mosby.

Interventions

Amnioinfusion. Amnioinfusion is infusion of room-temperature isotonic fluid (usually normal saline or lactated Ringer's solution) into the uterine cavity if the volume of amniotic fluid is low. Without the buffer of amniotic fluid the umbilical cord can easily become compressed during contractions or fetal movement, diminishing the flow of blood between the fetus and placenta. The purpose of amnioinfusion is to relieve intermittent umbilical cord compression that results in variable decelerations and transient fetal hypoxemia by restoring the amniotic fluid volume to a normal or near-normal level (Tucker et al., 2009). Women with an abnormally small amount of amniotic fluid (oligohydramnios) or no amniotic fluid (anhydramnios) are candidates for this procedure. Conditions that can result in oligohydramnios or anhydramnios are uteroplacental insufficiency and premature rupture of membranes.

In the past, amnioinfusion was also used to dilute moderate to thick meconium in an attempt to prevent meconium aspiration syndrome. However, a recent large research study found that amnioinfusion did not significantly reduce the incidence of meconium aspiration syndrome or perinatal death (Fraser et al., 2005). Therefore routine amnioinfusion for meconium-stained amniotic fluid without the presence of variable decelerations is not recommended by ACOG (2006b).

Risks of amnioinfusion are overdistention of the uterine cavity and increased uterine tone. Fluid will be administered through an IUPC either by gravity flow or by use of an infusion pump. Usually a bolus of fluid will be administered over 20 to 30 minutes, and then the infusion will be slowed to a maintenance rate. Likely no more than 1000 ml of fluid will need to be administered. The fluid may be warmed by infusing it through a blood warmer for the preterm fetus (Tucker et al., 2009).

Intensity and frequency of UCs should be continually assessed during the procedure. The recorded uterine resting tone during amnioinfusion will appear higher than normal because of resistance to outflow and turbulence at the end of the catheter. Uterine resting tone should not exceed 40 mm Hg during the procedure. The amount of fluid return must be estimated and documented during amnioinfusion to prevent overdistension of the uterus. The volume of fluid returned should be approximately the same as the amount infused (Tucker et al., 2009).

Tocolytic therapy. Tocolysis (relaxation of the uterus) can be achieved through the administration of drugs that inhibit UCs. This therapy can be used as an adjunct to other interventions in the management of fetal stress when the fetus is exhibiting abnormal patterns associated with increased UA. Tocolysis improves blood flow through the placenta by inhibiting UCs. Tocolysis may be considered by the primary health care provider and implemented when other interventions to reduce UA, such as maternal position change and discontinuance of an oxytocin infusion, have no effect on diminishing the UCs. Tocolytics are often administered when women are having excessive UCs spontaneously. Tocolytics are also frequently administered after a decision for cesarean birth has been made while preparations for surgery are underway. The most commonly used tocolytic in these situations is probably terbutaline (Brethine), given subcutaneously. Terbutaline works quickly and has been demonstrated to improve Apgar scores and cord pH values without apparent complications (Garite, 2007). If the FHR and UC patterns improve, then the woman may be allowed to continue labor; if no improvement is seen, immediate cesarean birth may be needed.

Patient and family teaching

Although the use of EFM can be reassuring to many parents, it can be a source of anxiety to some. Therefore the nurse must be particularly sensitive and respond appropriately to the emotional, informational, and comfort needs of the woman in labor and those of her family (Fig. 11-14 and Box 11-8).

Part of the nurse's role includes acting as a partner with the woman to achieve a high-quality birthing experience. In addition to teaching and supporting the woman and her family with understanding of the laboring and birth process, breathing techniques, use of equipment, and pain-management techniques, the nurse can assist with two factors that have an effect on fetal status: postioning and pushing. The nurse should solicit the woman's cooperation in avoiding the supine position. Instead, the woman should be encouraged to maintain a side-lying position or semi-Fowler's position with a lateral tilt to the uterus. In

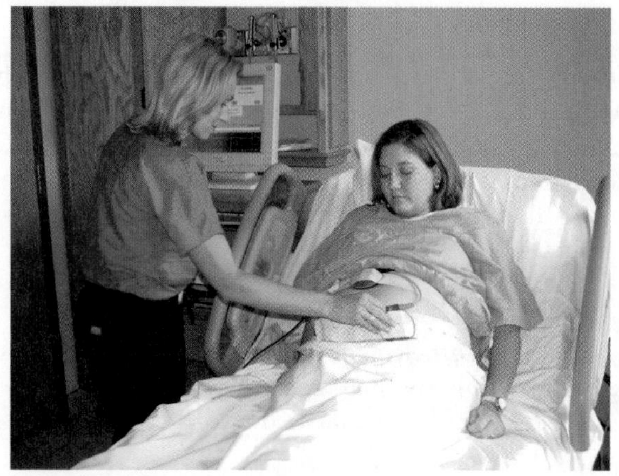

Fig. 11-14 Nurse explains electronic fetal monitoring as ultrasound transducer monitors the fetal heart rate. (Courtesy Julie Perry Nelson, Loveland, CO.)

BOX 11-8

Patient and Family Teaching when Electronic Fetal Monitor is Used

The following guidelines relate to patient teaching and the functioning of the monitor.

- Explain the purpose of monitoring.
- Explain each procedure.
- Provide rationale for maternal position other than supine.
- Explain that fetal status can be continuously assessed by electronic fetal monitoring (EFM), even during contractions.
- Explain that the lower tracing on the monitor strip paper shows uterine activity; the upper tracing shows the fetal heart rate (FHR).
- Reassure woman and partner that prepared childbirth techniques can be implemented without difficulty.
- Explain that, during external monitoring, effleurage can be performed on sides of abdomen or upper portion of thighs.
- Explain that breathing patterns based on the time and intensity of contractions can be enhanced by the observation of uterine activity on the monitor strip, which shows the onset of contractions.
- Note peak of contraction; knowing that contraction will not get stronger and is halfway over is usually helpful.
- Note diminishing intensity.
- Coordinate with appropriate breathing and relaxation techniques.
- Reassure woman and partner that the use of internal monitoring does not restrict movement, although she is confined to bed.*
- Explain that use of external monitoring usually requires the woman's cooperation during positioning and movement.
- Reassure woman and partner that use of monitoring does not imply fetal jeopardy.

*Portable telemetry monitors allow the FHR and uterine contraction patterns to be observed on centrally located display stations. These portable units permit ambulation during electronic monitoring.

addition, the nurse should instruct the woman to keep her mouth and glottis open and to let air escape from her lungs during the pushing process. Both of these interventions will help to improve fetal oxygenation. See Chapter 12 for further discussion of maternal positioning and pushing techniques.

Documentation

Clear and complete documentation in the woman's medical record is essential. Each FHR and UA assessment must be completely documented in the woman's medical record. Currently, more and more hospitals are moving to use of the electronic medical record and computerized charting. With computerized charting, each required component usually appears on the screen so that it will routinely be addressed. Computerized charting often includes forced choices that greatly increase the use of standardized FHR terminology by all members of the health care team. In the past, nurses were often encouraged to chart both on the monitor strip and in the medical record. However, charting directly on the monitor strip is unnecessary when an electronic medical record is used. Any information that is handwritten on the monitor strip will not be recorded in the computer record. Furthermore, given that the EFM tracing is stored on computer, the paper strips are destroyed after the woman is discharged. No permanent record of the handwritten charting exists.

In institutions that still use a paper chart, documentation on the woman's monitor strip is started before the initiation of monitoring and consists of identifying information plus other relevant data. This documentation is continued and updated according to institutional protocol as monitoring progresses. See Box 11-6 for a checklist that can be used for documentation in a paper medical record. In some institutions, observations noted and interventions implemented are recorded on the monitor strip to produce a comprehensive document that chronicles the course of labor and the care rendered. In other institutions, this documentation is confined to the labor flow record. Advocates of documenting on both the medical record and the EFM strip cite as advantages of this approach the ease of writing directly on the strip while at the bedside and the improved accuracy in documenting critical events and the interventions implemented. Others believe that charting on the EFM strip constitutes duplicate documentation of the same information noted in the medical record, and thus it is unnecessary additional paperwork for the nurse.

A disadvantage of documenting on both the EFM strip and the medical record is that the times noted for events and interventions on the EFM strip frequently do not correlate with what is later documented in the medical record. These inaccuracies can lead persons involved in the retrospective review process carried out during litigation to infer that documentation errors have occurred. Therefore, if institutional policy mandates documentation on both the monitor strip and the medical record, the nurse must make sure the times and notations of events and interventions recorded in each place agree. Many of the aspects of care and events that can be documented on the patient's medical record or the monitor strip are listed in Box 11-9.

BOX 11-9

Checklist for Fetal Heart Rate and Uterine Activity Assessment with Electronic Fetal Monitoring

Patient's name ______________________________

Date/time ______________________________

1. What is the baseline fetal heart rate (FHR)?

   ____________ Beats/min

   Check one of the following as observed on the monitor strip:

   ____________ Average baseline FHR (110-160 beats/min)

   ____________ Tachycardia (>160 beats/min)

   ____________ Bradycardia (<110 beats/min)

2. What is the baseline variability?

   ____________ Absent variability

   ____________ Minimal variability (detectable up to 5 beats/min)

   ____________ Moderate variability (6-25 beats/min)

   ____________ Marked variability (>25 beats/min)

3. Any periodic or episodic changes in FHR?

   ____________ Accelerations with fetal movement

   ____________ Accelerations with contractions

   ____________ Early decelerations (head compression)

   ____________ Late decelerations (uteroplacental insufficiency)

   ____________ Variable decelerations (cord compression)

   ____________ Prolonged deceleration (>2 minutes up to 10 minutes)

4. What is the uterine activity or contraction pattern?

   ____________ Frequency (beginning to end of UC)

   ____________ Duration (beginning of one UC to beginning of the next UC)

   Abdominal palpation method

   ____________ Strength (mild, moderate, strong)

   ____________ Resting tone (from end of one contraction to beginning of next one)

   Internal monitoring (intrauterine pressure catheter)

   ____________ Intensity (mm Hg pressure)

   ____________ Resting tone (mm Hg pressure)

   Comments: ______________________________

   ____

   Panel Number: ______________________________

   What can be or should have been done?

   ____

   ____

   ____

Modified from Tucker, S. (2004). *Pocket guide to fetal monitoring and assessment* (5th ed.). St. Louis: Mosby.

KEY POINTS

- Fetal well-being during labor is gauged by the response of the FHR to UCs.
- Standardized definitions for many common FHR patterns have been adopted for use in clinical practice by ACNM, ACOG, and AWHONN.
- The five essential components of the fetal heart rate tracing are baseline rate, baseline variability, accelerations, decelerations, and changes or trends over time.
- The monitoring of fetal well-being includes FHR and UA assessment, as well as assessment of maternal vital signs.
- Assessing FHR and UA patterns, implementing independent nursing interventions, and reporting abnormal patterns to the physician or nurse-midwife are the nurse's responsibilities.
- AWHONN and ACOG have established and published health care provider standards and guidelines for FHR monitoring.
- The emotional, informational, and comfort needs of the woman and her family must be addressed when the mother and her fetus are being monitored.
- Documentation of fetal assessment is initiated and updated according to institutional protocol.

Audio Chapter Summaries: Access an audio summary of these Key Points on evolve

References

Albers, L. L. (2007). The evidence for physiologic management of the active phase of the first stage of labor. *Journal of Midwifery & Women's Health, 52*(3), 207-215.

American Academy of Pediatrics (AAP) and American College of Obstetricians and Gynecologists (ACOG). (2007). *Guidelines for perinatal care* (6th ed.). Washington, DC: AAP & AGOG.

American College of Obstetricians and Gynecologists (ACOG). (2009). *Intrapartum fetal heart rate monitoring: Nomenclature, interpretation, and general management principles. ACOG Practice Bulletin No. 106.* Washington, DC: ACOG.

American College of Obstetricians and Gynecologists (ACOG). (2006a). *Umbilical cord blood gas and acid-base analysis. ACOG Committee Opinion.* Washington, DC: ACOG.

American College of Obstetricians and Gynecologists (ACOG). (2006b). *Amnioinfusion does not prevent meconium aspiration syndrome. ACOG Committee Opinion No. 346.* Washington, DC: ACOG.

Collard, T. D., Diallo, H., Habinsky, A., Hentschell, C., & Vezeau, T. M. (2008/2009). Elective cesarean section: Why women choose it and what nurses need to know. *Nursing for Women's Health, 12*(6), 480-488.

Fraser, W. D., Hofmeyr, J., Lede, R., Faron, G., Alexander, S., Goffinet, F., et al. (2005). Amnioinfusion Trial Group: Amnioinfusion for the prevention of the meconium aspiration syndrome. *New England Journal of Medicine, 353*(9), 909-917.

Garite, T. J. (2007). Intrapartum fetal evaluation. In S. Gabbe, J. Niebyl, & J. Simpson (Eds.), *Obstetrics: Normal and problem pregnancies* (5th ed.). Philadelphia: Churchill Livingstone.

Gilbert, E. S. (2007). *Manual of high risk pregnancy and delivery* (4th ed.). St. Louis: Mosby.

Macones, G. A., Hankins, G. D. V., Spong, C. Y., Hauth, J., & Moore, T. (2008). The 2008 National Institute of Child Health and Human Development Workshop Report on Electronic Fetal Monitoring: Update on definitions, interpretation, and research guidelines. *Journal of Obstetric, Gynecologic, and Neonatal Nursing, 37*(5), 510-515.

Nageotte, M. P., & Gilstrap, L. C. (2009). Intrapartum fetal surveillance. In R. K. Creasy, R. Resnik, & J. D. Iams (Eds.), *Creasy and Resnik's maternal-fetal medicine: Principles and practice* (6th ed.). Philadelphia: Saunders.

National Institute of Child Health and Human Development (NICHD) Research Planning Workshop. (1997). Electronic fetal heart rate monitoring: Research guidelines for interpretation. *American Journal of Obstetrics and Gynecology, 177*(6), 1385-1390; *Journal of Obstetric, Gynecologic, and Neonatal Nursing, 26*(6), 635-640.

Simpson, K., & James, D. (2005). Efficacy of intrauterine resuscitation techniques in improving fetal oxygen status during labor. *Obstetrics and Gynecology, 105*(6), 1362-1368.

Tucker, S. M., Miller, L. A, & Miller, D. A. (2009). *Mosby's pocket guide to fetal monitoring: A multidisciplinary approach* (6th ed.). St. Louis: Mosby.

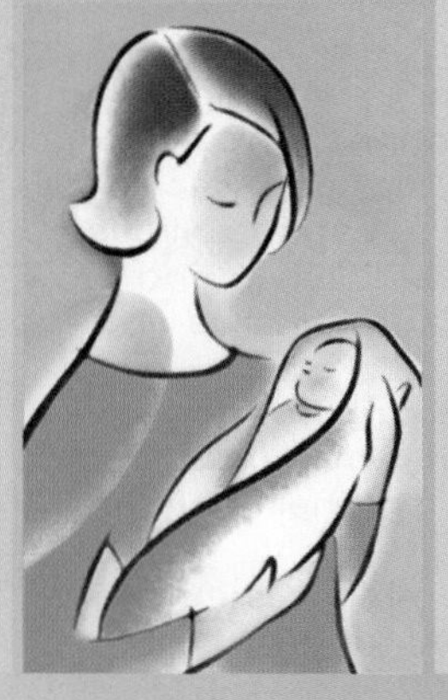

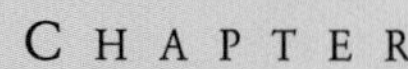

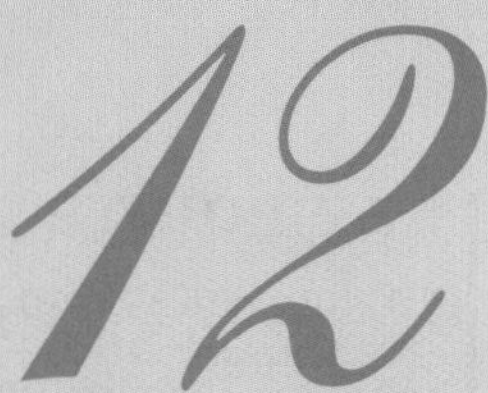

CHAPTER 12

Nursing Care of the Family during Labor and Birth

KITTY CASHION

LEARNING OBJECTIVES

- *Review the factors included in the initial assessment of the woman in labor.*
- *Describe the ongoing assessment of maternal progress during the first, second, third, and fourth stages of labor.*
- *Recognize the physical and psychosocial findings indicative of maternal progress during labor.*
- *Identify signs of developing complications during labor and birth.*
- *Identify nursing interventions for each stage of labor and birth.*
- *Examine the influence of cultural and religious beliefs and practices on the process of labor and birth.*
- *Describe the role and responsibilities of the nurse during an emergency childbirth.*
- *Discuss how the nurse can increase the use of evidence-based practices in caring for women during labor and birth.*

KEY TERMS AND DEFINITIONS

active phase Phase in the first stage of labor, when the cervix dilates from 4 to 7 cm

amniotomy Artificial rupture of the fetal membranes, using a plastic Amnihook or a surgical clamp

bloody show Blood-tinged mucoid vaginal discharge that originates in the cervix and indicates passage of the mucous plug (operculum) as the cervix ripens before labor and dilates during labor; increases as labor progresses

crowning Phase in the descent of the fetus when the top of the head can be seen at the vaginal orifice as the widest part of the head (biparietal diameter) distends the vulva just before birth

doula Experienced female assistant hired to give the woman support during labor and birth

episiotomy Surgical incision of the perineum at the end of the second stage of labor to facilitate birth and to prevent laceration of the perineum

fern test Appearance of a fernlike pattern found on microscopic examination of certain fluids such as amniotic fluid

first stage of labor Stage of labor from the onset of regular uterine contractions to full effacement and dilation of the cervix

fourth stage of labor First 1 to 2 hours after birth

latent phase Phase in the first stage of labor when the cervix dilates from 0 to 3 cm

Leopold maneuvers Four maneuvers for diagnosing the fetal position by external palpation of the mother's abdomen

lithotomy position Position in which the woman lies on her back with her knees flexed and with abducted thighs drawn up toward her chest; stirrups attached to an examination table can be used to facilitate assuming and maintaining this position

Nitrazine test Evaluation of body fluids using a test swab to determine the fluid's pH; urine exhibiting an acidic result and amniotic fluid exhibiting an alkaline result

nuchal cord Encircling of fetal neck by one or more loops of umbilical cord

Ritgen maneuver Technique used to control the birth of the head; upward pressure from the coccygeal region to extend the head during the actual birth

rupture of membranes (ROM) Integrity of the amniotic membranes is broken either spontaneously (SROM) or artificially (AROM) by amniotomy

second stage of labor Stage of labor from full dilation of the cervix to the birth of the baby

third stage of labor Stage of labor from the birth of the baby to the separation and expulsion of the placenta

transition phase Phase in the first stage of labor when the cervix dilates from 8 to 10 cm

uterine contractions Primary powers of labor that act involuntarily to dilate and efface the cervix, expel the fetus, facilitate separation of the placenta, and prevent hemorrhage

uterine resting tone Tension in the uterine muscle between contractions; relaxation of the uterus

Valsalva maneuver Any forced expiratory effort against a closed airway, such as holding one's breath and tightening the abdominal muscles (e.g., pushing during the second stage of labor)

WEB RESOURCES

Additional related content can be found on the companion website at evolve

http://evolve.elsevier.com/Lowdermilk/Maternity/

- NCLEX Review Questions
- Animation: Vaginal Birth
- Assessment Video: Leopold Maneuvers
- Case Study: First Stage of Labor
- Case Study: Second/Third Stages of Labor
- Critical Thinking Exercise: Positioning during Labor
- Nursing Care Plan: Labor and Birth
- Spanish Guidelines: Care during Labor
- Spanish Guidelines: Labor Assessment
- Video: Childbirth (Vaginal)

For most women, labor begins with the first uterine contraction, continues with hours of hard work during cervical dilation and birth, and ends as the woman begins to recover physically from birth and she and her significant others begin the attachment process with the newborn. Nursing care management focuses on assessment and support of the woman and her significant others throughout labor and birth, with the goal of ensuring the best possible outcome for all involved.

A woman often has lingering impressions of her childbirth experience. Caregivers who are respectful, supportive, and calm help the woman to remember her childbirth experience in positive terms. Involving the laboring woman as a partner in the formulation of an individualized plan of care helps preserve the woman's sense of control, facilitates her participation in her own childbirth experience, and enhances her self-esteem and level of satisfaction. A satisfactory view of childbirth may also enhance a woman's adaptation to her role as a mother.

FIRST STAGE OF LABOR

CARE MANAGEMENT

The **first stage of labor** begins with the onset of regular uterine contractions and ends with full cervical effacement and dilation. It consists of the following three phases: the **latent phase** (through 3 cm of dilation), the **active phase** (4 to 7 cm of dilation), and the **transition phase** (8 to 10 cm of dilation). Most nulliparous women seek admission to the hospital in the latent phase because they have not experienced labor before and are unsure of the "right" time to come in. Multiparous women usually do not come to the hospital until they are in the active phase of the first stage of labor.

Assessment

Assessment begins at the first contact with the woman, whether by telephone or in person. Many women still call the hospital or birthing center first for validation that coming in for evaluation or admission is acceptable. Many hospitals, however, now discourage this practice because of concerns related to legal liability. Nurses are often instructed to tell patients who call with questions "You need to call your primary care provider," or "If you think you need to be checked, come to the hospital." If advice is given over the telephone, it must be carefully documented in the patient's record or in a telephone triage logbook on the unit (Gilbert, 2007).

Some pregnant women call the primary health care provider or come to the hospital while in false labor or early in the latent phase of the first stage of labor. Some feel discouraged after learning that the contractions that feel so strong and regular are not true contractions because they are not causing cervical dilation or are still not strong or frequent enough for admission. During the third trimester of pregnancy, women should be instructed regarding the stages of labor and the signs indicating its onset. They should be informed of the possibility that they will not be admitted if they are 3 cm or less dilated (see Teaching Guidelines box).

If the woman lives near the hospital and has adequate support and transportation, she may be asked to stay home or return home to allow labor to progress (i.e., until the uterine contractions are more frequent and intense). The ideal setting for the low risk woman at this time is the familiar environment of her home. The woman who lives at a considerable distance from the hospital or has a history of rapid labors in the past, however, may be admitted in latent labor. A warm shower is often relaxing for the woman in early labor. Soothing back, foot, or hand massages or a warm drink of preferred liquids such as tea or milk can help the woman to rest and even to sleep, especially if false or early labor is occurring at night. Diversional activities such as walking outdoors or in the house, reading, watching television, doing needlework, or talking with friends can reduce the perception of early discomfort, help the time pass, and reduce anxiety.

Case Study: First Stage of Labor

When the woman arrives at the perinatal unit, assessment is the top priority (Fig. 12-1). The nurse first performs a screening assessment by using the techniques of interview and physical assessment and reviews the laboratory and diagnostic test findings to determine the health status of the woman and her fetus and the progress of her labor. The nurse also notifies the primary health care provider, and if the woman is admitted, a detailed systems assessment is performed.

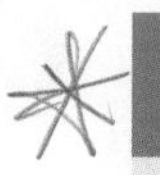

TEACHING GUIDELINES

How to Distinguish True Labor from False Labor

TRUE LABOR

- Contractions
  - Occur regularly, becoming stronger, lasting longer, and occurring closer together
  - Become more intense with walking
  - Usually felt in the lower back, radiating to lower portion of the abdomen
  - Continue despite use of comfort measures
- Cervix (by vaginal examination)
  - Shows progressive change (softening, effacement, and dilation signaled by the appearance of bloody show)
  - Moves to an increasingly anterior position
- Fetus
  - Presenting part usually becomes engaged in the pelvis, which results in increased ease of breathing; at the same time, the presenting part presses downward and compresses the bladder, resulting in urinary frequency

FALSE LABOR

- Contractions
  - Occur irregularly or become regular only temporarily
  - Often stop with walking or position change
  - Can be felt in the back or abdomen above the navel
  - Can often be stopped through the use of comfort measures
- Cervix (by vaginal examination)
  - May be soft but with no significant change in effacement or dilation or evidence of bloody show
  - Often in a posterior position
- Fetus
  - Presenting part is usually not engaged in the pelvis

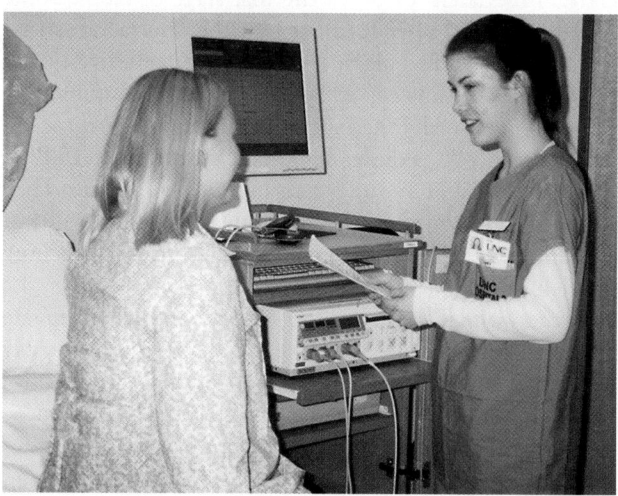

Fig. 12-1 Woman being assessed for admission to the labor and birth unit. (Courtesy Dee Lowdermilk, Chapel Hill, NC.)

LEGAL TIP Obstetric Triage and EMTALA

The Emergency Medical Treatment and Active Labor Act (EMTALA) is a federal regulation enacted to ensure that a woman gets emergency treatment or active labor care whenever such treatment is sought. According to the EMTALA, true labor is considered an emergency medical condition. Nurses working in labor and birth units must be familiar with their responsibilities according to the EMTALA regulations, which include providing services to pregnant women when they experience an urgent pregnancy problem (e.g., labor, decreased fetal movement, rupture of membranes, recent trauma) and fully documenting all relevant information (e.g., assessment findings, interventions implemented, patient responses to care measures provided). A pregnant woman presenting in an obstetric triage is considered to be in "true" labor until a qualified health care provider certifies that she is not. Agencies need to have specific policies and procedures in place so that compliance with the EMTALA regulations is achieved while providing safe and efficient care (Angelini & Mahlmeister, 2005; Tucker, Miller, & Miller, 2009).

When the woman is admitted, she is usually moved from an observation area to the labor room; the labor, delivery, and recovery (LDR) room; or the labor, delivery, recovery, and postpartum (LDRP) room. If the woman wishes, include her partner in the assessment and admission process. The nurse can direct significant others not participating in this process to the appropriate waiting area. The woman undresses and puts on her own gown or a hospital gown. The nurse places an admissions band on the woman's wrist. Her personal belongings are put away safely or given to family members, according to agency policy. Women who participate in expectant parents classes often bring a birth bag or Lamaze bag with them. The nurse then shows the woman and her partner the layout and operation of the unit and room, how to use the call light and telephone system, and how to adjust lighting in the room and the different bed positions.

The nurse assures the woman that she is in competent, caring hands and that she and her partner can ask questions related to her care and her status and those of her fetus at any time during labor. The nurse can minimize the woman's anxiety by explaining terms commonly used during labor. The woman's interest, response, and prior experience guide the depth and breadth of these explanations.

Most hospitals have specific forms, whether paper or electronic, that are used to obtain important assessment information when a woman in labor is being evaluated or admitted (Fig. 12-2). More and more hospitals now use an electronic medical record in which almost all charting is

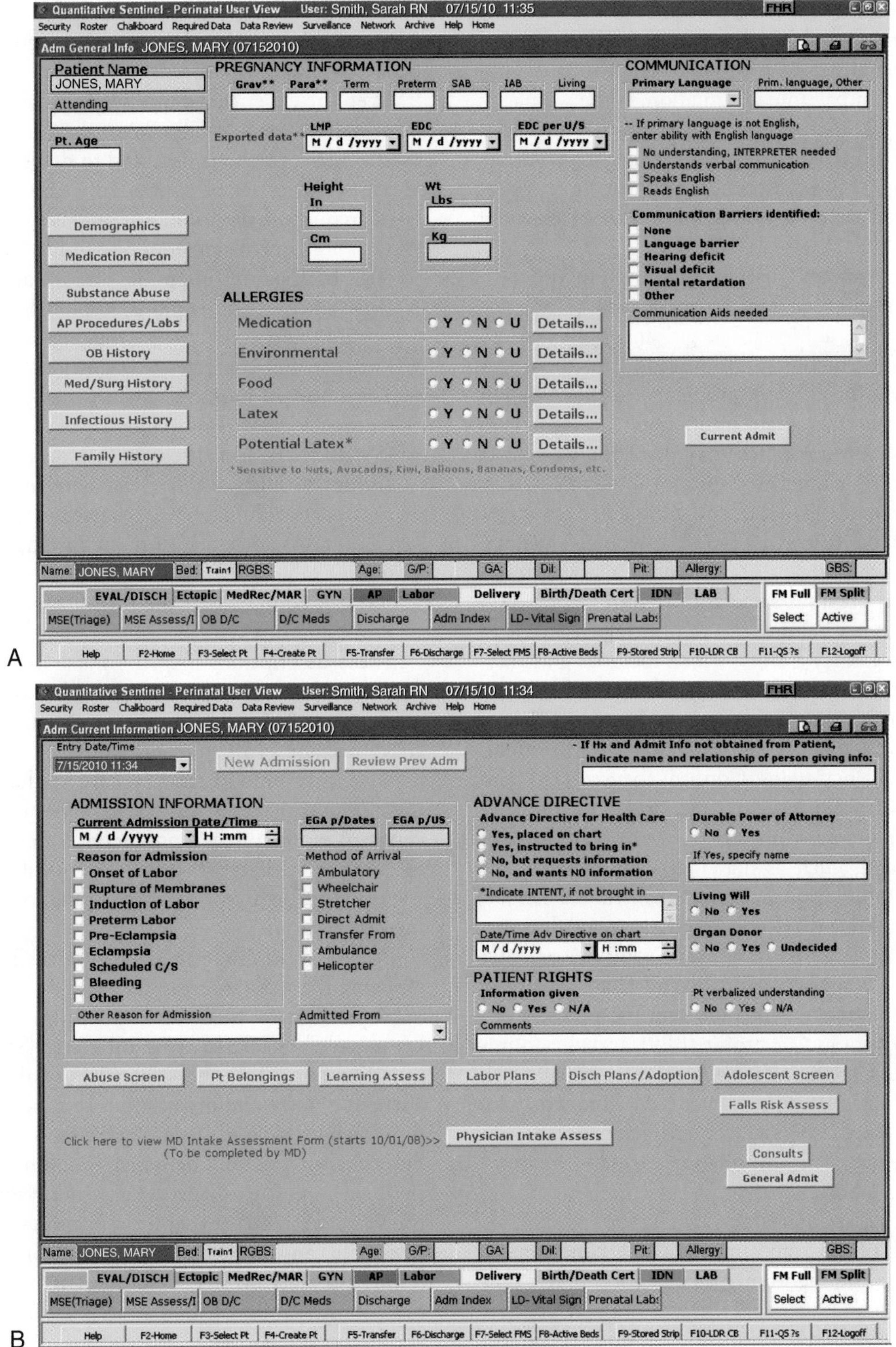

Fig. 12-2 Admission screens in an electronic patient record. **A**, General Admission screen. **B**, Current Admission screen. (Courtesy Kitty Cashion, Memphis, TN.)

done on computer. Sources of data include the prenatal record, the initial interview, physical examination to determine baseline physiologic parameters, laboratory and diagnostic test results, expressed psychosocial and cultural factors, and the clinical evaluation of labor status.

Prenatal data

The nurse reviews the prenatal record to identify the woman's individual needs and risks. Paper or electronic copies of prenatal records are generally filed in the perinatal unit at some time during the woman's pregnancy (usually in the third trimester) so that they are readily available on admission. If the woman has had no prenatal care or her prenatal record is unavailable, then the nurse must obtain certain baseline information. If the woman is having discomfort, then the nurse should ask questions between contractions when the woman can concentrate more fully on her answers. At times the partner or support person may need to be a secondary source of essential information.

Knowing the woman's age is important in order to individualize the plan of care to the needs of her age group. For example, a 14-year-old girl and a 40-year-old woman have different but specific needs, and their ages place them at risk for different problems. Accurate height and weight measurements are important. A weight gain greater than that recommended may place the woman at a higher risk for cephalopelvic disproportion and cesarean birth, especially if she is petite and has gained 16 kg or more. Other factors to consider are the woman's general health status, current medical conditions or allergies, respiratory status, and previous surgical procedures.

Thoroughly review her prenatal record. Take note of her obstetric and pregnancy history, which includes gravidity, parity, and problems such as history of vaginal bleeding, gestational hypertension, anemia, gestational diabetes, infections (e.g., bacterial, viral, or sexually transmitted), and immunodeficiency status. Confirm the expected date of birth (EDB). Other important data found in the prenatal record include patterns of maternal weight gain, physiologic measurements such as maternal vital signs (blood pressure, temperature, pulse, respirations), fundal height, baseline fetal heart rate (FHR), and laboratory and diagnostic test results. See Table 7-1 for a list of common prenatal laboratory tests. Common diagnostic and fetal assessment tests performed prenatally include amniocentesis, nonstress test (NST), biophysical profile (BPP), and ultrasound examination. See Chapter 19 for more information.

If this labor and birth experience is not the woman's first, the nurse needs to note the characteristics of her previous experiences. This information includes the duration of previous labors, the type of anesthesia used, the kind of birth (e.g., spontaneous vaginal, forceps-assisted, vacuum-assisted, or cesarean birth), and the condition of the newborn. Explore the woman's perception of her previous labor and birth experiences because this perception may influence her attitude toward her current experience.

Interview

The nurse determines the woman's chief complaint or reason for coming to the hospital in the interview. Her primary reason, for example, may be that her bag of waters (BOW, amniotic membranes) ruptured, with or without contractions. The woman may have come in for an obstetric check, a period of observation reserved for women who are unsure about the onset of their labor. This check allows time on the unit for the diagnosis of labor without official admission and minimizes or avoids cost to the patient when used by the hospital and approved by the woman's health insurance plan.

Even the experienced mother may have difficulty determining the onset of labor. Ask the woman to recall the events of the previous days and to describe the following:

- Time and onset of contractions and progress in terms of frequency, duration, and intensity
- Location and character of discomfort from contractions (e.g., back pain, suprapubic discomfort)
- Persistence of contractions despite changes in maternal position and activity (e.g., walking or lying down)
- Presence and character of vaginal discharge or show
- The status of amniotic membranes, such as a gush or seepage of fluid ([spontaneous] **rupture of membranes** [S] [ROM]). If a discharge has occurred that may be amniotic fluid, ask her the date and time she first noticed the fluid and its characteristics (e.g., amount, color, unusual odor). In many instances, a sterile speculum examination and a **Nitrazine (pH) test** or **fern test** can confirm that the membranes are ruptured (see Procedure box).

These descriptions help the nurse assess the degree of progress in the process of labor. **Bloody show** is distinguished from bleeding by the fact that it feels thick and sticky because of its mucoid nature.

Very little bloody show occurs in the beginning, but the amount increases with effacement and dilation of the cervix. A woman may report a small amount of brownish to bloody discharge that may be attributed to cervical trauma resulting from vaginal examination or coitus within the last 48 hours.

In case general anesthesia is needed in an emergency, assessing the woman's respiratory status is important. The nurse determines this status by asking the woman if she has a "cold" or related symptoms (e.g., "stuffy nose," sore throat, or cough). Recheck the status of allergies, including allergies to latex and medications routinely used in obstetrics, such as opioids (e.g., hydromorphone [Dilaudid], butorphanol [Stadol], fentanyl [Sublimaze], nalbuphine [Nubain], anesthetic agents (e.g., bupivacaine, lidocaine, ropivacaine), and antiseptics (Betadine). Some allergic responses cause swelling of the mucous membranes of the respiratory tract, which could interfere with breathing and the administration of inhalation anesthesia. Also, inquire about allergies to tape.

Because vomiting and subsequent aspiration into the respiratory tract can complicate an otherwise normal labor, the nurse records the time and type of the woman's most recent solid and liquid intake.

The nurse obtains any information not found in the prenatal record during the admission assessment. Pertinent data include the birth plan (Box 12-1), the choice of infant feeding method, the type of pain management preferred, and the name of the pediatric health care provider. Obtain a patient profile that identifies the woman's preparation

Procedure

Tests for Rupture of Membranes

NITRAZINE TEST FOR PH

- Explain procedure to the woman or couple.

Procedure

- Wash hands.
- Use a cotton-tipped applicator impregnated with Nitrazine dye for determining pH (differentiates amniotic fluid, which is slightly alkaline, from urine and purulent material [pus], which are acidic).
- Dip the cotton-tipped applicator deep into the vagina to pick up fluid. (Procedure may be performed during speculum examination.)

Read results

- Membranes probably intact: identifies vaginal and most body fluids that are acidic:

Yellow	pH 5.0
Olive-yellow	pH 5.5
Olive-green	pH 6.0

- Membranes probably ruptured: identifies amniotic fluid that is alkaline:

Blue-green	pH 6.5
Blue-gray	pH 7.0
Deep blue	pH 7.5

- Realize that false test results are possible because of presence of bloody show, insufficient amniotic fluid, or semen.
- Provide pericare as needed.
- Remove gloves and wash hands.

Document results

- Results are positive or negative.

TEST FOR FERNING OR FERN PATTERN

- Explain procedure to woman or couple.
- Wash hands, apply sterile gloves, obtain specimen of fluid (usually during sterile speculum examination).
- Spread a drop of fluid from the vagina on a clean glass slide with a sterile, cotton-tipped applicator.
- Allow fluid to dry.
- Examine the slide under microscope; observe for appearance of ferning (a frondlike crystalline pattern) (do not confuse with cervical mucus test, when high levels of estrogen cause the ferning).
- Observe for absence of ferning (alerts staff to possibility that amount of specimen was inadequate or that specimen was urine, vaginal discharge, or blood).
- Provide pericare as needed.
- Remove gloves and wash hands.

Document results

- Results are positive or negative.

for childbirth, the support person or family members desired during childbirth and their availability, and ethnic or cultural expectations and needs. Determine the woman's use of alcohol, drugs, and tobacco before or during pregnancy.

BOX 12-1

Birth Plan

The birth plan should include the woman's or the couple's preferences related to the following:

- Presence of birth companions such as the partner, older children, parents, friends, and doula and the role each will play
- Presence of other persons such as students, male attendants, and interpreters
- Clothing to be worn
- Environmental modifications such as lighting, music, privacy, focal point, and items from home such as pillows
- Labor activities such as preferred positions for labor and for birth, ambulation, birth balls, showers and whirlpool baths, and oral food and fluid intake
- List of comfort and relaxation measures
- Labor and birth medical interventions such as pharmacologic pain relief measures, intravenous therapy, electronic monitoring, induction or augmentation measures, and episiotomy
- Care and handling of the newborn immediately after birth, such as cutting of the cord, delaying eye care, and breastfeeding
- Cultural and religious requirements related to the care of the mother, newborn, and placenta

The childbirth.org website (www.childbirth.org) provides couples with an interactive birth plan along with examples of birth plans.

The nurse reviews the birth plan. If no written plan has been prepared, then the nurse helps the woman formulate a birth plan by describing options available and determining the woman's wishes and preferences. As caregiver and advocate the nurse integrates the woman's desires into the plan of care as much as possible. The nurse also prepares the woman for the possibility of change in her plan as labor progresses and assures her that the staff will provide information so that she can make informed decisions. The woman must also realize, however, that the longer her list of "wishes" is, the greater the likelihood that her expectations will not be met.

The nurse should discuss with the woman and her partner their plans for preserving childbirth memories by using photography and videotaping and provide information about the agency's policies regarding these practices and under what circumstances they are allowed. Protection of privacy and safety and infection control are major concerns for the expecting parents and the agency. The woman's record should reflect that the childbirth was recorded. Some hospitals and health care providers do not allow videotaping of the birth because of concerns related to legal liability.

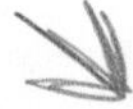

Psychosocial factors

The woman's general appearance and behavior (and that of her partner) provide valuable clues to the type of supportive care she will need. However, keep in mind that general appearance and behavior may vary, depending on the stage and phase of labor (Table 12-1 and Box 12-2).

Women with a history of sexual abuse. Labor can trigger memories of sexual abuse, especially during intrusive procedures such as vaginal examinations. Monitors, intravenous (IV) lines, and epidurals can make the woman feel a loss of control or feel as if she is being confined to bed and "restrained." Being watched by students and having intense sensations in the uterus and genital area, especially at the time when she must push the baby out, can also trigger memories.

The nurse can help the abuse survivor to associate the sensations she is experiencing with the process of childbirth and not with her past abuse. Help maintain her sense of control by explaining all procedures and why they are needed, validating her needs, and paying close attention to her requests. Wait for the woman to give permission before touching her, and accept her often extreme reactions to labor. Avoid words and phrases that can cause the woman to recall the words of her abuser (e.g., "open your legs," "relax and it won't hurt so much"). Limit the number of procedures that invade her body (e.g., vaginal examinations, urinary catheter, internal monitor, forceps or vacuum extractor) as much as possible. Encourage her to choose a person (e.g., doula, friend, family member) to be with her during labor to provide continuous support and comfort and to act as her advocate. Nurses are advised to care for all laboring women in this manner, because it is not unusual for a woman to choose not to reveal a history of sexual abuse. These care measures can help a woman to perceive her childbirth experience in positive terms.

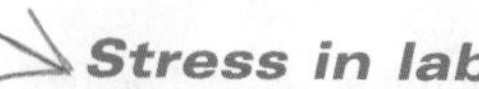

Stress in labor

The way in which women and their support person or family members approach labor is related to the manner in which they have been socialized to the childbearing process. Their reactions reflect their life experiences regarding childbirth–physical, social, cultural, and religious.

TABLE 12-1

Expected Maternal Progress in First Stage of Labor

CRITERION	PHASES MARKED BY CERVICAL DILATION*		
	LATENT (0-3 CM)	ACTIVE (4-7 CM)	TRANSITION (8-10 CM)
Duration†	Approx 6-8 hr	Approx 3-6 hr	Approx 20-40 min
Contractions			
Strength	Mild to moderate	Moderate to strong	Strong to very strong
Rhythm	Irregular	More regular	Regular
Frequency	5-30 min apart	3-5 min apart	2-3 min apart
Duration	30-45 sec	40-70 sec	45-90 sec
Descent			
Station of presenting part	Nulliparous: 0 Multiparous: −2 cm to 0	Varies: +1 to +2 cm Varies: +1 to +2 cm	Varies: +2 to +3 cm Varies: +2 to+3 cm
Show color	Brownish discharge, mucous plug, or pale pink mucus	Pink to bloody mucus	Bloody mucus
Amount	Scant	Scant to moderate	Copious
Behavior and appearance‡	Excited; thoughts center on self, labor, and baby; may be talkative or silent, calm or tense; some apprehension; pain controlled fairly well; alert, follows directions readily; open to instructions	Becomes more serious, doubtful of control of pain, more apprehensive; desires companionship and encouragement; attention more inwardly directed; fatigue evidenced; malar (cheeks) flush; has some difficulty following directions	Pain described as severe; backache common; frustration, fear of loss of control, and irritability may be voiced; vague in communications; amnesia between contractions; writhing with contractions; nausea and vomiting, especially if hyperventilating; hyperesthesia; circumoral pallor, perspiration of forehead and upper lip; shaking tremor of thighs; feeling of need to defecate, pressure on anus

*In the nullipara, effacement is often complete before dilation begins; in the multipara, effacement occurs simultaneously with dilation.

†Duration of each phase is influenced by such factors as parity, maternal emotions, position, level of activity, and fetal size, presentation, and position. For example, the labor of a nullipara tends to last longer, on average, than the labor of a multipara. Women who ambulate and assume upright positions or change positions frequently during labor tend to experience a shorter first stage. Descent is often prolonged in breech presentations and occiput posterior positions.

‡Women who have epidural analgesia for pain relief may not demonstrate some of these behaviors.

BOX 12-2

Psychosocial Assessment of the Laboring Woman

VERBAL INTERACTIONS

- Does the woman ask questions?
- Can she ask for what she needs?
- Does she talk to her support person or persons?
- Does she talk freely with the nurse or respond only to questions?

BODY LANGUAGE

- Is she relaxed or tense?
- What is her anxiety level?
- How does she react to being touched by the nurse or support person?
- Does she avoid eye contact?
- Does she look tired?

PERCEPTUAL ABILITY

- Does a language barrier exist?
- Are repeated explanations necessary because her anxiety level interferes with her ability to comprehend?
- Can she repeat what she has been told or otherwise demonstrate her understanding?

DISCOMFORT LEVEL

- To what degree does the woman describe what she is experiencing?
- How does she react to a contraction?
- Are any nonverbal pain messages noted?
- Does she ask for comfort measures?

Society communicates its expectations regarding acceptable and unacceptable maternal behaviors during labor and birth. Some women may use these expectations as the basis for evaluating their own actions during childbirth. An idealized perception of labor and birth may be a source of guilt and cause a sense of failure if the woman finds the process less than joyous, especially when the pregnancy is unplanned or is the product of a shaky or terminated relationship. In many instances, women have heard horror stories or have seen friends or relatives going through labors that appear anything but easy. Multiparous women will often base their expectations of the present labor on their previous childbirth experiences.

Discuss the feelings a woman has about her pregnancy and fears regarding childbirth. This discussion is especially important if the woman is a primigravida who has not attended childbirth classes or is a multiparous woman who has had a previous negative childbirth experience. Women in labor usually have a variety of concerns that they will voice if asked but rarely volunteer. Major fears and concerns relate to the process and effects of childbirth, maternal and fetal well-being, and the attitude and actions of the health care staff. Unresolved fears increase a woman's stress and can inhibit the process of labor as a result of the inhibiting effects of catecholamines associated with the stress response on uterine contractions (Zwelling, Johnson, & Allen, 2006).

The father, coach, or significant other also experiences stress during labor. The nurse can assist and support these individuals by identifying their needs and expectations and by helping make sure these are met. The nurse can determine what role the support person intends to fulfill and whether he or she is prepared for that role by making observations and asking her or himself such questions as, "Has the couple attended childbirth classes?" "What role does this person expect to play?" "Does he or she do all the talking?" "Is he or she nervous, anxious, aggressive, or hostile?" "Does he or she look hungry, tired, worried, or confused?" "Does he or she watch television, sleep, or stay out of the room instead of paying attention to the woman?" "Where does he or she sit?" "Does he or she touch the woman; what is the character of the touch?" Be sensitive to the needs of support persons and provide teaching and support as appropriate. In many instances the support these persons provide to the laboring woman is in direct proportion to the support they receive from the nurses and other health care providers.

Cultural factors

As the population in the United States and Canada becomes more diverse, noting the woman's ethnic or cultural and religious background is increasingly important so as to anticipate nursing interventions to add or eliminate from the individualized plan of care (Fig. 12-3). Nurses should be committed to providing culturally sensitive care and to developing an appreciation and respect for cultural diversity (Callister, 2005). Encourage the woman to request specific caregiving behaviors and practices that are important to her. If a special request contradicts usual practices in that setting, then the woman or the nurse can ask the woman's primary health care provider to write an order to accommodate the special request. For example, in many cultures, having a male caregiver examine a pregnant woman would be unacceptable. In some cultures, taking the placenta home is traditional; in other cultures the woman has only certain nourishments during labor. Some women believe that cutting the body, as with an episiotomy, allows the spirit to leave the body and that rupturing the membranes prolongs, not shortens, labor. The nurse should explain the rationale for required care measures carefully (see Cultural Considerations box).

Within cultures, women may have an idea of the "right" way to behave in labor and may react to the pain experienced in that way. These behaviors can range from total silence to moaning or screaming, but they do not necessarily indicate the degree of pain. A woman who moans with contractions may not be in as much physical pain as a woman who is silent but winces during contractions. Some women believe that screaming or crying out in pain is shameful if a man is present. If the woman's support person is her mother, she may perceive the need to

Cultural Considerations

Birth Practices in Different Cultures

Somalia: Because Somalis in general do not like to show any sign of weakness, women are extremely stoic during childbirth.

Japan: Natural childbirth methods practiced; may labor silently; may eat during labor; father may be present.

China: Stoic response to pain; fathers not usually present; side-lying position preferred for labor and birth because this position is thought to reduce infant trauma.

India: Natural childbirth methods preferred; father is not usually present; female relatives are usually present.

Iran: Fathers not present; female support and female caregivers preferred.

Mexico: May be stoic about discomfort until second stage, then may request pain relief; fathers and female relatives may be present.

Laos: May use squatting position for birth; fathers may or may not be present; female attendants preferred.

Source: D'Avanzo, C. E. (2008). *Mosby's pocket guide to cultural health assessment* (4th ed.). St. Louis: Mosby.

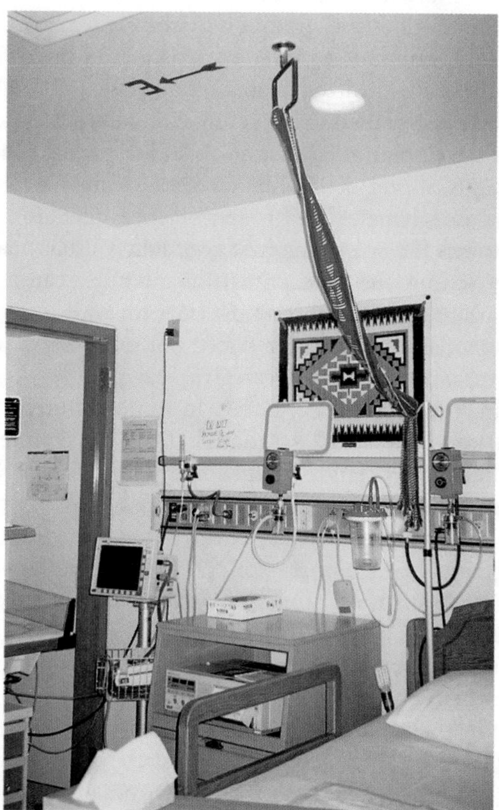

Fig. 12-3 Birthing room specific to a Native American population. Note the arrow pointing east, the rug on the wall, and the cord hanging from the ceiling. (Courtesy Patricia Hess, San Francisco, CA; Chinle Comprehensive Health Care Center, Chinle, AZ.)

"behave" more strongly than if her support person is the father of the baby. She will perceive herself as failing or succeeding based on her ability to follow these "standards" of behavior. Conversely, a woman's behavior in response to pain may influence the support received from significant others. In some cultures, women who lose control and cry out in pain are scolded, whereas in other cultures, support persons will become more helpful.

A companion is an important source of support, encouragement, and comfort for women during childbirth. The woman's cultural and religious background influences her choice of birth companion. Trends in the society in which she lives also influence her choice. For example, in Western societies the father is viewed as the ideal birth companion. For European-American couples, attending childbirth classes together has become a traditional, expected activity. Laotian (Hmong) husbands also traditionally participate actively in the labor process. In some other cultures the father may be available, but his presence in the labor room with the mother may not be considered appropriate, or he may be present but resist active involvement in her care. Such behavior could be perceived by the nursing staff to indicate a lack of concern, caring, or interest. Women from many cultures prefer female caregivers and want to have at least one female companion present during labor and birth. If couples from these cultures immigrate to the United States or Canada, their roles may change. The nurse will need to talk to the woman and her support persons to determine the roles they will assume.

The non–English-speaking woman in labor. A woman's level of anxiety in labor increases when she does not understand what is happening to her or what is being said. Non–English-speaking women often feel a complete loss of control over their situation if no health care provider is present who speaks their language. They can panic and withdraw or become physically abusive when someone tries to do something they perceive might harm them or their babies. A support person is sometimes able to serve as an interpreter. However, caution is warranted because the interpreter may not be able to convey exactly what the nurse or others are saying or what the woman is saying, which can increase the woman's stress level even more.

Ideally, a bilingual nurse will care for the woman. Alternatively, contact a hospital employee or volunteer interpreter for assistance (see Box 1-7). Ideally, the interpreter is from the woman's culture. For some women a female interpreter is more acceptable than a male interpreter. If no one in the hospital is able to interpret, call a service so that interpretation can take place over the telephone. Even when the nurse has limited ability to communicate verbally with the woman, in most instances the woman appreciates the nurse's efforts to do so. Speaking slowly and avoiding complex words and medical terms can help a woman and her partner to understand.

Physical examination

The initial physical examination includes a general systems assessment and an assessment of fetal status. During the examination, uterine contractions are assessed and a vaginal examination is performed. The findings of the admission physical examination serve as a baseline for assessing the woman's progress from that point.

The information obtained from a complete and accurate assessment during the initial examination serves as the basis for determining whether the woman should be admitted and what her ongoing care should be. Expected maternal progress and minimal assessment guidelines during the first stage of labor are presented in Table 12-1 and the Care Path for the Low Risk Woman in the First Stage of Labor.

Standard Precautions should guide all assessment and care measures (Box 12-3). Explain the assessment findings to the woman whenever possible. Throughout labor, accurately document any procedure as soon as possible after it has been performed (Fig. 12-4).

General systems assessment. A brief systems assessment is performed, which includes an assessment of the heart, lungs, and skin and an examination to determine the presence and extent of edema of the legs, face, hands, and sacrum. It also includes testing of deep tendon reflexes and for clonus.

Vital signs. Assess vital signs (temperature, pulse, respirations, and blood pressure) on admission. The initial

BOX 12-3

Standard Precautions during Childbirth

- Wash hands or use cleansing foam before and after putting on gloves and performing procedures.
- Wear gloves (clean or sterile, as appropriate) when performing procedures that require contact with the woman's genitalia and body fluids, including bloody show (e.g., during vaginal examination, amniotomy, hygienic care of the perineum, insertion of an internal scalp electrode and intrauterine pressure monitor, urinary catheterization).
- Wear a mask that has a shield or protective eyewear and a cover gown when assisting with the birth. Cap and shoe covers are worn for cesarean birth but are optional for vaginal birth in a birthing room. Gowns worn by the primary health care provider who is attending the birth should have a waterproof front and sleeves and should be sterile.
- Drape the woman with sterile towels and sheets as appropriate. Explain to the woman what can and cannot be touched.
- Help the woman's partner put on appropriate coverings for the type of birth, such as cap, mask, gown, and shoe covers. Show the partner where to stand and what can and cannot be touched.
- Wear gloves and gown when handling the newborn immediately after birth.
- Use an appropriate method to suction the newborn's airway, such as a bulb syringe or mechanical wall suction.

Spanish Guidelines: Labor Assessment

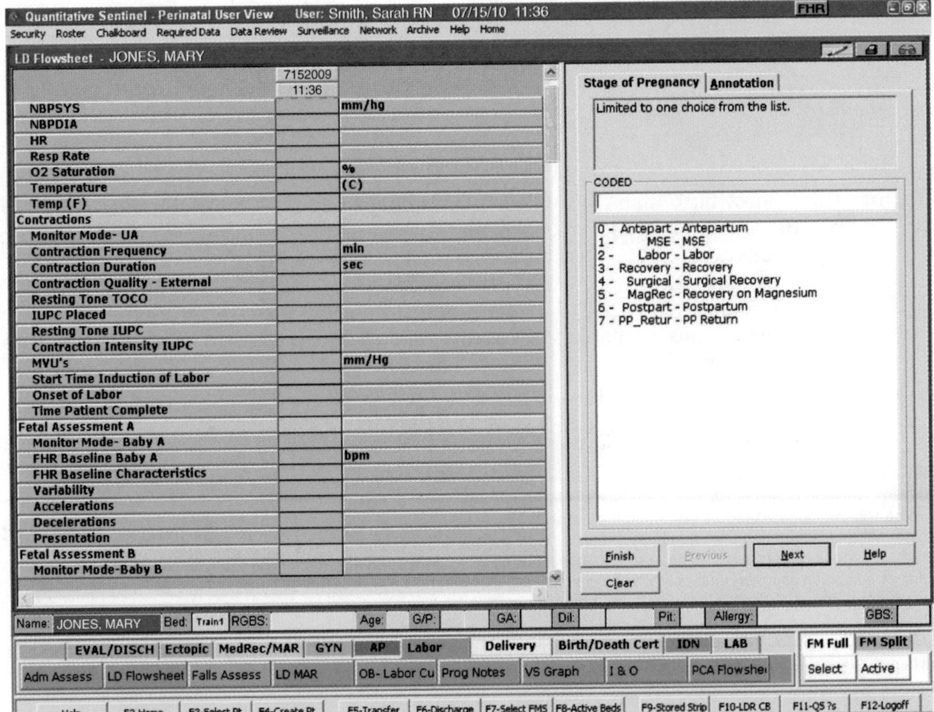

Fig. 12-4 Portion of the Labor Flowsheet screen in an electronic patient record. (Courtesy Kitty Cashion, Memphis, TN.)

CARE PATH Low Risk Woman in First Stage of Labor

CARE MANAGEMENT	CERVICAL DILATION		
	0-3 cm (latent)	4-7 cm (active)	8-10 cm (transition)
I. ASSESSMENT MEASURES*	FREQUENCY		
Blood pressure, pulse, respirations	Every 30-60 min	Every 30 min	Every 15-30 min
Temperature†	Every 4 hr	Every 4 hr	Every 4 hr
Uterine activity	Every 30-60 min	Every 15-30 min	Every 10-15 min
Fetal heart rate	Every 30-60 min	Every 15-30 min	Every 15-30 min
Vaginal show	Every 30-60 min	Every 30 min	Every 15 min
Behavior, appearance, mood, energy level of woman; condition of partner	Every 30 min	Every 15 min	Every 5 min
Vaginal examination‡	As needed to identify progress	As needed to identify progress	As needed to identify progress
II. Physical Care Measures§	Stay at home for as long as possible Relaxation measures; rest and sleep if at night Activity—ambulation; emphasize upright positions Diversional activities Nourishment—light foods and full liquids Encourage to void every 2 hr Perform basic hygiene measures	Coach breathing techniques Encourage effleurage Assist in using relaxation techniques between contractions Encourage ambulation, upright positions Assist with position changes Use comfort measures desired by woman: massage, hot or cold packs, touch, etc. Initiate hydrotherapy (shower, bath, Jacuzzi) Provide nourishment as desired Encourage voiding every 2 hr Assist with hygiene, perineal care Provide pharmacologic pain relief as requested by the woman and ordered by the primary health care provider Provide relief for partner	Coach breathing techniques Reduce touch if increased sensitivity is noted Help to relax between contractions Assist with position changes Use comfort measures according to acceptance level Continue hydrotherapy if effective Provide sips of clear liquids or ice chips Encourage voiding every 2 hr Provide hygiene measures, emphasizing mouth and perineal care Provide pharmacologic pain relief as requested by the woman and ordered by the primary health care provider Prepare for birth
III. Emotional Support	Review birth plan Review process of labor—what to expect, pain management techniques available Redemonstrate breathing techniques Keep informed: progress, procedures	Provide feedback about performance Reduce distractions during contractions Role model comfort measures Reassure, encourage, praise Take charge as needed, talk through contraction until control regained Continue to keep informed	Provide continuous support Reduce distractions Role model care measures to assist partner Continue reassurance, praise, and encouragement Keep informed Take charge as needed

*Full assessment using interview, physical examination, and laboratory testing is initiated on admission. Subsequently, frequency of assessment is determined by the risk status of the maternal-fetal unit. More frequent assessment is required in high risk situations. Frequency of assessment and method of documentation are also determined by agency policy, which is usually based on the recommended care standards of medical and nursing organizations.

†If membranes have ruptured, then the temperature should be assessed at least every 2 hr; assess orally or tympanically between contractions.

‡Perform vaginal examination at admission and thereafter only when signs indicate that progress has occurred (e.g., significant increase in frequency, duration, and intensity of contractions; rupture of membranes; perineal pressure); strict aseptic technique should be used. In the presence of vaginal bleeding, ultrasound examination is performed to determine placental location.

§Physical care measures are performed by the nurse working together with the woman's partner and significant others. The woman is capable of greater independence in the latent phase but needs more assistance during the active and transition phases.

values are used as the baseline for comparison for all future measurements. If the blood pressure is elevated, reassess it 30 minutes later, between contractions, using a correct-size blood pressure cuff to obtain a reading after the woman has relaxed. Encourage the woman to lie on her side to prevent supine hypotension and fetal distress (Fig. 12-5). Monitor her temperature so that you can identify signs of infection or a fluid deficit (e.g., dehydration associated with inadequate intake of fluids).

Leopold maneuvers (abdominal palpation). Leopold maneuvers are performed with the woman briefly lying on her back (see Procedure box). These maneuvers help identify the (1) number of fetuses; (2) presenting part, fetal lie, and fetal attitude; (3) degree of the presenting part's descent into the pelvis; and (4) expected location of the point of maximal intensity (PMI) of the fetal heart rate (FHR) on the woman's abdomen.

Assessment of fetal heart rate. The point of maximal intensity (PMI) of the FHR is the location on the maternal abdomen at which the FHR is heard the loudest. It is usually directly over the fetal back (Fig. 12-6). In a vertex presentation, you can usually hear the FHR below the mother's umbilicus in either the right or the left lower quadrant of the abdomen. In a breech presentation, you usually hear the FHR above the mother's umbilicus. The Care Path for Low Risk Woman in First Stage of Labor summarizes assessments recommended for determining fetal status. In addition, you must assess the FHR after ROM because this is the most common time for the umbilical cord to prolapse, after any change in the contraction pattern or maternal status, and before and after the woman receives medication or a procedure is performed (Tucker et al., 2009).

Assessment of uterine contractions. A general characteristic of effective labor is regular uterine

Procedure

Assessment Video: Leopold Maneuvers

Leopold Maneuvers

- Wash hands.
- Ask woman to empty bladder.
- Position woman supine with one pillow under her head and with her knees slightly flexed.
- Place small, rolled towel under woman's right or left hip to displace uterus off major blood vessels (prevents supine hypotensive syndrome; see Fig. 12-5, *D*).
- *If right-handed, stand on woman's right, facing her:*
  1. Identify fetal part that occupies the fundus. The head feels round, firm, freely movable, and palpable by ballottement; the breech feels less regular and softer. This maneuver identifies fetal lie (longitudinal or transverse) and presentation (cephalic or breech) (Fig. A).
  2. Using palmar surface of one hand, locate and palpate the smooth convex contour of the fetal back and the irregularities that identify the small parts (feet, hands, elbows). This maneuver helps identify fetal presentation (Fig. B).
  3. With right hand, determine which fetal part is presenting over the inlet to the true pelvis. Gently grasp the lower pole of the uterus between the thumb and fingers, pressing in slightly (Fig. C). If the head is presenting and not engaged, determine the attitude of the head (flexed or extended).
  4. Turn to face the woman's feet. Using both hands, outline the fetal head (Fig. D) with the palmar surface of the fingertips. When the presenting part has descended deeply, only a small portion of it may be outlined. Palpation of the cephalic prominence helps identify the attitude of the head. If the cephalic prominence is found on the same side as the small parts, this means that the head must be flexed and the vertex is presenting (see Fig. D). If the cephalic prominence is on the same side as the back, this indicates that the presenting head is extended and the face is presenting.
- Document fetal presentation, position, and lie and whether presenting part is flexed or extended, engaged, or free floating. Use agency's protocol for documentation (e.g., "Vtx, LOA, floating").

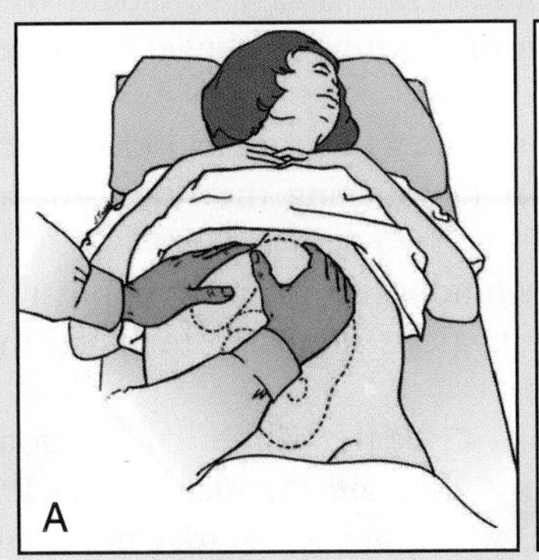

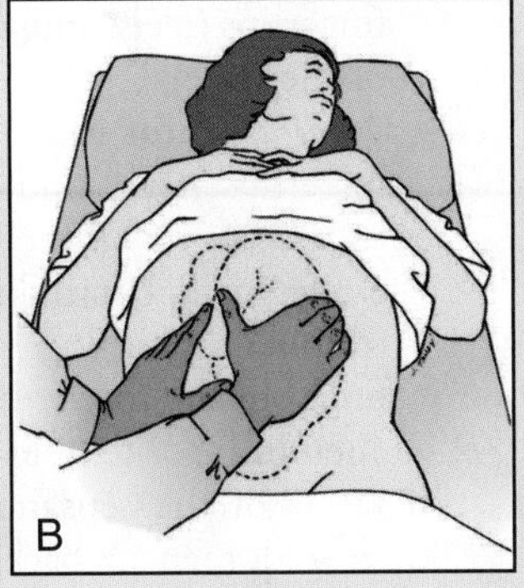

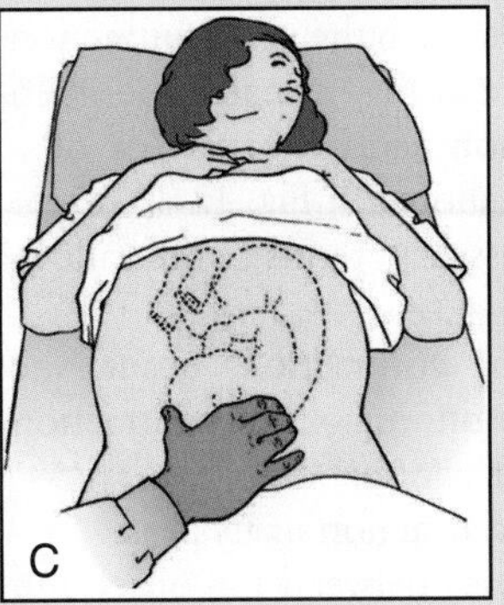

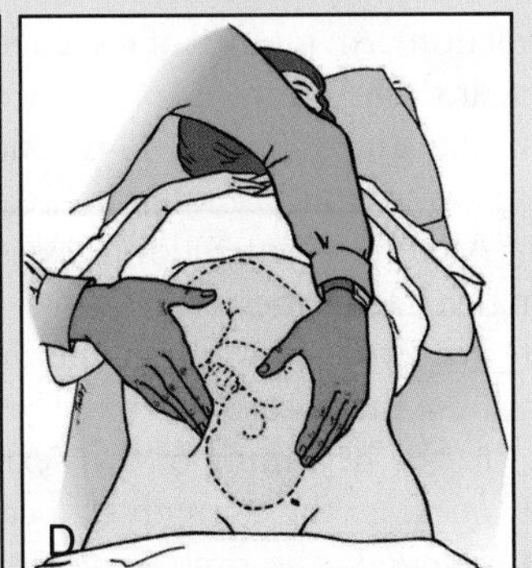

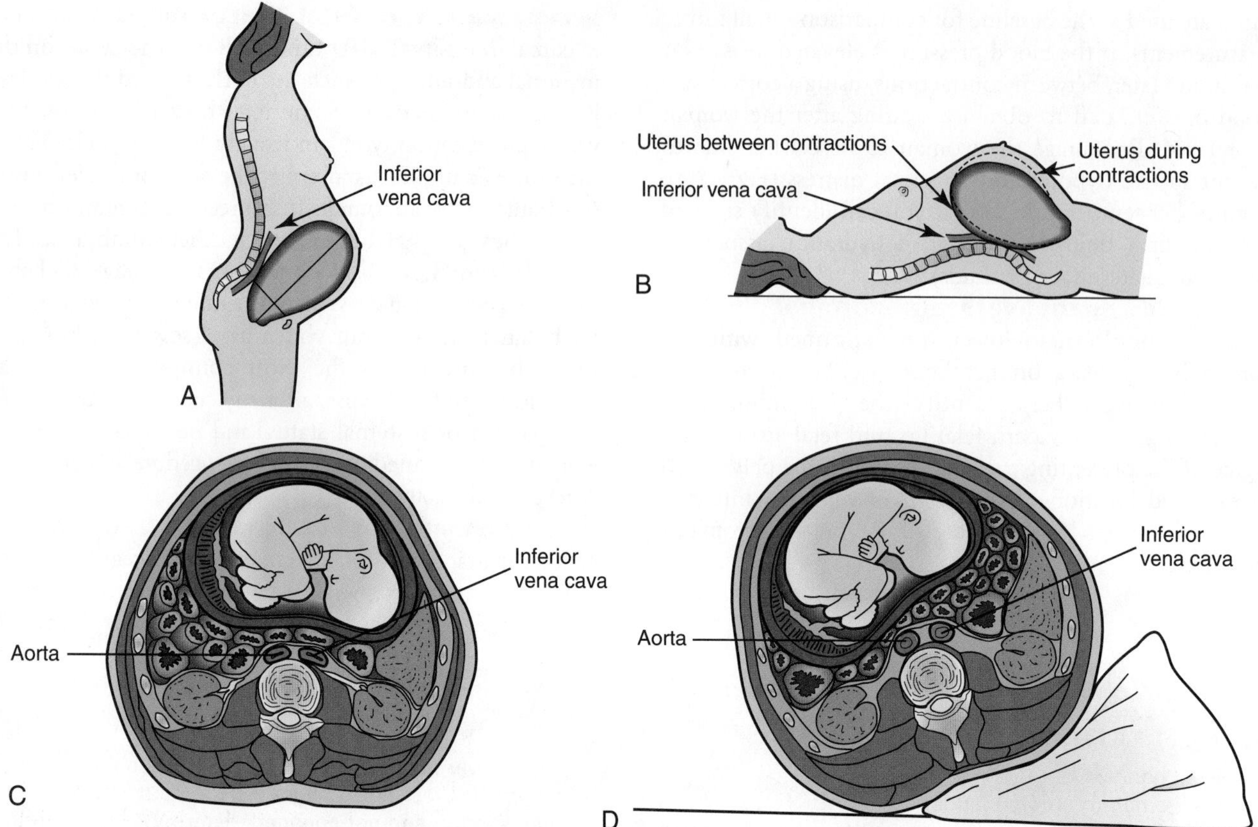

Fig. 12-5 Supine hypotension. Note relation of pregnant uterus to ascending vena cava in standing position (**A**), and in the supine position (**B**). **C**, Compression of aorta and inferior vena cava with woman in supine position. **D**, Compression of these vessels is relieved by placement of a wedge pillow under the woman's right side.

activity (i.e., contractions becoming more frequent with increased duration), but uterine activity is not directly related to labor progress. **Uterine contractions** are the primary powers that act involuntarily to expel the fetus and the placenta from the uterus. Several methods can be used to evaluate uterine contractions, including the woman's subjective description, palpation and timing of contractions by a health care provider, and electronic monitoring.

Each contraction exhibits a wavelike pattern. It begins with a slow increment (the "building up" of a contraction from its onset), gradually reaches a peak, and then diminishes rapidly (decrement, the "letting down" of the contraction). An interval of rest ends when the next contraction begins. The outward appearance of the woman's abdomen during and between contractions and the pattern of a typical uterine contraction are shown in Fig. 12-7.

A uterine contraction is assessed in terms of the following characteristics:

- *Frequency:* how often uterine contractions occur; the time that elapses from the beginning of one contraction to the beginning of the next contraction
- *Intensity:* the strength of a contraction at its peak
- *Duration:* the time that elapses between the onset and the end of a contraction
- *Resting tone:* the tension in the uterine muscle between contractions; relaxation of the uterus

You assess uterine contractions by palpation or by using an external or internal electronic monitor (see Chapter 11 for further discussion). You measure frequency and duration by all three methods of uterine activity monitoring. The accuracy of determining intensity varies by the method used. The woman's description and palpation are more subjective and a less precise way of determining the intensity of uterine contractions than is the electronic fetal monitor. The following terms describe what is felt on palpation:

- *Mild:* slightly tense fundus that is easy to indent with fingertips (feels similar to touching the finger to the tip of the nose)
- *Moderate:* firm fundus that is difficult to indent with fingertips (feels similar to touching the finger to the chin)
- *Strong:* rigid, boardlike fundus that is almost impossible to indent with fingertips (feels similar to touching the finger to the forehead)

Women in labor tend to describe the pain of contractions in terms of the sensations they are experiencing in the lower abdomen or back, which are sometimes unrelated to the firmness of the uterine fundus. Therefore their

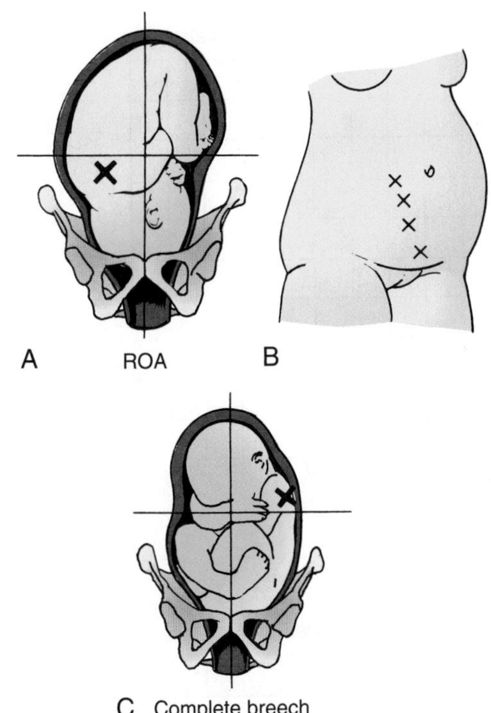

Fig. 12-6 Location of the fetal heart tones (FHTs). **A**, FHTs with fetus in right occipitoanterior (ROA) position. **B**, Changes in location of point of maximal intensity of FHTs as fetus undergoes internal rotation from ROA to OA and descent for birth. **C**, FHTs with fetus in left sacrum posterior position. (**A** and **C**, Courtesy Ross Laboratories, Columbus, OH.)

assessment of the strength of their contractions can be less accurate than that of the health care provider, although the amount of discomfort reported is valid.

External electronic monitoring provides some information about the relative strength of the uterine contractions. Internal electronic monitoring with an intrauterine pressure catheter, however, is the most accurate way of assessing the intensity of uterine contractions.

The Care Path for Low Risk Woman in First Stage of Labor summarizes assessments recommended for determining the status of contractions.

NURSING ALERT If you find the characteristics of contractions to be abnormal, either exceeding or falling below what is considered acceptable in terms of the standard characteristics, report this finding to the primary health care provider.

You must consider uterine activity in the context of its effect on cervical effacement and dilation and on the degree of descent of the presenting part (see Chapter 9). You must also consider the effect on the fetus. You can verify the progress of labor effectively through the use of graphic charts (partograms) on which you plot cervical dilation and station (descent). This type of graphic charting assists in early identification of deviations from expected labor patterns. Fig. 12-8 provides examples of partograms. Hospitals and birthing centers may develop their own graphs for recording assessments. Such graphs may include not only data on dilation and descent, but also data on maternal vital signs, FHR, and uterine activity.

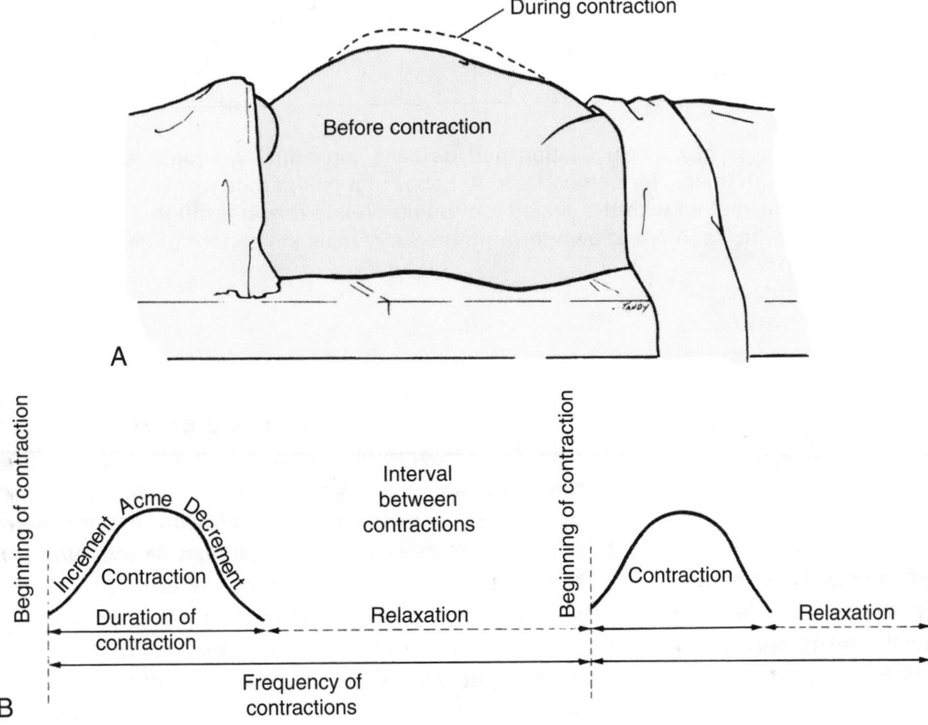

Fig. 12-7 Assessment of uterine contractions. **A**, Abdominal contour before and during uterine contraction. **B**, Wavelike pattern of contractile activity.

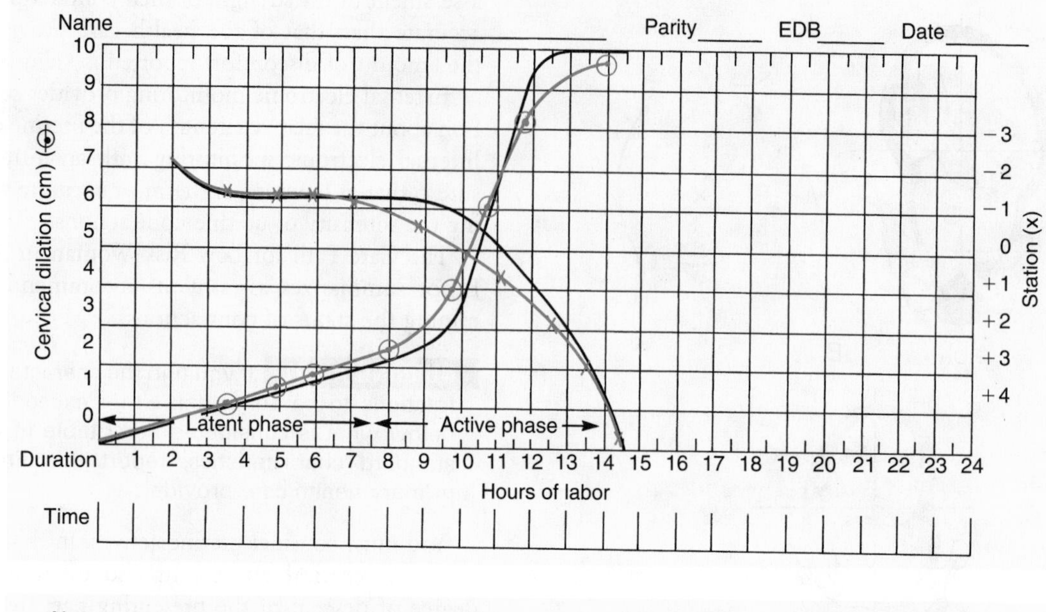

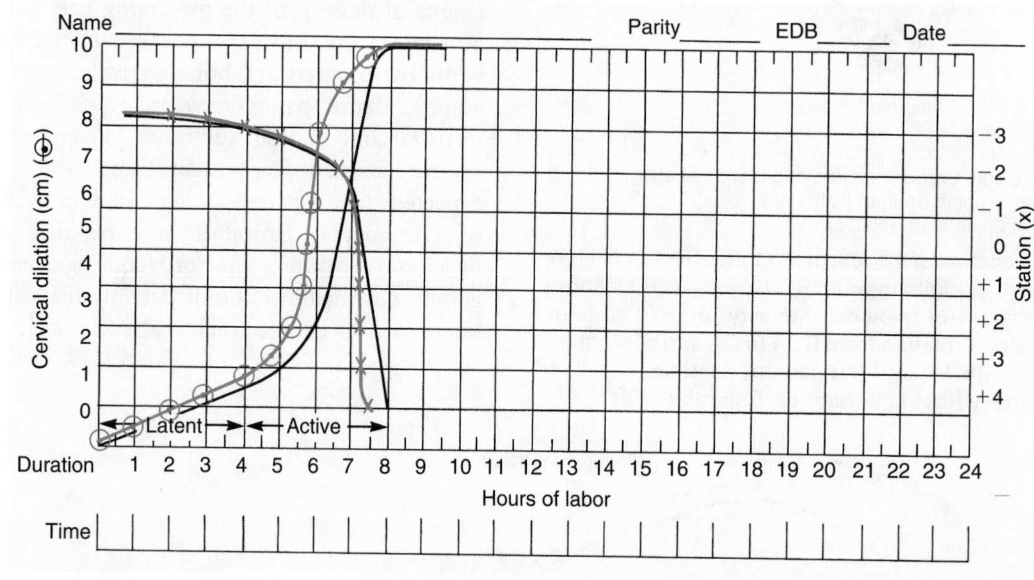

Fig. 12-8 Partograms for assessment of patterns of cervical dilation and descent. Individual woman's labor patterns (colored) are superimposed on prepared labor graph (black) for comparison. **A**, Labor of a nulliparous woman. **B**, Labor of a multiparous woman. The rate of cervical dilation is plotted with the circled plot points. A line drawn through these symbols depicts the slope of the curve. Station is plotted with Xs. A line drawn through the Xs reveals the pattern of descent.

NURSING ALERT The nurse should recognize that active labor can actually last longer than the expected labor patterns because all women are different. This finding is not a cause for concern unless the maternal-fetal unit exhibits signs of stress (e.g., nonreassuring FHR patterns, maternal fever).

Vaginal examination. The vaginal examination reveals whether the woman is in true labor and enables the examiner to determine whether the membranes have ruptured (Fig. 12-9). Because this examination is often stressful and uncomfortable for the woman, perform it only when indicated by the status of the woman and her fetus. For example, you should perform a vaginal examination on admission, when significant change has occurred in uterine activity, on maternal perception of perineal pressure or the urge to bear down, when membranes rupture, or when you note variable decelerations of the FHR. A full explanation of the examination and support of the woman are important factors in reducing the stress and discomfort associated with the examination. (See Procedure Box: Vaginal Examination of the Laboring Woman.)

Laboratory and diagnostic tests

Analysis of urine specimen. A clean-catch urine specimen may be obtained to gather further data about the pregnant woman's health. It is a convenient and simple procedure that can provide information about her hydration status (e.g., specific gravity, color, amount), nutritional status (e.g., ketones), infection status (e.g., leukocytes), and the status of possible complications such as preeclampsia, shown by finding protein in the urine. In most hospitals this test must be performed in the laboratory rather than at the bedside, even if a urine "dip stick" is used.

Blood tests. The blood tests performed vary with the hospital protocol and the woman's health status. Currently, all blood tests must be performed in the hospital laboratory rather than on the perinatal unit. Blood samples are often obtained from the hub of the catheter when IV access is obtained. A hematocrit evaluation will likely be ordered. More comprehensive blood assessments such as white blood cell count, red blood cell count, the hemoglobin level, hematocrit, and platelet values are included in a complete blood cell count (CBC). A CBC may be ordered for women with a history of infection, anemia, gestational hypertension, or other disorders. If human immunodeficiency virus (HIV) testing was not performed during the third trimester of pregnancy, a rapid HIV test should be performed on admission.

Most hospitals require that a "type and screen," to determine the woman's blood type and Rh status, be performed on admission. Even if these tests have already been performed during pregnancy the hospital's laboratory or blood bank must verify the results in-house.

If the woman had no prenatal care or if her prenatal records are not available, then a "prenatal screen" will probably be drawn on admission. The prenatal screen includes laboratory tests that would normally have been drawn at the initial prenatal visit (see Table 7-1).

Other tests. If the woman's group B *Streptococcus* status is not known, a rapid test may be performed on admission. The rapid test results are usually available within an hour or so and will determine if the woman must be given antibiotics during labor.

Assessment of amniotic membranes and fluid. Labor is initiated at term by SROM in approximately 25% of pregnant women. A lag period, rarely exceeding 24 hours, may precede the onset of labor. Membranes (the BOW) also can rupture spontaneously at any time during labor but most commonly in the transition phase of the first stage of labor. The Procedure Box called Tests for Rupture of Membranes explains how to determine if membranes are ruptured. If the membranes do not rupture spontaneously, the BOW will be ruptured artificially at some time during labor. Artificial rupture of membranes (AROM), called an **amniotomy,** is performed by the physician or certified nurse midwife using a plastic Amnihook or a surgical clamp.

Whether the membranes rupture spontaneously or artificially, the time of rupture should be recorded. Other necessary documentation includes information regarding the color (clear or meconium-stained), estimated amount, and odor of the fluid. See Chapter 22 for additional information.

Procedure

Vaginal Examination of the Laboring Woman

- Use a sterile glove and antiseptic solution or soluble gel for lubrication.
- Position the woman to prevent supine hypotension.
- Cleanse the perineum and vulva if needed.
- After obtaining the woman's permission to touch her, gently insert the index and middle fingers into the woman's vagina.
- Determine:
  - Dilation, effacement, and position of the cervix
  - Presenting part, position, and station
  - Status of membranes (intact, bulging, or ruptured)
  - If membranes are ruptured, color, estimated amount, and odor of fluid
- Explain findings of the examination to the woman.
- Document findings and report to primary health care provider.

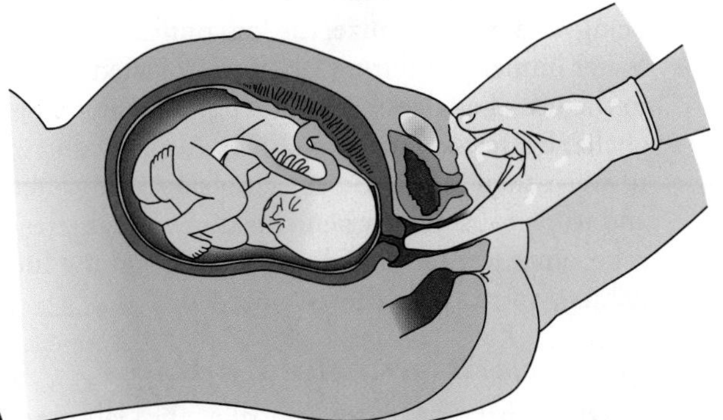

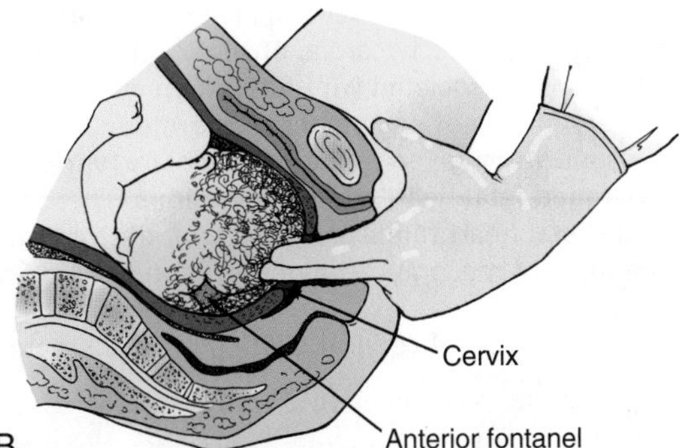

Fig. 12-9 Vaginal examination. **A,** Undilated, uneffaced cervix; membranes intact. **B,** Palpation of sagittal suture line. Cervix effaced and partially dilated.

NURSING ALERT The umbilical cord may prolapse when the membranes rupture. Monitor the FHR and pattern closely for several minutes immediately after ROM to ensure fetal well-being, and document the findings.

When membranes rupture, microorganisms from the vagina can then ascend into the amniotic sac, causing chorioamnionitis and placentitis to develop. For this reason, assess maternal temperature and vaginal discharge frequently (at least every 2 hours) so that you can quickly identify an infection developing after ROM. Even when membranes are intact, however, microorganisms may ascend and cause infection.

Signs of potential problems

Assessment findings serve as a baseline for evaluating the woman's subsequent progress during labor. Although you should anticipate some problems of labor, others may appear unexpectedly during the clinical course of labor (see Signs of Potential Complications box).

Nursing Diagnoses

Possible nursing diagnoses appropriate for the woman in the first stage of labor include:

- *Anxiety* related to:
  - Negative experience with previous childbirth
  - Triggering of memories associated with history of sexual abuse
  - Cultural differences
- *Acute pain* related to:
  - Effects of uterine contractions and fetal descent
- *Impaired urinary elimination* related to:
  - Reduced intake of oral fluids
  - Diminished sensation of bladder fullness associated with epidural anesthesia or analgesia
- *Impaired fetal gas exchange* related to:
  - Maternal hypotension
  - Maternal position
  - Intense and frequent uterine contractions
  - Compression of the umbilical cord
- *Situational low self-esteem (maternal)* related to:
  - Inability to meet self-expectations regarding performance during childbirth
  - Loss of control during labor
- *Situational low self-esteem (father or partner)* related to:
  - Unrealistic expectations regarding role as labor coach
  - Perceived ineffectiveness in meeting the needs of the laboring woman

Expected Outcomes of Care

Expected outcomes for the woman in the first stage of labor are that she will accomplish the following:

- Continue normal progression of labor while the FHR and pattern remain reassuring.
- Maintain adequate hydration status through oral or IV intake (or both).
- Actively participate in the labor process.
- Verbalize discomfort and indicate the need for measures that help reduce discomfort and promote relaxation.
- Accept comfort and support measures from significant others and health care providers as needed.
- Sustain no injury to herself or the fetus.

Plan of Care and Interventions

The various physical needs, the required interventions, and the rationale for care are presented in Table 12-2, the Nursing Care Plan on p. 353, and the Care Path: Low Risk Woman in First Stage Labor, on p. 346.

General hygiene

Offer women in labor the use of showers or warm water baths, if they are available, to enhance the feeling of well-being and to minimize the discomfort of contractions. Water immersion during labor is associated with decreases in the use of analgesia and in reported maternal pain (Berghella, Baxter, & Chauhan, 2008). Also, encourage women to wash their hands or use cleansing foam after voiding and to perform self-hygiene measures. Change the linen if it becomes wet or stained with blood, and use linen savers (Chux), and change them as needed.

Nutrient and fluid intake

Oral intake. Traditionally the laboring woman could only have clear liquids or ice chips or was given nothing by mouth during the active phase of labor to

signs of POTENTIAL COMPLICATIONS

Labor

- Intrauterine pressure of ≥80 mm Hg (determined by intrauterine pressure catheter monitoring) or resting tone of ≥20 mm Hg
- Contractions lasting ≥90 sec
- More than 5 contractions in a 10-minute period
- Relaxation between contractions lasting <30 sec
- Fetal bradycardia; tachycardia; absent or minimal variability not associated with fetal sleep cycle or temporary effects of central nervous system depressant drugs given to the woman; late, variable, or prolonged fetal heart rate decelerations
- Irregular fetal heart rate; suspected fetal dysrhythmias
- Appearance of meconium-stained or bloody fluid from the vagina
- Arrest in progress of cervical dilation or effacement, descent of the fetus, or both
- Maternal temperature of ≥38° C
- Foul-smelling vaginal discharge
- Continuous bright- or dark-red vaginal bleeding

NURSING CARE PLAN *Labor and Birth*

NURSING DIAGNOSIS Anxiety related to labor and the birthing process

Expected Outcome *Woman exhibits decreased signs of anxiety.*

Nursing Interventions/*Rationales*

- Orient the woman and significant others to the labor and birth unit and explain the admission protocol *to allay initial feelings of anxiety.*
- Assess the woman's knowledge, experience, and expectations of labor; note any signs or expressions of anxiety, nervousness, or fear *to establish a baseline for intervention.*
- Discuss the expected progression of labor, and describe what to expect during the process *to allay anxiety associated with the unknown.*
- Actively involve the woman in care decisions during labor, interpret sights and sounds of the environment (monitor sights and sounds, unit activities), and share information on the progression of labor (vital signs, fetal heart rate, dilation, effacement) *to increase her sense of control and allay fears.*

NURSING DIAGNOSIS Acute pain related to increasing frequency and intensity of contractions

Expected Outcome *Woman exhibits signs of ability to cope with discomfort.*

Nursing Interventions/*Rationales*

- Assess the woman's level of pain and strategies that she has used to cope with pain *to establish a baseline for intervention.*
- Encourage the significant other to remain as a support person during the labor process *to assist with support and comfort measures because measures are often more effective when delivered by a familiar person.*
- Instruct the woman and support person in use of specific techniques such as conscious relaxation, focused breathing, effleurage, massage, and application of sacral pressure *to increase relaxation, decrease the intensity of contractions, and promote the use of controlled thought and direction of energy.*
- Provide comfort measures such as frequent mouth care *to prevent dry mouth;* application of damp cloth to the forehead and changing of damp gown or bed covers *to relieve discomfort associated with diaphoresis.*
- Help the woman change position *to reduce stiffness and promote comfort.*
- Explain the analgesics and anesthesia that are available for use during labor and birth *to provide knowledge to help the woman make decisions about pain control.*
- Administer analgesics and assist with regional anesthesia (e.g., epidural) as ordered or desired *to provide effective pain relief during labor and birth.*

NURSING DIAGNOSIS Risk for impaired urinary elimination related to sensory impairment secondary to labor

Expected Outcome *Bladder does not show signs of distention.*

Nursing Interventions/*Rationales*

- Palpate the bladder superior to the symphysis on a frequent basis (at least every 2 hours) *to detect a full bladder that occurs from increased fluid intake and the inability to feel the urge to void.*
- Encourage frequent voiding (at least every 2 hours), and catheterize if necessary *to prevent bladder distention because it impedes the progress of the fetus down the birth canal and may result in trauma to the bladder.*
- Assist to the bathroom or bedside commode to void if appropriate, provide privacy, and use techniques to stimulate voiding such as running water *to facilitate bladder emptying with an upright position (natural) and relaxation.*

NURSING DIAGNOSIS Risk for ineffective individual coping related to birthing process

Expected Outcome *Woman actively participates in the birth process with no evidence of injury to her or her fetus.*

Nursing Interventions/*Rationales*

- Constantly monitor events of labor and birth, including physiologic responses of the woman and fetus and emotional responses of the woman and partner, *to ensure maternal, partner, and fetal well-being.*
- Provide ongoing feedback to the woman and partner *to allay anxiety and enhance participation.*
- Continue to provide comfort measures and minimize distractions *to decrease discomfort and aid in the focus on the birth process.*
- Encourage the woman to experiment with various positions *to assist downward movement of the fetus.*
- Ensure that the woman takes deep cleansing breaths before and after each contraction *to enhance gas exchange and oxygen transport to the fetus.*
- Encourage the woman to push spontaneously when the urge to bear down is perceived during a contraction *to aid the descent and rotation of the fetus.*
- Encourage the woman to exhale, holding breath for short periods while bearing down, *to avoid holding breath and triggering the Valsalva maneuver, thereby increasing intrathoracic and cardiovascular pressure and decreasing perfusion of placental oxygen, placing the fetus at risk.*
- Have the woman take deep breaths and relax between contractions *to reduce fatigue and increase the effectiveness of the pushing efforts.*
- Have the woman pant as the fetal head crowns *to control birth of the head.*
- Explain to the woman and labor partner what is expected in the third stage of labor *to enlist cooperation.*
- Have the woman maintain her position *to facilitate delivery of the placenta.*

NURSING DIAGNOSIS Fatigue related to energy expenditure during labor and birth

Expected Outcome *Woman's energy level is restored.*

Nursing Interventions/*Rationales*

- Educate the woman and partner about the need for rest, and help them plan strategies (e.g., restricting visitors, increasing role of support systems performing functions associated with daily routines) that allow specific times for rest and sleep *to ensure that woman can restore depleted energy levels in preparation for caring for a new infant.*
- Monitor the woman's fatigue level and the amount of rest received *to ensure the restoration of energy.*
- Group care activities as much as possible *to allow for uninterrupted periods of rest.*

NURSING DIAGNOSIS Risk for deficient fluid volume related to decreased fluid intake and increased fluid loss during labor and birth

Expected Outcome *Fluid balance is maintained, with no signs of dehydration.*

Nursing Interventions/*Rationales*

- Monitor fluid loss (i.e., blood, urine, perspiration) and vital signs; inspect skin turgor and mucous membranes for dryness *to evaluate hydration status.*
- Administer parenteral fluid per physician or nurse-midwife orders *to maintain hydration.*
- Monitor the fundus for firmness after placental separation *to ensure adequate contraction and prevent further blood loss.*
- Offer oral fluids following orders of physician or nurse-midwife and desire of the woman *to provide hydration.*

TABLE 12-2

Physical Nursing Care during Labor

NEED	NURSING ACTIONS	RATIONALE
GENERAL HYGIENE		
Showers or bed baths, Jacuzzi bath	Assess for progress in labor	Determines appropriateness of the activity
	Supervise showers closely if woman is in true labor	Prevents injury from fall; labor may be accelerated
	Suggest allowing warm water to flow over back	Aids relaxation; increases comfort
Perineum	Cleanse frequently, especially after rupture of membranes and when show increases	Enhances comfort and reduces risk of infection
Oral hygiene	Offer toothbrush or mouthwash, or wash the teeth with an ice-cold wet washcloth as needed	Refreshes mouth; helps counteract dry, thirsty feeling
Hair	Brush, braid per woman's wishes	Improves morale; increases comfort
Handwashing	Offer washcloths or cleansing foam before and after voiding and as needed	Maintains cleanliness; prevents infection
Face	Offer cool washcloth	Provides relief from diaphoresis; cools and refreshes
Gowns and linens	Change as needed	Improves comfort; enhances relaxation
NUTRIENT AND FLUID INTAKE		
Oral	Offer fluids and solid foods as ordered by primary health care provider and desired by laboring woman	Provides hydration and calories; enhances positive emotional experience and maternal control
Intravenous (IV)	Establish and maintain IV line as ordered	Maintains hydration; provides venous access for medications
ELIMINATION		
Voiding	Encourage voiding at least every 2 hr	A full bladder may impede descent of presenting part; overdistention may cause bladder atony and injury, as well as postpartum voiding difficulty
Ambulatory woman	Allow ambulation to bathroom according to orders of primary health care provider, if:	
	The presenting part is engaged	Reinforces normal process of urination
	The membranes are not ruptured	Precautionary measure to protect against prolapse of umbilical cord
	The woman is not medicated	Precautionary measure to protect against injury
Woman on bed rest	Offer bedpan	Prevents complications of bladder distention and ambulation
	Encourage upright position on bedpan, allow tap water to run; place woman's hands in warm water; pour warm water over the vulva; give positive suggestion	Encourages voiding
	Provide privacy	Shows respect for woman
	Put up side rails on bed	Prevents injury from fall
	Place call bell and telephone within reach	Reinforces safe care
	Offer washcloth or cleansing foam for hands	Maintains cleanliness; prevents infection
	Wash vulvar area	Maintains cleanliness; enhances comfort; prevents infection
Catheterization	Catheterize according to orders of primary health care provider or hospital protocol if measures to facilitate voiding are ineffective	Prevents complications of bladder distention
	Insert catheter between contractions	Minimizes discomfort
	Avoid force if obstacle to insertion is noted	"Obstacle" may be caused by compression of urethra by presenting part
Bowel elimination—sensation of rectal pressure	Perform vaginal examination	Prevents misinterpretation of rectal pressure from the presenting part as the need to defecate
		Determine degree of descent of presenting part
	Help the woman ambulate to bathroom, or offer bedpan if rectal pressure is not from presenting part	Reinforce normal process of bowel elimination and safe care
	Cleanse perineum immediately after passage of stool	Reduces risk of infection and sense of embarrassment

minimize the risk of anesthesia complications and their secondary effects if general anesthesia were required in an emergency. No randomized trials have been conducted evaluating the ingestion of solid foods in labor; therefore current management is based mostly on expert opinion. Ice chips and sips of clear liquids are still the only oral intake recommended during labor in the United States by the American Society of Anesthesiologists Task Force on Obstetrical Anesthesia (Berghella et al., 2008). This practice is being challenged today by some health care providers, however, because regional anesthesia is used more often than general anesthesia, even for emergency cesarean births. Women are awake during regional anesthesia and are able to participate in their own care and protect their airway.

Intravenous Intake. Fluids are usually administered intravenously to the laboring woman to maintain hydration, especially when a labor is long and the woman is unable to ingest a sufficient amount of fluid orally or if she is receiving epidural or intrathecal anesthesia. In most cases an electrolyte solution without glucose is adequate and does not introduce excess glucose into the bloodstream. The latter is important because an excessive maternal glucose level results in fetal hyperglycemia and fetal hyperinsulinism. After birth the neonate's high levels of insulin will then reduce his or her glucose stores, and hypoglycemia will result. Infusions containing glucose can also reduce sodium levels in both the woman and the fetus, leading to transient neonatal tachypnea. If maternal ketosis occurs, the primary health care provider may order an IV solution containing a small amount of dextrose to provide the glucose needed to assist in fatty acid metabolism.

NURSING ALERT Carefully monitor the intake and output of laboring women receiving IV fluids because they also face an increased danger of hypervolemia as a result of the fluid retention that occurs during pregnancy.

Elimination

Voiding. Encourage voiding every 2 hours. A distended bladder may impede descent of the presenting part, slow or stop uterine contractions, and lead to decreased bladder tone or uterine atony after birth. Women who receive epidural analgesia or anesthesia are especially at risk for the retention of urine.

Assist the woman to the bathroom to void, unless any of the following apply: the primary health care provider has ordered bed rest; the woman is receiving epidural analgesia or anesthesia; internal monitoring is being used; ambulation will compromise the status of the laboring woman or her fetus. You can usually interrupt external monitoring long enough for the woman to go to the bathroom.

If using a bedpan is necessary, encourage spontaneous voiding by providing privacy and having the woman sit upright (as she would on a toilet). Other interventions to encourage urination are having the woman listen to the sound of water slowly running from a faucet or placing her hands in warm water.

Catheterization. If the woman is unable to void and her bladder is distended, she may need a catheter. Many hospitals have protocols that rely on the nurse's judgment concerning the need for catheterization. Before performing the catheterization, clean the vulva and perineum because vaginal show and amniotic fluid may be present. If an obstacle that prevents advancement of the catheter is present, this obstacle is most likely the presenting part. If you cannot advance the catheter, stop the procedure and notify the primary health care provider of the difficulty.

Bowel elimination. Most women do not have bowel movements during labor because of decreased intestinal motility. Stool that has formed in the large intestine often moves downward toward the anorectal area through the pressure exerted by the fetal presenting part as it descends. This stool is often expelled during second-stage pushing and birth. However, the passage of stool with bearing-down efforts increases the risk of infection and may embarrass the woman, thereby reducing the effectiveness of her pushing efforts. To prevent these problems, immediately cleanse the perineal area to remove any stool, while reassuring the woman that the passage of stool at this time is a normal and expected event because the same muscles used to expel the baby also expel stool.

Routine use of enemas on admission for women at term has shown modest benefits. A trend has been noted toward lower infection rates and the newborns have fewer lower respiratory tract infections and less need for antibiotics. However, because enemas cause discomfort for women and increase the costs of giving birth, the small benefits do not outweigh the disadvantages of this practice (Berghella et al., 2008). In addition, a recent Cochrane review of this topic found that the evidence does not support the routine use of enemas during labor (Reveiz, Gaitan, & Cuervo, 2007).

When the presenting part is deep in the pelvis, even in the absence of stool in the anorectal area, the woman may feel rectal pressure and think she needs to defecate. If the woman expresses the urge to defecate, perform a vaginal examination to assess cervical dilation and station. If a multiparous woman experiences the urge to defecate, it often means that birth will follow quickly.

Ambulation and positioning

Confinement to bed is the norm for labor management in the United States. The increased use of epidurals during childbirth, accompanied by multiple medical interventions (e.g., monitors, intravenous infusions) and reduced motor control, contributes to this practice. Upright positions and mobility during labor, however, may be more pleasant for laboring women. These practices have also

Critical Thinking Exercise: Positioning during Labor

been associated with improved uterine contraction intensity and shorter labors, reduced need for pain medications, and increased maternal autonomy and control. No harmful effects have been observed from maternal activity and position change (Albers, 2007). Encourage ambulation if membranes are intact, if the fetal presenting part is engaged after ROM, and if the woman has not received medication for pain (Fig. 12-10). The woman also may prefer to stand and lean forward on her partner, doula, or nurse for support at times during labor (Fig. 12-11, *A*). Ambulation may be contraindicated, however, because of maternal or fetal status.

When the woman lies in bed, she will usually change her position spontaneously as labor progresses. If she does not change position every 30 to 60 minutes, assist her to do so. The side-lying (lateral) position is preferred because it promotes optimal uteroplacental and renal blood flow and increases fetal oxygen saturation (Fig. 12-12, *B*). If the woman wants to lie supine, place a pillow under one hip as a wedge to prevent the uterus from compressing the aorta and vena cava (see Fig. 12-5). Sitting is not contraindicated unless fetal status is adversely affected, which you can determine by checking the FHR and pattern. If the fetus is in the occiput posterior position, encouraging the woman to squat during contractions is often helpful because this position increases the pelvic diameter, allowing the head to rotate to a more anterior position (Fig. 12-12, *A*). A hands-and-knees position during contractions is also recommended to facilitate the rotation of the fetal occiput from a posterior to an anterior position, as gravity pulls the fetal back forward (Fig. 12-11, *B*). Women with epidural anesthesia will likely not be able to squat but may be able to assume a hands-and-knees position.

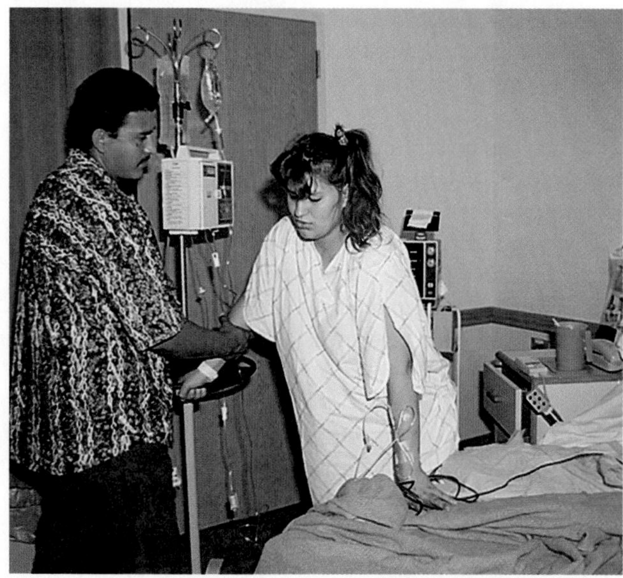

Fig. 12-10 Woman preparing to walk with partner. (Courtesy Marjorie Pyle, RNC, Lifecircle, Costa Mesa, CA.)

Much research continues to focus on acquiring a better understanding of the physiologic and psychologic effects of maternal position in labor. Box 12-4 describes a variety of positions that are recommended for the laboring woman.

The woman can use a birth ball (gymnastic ball, physical therapy ball) to support her body as she assumes a variety of labor and birth positions (Fig. 12-13). The woman can sit on the ball while leaning over the bed, or she can lean over the ball to support her upper body and reduce stress on her arms and hands when she assumes a hands-and-knees position. The birth ball can encourage pelvic mobility and pelvic and perineal relaxation when the woman sits on the firm yet pliable ball and rocks in rhythmic movements. Warm compresses applied to the

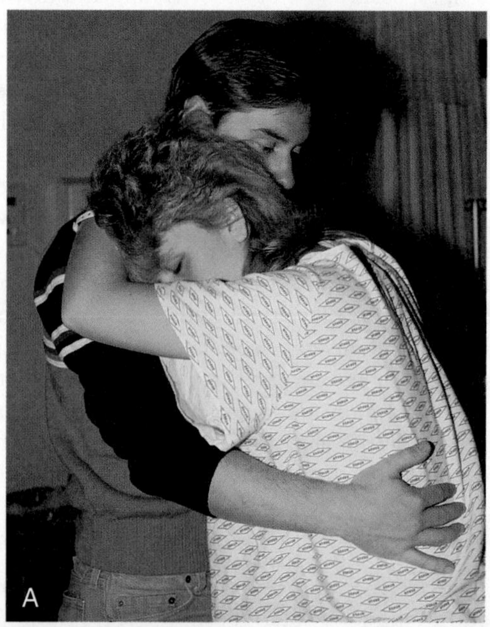

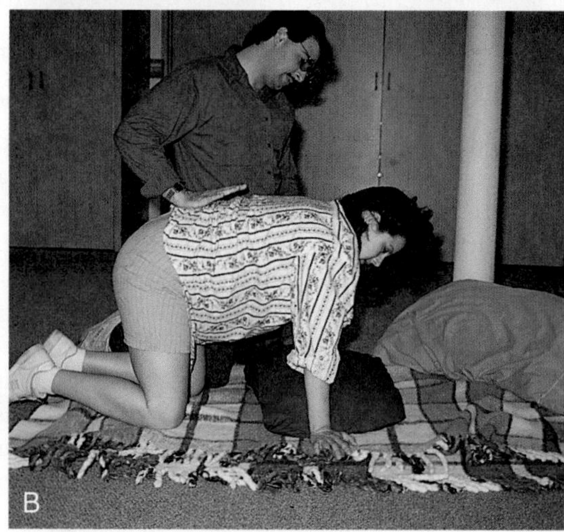

Fig. 12-11 **A,** Woman standing and leaning forward with support. **B,** Woman in hands-and-knees position. (Courtesy Marjorie Pyle, RNC, Lifecircle, Costa Mesa, CA.)

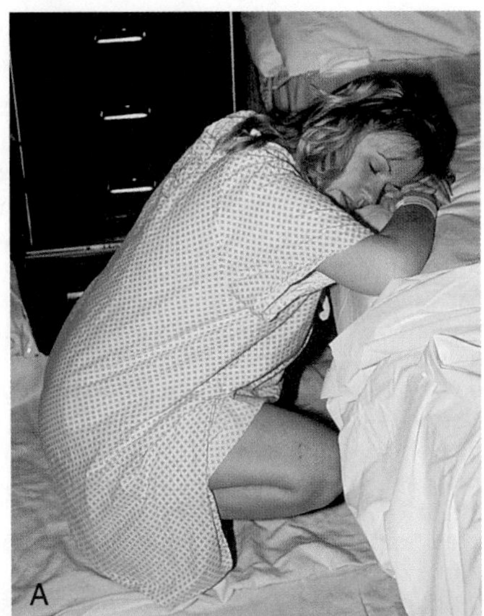
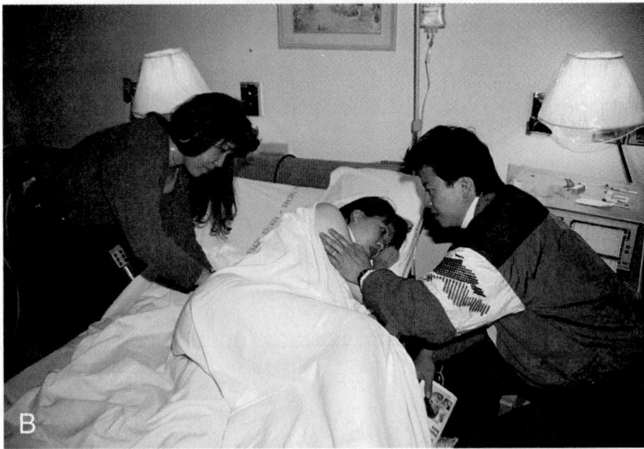

Fig. 12-12 Maternal positions for labor. **A**, Squatting. **B**, Lateral position. Support person is applying sacral pressure while partner provides encouragement. (Courtesy Marjorie Pyle, RNC, Lifecircle, Costa Mesa, CA.)

perineum and lower back can maximize this relaxation and comfort effect. The birth ball should be large enough so that when the woman sits, her knees are bent at a 90-degree angle and her feet are flat on the floor and approximately 2 feet apart.

Supportive care during labor and birth

Support during labor and birth involves emotional support, physical care and comfort measures, and provision of advice and information. The value of the continuous supportive presence of a person (e.g., doula, childbirth educator, family member, friend, nurse, partner) during labor has long been known. Women who have continuous support beginning early in labor are less likely to use pain medication or epidurals, more likely to have a spontaneous vaginal birth, and less likely to report dissatisfaction with their birth experience. No harmful effects from continuous labor support have been identified. To the contrary, good evidence has been found that labor support improves

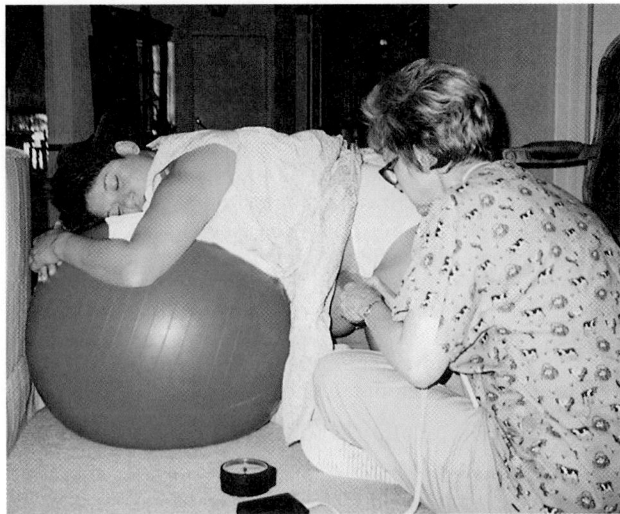

FIG. 12-13 Woman laboring using birth ball. (Courtesy Polly Perez, Cutting Edge Press, Johnson, VT.)

important health outcomes (Albers, 2007; Berghella et al., 2008; Hodnett, Gates, Hofmeyr, & Sakala, 2007).

Labor rooms should be airy, clean, and homelike. The laboring woman should feel safe in this environment and free to be herself and to use the comfort and relaxation measures she prefers. To enhance relaxation, turn off bright overhead lights when not needed, and keep noise and intrusions to a minimum. Control the temperature to ensure the laboring woman's comfort. The room should be large enough to accommodate a comfortable chair for the woman's partner, the monitoring equipment, and hospital personnel. Encourage couples to bring their own pillows to make the hospital surroundings more homelike and to facilitate position changes. Environmental modifications should reflect the preferences of the woman, including the number of visitors and availability of a telephone, television, and music.

Labor support by the nurse. Supportive nursing care for a woman in labor includes the following:

- Helping the woman maintain control and participate to the extent she wishes in the birth of her infant
- Meeting the woman's expected outcomes for her labor
- Acting as the woman's advocate, supporting her decisions and respecting her choices as appropriate and relating her wishes as needed to other health care providers
- Helping the woman conserve her energy
- Helping control the woman's discomfort
- Acknowledging the woman's efforts, as well as those of her partner, during labor and providing positive reinforcement
- Protecting the woman's privacy and modesty

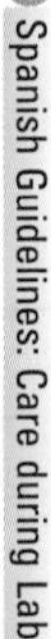

Couples who have attended childbirth education programs that teach the psychoprophylactic approach will know something about the labor process, coaching techniques, and comfort measures. The nurse should play a supportive role and keep such a couple informed of

BOX 12-4

Some Maternal Positions* during Labor and Birth

SEMIRECUMBENT POSITION

With woman sitting with her upper body elevated to at least a 30-degree angle, place a wedge or small pillow under hip to prevent vena caval compression and reduce likelihood of supine hypotension (see Fig. 12-5).

- The greater the angle of elevation is, the more gravity or pressure is exerted that promotes fetal descent, the progress of contractions, and the widening of pelvic dimensions.
- Position is convenient for rendering care measures and for external fetal monitoring.

LATERAL POSITION (SEE FIG. 12-12, *B*)

Have woman alternate between left and right side-lying positions, and provide abdominal and back support as needed for comfort.

- Removes pressure from the vena cava and back, enhances uteroplacental perfusion, and relieves backache
- Makes performing back massage or counterpressure easier
- Associated with less frequent, but more intense, contractions
- May be more difficult to obtain good external fetal monitor tracings
- May be used as a birthing position
- Takes pressure off perineum, allowing it to stretch gradually
- Reduces risk for perineal trauma

UPRIGHT POSITION

The gravity effect enhances the contraction cycle and fetal descent: The weight of the fetus places increasing pressure on the cervix; the cervix is pulled upward, facilitating effacement and dilation; impulses from the cervix to the pituitary gland increase, causing more oxytocin to be secreted; and contractions are intensified, thereby applying more forceful downward pressure on the fetus, but they are less painful.

- Fetus is aligned with pelvis, and pelvic diameters are widened slightly.
- Effective upright positions include the following:
  - Ambulation (see Fig. 12-10)
  - Standing and leaning forward with support provided by coach (see Fig. 12-11, *A*), end of bed, back of chair, or birth ball (see Fig. 12-13); relieves backache and facilitates application of counterpressure or back massage
  - Sitting up in bed, chair, or birthing chair, on toilet, or on bedside commode
  - Squatting (see Figs. 12-12, *A* and 12-17, *E*)

HANDS-AND-KNEES POSITION—IDEAL POSITION FOR POSTERIOR POSITIONS OF THE PRESENTING PART (SEE FIG. 12-11, *B*)

Assume an "all-fours" position in bed or on a covered floor; allows for pelvic rocking.

- Relieves backache characteristic of "back labor"
- Facilitates internal rotation of the fetus by increasing mobility of the coccyx, increasing the pelvic diameters, and using gravity to turn the fetal back and rotate the head (NOTE: A side-lying position, double hip squeeze, or knee squeeze can also facilitate internal rotation.)

* Assess the effect of each position on the laboring woman's comfort and anxiety level, progress of labor, and fetal heart rate pattern. Alternate positions every 30 to 60 min, allowing woman to take control of her position changes.

labor progress. If necessary, review the methods learned in class.

Even when expectant parents have not attended childbirth classes, the nurse can teach them simple breathing and relaxation techniques during the early phase of labor. In this case the nurse may provide more of the coaching and supportive care. (See Chapter 10.)

Comfort measures vary with the situation (Fig. 12-14). The nurse can draw on the couple's list of comfort measures learned during the pregnancy. Such measures include maintaining a comfortable, supportive atmosphere in the labor and birth area, using touch therapeutically (e.g., heat or cold applied to the lower back in the event of back labor, a cool cloth applied to the forehead), providing nonpharmacologic measures to relieve discomfort (e.g., massage, hydrotherapy), administering analgesics when necessary, and, most important of all, just being there (MacKinnon, McIntyre, & Quance, 2005) (see Table 12-2; see also the Care Path: Low Risk Woman in First Stage Labor). See Chapter 10 for a full discussion of both pharmacologic and nonpharmacologic comfort measures.

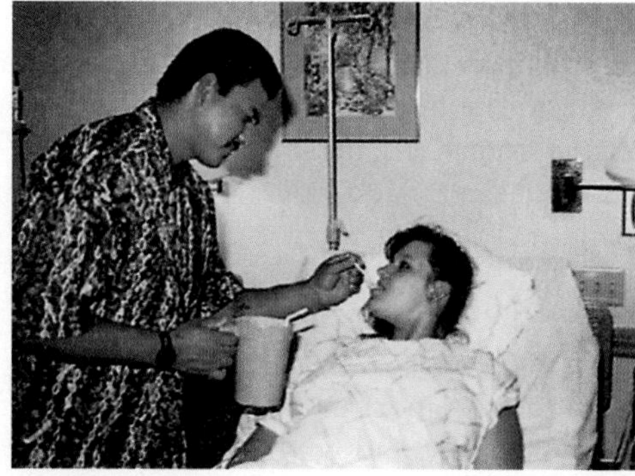

Fig. 12-14 Partner providing comfort measures. (Courtesy Marjorie Pyle, RNC, Lifecircle, Costa Mesa, CA.)

Most women in labor respond positively to touch, but you should obtain permission before using any touching measures. Women appreciate gentle handling by staff members. Offer back rubs and counterpressure, especially if the woman is experiencing back labor. Teach the support person to exert counterpressure against the woman's sacrum over the occiput of the head of a fetus in a posterior position (see Fig. 12-12, *B*). The back pain is caused by the occiput pressing on spinal nerves, and counterpressure lifts the occiput off these nerves, thereby providing some relief from pain. The partner will need to be relieved after a while, however, because exerting counterpressure is hard work. Hand and foot massage can also be soothing and relaxing. The woman's perception of the soothing qualities of touch may change as labor progresses. Many women become more sensitive to touch (hyperesthesia) as labor progresses. This response is typical during the transition phase (see Table 12-1). They may tell their coach to leave them alone or not to touch them. The partner who is unprepared for this normal response may feel rejected and may react by withdrawing active support. The nurse can reassure him or her that this response is a positive indication that the first stage is ending and the second stage is approaching. Women with increased sensitivity to touch may tolerate it better on surfaces of the body where hair does not grow, such as the forehead, the palms of the hands, and the soles of the feet.

Labor support by the father or partner. Although another woman or a man other than the father may be the woman's partner, the father of the baby is usually the support person during labor. He is often able to provide the comfort measures and touch that the laboring woman needs. When the woman becomes focused on her pain, the partner can sometimes persuade her to try nonpharmacologic variations of comfort measures. In addition, he is usually able to interpret the woman's needs and desires for staff members.

The feelings of a first-time father change as labor progresses. Although he is often calm at the onset of labor, feelings of fear and helplessness begin to dominate as labor becomes more active and the father realizes that labor is more work than he anticipated. The first-time father may feel excluded as birth preparations begin during the transition phase. Once the second stage begins and birth nears, the father's focus changes from the woman to the baby who is about to be born. The father will be exposed to many sights and smells he may never before have experienced. Therefore the nurse needs to tell him what to expect and to make him comfortable about leaving the room to regain his composure should something occur that surprises him. Before he leaves the room, make sure that someone else is available to support the woman during his absence. Staff members should tell the father that his presence is helpful and encourage him to be involved in the care of the woman to the extent to which he is comfortable. Box 12-5 details ways in which the nurse can support the father-partner. A well-informed father can make an important contribution to the health and well-being of the mother and child, their family interrelationship, and his self-esteem.

Labor support by doulas. Continuity of care has been cited by women as a critical component of a satisfying childbirth experience. A specially trained, experienced female labor attendant called a **doula** can meet this need. The doula provides a continuous, one-on-one caring presence throughout the labor and birth of the woman she is attending. The primary role of the doula is to focus on the laboring woman and provide physical and emotional support by using soft, reassuring words: touching, stroking, and hugging. The doula also administers comfort measures to reduce pain and enhance relaxation, walks with the woman, helps her to change positions, and coaches her bearing-down efforts. Doulas provide information and explain procedures and events. They advocate for the woman's right to participate actively in the management of her labor.

The doula also supports the woman's partner, who often feels unqualified to be the sole labor support. The doula can encourage and praise the partner's efforts, create a partnership as caregivers, and provide respite care. Doulas also facilitate communication between the laboring woman and her partner, as well as between the couple and the health care team.

Doula support during labor is associated with decreased use of analgesia, decreased incidence of operative birth, increased incidence of spontaneous vaginal birth, and increased maternal satisfaction (Berghella et al., 2008).

BOX 12-5

Guidelines for Supporting the Father or Significant Other

- Orient him to the labor room and the unit; explain the location of the cafeteria, toilet, waiting room, and nursery; give information about visiting hours; introduce personnel by name, and describe their functions.
- Inform him of the sights and smells he can expect to encounter; encourage him to leave the room if necessary.
- Respect his or the couple's decision about the degree of his involvement. Offer them freedom to make decisions.
- Tell him when his presence has been helpful, and continue to reinforce his efforts throughout labor.
- Offer to teach him comfort measures.
- Inform him frequently of the progress of the labor and the woman's needs. Keep him informed about procedures to be performed.
- Prepare him for changes in the woman's behavior and physical appearance.
- Remind him to eat; offer him snacks and fluids if possible.
- Relieve him of the job of support person as necessary. Offer him blankets if he is to sleep in a chair by the bedside.
- Acknowledge the stress experienced by each partner during labor and birth, and identify normal responses.
- Attempt to modify or eliminate unsettling stimuli, such as extra noise and extra light.

The roles of the nurse and the doula are complementary. They should work together as a team, with the doula providing supportive nonmedical care measures while the nurse focuses on monitoring the status of the maternal-fetal unit, implementing clinical care protocols (including pharmacologic interventions), and documenting assessment findings, actions, and responses.

Labor support by the grandparents. When grandparents act as labor coaches, supporting and treating them with respect is especially important. They may have a way to deal with pain relief based on their experience. Encourage them to help as long as their actions do not compromise the status of the mother or the fetus. The nurse acts as a role model for the parents-to-be by treating grandparents with dignity and respect, by acknowledging the value of the grandparents' contributions to parental support, and by recognizing the difficulty grandparents have in witnessing the woman's discomfort or crisis. If they have never witnessed a birth, the nurse may need to provide explanations of what is happening. Many of the activities used to support fathers also are appropriate for grandparents.

Siblings during labor and birth

The preparation of siblings for acceptance of the new child helps promote the attachment process. Such preparation and participation during pregnancy and labor may help the older children accept this change. The older child or children who know themselves to be important to the family become active participants. Rehearsal for the event before labor is essential.

The age and developmental level of children influence their responses; therefore adjust preparation for the children to be present during labor to meet each child's needs. The child younger than 2 years shows little interest in pregnancy and labor. However, for the older child, such preparation may reduce fears and misconceptions. Parents need to be prepared for labor and birth themselves and feel comfortable about the process and the presence of their children. Most parents have a "feel" for their children's maturational level and their physical and emotional ability to observe and cope with the events of the labor and birth process. Preparation often includes a description of the anticipated sights, events (e.g., ROM, monitors, IV infusions), smells, and sounds; a labor and birth demonstration; a tour of the birthing unit; and an opportunity to be around a real newborn. Children must learn that their mother will be working hard during labor and birth. She will not be able to talk to them during contractions. She may groan, scream, grunt, and pant at times, as well as say things she would not say otherwise (e.g., "I can't take this anymore," "Take this baby out of me," or "This pain is killing me"). You can tell them that labor is uncomfortable, but that their mother's body is made for the job. Storybooks about the birth process can be read to or by children to prepare them for the event. Films are available for preparing preschool and school-age children to participate in the labor and birth experience. Most agencies require that a specific person watch over the children who are participating in their mother's childbirth experience, to provide them with support, explanations, diversions, and comfort as needed. Health care providers involved in attending women during birth must be comfortable with the presence of children and the unpredictability of their questions, comments, and behaviors.

Emergency interventions

Emergency conditions that require immediate nursing intervention can arise with startling speed. The Emergency box lists interventions for a nonreassuring FHR, inadequate uterine relaxation, vaginal bleeding, infection, and prolapse of the cord.

Evaluation

The expected outcomes of care are used to evaluate the effectiveness of care.

SECOND STAGE OF LABOR

CARE MANAGEMENT

The **second stage of labor** is the stage in which the infant is born. This stage begins with full cervical dilation (10 cm) and complete effacement (100%) and ends with the baby's birth. The median duration of second stage labor is 50 minutes in nulliparous women and 20 minutes in multiparous women. In addition to parity, maternal size and fetal weight, position, and descent influence the length of this stage. The use of epidural anesthesia during labor often increases the length of second stage labor because the epidural blocks or reduces the woman's urge to bear down and limits her ability to attain an upright position to push. Currently the second stage of labor is considered to be prolonged if its duration exceeds the following time frames (Battista & Wing, 2007):

Nulliparous women	>2 hours with no regional anesthesia use
	>3 hours with use of regional anesthesia
Multiparous women	>1 hour with no regional anesthesia use
	>2 hours with use of regional anesthesia

The second stage of labor is composed of three phases: the latent, descent, and transition phases. Maternal verbal and nonverbal behaviors, uterine activity, the urge to bear down, and fetal descent characterize these phases.

The latent phase is a period of rest and relative calm (i.e., "laboring down"). During this early phase the fetus continues to descend passively through the birth canal and rotate to an anterior position as a result of ongoing uterine

Interventions for Emergencies during Labor

SIGNS	INTERVENTIONS (PRIORITIES ARE BASED ON WHAT SIGN IS PRESENT)*
NONREASSURING OR ABNORMAL FETAL HEART RATE PATTERN	
• Fetal bradycardia (FHR <110 beats/min for >10 min) • Fetal tachycardia (FHR >160 beats/min for >10 min in term pregnancy) • Irregular FHR, abnormal sinus rhythm shown by internal monitor • Absent or minimal baseline FHR variability without an identified cause • Late, variable, and prolonged deceleration patterns • Absence of FHTs	• Notify primary health care provider.† • Change maternal position. • Discontinue oxytocin (Pitocin) infusion if tachysystole is occurring. • Start an IV line if one is not in place. • Increase IV fluid rate if fluid is being infused per protocol or order. • Administer oxygen at 8 to 10 L/min by non-rebreather facemask. • Check maternal temperature for elevation. • Assist with amnioinfusion if ordered. • Perform fetal scalp stimulation or vibroacoustic stimulation as ordered or per protocol.
INADEQUATE UTERINE RELAXATION	
• Intrauterine pressure >80 mm Hg (shown by intrauterine pressure catheter monitoring) • Contractions consistently lasting >90 sec • More than five contractions in 10 minutes	• Notify primary health care provider.† • Discontinue oxytocin infusion if being infused. • Change woman to side-lying position. • Start an IV line if one is not in place. • Increase IV fluid rate if fluid is being infused. • Administer oxygen at 8 to 10 L/min by non-rebreather facemask. • Palpate and evaluate contractions. • Give tocolytic (terbutaline) as ordered or per protocol.
VAGINAL BLEEDING	
• Vaginal bleeding (bright red, dark red, or in an amount in excess of that expected during normal cervical dilation) • Continuous vaginal bleeding with FHR changes • Pain; may or may not be present	• Notify primary health care provider.† • Assist with ultrasound examination if performed. • Start an IV line if one is not in place. • Begin continuous FHR and contraction monitoring if not already in progress. • Anticipate emergency (stat) cesarean birth. • *Do NOT perform a vaginal examination.*
INFECTION	
• Foul-smelling amniotic fluid • Maternal temperature >38° C in presence of adequate hydration (straw-colored urine) • Fetal tachycardia >160 beats/min for >10 min	• Notify primary health care provider.† • Institute cooling measures for laboring woman. • Start an IV line if one is not in place. • Assist with or perform collection of catheterized urine specimen and amniotic fluid sample, and send to the laboratory for urinalysis and cultures. • Administer antibiotics as ordered.
PROLAPSE OF CORD	

• Fetal bradycardia with variable deceleration during uterine contraction
• Woman reporting feeling the cord after membranes rupture
• Cord lying alongside or below the presenting part of the fetus; can be seen or felt in or protruding from the vagina
• Major predisposing factors:
  • Rupture of membranes with a gush
  • Loose fit of presenting part in lower uterine segment
  • Presenting part not yet engaged
  • Breech presentation
	• Call for assistance. Do not leave woman alone.
	• Have someone notify the primary health care provider immediately.
	• Glove the examining hand quickly and insert two fingers into the vagina to the cervix; with one finger on either side of the cord or both fingers to one side, exert upward pressure against the presenting part to relieve compression of the cord.
	• Place a rolled towel under the woman's hip.
	• Place woman in extreme Trendelenburg or modified Sims position or knee-chest position.
	• Wrap the cord loosely in a sterile towel saturated with warm sterile normal saline if the cord is protruding from the vagina.
	• Administer oxygen at 8-10 L/min by non-rebreather facemask until birth is accomplished.
	• Start IV fluids or increase existing drip rate.
	• Continue to monitor FHR by internal fetal scalp electrode, if possible.
	• Do not attempt to replace cord into cervix.
	• Prepare for immediate birth (vaginal or cesarean).

FHR, Fetal heart rate; *FHT,* fetal hear tones; *IV,* intravenous.

*Because emergency situations are often frightening events, the nurse needs to explain to the woman and her support person what is happening and how it is being managed.

†In most emergency situations, nurses take immediate action following a protocol and standards of nursing practice. The nurse or another person must notify the primary health care provider as soon as possible.

Case Study: Second/Third Stages of Labor

contractions. The woman is quiet and often relaxes with her eyes closed between contractions. The urge to bear down is not strong, and some women do not experience it at all or only during the acme (peak) of a contraction. Allowing a woman to rest during this phase and waiting until the urge to push intensifies reduces maternal fatigue and conserves energy for bearing-down efforts. Delayed pushing is associated with a longer second stage of labor but a significantly higher incidence of spontaneous vaginal birth. Other benefits of delayed pushing include less FHR decelerations, fewer forceps- and vacuum-assisted births, and less perineal damage (lacerations and episiotomies). Careful monitoring with assurance of reassuring fetal status should be used during delayed pushing. The length of second stage labor is not associated with poor neonatal outcome, as long as the fetal status during this time is reassuring (Berghella et al., 2008; Brancato, Church, & Stone, 2008; Roberts & Hanson, 2007; Simpson & James, 2005).

During the descent phase or the phase of active pushing the woman has strong urges to bear down as the reflex called the *Ferguson reflex* is activated when the presenting part presses on the stretch receptors of the pelvic floor. At this point the fetal station is usually +1, and the position is anterior. This stimulation causes the release of oxytocin from the posterior pituitary gland, which provokes stronger expulsive uterine contractions. The woman becomes more focused on bearing-down efforts, which become rhythmic. She changes positions frequently to find a more comfortable pushing position. The woman often announces the onset of contractions and becomes more vocal as she bears down. The urge to bear down intensifies as descent progresses.

In the transition phase the presenting part is on the perineum, and bearing-down efforts are most effective for promoting birth. The woman may be more verbal about the pain she is experiencing; she may scream or swear and may act out of control.

The nurse encourages the woman to "listen" to her body as she progresses through the phases of the second stage of labor. When a woman listens to her body to tell her when to bear down, she is using an internal locus of control and often feels more satisfied with her efforts to give birth to her baby. This feeling enhances her sense of self-esteem and accomplishment, and her efforts become more effective. Always encourage the woman's trust in her own body and her ability to give birth to her baby.

If a woman is confined to bed, especially in a recumbent position, the rhythmic urge to bear down is delayed because gravity is not being used to press the presenting part against the pelvic floor. Being moved to another room and placed on a delivery table in the lithotomy position, as has been the custom in North America, also has an inhibiting effect on the urge to bear down. Today, Western societies have incorporated the birthing practice of most non-Western societies in which labor and birth occur in the same room and women use various positions for bearing down, such as the side-lying position, kneeling, squatting, sitting, or standing.

Assessment

The only certain objective sign that the second stage of labor has begun is the inability to feel the cervix during vaginal examination, indicating that the cervix is fully dilated and effaced. The precise moment that this sign occurs is not easy to determine because it depends on when a vaginal examination is performed to validate full dilation and effacement. This situation makes timing of the actual duration of the second stage difficult. Other signs that suggest the onset of the second stage include the following:

- Urge to push or feeling the need to have a bowel movement
- Involuntary bearing-down efforts
- Sudden appearance of sweat on upper lip
- An episode of vomiting
- Increased bloody show
- Shaking of extremities
- Increased restlessness; verbalization (e.g., "I can't go on.")

These signs commonly appear at the time the cervix reaches full dilation. However, women with an epidural block may not exhibit such signs. Table 12-3 gives other indicators for each phase of the second stage.

Some women begin to experience an irresistible urge to bear down before full dilation. For some women, this urge occurs as early as 5 cm of dilation and is most often related to the station of the presenting part below the level of the ischial spines of the maternal pelvis. This occurrence creates a conflict between the woman, whose body is telling her to push, and her health care providers, who believe that pushing the fetal presenting part against an incompletely dilated cervix will result in cervical edema and lacerations, as well as a slowing of labor progress. Evaluate the premature urge to bear down as a sign of labor progress possibly indicating the onset of the second stage of labor. Base the timing of when a woman pushes in relation to whether or not her cervix is fully dilated on research evidence rather than on tradition or routine practice. Pushing with the urge to bear down at the acme of a contraction may be safe and effective for a woman if her cervix is soft, retracting, and 8 cm or more dilated and if the fetus is at +1 station and rotating to an anterior position (Roberts, 2002).

Assessment is continuous during the second stage of labor. Professional standards and agency policy determine the specific type and timing of assessments, as well as the way in which you document findings. The Care Path: Low Risk Woman in Second Stage Labor indicates typical assessments and the recommended frequency for their performance. Signs and symptoms of impending birth (see Table 12-3) may appear unexpectedly, requiring immediate action by the nurse (Box 12-6).

TABLE 12-3

Expected Maternal Progress in Second Stage of Labor

CRITERION	LATENT PHASE (AVERAGE DURATION, 10-30 MIN)	DESCENT PHASE (AVERAGE DURATION VARIES)*	TRANSITION PHASE (AVERAGE DURATION 5-15 MIN)
Contractions	Period of physiologic lull for all criteria; period of peace and rest; "laboring down"	Significant increase	Overwhelmingly strong
Magnitude (intensity)			Expulsive
Frequency		2-2.5 min	1-2 min
Duration		90 sec	90 sec
Descent, station	0 to +2	Increases and Ferguson reflex† activated, +2 to +4	Rapid, +4 to birth Fetal head visible at introitus
Show: color and amount		Significant increase in dark red bloody show	Bloody show accompanies birth of head
Spontaneous bearing-down efforts	Slight to absent, except during acme of strongest contractions	Increased urge to bear down	Greatly increased
Vocalization	Quiet; concern over progress	Grunting sounds or expiratory vocalization; announces contractions	Grunting sounds and expiratory vocalizations continue; may scream or swear
Maternal behavior	Experiences sense of relief that transition to second stage is finished	Senses increased urge to push	Describes extreme pain Expresses feelings of powerlessness
	Feels fatigued and sleepy	Alters respiratory pattern: has short 4- to 5-sec breath holds with regular breaths in between, five to seven times per contraction	Shows decreased ability to listen or concentrate on anything but giving birth
	Feels a sense of accomplishment and optimism, because the "worst is over"	Makes grunting sounds or expiratory vocalizations	Describes ring of fire (burning sensation of acute pain as vagina stretches and fetal head crowns)
	Feels in control	Frequent repositioning	Often shows excitement immediately after birth of head

Source: Roberts, J. (2002). The "push" for evidence: Management of the second stage. *Journal of Midwifery & Women's Health, 47*(1), 2-15; Simkin, P., & Ancheta, R. (2000). *The labor progress handbook.* Malden, MA: Blackwell Science.

*Duration of descent phase can vary depending on maternal parity, effectiveness of bearing-down effort, and presence of spinal anesthesia or epidural analgesia.

†Pressure of presenting part on stretch receptors of pelvic floor stimulates release of oxytocin from posterior pituitary, resulting in more intense uterine contractions.

Nursing Diagnoses

Possible nursing diagnoses appropriate for the woman in the second stage of labor include the following:

- *Risk for injury to mother and fetus* related to:
  - Persistent use of Valsalva maneuver
- *Situational low self-esteem* related to:
  - Deficient knowledge of normal, beneficial effects of vocalization during bearing-down efforts
  - Inability to carry out plan for birth without medication
- *Ineffective coping* related to:
  - Coaching that contradicts woman's physiologic urge to push
- *Anxiety* related to:
  - Inability to control defecation with bearing-down efforts
  - Lack of knowledge regarding perineal sensations associated with the urge to bear down
- *Risk for infection* related to:
  - Multiple invasive procedures such as vaginal examinations
  - Tissue trauma (episiotomy or lacerations) during birth

CARE PATH Low Risk Woman in the Second Stage of Labor

I. ASSESSMENT MEASURES*	FREQUENCY
Blood pressure, pulse, respirations	Every 5-30 min
Uterine activity	Assess every contraction
Bearing-down effort	Assess each effort
Fetal heart rate	Every 5-15 min
Vaginal show	Every 15 min
Signs of fetal descent: urge to bear down, perineal bulging, crowning	Every 10-15 min
Behavior, appearance, mood, energy level of woman; condition of partner	Every 10-15 min
II. PHYSICAL CARE MEASURES†	**TIMING**
Assist to rest in position of comfort.	Latent phase
Encourage relaxation to conserve energy.	
Promote urge to push; if delayed: ambulation, shower, pelvic rock, position changes.	
Assist to bear down effectively.	Descent phase
Help to use recommended positions that facilitate descent.	
Encourage correct breathing during bearing-down efforts.	
Help to relax between contractions.	
Provide comfort measures as needed.	
Cleanse perineum immediately if fecal material is expelled.	
Assist to pant during contraction to avoid rapid birth of head.	Transition phase
Coach to gently bear down between contractions.	
III. EMOTIONAL SUPPORT	
Keep informed of progress of fetal descent.	
Provide feedback for bearing-down efforts.	
Explain purpose if medications given.	
Role model comfort measures.	
Provide continuous nursing presence.	
Create a quiet, calm environment.	
Reassure, encourage, praise.	
Take charge as needed until woman regains confidence in ability to birth her baby.	
Offer mirror to watch birth.	

*Frequency of assessment is determined by the risk status of the maternal-fetal unit. More frequent assessment is required in high risk situations. Frequency of assessment and method of documentation are also determined by agency policy, which is usually based on the recommended care standards of medical and nursing organizations.
†Physical care measures are performed by the nurse working together with the woman's partner and significant others.

Expected Outcomes of Care

Expected outcomes for the woman in the second stage of labor are that the woman will accomplish the following:

- Continue normal progression of labor while the FHR and pattern remain reassuring.
- Maintain adequate hydration status through oral or IV intake (or both).
- Actively participate in the labor process.
- Verbalize discomfort and indicate the need for measures that help reduce discomfort and promote relaxation.
- Accept comfort and support measures from significant others and health care providers as needed.
- Sustain no injury to herself or the fetus during labor and birth.
- Initiate, along with the partner and family, the processes of bonding and attachment with the newborn.
- Express satisfaction with her performance during labor and birth.

Plan of Care and Interventions

The nurse continues to monitor maternal-fetal status and events of the second stage and provide comfort measures for the mother. This task includes helping her change position; providing mouth care; maintaining clean, dry bedding; and keeping extraneous noise, conversation, and other distractions (e.g., laughing, talking of attending personnel in or outside the labor area) to a minimum. Encourage the woman to indicate other support measures she would like (see Table 12-3; also see Care Path for Low Risk Woman in Second Stage of Labor, above, and Nursing Care Plan on p. 353).

In the hospital, birth may occur in an LDR, LDRP, or delivery room. If the mother is going to be transferred to the delivery room for birth, perform the transfer early enough to avoid rushing her.

Maternal position

No single position for childbirth exists. Labor is a dynamic, interactive process involving the woman's uterus,

BOX 12-6

Guidelines for Assistance at the Emergency Birth of a Fetus in the Vertex Presentation

1. The woman usually assumes the position most comfortable for her. A lateral position is often recommended.
2. Reassure the woman that birth is usually uncomplicated and easy in these situations. Use eye-to-eye contact and a calm, relaxed manner. If someone else is available, such as the partner, that person could help support the woman in the position, assist with coaching, and compliment her on her efforts.
3. Wash your hands and put on gloves, if available.
4. Place under woman's buttocks whatever clean material is available.
5. Avoid touching the vaginal area to decrease the possibility of infection.
6. As the head begins to crown, you should perform the following tasks:
   a. Tear the amniotic membrane if it is still intact.
   b. Instruct the woman to pant or pant-blow, thus minimizing the urge to push.
   c. Place the flat side of your hand on the exposed fetal head and apply *gentle* pressure toward the vagina to prevent the head from "popping out." The mother may participate by placing her hand under yours on the emerging head. NOTE: Rapid delivery of the fetal head must be prevented because a rapid change of pressure within the molded fetal skull follows, which may result in dural or subdural tears. Rapid delivery of the head may also cause vaginal or perineal lacerations.
7. After the birth of the head, check for the umbilical cord. If the cord is around the baby's neck, try to slip it over the baby's head or pull it gently to get some slack so that you can slip it over the shoulders.
8. Support the fetal head as external rotation occurs. Then, with one hand on each side of the baby's head, exert gentle pressure downward so that the anterior shoulder emerges under the symphysis pubis and acts as a fulcrum; then, as gentle pressure is exerted in the opposite direction, the posterior shoulder, which has passed over the sacrum and coccyx, emerges.
9. Be alert! Hold the baby securely because the rest of the body may emerge quickly. The baby will be slippery!
10. Cradle the baby's head and back in one hand and the buttocks in the other. Keep the head down to drain away the mucus. Use a bulb syringe, if one is available, to remove mucus from the baby's mouth and nose.
11. Dry the baby quickly to prevent rapid heat loss. Keep the baby at the same level as the mother's uterus until the end of the cord stops pulsating. NOTE: The baby should be kept at the same level as the mother's uterus to prevent the baby's blood from flowing to or from the placenta and the resultant hypovolemia or hypervolemia. Also, do not "milk" the cord.
12. Place the baby on the mother's abdomen, cover the baby (remember to keep the head warm too) with the mother's clothing, and have her cuddle the baby. Compliment her (them) on a job well done and on the baby, if appropriate.
13. Wait for the placenta to separate; do not tug on the cord. NOTE: Inappropriate traction may tear the cord, separate the placenta, or invert the uterus. Signs of placental separation include a slight gush of dark blood from the introitus, lengthening of the cord, and change in the uterine contour from a discoid to globular shape.
14. Instruct the mother to push to deliver the separated placenta. Gently ease out the placental membranes using an up-and-down motion until the membranes are removed. If birth occurs outside a hospital setting, to minimize complications, do not cut the cord without proper clamps and a sterile cutting tool. Inspect the placenta for intactness. Place the baby on the placenta and wrap the two together for additional warmth.
15. Check the firmness of the uterus. Gently massage the fundus and demonstrate to the mother how she can massage her own fundus properly.
16. If supplies are available, clean the mother's perineal area and apply a peripad.
17. In addition to gentle massage of the fundus, the following measures can be taken to prevent or minimize hemorrhage:
   a. Put the baby to the mother's breast as soon as possible. Sucking or nuzzling and licking the nipple stimulates the release of oxytocin from the posterior pituitary. NOTE: If the baby does not or cannot nurse, manually stimulate the mother's nipples.
   b. Do not allow the mother's bladder to become distended. Assess the bladder for fullness and encourage her to void if fullness is found.
   c. Expel any clots from the mother's uterus.
18. Comfort or reassure the mother and her family or friends. Keep the mother and the baby warm. Give her fluids if available and tolerated.
19. If this birth is multifetal, identify the infants in order of birth (using letters A, B, C, etc.).
20. Make notations regarding the following aspects of the birth:
   a. Fetal presentation and position
   b. Presence of cord around neck (nuchal cord) or other parts and number of times cord encircled part
   c. Color and estimated amount of amniotic fluid, if rupture of membranes occurs immediately before birth
   d. Time of birth
   e. Estimated time of determination of Apgar score (e.g., 1 and 5 min after birth), resuscitation efforts implemented, and ultimate condition of baby
   f. Gender of baby
   g. Time of placental expulsion, as well as the appearance and completeness of the placenta
   h. Maternal condition: affect, amount of bleeding, and status of uterine tonicity
   i. Any unusual occurrences during the birth (e.g., maternal or paternal response, verbalizations, gestures in response to birth of baby)

pelvis, and voluntary muscles. In addition, angles between the baby and the woman's pelvis constantly change as the infant turns and flexes down the birth canal. The woman may want to assume various positions for childbirth, and you should encourage and assist her in attaining and maintaining her position or positions of choice (Fig. 12-15). Supine, semirecumbent, or lithotomy positions are still widely used in Western societies despite evidence that women prefer upright positions for their bearing-down efforts and birth (Roberts & Hanson, 2007).

Birth attendants play a major role in influencing a woman's choice of positions for birth, with nurse-midwives tending to advocate nonlithotomy positions for

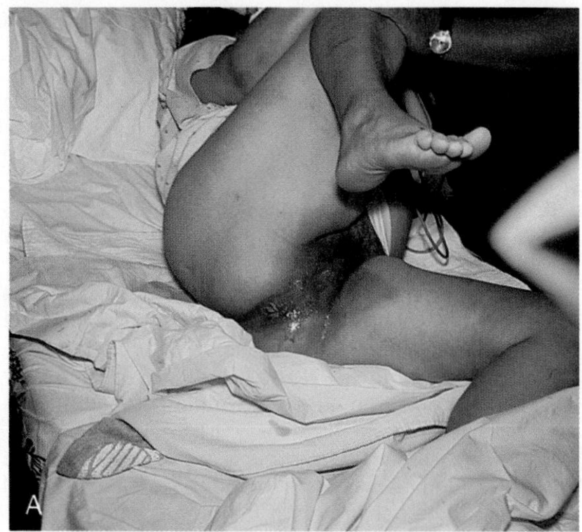

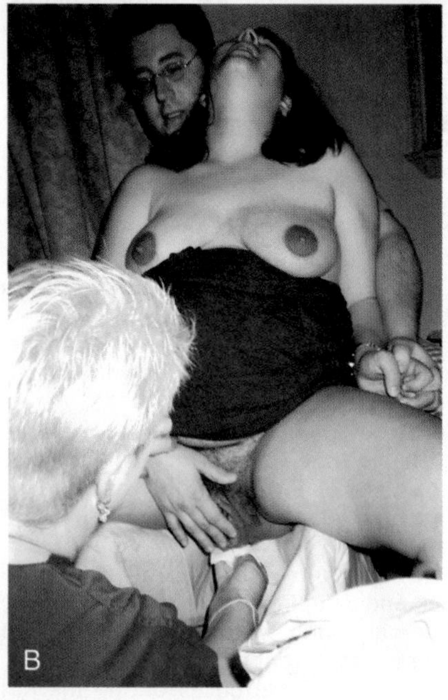

Fig. 12-15 **A**, Pushing, side-lying position. Perineal bulging can be seen. **B**, Pushing, semi-sitting position. Midwife assists mother to feel top of fetal head. (**A**, Courtesy Michael S. Clement, MD, Mesa, AZ. **B**, Courtesy Roni Wernik, Palo Alto, CA.)

the second stage of labor. The use of upright positions for birth is associated with a shorter interval to the birth, less pain and perineal damage, and less operative vaginal births (Roberts & Hanson, 2007). The benefits of upright positions may be related to gravity, less aortovagal compression, improved fetal alignment, and larger anterior-posterior and transverse pelvic outlets (Berghella et al., 2008).

Squatting is highly effective in facilitating the descent and birth of the fetus. It is one of the best positions for the second stage of labor (Mayberry, Wood, Strange, Lee, Heisler, & Nielsen-Smith, 2000; Roberts, 2002). Women should assume a modified, supported squat until the fetal head is engaged, at which time a deep squat can be used. A firm surface is required for this position, and the woman will need side support (see Fig. 12-12, *A*). In a birthing bed a squat bar is available that she can use to help support herself (see Fig. 12-17, *E*). A birth ball also can be used to help a woman maintain the squatting position. The fetus will be aligned with the birth canal, and pelvic and perineal relaxation will be facilitated as she sits on the ball or holds it in front of her for support as she squats. Women may want to sit on the toilet or bedside commode during pushing because they are concerned about stool incontinence during this stage. You must closely monitor these women, however, and remove them from the toilet before birth occurs.

The side-lying, or lateral, position, with the upper part of the woman's leg held by the nurse or coach or placed on a pillow, is an effective position for the second stage of labor (Fig. 12-15, *A*). Women using the lateral position have more control over their bearing-down efforts. In addition, a slower, more controlled descent of the fetus results in a reduced risk of perineal trauma. Some women prefer a semi-sitting (semirecumbent) position. To maintain good uteroplacental circulation and to enhance the woman's bearing-down efforts in this position, elevate the woman's back and shoulders to at least a 30-degree angle, and place a wedge under one hip (Fig. 12-15, *B*).

The hands-and-knees position, along with pelvic rocking and abdominal stroking, is an effective position for birth because it enhances placental perfusion, helps rotate the fetus from a posterior to an anterior position, and may facilitate the birth of the shoulders, especially if the fetus is large. It also reduces perineal trauma (Simkin & Ancheta, 2000) (see Fig. 12-11, *B*).

The birthing bed is commonly used today and can be set for different positions according to the woman's needs (Figs. 12-16 and 12-17). The woman can squat, kneel, sit, recline, or lie on her side, choosing the position most comfortable for her without having to climb into bed for the birth. At the same time, the birthing bed provides excellent exposure for examinations, electrode placement, and birth. You can also position the bed for the administration of anesthesia, and it is ideal to help women receiving an epidural to assume different positions to facilitate birth. You can also use the bed to transport the woman to

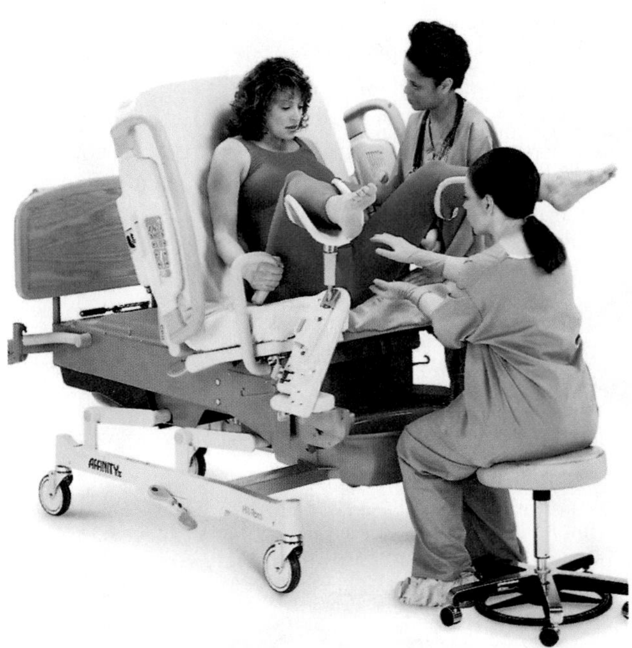

Fig. 12-16 Birthing bed. (Courtesy Hill-Rom, Batesville, IN.)

Critical Thinking/Clinical Decision Making

Delayed Pushing in Second Stage Labor

You are the nurse assigned to care for Emily, a 25-year-old G1 P0 at 38 weeks of gestation. You have just performed a vaginal examination and found that Emily's cervix is completely dilated. She has an epidural, which is working well. Currently, Emily is feeling neither pressure nor pain. On learning that Emily's cervix is completely dilated, her physician exclaims, "Good! Get in there and help her push so we can have this baby! I'm ready to go home. I've had a long day!"

1. Is evidence sufficient to draw conclusions about effective management of second stage labor?
2. What assumptions can be made about the following practices during second stage labor:
   a. "Laboring down"
   b. Delayed pushing
   c. Positioning for pushing
   d. Spontaneous versus directed pushing efforts
3. What are the priority nursing interventions for supporting Emily as she pushes in second stage labor?
4. Does the evidence objectively support your conclusion?
5. Do alternative perspectives to your conclusion exist?

the operating room if a cesarean birth is necessary. The woman can use squat bars, over-the-bed tables, birth balls, and pillows for support.

Bearing-down efforts

As the fetal head reaches the pelvic floor, most women experience the urge to bear down. Reflexively the woman will begin to exert downward pressure by contracting her abdominal muscles while relaxing her pelvic floor. This bearing down is an involuntary response to the Ferguson reflex. A strong expiratory grunt or groan (vocalization) often accompanies pushing when the woman exhales as she pushes. This natural vocalization by women during open-glottis bearing-down efforts should not be discouraged.

When coaching women to push, encourage them to push as they feel like pushing (instinctive, spontaneous pushing) rather than to give a prolonged push on command. Prolonged breath-holding, or sustained, directed bearing down, which is still a common practice, may trigger the **Valsalva maneuver**, which occurs when the woman closes the glottis (closed-glottis pushing), thereby increasing intrathoracic and cardiovascular pressure. This increased pressure reduces cardiac output and decreases perfusion of the uterus and the placenta. Adverse effects associated with prolonged breath holding and forceful pushing efforts include fetal hypoxia and subsequent acidosis (Simpson & James, 2005). Pelvic floor problems also have been associated with directed pushing (Schaffer, Bloom, Casey, McIntire, Nihira, & Leveno, 2005). The benefits of spontaneous pushing efforts rather than sustained Valsalva pushes include less hypoxic stress for the fetus and less pelvic or perineal damage for the woman (Roberts & Hanson, 2007).

A woman can become confused and anxious when she is being told to do something in conflict with what her body is telling her. Using phrases such as "you are doing so well," "you are moving the baby down," and "follow what your body is telling you" rather than "Push, push, push," encourages a woman to feel confident in her body and what she is feeling (Sampselle, Miller, Luecha, Fischer, & Rosten, 2005).

Women will usually begin to push naturally as the contraction increases in intensity and the Ferguson reflex strengthens. Monitor the woman's breathing so that she does not hold her breath for more than 5 to 7 seconds at a time, and remind her to ventilate her lungs fully by taking deep cleansing breaths before and after each contraction. Bearing down while exhaling (open-glottis pushing) and taking breaths between bearing-down efforts help maintain adequate oxygen levels for the mother and fetus and result in approximately five pushes during a contraction, with each push lasting approximately 5 seconds (Mayberry et al., 2000).

A woman may reach the second stage of labor and then experience a lack of readiness to complete the process and give birth to her child. She may have doubts about her readiness to be a mother or may desire to wait for her support person or primary health care provider to arrive. Fear, anxiety, or embarrassment regarding unfamiliar or painful sensations and behaviors during pushing (e.g., sounds made, passage of stool) may be other inhibiting factors. By recognizing that a woman may experience a

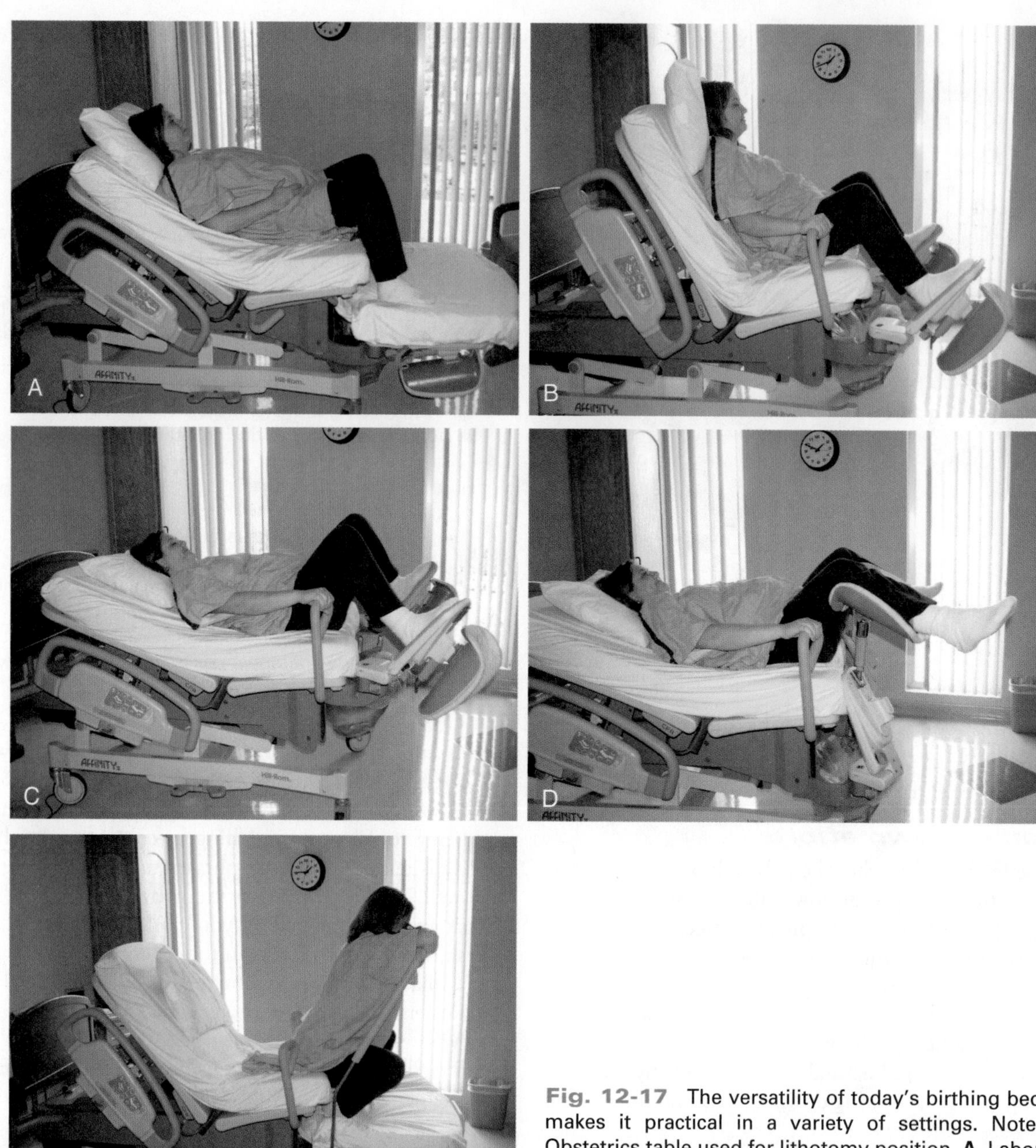

Fig. 12-17 The versatility of today's birthing bed makes it practical in a variety of settings. Note: Obstetrics table used for lithotomy position. **A**, Labor bed. **B**, Birth chair. **C**, Birth bed. **D**, Obstetrics table. **E**, Squatting or birth bar. (Courtesy Julie Perry Nelson, Loveland, CO.)

need to hold back the birth of her baby, you can address her concerns and effectively coach her during this stage of labor.

To ensure the slow birth of the fetal head, encourage the woman to control the urge to bear down by coaching her to take panting breaths or to exhale slowly through pursed lips as the baby's head crowns. At this point the woman needs simple, clear directions from one person. Amnesia between contractions often occurs in the second stage; therefore you may have to rouse the woman to get her to cooperate in the bearing-down process.

Fetal heart rate and pattern

As noted previously, you must check the FHR regularly (see Chapter 11 for further discussion). If the baseline rate begins to slow, if a loss of variability occurs, or if deceleration patterns develop (e.g., late, variable, or prolonged), initiate interventions promptly. Turn the woman on her side to reduce the pressure of the uterus against the ascending vena cava and descending aorta (see Fig. 12-5), and administer oxygen by non-rebreather face mask at 8 to 10 L/min (Tucker et al., 2009). These interventions are often all that is necessary to restore a reassuring pattern. If the FHR and pattern do not become reassuring immediately, notify the primary health care provider because the woman may need medical intervention to birth the baby. See Emergency box for more interventions related to non-reassuring FHR.

Support of the father or partner

During the second stage the woman needs continuous support and coaching (see Care Path: Low Risk Woman in Second Stage Labor). Because the coaching process is often physically and emotionally tiring for support persons, the nurse encourages them to take short breaks as needed. If birth occurs in an LDR or LDRP room, then the support person usually wears street clothes. Instruct the support person who attends the birth in a delivery room to put on a cover gown or scrub clothes, mask, cap, and shoe covers, as required by agency policy. The nurse also specifies support measures to be used for the laboring woman and points out areas of the room in which the partner can move freely.

Encourage partners to be present at the birth of their infants if doing so is in keeping with their cultural and personal expectations and beliefs. The presence of partners maintains the psychologic closeness of the family unit, and the partner can continue to provide the supportive care given during labor. The woman and her partner need to

EVIDENCE-BASED PRACTICE

Benefits of Continuous Labor Support

Pat Gingrich

ASK THE QUESTION

How does continuous labor support benefit laboring patients? Who should provide this support? Is this type of support a nursing role?

SEARCH FOR EVIDENCE

Search Strategies: Professional organization guidelines, meta-analyses, systematic reviews, randomized controlled trials, nonrandomized prospective studies, and retrospective studies since 2006.

Databases Searched: CINAHL, Cochrane, Medline, National Guideline Clearinghouse, and the websites for Association of Women's Health, Obstetric and Neonatal Nurses; National Practice Guidelines; Lamaze International; Society of Obstetricians and Gynaecologists of Canada; and World Health Organization.

CRITICALLY ANALYZE THE EVIDENCE

For millennia, women have labored in the company of other women, usually family or friends who have experienced birth themselves. In the last century, Western women in labor became more isolated in institutional, high-technology settings. Loss of dedicated labor support coincided with increasing technology, pain management, and operative birth. Observers now question whether returning the human touch of birthing assistants could improve outcomes. Lamaze International defines labor support as a trusted friend or doula who is not employed by the facility, offering to the laboring women and her partner physical and emotional support, information, and advocacy but never medical advice. The Lamaze Practice Guideline recommends that all women should have access to doula care covered under insurance (Green, Amis, Hotelling, 2007).

A Cochrane systematic analysis reviewed 16 randomized controlled trials involving 13,391 women from 11 countries. Taken as a whole the studies demonstrated that continuous labor support leads to shorter labors, increased vaginal birth, decreased analgesia, and decreased dissatisfaction (Hodnett, Gates, Hofmeyr, Sakal, 2007). These associations were especially true if the labor support was not an employee of the facility, the support was begun early in labor, and the setting did not typically use epidural analgesia.

In a randomized controlled trial of 420 women, continuous labor support was associated with decreased cesarean and instrumental birth, decreased need for pain medication or regional analgesia, and 100% positive feelings about birth (McGrath & Kennell, 2008).

Finally, a retrospective study of 11,471 women found that doula support was associated with increased breastfeeding intention and initiation and decreased caesarean birth (Motti-Santiago, Walker, Ewna, Vragovic, Winder, Stubblefield, 2008). This study did not randomize, however, thus the use of doulas and intention to breastfeed may represent prior related preferences of a certain population of women.

IMPLICATIONS FOR PRACTICE

Nurses and midwives provide attentive care for laboring women, but their workload usually precludes their continuous presence at the bedside. Partners might be well intentioned but may find the powerful reality of birth to be overwhelming. An experienced doula or birth attendant can keep the laboring woman calm and comfortable, which not only improves the experience emotionally, but also reduces pain, stress hormones, and muscular tension, thereby facilitating vaginal birth. Doulas are not there to replace the nurse or the partner but rather to provide support as needs arise. Insurance companies and institutions that see the measurable benefits of doulas are wise to value and encourage their contribution.

References:

Green, J., Amis, D., & Hotelling, B. A. (2007). Care practice no. 3: Continuous labor support. *Journal of Perinatal Education, 16*(3), 25-28.

Hodnett, E. D., Gates, S., Hofmyer, G. J., & Sakal, C. (2007). Continuous support for women during childbirth. In *The Cochrane Database of Systematic Reviews*, 2007, Issue 3, CD 003766.

McGrath, S. K., & Kennell, J. N. (2008). A randomized controlled trial of continuous labor support: Effect on cesarean delivery rates. *Birth, 35*(2), 92-97.

Motti-Santiago, J., Walker, C., Ewna, J., Vragovic, O., Winder, S., & Stubblefield, P. (2008). A hospital-based doula program and childbirth outcomes in an urban, multicultural setting. *Maternal and Child Health Journal, 35*(3), 372-377.

have an equal opportunity to initiate the attachment process with the baby.

LEGAL TIP Documentation

Document all observations (e.g., maternal vital signs, FHR and pattern, progress of labor) and nursing interventions, including patient response, concurrent with care. The course of labor and the maternal-fetal response may change without warning. All documentation should be accurate, complete, timely, and according to agency policy

Supplies, instruments, and equipment

To prepare for birth in any setting, the birthing area is usually set up during the transition phase for nulliparous women and during the active phase for multiparous women.

Prepare the birthing bed or table, and arrange instruments on the instrument table or delivery cart (Fig. 12-18). Follow standard procedures for gloving, identifying and opening sterile packages, adding sterile supplies to the instrument table, unwrapping sterile instruments, and handing them to the primary health care provider. Ready the crib or radiant warmer and equipment for the support and stabilization of the infant (Fig. 12-19).

Video: Childbirth (Vaginal)

The items used for birth may vary among different facilities; therefore consult each facility's procedure manual to determine the protocols specific to that facility.

The nurse estimates the time until the birth will occur and notifies the primary health care provider if he or she is not in the patient's room. Even the most experienced nurse can miscalculate the time left before birth occurs; therefore every nurse who attends a woman in labor must be prepared to assist with an emergency birth if the primary health care provider is not present (see Box 12-6).

Animation: Vaginal Birth

Birth in a delivery room or birthing room

The woman will need assistance if she must move from the labor bed to the delivery table (Fig. 12-20). The various positions assumed for birth in a delivery room are the Sims or lateral position in which the attendant supports the upper part of the woman's leg, the dorsal position (supine position with one hip elevated), and the lithotomy position.

The **lithotomy position** makes dealing with complications that arise more convenient for the primary health care provider (see Fig. 12-17, *D*). To place the woman in this position, bring her buttocks to the edge of the bed or table and place her legs in stirrups. Take care to pad the stirrups, to raise and place both legs simultaneously, and to adjust the shanks of the stirrups so that the calves of the legs are supported. No pressure should be placed on the popliteal space. Stirrups that are not the same height will strain ligaments in the woman's back as she bears down, leading to considerable discomfort in the postpartum period. The lower portion of the table may be dropped down and rolled back under the table.

The maternal position for birth in a birthing room varies from a lithotomy position, with the woman's feet in stirrups or resting on footrests or with her legs held and supported by the nurse or support person, to one in which her feet rest on footrests while she holds onto a squat bar, to a side-lying position with the woman's upper leg supported by the coach, nurse, or squat bar. Once the woman is positioned, the foot of the bed is removed so that the

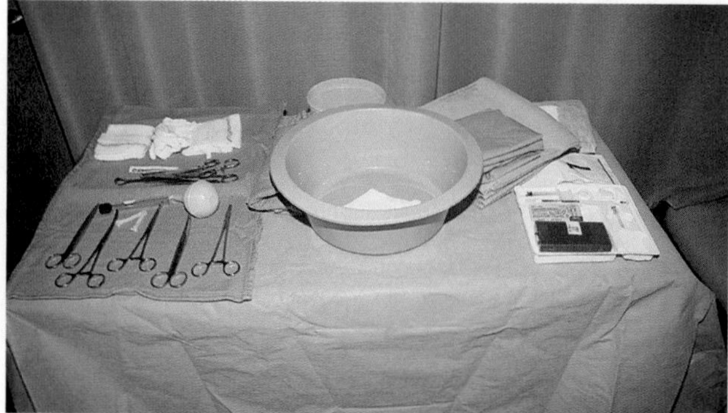

Fig. 12-18 Instrument table. (Courtesy Marjorie Pyle, RNC, Lifecircle, Costa Mesa, CA.)

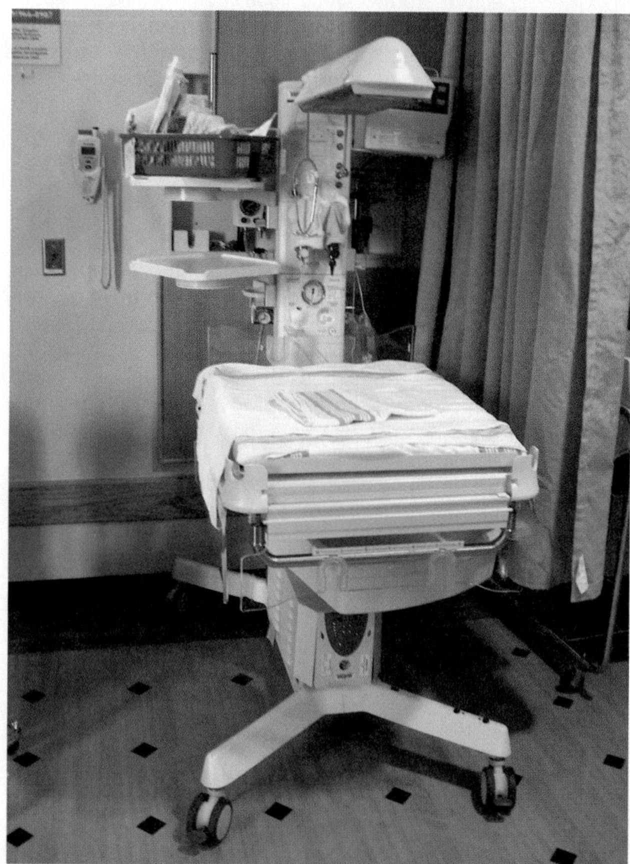

Fig. 12-19 Radiant warmer for newborn. (Courtesy Dee Lowdermilk, Chapel Hill, NC.)

primary health care provider attending the birth can gain better perineal access for performing an episiotomy, delivering a large baby, using forceps or vacuum extractor, or getting access to the emerging head to facilitate suctioning. Alternatively, the foot of the bed can be left in place and lowered slightly to form a ledge that allows access for birth and that also serves as a place to lay the newborn (see Fig. 12-17, *A*).

Once the woman is positioned for birth either in a delivery room or in a birthing room, the vulva and perineum are cleansed. Hospital protocols and the preferences of primary health care providers for cleansing may vary.

The nurse continues to coach and encourage the woman. The nurse auscultates the FHR or evaluates the monitor tracing every 5 to 15 minutes, depending on whether the woman is at low or high risk for problems or per protocol of the birthing facility, or continuously monitors the FHR with electronic monitoring. Keep the primary health care provider informed of the FHR and pattern (Tucker et al., 2009). Prepare or obtain an oxytocic medication such as oxytocin (Pitocin) so that it is ready to be administered immediately after expulsion of the placenta. Always follow Standard Precautions as you provide care during the process of labor and birth (see Box 12-3).

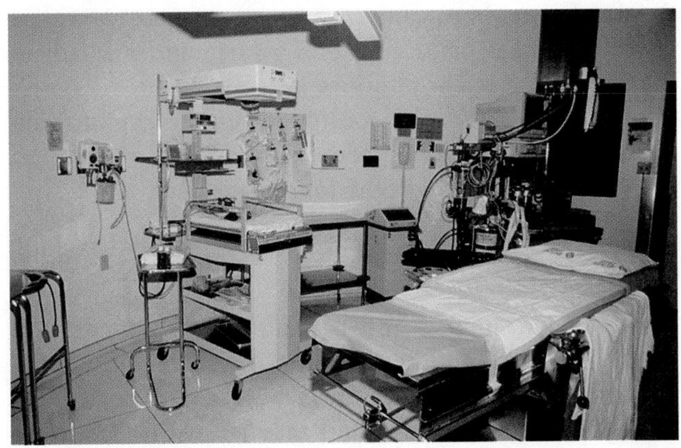

Fig. 12-20 Delivery room. (Courtesy Michael S. Clement, MD, Mesa, AZ.)

In the delivery room the primary health care provider puts on a cap, a mask that has a shield or protective eyewear, and shoe covers. After washing hands the provider puts on a sterile gown (with waterproof front and sleeves) and gloves. Nurses attending the birth also may need to wear caps, protective eyewear, masks, gowns, and gloves. The woman may then be draped with sterile drapes. In the birthing room, Standard Precautions are observed, but the amount and types of protective coverings worn by those in attendance often varies.

Maintain contact with the parents by touching, verbal comforting, explaining the reasons for care, and sharing in the parents' joy at the birth of their child.

Mechanism of birth: vertex presentation. The three phases of the spontaneous birth of a fetus in a vertex presentation are (1) birth of the head, (2) birth of the shoulders, and (3) birth of the body and extremities (see Chapter 9).

With voluntary bearing-down efforts the head appears at the introitus (Fig. 12-21). **Crowning** occurs when the widest part of the head (the biparietal diameter) distends the vulva just before birth. The birth attendant may apply mineral oil to the perineum and stretch it as the head is crowning. Immediately before birth the perineal musculature becomes greatly distended. If an episiotomy (incision into the perineum to enlarge the vaginal outlet) is necessary, it is performed at this time to minimize soft-tissue damage. Local anesthetic may be administered if necessary before the episiotomy. Box 12-7 shows the process of normal vaginal childbirth using a series of photographs.

The physician or nurse-midwife may use a hands-on approach to control the birth of the head, believing that guarding the perineum results in a gradual birth that will prevent fetal intracranial injury, protect maternal tissues, and reduce postpartum perineal pain. This approach involves (1) applying pressure against the rectum, drawing it downward to aid in flexing the head as the back of the

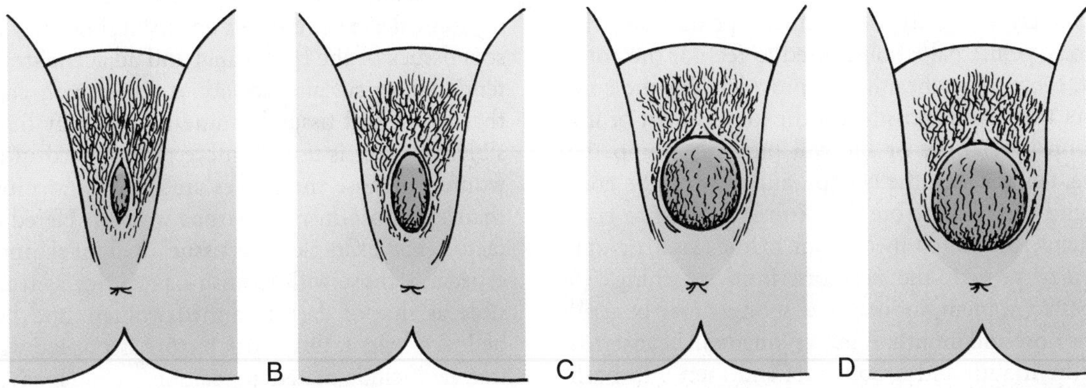

Fig. 12-21 Beginning birth with vertex presenting. **A**, Anteroposterior slit. **B**, Oval opening. **C**, Circular shape. **D**, Crowning.

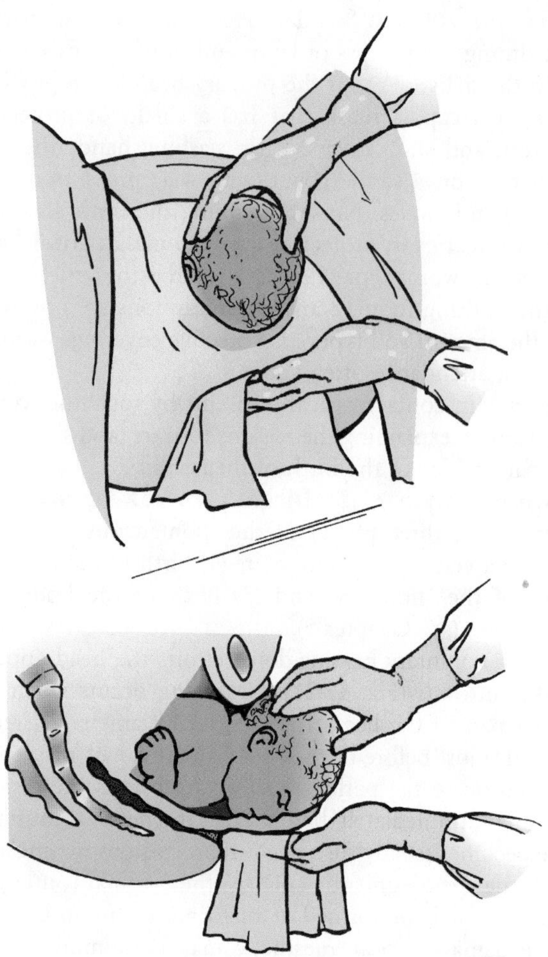

Fig. 12-22 Birth of head with modified Ritgen maneuver. Note control to prevent too rapid birth of head.

neck catches under the symphysis pubis, (2) then applying upward pressure from the coccygeal region (modified **Ritgen maneuver**) (Fig. 12-22) to extend the head during the actual birth, thereby protecting the musculature of the perineum, and (3) assisting the mother with voluntary control of the bearing-down efforts by coaching her to pant while letting uterine forces expel the fetus.

The umbilical cord often encircles the neck (**nuchal cord**) but rarely so tightly as to cause hypoxia. After the head is born, gentle palpation is used to feel for the cord. If present, the primary health care provider slips the cord gently over the head if possible. If the loop is tight or if a second loop is seen, he or she will probably clamp the cord twice, cut between the clamps, and unwind the cord from around the neck before the birth is allowed to continue. Mucus, blood, or meconium in the nasal or oral passages may prevent the newborn from breathing. To eliminate this problem, moist gauze sponges may be used to wipe the nose and mouth. A bulb syringe will be inserted first into the mouth and oropharynx and then into both nares to aspirate these fluids as needed.

Immediate assessments and care of the newborn

The time of birth is the precise time when the entire body is out of the mother. In case of multiple births, each birth would be noted in the same way. You must record the time of birth. If the newborn's condition is not compromised, he or she may be placed on the mother's abdomen immediately after birth and covered with a warm, dry blanket. The cord may be clamped at this time, and the primary health care provider may ask if the woman's partner would like to cut the cord. If so, then the partner is given a sterile pair of scissors and instructed to cut the cord 1 inch (2.5 cm) above the clamp.

The care given immediately after the birth focuses on assessing and stabilizing the newborn. The nurse's main responsibility at this time is the infant because the primary health care provider is involved with the delivery of the placenta and the care of the mother. The nurse must watch the infant for any signs of distress and initiate appropriate interventions should any appear.

Perform a brief assessment of the newborn immediately, even while the mother is holding the infant. This assessment includes assigning Apgar scores at 1 and 5 minutes after birth (see Table 17-1). Maintaining a patent airway, supporting respiratory effort, and preventing cold stress by drying the newborn and covering the newborn with a warmed blanket or placing him or her under a radiant warmer are the major priorities in terms of the newborn's immediate care. You can postpone further examination, identification procedures, and care until later in the third stage of labor or early in the fourth stage.

Perineal trauma related to childbirth

Most acute injuries and lacerations of the perineum, vagina, uterus, and their support tissues occur during childbirth. Alternative measures for perineal management, such as warm compresses and massage with a lubricant (e.g., prenatal and intrapartum), have demonstrated limited effectiveness in reducing perineal trauma, though they may lessen the degree of perineal lacerations. Therefore further research is recommended (Berghella et al., 2008; Albers, Sedler, Bedrick, Teaf, & Peralta, 2005).

Some degree of damage occurs during every birth to the soft tissues of the birth canal and adjacent structures. The tendency to sustain lacerations varies with each woman; that is, the soft tissue in some women may be less distensible. Damage is usually more pronounced in nulliparous women because the tissues are firmer and more resistant than are those in multiparous women. Heredity is also a factor. For example, the tissue of light-skinned women, especially those with reddish hair, is not as readily distensible as that of darker-skinned women, and healing may be less efficient. Other risk factors associated with perineal trauma include maternal position, pelvic inadequacy (e.g., narrow subpubic arch with a constricted outlet), fetal mal-

BOX 12-7

Normal Vaginal Childbirth

FIRST STAGE

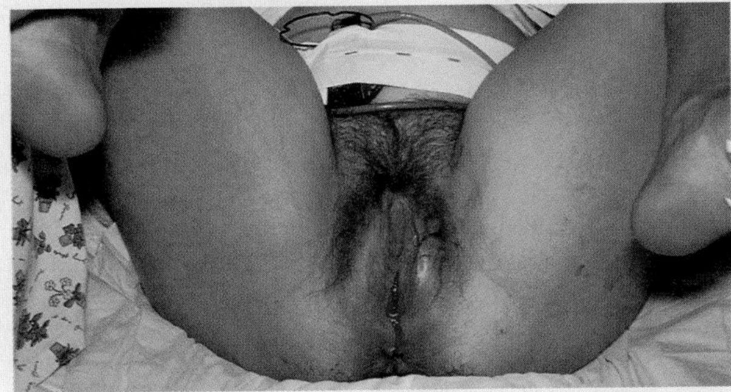

Anteroposterior slit; vertex is visible during contraction.

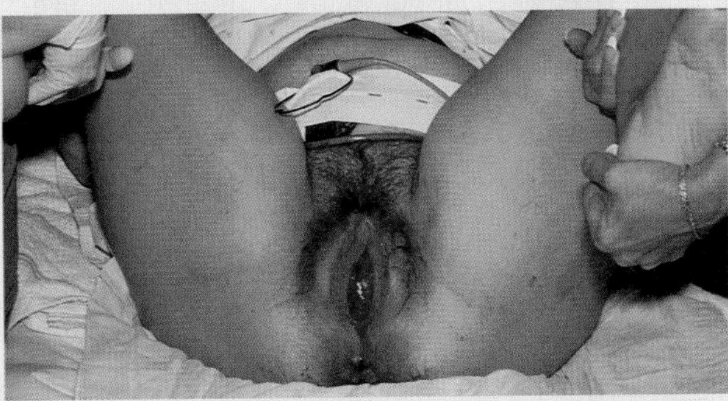

Oval opening; vertex is presenting. Note: Nurse (on left) is wearing gloves, but support person (on right) is not.

SECOND STAGE

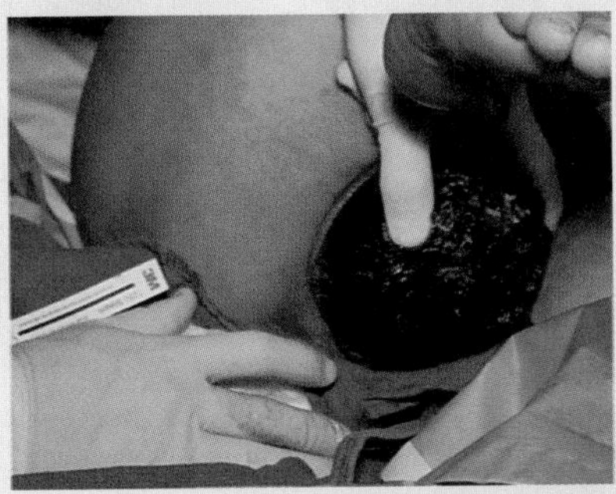

Crowning occurs.

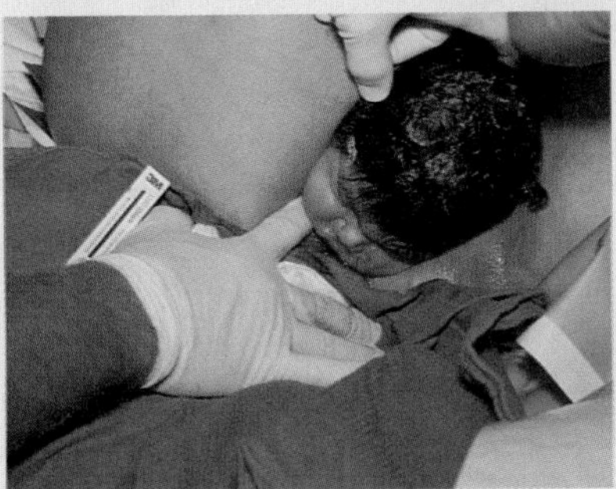

Nurse-midwife uses Ritgen maneuver as head is born by extension.

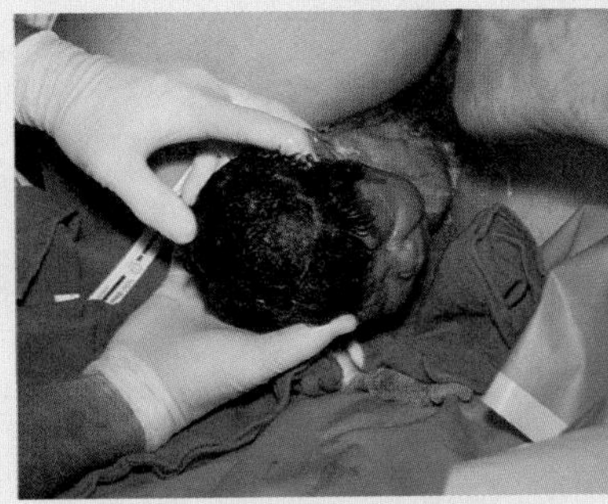

After nurse-midwife checks for nuchal cord, she supports head during external rotation and restitution.

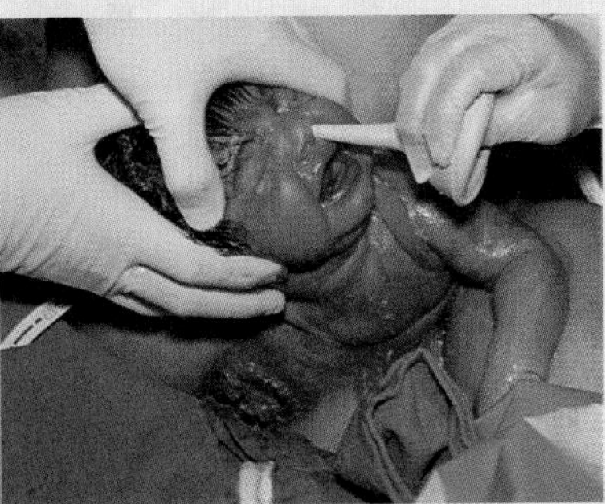

Bulb syringe is used to suction mucus.

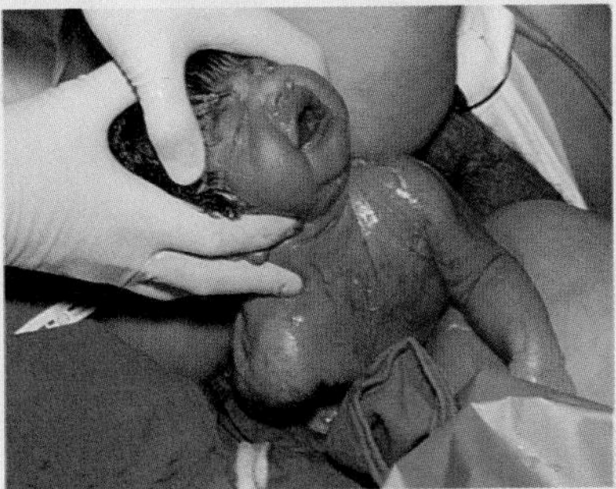

Birth of posterior shoulder occurs.

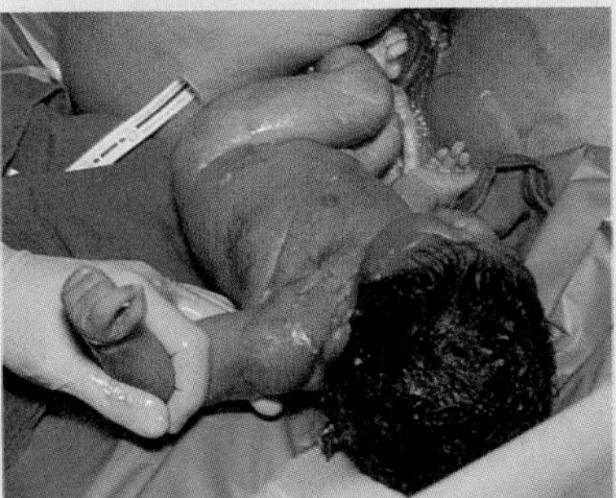

Birth of newborn occurs by slow expulsion.

Continued

BOX 12-7

Normal Vaginal Childbirth—cont'd

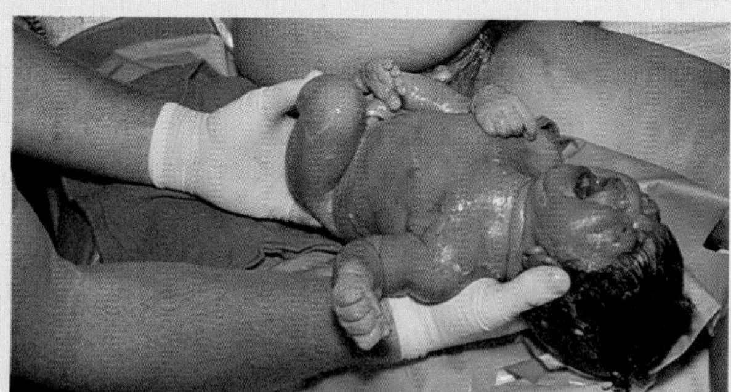

Second stage complete. Note that newborn is not completely pink yet.

THIRD STAGE

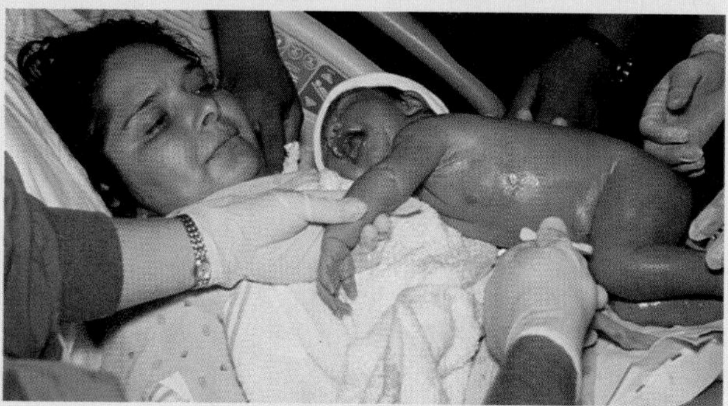

Newborn is placed on mother's abdomen while cord is clamped and cut.

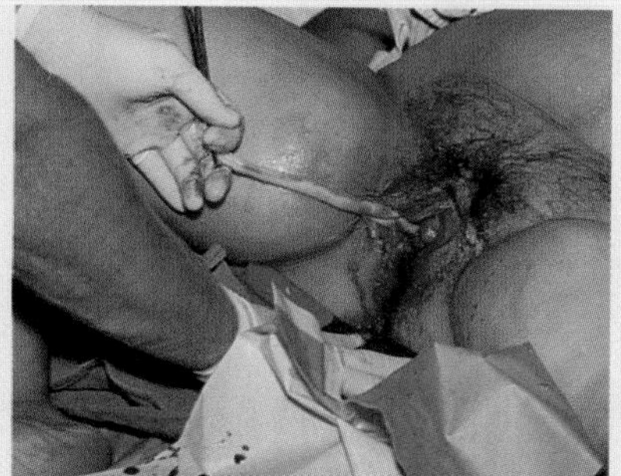

Note increased bleeding as placenta separates.

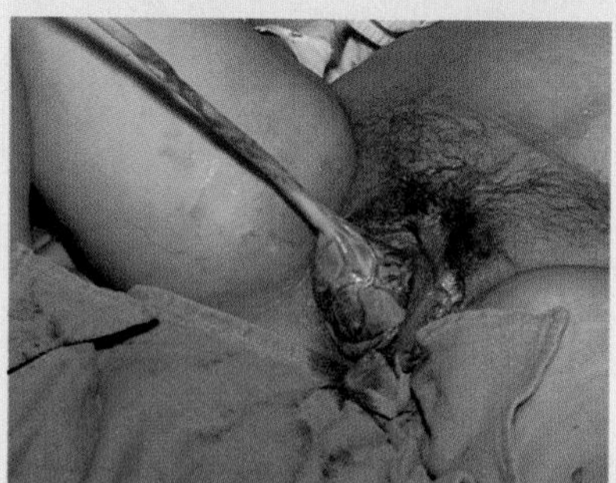

Expulsion of placenta occurs.

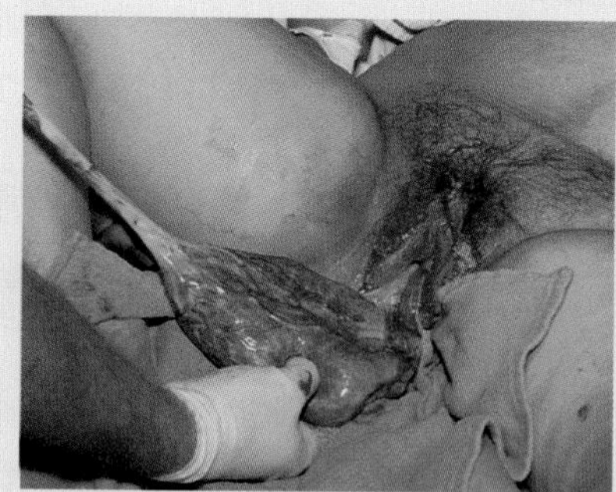

Expulsion is complete, marking the end of the third stage.

THE NEWBORN

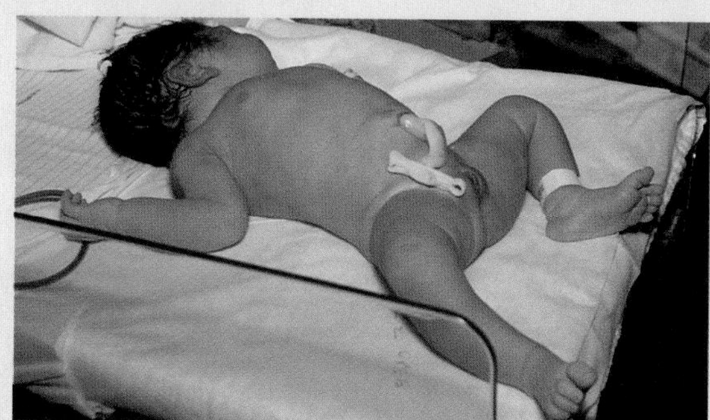

Newborn awaiting assessment: Note that color is almost completely pink.

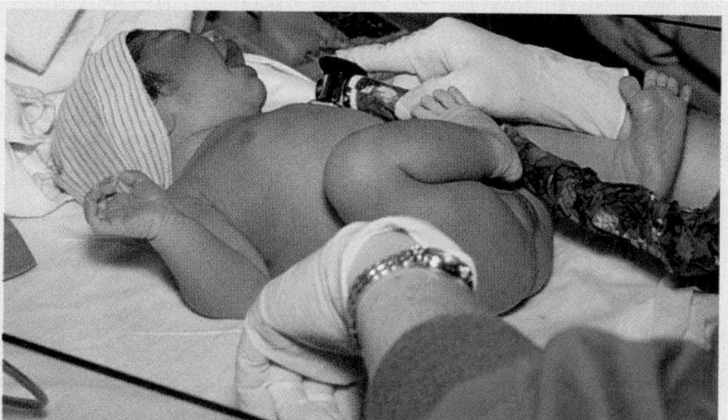

Assessment takes place while the newborn is under radiant warmer.

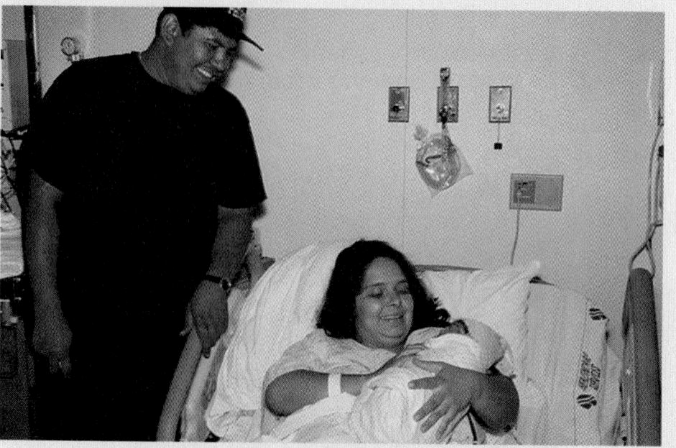

Parents are admiring their newborn.

Courtesy Michael S. Clement, MD, Mesa, AZ.

presentation and position (e.g., breech, occiput posterior position), large (macrosomic) infants, use of forceps or vacuum to facilitate birth, prolonged second stage of labor, fetal distress, and rapid labor in which there is insufficient time for the perineum to stretch.

Some injuries to the supporting tissues, whether they were acute or nonacute and whether they were repaired or not, may lead to genitourinary and sexual problems later in life (e.g., pelvic relaxation, uterine prolapse, cystocele, rectocele, dyspareunia, urinary and bowel dysfunction). Use of Kegel exercises in the prenatal and postpartum periods improves and restores the tone and strength of the perineal muscles. Health practices, including good nutrition and appropriate hygienic measures, help maintain the integrity and suppleness of the perineal tissue, enhance healing, and prevent infection.

Perineal lacerations. Perineal lacerations usually occur as the fetal head is being born. The extent of the laceration is defined in terms of its depth:

First degree: laceration that extends through the skin and structures superficial to muscles

Second degree: laceration that extends through muscles of the perineal body

Third degree: laceration that continues through the anal sphincter muscle

Fourth degree: laceration that also involves the anterior rectal wall

Perineal injury is often accompanied by small lacerations on the medial surfaces of the labia minora below the pubic rami and to the sides of the urethra (periurethral) and clitoris. Lacerations in this highly vascular area often result in profuse bleeding. Third- and fourth-degree lacerations must be carefully repaired so that the woman retains fecal continence. Take measures to promote soft stools (e.g., roughage, fluid, activity, stool softeners) to increase the woman's comfort and foster healing. Antimicrobial therapy may be instituted in some cases. Enemas and suppositories are contraindicated for these women.

Simple perineal injuries usually heal without permanent disability, regardless of whether they were repaired. However, repairing a new perineal injury to prevent future complications is easier than correcting long-term damage.

Vaginal lacerations. Vaginal lacerations often occur in conjunction with perineal lacerations. Vaginal lacerations tend to extend up the lateral walls (sulci) and, if deep enough, involve the levator ani muscle. Additional injury may occur high in the vaginal vault near the level of the ischial spines. Vaginal vault lacerations are often circular and may result from use of forceps to rotate the fetal head, rapid fetal descent, or precipitous birth.

Cervical injuries. Cervical injuries occur when the cervix retracts over the advancing fetal head. These cervical lacerations occur at the lateral angles of the external os. Most lacerations are shallow, and bleeding is minimal. Larger lacerations may extend to the vaginal vault or beyond it into the lower uterine segment; serious bleeding may occur. Extensive lacerations may occur after hasty attempts to enlarge the cervical opening artificially or to deliver the fetus before full cervical dilation is achieved. Injuries to the cervix can have adverse effects on future pregnancies and childbirths.

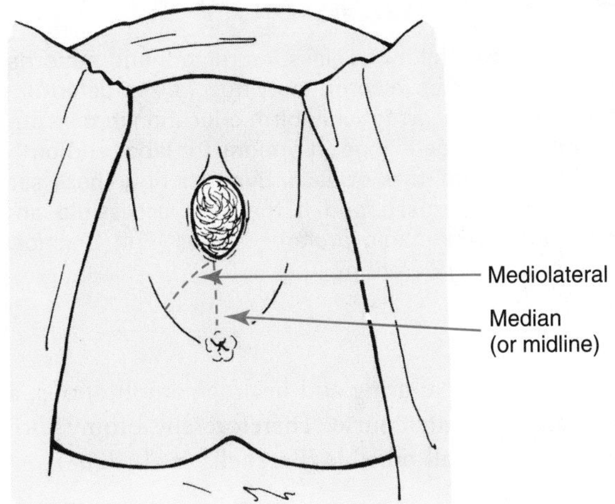

Fig. 12-23 Types of episiotomies.

Episiotomy

An **episiotomy** is an incision made in the perineum to enlarge the vaginal outlet (Fig. 12-23). It is performed more commonly in the United States and Canada than in Europe. The side-lying position for birth, used routinely in Europe, reduces tension on the perineum, making possible a gradual stretching of the perineum with fewer indications for episiotomies. Different types of episiotomies are performed, depending on the site and direction of the incision (see Fig. 12-23). The type of episiotomy that provides the best outcome is unknown (Berghella et al., 2008). Midline (median) episiotomy is most commonly used in the United States. It is effective, easily repaired, and generally the least painful. However, midline episiotomies also are associated with an increased incidence of third- and fourth-degree lacerations. Sphincter tone is usually restored after primary healing and a good repair. Mediolateral episiotomy is used in operative births when the need for posterior extension is likely. Although a fourth-degree laceration can be prevented using this technique, a third-degree laceration may occur. The blood loss is also greater and the repair more difficult and painful than with midline episiotomies. It is also more painful in the postpartum period, and the pain lasts longer.

Routine performance of episiotomies has declined in the United States since the 1990s. The practice in many settings now is to support the perineum manually during birth and allow the perineum to tear rather than perform an episiotomy. Tears are often smaller than an episiotomy, are repaired easily or not at all, and heal quickly. Routine use of episiotomy is associated with increased posterior

COMMUNITY ACTIVITY

Contact local childbirth class instructors and maternal infant care nurses in community hospitals to determine the level of support for childbirth education in the community. Investigate support options for labor and birth, and specify the roles of each. Evaluate how these services are advertised and if they are accessible and affordable. Are ethnic preferences for birth practices taken into consideration?

perineal trauma, suturing and healing complications, and later pain with intercourse. Therefore episiotomy should be avoided if at all possible (Berghella et al., 2008).

Evaluation

The expected outcomes of care are used to evaluate the effectiveness of care.

THIRD STAGE OF LABOR

CARE MANAGEMENT

The **third stage of labor** lasts from the birth of the baby until the placenta is expelled. The goal in the management of the third stage of labor is the prompt separation and expulsion of the placenta achieved in the easiest, safest manner. The third stage is generally by far the shortest stage of labor. The placenta is usually expelled within 10 to 15 minutes after the birth of the baby. If the third stage of labor has not been completed within 30 minutes, then the placenta is considered to be retained and interventions to hasten delivery are usually instituted (Battista & Wing, 2007).

Under normal circumstances the placenta is attached to the decidual layer of the basal plate's thin endometrium by numerous fibrous anchor villi—much in the same way as a postage stamp is attached to a sheet of postage stamps. After the birth of the fetus the sudden decrease in uterine volume and strong uterine contractions cause the placental site to shrink. This event causes the anchor villi to break and the placenta to separate from its attachments. Normally the first few strong contractions that occur after the baby's birth cause the placenta to shear away from the basal plate. A placenta cannot detach itself from a flaccid (relaxed) uterus because the placental site is not reduced in size.

Assessment

Placental separation and expulsion

The following signs indicate placental separation (Fig. 12-24):

- A firmly contracting fundus
- A change in the uterus from a discoid to a globular ovoid shape as the placenta moves into the lower uterine segment
- A sudden gush of dark blood from the introitus
- Apparent lengthening of the umbilical cord as the placenta descends to the introitus
- The finding of vaginal fullness (the placenta) on vaginal or rectal examination or of fetal membranes at the introitus

Depending on preference the primary health care provider may use an expectant or active approach to manage the third stage of labor. Research is currently under way to determine which approach is better. Expectant management (watchful waiting) involves the natural, spontaneous separation and expulsion of the placenta by efforts of the mother with clamping and cutting of the cord after pulsation ceases. It may involve the use of gravity or nipple stimulation to facilitate separation and expulsion, but no oxytocic (uterotonic) medications are given. A quiet, relaxed environment that supports close skin-to-skin contact between mother and newborn also promotes the release of endogenous oxytocin.

Active management encourages placental separation and expulsion with administration of one or more oxytocic (uterotonic) medications after the birth of the anterior shoulder of the fetus. Immediately after clamping and cutting the umbilical cord the primary health care provider delivers the placenta by application of controlled cord traction when signs of separation are noted.

Nursing Diagnoses

Possible nursing diagnoses appropriate for the woman in the third stage of labor include:

- *Risk for deficient fluid volume* related to:
  - Blood loss occurring after placental separation and expulsion
  - Inadequate contraction of the uterus
- *Anxiety* related to:
  - Lack of knowledge regarding separation and expulsion of the placenta
  - Occurrence of perineal trauma and the need for repair
- *Fatigue* related to:
  - Energy expenditure associated with childbirth and the bearing-down efforts of the second stage

Expected Outcomes of Care

Expected outcomes for the woman in the third stage of labor are that the woman will accomplish the following:

- Continue normal progression of labor.
- Maintain adequate hydration status through oral or IV intake (or both).
- Actively participate in the labor and birth process.
- Verbalize discomfort and indicate the need for measures that help reduce discomfort and promote relaxation.
- Accept comfort and support measures from significant others and health care providers as needed.
- Expel the placenta with a blood loss of less than 500 ml.

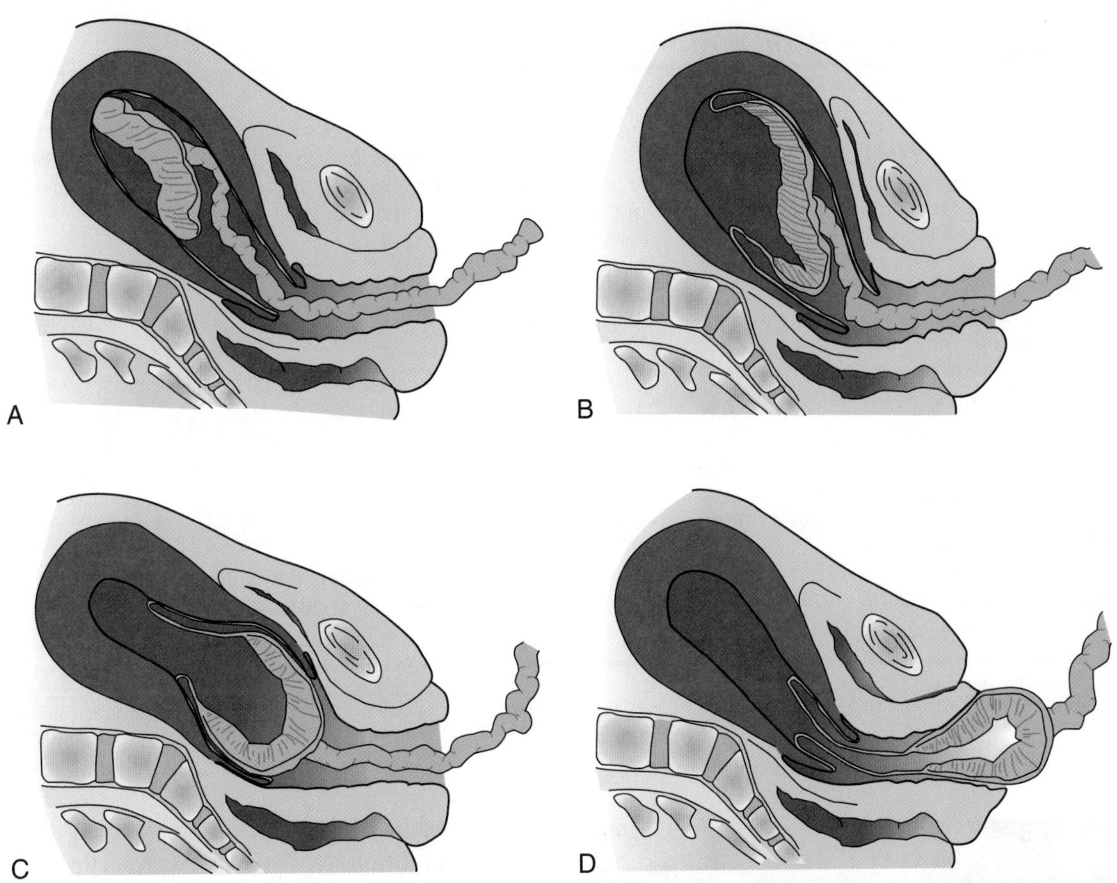

Fig. 12-24 Third stage of labor. **A**, Placenta begins to separate in central portion, accompanied by retroplacental bleeding. Uterus changes from discoid to globular shape. **B**, Placenta completes separation and enters lower uterine segment. Uterus is globular shape. **C**, Placenta enters vagina, cord is seen to lengthen, and an increase in bleeding may be seen. **D**, Expulsion (delivery) of placenta and completion of third stage.

- Initiate, along with the partner and family, the processes of bonding and attachment with the newborn.
- Express satisfaction with her performance during labor and birth.

Plan of Care and Interventions

To assist in the delivery of the placenta, instruct the woman to push when signs of separation have occurred. If possible, the woman should expel the placenta during a uterine contraction. Alternate compression and elevation of the fundus, plus minimal, controlled traction on the umbilical cord, may also be used to facilitate delivery of the placenta and amniotic membranes. Oxytocics are usually administered after the placenta is removed because they stimulate the uterus to contract, thereby helping to prevent hemorrhage. Oxytocics may be given earlier, however, if the third stage of labor is actively managed. The Care Path: Low Risk Woman in Third Stage of Labor on p. 378 lists appropriate assessments and care measures. Also see Nursing Care Plan on p. 353.

Whether the placenta first appears by its shiny fetal surface (Schultze mechanism) or turns to show its dark roughened maternal surface first (Duncan mechanism) is of no clinical importance.

After the placenta and the amniotic membranes emerge the primary health care provider examines them for intactness to ensure that no portion remains in the uterine cavity (i.e., no fragments of the placenta or membranes are retained) (Fig. 12-25).

When the third stage of labor has been completed the primary health care provider examines the woman for any perineal, vaginal, or cervical lacerations requiring repair. If an episiotomy was performed, it will be sutured. Immediate repair promotes healing, limits residual damage, and decreases the possibility of infection. The woman usually feels some discomfort while the primary health care provider carries out the postbirth vaginal examination. Help the woman to use breathing and relaxation or distraction techniques to assist her in dealing with the discomfort. During this time the nurse performs a quick assessment of the newborn's physical condition, weighs the baby, and places matching identification bands on baby and mother. The baby may also receive eye prophylaxis and a vitamin K injection at this time.

CARE PATH Low Risk Woman in Third Stage of Labor

I. ASSESSMENT MEASURES*	FREQUENCY
Blood pressure, pulse, respirations	Every 15 min
Uterine activity	Assess for signs of placental separation
Vaginal show	Assess bleeding until placental expulsion occurs
Behavior, appearance, mood, energy level of woman; condition of partner	As needed

II. PHYSICAL CARE MEASURES†

- Assist to bear down to facilitate delivery of separated placenta.
- Administer oxytocic as ordered.
- Provide pain relief as needed.
- Provide hygiene and comfort measures as needed.

III. EMOTIONAL SUPPORT

- Keep informed about progress of placental separation.
- Explain purpose if medication given.
- Describe status of perineal tissue, and inform if repair is needed.
- Introduce parents to their baby.
- Assess and care for newborn within view of parents; delay eye prophylaxis to facilitate eye contact.
- Provide private time for family to bond with their new baby and help them to create memories.
- Encourage breastfeeding if desired.

*Frequency of assessment is determined by the risk status of the maternal-fetal unit. More frequent assessment is required in high risk situations. Frequency of assessment and method of documentation are also determined by agency policy, which is usually based on the recommended care standards of medical and nursing organizations.
†Physical care measures are performed by the nurse working together with the woman's partner and significant others.

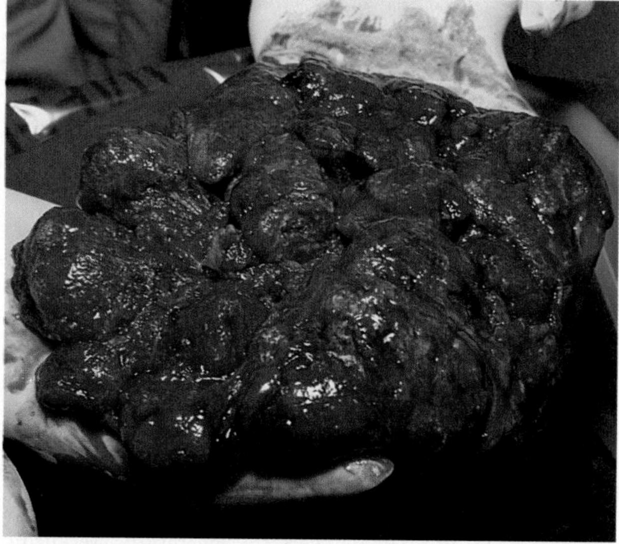

Fig. 12-25 Examination of the placenta. (Courtesy Michael S. Clement, MD, Mesa, AZ.)

After any necessary repairs have been completed, cleanse the vulvar area gently with warm water or normal saline, and apply a perineal pad or an ice pack to the perineum. Reposition the birthing bed or table, and lower the woman's legs simultaneously from the stirrups if she gave birth in a lithotomy position. Remove any drapes, and place dry linen under the woman's buttocks. Provide the woman with a clean gown and a blanket, which is warmed, if needed.

Some women and their families may have culturally based beliefs regarding the care of the placenta and the manner of its disposal after birth, viewing the care and disposal of the placenta as a way of protecting the newborn from bad luck and illness. Requests by the woman to take the placenta home and dispose of it according to her customs sometimes conflict with health care agency policies, especially those related to infection control and the disposal of biologic wastes. Many cultures follow specific rules regarding the disposal of the placenta in terms of method (burning, drying, burying, eating), site for disposal (in or near the home), and timing of disposal (immediately after birth, time of day, astrologic signs). Disposal rituals may vary according to the gender of the child and the length of time before another child is desired. Some cultures believe that eating the placenta is a means of restoring a woman's well-being after birth or ensuring high-quality breast milk. Health care providers can provide culturally sensitive health care by encouraging women and their families to express their wishes regarding the care and disposal of the placenta and by establishing a policy to fulfill these requests (D'Avanzo, 2008).

Evaluation

The expected outcomes of care are used to evaluate the effectiveness of care.

FOURTH STAGE OF LABOR

CARE MANAGEMENT

The first 1 to 2 hours after birth, sometimes called the **fourth stage of labor**, is a crucial time for mother and newborn. Both are not only recovering from the physical process of birth, but also becoming acquainted with each other and additional family members. During this time, maternal organs undergo their initial readjustment to the nonpregnant state, and the functions of body systems begin to stabilize.

In most hospitals the mother remains in the labor and birth area during this recovery time. In an institution in which LDR rooms are used the woman stays in the same room where she gave birth. In traditional settings, women are taken from the delivery room to a separate recovery area for observation. Arrangements for care of the newborn vary during the fourth stage of labor. In many settings the baby remains at the mother's bedside, and the labor or birth nurse cares for both of them. In other institutions the baby is taken to the nursery for several hours of observation after an initial bonding period with the parents and perhaps other family members (Fig. 12-26).

Assessment

If the recovery nurse has not previously cared for the new mother, her assessment begins with an oral report from the nurse who attended the woman during labor and birth and a review of the prenatal, labor, and birth records. Of primary importance are conditions that can predispose the mother to hemorrhage, such as precipitous labor, a large baby, grand multiparity (i.e., having given birth to six or more viable infants), induced labor, or a magnesium infusion during labor. For healthy women, hemorrhage is the most dangerous potential complication during the fourth stage of labor.

During the first hour after birth the mother is assessed frequently. Box 12-8 and Fig. 14-2 on p. 401 describe the physical assessment of the mother during the fourth stage of labor. All factors except temperature are assessed every 15 minutes for 1 hour. Temperature is assessed at the beginning and end of the recovery period. After the fourth 15-minute assessment, if all parameters have stabilized within the normal range, the process is usually repeated once in the second hour.

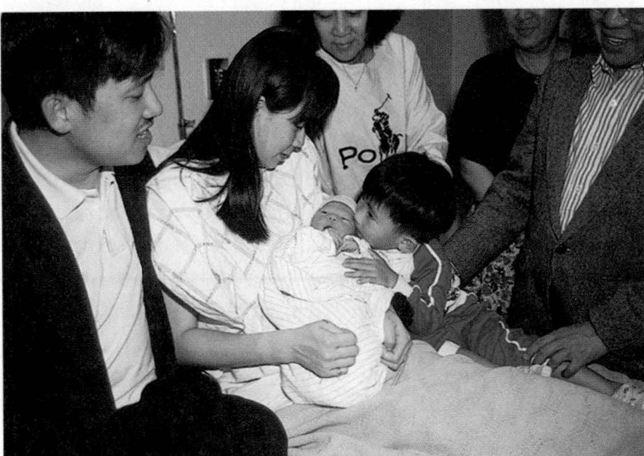

Fig. 12-26 Big brother becomes acquainted with new baby sister. (Courtesy Marjorie Pyle, RNC, Lifecircle, Costa Mesa, CA.)

Postanesthesia recovery

The woman who has given birth by cesarean or has received regional anesthesia for a vaginal birth requires special attention during the recovery period. Obstetric recovery areas are held to the same standard of care that would be expected of any other postanesthesia recovery (PAR) room (American Academy of Pediatrics [AAP] & American College of Obstetricians and Gynecologists [ACOG], 2007). A PAR score is determined for each woman on arrival and is updated as part of every 15 minute assessment. Components of the PAR score include activity, respirations, blood pressure, level of consciousness, and color.

NURSING ALERT Regardless of her obstetric status, no woman should be discharged from the recovery area until she has completely recovered from the effects of anesthesia.

If the woman received general anesthesia, she should be awake and alert and oriented to time, place, and person. Her respiratory rate should be within normal limits, and her oxygen saturation level at least 95%, as measured by a pulse oximeter. If the woman received epidural or spinal anesthesia, she should be able to raise her legs, extended at the knees, off the bed, or to flex her knees, place her feet flat on the bed, and raise her buttocks well off the bed. The numb or tingling, prickly sensation should be entirely gone from her legs. The length of time required to recover from regional anesthesia varies greatly among women. Several hours are often needed for these anesthetic effects to disappear completely.

Nursing Diagnoses

Possible nursing diagnoses appropriate for the woman in the fourth stage of labor include:

- *Risk for deficient fluid volume (hemorrhage)* related to:
    - Uterine atony after childbirth
- *Acute pain* related to:
    - Uterine involution
    - Trauma to perineum, episiotomy
    - Hemorrhoids

Expected Outcomes of Care

Expected outcomes for the woman in the fourth stage of labor are that the woman will accomplish the following:

- Successfully adapt physiologically from being pregnant to being "not pregnant."
- Maintain adequate hydration status through oral or IV intake (or both).
- Verbalize discomfort and indicate the measures that help reduce discomfort an relaxation.

BOX 12-8

Assessment during Fourth Stage of Labor

BLOOD PRESSURE
- Measure blood pressure every 15 minutes for the first hour.

PULSE
- Assess rate and regularity. Measure every 15 minutes for the first hour.

TEMPERATURE
- Determine temperature at the beginning of the recovery period and after the first hour of recovery.

FUNDUS
- Position the woman with knees flexed and head flat.
- Just below umbilicus, cup the hand and press firmly into the abdomen. At the same time, stabilize the uterus at the symphysis with the opposite hand (Fig. 14-2).
- If the fundus is firm (and the bladder is empty), with uterus in midline, measure its position relative to woman's umbilicus. Lay fingers flat on abdomen under the umbilicus; measure how many fingerbreadths (fb) or centimeters (cm) fit between the umbilicus and the top of the fundus. If the fundus is above the umbilicus, the value is recorded as plus (+) fb or cm; if below, as minus (−) fb or cm.
- If the fundus is not firm, massage it gently to contract and expel any clots before measuring distance from umbilicus.
- Place the hands appropriately; massage gently only until firm.
- Expel clots while keeping hands placed as in Fig. 14-2. With upper hand, firmly apply pressure downward toward the vagina; observe the perineum for amount and size of expelled clots.

BLADDER
- Assess distention by noting the location and firmness of the uterine fundus and by observing and palpating the bladder. A distended bladder is seen as a suprapubic rounded bulge that is dull to percussion and fluctuates similar to a water-filled balloon. When the bladder is distended, the uterus is usually boggy in consistency, well above the umbilicus, and to the woman's right side.
- Assist the woman to void spontaneously. Measure the amount of urine voided.
- Catheterize if the bladder is distended and the woman is unable to void spontaneously.
- Reassess after voiding or catheterization to make sure the bladder is not palpable and the fundus is firm and in the midline.

LOCHIA
- Observe lochia on perineal pads and on linen under the mother's buttocks. Determine the amount and color; note the size and number of clots; note any odor.
- Observe perineum for source of bleeding (e.g., episiotomy, lacerations).

PERINEUM
- Ask or assist the woman to turn on her side and flex the upper leg on the hip.
- Lift the upper buttock.
- Observe the perineum in good lighting.
- Assess episiotomy or laceration repair for intactness, hematoma, edema, bruising, redness, and drainage.
- Assess for the presence of hemorrhoids.

- Accept comfort and support measures from significant others and health care providers as needed.
- Initiate, along with the partner and family, the processes of bonding and attachment with the newborn.
- Express satisfaction with her performance during labor and birth.

Plan of Care and Interventions

Care of the new mother

Restriction of food and fluid intake and the loss of fluids (blood, perspiration, or emesis) during labor cause many women to be very hungry and thirsty soon after birth. In the absence of complications a woman who has given birth vaginally, who has recovered from the effects of the anesthetic, and who has stable vital signs, a firm uterus, and small to moderate lochial flow may have fluids and a regular diet as desired (AAP & ACOG, 2007). In the immediate postpartum period, women who give birth by cesarean are usually restricted to clear liquids and ice chips.

As soon as they have had a chance to bond with the new baby and eat, most new mothers are ready for a nap, or at least a quiet period of rest. After this rest period the woman may want to shower and change clothes. Most new mothers are capable of self-management or are assisted in these activities by family members or support persons. See the Nursing Care Plan on p. 353.

Care of the family

Most parents enjoy being able to handle, hold, explore, and examine the baby immediately after birth. Both parents can assist with the thorough drying of the infant. The infant is usually wrapped in a receiving blanket and given to the woman to hold. If skin-to-skin contact is desired, place the unwrapped infant on the woman's chest or abdomen, and then cover the baby with a warm blanket. Holding the newborn next to her skin helps the mother maintain the baby's body heat and provides skin-to-skin contact. Take care to keep the baby's head warm. Stockinette caps are often used to cover the newborn's head.

Many women wish to begin breastfeeding their newborns at this time to take advantage of the infant's alert state (*first period of reactivity*) and to stimulate the production of oxytocin that promotes contraction of the uterus. The nurse encourages and assists the woman to breastfeed at this time if she desires to do so. In some cultures, however (e.g., Vietnamese, Hispanic), breastfeeding is not acceptable to some women until the milk comes in.

Family-newborn relationships. The woman's reaction to the sight of her newborn may range from excited outbursts of laughing, talking, and even crying to apparent apathy. A polite smile and nod may be her only acknowledgment of the comments of nurses and the primary health care provider. Occasionally, the reaction is one of anger or indifference; the woman turns away from the baby, concentrates on her own pain, and sometimes makes hostile comments. These varied reactions can arise from pleasure, exhaustion, or deep disappointment. When evaluating parent-newborn interactions after birth, consider the cultural characteristics of the woman and her family and the expected behaviors of that culture. In some cultures the birth of a male child is preferred, and women may grieve when a female child is born (D'Avanzo, 2008).

Whatever the reaction and its cause may be, the woman needs continuing acceptance and support from all staff. Make a notation regarding the parents' reaction to the newborn in the recovery record. Assess this reaction by asking yourself such questions as, "How do the parents look?" "What do they say?" "What do they do?" Conduct further assessment of the parent-newborn relationship as you give care during the period of recovery. This assessment is especially important if you notice warning signs (e.g., passive or hostile reactions to the newborn, disappointment with sex or appearance of the newborn, absence of eye contact, limited interaction of parents with each other) immediately after birth. Nurses often find it helpful to discuss any warning signs with the woman's primary health care provider.

Siblings, who may have appeared only remotely interested in the final phases of the second stage, tend to experience renewed interest and excitement when the newborn appears. They may wish to touch or hold the new baby immediately (see Fig. 12-26).

Parents usually respond to praise of their newborn. Many need reassurance that the dusky appearance of their baby's extremities immediately after birth is normal until circulation is well established. If appropriate, explain the reason for the molding of the newborn's head. Communicate information about hospital routine. Recognize, however, that the cultural background of the parents may influence their expectations regarding the care and handling of their newborn immediately after birth. For example, some traditional Southeast Asians believe that the head should not be touched because it is the most sacred part of a person's body. They also believe that praise of the baby is dangerous because jealous spirits may then cause the baby harm or take it away (D'Avanzo, 2008).

Evaluation

The expected outcomes of care are used to evaluate the effectiveness of care. Determining a woman's satisfaction with and impressions of her total childbirth experience is a critical component in the provision of high-quality maternal-newborn health care that meets the individual needs of women and families using these services.

KEY POINTS

- The onset of labor is sometimes difficult to determine for both nulliparous and multiparous women.
- The familiar environment of her home is most often the ideal place for a woman during the latent phase of the first stage of labor.
- The nurse assumes much of the responsibility for assessing the progress of labor and for keeping the primary health care provider informed about progress in labor and deviations from expected findings.
- Assessment of the laboring woman's urinary output and bladder is critical to ensure her progress and to prevent injury to the bladder.
- Regardless of the actual labor and birth experience, the woman's or couple's perception of the birth experience is most likely to be positive when events and performances are consistent with expectations, especially in terms of maintaining control and adequacy of pain relief.
- The woman's level of anxiety may increase when she does not understand what is being said to her about her labor because of the medical terms used or because of a language barrier.
- Coaching, emotional support, and comfort measures assist the woman to use her energy constructively in relaxing and working with the contractions.
- The progress of labor is enhanced when a woman changes her position frequently during the first stage of labor.
- Doulas provide a continuous supportive presence during labor that can have a positive effect on the process of childbirth and its outcome.
- The cultural beliefs and practices of a woman and her significant others, including her partner, can have a profound influence on their approach to labor and birth.
- The quality of the nurse-patient relationship is a factor in the woman's ability to cope with the stressors of the labor process.
- Women with a history of sexual abuse often experience profound stress and anxiety during childbirth.

Continued

KEY POINTS—cont'd

- The inability to palpate the cervix during vaginal examination indicates that complete effacement and full dilation have occurred and is the only certain, objective sign that the second stage has begun.
- Women may have an urge to bear down at various times during labor; for some, it may be before the cervix is fully dilated, and for others it may not occur until the active phase of the second stage of labor.
- When encouraged to respond to the rhythmic nature of the second stage of labor the woman normally changes body positions, bears down spontaneously, and vocalizes (open-glottis pushing) when she perceives the urge to push (Ferguson reflex).
- Women should bear down several times during a contraction using the open-glottis pushing method. They should avoid sustained closed-glottis pushing because this will prevent oxygen transport to the fetus.
- Siblings present for labor and birth need preparation and support for the event.
- Objective signs indicate that the placenta has separated and is ready to be expelled; excessive traction (pulling) on the umbilical cord, before the placenta has separated, can result in maternal injury.
- During the fourth stage of labor, frequently assess the woman's fundal tone, lochial flow, and vital signs to ensure that she is physically recovering well after giving birth.
- Most parents and families enjoy being able to handle, hold, explore, and examine the baby immediately after the birth.
- Nurses should observe the progress in the development of parent-child relationships and be alert for warning signs that may appear during the immediate postpartum period.

Audio Chapter Summaries: Access an audio summary of these Key Points on evolve

References

Albers, L. L. (2007). The evidence for physiologic management of the active phase of the first stage of labor. *Journal of Midwifery & Women's Health, 52*(3), 207-215.

Albers, L., Sedler, K., Bedrick, E., Teaf, D., & Peralta, P. (2005). Midwifery care measures in the second stage of labor and reduction of genital tract trauma at birth: A randomized trial. *Journal of Midwifery & Women's Health, 50*(5), 365-372.

American Academy of Pediatrics (AAP) & American College of Obstetricians and Gynecologists (ACOG). (2007). *Guidelines for perinatal care* (6th ed.). Washington, DC: ACOG.

Angelini, D., & Mahlmeister, L. (2005). Liability in triage: Management of EMTALA regulations and common obstetric risks. *Journal of Midwifery & Women's Health, 50*(6), 472-478.

Battista, L. R., & Wing, D. A. (2007). Abnormal labor and induction of labor. In S. Gabbe, J. Niebyl, & J. Simpson (Eds.), *Obstetrics: Normal and problem pregnancies* (5th ed.). Philadelphia: Churchill Livingstone.

Berghella, V., Baxter, J. K., & Chauhan, S. P. (2008). Evidence-based labor and delivery management. *American Journal of Obstetrics & Gynecology, 199*(5), 445-454.

Brancato, R. M., Church, S., & Stone, P. W. (2008). A meta-analysis of passive descent versus immediate pushing in nulliparous women with epidural analgesia in the second stage of labor. *Journal of Obstetric, Gynecologic, and Neonatal Nursing, 37*(1), 4-12.

Callister, L. (2005). What has the literature taught us about culturally competent care of women and children. *MCN American Journal of Maternal Child Nursing, 30*(6), 380-388.

D'Avanzo, C. E. (2008). *Mosby's pocket guide to cultural health assessment* (4th ed.). St. Louis: Mosby.

Gilbert, E. S. (2007). *Manual of high risk pregnancy & delivery* (4th ed.). St. Louis: Mosby.

Hodnett, E. D., Gates, S., Hofmeyr, G. J., & Sakala, C. (2007). Continuous support for women during childbirth. In *The Cochrane Database of Systematic Reviews*, 2007, Issue 3, CD 003766.

MacKinnon, K., McIntyre, M., & Quance, M. (2005). The meaning of the nurse's presence during childbirth. *Journal of Obstetric, Gynecologic, and Neonatal Nursing, 34*(1), 28-36.

Mayberry, L., Wood, S. H., Strange, L. B., Lee, L., Heisler, D. R., & Nielsen-Smith K. (2000). *Second stage labor management: Promotion of evidence-based practice and a collaborative approach to patient care.* Washington, DC: Association of Women's Health, Obstetric and Neonatal Nurses.

Reveiz, L., Gaitan, H. G., & Cuervo, L. G. (2007). Enemas during labour. In *The Cochrane Database of Systemic Reviews*, 2007, Issue 4, CD 000330.

Roberts, J. (2002). The "push" for evidence: Management of the second stage. *Journal of Midwifery & Women's Health, 47*(1), 2-15.

Roberts, J., & Hanson, L. (2007). Best practices in second stage labor care: Maternal bearing down and positioning. *Journal of Midwifery & Women's Health, 52*(3), 238-245.

Sampselle, C., Miller, J., Luecha, Y., Fischer, K., & Rosten, L. (2005). Provider support of spontaneous pushing during the second stage of labor. *Journal of Obstetric, Gynecologic, and Neonatal Nursing, 34*(6), 695-702.

Schaffer, J. L., Bloom, S. L., Casey, B. M., McIntire, D. D., Nihira, M. A., & Leveno, K. J. (2005). A randomized control trial of the effects of coached vs uncoached maternal pushing during the second-stage of labor on postpartum pelvic floor structure and function. *American Journal of Obstetrics & Gynecology, 192*(5), 1692-1696.

Simkin, P., & Ancheta, R. (2000). *The labor progress handbook.* Malden, MA: Blackwell Science.

Simpson, K., & James, D. (2005). Effects of immediate versus delayed pushing during second-stage labor on fetal well-being: A randomized clinical trial. *Nursing Research, 54*(3), 149-157.

Tucker, S. M., Miller, L. A, & Miller, D. A. (2009). *Mosby's pocket guide to fetal monitoring: A multidisciplinary approach* (6th ed.). St. Louis: Mosby.

Zwelling, E., Johnson, K., & Allen, J. (2006). How to implement complementary therapies for laboring women. *MCN American Journal of Maternal Child Nursing, 31*(6), 364-372.

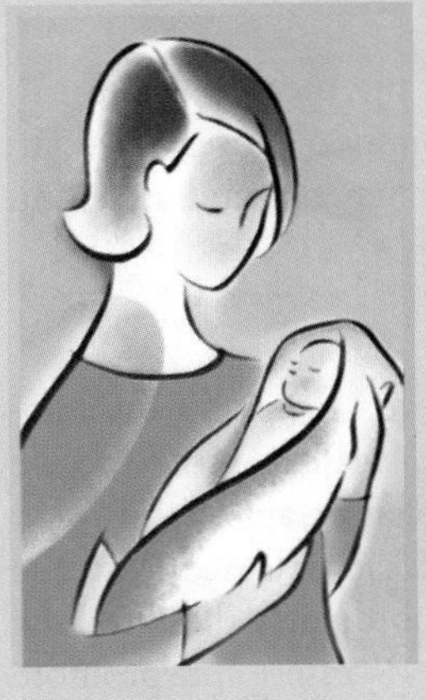

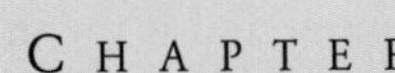

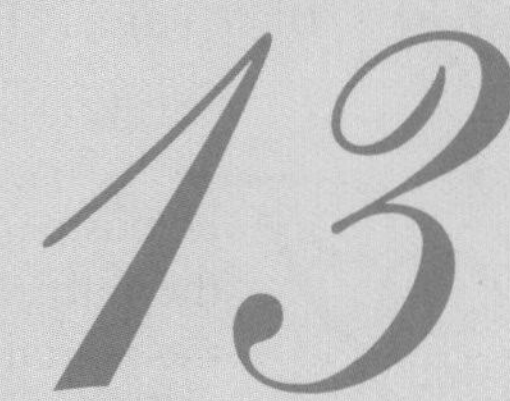

CHAPTER 13

Maternal Physiologic Changes

KITTY CASHION

LEARNING OBJECTIVES

- *Describe the anatomic and physiologic changes that occur during the postpartum period.*
- *Identify characteristics of uterine involution and lochial flow, and describe ways to measure them.*
- *List expected values for vital signs, deviations from normal findings, and probable causes of the deviations.*

KEY TERMS AND DEFINITIONS

afterpains (afterbirth pains) Painful uterine cramps that occur intermittently for approximately 2 or 3 days after birth and that result from contractile efforts of the uterus to return to its normal involuted condition

autolysis The self-destruction of excess hypertrophied tissue

diastasis recti abdominis Separation of the two rectus muscles along the median line of the abdominal wall

involution Return of the uterus to a nonpregnant state after birth

lochia Vaginal discharge during the puerperium consisting of blood, tissue, and mucus

- **lochia alba** Thin, yellowish to white, vaginal discharge that follows lochia serosa on approximately the tenth day after birth and that may last from 2 to 6 weeks postpartum
- **lochia rubra** Red, distinctly blood-tinged vaginal flow that follows birth and lasts 2 to 4 days
- **lochia serosa** Serous, pinkish brown, watery vaginal discharge that follows lochia rubra until approximately the tenth day after birth

pelvic relaxation Lengthening and weakening of the fascial supports of pelvic structures

puerperium Period between the birth of the newborn and the return of the reproductive organs to their normal nonpregnant state; fourth trimester of pregnancy

subinvolution Failure of the uterus to reduce to its normal size and condition after pregnancy

WEB RESOURCES

Additional related content can be found on the companion website at evolve

http://evolve.elsevier.com/Lowdermilk/Maternity/

- NCLEX Review Questions
- Spanish Guidelines: Postpartum Physical Examination

The postpartum period is the interval between the birth of the newborn and the return of the reproductive organs to their normal nonpregnant state. This period is sometimes called the **puerperium**, or fourth trimester of pregnancy. Although the puerperium has traditionally been considered as lasting 6 weeks, this time frame varies among women. The distinct physiologic changes that occur as the processes of pregnancy are reversed are normal. To provide care during the recovery period that is beneficial to the mother, her infant, and her family, the nurse must synthesize knowledge of maternal anatomy and physiology of the recovery period, the newborn's physical and behavioral characteristics, infant care activities, and family response to the birth of the infant. This chapter focuses on anatomic and physiologic changes that occur in the mother during the postpartum period.

REPRODUCTIVE SYSTEM AND ASSOCIATED STRUCTURES

Uterus

Involution process

The return of the uterus to a nonpregnant state after birth is known as **involution**. This process begins immediately after expulsion of the placenta with contraction of the uterine smooth muscle.

At the end of the third stage of labor the uterus is in the midline, approximately 2 cm below the level of the umbilicus, with the fundus resting on the sacral promontory. At this time the uterus weighs approximately 1000 g.

Within 12 hours the fundus rises to the level of the umbilicus, or slightly above or below (Fig. 13-1). Thereafter the fundus descends approximately 1 cm every day. By 1 week after birth the fundus is located 4 to 5 fingerbreadths below the umbilicus. The uterus should not be palpable abdominally after 2 weeks and should have returned to its nonpregnant location by 6 weeks after birth (Blackburn, 2007).

The uterus, which at full term weighs approximately 11 times its prepregnancy weight, involutes to approximately 500 g by 1 week after birth and to 350 g by 2 weeks after birth. At 6 weeks, it weighs 60 to 80 g (see Fig. 13-1).

Increased estrogen and progesterone levels are responsible for stimulating the massive growth of the uterus during pregnancy. Prenatal uterine growth results from both hyperplasia, an increase in the number of muscle cells, and from hypertrophy, an enlargement of the existing cells. Postpartally, the decrease in these hormones causes **autolysis**, the self-destruction of excess hypertrophied tissue. The additional cells laid down during pregnancy remain, however, and account for the slight increase in uterine size after each pregnancy.

Subinvolution is the failure of the uterus to return to a nonpregnant state. The most common causes of subinvolution are retained placental fragments and infection (see Chapter 23).

Contractions

Postpartum hemostasis is achieved primarily by compression of intramyometrial blood vessels as the uterine muscle contracts rather than by platelet aggregation and clot formation. The hormone oxytocin, released from the pituitary gland, strengthens and coordinates these uterine contractions, which compress blood vessels and promote hemostasis. During the first 1 to 2 postpartum hours, uterine contractions may decrease in intensity and become uncoordinated. Because the uterus must remain firm and well contracted, exogenous oxytocin (Pitocin) is usually administered intravenously or intramuscularly immediately after expulsion of the placenta. Women who plan to breastfeed should also be encouraged to put the baby to the breast immediately after birth because suckling stimulates oxytocin release.

Afterpains

In first-time mothers, uterine tone is good, the fundus generally remains firm, and the mother usually perceives only mild uterine cramping. Periodic relaxation and vigorous contraction are more common in subsequent pregnancies and may cause uncomfortable cramping called **afterpains (afterbirth pains)** that persist throughout the early puerperium. Afterpains are more noticeable after births in which the uterus was overdistended (e.g., large baby, multifetal gestation, polyhydramnios). Breastfeeding and exogenous oxytocic medication usually intensify these afterpains because both stimulate uterine contractions.

Placental site

Immediately after the placenta and membranes are expelled, vascular constriction and thromboses reduce the placental site to an irregular nodular and elevated area. Upward growth of the endometrium causes sloughing of necrotic tissue and prevents the scar formation that is characteristic of normal wound healing. This unique healing process enables the endometrium to resume its usual cycle of changes and to permit implantation and placentation in future pregnancies. Endometrial regeneration is completed by postpartum day 16, except at the placental site. Regeneration at the placental site occurs gradually and is not usually complete until 6 weeks after birth (Blackburn, 2007).

Lochia

Post-childbirth uterine discharge, commonly called **lochia**, is initially bright red (lochia rubra) and may contain small clots. For the first 2 hours after birth the amount of uterine discharge should be approximately that of a heavy

Spanish Guidelines: Postpartum Physical Examination

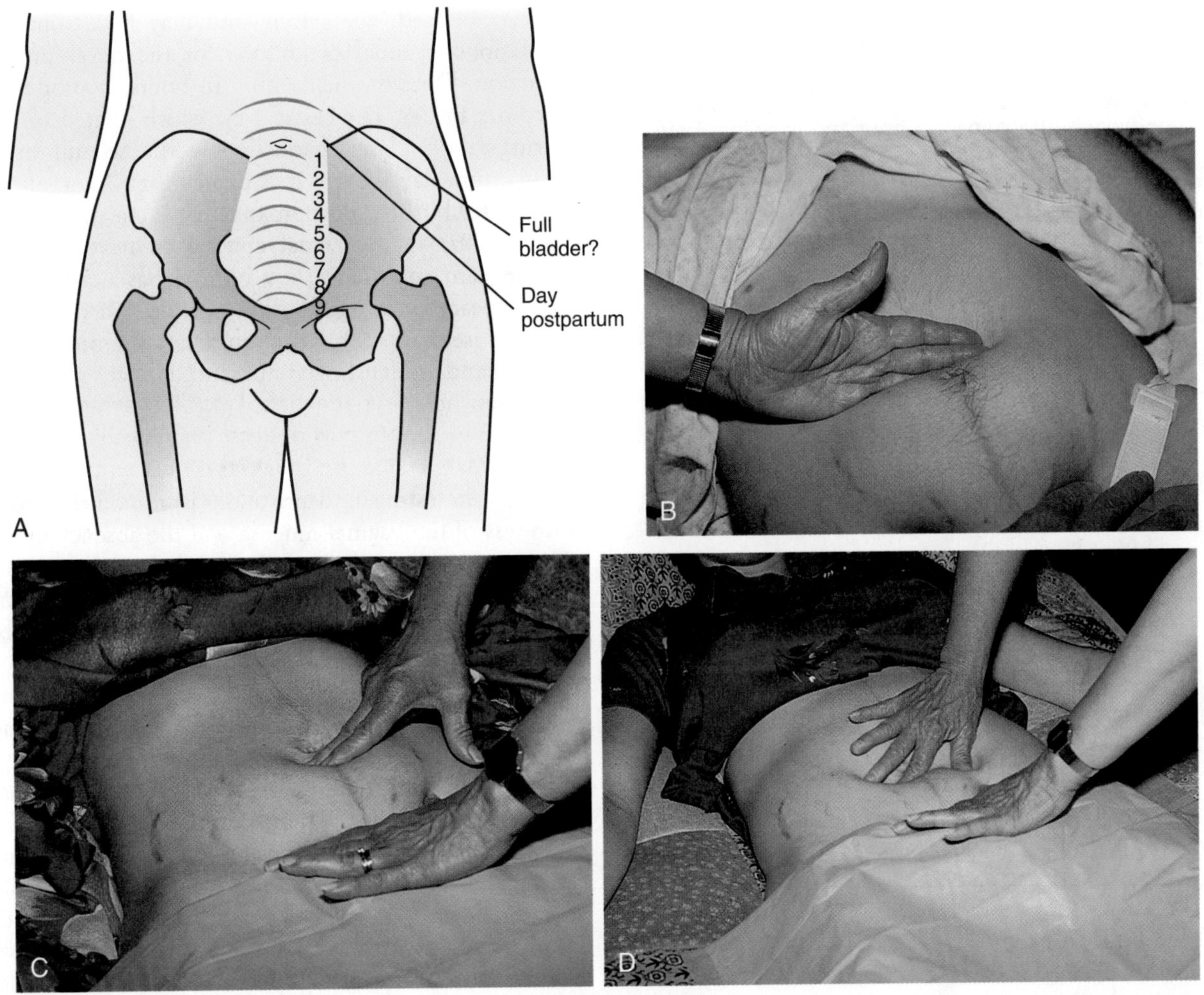

Fig. 13-1 Assessment of involution of uterus after childbirth. **A**, Normal progress, days 1 through 9. **B**, Size and position of uterus 2 hours after childbirth. **C**, Two days after childbirth. **D**, Four days after childbirth. (**B**, **C**, **D**, Courtesy Marjorie Pyle, RNC, Lifecircle, Costa Mesa, CA.)

menstrual period. After that time the lochial flow should steadily decrease.

Lochia rubra consists mainly of blood and decidual and trophoblastic debris. The flow pales, becoming pink or brown (lochia serosa) after 3 to 4 days. **Lochia serosa** consists of old blood, serum, leukocytes, and tissue debris. The median duration for lochia serosa discharge is 22 to 27 days (Katz, 2007). In most women, approximately 10 days after childbirth the drainage becomes yellow to white (**lochia alba**). Lochia alba consists primarily of leukocytes and decidual cells but also contains epithelial cells, mucus, serum, and bacteria. Lochia alba may last until 6 weeks after birth (Blackburn, 2007).

If the woman receives an oxytocic medication, the flow of lochia is often scant until the effects of the medication wear off. The amount of lochia is typically smaller after cesarean births. Flow of lochia usually increases with ambulation and breastfeeding. Lochia tends to pool in the vagina when the woman is lying in bed; on standing the woman may experience a gush of blood. This gush should not be confused with hemorrhage.

Persistence of lochia rubra early in the postpartum period suggests continued bleeding as a result of retained fragments of the placenta or membranes. Recurrence of bleeding approximately 7 to 14 days after birth is from the healing placental site. Approximately 10% to 15% of women will still be experiencing normal lochia serosa discharge at the 6-week postpartum examination (Katz, 2007). In the majority of women, however, a continued flow of lochia serosa or lochia alba by 3 to 4 weeks after birth may indicate endometritis, particularly if fever, pain, or abdominal tenderness is associated with the discharge. Lochia should smell similar to normal menstrual flow; an offensive odor usually indicates infection.

Not all postpartal vaginal bleeding is lochia; vaginal bleeding after birth may be a result of unrepaired vaginal or cervical lacerations. Table 13-1 distinguishes between lochial and nonlochial bleeding.

Cervix

The cervix is soft immediately after birth. The ectocervix (portion of the cervix that protrudes into the vagina)

Critical Thinking/Clinical Decision Making

Assessment of Postpartum Bleeding

You are the nurse assigned to care for Margarita, a G9 P9 who gave birth vaginally 1 hour ago to twins. Twin A weighed 7 pounds, 4 ounces, and Twin B weighed 6 pounds, 12 ounces. Margarita did not have an episiotomy and sustained no lacerations requiring repair. You are at the nurse's station when Margarita calls and asks for her nurse to "come quick!" When you arrive in her room, you find Margarita lying in a puddle of blood. The disposable pad underneath her, as well as Margarita's perineal pad, are completely soaked with blood.

1. What other immediate assessment is necessary to determine the cause and management of Margarita's excessive bleeding?
2. What assumptions can be made about the following issues:
   a. Normal amount of lochia expected at this time (1 hour after birth)
   b. Margarita's risk factors for uterine atony
   c. Immediate nursing interventions for Margarita
   d. Other possible causes for Margarita's excessive bleeding
3. Using the situation-background-assessment-recommendation (SBAR) technique, how would you report to Margarita's health care provider about her current status?
4. Does the evidence objectively support your conclusion?
5. Do alternative perspectives to your conclusion exist?

TABLE 13-1

Lochial and Nonlochial Bleeding

LOCHIAL BLEEDING	NONLOCHIAL BLEEDING
Lochia usually trickles from the vaginal opening. The steady flow increases as the uterus contracts.	If the bloody discharge spurts from the vagina, damage to a blood vessel may have occurred during birth. If so, some of the bleeding is not just normal lochial flow.
A gush of lochia may result as the uterus is massaged. If the lochia is dark in color, it has been pooled in the relaxed vagina, and the amount soon lessens to a trickle of bright red lochia (in the early puerperium).	If the amount of bleeding continues to be excessive and bright red, a vaginal or cervical tear may be the source.

appears bruised, edematous, and may have some small lacerations–optimal conditions for the development of infection. Over the next 12 to 18 hours, it shortens and becomes firmer. The cervical os, which dilated to 10 cm during labor, closes gradually. By the second or third postpartum day the cervix is dilated 2 to 3 cm, and by 1 week after birth, it is approximately 1 cm dilated (Blackburn, 2007). The external cervical os never regains its prepregnant appearance; it no longer has a circular shape but appears as a jagged slit often described as a "fish mouth" (see Fig. 6-2). Lactation delays the production of cervical and other estrogen-influenced mucus and mucosal characteristics.

Vagina and Perineum

Postpartum estrogen deprivation is responsible for the thinness of the vaginal mucosa and the absence of rugae. The greatly distended, smooth-walled vagina gradually decreases in size and regains tone, although it never completely returns to its prepregnancy state (Blackburn, 2007). Rugae reappear within 3 to 4 weeks, but they are never as prominent as they are in the nulliparous woman. Most rugae are permanently flattened. The mucosa remains atrophic in the lactating woman, at least until menstruation resumes. Thickening of the vaginal mucosa occurs with the return of ovarian function. Estrogen deficiency is also responsible for a decreased amount of vaginal lubrication. Localized dryness and coital discomfort (dyspareunia) may persist until ovarian function returns and menstruation resumes. The use of a water-soluble lubricant during sexual intercourse is usually recommended.

Initially, the introitus is erythematous and edematous, especially in the area of the episiotomy or laceration repair. It is usually barely distinguishable from that of a nulliparous woman if lacerations and an episiotomy have been carefully repaired, hematomas are prevented or treated early, and the woman observes good hygiene during the first 2 weeks after birth.

Most episiotomies and laceration repairs are visible only if the woman is lying on her side with her upper buttock raised or if she is placed in the lithotomy position. A good light source is essential for visualization of some repairs. Healing of an episiotomy or laceration is the same as any surgical incision. Signs of infection (pain, redness, warmth, swelling, or discharge) or loss of approximation (separation of the incision edges) may occur. Initial healing occurs within 2 to 3 weeks, but 4 to 6 months may be required for the repair to heal completely (Blackburn, 2007).

Hemorrhoids (anal varicosities) are commonly seen (see Fig. 6-10). Internal hemorrhoids may evert while the woman is pushing during birth. Women often experience associated symptoms such as itching, discomfort, and bright-red bleeding with defecation. Hemorrhoids usually decrease in size within 6 weeks of childbirth.

Pelvic Muscular Support

The supporting structure of the uterus and vagina may be injured during childbirth and may contribute to later gynecologic problems. Supportive tissues of the pelvic floor that are torn or stretched during childbirth may require up to 6 months to regain tone. Kegel exercises, which help to strengthen perineal muscles and encourage healing, are recommended after childbirth (see Teaching Guidelines, Chapter 2, p. 55). Later in life, women can experience pelvic relaxation, the lengthening and weakening of the fascial supports of pelvic structures. These structures include the uterus, upper posterior vaginal wall, urethra, bladder, and rectum. Although pelvic relaxation can occur in any woman, it is usually a direct but delayed complication of childbirth (see Chapter 23).

ENDOCRINE SYSTEM

Placental Hormones

Significant hormonal changes occur during the postpartal period. Expulsion of the placenta results in dramatic decreases of the hormones produced by that organ. Decreases in human chorionic somatomammotropin, estrogens, cortisol, and the placental enzyme insulinase reverse the diabetogenic effects of pregnancy, resulting in significantly lower blood sugar levels in the immediate puerperium. Mothers with type 1 diabetes will likely require much less insulin than they did at the end of pregnancy for several days after birth. Because these normal hormonal changes make the puerperium a transitional period for carbohydrate metabolism, interpreting glucose tolerance tests is difficult during this time.

Estrogen and progesterone levels drop markedly after expulsion of the placenta and reach their lowest levels 1 week after childbirth. Decreased estrogen levels are associated with breast engorgement and with the diuresis of excess extracellular fluid accumulated during pregnancy. In nonlactating women, estrogen levels begin to rise by 2 weeks after birth and by postpartum day 17 are significantly higher than in women who breastfeed (Katz, 2007).

Human chorionic gonadotropin (hCG) disappears fairly quickly from maternal circulation. However, because removing hCG from the extravascular and intracellular spaces takes additional time, the hormone can be detected for 3 to 4 weeks after birth in the maternal system (Blackburn, 2007).

Pituitary Hormones and Ovarian Function

Lactating and nonlactating women differ considerably in the time when the first ovulation occurs and when menstruation resumes. The persistence of elevated serum prolactin levels in breastfeeding women appears to be responsible for suppressing ovulation (Katz, 2007). Prolactin levels in blood rise progressively throughout pregnancy and remain elevated in women who breastfeed (Lawrence & Lawrence, 2009). The duration of anovulation is influenced by the frequency of breastfeeding, the duration of each feeding, and the degree to which supplementary feedings are used (Katz, 2007). Individual differences in the strength of an infant's sucking stimulus probably also affect prolactin levels. In nonlactating women, prolactin levels decline after birth and reach the prepregnant range by the third postpartum week (Katz, 2007).

Ovulation occurs as early as 27 days after birth in nonlactating women, with a mean time of approximately 70 to 75 days. Menstruation usually resumes by 4 to 6 weeks after childbirth in nonlactating women. In women who breastfeed the mean length of time to initial ovulation is approximately 6 months (Blackburn, 2007; Katz, 2007). In lactating women, both resumption of ovulation and return of menses are determined in large part by the duration and frequency of breastfeeding (Blackburn, 2007). Some women ovulate before their first postpartum menstrual period occurs; therefore contraceptive options should be discussed early in the puerperium (Blackburn, 2007; Cunningham, Leveno, Bloom, Hauth, Gilstrap, & Wenstrom, 2005).

The first menstrual flow after childbirth is usually heavier than normal. Within three to four cycles the amount of menstrual flow returns to the woman's prepregnancy volume.

ABDOMEN

When the woman stands up during the first days after birth, her abdomen protrudes and gives her a still-pregnant appearance. During the first 2 weeks after birth the abdominal wall is relaxed. Approximately 6 weeks are required for the abdominal wall to return almost to its nonpregnant state (Fig. 13-2). The skin regains most of its previous

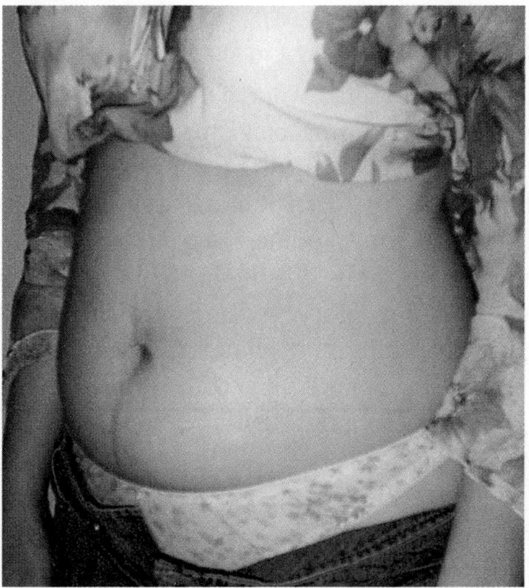

Fig. 13-2 Abdominal wall 6 weeks after vaginal birth is almost back to prepregnancy appearance. Note that the linea nigra is still visible. (Courtesy Jodi Brackett, Phoenix, AZ.)

elasticity, but some striae may persist. The return of muscle tone depends on previous tone, proper exercise, and the amount of adipose tissue present. Occasionally, with or without overdistention because of a large fetus or multiple fetuses, the abdominal wall muscles separate, a condition termed **diastasis recti abdominis** (see Fig. 6-13). Persistence of this defect may be disturbing to the woman, but surgical correction rarely is necessary. With time the defect becomes less apparent.

URINARY SYSTEM

The hormonal changes of pregnancy (i.e., high steroid levels) contribute to an increase in renal function; diminishing steroid levels after childbirth may partly explain the reduced renal function that occurs during the puerperium. Kidney function returns to normal within 1 month after birth. From 2 to 8 weeks are required for the pregnancy-induced hypotonia and dilation of the ureters and renal pelves to return to the nonpregnant state (Cunningham et al., 2005). In a small percentage of women, dilation of the urinary tract may persist for 3 months, which increases the chance of developing a urinary tract infection.

Urine Components

The renal glycosuria induced by pregnancy disappears by 1 week postpartum (Blackburn, 2007), but lactosuria may occur in lactating women. The blood urea nitrogen (BUN) increases during the puerperium as autolysis of the involuting uterus occurs. This breakdown of excess protein in the uterine muscle cells also contributes to pregnancy-associated proteinuria, which resolves by 6 weeks after birth. The BUN returns to a nonpregnant level by 2 to 3 months after childbirth (Blackburn, 2007). Ketonuria may occur in women with an uncomplicated birth or after a prolonged labor with dehydration.

Postpartal Diuresis

Within 12 hours of birth, women begin to lose excess tissue fluid accumulated during pregnancy. Profuse diaphoresis often occurs, especially at night, for the first 2 or 3 days after childbirth. Postpartal diuresis, caused by decreased estrogen levels, removal of increased venous pressure in the lower extremities, and loss of the remaining pregnancy-induced increase in blood volume, also aids the body in ridding itself of excess fluid. Fluid loss through perspiration and increased urinary output accounts for a weight loss of approximately 2.25 kg during the puerperium.

Urethra and Bladder

Birth-induced trauma, increased bladder capacity after childbirth, and the effects of conduction anesthesia combine to cause a decreased urge to void. In addition, pelvic soreness caused by the forces of labor, vaginal lacerations, or an episiotomy reduces or alters the voiding reflex. Decreased voiding combined with postpartal diuresis may result in bladder distention. Immediately after birth, excessive bleeding can occur if the bladder becomes distended because it pushes the uterus up and to the side and prevents the uterus from contracting firmly. Later in the puerperium, overdistention can make the bladder increasingly susceptible to infection and impede the resumption of normal voiding (Cunningham et al., 2005). With adequate emptying of the bladder, bladder tone is usually restored 5 to 7 days after childbirth.

GASTROINTESTINAL SYSTEM

Appetite

The mother is usually hungry shortly after the birth and can tolerate a light diet. Most new mothers are very hungry after full recovery from analgesia, anesthesia, and fatigue. Requests for double portions of food and frequent snacks are not uncommon.

Bowel Evacuation

A spontaneous bowel evacuation may not occur for 2 to 3 days after childbirth. This delay can be explained by decreased muscle tone in the intestines during labor and the immediate puerperium, prelabor diarrhea, lack of food, or dehydration. The mother often anticipates discomfort during the bowel movement because of perineal tenderness as a result of episiotomy, lacerations, or hemorrhoids and resists the urge to defecate. Regular bowel habits should be reestablished when bowel tone returns.

Operative vaginal birth (forceps use) and anal sphincter lacerations are associated with an increased risk of postpartum anal incontinence. Women with this problem are more often incontinent of flatus than of stool. If anal incontinence lasts more than 6 months, studies should be conducted to determine the specific cause and appropriate treatment (Katz, 2007).

BREASTS

Promptly after birth, a decrease occurs in the concentrations of hormones (i.e., estrogen, progesterone, hCG, prolactin, cortisol, and insulin) that stimulated breast development during pregnancy. The time required for these hormones to return to prepregnancy levels is determined in part by whether the mother breastfeeds her infant.

Breastfeeding Mothers

During the first 24 hours after birth, little, if any, change occurs in the breast tissue. Colostrum, a clear yellow fluid, may be expressed from the breasts. The breasts gradually become fuller and heavier as the colostrum transitions to milk by approximately 72 to 96 hours after birth; this breast change is often referred to as the "milk coming in." The breasts may feel warm, firm, and somewhat tender. Bluish-white milk with a skim-milk appearance (true milk) can be expressed from the nipples. As milk glands and milk ducts fill with milk, breast tissue may feel somewhat nodular or lumpy. Unlike the lumps associated with fibrocystic breast disease or cancer, which may be consistently palpated in the same location, the nodularity associated with milk production tends to shift in position. Some women experience engorgement, but with frequent breastfeeding and proper care, this condition is temporary and typically lasts only 24 to 48 hours (see Chapter 18).

Non-Breastfeeding Mothers

The breasts generally feel nodular in contrast to the granular feel of breasts in nonpregnant women. The nodularity is bilateral and diffuse. Prolactin levels drop rapidly. Colostrum is present for the first few days after childbirth. Palpation of the breasts on the second or third day, as milk production begins, may reveal tissue tenderness in some women. On the third or fourth postpartum day, engorgement may occur. The breasts are distended (swollen), firm, tender, and warm to the touch (because of vasocongestion). Breast distention is caused primarily by the temporary congestion of veins and lymphatics rather than by an accumulation of milk. Milk is present but should not be expressed. Axillary breast tissue (the tail of Spence) and any accessory breast or nipple tissue along the milk line may be involved. Engorgement resolves spontaneously, and discomfort decreases usually within 24 to 36 hours. A breast binder or well-fitted, supportive bra, ice packs, fresh cabbage leaves, and mild analgesics may be used to relieve discomfort. Nipple stimulation is avoided. If suckling is never begun (or is discontinued), lactation ceases within a few days to a week.

CARDIOVASCULAR SYSTEM

Blood Volume

Changes in blood volume after birth depend on several factors, such as blood loss during childbirth and the amount of extravascular water (physiologic edema) mobilized and excreted. Pregnancy-induced hypervolemia (an increase in blood volume of at least 35% more than prepregnancy values near term) allows most women to tolerate considerable blood loss during childbirth. Although the average loss is less, up to 500 ml (10% of blood volume) may be lost during a vaginal birth and 1000 ml (15% to 30% of blood volume) during a cesarean birth. During the first few days after delivery the plasma volume decreases further as a result of diuresis (Blackburn, 2007).

The woman's response to blood loss during the early puerperium differs from that in a nonpregnant woman. Three postpartal physiologic changes protect the woman by increasing the circulating blood volume: (1) Elimination of uteroplacental circulation reduces the size of the maternal vascular bed by 10% to 15%, (2) loss of placental endocrine function removes the stimulus for vasodilation, and (3) mobilization of extravascular water stored during pregnancy occurs. In fact, by the third postpartum day the plasma volume has been replenished as extravascular fluid returns to the intravascular space (Katz, 2007).

Cardiac Output

Pulse rate, stroke volume, and cardiac output increase throughout pregnancy. Cardiac output remains increased for at least the first 48 hours postpartum because of an increase in stroke volume. This increased stroke volume is caused by the return of blood to the maternal systemic venous circulation, a result of rapid decrease in uterine blood flow and mobilization of extravascular fluid (Blackburn, 2007). Cardiac output decreases by 30% by 2 weeks after childbirth and then gradually decreases to nonpregnant values by 6 to 12 weeks postpartum in most women. However, cardiac output, stroke volume, end diastolic volume, and systemic vascular resistance remain elevated over nonpregnant values in some women for up to 12 weeks or longer (Blackburn, 2007).

Vital Signs

Few alterations in vital signs are seen under normal circumstances. Heart rate and blood pressure return to nonpregnant levels within a few days (Katz, 2007) (Table 13-2). Respiratory function rapidly returns to nonpregnant levels after birth (Blackburn, 2007). After the uterus is emptied, the diaphragm descends, the normal cardiac axis is restored, and the point of maximal impulse and the electrocardiogram are normalized.

Blood Components

Hematocrit and hemoglobin

After childbirth the total blood volume declines by approximately 16% from its predelivery value, resulting in a transient anemia. By 8 weeks after childbirth, however, the number of red blood cells has increased and the majority of women have a normal hematocrit (Katz, 2007).

White blood cell count

Normal leukocytosis of pregnancy averages approximately 12,000/mm^3. During the first 10 to 12 days after childbirth, values between 20,000 and 25,000/mm^3 are common. Neutrophils are the most numerous white blood cells. Leukocytosis coupled with the normal increase in erythrocyte sedimentation rate may obscure the diagnosis of acute infection at this time.

Coagulation factors

Clotting factors and fibrinogen are normally increased during pregnancy and remain elevated in the immediate puerperium. When combined with vessel damage and immobility, this hypercoagulable state causes an increased risk of thromboembolism, especially after a cesarean birth. Fibrinolytic activity also increases during the first 1 to 4 days after childbirth (Katz, 2007).

TABLE 13-2
Vital Signs after Childbirth

NORMAL FINDINGS	DEVIATIONS FROM NORMAL (FINDINGS AND PROBABLE CAUSES)
TEMPERATURE	
Temperature during first 24 hours may rise to 38° C (100.4° F) as a result of dehydrating effects of labor or a consequence of epidural anesthesia. After 24 hours the woman should be afebrile.	A diagnosis of puerperal sepsis is suggested if a rise in maternal temperature to 38° C (100.4° F) is noted after the first 24 hours after childbirth and recurs or persists for 2 days. Other possible diagnoses are mastitis, endometritis, urinary tract infection, and other systemic infections.
PULSE	
Pulse returns to nonpregnant levels within a few days postpartum, although the rate of return varies among individual women.	A rapid pulse rate or one that is increasing may indicate hypovolemia as a result of hemorrhage.
RESPIRATIONS	
Respirations should decrease to within the woman's normal prepregnancy range by 6 to 8 weeks after birth.	Hypoventilation (respiratory depression) may follow an unusually high subarachnoid (spinal) block or epidural narcotic after a cesarean birth.
BLOOD PRESSURE	
Blood pressure is altered slightly if at all. Orthostatic hypotension, as indicated by feelings of faintness or dizziness immediately after standing up, can develop in the first 48 hours as a result of the splanchnic engorgement that may occur after birth.	A low or decreasing blood pressure may reflect hypovolemia secondary to hemorrhage. However, it is a late sign, and other symptoms of hemorrhage usually alert the staff. An increased reading may result from excessive use of vasopressor or oxytocic medications. Because preeclampsia can persist into or occur first in the postpartum period, routine evaluation of blood pressure is needed. If a woman complains of headache, hypertension must be ruled out as a cause before analgesics are administered.

Varicosities

Varicosities (varices) of the legs (Fig. 13-3) and around the anus (hemorrhoids) are common during pregnancy. Varices, even the less common vulvar varices, regress (empty) rapidly immediately after childbirth. Surgical repair of varicosities is not considered during pregnancy. Total or nearly total regression of varicosities is expected after childbirth.

NEUROLOGIC SYSTEM

Neurologic changes during the puerperium are those that result from a reversal of maternal adaptations to pregnancy and those resulting from trauma during labor and childbirth.

Pregnancy-induced neurologic discomforts disappear after birth. Elimination of physiologic edema through the diuresis that follows childbirth relieves carpal tunnel syndrome by easing compression of the median nerve. The periodic numbness and tingling of fingers that afflicts 5% of pregnant women usually disappears after the birth unless lifting and carrying the baby aggravates the condition. Headache requires careful assessment. Postpartum headaches may be caused by various conditions, including postpartum-onset preeclampsia, stress, and leakage of cerebrospinal fluid into the extradural space during placement of the needle for epidural or spinal anesthesia. Depending on the cause and effectiveness of the treatment, the duration of the headaches can vary from 1 to 3 days to several weeks.

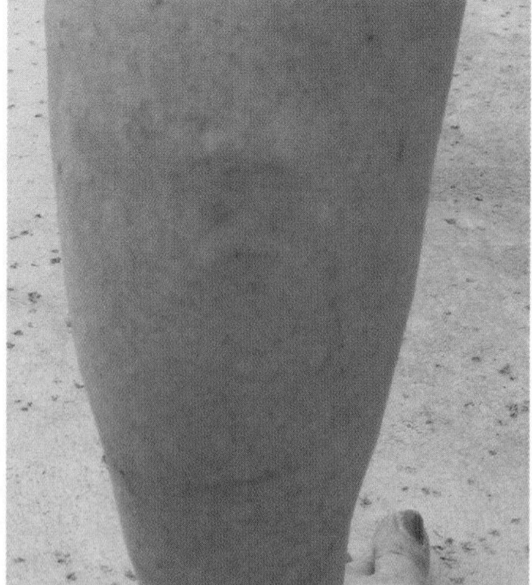

Fig. 13-3 Varicosities in legs. (Courtesy Bernadine Cunningham, Phoenix, AZ.)

MUSCULOSKELETAL SYSTEM

Adaptations of the mother's musculoskeletal system that occur during pregnancy are reversed in the puerperium. These adaptations include the relaxation and subsequent hypermobility of the joints and the change in the mother's center of gravity in response to the enlarging uterus. The joints are completely stabilized by 6 to 8 weeks after birth. Although all other joints return to their normal prepregnancy state, those in the parous woman's feet do not. The new mother may notice a permanent increase in her shoe size.

INTEGUMENTARY SYSTEM

Chloasma of pregnancy (mask of pregnancy) usually disappears at the end of pregnancy. Hyperpigmentation of the areolae and linea nigra may not regress completely after childbirth. Some women will have permanent darker pigmentation of those areas (see Fig. 13-2). Striae gravidarum (stretch marks) on the breasts, the abdomen, the hips, and the thighs may fade but usually do not disappear.

Vascular abnormalities such as spider angiomas (nevi), palmar erythema, and epulis generally regress in response to the rapid decline in estrogen after pregnancy. For some woman, spider nevi persist indefinitely.

Hair growth slows during the postpartum period. Some women actually experience hair loss because the amount of hair lost is temporarily more than the amount regrown. The abundance of fine hair seen during pregnancy usually disappears after giving birth; however, any coarse or bristly hair that appears during pregnancy usually remains. Fingernails return to their nonpregnant consistency and strength.

Profuse diaphoresis that occurs in the immediate postpartum period is the most noticeable change in the integumentary system.

IMMUNE SYSTEM

No significant changes in the maternal immune system occur during the postpartum period. The mother's need for a rubella vaccination or for prevention of Rh isoimmunization is determined.

KEY POINTS

- The uterus involutes rapidly after birth and returns to the true pelvis within 2 weeks.
- The rapid drop in estrogen and progesterone levels after expulsion of the placenta is responsible for triggering many of the anatomic and physiologic changes in the puerperium.
- The return of ovulation and menses is determined in part by whether the woman breastfeeds her baby.
- Assessment of lochia and fundal height is essential to monitor the progress of normal involution and to identify potential problems.
- Under normal circumstances, few alterations in vital signs are seen after birth.
- Hypercoagulability, vessel damage, and immobility predispose the woman to thromboembolism.
- Marked diuresis, decreased bladder sensitivity, and overdistention of the bladder can lead to problems with urinary elimination.
- Pregnancy-induced hypervolemia and postpartum physiologic changes allow the woman to tolerate considerable blood loss at birth.

Audio Chapter Summaries: Access an audio summary of these Key Points on evolve

References

Blackburn, S.T. (2007). *Maternal, fetal, and neonatal physiology: A clinical perspective* (3rd ed.). St. Louis: Saunders.

Cunningham, F., Leveno, K., Bloom, S., Hauth, J., Gilstrap, L., & Wenstrom, K. (2005). *Williams obstetrics* (22nd ed.). New York: McGraw-Hill.

Katz, V.L. (2007). Postpartum care. In S. Gabbe, J. Niebyl, & J. Simpson (Eds.), *Obstetrics: Normal and problem pregnancies* (5th ed.). Philadelphia: Churchill Livingstone.

Lawrence, R.M. & Lawrence, R.A. (2009). The breast and the physiology of lactation. In R. K. Creasy, R. Resnik, & J. D. Iams (Eds.), *Creasy and Resnik's maternal-fetal medicine: Principles and practice* (6th ed.). Philadelphia: Saunders.

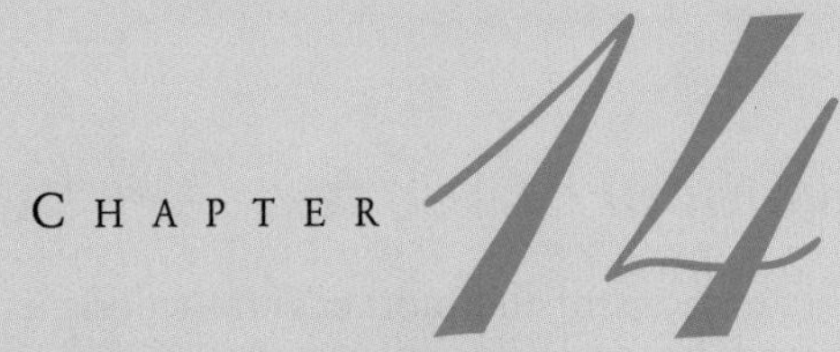

CHAPTER 14

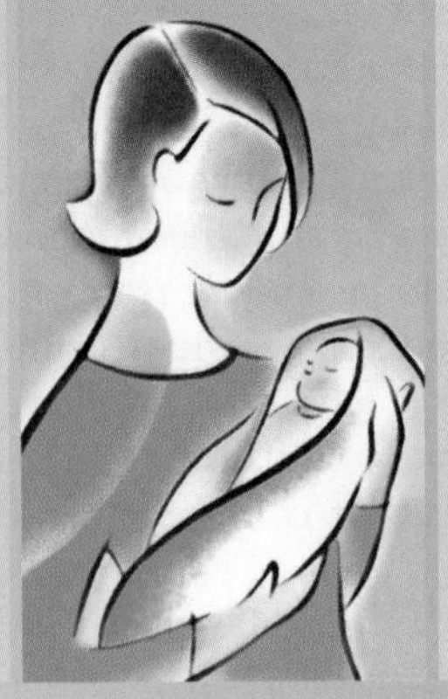

Nursing Care of the Family during the Fourth Trimester

KATHRYN RHODES ALDEN

LEARNING OBJECTIVES

- *Describe components of a systematic postpartum assessment.*
- *Recognize signs of potential complications in the postpartum woman.*
- *Identify common selection criteria for safe early postpartum discharge.*
- *Discuss nursing management of women in the postpartum period.*
- *Explain the influence of cultural beliefs and practices on postpartum care.*
- *Discuss postpartum teaching for self-management.*
- *Describe the nurse's role in these postpartum follow-up strategies: home visits, telephone follow-up, warm lines and help lines, support groups, and referrals to community resources.*

KEY TERMS AND DEFINITIONS

couplet care One nurse, educated in both maternal and newborn care, functions as the primary nurse for both mother and neonate (also known as mother-baby care or single-room maternity care)

engorgement Swelling of the breast tissue brought about by an increase in blood and lymph supplied to the breast, occurring as early milk (colostrum) transitions to mature milk, at approximately 72 to 96 hours after birth

uterine atony Relaxation of uterine muscle possibly leading to excessive postpartum bleeding and postpartum hemorrhage

warm line A help line, or consultation service, for families to access, most often for support of newborn care and postpartum care after hospital discharge

WEB RESOURCES

Additional related content can be found on the companion website at evolve

http://evolve.elsevier.com/Lowdermilk/Maternity/

- NCLEX Review Questions
- Case Study: Fourth Trimester
- Critical Thinking Exercise: Priority Nursing Care: Postpartum Unit
- Nursing Care Plan: Postpartum Care: Vaginal Birth
- Spanish Guidelines: Assessing for Hemorrhage
- Spanish Guidelines: Assessing for Infection
- Spanish Guidelines: Discharge Teaching
- Spanish Guidelines: Postpartum Adjustment

At no other time is family-centered maternity care more important than in the postpartum period. Nursing care is provided in the context of the family unit and focuses on assessment and support of the woman's physiologic and emotional adaptation after birth. During the early postpartum period, components of nursing care include assisting the mother with rest and recovery from the process of labor and birth, assessment of physiologic and psychologic adaptation after birth, prevention of complications, education regarding self-care and infant care, and support of the mother and her partner during the initial transition to parenthood. In addition, the nurse considers the needs of other family members and includes strategies in the plan of care to assist the family in adjusting to the new baby.

The approach to the care of women after birth is wellness oriented. Most women in the United States remain hospitalized no more than 1 or 2 days after vaginal birth and some for as few as 6 hours. Because so much important information needs to be shared with these women in a very short time, their care must be thoughtfully planned and provided. Care during the first 1 to 2 hours after birth, also known as the fourth stage of labor, is covered in Chapter 12. This chapter discusses nursing care of the postpartum woman and her family subsequent to the initial recovery period after birth, extending into the fourth trimester–the first 3 months after birth.

TRANSFER FROM THE RECOVERY AREA

After the initial recovery period has been completed, and provided that her condition is stable, the woman may be transferred to a postpartum room in the same or another nursing unit. In facilities with labor, delivery, recovery, and postpartum (LDRP) rooms the nurse who provides care during the recovery period usually continues caring for the woman. Women who have received general or regional anesthesia must be cleared for transfer from the recovery area by a member of the anesthesia care team.

In preparing the transfer report the recovery nurse uses information from the records of admission, labor and birth, and recovery. Information that must be communicated to the postpartum nurse includes the identity of the health care provider; gravidity and parity; age; anesthetic used; any medications given; duration of labor and time of rupture of membranes; whether labor was induced or augmented; type of birth and repair; blood type and Rh status; group B streptococci status; status of rubella immunity; syphilis, hepatitis B, and human immunodeficiency virus (HIV) test results (if positive); intravenous infusion of any fluids; physiologic status since birth; description of the fundus, lochia, bladder, and perineum; sex and weight of the infant; time of birth; name of the pediatric care provider, chosen method of feeding; any abnormalities noted; and assessment of initial parent-infant interaction.

Most of this information is also documented for the nursing staff in the newborn nursery if the infant is transferred to that unit (in some settings the newborn never leaves the mother's room). In addition, specific information should be provided regarding the newborn's Apgar scores, weight, voiding, stooling, and any feedings since birth. Nursing interventions that have been completed (e.g., eye prophylaxis, vitamin K injection) are also recorded.

PLANNING FOR DISCHARGE

From their initial contact with the postpartum woman, nurses are preparing the new mother for the time when she will return home. The length of hospital stay after giving birth depends on many factors, including the physical condition of the mother and the newborn, mental and emotional status of the mother, social support at home, patient education needs for self-care management and infant care, and financial constraints.

Women who give birth in birthing centers may be discharged within a few hours, after the woman's and the infant's conditions are stable. Mothers and newborns who are at low risk for complications may be discharged from the hospital within 24 to 36 hours after vaginal birth, often called *early postpartum discharge, shortened hospital stay,* or *1-day maternity stay.* The trend of shortened hospital stays is based largely on efforts to reduce health care costs coupled with consumer demands to have fewer medical interventions and more family-focused experiences. Although some advantages to early postpartum discharge can be found, disadvantages also exist (Box 14-1).

Laws Relating to Discharge

The trend toward early postpartum discharge in the early 1990s raised serious concerns among health care providers because some medical problems do not show up in the first 24 hours after birth. The greatest risk associated with early discharge is for the infant who may develop jaundice, feeding difficulties, infection, gastrointestinal obstruction, or unrecognized respiratory or cardiac problems. In addition, new mothers have not had sufficient time to learn how to care for their newborns, and breastfeeding may not be well established (AAP Committee on Fetus and Newborn, 2010).

The concern for the potential increase in adverse maternal-infant outcomes from early discharge practices led the American College of Obstetricians and Gynecologists (ACOG), the American Academy of Pediatrics (AAP), and other professional health care organizations to promote the enactment of federal and state maternity length-of-stay bills to ensure adequate care for both the mother and the newborn. The passage of the Newborns' and Mothers'

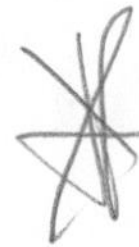

BOX 14-1

Advantages and Disadvantages of Early Postpartum Discharge

ADVANTAGES

- Reinforces the concept of childbirth as a normal physiologic event
- Allows shorter separations between mothers and other children
- Extends a couple's sense of control and participation beyond the birth itself
- Capitalizes on the security of the home environment during the stressors of early parenting
- Decreases unnecessary exposure to the pathogens in the hospital environment
- Allows beds on the maternity service to be used more effectively (i.e., quick turnover in patients or greater availability for patients with a complication)
- Allows more time for mother, father, partner, infant, and other family members to bond
- Creates less disruption in the daily life of the family
- Promotes active involvement of family and support persons in assisting the mother and newborn

DISADVANTAGES

- Complications (maternal or newborn) may go unrecognized.
- Families may be or feel unprepared for the reality they face once the baby is at home.
- The mother is fatigued from the labor and childbirth process.
- The mother is experiencing postpartum pain or discomfort.
- The length of time for learning after the birth in the hospital setting is decreased.
- A vulnerability and crisis potential exists for both women and families.

BOX 14-2

Minimum Criteria for Discharge of a Healthy Term Newborn

INFANT

- Normal physical examination and clinical course
- Vital signs (temperature, heart rate, respirations) within normal limits and stable for 12 hr prior to discharge
- Minimum of two successful feedings and able to coordinate sucking, swallowing, and breathing during feeding
- Urinated regularly and spontaneously stooled at least once
- Risk of hyperbilirubinemia assessed and follow-up plans in place as needed
- Circumcision site without significant bleeding
- Evaluated and monitored for sepsis (e.g., group B streptococcus)
- Maternal laboratory data reviewed (syphilis, hepatitis B; HIV if performed)
- Infant blood type and Coombs test results reviewed
- Hepatitis B immunization administered
- Newborn hearing and metabolic screening completed

MOTHER

- Knowledgeable, able, and competent to provide care

FAMILY/GENERAL

- Risk factors assessed
- Mother and family educated about safe environment

FOLLOW-UP CARE

- Plan in place for continuing medical care
- If discharged before 48 hr, follow-up within 72 hr by health care professional

Source: American Academy of Pediatrics (AAP) Committee on Fetus and Newborn. (2010). Hospital stay for healthy term infants. *Pediatrics, 125*(2), 405-409.

Health Protection Act of 1996 provided minimal federal standards for health plan coverage for mothers and their newborns. Under this act, all health plans are required to allow the new mother and newborn to remain in the hospital for a minimum of 48 hours after a normal vaginal birth and for 96 hours after a cesarean birth unless the attending provider, in consultation with the mother, decides on early discharge (AAP Committee on Fetus and Newborn, 2010).

Criteria for Discharge

The American Academy of Pediatrics (2010) recommends that the hospital stay for a mother with a healthy term newborn should be of sufficient length to identify early problems and determine that the mother and family are prepared and able to care for the newborn at home. The health of the mother and newborn should be stable. There should be adequate support systems in place and access to follow-up care (AAP Committee on Fetus and Newborn, 2010).

Ideally, hospital stays are long enough to identify problems and to ensure that the woman is sufficiently recovered and is prepared to care for herself and the baby at home. Nurses must consider the medical needs of the woman and her baby and provide care that is coordinated to meet those needs so as to provide timely physiologic interventions and treatment to prevent morbidity and hospital readmission. With predetermined criteria for identifying low risk mothers and newborns (Box 14-2) the length of hospitalization can be based on the medical need for care in an acute care setting or in consideration of the ongoing care needed in the home environment. Early follow-up visits are key to reduce readmissions of newborns.

Hospital-based maternity nurses continue to play invaluable roles as caregivers, teachers, and patient and family advocates in developing and implementing effective home care strategies. Postpartum order sets and maternal-newborn teaching checklists (Box 14-3) can be used to accomplish patient care tasks and educational outcomes. With coordination, clinical care and education can be planned and provided throughout pregnancy, during the hospital stay, and in the home after discharge to ensure the family's continued well-being.

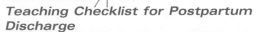

BOX 14-3

Teaching Checklist for Postpartum Discharge

MATERNAL SELF-MANAGEMENT
- Episiotomy or laceration and perineal care
- Vaginal bleeding or discharge
- Breast care
- Nutrition
- Activity
- Exercise
- Return of menstruation
- Postpartum emotions: baby blues, postpartum depression
- Postpartum warning signs: when to call health care provider

INFANT CARE
- Diapering
- Bathing, skin care, cord care
- Circumcised or uncircumcised care
- Burping
- Bowel movements and wet diapers
- Sleeping habits
- Newborn behavior
- Jaundice
- Signs of illness and when to call health care provider
- Car seat safety
- General infant safety and poison control
- Signs and symptoms of dehydration
- Bulb syringe

BREASTFEEDING
- Positioning
- Latch
- Feeding frequency and duration
- Signs of effective feeding: maternal and infant
- Sore nipples
- Engorgement
- Expression and storage of breast milk
- Nursing while working
- Weaning

BOTTLE-FEEDING
- Types of formulas
- Preparing and storing formula
- Frequency of feeding

LEGAL TIP **Early Discharge**

Whether or not the woman and her family have chosen early discharge, the nurse and the primary health care provider are held responsible if the woman is discharged before her condition has stabilized within normal limits. If complications occur, the medical and nursing staff could be sued for abandonment.

CARE MANAGEMENT—PHYSIOLOGIC NEEDS

Case Study: Fourth Trimester

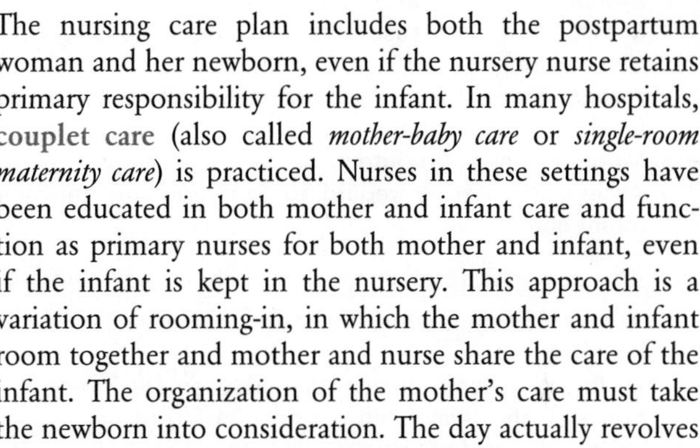

The nursing care plan includes both the postpartum woman and her newborn, even if the nursery nurse retains primary responsibility for the infant. In many hospitals, **couplet care** (also called *mother-baby care* or *single-room maternity care*) is practiced. Nurses in these settings have been educated in both mother and infant care and function as primary nurses for both mother and infant, even if the infant is kept in the nursery. This approach is a variation of rooming-in, in which the mother and infant room together and mother and nurse share the care of the infant. The organization of the mother's care must take the newborn into consideration. The day actually revolves around the baby's feeding and care times.

A focused physical assessment, including vital signs, is performed on admission to the postpartum unit. If the woman's vital signs are stable, they are usually assessed every 4 to 8 hours while she is hospitalized. Other components of the initial assessment include the mother's emotional status, energy level, physical discomfort, hunger, and thirst. Intake and output assessments are performed if an intravenous infusion or urinary catheter is in place. For the woman who gave birth by cesarean the incisional dressing is also assessed.

Ongoing assessments are performed throughout hospitalization. In addition to vital signs, physical assessment of the postpartum woman focuses on evaluation of breasts, uterine fundus, lochia, perineum, bladder and bowel function, and legs (Table 14-1).

Critical Thinking Exercise: Priority Nursing Care: Postpartum Unit

Several laboratory tests may be performed in the early postpartum period. Hemoglobin and hematocrit values are often evaluated on the first postpartum day to assess the effects of blood loss during birth, especially after cesarean birth. In some hospitals, a clean-catch or catheterized urine specimen is obtained and sent to the laboratory for routine urinalysis or culture and sensitivity, especially if an indwelling catheter was inserted during the intrapartum period. In addition, if the woman's rubella and Rh status are unknown, tests to determine her status and the need for possible treatment should be performed at this time.

Plan of Care and Interventions

Once the nursing diagnoses are formulated the nurse plans with the woman what nursing measures are appropriate and which are to be given priority. The nursing plan of care includes periodic assessments to detect deviations

NURSING PROCESS *Physiologic Postpartum Concerns*

ASSESSMENT

Initial Assessment

- Obtain information from the nursing staff report and medical record regarding the length and difficulty of the labor, type of birth (i.e., vaginal or cesarean), presence of perineal lacerations or episiotomy, gravidity, parity, and whether the mother plans to breastfeed or bottle-feed.
- Assess vital signs.
- Conduct a general systems assessment, including a systematic postpartum assessment.
- For cesarean birth assess the abdominal dressing over the incision.
- Assess discomfort, emotional status, fatigue, energy level, hunger, and thirst.
- Monitor intake and output.
- Assess knowledge regarding self-management and infant care.

Ongoing Assessment

- Assess vital signs every 4-8 hours or once each shift per hospital protocol.
- Perform focused postpartum assessment every 4-8 hours or once each shift per hospital protocol.
- Assess discomfort, fatigue, and emotional status.
- Monitor intake and output.
- Monitor laboratory values, especially hemoglobin and hematocrit; collect urine for routine urinalysis and culture or sensitivity; note rubella and Rh status.

NURSING DIAGNOSES

Examples of nursing diagnoses for meeting physical needs in the postpartum period include:

- *Risk for deficient fluid volume (hemorrhage)* related to:
  - Uterine atony after childbirth
- *Risk for constipation* related to:
  - Postchildbirth discomfort
  - Childbirth trauma to tissues
  - Decreased intake of solid food or fluids
  - Side effects of narcotic analgesics
- *Acute pain* related to:
  - Uterine involution
  - Trauma to perineum (laceration or episiotomy)
  - Hemorrhoids
  - Sore nipples
  - Engorged breasts
- *Disturbed sleep pattern* related to:
  - Discomforts of the postpartum period
  - Long labor process
  - Infant care needs and hospital routine
- *Ineffective breastfeeding* related to:
  - Maternal discomfort
  - Insufficient knowledge regarding breastfeeding techniques
  - Lack of support from spouse, partner, family, or friends
  - Lack of maternal self-confidence, anxiety, and fear of failure
  - Infant sucking difficulties
  - Difficulty waking the sleepy baby

EXPECTED OUTCOMES OF CARE

Expected outcomes for the postpartum period are based on the nursing diagnoses identified for the individual patient. Examples of expected outcomes are:

- Vital signs are within normal limits.
- Fundus is firm, midline, and demonstrates normal involution.
- Lochia has changed color and decreased in amount; no foul odor is noted.
- Bowel function will return to normal (bowel movement by day 2-3 after vaginal birth, by day 3-5 after cesarean).
- Bladder function will return to normal; no dysuria is noted; bladder feels empty after voiding.
- Pain is resolved and relieved or controlled by oral analgesic medications.
- Woman verbalizes or demonstrates knowledge of self management, signs of potential complications, and when to notify health care provider.
- The newborn is integrated into the family.

PLAN OF CARE AND INTERVENTIONS

Many of the interventions in the postpartum period are focused on preventing potential complications through thorough assessment and patient education. Major areas of focus include: prevention of infection; prevention of excessive bleeding; maintenance of uterine tone; prevention of bladder distention; promotion of rest, comfort, and ambulation, and exercise; promotion of nutrition; promotion of normal bladder and bowel patterns; breastfeeding promotion and support; and health promotion for future pregnancies and children (see text).

EVALUATION

The nurse can be reasonably assured that care was effective when the expected outcomes of care for physical needs have been achieved.

from normal physical changes, measures to relieve discomfort or pain, safety measures to prevent injury or infection, and teaching and counseling measures designed to promote the woman's feelings of competence in self-management and infant care. The spouse or partner and other family members who are present may be included in the teaching. The nurse evaluates continuously and is ready to change the plan if indicated. Almost all hospitals use standardized care plans or care paths as a basis for planning. Nurses individualize care of the postpartum woman and neonate according to their specific needs (see Nursing Care Plan box). Signs of potential problems that may be identified during the assessment process are listed in Table 14-1.

TABLE 14-1

Postpartum Assessment and Signs of Potential Complications

ASSESSMENT	NORMAL FINDINGS	SIGNS OF POTENTIAL COMPLICATIONS
Blood pressure (BP)	Consistent with BP baseline during pregnancy; may have orthostatic hypotension for 48 hours	Hypertension: anxiety, preeclampsia, essential hypertension Hypotension: hemorrhage
Temperature	36.2°-38° C	>38° C after 24 hours: infection
Pulse	50-90 beats/min	Tachycardia: pain, fever, dehydration, hemorrhage
Respirations	16-24 breaths/min	Bradypnea: effects of narcotic medications Tachypnea: anxiety; may be sign of respiratory disease
Breath sounds	Clear to auscultation	Crackles: possible fluid overload
Breasts	Day 1-2: soft Day 2-3: filling Day 3-5: full, soften with breastfeeding (milk is "in")	Firmness, heat, pain: engorgement Redness of breast tissue, heat, pain, fever, body aches: mastitis
Nipples	Skin intact; no soreness reported	Redness, bruising, cracks, fissures, abrasions, blisters: usually associated with latch problems
Uterus (fundus)	Firm, midline; first 24 hours at level of umbilicus; involutes ~1 cm/day	Soft, boggy, higher than expected level: uterine atony Lateral deviation: overdistended bladder
Lochia	Day 1-3: rubra (dark red) Day 4-10: serosa (brownish red or pink) After 10 days: alba (yellowish white) Amount: scant to moderate Few clots Fleshy odor	Large amount of lochia: uterine atony, vaginal or cervical laceration Foul odor: infection
Perineum	Minimal edema Laceration or episiotomy: edges approximated Pain minimal to moderate: controlled by analgesics, nonpharmacologic techniques, or both	Pronounced edema, bruising, hematoma Redness, warmth, drainage: infection Excessive discomfort first 1-2 days: hematoma; after day 3: infection
Rectal area	No hemorrhoids; if hemorrhoids are present, soft and pink	Discolored hemorrhoidal tissue, severe pain: thrombosed hemorrhoid
Bladder	Able to void spontaneously; no distention; able to empty completely; no dysuria Diuresis begins ~12 hr after birth; may void 3000 ml/day	Overdistended bladder possibly causing uterine atony, excessive lochia Dysuria, frequency, urgency: infection
Abdomen and bowels	Abdomen soft, active bowel sounds in all quadrants Bowel movement by day 2-3 after birth Cesarean: incision dressing clean and dry; suture line intact	No bowel movement by day 3-4: constipation; diarrhea Abdominal incision—redness, edema, warmth, drainage: infection
Legs	Deep tendon reflexes (DTRs) 1+-2+ Peripheral edema possibly present Homans sign negative	DTRs ≥3+: preeclampsia Redness, tenderness, pain, positive Homans sign: thrombophlebitis
Energy level	Able to care for self and infant; able to sleep	Lethargy, extreme fatigue, difficulty sleeping: postpartum depression
Emotional status	Excited, happy, interested or involved in infant care	Sad, tearful, disinterested in infant care: postpartum blues or depression

NURSING CARE PLAN Postpartum Care: Vaginal Birth

NURSING DIAGNOSIS Risk for deficient fluid volume related to uterine atony and hemorrhage

Expected outcome *Fundus is firm and midline, lochia is moderate, and no evidence of hemorrhage is seen.*

Nursing Interventions/*Rationales*

- Monitor lochia (color, amount, consistency), and count and weigh sanitary pads if lochia is heavy *to evaluate amount of bleeding.*
- Monitor and palpate fundus for location and tone *to determine status of uterus and dictate further interventions because uterine atony is most common cause of postpartum hemorrhage.*
- Monitor intake and output, assess for bladder fullness, and encourage voiding *because a full bladder interferes with involution of the uterus.*
- Monitor vital signs (increased pulse and respirations, decreased blood pressure) and skin temperature and color *to detect signs of hemorrhage or shock.*
- Monitor postpartum hematology studies *to assess effects of blood loss.*
- If fundus is boggy, apply gentle massage and assess tone response *to promote uterine contractions and increase uterine tone.* (Do not overstimulate because doing so can cause fundal relaxation.)
- Express uterine clots *to promote uterine contraction.*
- Explain to the woman the process of involution and teach her to assess and massage the fundus and to report any persistent bogginess *to involve her in self-management and increase sense of self-control.*
- Administer oxytocic agents per physician or nurse-midwife order and evaluate effectiveness *to promote continuing uterine contraction.*
- Administer fluids, blood, blood products, or plasma expanders as ordered *to replace lost fluid and lost blood volume.*

NURSING DIAGNOSIS Acute pain related to postpartum physiologic changes (hemorrhoids, episiotomy, breast engorgement, cracked and sore nipples)

Expected outcome *Woman exhibits signs of decreased discomfort.*

Nursing Interventions/*Rationales*

- Assess location, type, and quality of pain *to direct intervention.*
- Explain to the woman the source and reasons for the pain, its expected duration, and treatments *to decrease anxiety and increase sense of control.*
- Administer prescribed pain medications *to provide pain relief.*
- If pain is perineal (laceration episiotomy, hemorrhoids), apply ice packs in the first 24 hours *to reduce edema and vulvar irritation and reduce discomfort;* encourage sitz baths using cool water for first 24 hours *to reduce edema* and warm water thereafter *to promote circulation;* apply witch hazel compresses *to reduce edema;* teach the woman to use prescribed perineal creams, sprays, or ointments *to depress response of peripheral nerves;* teach the woman to tighten buttocks before sitting and to sit on flat, hard surfaces *to compress buttocks and reduce pressure on the perineum.* (Avoid donuts and soft pillows because they separate the buttocks and decrease venous blood flow, increasing pain.)
- If nipples are sore, have the woman rub breast milk into nipples after feeding and air-dry nipples, apply purified lanolin or other breast creams as prescribed or hydrogel pads, and wear breast shields in her bra *to minimize nipple irritation.* Assist the woman to correct latch problem *to prevent further nipple soreness.*
- If breasts are engorged, have woman apply ice packs to breasts (15 minutes on, 45 minutes off), and apply cabbage leaves in same manner *to relieve discomfort* (use only two to three times). Use warm compresses or take a warm shower before breastfeeding *to stimulate milk flow and relieve stasis.* Hand express milk or pump milk *to relieve discomfort if infant is unable to latch on and feed.*
- If pain is from breast and woman is not breastfeeding, encourage the use of a well-fitted, supportive bra or breast binder and application of ice packs and cabbage leaves *to suppress milk production and decrease discomfort.*

NURSING DIAGNOSIS Disturbed sleep pattern related to excitement, discomfort, and environmental interruptions

Expected outcome *Woman sleeps for uninterrupted periods and states she feels rested after waking.*

Nursing Interventions/*Rationales*

- Establish the woman's routine sleep patterns and compare with current sleep patterns, exploring factors that interfere with sleep, *to determine scope of problem and direct interventions.*
- Individualize nursing routines to fit the woman's natural body rhythms (i.e., wake-sleep cycles), provide a sleep-promoting environment (i.e., darkness, quiet, adequate ventilation, appropriate room temperature), prepare for sleep using the woman's usual routines (i.e., back rub, soothing music, warm milk), and teach the use of guided imagery and relaxation techniques *to promote optimum conditions for sleep.*
- Avoid circumstances or routines that may interfere with sleep (e.g., caffeine, foods that induce heartburn, fluids, strenuous mental or physical activity) *to promote healthy sleep patterns.*
- Administer sedation or pain medication as prescribed *to enhance quality of sleep.*
- Advise the woman or partner to limit visitors and activities *to prevent fatigue.*
- Teach the woman to use infant nap time as a time for her also *to nap and replenish energy and decrease fatigue.*

NURSING DIAGNOSIS Risk for impaired urinary elimination related to perineal trauma and effects of anesthesia

Expected outcome *Woman will void within 6 to 8 hours after birth and will empty bladder completely.*

Nursing Interventions/*Rationales*

- Assess position and character of the uterine fundus and bladder *to determine if any further interventions are indicated because of displacement of the fundus or distention of the bladder.*
- Measure intake and output *to assess for evidence of dehydration and subsequent anticipated decrease in urine output.*
- Encourage voiding by walking the woman to bathroom, running water over the perineum, running water in the sink, providing privacy *to encourage voiding.*
- Encourage oral intake *to replace fluids lost during childbirth and prevent dehydration.*
- Catheterize as necessary by indwelling or straight method *to ensure bladder emptying and allow uterine involution.*

Nurses assume many roles while implementing the nursing care plan. They provide direct physical care, teach mother-baby care, and provide anticipatory guidance and counseling. Perhaps most important of all, they nurture the woman by providing encouragement and support as she begins to assume the many tasks of motherhood. Nurses who take the time to "mother the mother" do much to increase feelings of self-confidence in new mothers.

The first step in providing individualized care is to confirm the woman's identity by checking her wristband. At the same time the infant's identification number is matched with the corresponding band on the mother's wrist and, in some instances, the father's wrist. The nurse determines how the mother wishes to be addressed and then notes her preference in her record and in her nursing care plan.

The woman and her family are oriented to their surroundings. Familiarity with the unit, routines, resources, and personnel reduces one potential source of anxiety–the unknown. The mother is reassured through knowing whom and how she can call for assistance and what she can expect in the way of services and supplies. If the woman's usual daily routine before admission differs from the facility's routine, then the nurse works with the woman to develop a mutually acceptable routine.

As part of orientation to the environment, nurses provide information about unit policies and procedures related to infant security. Infant abduction from hospitals in the United States is an ongoing concern. As a result, many units now have special limited-entry systems in place. Nurses teach mothers to check the identity of any person who comes to remove the baby from her room. Hospital personnel usually wear picture identification badges. On some units, all staff members wear matching scrubs or special badges. Other units use closed-circuit television, computer monitoring systems, or fingerprint identification pads. As a rule the neonate is never carried in a staff member's arms between the mother's room and the nursery but is always wheeled in a bassinet. Patients and nurses must work together to ensure the safety of newborns in the hospital environment.

Prevention of infection

Nurses in the postpartum setting are acutely aware of the importance of preventing infection in their patients. One important means of preventing infection involves maintaining a clean environment. Bed linens should be changed as needed, and disposable pads and draw sheets are changed frequently. Women should wear slippers when walking about to prevent contaminating the linens when they return to bed. Personnel must be conscientious about their hand hygiene to prevent cross-infection. Standard Precautions must be practiced. Staff members with colds, coughs, or skin infections (e.g., a cold sore on the lips [herpes simplex virus type 1]) must follow hospital protocol when in contact with postpartum patients. In many hospitals, staff members with open herpetic lesions, strep throat, conjunctivitis, upper respiratory infections, or diarrhea are encouraged to avoid contact with mothers and infants by staying home until the condition is no longer contagious.

Perineal lacerations and episiotomies increase the risk of infection as a result of interruption in skin integrity. Proper perineal care helps to prevent infection in the genitourinary area and aids the healing process. Educating the woman to wipe from front to back (urethra to anus) after voiding or defecating is a simple first step. In many hospitals, a squeeze bottle filled with warm water or an antiseptic solution is used after each voiding to cleanse the perineal area. The woman should change her perineal pad from front to back each time she voids or defecates and should wash her hands thoroughly before and after doing so (Box 14-4).

Prevention of excessive bleeding

ⓔ Spanish Guidelines: Assessing for Hemorrhage

Although a moderate amount of vaginal bleeding (lochia) in the immediate postpartum period is to be expected, nurses are aware of the need to assess for and prevent excessive bleeding. The most common cause of excessive bleeding after birth is **uterine atony**, failure of the uterine muscle to contract firmly. The two most important interventions for preventing excessive bleeding are maintaining good uterine tone and preventing bladder distention. If uterine atony occurs the relaxed uterus distends with blood and clots, blood vessels in the placental site are not clamped off, and excessive bleeding results. Although the cause of uterine atony is not always clear, it often results from retained placental fragments.

Excessive blood loss after birth can also be caused by vaginal or vulvar hematomas or unrepaired lacerations of the vagina or cervix. These potential sources might be suspected if excessive vaginal bleeding occurs in the presence of a firmly contracted uterus.

NURSING ALERT A perineal pad saturated in 15 minutes or less and pooling of blood under the buttocks are indications of excessive blood loss, requiring immediate assessment, intervention, and notification of the primary health care provider.

ⓔ Spanish Guidelines: Assessing for Infection

Accurate visual estimation of blood loss is an important nursing responsibility. Blood loss is usually described subjectively as scant, light, moderate, or heavy (profuse). Fig. 14-1 shows examples of perineal pad saturation corresponding to each of these descriptions.

Although postpartal blood loss may be estimated by observing the amount of staining on a perineal pad, judging the amount of lochial flow is difficult based only on observation of perineal pads. More objective estimates of blood loss include measuring serial hemoglobin or hematocrit values, weighing blood clots and items saturated with blood (1 ml equals 1 g), and establishing how many milliliters are required to saturate perineal pads being used.

BOX 14-4

Interventions for Episiotomy, Lacerations, and Hemorrhoids

Explain both procedure and rationale before implementation.

CLEANSING

- Wash hands before and after cleansing perineum and changing pads.
- Wash perineum with mild soap and warm water at least once daily.
- Cleanse from symphysis pubis to anal area.
- Apply peripad from front to back, protecting inner surface of pad from contamination.
- Wrap soiled pad and place in covered waste container.
- Change pad with each void or defecation or at least four times per day.
- Assess amount and character of lochia with each pad change.

ICE PACK

- Apply a covered ice pack to perineum from front to back.
- During first 24 hours after birth to decrease edema formation and increase comfort
- After the first 24 hours to provide anesthetic effect

SQUEEZE BOTTLE

- Demonstrate for and assist woman; explain rationale.
- Fill bottle with tap water warmed to approximately 38° C (comfortably warm on the wrist).
- Instruct woman to position nozzle between her legs so that squirts of water reach perineum as she sits on toilet seat. Explain that the whole bottle of water is used to cleanse perineum.
- Remind her to blot dry with toilet paper or clean wipes.
- Remind her to avoid contamination from anal area.
- Apply clean pad.

SITZ BATH

Built-in type

- Prepare bath by thoroughly scrubbing with cleaning agent and rinsing.
- Pad with towel before filling.
- Fill one half to one third with water of correct temperature (38°-40.6° C). Some women prefer cool sitz baths. Ice is added to water to lower the temperature to the level comfortable for the woman.
- Encourage woman to use at least twice a day for 20 minutes.
- Teach woman to enter bath by tightening gluteal muscles and keeping them tightened and then relaxing them after she is in the bath.
- Place dry towels within reach.
- Ensure privacy.
- Place call light within easy reach.
- Check woman in 15 minutes; assess pulse as needed.

Disposable type

- Clamp tubing and fill bag with warm water.
- Raise toilet seat, place bath in bowl with overflow opening directed toward back of toilet.
- Place container above toilet bowl.
- Attach tube into groove at front of bath.
- Loosen tube clamp to regulate rate of flow; fill bath to approximately one half full; continue as above for built-in sitz bath.

TOPICAL APPLICATIONS

- Apply anesthetic cream or spray after cleansing perineal area: use sparingly three to four times per day.
- Offer witch hazel pads (Tucks) after voiding or defecating; woman pats perineum dry from front to back, then applies witch hazel pads.

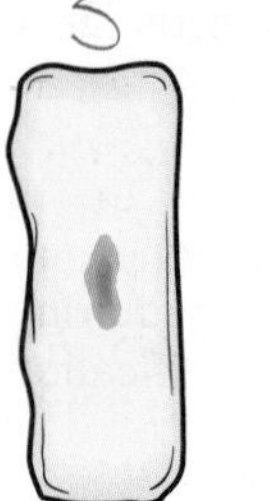
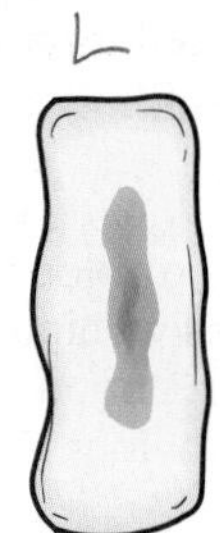
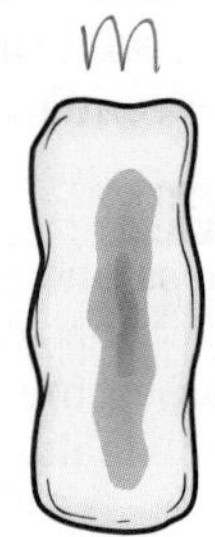
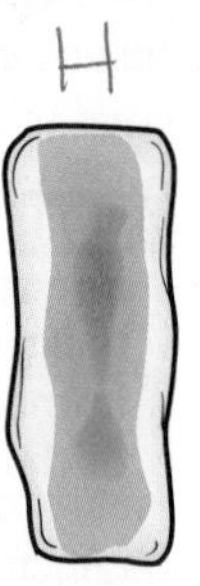

Fig. 14-1 Blood loss after birth is assessed by the extent of perineal pad saturation as (from left to right) scant (<2.5 cm), light (<10 cm), moderate (>10 cm), or heavy (one pad saturated within 2 hours).

Any estimation of lochial flow is inaccurate and incomplete without consideration of the time factor. The woman who saturates a perineal pad in 1 hour or less is bleeding much more heavily than the woman who saturates one perineal pad in 8 hours.

In general, nurses tend to overestimate, rather than underestimate, blood loss. Different brands of perineal pads vary in their saturation volume and soaking appearance. For example, blood placed on some brands tends to soak down into the pad, whereas, on other brands, it tends to spread outward. Nurses should determine saturation volume and soaking appearance for the brands used in their institution so that they can improve accuracy of blood loss estimation.

NURSING ALERT The nurse always checks for bleeding under the mother's buttocks, as well as on the perineal pad. Blood can flow between the buttocks onto the linens under the mother, although the amount on the perineal pad is slight; thus excessive bleeding may go undetected.

When excessive bleeding occurs, vital signs are closely monitored. An important factor to realize is that blood pressure is not a reliable indicator of impending shock from early hemorrhage. More sensitive means of identifying hypovolemic shock are provided by respirations, pulse, skin condition, urinary output, and level of consciousness (see Emergency box). The frequent physical assessments performed during the fourth stage of labor are designed to provide prompt identification of excessive bleeding.

EMERGENCY

Hypovolemic Shock

SIGNS AND SYMPTOMS

- Persistent significant bleeding—perineal pad soaked within 15 minutes; may not be accompanied by a change in vital signs or maternal color or behavior.
- Woman states that she feels weak, light-headed, "funny," or "sick to my stomach" or that she "sees stars."
- Woman begins to act anxious or exhibits air hunger.
- Woman's skin turns ashen or grayish.
- Skin feels cool and clammy.
- Pulse rate increases.
- Blood pressure decreases.

INTERVENTIONS

- If uterus is atonic, massage gently and expel clots to cause uterus to contract. Add oxytocic agent to intravenous drip, as ordered.
- Notify primary health care provider.
- Give oxygen by nonrebreathing facemask or nasal prongs at 8 to 10 L/min.
- Tilt the woman onto her side or elevate the right hip; elevate her legs to at least a 30-degree angle.
- Provide additional or maintain existing intravenous infusion of lactated Ringer's solution or normal saline solution to restore circulatory volume.
- Administer blood or blood products, as ordered.
- Monitor vital signs.
- Insert an indwelling urinary catheter to monitor perfusion of kidneys.
- Administer emergency drugs, as ordered.
- Prepare for possible surgery or other emergency treatments or procedures.
- Chart incident, medical and nursing interventions instituted, and results of treatments.

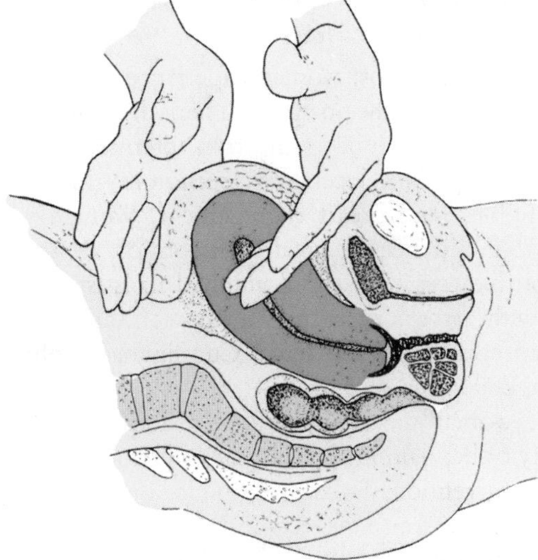

Fig. 14-2 Palpating the uterine fundus. Note that upper hand is cupped over fundus; lower hand dips in above symphysis pubis and supports uterus while it is massaged gently.

Nurses are alert for excessive bleeding throughout the hospital stay as they perform periodic assessment of the uterine fundus and lochia.

Maintenance of uterine tone

A major intervention to alleviate uterine atony and restore uterine muscle tone is stimulation by gently massaging the fundus until firm (Fig. 14-2). Fundal massage may cause a temporary increase in the amount of vaginal bleeding seen as pooled blood leaves the uterus. Clots may also be expelled. The uterus may remain boggy even after massage and expulsion of clots.

Fundal massage can be a very uncomfortable procedure. If the nurse explains the purpose of fundal massage, as well as the causes and dangers associated with uterine atony, then the woman will likely be more cooperative. Teaching the woman to massage her own fundus enables her to maintain some control and decreases her anxiety.

When uterine atony and excessive bleeding occur, additional interventions likely to be used are administration of intravenous fluids and oxytocic medications (drugs that stimulate contraction of the uterine smooth muscle). See Table 23-1 for information about common oxytocic medications.

Prevention of bladder distention

Uterine atony and excessive bleeding after birth may be the result of bladder distention. A full bladder causes the uterus to be displaced above the umbilicus and well to one side of the abdominal midline. It also prevents the uterus from contracting normally.

Women may be at risk of bladder distention resulting from urinary retention based on intrapartum factors. These risk factors include epidural anesthesia, episiotomy, extensive vaginal or perineal lacerations, instrument-assisted birth, or prolonged labor. Women who have had indwelling catheters, such as with cesarean birth, may experience some difficulty as they initially attempt to void after the catheter is removed. Nurses who are aware of these risk factors may be proactive in preventing complications.

Nursing interventions for all postpartum women focus on helping the woman to empty her bladder spontaneously as soon as possible after birth. The first priority is to assist the woman to the bathroom or onto a bedpan if she is unable to ambulate. Having the woman listen to running water, placing her hands in warm water, or pouring water from a squeeze bottle over her perineum may stimulate voiding. Other techniques include assisting the woman into the shower or sitz bath and encouraging her to void; relaxation techniques may also be helpful. Administering analgesics, if ordered, may be indicated because some women may fear voiding because of anticipated pain. If these measures are unsuccessful, a sterile catheter may be inserted to drain the urine.

Promotion of comfort, rest, ambulation, and exercise

Comfort. Most women experience some degree of discomfort during the postpartum period. Common causes of discomfort include pain from uterine contractions (afterpains), perineal lacerations, episiotomy, hemorrhoids, sore nipples, and breast engorgement. Women who are likely to experience the greatest discomfort are those who gave birth by cesarean, those who had an assisted operative birth with forceps or vacuum extraction, and those who have an episiotomy (Declercq, Cunningham, Johnson, & Sakala, 2008).

The woman's description of the location, type, and severity of her pain is the best guide in choosing an appropriate intervention. To confirm the location and extent of discomfort the nurse inspects and palpates areas of pain as appropriate for redness, swelling, discharge, and heat and observes for body tension, guarded movements, and facial tension. Blood pressure, pulse, and respirations may be elevated in response to acute pain. Diaphoresis may accompany severe pain. A lack of objective signs does not necessarily mean pain is nonexistent because a cultural component may be factor in the expression of pain. Nursing interventions are intended to eliminate the discomfort entirely or reduce it to a tolerable level that allows the woman to care for herself and her baby. Nurses may use both nonpharmacologic and pharmacologic interventions to promote comfort. Pain relief is often enhanced by using more than one method or route.

A variety of nonpharmacologic measures may be used to reduce postpartum discomfort. These measures include relaxation, distraction, therapeutic touch, imagery, acupressure, aromatherapy, hydrotherapy, massage therapy, music therapy, and transcutaneous electrical nerve stimulation (TENS).

For women who are experiencing discomfort associated with uterine contractions (afterpains), application of warmth (e.g., heating pad) or lying prone may be helpful. Because afterpains are more severe during and after breastfeeding, the timing of interventions may be planned to provide the most timely and effective relief.

Simple interventions that can decrease the discomfort associated with perineal lacerations or episiotomy include encouraging the woman to lie on her side whenever possible. Other interventions include application of an ice pack, topical application (if ordered) of anesthetic spray or cream, dry heat, cleansing with a squeeze bottle, and a cleansing shower, tub bath, or sitz bath. Many of these interventions are also effective for hemorrhoids, especially ice packs, sitz baths, and topical applications (e.g., witch hazel pads). Box 14-4 gives additional specific information about these interventions.

Sore nipples in breastfeeding mothers are most likely related to ineffective latch technique. Assessment and assistance with feeding can help to alleviate the cause. To ease the discomfort associated with sore nipples the mother may apply topical preparations such as purified lanolin or hydrogel pads (see Chapter 18).

Breast engorgement may occur, whether the woman is breastfeeding or formula feeding. The discomfort associated with engorged breasts may be reduced by applying ice packs or cabbage leaves (or both) to the breasts and wearing a well-fitted support bra. Antiinflammatory medications may also be helpful in relieving some of the discomfort. Decisions about specific interventions for engorgement are based on whether the woman chooses breastfeeding or bottle-feeding (see Chapter 18).

Pharmacologic interventions are commonly used to relieve or reduce postpartum discomfort. Most health care providers routinely order a variety of analgesics to be administered as needed, including both opioid and nonopioid (e.g., nonsteroidal antiinflammatory drugs [NSAIDs]). In some hospitals, NSAIDs are administered on a scheduled basis, especially if the woman has had perineal repair. Topical application of antiseptic or anesthetic ointment or spray can be used for perineal pain. Patient-controlled analgesia pumps and epidural analgesia are technologies commonly used to provide pain relief after cesarean birth.

NURSING ALERT The nurse should carefully monitor all women receiving opioid analgesics because respiratory depression and decreased intestinal motility are side effects.

Many women want to participate in decisions about analgesia. Severe pain, however, can interfere with active participation in choosing pain relief measures. If an analgesic is to be given, the nurse must make a clinical judgment of the type, appropriate dosage, and frequency from the medications ordered. The woman is informed of the prescribed analgesic and its common side effects; this teaching is documented.

Breastfeeding mothers often have concerns about the effects of an analgesic on the infant. Although nearly all drugs present in maternal circulation are also found in breast milk, many analgesics commonly used during the postpartum period are considered relatively safe for breastfeeding mothers. In many instances the timing of medications can be adjusted to minimize infant exposure. A mother may be given pain medication immediately after breastfeeding so that the interval between medication administration and the next nursing period is as long as possible. The decision to administer medications of any type to a breastfeeding mother must always be made by carefully weighing the woman's need against actual or potential risks to the infant.

If acceptable pain relief has not been obtained in 1 hour and no change in the initial assessment is seen, the nurse may need to contact the primary care provider for additional pain relief orders or further directions. Unrelieved pain results in fatigue, anxiety, and a worsening perception of the pain. It might also indicate the presence of a previously unidentified or untreated problem.

Rest. Postpartum fatigue (PPF) is more than just feeling tired; it is a complex phenomenon affected by a combination of physiologic, psychologic, and situational variables. Fatigue is common in the early postpartum period and involves both physiologic and psychologic components. Physical fatigue or exhaustion may be associated with long labors or cesarean birth; hospital routines and infant care demands such as breastfeeding also contribute to maternal fatigue. Fatigue can also be associated with anemia, infection or thyroid dysfunction (Corwin & Arbour, 2007). The excitement and exhilaration experienced after the birth of the infant may make resting difficult. Physical discomfort may interfere with sleep. Well-intentioned visitors may interrupt periods of rest in the hospital and at home. Mothers may also experience psychologic fatigue related to anxiety or depression. PPF is a recognized risk factor for postpartum depression (Kuo, Yang, Kuo, et al., 2012).

Fatigue is likely to worsen over the first 6 weeks after birth, often because of situational factors. After discharge from the hospital, fatigue increases as the woman provides care and feeding for the newborn in combination with other family and household responsibilities such as caring for other children, preparing meals, and doing laundry. Many women have partners, family members, or friends to provide much-needed assistance, whereas others may be without any help at all. The nurse needs to inquire about resources available to the woman after discharge and help her plan accordingly (Runquist, 2007).

Interventions are planned to meet the woman's individual needs for sleep and rest while she is in the hospital. Back rubs, other comfort measures, and medication for sleep for the first few nights may be necessary. The side-lying position for breastfeeding helps minimize fatigue in nursing mothers. Support and encouragement of mothering behaviors help reduce anxiety. Hospital and nursing routines may be adjusted to meet individual needs. In addition, the nurse can help the family limit visitors and provide a comfortable chair or bed for the partner or other family member who may be staying with the new mother.

Because PPF can be very debilitating, follow-up after hospital discharge is important. Screening for PPF can be accomplished with a nurse-initiated telephone call at 2 weeks, as well as at the routine 6-week postpartum visit with the health care provider (Corwin & Arbour, 2007).

Physiologic factors contributing to postpartum fatigue are amenable to intervention and may be identified even before birth. Women with anemia, infection or inflammation, or thyroid dysfunction can be identified as having increased risk for postpartum fatigue. Other physical conditions and psychologic or situational factors that might contribute to PPF can also be identified during the prenatal period. The medical records of women with known risk factors can be red-flagged to alert hospital staff to their special needs.

Ambulation. Early ambulation is associated with a reduced incidence of venous thromboembolism (VTE); it also promotes the return of strength. Free movement is encouraged once anesthesia wears off, unless a narcotic analgesic has been administered. After the initial recovery period is over the mother is encouraged to ambulate frequently.

In the early postpartum period, women may feel lightheaded or dizzy on standing. The rapid decrease in intraabdominal pressure after birth results in dilation of blood vessels supplying the intestines (splanchnic engorgement) and causes blood to pool in the viscera. This condition contributes to the development of orthostatic hypotension when the woman who has recently given birth sits or stands up, first ambulates, or takes a warm shower or sitz bath. When assisting a woman to ambulate the nurse needs to consider the baseline blood pressure, amount of blood loss, and type, amount, and timing of analgesic or anesthetic medications administered.

Women who have had epidural anesthesia may have slow return of sensory and motor function in their lower extremities, increasing the risk of falls with early ambulation. Careful assessment by the postpartum nurse can prevent falls. Factors that the nurse should consider are the time lapse since epidural medication was given; the woman's ability to bend both knees, place both feet flat on the bed, and lift buttocks off the bed without assistance; medications since birth; vital signs; and estimated blood loss with birth. Before allowing the woman to ambulate the nurse assesses the ability of the woman to stand unassisted beside her bed, simultaneously bending both knees slightly, and then standing with knees locked. If the patient is unable to balance herself, she can be safely eased back into bed without injury (Frank, Lane, & Hokanson, 2009).

NURSING ALERT Having a hospital staff or family member present the first time the woman gets out of bed after birth is wise because she may feel weak, dizzy, faint, or light-headed.

Prevention of VTE is important in the postpartum period. Women who must remain in bed after giving birth are at increased risk for the development of a thromboembolism. Antiembolic stockings (TED hose) or a sequential compression device (SCD) may be ordered prophylactically. If a woman remains in bed longer than 8 hours (e.g., for postpartum magnesium sulfate therapy for preeclampsia), exercise to promote circulation in the legs is indicated using the following routine:

- Alternate flexion and extension of feet.
- Rotate the ankle in circular motion.
- Alternate flexion and extension of the legs.
- Press the back of the knee to the bed surface; relax.

If the woman is susceptible to thromboembolism, she is encouraged to walk about actively for true ambulation and is discouraged from sitting immobile in a chair. Women with varicosities are advised to wear support hose. If a thrombus is suspected, as evidenced by complaint of pain in calf muscles, warmth, redness, or tenderness in the suspected leg, or a positive Homans sign, the primary health care provider should be notified immediately; meanwhile the woman should be confined to bed, with the affected limb elevated on pillows.

Exercise. Postpartum exercise can begin soon after birth, although the woman should be encouraged to start with simple exercises and gradually progress to more strenuous ones. Fig. 14-3 illustrates several exercises appropriate for the new mother. Abdominal exercises are postponed until approximately 4 weeks after cesarean birth.

Kegel exercises to strengthen pelvic muscle tone are extremely important, particularly after vaginal birth. Kegel exercises help women regain the muscle tone that is often lost as pelvic tissues are stretched and torn during pregnancy and birth. Improved pelvic muscle strength may help to prevent issues with urinary continence in later years.

Women must learn to perform Kegel exercises correctly (see Teaching Guidelines box in Chapter 2, p. 55). Some women who learn Kegel exercises perform them incorrectly and may increase their risk of incontinence, which may occur when women inadvertently bear down on the pelvic floor muscles, thrusting the perineum outward. The woman's technique can be assessed during the pelvic examination at her checkup by inserting two fingers intravaginally and checking whether the pelvic floor muscles correctly contract and relax.

Promotion of nutrition

During the hospital stay, most women display a good appetite and eat well. Women may request that family members bring in favorite or culturally appropriate foods. Cultural dietary preferences must be respected. This interest in food presents an ideal opportunity for nutritional counseling about dietary needs after birth, with specific information related to breastfeeding, preventing constipation and anemia, promoting weight loss, and promoting healing and well-being (see Chapter 8). Prenatal vitamins and iron supplements are often continued until 6 weeks after childbirth or until the ordered supply has been used.

The recommended caloric intake for the moderately active, nonlactating postpartum woman is 1800 to 2200 kcal/day. According to the Institute of Medicine (2005) the estimated energy requirement (EER) for a lactating woman during the first 6 months is 2700 kcal/day; during the next 6 months the EER is 2768 kcal/day. Higher-than-normal caloric intake is recommended for lactating women who are underweight or who exercise vigorously and those who are breastfeeding more than one infant. Although most women desire to return to their prepregnancy weight as soon as possible, gradual weight loss is recommended. (Becker & Scott, 2008)

Promotion of normal bladder and bowel patterns

Bladder function. After giving birth the mother should void spontaneously within 6 to 8 hours. The first several voidings should be measured to document adequate emptying of the bladder. A volume of at least 150 ml is expected for each voiding. Some women experience difficulty in emptying the bladder, possibly a result of diminished bladder tone, edema from trauma, or fear of discomfort. Nursing interventions for inability to void and bladder distention are discussed on p. 401.

Bowel function. After birth, women may be at risk for constipation related to side effects of medications (narcotic analgesics, iron supplements, magnesium sulfate), dehydration, immobility, or the presence of episiotomy, perineal lacerations, or hemorrhoids. The woman may have a fear of pain with having the first bowel movement after birth. Interventions to promote normal bowel elimination include educating the woman about measures to prevent constipation, such as exercise and intake of adequate roughage and fluids. Alerting the woman to side effects of medications such as opioid analgesics (e.g., decreased gastrointestinal tract motility) may encourage her to implement measures to reduce the risk of constipa-

Critical Thinking/Clinical Decision Making

Weight Loss after Birth

Wendy, a primipara, is postpartum 3 days after giving birth by cesarean to a 9-pound son. She has had an uncomplicated recovery thus far, and breastfeeding is going well. During a discharge teaching session, Wendy expresses concern to the nurse about regaining her figure after childbirth and states that she is worried that she cannot fit into her business clothes when she returns to her job as an administrative assistant in 6 weeks. Before pregnancy, her weight was appropriate for her height. However, during pregnancy, she gained 46 pounds.

1. Evidence—Is evidence sufficient to draw conclusions about counseling women with regard to regaining their nonpregnant appearance?
2. Assumptions—What assumptions can be made about the following issues?
   a. Appropriate diet for the postpartum mother who wants to improve her appearance
   b. The relationship between breastfeeding and postpartum weight loss
   c. Exercises for the postpartum woman who wants to improve her appearance
   d. The relationship between perceived body image and self-esteem in postpartum women
3. What implications and priorities for nursing care can be drawn at this time?
4. Does the evidence objectively support your conclusion?
5. Do alternative perspectives to your conclusion exist?

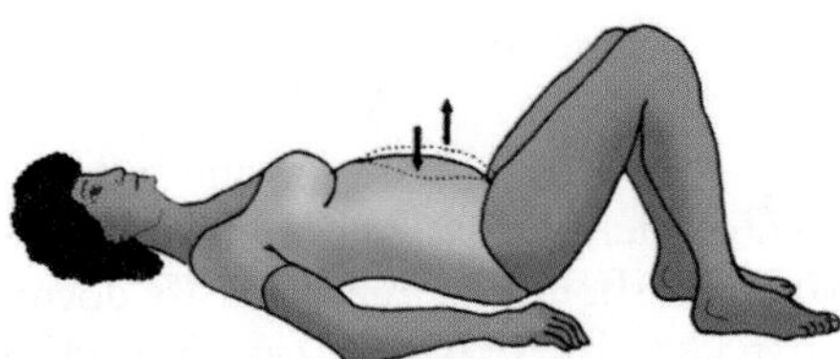

Abdominal Breathing. Lie on back with knees bent. Inhale deeply through nose. Keep ribs stationary and allow abdomen to expand upward. Exhale slowly but forcefully while contracting the abdominal muscles; hold for 3 to 5 seconds while exhaling. Relax.

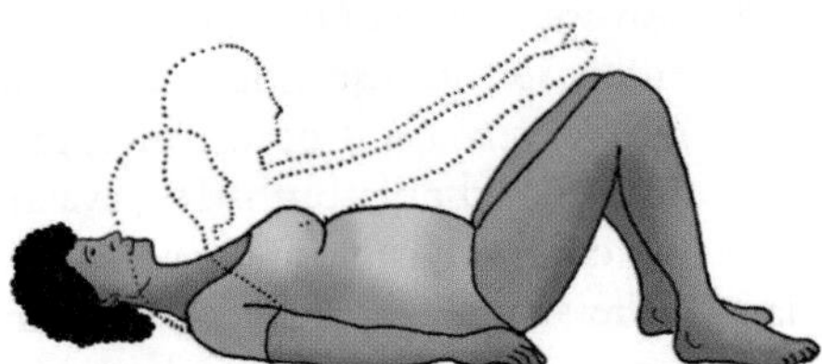

Reach for the Knees. Lie on back with knees bent. While inhaling, deeply lower chin onto chest. While exhaling, raise head and shoulders slowly and smoothly and reach for knees with arms outstretched. The body should rise only as far as the back will naturally bend while waist remains on floor or bed (about 6 to 8 inches). Slowly and smoothly lower head and shoulders back to starting position. Relax.

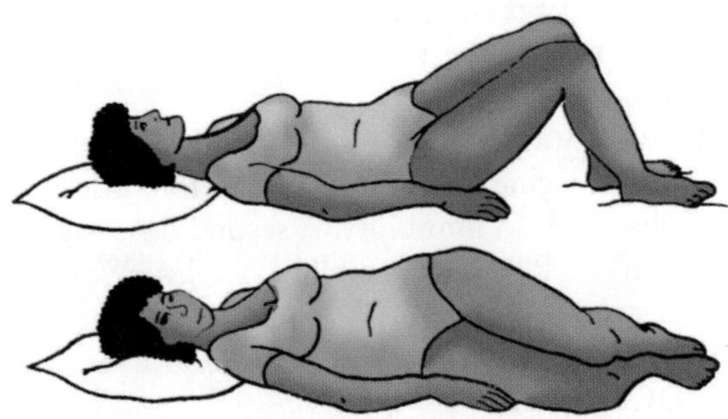

Double Knee Roll. Lie on back with knees bent. Keeping shoulders flat and feet stationary, slowly and smoothly roll knees over to the left to touch floor or bed. Maintaining a smooth motion, roll knees back over to the right until they touch floor or bed. Return to starting position and relax.

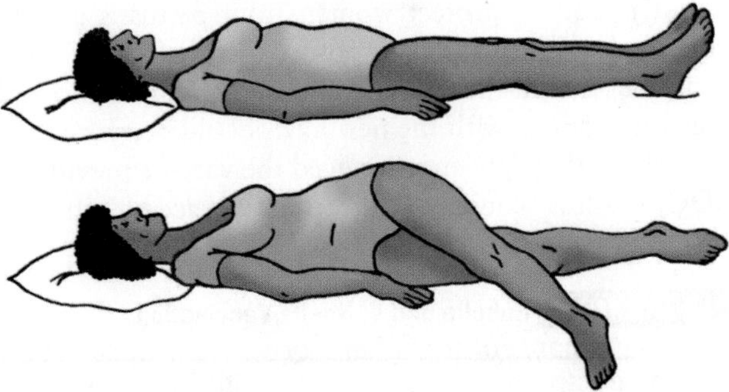

Leg Roll. Lie on back with legs straight. Keeping shoulders flat and legs straight, slowly and smoothly lift left leg and roll it over to touch the right side of floor or bed and return to starting position. Repeat, rolling right leg over to touch left side of floor or bed. Relax.

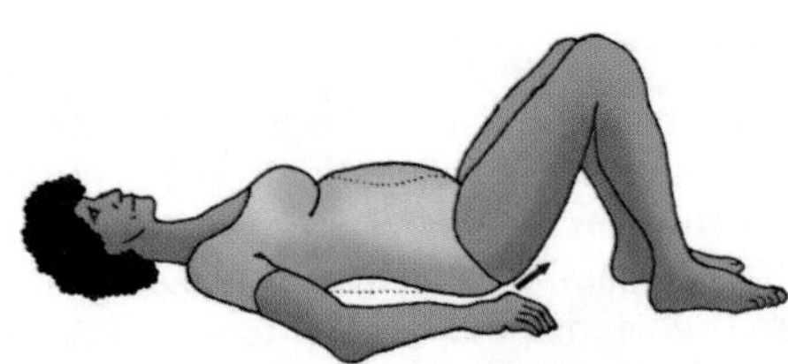

Combined Abdominal Breathing and Supine Pelvic Tilt (Pelvic Rock). Lie on back with knees bent. While inhaling deeply, roll pelvis back by flattening lower back on floor or bed. Exhale slowly but forcefully while contracting abdominal muscles and tightening buttocks. Hold for 3 to 5 seconds while exhaling. Relax.

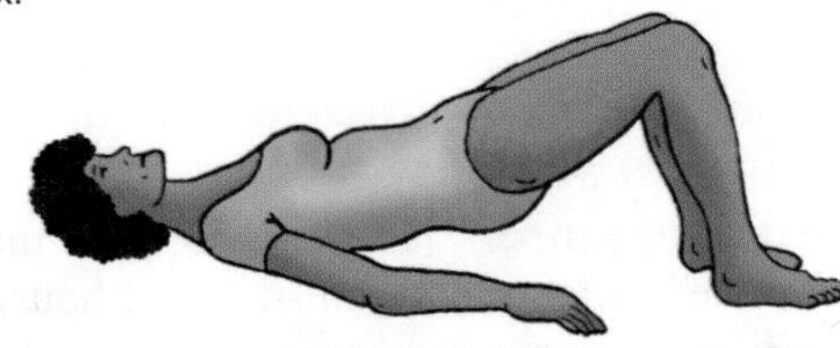

Buttocks Lift. Lie on back with arms at sides, knees bent, and feet flat. Slowly raise buttocks and arch back. Return slowly to starting position.

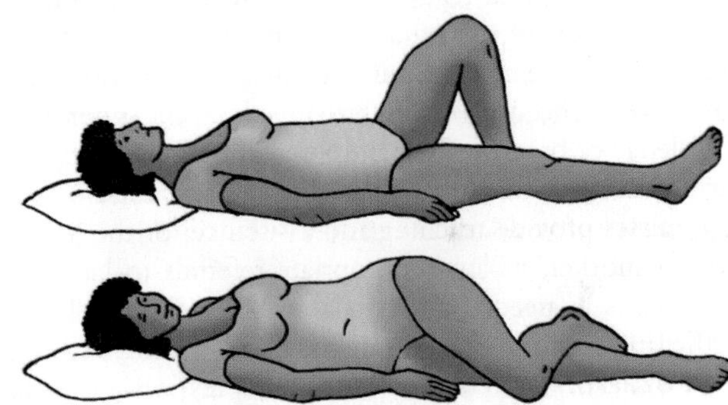

Single Knee Roll. Lie on back with right leg straight and left leg bent at the knee. Keeping shoulders flat, slowly and smoothly roll left knee over to the right to touch floor or bed and then back to starting position. Reverse position of legs. Roll right knee over to the left to touch floor or bed and return to starting position. Relax.

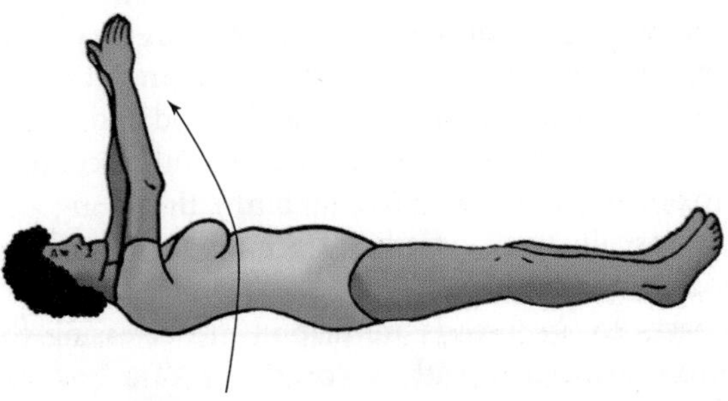

Arm Raises. Lie on back with arms extended at 90-degree angle from body. Raise arms so they are perpendicular and hands touch. Lower slowly.

Fig. 14-3 Postpartum exercise should begin as soon as possible. The woman should start with simple exercises and gradually progress to more strenuous ones.

tion. Stool softeners or laxatives may be necessary during the early postpartum period. With early discharge a new mother may be home before having a bowel movement.

NURSING ALERT Rectal suppositories or enemas should not be administered to women with third- or fourth-degree perineal lacerations. These measures to treat constipation may be very uncomfortable and can cause hemorrhage or damage to the suture line. They can also predispose the woman to infection (Association of Women's Health, Obstetric and Neonatal Nurses, 2006).

Some mothers experience gas pains, especially after cesarean birth. Antigas medications may be ordered. Ambulation or rocking in a rocking chair may stimulate passage of flatus and relieve discomfort.

Breastfeeding promotion and lactation suppression

Breastfeeding promotion. The ideal time to initiate breastfeeding is within the first 1 to 2 hours after birth. Baby-friendly hospitals mandate that the infant be put to the breast within the first hour after birth (Baby-Friendly Hospital Initiative, 2010). At this time, most infants are alert and ready to nurse. Breastfeeding aids in the contraction of the uterus and prevention of maternal hemorrhage. The first hour after birth is also an opportune time to assist the mother with breastfeeding, assess her basic knowledge of breastfeeding and assess the physical appearance of the breasts and nipples. Throughout the hospital stay, nurses provide teaching and assistance for the breastfeeding mother, making appropriate referrals to lactation consultants as needed and available. (See Chapter 18 for further information on assisting the breastfeeding woman.)

Lactation suppression. Suppression of lactation is initiated when the woman has decided not to breastfeed or in the case of neonatal death. It is important for the woman to wear a well-fitted support bra or breast binder continuously for at least the first 72 hours after birth. Women should avoid breast stimulation, including massage, running warm water over the breasts, newborn suckling, or pumping of the breasts. Some non-breastfeeding mothers experience severe breast **engorgement** (swelling of breast tissue caused by increased blood and lymph supply to the breasts as the body produces milk, occurring at approximately 72 to 96 hours after birth). Breast engorgement can usually be managed satisfactorily with nonpharmacologic interventions.

Ice packs to the breasts are helpful in decreasing the discomfort associated with engorgement. The woman should use a 15-minutes-on, 45-minutes-off schedule (to prevent the rebound swelling that can occur if ice is used continuously), or she can place fresh cabbage leaves inside her bra and replace them when wilted. A mild analgesic or antiinflammatory medication may aid in decreasing the discomfort associated with engorgement. Medications that were once prescribed for lactation suppression (e.g., estrogen, estrogen and testosterone, bromocriptine) are no longer used.

Health promotion for future pregnancies and children

Rubella vaccination. For women who have not had rubella (10%-20% of all women) or women who are serologically not immune (titer of 1:8 or enzyme immunoassay level less than 0.8) a subcutaneous injection of rubella vaccine is recommended in the postpartum period to prevent the possibility of contracting rubella in future pregnancies (Centers for Disease Control and Prevention [CDC], 2012a). Seroconversion occurs in approximately 90% of women vaccinated after birth. The live attenuated rubella virus is not communicable in breast milk; therefore breastfeeding mothers can be vaccinated. However, because the virus is shed in urine and other body fluids, the vaccine should not be given if the mother or other household members are immunocompromised. Rubella vaccine is made from duck eggs; therefore women who have allergies to these eggs may develop a hypersensitivity reaction to the vaccine, for which they will need adrenaline. A transient arthralgia or rash is common in vaccinated women but is benign. Because the vaccine may be teratogenic, women who receive the vaccine should avoid pregnancy for a month.

Varicella vaccination. The CDC recommends that varicella vaccine be administered before discharge in women who have no immunity. A second dose is given at the postpartum follow-up visit (4-8 weeks). Women are instructed not to conceive for 1 month after each dose because of potential teratogenic effects on a developing fetus (CDC, 2012c).

Tetanus-diphtheria-acellular pertussis vaccine. Tetanus-diphtheria-acellular pertussis (Tdap) vaccine is recommended for postpartum women who have not previously received the vaccine; it is given before discharge from the hospital or as early as possible in the postpartum period to protect women from pertussis and to decrease the risk of infant exposure to pertussis. Women should be advised that other adults and children who will come into contact with the newborn should be vaccinated with Tdap if they have not received the vaccine previously (CDC, 2012b). Women who receive the vaccine can continue to breastfeed.

LEGAL TIP **Rubella and Varicella Vaccination**
Informed consent for rubella or varicella vaccination in the postpartum period includes information about possible side effects and the risk of teratogenic effects. Women must understand that they must practice contraception to prevent pregnancy for 1 month after being vaccinated (CDC, 2012c).

Prevention of Rh isoimmunization. Injection of Rh immune globulin (RhIg) (a solution of gamma globulin that contains Rh antibodies) within 72 hours after birth prevents sensitization in the Rh-negative woman who has had a fetomaternal transfusion of Rh-positive fetal red blood cells (RBCs) (see Medication Guide box). RhIg promotes lysis of fetal Rh-positive blood cells before the mother forms her own antibodies against them.

NURSING ALERT After birth, RhIg is administered to all Rh-negative, antibody (Coombs)-negative women who give birth to Rh-positive infants. Rh immune globulin is administered to the mother intramuscularly (RhoGam, Gamulin RH, HypRho-D, Rhophylac) or intravenously (Rhophylac). It should never be given to an infant.

The administration of 300 mcg (1 vial) of Rh immune globulin is usually sufficient to prevent maternal sensitization. If a large fetomaternal transfusion is suspected, however, the dose needed should be determined by performing a Kleihauer-Betke test, which detects the amount of fetal blood in the maternal circulation. If more than 15 ml of fetal blood is present in maternal circulation, the dose of Rh immune globulin must be increased.

A 1:1000 dilution of Rh immune globulin is crossmatched to the mother's RBCs to ensure compatibility. Because Rh immune globulin is usually considered a blood product, precautions similar to those used for transfusing blood are necessary when it is given. The identification number on the patient's hospital wristband should correspond to the identification number found on the laboratory slip. The nurse must also check to see that the lot number on the laboratory slip corresponds to the lot number on the vial. Finally, the expiration date on the vial should be checked to ensure a usable product.

Rh immune globulin suppresses the immune response. Therefore the woman who receives both Rh immune globulin and rubella vaccine must be tested at 3 months to see if she has developed rubella immunity. If not, the woman will need another dose of rubella vaccine.

Some disagreement exists about whether Rh immune globulin should be considered a blood product. Health care providers need to discuss the most current information about this issue with women whose religious beliefs conflict with having blood products administered to them (e.g., Jehovah's Witnesses).

CARE MANAGEMENT—PSYCHOSOCIAL NEEDS

Meeting the psychosocial needs of new mothers involves assessing the parents' reactions to the birth experience, feelings about themselves, and interactions with the new baby and other family members. Specific interventions are then planned to increase the parents' knowledge and self-confidence as they assume the care and responsibility of the new baby and integrate this new member into their existing family structure in a way that meets their cultural

Medication Guide

Rh Immune Globulin (RhIg), RhoGAM, Gamulin Rh, HypRho-D, Rhophylac

ACTION

Suppression of immune response in nonsensitized women with Rh-negative blood who receive Rh-positive blood cells because of fetomaternal hemorrhage, transfusion, or accident

INDICATIONS

Routine antepartum prevention at 20 to 30 weeks of gestation in women with Rh-negative blood; to suppress antibody formation after birth, miscarriage or pregnancy termination, abdominal trauma, ectopic pregnancy, amniocentesis, version, or chorionic villi sampling

DOSAGE AND ROUTE

Standard dose 1 vial (300 mcg) intramuscularly in deltoid or gluteal muscle; microdose 1 vial (50 mcg) intramuscularly in deltoid muscle; Rhophylac can be given intramuscularly or intravenously (available in prefilled syringes)

ADVERSE EFFECTS

Myalgia, lethargy, localized tenderness and stiffness at injection site, mild and transient fever, malaise, headache, rarely nausea, vomiting, hypotension, tachycardia, possible allergic response

NURSING CONSIDERATIONS

- Give standard dose to mother at 28 weeks of gestation as prophylaxis or after an incident or exposure risk that occurs after 28 weeks of gestation (e.g., amniocentesis, second-trimester miscarriage or abortion, after external version attempt) and within 72 hours after birth if baby is Rh positive.
- Give microdose for first-trimester miscarriage or abortion, ectopic pregnancy, chorionic villus sampling.
- Verify that the woman is Rh negative and has not been sensitized, that Coombs test is negative, and that baby is Rh positive. Provide explanation to the woman about procedure, including the purpose, possible side effects, and effect on future pregnancies. Have the woman sign a consent form if required by agency. Verify correct dose and confirm lot number and woman's identity before giving injection (verify with another registered nurse or use other procedure per agency policy); document administration per agency policy. Observe patient for at least 20 minutes after administration for allergic response.
- The medication is made from human plasma (a consideration if the woman is a Jehovah's Witness). The risk of transmitting infectious agents, including viruses, cannot be completely eliminated.

expectations (see Chapter 15 and Nursing Process box: Psychosocial Needs).

There is evidence that nurses and other health care providers do not adequately address maternal psychosocial needs, instead focusing their attention on postpartum physical changes and care that is medically based (Cheung, Fowles, & Walker, 2006). Taking time to assess maternal emotional needs and to address concerns before discharge may promote better psychologic health and adjustment to parenting. Ongoing support for postpartum women is also needed. Even though issues such as fatigue are often evident during the hospital stay, clearly this type of support will likely be an ongoing concern after discharge when the woman is providing care for the newborn, herself, and other family members. Postpartum support is especially beneficial to at risk populations such as low-income primiparas, those at risk for family dysfunction and child abuse, and those at risk for postpartum depression (Shaw, Levitt, Wong, & Kaczorowski, 2006).

Spanish Guidelines: Postpartum Adjustment

Sometimes the psychosocial assessment indicates serious actual or potential problems that must be addressed. The Signs of Potential Complications box identifies psychosocial characteristics and behaviors that may be signs of potential complications and warrant ongoing evaluation after hospital discharge. Patients exhibiting these needs should be referred to appropriate community resources for assessment and management.

Impact of the birth experience

Many women indicate a need to examine the birth process itself and look retrospectively at their own behavior during labor and birth. Their partners may express similar desires. If their birth experience deviated from their birth plan (e.g., induction, epidural anesthesia, cesarean birth), both partners may need to mourn the loss of their expectations before they can adjust to the reality of their actual birth experience. Inviting them to review the events

NURSING PROCESS *Psychosocial Postpartum Concerns*

ASSESSMENT

- Obtain information from the medical record and nursing staff regarding any risk factors for psychologic problems after birth (e.g., history of depression, anxiety, panic disorders); review the history and current list of medications to identify any that are used for psychologic conditions.
- Assess emotional status.
- Assess reaction to the labor and birth.
- Observe interactions with the neonate.
- Observe interactions with the partner.
- Identify cultural beliefs and practices.
- Assess maternal self-concept and body image.
- Assess the support system.

NURSING DIAGNOSES

Examples of nursing diagnoses for meeting psychosocial needs during the postpartum period include:

- *Readiness for enhanced family processes* related to:
  - Excitement about newborn
- *Risk for impaired parenting* related to:
  - Long, difficult labor
  - Unmet expectations of labor and birth
- *Anxiety* related to:
  - Newness of parenting role, sibling rivalry, or response of grandparent
- *Risk for situational low self-esteem* related to:
  - Body image changes
- *Risk for caregiver role strain* related to:
  - Postpartum fatigue
- *Risk for ineffective coping* related to:
  - Lack of support
  - Postpartum fatigue

EXPECTED OUTCOMES OF CARE

Examples of common expected outcomes include that the mother (family) will do the following:

- Identify measures that promote a healthy personal adjustment in the postpartum period.
- Maintain healthy family functioning based on cultural norms and personal expectations.
- Discuss the events of her birth experience.
- Demonstrate an attachment to the newborn.
- Express positive feelings about the birth, her role, or the newborn.
- Indicates that she feels safe at home.
- Rests or sleeps in between infant feedings.
- Identifies sources of support and assistance at home.
- Demonstrates knowledge of resources to call after discharge (physician, clinic, lactation consultant, social worker, etc.).

PLAN OF CARE AND INTERVENTIONS

The nurse functions in the roles of a teacher, encourager, and supporter rather than a doer while implementing the psychosocial plan of care for a postpartum woman. Implementation of the psychosocial care plan involves carrying out specific activities to achieve the expected outcome of care planned for each individual woman. Topics that should be included in the psychosocial plan of care include promotion of parenting skills and family member adjustment to the newborn infant (see text).

EVALUATION

The nurse can be reasonably assured that care was effective if expected outcomes of care for psychosocial needs have been met.

and describe how they feel helps the nurse assess how well they understand what happened and how well they have been able to put their childbirth experience into perspective.

Maternal self-image

An important assessment involves the woman's self-concept, body image, and sexuality. How the new mother feels about herself and her body during the postpartum period can affect her behavior and adaptation to parenting. The woman's self-concept and body image can also affect her sexuality.

Feelings related to sexual adjustment after childbirth are often a cause of concern for new parents. Women who have recently given birth may be reluctant to resume sexual intercourse for fear of pain or may worry that coitus could damage healing perineal tissue. Because many new parents are anxious for information but reluctant to bring up the subject, postpartum nurses should matter-of-factly include the topic of postpartum sexuality during their routine physical assessment and teaching. Partners often have questions and concerns as well; it is helpful to include them in teaching sessions or discussions regarding sexuality in the postpartum period.

Adaptation to parenthood and parent-infant interactions

The psychosocial assessment also includes evaluating adaptation to parenthood. This task is accomplished by observing maternal and paternal reactions to the newborn and their interactions with the infant. Clues indicating successful adaptation begin to appear early after birth as parents react positively to the newborn infant and continue the process of establishing a relationship with their infant. In nontraditional families, such as lesbian couples, it is important to observe the partner's reactions and interactions with the neonate.

Parents are adapting well to their new roles when they exhibit a realistic perception and acceptance of their newborn's needs and limited abilities, immature social responses, and helplessness. Examples of positive parent-infant interactions include taking pleasure in the infant and in providing care, responding appropriately to infant cues, providing comfort, and reading the infant's cues for new experiences and sensing the infant's fatigue level (see Chapter 15). Should these indicators be missing, the nurse needs to investigate further what is hindering the normal adaptation process.

Family structure and functioning

A woman's adjustment to her role as mother is affected greatly by her relationships with her partner, her mother, and other relatives, and any other children (Fig. 14-4). Nurses can help ease the new mother's return home by identifying possible conflicts among family members and helping the woman plan strategies for dealing with these problems before discharge. Such a conflict could arise when couples have very different ideas about parenting. Dealing with the stresses of sibling rivalry and unsolicited grandparent advice can also affect the woman's psychological well-being. Only by asking about other nuclear and extended family members can the nurse discover potential

signs of POTENTIAL COMPLICATIONS

Postpartum Psychosocial Concerns

The following signs may suggest potentially serious complications and should be reported to the health care provider or clinic (these may be noticed by the partner or other family members):

- Unable or unwilling to discuss labor and birth experience
- Refers to self as ugly and useless
- Excessively preoccupied with self (body image)
- Markedly depressed
- Lacks a support system
- Partner or other family members react negatively to the baby
- Refuses to interact with or care for baby. For example, does not name baby, does not want to hold or feed baby, is upset by vomiting and wet or dirty diapers. (Cultural appropriateness of actions needs to be considered.)
- Expresses disappointment over baby's sex
- Sees baby as messy or unattractive
- Baby reminds mother of family member or friend she does not like
- Has difficulty sleeping
- Experiences loss of appetite

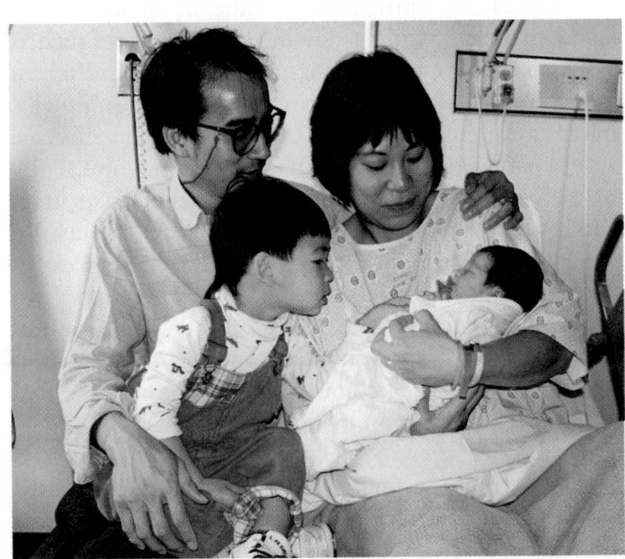

Fig. 14-4 Mother, father, and sibling get acquainted with the newborn. (Courtesy Kim Molloy, Knoxville, IA.)

problems in such relationships and help plan workable solutions for them.

Impact of cultural diversity

The final component of a complete psychosocial assessment is the woman's cultural beliefs, values, and practices. Much of a woman's behavior during the postpartum period is strongly influenced by her cultural background. Nurses are likely to come into contact with women from many different countries and cultures. Within the North American population, varied traditional health beliefs and practices can be found. All cultures have developed safe and satisfying methods of caring for new mothers and babies. Only by understanding and respecting the values and beliefs of each woman can the nurse design a plan of care to meet her individual needs (see Cultural Considerations box).

To identify cultural beliefs and practices when planning and implementing care the nurse conducts a cultural assessment. This assessment is ongoing; it is ideally begun during pregnancy and continued into the postpartum period. It can be accomplished most easily through conversation with the mother and her partner. Some hospitals have assessment tools designed to identify cultural beliefs and practices that may influence care (Cooper, Grywalski, Lamp, Newhouse, & Studlien, 2007). Components of the cultural assessment include the ability to read and write English, family involvement and support, dietary preferences, infant care, attachment, circumcision, religious or cultural beliefs, folk medicine practices, nonverbal communication, and personal space preferences.

Women from various cultures may view health as a balance between opposing forces (e.g., cold versus hot, yin versus yang), being in harmony with nature, or just "feeling good." Traditional practices may include the observance of certain dietary restrictions, clothing, or taboos for balancing the body; participation in certain activities such as sports and art for maintaining mental health; and use of silence, prayer, or meditation for developing spiritually. Practices (e.g., using religious objects or eating garlic) are used to protect oneself from illness and may involve avoiding people who are believed to create hexes or spells or who have an "evil eye." Restoration of health may involve taking folk medicines (e.g., herbs, animal substances) or using a traditional healer.

Childbirth occurs within this sociocultural context. Rest, seclusion, dietary constraints, and ceremonies honoring the mother are all common traditional practices that are followed for the promotion of the health and well-being of the mother and baby.

Several common traditional health practices are used and beliefs are held by women and their families during the postpartum period. In Asia, for example, pregnancy is considered to be a "hot" state, and childbirth results in a sudden loss of this state. Therefore balance must be restored by facilitating the return of the hot state, which is present physically or symbolically in hot food, hot water, and warm air.

Another common belief is that the mother and baby remain in a weak and vulnerable state for a period of several weeks after birth. During this time the mother

Cultural Considerations

Postpartum Period and Family Planning

POSTPARTUM CARE

- *Chinese, Latina, Korean, and Southeast Asian women* may wish to eat only warm foods and drink hot drinks to replace blood loss and to restore the balance of hot and cold in their bodies. These women may also wish to stay warm and avoid bathing, exercising, and hair washing for 7 to 40 days after childbirth. Self-management may not be a priority; care by family members is preferred. The woman has respect for elders and authority. These women may wear abdominal binders. They may prefer not to give their babies colostrum.
- *Arabic women* eat special meals designed to restore their energy. They are expected to stay at home for 40 days after childbirth to prevent illness resulting from exposure to the outside air.
- *Haitian women* may request to take the placenta home to bury or burn.
- *Muslim women* follow strict religious laws on modesty and diet. A Muslim woman must keep her hair, body, arms to the wrist, and legs to the ankles covered at all times. She cannot be alone in the presence of a man other than her husband or a male relative. Observant Muslims will not eat pork or pork products and are obligated to eat meat slaughtered according to Islamic laws (halal meat). If halal meat is not available, kosher meat, seafood, or a vegetarian diet is usually accepted.

FAMILY PLANNING

- Birth control is government mandated in mainland *China*. Most *Chinese women* will have an intrauterine device inserted after the birth of their first child. Women do not want hormonal methods of contraception because they fear putting these medications in their bodies.
- *Latina women* will likely choose the natural family planning method because most are Catholic.
- *(East) Indian* men are encouraged to have voluntary sterilization by vasectomy.
- *Muslim couples* may practice contraception by mutual consent as long as its use is not harmful to the woman. Acceptable contraceptive methods include foam and condoms, the diaphragm, and natural family planning.
- *Hmong women* highly value and desire large families, which limits birth control practices.
- *Arabic women* value large families, and sons are especially prized.

Critical Thinking/Clinical Decision Making

Cultural Influences during the Postpartum Period

Mingyu is a 29 year old from China who gave birth to her first child last evening. Her husband is completing postdoctoral study at the local university. Both Mingyu and her husband speak some English, although he is more fluent than she is. Her mother and father have come from China to be with her for 3 months. When the nurse enters the room, she notices immediately that the room temperature is rather warm and Mingyu is lying in bed with several layers of covers pulled up to her neck. She also has a blanket around her head. She has eaten nothing from the breakfast tray. The nursing assistant had reported that Mingyu refused to shower this morning. Although Mingyu's chart indicates that she intends to breastfeed, she requests formula for her baby.

1. Evidence—Is evidence sufficient to draw conclusions about the cultural beliefs of Asians as they relate to the postpartum period and breastfeeding?
2. Assumptions—What assumptions can be made about the following issues?
   a. Culturally appropriate diet, activity, and hygiene for the postpartum Asian woman
   b. Providing appropriate care for the newborn, including breastfeeding, in the Asian culture
   c. Role of other family members and friends in providing care to the postpartum woman and newborn
   d. Difficulty in establishing lactation if breastfeeding is not begun immediately
3. What implications and priorities for nursing care can be drawn at this time?
4. Does the evidence objectively support your conclusion?
5. Do alternative perspectives to your conclusion exist?

may remain in a passive role, taking no baths or showers, and may stay in bed to prevent cold air from entering her body.

Women who have immigrated to the United States or other Western nations without their extended families may have little help at home, which makes observing these activity restrictions difficult for them. The Cultural Considerations box lists some common cultural beliefs about the postpartum period and family planning.

Nurses need to consider all cultural aspects when planning care and to avoid using their own cultural beliefs as the framework for that care. Although the beliefs and behaviors of other cultures may seem different or strange, they should be encouraged as long as the mother wants to conform to them and she and the baby suffer no ill effects. The nurse also needs to determine whether a woman is using any folk medicine during the postpartum period because active ingredients in folk medicine may have adverse physiologic effects on the woman when ingested with prescribed medicines. The nurse should not assume that a mother desires to use traditional health practices that represent a particular cultural group merely because she is a member of that culture. Many young women who are first- or second-generation Americans follow their cultural traditions only when older family members are present or not at all.

DISCHARGE TEACHING

Self-Management and Signs of Complications

Discharge planning begins at the time of admission to the unit and should be reflected in the nursing care plan developed for each individual woman. For example, a great deal of time during the hospital stay is usually spent in teaching about maternal self-care management and newborn care because the goal is for all women to be capable of providing basic care for themselves and their infants at the time of discharge. In addition, every woman must be taught to recognize the physical and psychologic signs and symptoms that might indicate problems and how to obtain advice and assistance quickly if these signs appear. Table 14-1 and the Signs of Potential Complications box on p. 409 list several common indications of maternal physical and psychosocial complications in the postpartum period. (See Chapter 23 for more information on postpartum complications.) Before discharge, women need basic instruction regarding a variety of self-care topics such as nutrition, exercise, family planning, resumption of sexual intercourse, prescribed medications, and routine mother-baby checkups (see Box 14-3). Because of the limited time available for teaching, nurses must target their teaching on expressed needs of the woman. Giving the woman a list of topics and asking her to indicate her teaching needs will help the nurse maximize teaching efforts and may increase retention of information by the woman. Providing written materials on postpartum self-care, breastfeeding, and infant care that the woman may consult after discharge is helpful.

Ⓔ Spanish Guidelines: Discharge Teaching

Just before the time of discharge the nurse reviews the woman's medical record to see that laboratory reports, medications, signatures, and other items are in order. Some hospitals have a checklist to use before the woman's discharge. The nurse verifies that medications, if ordered, have arrived on the unit, that any valuables kept secured during the woman's stay have been returned to her and that she has signed a receipt for them, and that the infant is ready to be discharged. The woman's and the baby's identification bands are carefully checked.

Any medication that may cause drowsiness should not be administered to the mother before discharge if she is the one who will be holding the baby on the way out of the hospital. In most instances the woman is seated in a wheelchair and is given the baby to hold. Some families

EVIDENCE-BASED PRACTICE

How Soon is Too Soon? Early Discharge after Birth

Pat Gingrich

ASK THE QUESTION

What are the risks and benefits of early postpartum discharge for mother and baby? What do women want from their postpartum hospital experience?

SEARCH FOR EVIDENCE

Search Strategies: Professional organization guidelines, meta-analyses, systematic reviews, randomized controlled trials, nonrandomized prospective studies, and retrospective studies since 2006.

Search Databases: Cumulative Index to Nursing and Allied Health Literature, Cochrane, Medline, National Guideline Clearinghouse, TRIP Database Plus, and the websites for the Association of Women's Health, Obstetric and Neonatal Nurses, the Society of Obstetricians and Gynaecologists of Canada, and the National Institute for Health and Clinical Excellence.

CRITICALLY ANALYZE THE EVIDENCE

The optimal length of postpartum hospitalization has been debated for decades. After a period of shortened stays in the early 1990s, which critics dubbed *drive-through deliveries,* research demonstrated an increase in infant problems and readmissions. New laws required insurance and Medicaid to cover 48 hours for vaginal birth and 72 hours for cesarean birth, which has decreased readmission rates.

Length of hospital stay after giving birth depends on many factors: the physical condition of the mother and baby, social support at home, patient education needs for self-care and infant care, mental and emotional status of the mother, and financial constraints.

Women who greatly prefer to go home will probably do better there. The professional recommendation by the National Institute of Clinical Excellence (2004) is to allow early discharge at 24 hours after vaginal or cesarean birth, as long as fever and complications do not exist and close follow-up is maintained. According to a survey of 2583 Canadian women, effective follow-up, such as office or home visit or telephone contact with a health care provider within 72 hours of discharge, can significantly decrease infant readmissions and maternal postpartum depression (Goulet, D'Amour, & Pineault, 2007).

According to the professional guidelines published by the Society of Obstetricians and Gynaecologists of Canada (SOGC) the risk with early discharge is mainly for the infant, who may develop jaundice, infection, unrecognized heart or respiratory problems, or feeding problems (Cargill, Martel, & Society of Obstetricians and Gynaecologists of Canada, 2007). The rate of emergency room visits and readmissions was especially high for infants with young, primiparous, unmarried mothers.

IMPLICATIONS FOR PRACTICE

In an ongoing population-based survey of 16,000 U.S. women, a qualitative analysis found six major themes for postpartum concerns of the women at 2 to 9 months after childbirth: (1) the need for social support, (2) breastfeeding issues, (3) newborn care, (4) postpartum depression, (5) perceived need to extend hospital stay, and (6) need for insurance beyond delivery (Kanotra, D'Angelo, Phares, Morrow, Barfield, & Lansky, 2007). Nurses have the most opportunity to assess the physical, psychologic, and social well-being of their patients. Postpartum women deserve individualized patient education that includes comprehensive information and resources about infant care, breastfeeding, and postpartum depression. Educational information should be offered in many formats and include hands-on demonstrations. Written material should include 24-hour numbers to call for problems with infant care and breastfeeding, as well as contact information for community parenting groups. All patients should go home with a realistic expectation of the social and financial support they will need. Finally, nurses can advocate for policies that support flexible lengths of hospital stays, and programs recommended by the SOGC: early home visits, outpatient breastfeeding clinics, and early physician visits (Cargill et al., 2007).

References:

Cargill, Y., Martel, M. J., & Society of Obstetricians and Gynaecologists of Canada. (2007). Postpartum maternal and newborn discharge. SGOC Policy Statement No. 190. *Journal of Obstetrics and Gynaecology Canada, 29*(4), 357–363.

Goulet, L., D'Amour, D., & Pineault, R. (2007). Type and timing of services following postnatal discharge: Do they make a difference? *Women & Health, 45*(4), 19–39.

Kanotra, S., D'Angelo, D., Phares, T. M., Morrow, B., Barfield, W. D., & Lansky, A. (2007). Challenges faced by new mothers in the early postpartum period: An analysis of comment data from the 2000 Pregnancy Risk Assessment Monitoring System (PRAMS) survey. *Maternal and Child Health Journal, 11*(6), 549–558.

National Institute for Health and Clinical Excellence (NICE). (2004). *Caesarean section. NICE Clinical Guideline 13.* London: NICE. Retrieved June 3, 2009.

leave unescorted and ambulatory, depending on hospital protocol. Newborns must be secured in a car seat for the drive home.

In some hospitals, diaper bags or other items containing infant formula are routinely given to all mothers before discharge. Even though these bags are designated for breastfeeding and bottle-feeding mothers, all contain infant formula. Concern has surfaced that giving infant formula to breastfeeding mothers may undermine self-confidence in the ability to breastfeed.

NURSING ALERT Prepackaged formula should not be given to mothers who are breastfeeding. Such "gifts" are associated with earlier cessation of breastfeeding.

Sexual Activity and Contraception

Discussing sexual activity and family planning with the woman and her partner is important before they leave the hospital because many couples resume sexual activity before the traditional postpartum checkup 6 weeks after birth. For most women the risk of hemorrhage or infection is minimal by approximately 2 weeks postpartum. Couples may be anxious about the topic but uncomfortable and unwilling to bring it up. The nurse needs to discuss the physical and psychologic effects that giving birth can have on sexual activity (see Patient Instructions for Self-Management box). Contraceptive options should also be discussed with women (and their partners, if present) before discharge so that they can make informed decisions about fertility management before resuming sexual activity. Waiting to discuss contraception at the 6-week checkup may be too late. Ovulation can occur as soon as 1 month after birth, particularly in women who bottle-feed. Breastfeeding mothers should be informed that breastfeeding is not a reliable means of contraception and that other methods should be used; nonhormonal methods are best, given that oral contraceptives can interfere with milk production. Women who are undecided about contraception at the time of discharge need information about using condoms with foam or creams until the first postpartum checkup. Current contraceptive options are discussed in detail in Chapter 4.

Prescribed Medications

Women routinely continue to take their prenatal vitamins during the postpartum period. Breastfeeding mothers may be told to continue prenatal vitamins for the duration of breastfeeding. Supplemental iron may be prescribed for mothers with lower-than-normal hemoglobin levels. Women with extensive episiotomies or vaginal lacerations (third or fourth degree) are usually prescribed stool softeners to take at home. Pain relief medications (analgesics or NSAIDs) may be prescribed, especially for women who had cesarean birth. The nurse should make certain that the woman knows the route, dose, frequency, and common side effects of all medications that she may be taking at home.

Follow-Up after Discharge

Routine mother and baby follow-up visits

Women who have experienced uncomplicated vaginal births are commonly scheduled for the traditional 6-week postpartum follow-up examination. Women who have had a cesarean birth are often seen in the health care provider's office or clinic 2 weeks after hospital discharge. The date and time for the follow-up appointment should be included in the discharge instructions. If an appointment has not been made before the woman leaves the hospital, she should be encouraged to call the office or clinic and schedule an appointment.

Parents who have not already done so need to make plans for newborn follow-up at the time of discharge. Breastfeeding infants are routinely seen by the pediatric health care provider or clinic within 3-5 days after discharge and again at approximately 2 weeks of age (AAP Section on Breastfeeding, 2012). Formula-feeding infants may be seen for the first time at 2 weeks of age. If an appointment for a specific date and time was not made for the infant before leaving the hospital, the parents should be encouraged to call the office or clinic right away.

PATIENT INSTRUCTIONS FOR SELF-MANAGEMENT

Resumption of Sexual Intercourse

- You can safely resume sexual intercourse by the second to fourth week after birth when bleeding has stopped and the laceration or episiotomy has healed. For the first 6 weeks to 6 months the vagina does not lubricate well.
- Your physiologic reactions to sexual stimulation for the first 3 months after birth will likely be slower and less intense than before birth. The strength of the orgasm may be reduced.
- A water-soluble gel, cocoa butter, or a contraceptive cream or jelly might be recommended for lubrication. If some vaginal tenderness is present, your partner can be instructed to insert one or more clean, lubricated fingers into the vagina and rotate them within the vagina to help relax it and to identify possible areas of discomfort. A position in which you have control of the depth of the insertion of the penis is also useful. The side-by-side or female-on-top position may be more comfortable than other positions.
- The presence of the baby influences postbirth lovemaking. Parents hear every sound that the baby makes; conversely, you may be concerned that the baby hears every sound you make. In either case, any phase of the sexual response cycle may be interrupted by hearing the baby cry or move, leaving both of you frustrated and unsatisfied. In addition, the amount of psychologic energy expended by you in child care activities may lead to fatigue. Newborns require a great deal of attention and time.
- Some women have reported feeling sexual stimulation and orgasms when breastfeeding their babies. Breastfeeding mothers are often interested in returning to sexual activity before non-breastfeeding mothers.
- You should be instructed to perform the Kegel exercises correctly so as to strengthen your pubococcygeal muscle. This muscle is associated with bowel and bladder function and with vaginal feeling during intercourse.

Home visits

Home visits to mothers and newborns within a few days of discharge can help bridge the gap between hospital care and routine visits to health care providers. Nurses are able to assess the mother, infant, and home environment, as well as answer questions, provide education and emotional support, and make referrals to community resources if necessary. Home visits have been shown to reduce the need for more expensive health care, such as emergency department visits and rehospitalization; they may also reduce the incidence of postpartum depression in women who are at risk (Goulet et al., 2007). The support provided by nurses and other trained community health workers can enhance parent-infant interaction and parenting skills; home visits also help to promote mutual support between the mother and her partner (De La Rosa, Perry, & Johnson, 2009). Breastfeeding outcomes can be enhanced through home visitation programs (Mannan et al., 2008).

Home nursing care may not be available even if needed because no agencies are available to provide the service or no coverage is in place for payment by third-party payers. If care is available, a referral form containing information about both mother and baby should be completed at hospital discharge and sent immediately to the home care agency.

The home visit is most commonly scheduled on the woman's second day home from the hospital, but it can be scheduled on any of the first 4 days at home, depending on the individual family's situation and needs. Additional visits are planned throughout the first week, as needed. The home visits may be extended beyond that time if the family's needs warrant it and if a home visit is the most appropriate option for carrying out the follow-up care required to meet the specific needs identified.

During the home visit the nurse conducts a systematic assessment of the mother and newborn to determine physiologic adjustment and to identify any existing complications. The assessment also focuses on the mother's emotional adjustment and her knowledge of self-management and infant care. Conducting the assessment in a private area of the home provides an opportunity for the mother to ask questions on potentially sensitive topics such as breast care, constipation, sexual activity, or family planning. Family adjustment to the newborn is assessed and concerns are addressed during the home visit.

During the newborn assessment the nurse can demonstrate and explain normal newborn characteristics and behaviors, encouraging the mother and family to ask questions or express concerns they may have. The home care nurse verifies if the newborn screen for phenylketonuria and other inborn errors of metabolism has been drawn. If the infant was discharged from the hospital before 24 hours of age, a blood sample for the newborn screen may be drawn by the home care nurse or the family will need to take the infant to the health care provider's office or clinic.

Telephone follow-up

In addition to or instead of a home visit, many providers are implementing one or more postpartum telephone follow-up calls to their patients for assessment, health teaching, and identification of complications to effect timely intervention and referrals. Telephone follow-up may be offered by hospitals, private physicians, clinics, or private agencies. It may be either a separate service or combined with other strategies for extending postpartum care. Telephone nursing assessments are frequently used as follow-up to postpartum home visits.

Warm lines

The **warm line** is another type of telephone link between the new family and concerned caregivers or experienced parent volunteers. A warm line is a helpline or consultation service, not a crisis-intervention line. The warm line is appropriately used for dealing with less-extreme concerns that may seem urgent at the time the call is placed but are not actual emergencies. Calls to warm lines commonly relate to infant feeding, prolonged crying, or sibling rivalry. Families are encouraged to call when concerns arise; telephone numbers for warm lines should be provided for parents before hospital discharge.

Support groups

The woman adjusting to motherhood may desire interaction and conversation with other women who are having similar experiences. Postpartum women who have met earlier in prenatal clinics or on the hospital unit may begin to associate for mutual support. Members of childbirth classes who attend a postpartum reunion may decide to extend their relationship during the fourth trimester. Fathers or partners may also benefit from participation in support groups.

A postpartum support group enables mothers and fathers to share experiences and support each other as they adjust to parenting. Many new parents discover that they are not alone in their feelings of confusion and uncertainty, which can be reassuring. An experienced parent can often impart concrete information that can be valuable to other members in a postpartum support group. Inexperienced parents may find themselves imitating the behavior of others in the group whom they perceive as particularly capable.

Referral to community resources

To develop an effective referral system the nurse should have an understanding of the needs of the woman and family and of the organization and community resources available for meeting those needs. Locating and compiling information about available community services contributes to the development of a referral system. The nurse also needs to develop his or her own resource file of local and national services that are used commonly by health care providers (see Resources on this book's Evolve website).

KEY POINTS

- Postpartum care is family-centered and modeled on the concept of health.
- Cultural beliefs and practices affect maternal and family responses to the postpartum period.
- The nursing care plan includes assessments to detect deviations from normal, comfort measures to relieve discomfort or pain, and safety measures to prevent injury or infection.
- Teaching and counseling measures are designed to promote the woman's feelings of competence in self-management and infant care.
- Common nursing interventions in the postpartum period focus on prevention of excessive bleeding, bladder distention, infection; nonpharmacologic and pharmacologic relief of discomfort associated with the episiotomy, lacerations, or breastfeeding; and instituting measures to promote or suppress lactation.
- Meeting the psychosocial needs of new mothers involves taking into consideration the composition and functioning of the entire family.
- Early postpartum discharge will continue to be the trend as a result of consumer demand, medical necessity, discharge criteria for low risk childbirth, and cost-containment measures.
- Early discharge classes, telephone follow-up, home visits, warm lines, and support groups are effective means of facilitating physiologic and psychological adjustments in the postpartum period.

Audio Chapter Summaries Access an audio summary of these Key Points on evolve

References

American Academy of Pediatrics Committee on Psychological Aspects of Child and Family Health. (2010). Incorporating recognition and management of perinatal and postpartum depression into pediatric practice. *Pediatrics*, *126*(5), 1032-1039.

American Academy of Pediatrics Section on Breastfeeding. (2012). Breastfeeding and the use of human milk. *Pediatrics 129*(3), e829-e841.

Association of Women's Health, Obstetric, and Neonatal Nurses (AWHONN). (2006). *The compendium of postpartum care.* Washington, DC: AWHONN.

Baby Friendly Hospital Initiative USA. (2010). *The ten steps to successful breastfeeding.* Retrieved June 14, 2013 from www.babyfriendlyusa.org/eng/10steps.html.

Becker, G., & Scott, M. (2008). Chapter 16: Nutrition for lactating women. In R. Mannel, P.J. Martens, & M. Walker (Ed.), *Core curriculum for lactation consultant practice* (2nd ed.). Sudbury, MA: Jones and Bartlett.

Centers for Disease Control and Prevention. (2012a). Recommended adult immunization schedule. *MMWR Recommendations and Reports*, *61*(4), 1-9.

Centers for Disease Control and Prevention. (2012b). Tdap for pregnant women: Information for providers. Retrieved June 14, 2013 from www.cdc.gov/vaccines/vpd-vac/pertussis/tdap-pregnancy-hcp.htm#postpartum.

Centers for Disease Control and Prevention. (2012c). Varicella vaccination recommendations for specific age groups. Retrieved June 14, 2013 from www.cdc.gov/vaccines/vpd-vac/vricella/hcp-rec-spec-groups.htm.

Cheung, C., Fowles, E.R., & Walker, L.O. (2006). Postpartum maternal health care in the United States: A critical review. *Journal of Perinatal Education*, *15*(3), 34-42.

Cooper, M., Grywalski, M., Lamp, J., Newhouse, L., & Studlien, R. (2007). Enhancing cultural competence: A model for nurses. *Nursing for Women's Health*, *11*(2), 148-160.

Corwin, E.J., & Arbour, M. (2007). Postpartum fatigue and evidence-based interventions. *MCN American Journal of Maternal/Child Nursing*, *32*(4), 215-220.

De La Rosa, I.A., Perry, J., & Johnson, V. (2009). Benefits of increased home-visitation services: Exploring a case management model. *Family and Community Health*, *32*(10) 58-75.

Declercq, E., Cunningham, D. K., Johnson, C., & Sakala, C. (2008). Mothers' reports of postpartum pain associated with vaginal and cesarean deliveries: Results of a national survey. *Birth*, *35*(1), 16-24.

Frank, B.J., Lane, C., & Hokanson, H. (2009). Designing a postepidural fall risk assessment score for the obstetric patient. *Journal of Nursing Care Quality*, *24*(1), 50-54.

Goulet, L., D'Amour, D., Pineault, R. (2007). Type and timing of services following postnatal discharge: Do they make a difference? *Women & Health*, *45*(4), 19-39.

Institute of Medicine. (2005). *Dietary reference intakes for energy, carbohydrate, fiber, fatty acids, cholesterol, protein, and amino acids.* Washington, DC: Food and Nutrition Board, Institute of Medicine, National Academies Press.

Mannan, I., Rahman, S.M., Sania, A., Seraji, H.R., Arifeen, S.E., Winch, P.J., et al. (2008). Can early postpartum visits by trained community health workers improve breastfeeding of newborns? *Journal of Perinatology*, *28*(9), 632-640.

Runquist, J. (2007). Persevering through postpartum fatigue. *Journal of Obstetric, Gynecologic, and Neonatal Nursing*, *36*(1), 28-37.

Shaw, E., Levitt, C., Wong, S., Kaczorowski, J. (2006). Systematic review of the literature on postpartum care: Effectiveness of postpartum support to improve maternal parenting, mental health, quality of life, and physical health. *Birth*, *33*(3), 210-220.

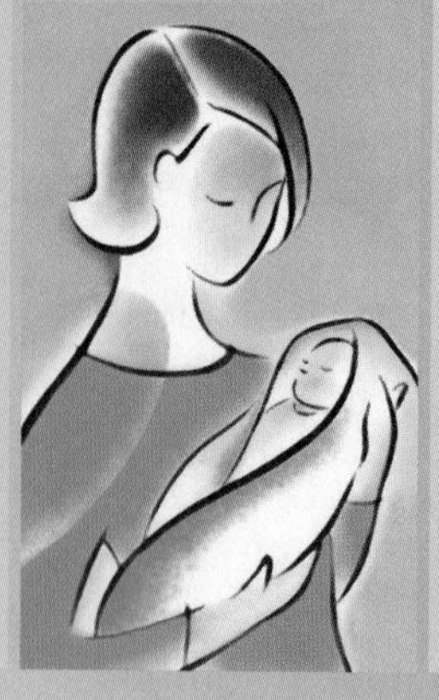

CHAPTER 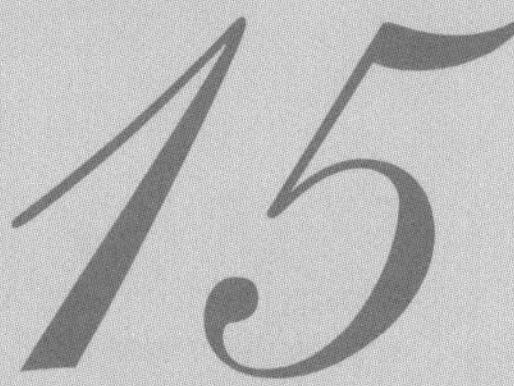

Transition to Parenthood

KATHRYN RHODES ALDEN

LEARNING OBJECTIVES

- *Identify parental and infant behaviors that facilitate and those that inhibit parental attachment.*
- *Describe sensual responses that strengthen attachment.*
- *Examine the process of becoming a mother and becoming a father.*
- *Compare maternal adjustment and paternal adjustment to parenthood.*
- *Describe how the nurse can facilitate parent-infant adjustment.*
- *Examine the effects of the following on parental response: parental age (i.e., adolescence and older than 35 years), social support, culture, socioeconomic conditions, personal aspirations, and sensory impairment.*
- *Describe sibling adjustment.*
- *Discuss grandparent adaptation.*

KEY TERMS AND DEFINITIONS

acquaintance Process that parents use to get to know or become familiar with their new infant; an important step in attachment

attachment A specific and enduring affective tie to another person

becoming a mother Transformation and growth of the mother identity

biorhythmicity Cyclic changes that occur with established regularity, such as sleeping and eating patterns

bonding A process by which parents, over time, form an emotional relationship with their infant

claiming process Process by which the parents identify their new baby in terms of likeness to other family members, differences, and uniqueness

en face Face-to-face position in which the parent's and the infant's faces are approximately 20 cm apart and on the same plane

engrossment A parent's absorption, preoccupation, and interest in his or her infant; term typically used to describe the father's intense involvement with his newborn

entrainment Phenomenon observed in the microanalysis of sound films in which the speaker moves several parts of the body and the listener responds to the sounds by moving in ways that are coordinated with the rhythm of the sounds (infants have been observed moving in time to the rhythms of adult speech but not to random noises or disconnected words or vowels); believed to be an essential factor in the process of maternal-infant bonding

letting-go phase Interdependent phase after birth in which the mother and family move forward as a system with interacting members

maternal sensitivity The quality of a mother's sensitive behaviors that are based on her awareness, perception, and responsiveness to infant cues and behaviors

mutuality Parent-infant interaction in which the infant's behaviors and characteristics call forth a corresponding set of paternal behaviors and characteristics

postpartum blues A let-down feeling, accompanied by irritability and anxiety, which usually begins 2 to 3 days after giving birth and disappears within a week or two; sometimes called "baby blues"

reciprocity Type of body movement or behavior that provides the observer with cues, such as the behavioral cues infants provide to parents and parents' responses to cues

sibling rivalry A sibling's jealousy of and resentment toward a new child in the family

synchrony Fit between the infant's cues and the parent's response

KEY TERMS AND DEFINITIONS—cont'd

taking-hold phase Period after birth characterized by a woman becoming more independent and more interested in learning infant care skills

taking-in phase Period after birth characterized by the woman's dependency; maternal needs are dominant, and talking about the birth is an important task

transition to parenthood Period from the preconception parenthood decision through the first months after birth of the baby during which parents define their parental roles and adjust to parenthood

WEB RESOURCES

Additional related content can be found on the companion website at evolve

http://evolve.elsevier.com/Lowdermilk/Maternity/

- NCLEX Review Questions
- Critical Thinking Exercise: Postpartum Home Care
- Nursing Care Plan: Home Care Follow-Up: Transition to Parenthood
- Nursing Care Plan: The Multiparous Woman and Family

Becoming a parent creates a period of change and instability for men and women who decide to have children. This period occurs whether parenthood is biologic or adoptive and whether the parents are married husband-wife couples, cohabiting couples, single mothers, single fathers, lesbian couples with one woman as biologic mother, or gay male couples who adopt a child. Parenting is as a process of role attainment and role transition that begins during pregnancy. The transition is an ongoing process as the parents and infant develop and change.

PARENTAL ATTACHMENT, BONDING, AND ACQUAINTANCE

The process by which a parent comes to love and accept a child and a child comes to love and accept a parent is known as **attachment**. Using the terms *attachment* and *bonding,* Klaus and Kennell proposed that the period shortly after birth is important to mother-to-infant attachment. They defined the phenomenon of **bonding** as a sensitive period in the first minutes and hours after birth when mothers and fathers must have close contact with their infants for optimal later development (Klaus & Kennell, 1976). Klaus and Kennell (1982) later revised their theory of parent-infant bonding, modifying their claim of the critical nature of immediate contact with the infant after birth. They acknowledged the adaptability of human parents, stating that more than minutes or hours were needed for parents to form an emotional relationship with their infants. The terms *attachment* and *bonding* continue to be used interchangeably.

Attachment is developed and maintained by proximity and interaction with the infant, through which the parent becomes acquainted with the infant, identifies the infant as an individual, and claims the infant as a member of the family. Positive feedback between the parent and the infant through social, verbal, and nonverbal responses (whether real or perceived) facilitates the attachment process. Attachment occurs through a mutually satisfying experience. A mother commented on her son's grasp reflex, "I put my finger in his hand, and he grabbed right on. It is just a reflex, I know, but it felt good anyway" (Fig. 15-1).

The concept of attachment includes **mutuality**; that is, the infant's behaviors and characteristics elicit a corresponding set of parental behaviors and characteristics. The infant displays signaling behaviors such as crying, smiling, and cooing that initiate the contact and bring the caregiver to the child. These behaviors are followed by executive behaviors such as rooting, grasping, and postural adjustments that maintain the contact. Most caregivers are attracted to an alert, responsive, cuddly infant and repelled by an irritable, apparently disinterested infant. Attachment occurs more readily with the infant whose temperament,

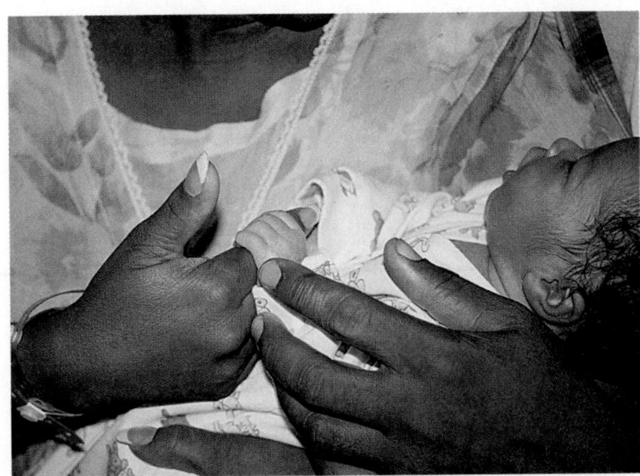

Fig. 15-1 Hands. (Courtesy Marjorie Pyle, RNC, Lifecircle, Costa Mesa, CA.)

social capabilities, appearance, and gender fit the parent's expectations. If the infant does not meet these expectations, the parent's disappointment can delay the attachment process. Table 15-1 presents a comprehensive list of classic infant behaviors affecting parental attachment. Table 15-2 presents a corresponding list of parental behaviors that affect infant attachment.

An important part of attachment is **acquaintance.** Parents use eye contact (Fig. 15-2), touching, talking, and exploring to become acquainted with their infant during the immediate postpartum period. Adoptive parents undergo the same process when they first meet their new child. During this period, families engage in the **claiming process,** which is the identification of the new baby (Fig. 15-3). The child is first identified in terms of "likeness" to other family members, then in terms of "differences," and finally in terms of "uniqueness." The unique newcomer is thus incorporated into the family. Mothers and fathers examine their infant carefully and point out characteristics that the child shares with other family members and that are indicative of a relationship between them. Maternal comments such as the following reveal the claiming process: "Everyone says, 'He's the image of his father,' but I found one part like me–his toes are shaped like mine."

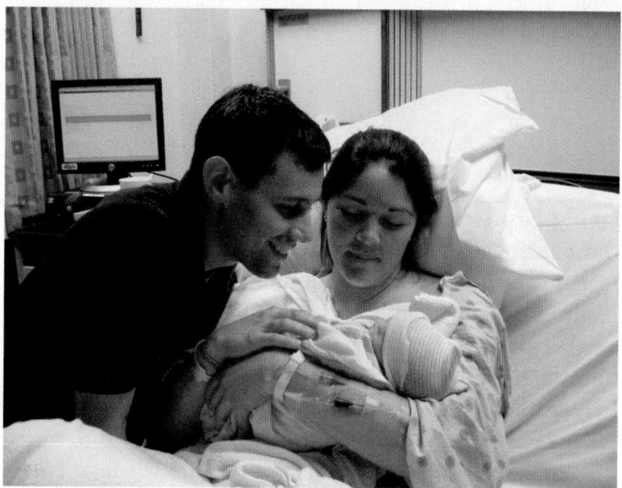

Fig. 15-2 Early acquaintance between parents and newborn as mother holds infant in en face position. (Courtesy Kathryn Alden, Chapel Hill, NC.)

On the other hand, some mothers react negatively. They "claim" the infant in terms of the discomfort or pain the baby causes. The mother interprets the infant's normal responses as being negative toward her and reacts to her child with dislike or indifference. She does not hold the child close or touch the child to be comforting. For example, "The nurse put the baby into Lydia's arms. She promptly laid him across her knees and glanced up at the television. 'Stay still until I finish watching; you've been enough trouble already.'"

Nursing interventions related to the promotion of parent-infant attachment are numerous and varied (Table 15-3). They can enhance positive parent-infant contacts by heightening parental awareness of an infant's responses and ability to communicate. As the parent attempts to become competent and loving in that role, nurses can bolster the parent's self-confidence and ego. Nurses are in prime positions to identify actual and potential problems and collaborate with other health care professionals who will provide care for the parents after discharge. Nursing considerations for fostering maternal-infant bonding

TABLE 15-1

Infant Behaviors Affecting Parental Attachment

FACILITATING BEHAVIORS	INHIBITING BEHAVIORS
Visually alert; eye-to-eye contact; tracking or following of parent's face	Sleepy; eyes closed most of the time; gaze aversion
Appealing facial appearance; randomness of body movements reflecting helplessness	Resemblance to person parent dislikes; hyperirritability or jerky body movements when touched
Smiles	Bland facial expression; infrequent smiles
Vocalization; crying only when hungry or wet	Crying for hours on end; colicky
Grasp reflex	Exaggerated motor reflex
Anticipatory approach behaviors for feedings; sucks well; feeds easily	Feeds poorly; regurgitates; vomits often
Enjoys being cuddled and held	Resists holding and cuddling by crying, stiffening body
Easily consolable	Inconsolable; unresponsive to parenting, caretaking tasks
Activity and regularity somewhat predictable	Unpredictable feeding and sleeping schedule
Attention span sufficient to focus on parents	Inability to attend to parent's face or offered stimulation
Differential crying, smiling, and vocalizing; recognizes and prefers parents	Shows no preference for parents over others
Approaches through locomotion	Unresponsive to parent's approaches
Clings to parent; puts arms around parent's neck	Seeks attention from any adult in room
Lifts arms to parents in greeting	Ignores parents

Source: Gerson, E. (1973). *Infant behavior in the first year of life.* New York: Raven Press.

TABLE 15-2

Parental Behaviors Affecting Infant Attachment

FACILITATING BEHAVIORS	INHIBITING BEHAVIORS
Looks; gazes; takes in physical characteristics of infant; assumes en face position; eye contact	Turns away from infant; ignores infant's presence
Hovers; maintains proximity; directs attention to, points to infant	Avoids infant; does not seek proximity; refuses to hold infant when given opportunity
Identifies infant as unique individual	Identifies infant with someone parent dislikes; fails to recognize any of infant's unique features
Claims infant as family member; names infant	Fails to place infant in family context or identify infant with family member; has difficulty naming
Touches; progresses from fingertip to fingers to palms to encompassing contact	Fails to move from fingertip touch to palmar contact and holding
Smiles at infant	Maintains bland countenance or frowns at infant
Talks to, coos, or sings to infant	Wakes infant when infant is sleeping; handles roughly; hurries feeding by moving nipple continuously
Expresses pride in infant	Expresses disappointment, displeasure in infant
Relates infant's behavior to familiar events	Does not incorporate infant into life
Assigns meaning to infant's actions and sensitively interprets infant's needs	Makes no effort to interpret infant's actions or needs
Views infant's behaviors and appearance in positive light	Views infant's behavior as exploiting, deliberately uncooperative; views appearance as distasteful, ugly

Source: Mercer, R. (1983). Parent-infant attachment. In L. Sonstegard, K. Kowalski, & B. Jennings (Eds.), *Women's health* (Vol. 2), *Childbearing*. New York: Grune & Stratton.

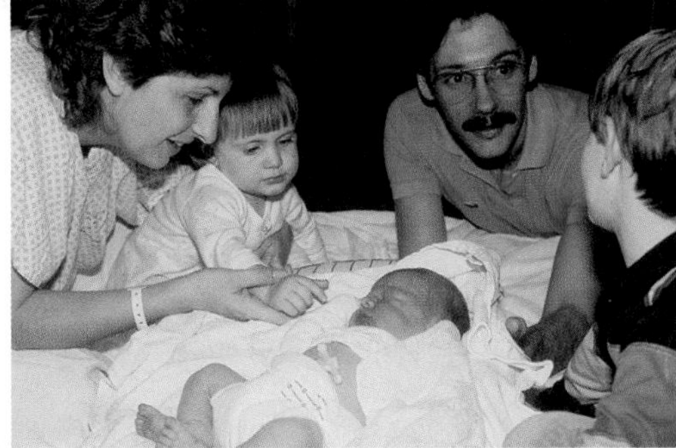

Fig. 15-3 Family members examine the new baby. They discuss how she resembles them and other family members. (Courtesy Marjorie Pyle, RNC, Lifecircle, Costa Mesa, CA.)

among special populations may vary (Cultural Considerations box).

Assessment of Attachment Behaviors

One of the most important areas of assessment is careful observation of specific behaviors thought to indicate the formation of emotional bonds between the newborn and the family, especially the mother. Unlike physical assessment of the neonate, which has concrete guidelines to follow, assessment of parent-infant attachment relies more on skillful observation and interviewing. Rooming-in of mother and infant and liberal visiting privileges for father or partner, siblings, and grandparents provide nurses with excellent opportunities to observe interactions and identify behaviors that demonstrate positive or negative attachment. Attachment behaviors can be easily observed during infant feeding sessions. Box 15-1 presents guidelines for assessment of attachment behaviors.

During pregnancy, and often even before conception occurs, parents develop an image of the "ideal" or "fantasy"

Cultural Considerations

Fostering Bonding in Women of Varying Ethnic and Cultural Groups

Childbearing practices and rituals of other cultures are not always congruent with standard practices associated with bonding in the Anglo-American culture. For example, Chinese families traditionally use extended family members to care for the newborn so that the mother can rest and recover, especially after a cesarean birth. Some Native-American, Asian, and Latina women do not initiate breastfeeding until their breast milk comes in. Haitian families do not name their babies until after the confinement month. Amount of eye contact varies among cultures as well. Yup'ik Eskimo mothers almost always position their babies so that they can make eye contact.

Nurses should become knowledgeable about the childbearing beliefs and practices of diverse cultural and ethnic groups. Because individual cultural variations exist within groups, nurses need to clarify with the patient and family members or friends what cultural norms they follow. Incorrect judgments may be made about parent-infant bonding if nurses do not practice culturally sensitive care.

Modified from Giger, J.N. (2012). *Transcultural nursing: Assessment and intervention* (6th ed.). St. Louis: Mosby.

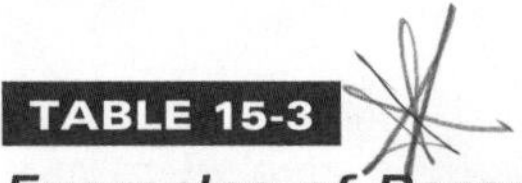

TABLE 15-3

Examples of Parent-Infant Attachment Interventions

INTERVENTION LABEL AND DEFINITION	ACTIVITIES
ATTACHMENT PROMOTION	
Facilitation of development of parent-infant relationship	Provide opportunity for parent or parents to see, hold, and examine newborn immediately after birth. Encourage parent or parents to hold infant close to body. Assist parent or parents to participate in infant care. Provide rooming-in in hospital.
ENVIRONMENTAL MANAGEMENT: ATTACHMENT PROCESS	
Manipulation of individuals' surroundings to facilitate development of parent-infant relationship	Create environment that fosters privacy. Individualize daily routine to meet parents' needs. Permit father or significant other to sleep in room with mother. Develop policies that permit presence of significant others as much as desired.
FAMILY INTEGRITY PROMOTION: CHILDBEARING FAMILY	
Facilitation of growth of individuals or families who are adding infant to family unit	Prepare parent or parents for expected role changes involved in becoming a parent. Prepare parent or parents for responsibilities of parenthood. Monitor effects of newborn on family structure. Reinforce positive parenting behaviors.
LACTATION COUNSELING	
Use of interactive helping process to assist in maintenance of successful breastfeeding	Correct misconceptions, misinformation, and inaccuracies about breastfeeding. Assess feeding techniques and assist as needed. Evaluate parents' understanding of infant's feeding cues (e.g., rooting, sucking, alertness). Determine frequency of feedings in relation to infant's needs. Demonstrate breast massage and discuss its advantages to increasing milk supply. Provide education, encouragement, and support.
PARENT EDUCATION: INFANT	
Instruction on nurturing and physical care needed during first year of life	Determine parents' knowledge, readiness, and ability to learn about infant care. Provide anticipatory guidance about developmental changes during first year of life. Teach parent or parents skills to care for newborn. Demonstrate ways in which parent or parents can stimulate infant's development. Discuss infant's capabilities for interaction. Demonstrate quieting techniques.
RISK IDENTIFICATION: CHILDBEARING FAMILY	
Identification of individual or family likely to experience difficulties in parenting and assigning priorities to strategies to prevent parenting problems	Determine developmental stage of parent or parents. Review prenatal history for factors that predispose individuals or family to complications. Ascertain understanding of English or other language used in community. Monitor behavior that may indicate problem with attachment. Plan for risk-reduction activities in collaboration with individual or family.

Modified from Bulechek, G. M., Butcher, H. K., & Dochterman, J. M. (2008). *Nursing interventions classification (NIC)* (5th ed.). St. Louis: Mosby.

BOX 15-1

Assessing Attachment Behavior

- When the infant is brought to the parents, do they reach out for the infant and call the infant by name? (Recognize that, in some cultures, parents may not name the infant in the early newborn period.)
- Do the parents speak about the infant in terms of identification—whom the infant resembles, and what appears special about their infant over other infants?
- When parents are holding the infant, what kind of body contact is seen—do parents feel at ease in changing the infant's position, are fingertips or whole hands used, and does the infant have parts of the body they avoid touching or parts of the body they investigate and scrutinize?
- When the infant is awake, what kinds of stimulation do the parents provide—do they talk to the infant, to each other, or to no one, and how do they look at the infant—direct visual contact, avoidance of eye contact, or looking at other people or objects?
- How comfortable do the parents appear in terms of caring for the infant? Do they express any concern regarding their ability or disgust for certain activities, such as changing diapers?
- What type of affection do they demonstrate to the newborn, such as smiling, stroking, kissing, or rocking?
- If the infant is fussy, what kinds of comforting techniques do the parents use, such as rocking, swaddling, talking, or stroking?

infant. At birth the fantasy infant becomes the real infant. How closely the dream child resembles the real child influences the bonding process. Assessing such expectations during pregnancy and at the time of the infant's birth allows identification of discrepancies in the parents' view of the fantasy child versus the real child.

The labor process significantly affects the immediate attachment of mothers to their newborn infants. Factors such as a long labor, feeling tired or "drugged" after birth, and problems with breastfeeding can delay the development of initial positive feelings toward the newborn.

PARENT-INFANT CONTACT

Early Contact

Early skin-to-skin contact between the mother and newborn immediately after birth and during the first hour facilitates maternal affectionate and attachment behaviors (Flacking, Lehtonen, Thomson, et al., 2012; Hung & Berg, 2011; Moore, Anderson, Bergman, et al., 2012). It also enhances breastfeeding and is associated with improved thermoregulation.

Parents who are unable to have early contact with their newborn (e.g., the infant was transferred to the intensive care nursery) can be reassured that such contact is not essential for optimal parent-infant interactions. Otherwise, adopted infants would not form affectionate ties with their parents. Nurses need to stress that the parent-infant relationship is a process that occurs over time.

Extended Contact

Rooming-in is common in family-centered care. With this practice the infant stays in the room with the mother. In some facilities the newborn never leaves the mother's presence; nursery nurses perform the initial assessment and care in the room with the parents. In other hospitals the infant is transferred to the postpartum or mother-baby unit from the transitional nursery (if the facility uses one) after showing satisfactory extrauterine adjustment. Nurses encourage the father or partner to participate in caring for the infant in as active a role as desired. They can also encourage siblings and grandparents to visit and become acquainted with the infant. Whether the method of family-centered care is rooming-in, mother-baby or couplet care, or a family birth unit, mothers and their partners are equal and integral parts of the developing family.

Extended contact with the infant should be available for all parents but especially for those at risk for parenting inadequacies, such as adolescents and low-income women. Postpartum nurses need to consider and encourage activities that optimize family-centered care.

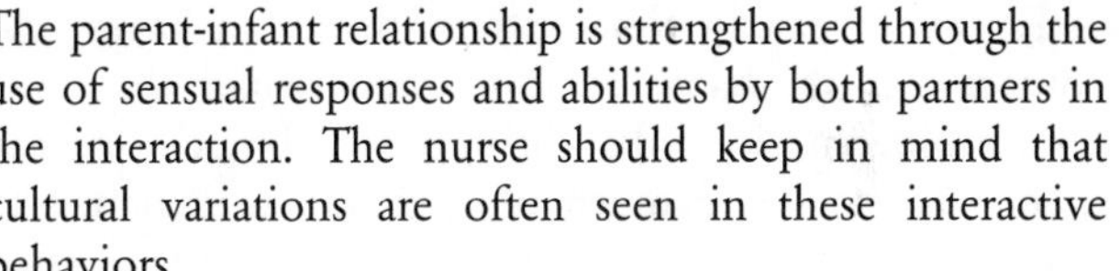

COMMUNICATION BETWEEN PARENT AND INFANT

The parent-infant relationship is strengthened through the use of sensual responses and abilities by both partners in the interaction. The nurse should keep in mind that cultural variations are often seen in these interactive behaviors.

The Senses

Touch

Touch, or the tactile sense, is used extensively by parents as a means of becoming acquainted with the newborn. Many mothers reach out for their infants as soon as they are born and the cord is cut. Mothers lift their infants to their breasts, enfold them in their arms, and cradle them. Once the infant is close, the mother begins the exploration process with her fingertips, one of the most touch-sensitive areas of the body. Within a short time she uses her palm to caress the baby's trunk and eventually enfolds the infant. Similar progression of touching is demonstrated by fathers, partners, and other caregivers. Gentle stroking motions are used to soothe and quiet the infant; patting or gently rubbing the infant's back is a comfort after feedings. Infants also pat the mother's breast as they nurse. Both seem to enjoy sharing each other's body warmth. Parents seem to have an innate desire to touch, pick up, and hold the infant (Fig. 15-4). They comment on the softness of the baby's skin and note details of the baby's appearance. As parents become increasingly sensi-

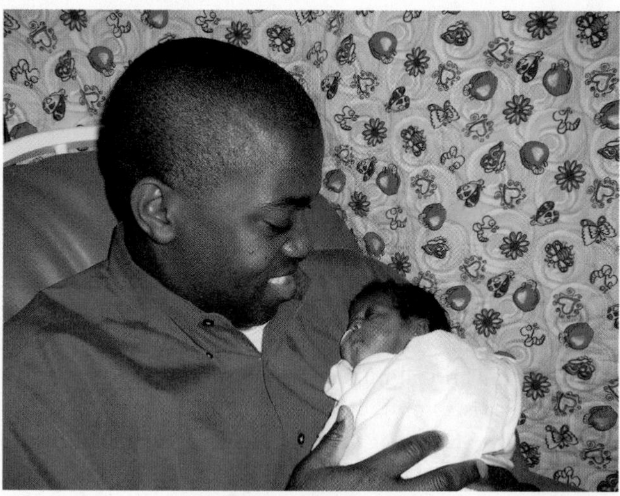

Fig. 15-4 Father interacts with his newborn son. (Cheryl Briggs, RN, Annapolis, MD.)

tive to the infant's like or dislike for different types of touch, they draw closer to the baby.

Touching behaviors by mothers vary in different cultural groups. For example, minimal touching and cuddling is a traditional Southeast Asian practice thought to protect the infant from evil spirits. Because of tradition and spiritual beliefs, women in India and Bali have practiced infant massage since ancient times (Giger, 2012).

Eye contact

Parents repeatedly demonstrate interest in having eye contact with the baby. Some mothers remark that once their babies have looked at them, they feel much closer to them. Parents spend much time getting their babies to open their eyes and look at them. In the United States, eye contact appears to reinforce the development of a trusting relationship and is an important factor in human relationships at all ages. In other cultures, eye contact is perceived differently. For example, in Mexican culture, sustained direct eye contact is considered rude, immodest, and dangerous for some. This danger may arise from the *mal de ojo* (evil eye), resulting from excessive admiration. Women and children are thought to be more susceptible to the *mal de ojo* (Giger, 2012).

As newborns become functionally able to sustain eye contact with their parents, they spend time in mutual gazing, often in the **en face** position, a position in which the parent's face and the infant's face are approximately 20 cm apart and on the same plane (see Fig. 15-2). Nurses and physicians or midwives can facilitate eye contact immediately after birth by positioning the infant on the mother's abdomen or breasts with the mother's and the infant's faces on the same plane. Dimming the lights encourages the infant's eyes to open. To promote eye contact, instillation of prophylactic antibiotic ointment in the infant's eyes can be delayed until the infant and parents have had some time together in the first hour after birth.

Voice

The shared response of parents and infants to each other's voices is remarkable. Parents wait tensely for the first cry. Once that cry has reassured them of the baby's health, they begin comforting behaviors. As the parents talk in high-pitched voices, the infant is alerted and turns toward them.

Infants respond to higher-pitched voices and can distinguish their mother's voice from others soon after birth. Infants use their cries to signal hunger, discomfort, boredom, and tiredness. With experience, parents learn to distinguish among such cries.

Odor

Another behavior shared by parents and infants is a response to each other's odor. Mothers comment on the smell of their babies when first born and have noted that each infant has a unique odor. Infants learn rapidly to distinguish the odor of their mother's breast milk.

Entrainment

Newborns move in time with the structure of adult speech, which is termed **entrainment**. They wave their arms, lift their heads, and kick their legs, seemingly "dancing in tune" to a parent's voice. Culturally determined rhythms of speech are ingrained in the infant long before he or she uses spoken language to communicate. This shared rhythm also gives the parent positive feedback and establishes a positive setting for effective communication.

Biorhythmicity

The fetus is in tune with the mother's natural rhythms—**biorhythmicity**—such as her heartbeat. After birth the mother's heartbeat or a recording of a heartbeat can soothe a crying infant. One of the newborn's tasks is to establish a personal biorhythm. Parents can help in this process by giving consistent loving care and using their infant's alert state to develop responsive behavior and thereby increase social interactions and opportunities for learning (Fig. 15-5). The more quickly parents become competent in child care activities, the more quickly they can direct their psychologic energy toward observing and responding to the communication cues the infant gives them.

Reciprocity and Synchrony

Reciprocity is a type of body movement or behavior that provides the observer with cues. The observer or receiver interprets those cues and responds to them. Reciprocity often takes several weeks to develop with a new baby. For example, when the newborn fusses and cries, the mother responds by picking up and cradling the infant; the baby becomes quiet and alert and establishes eye contact; the mother verbalizes, sings, and coos while the baby maintains eye contact. The baby then averts the eyes and yawns; the mother decreases her active response. If the parent continues to stimulate the infant, the baby may become fussy.

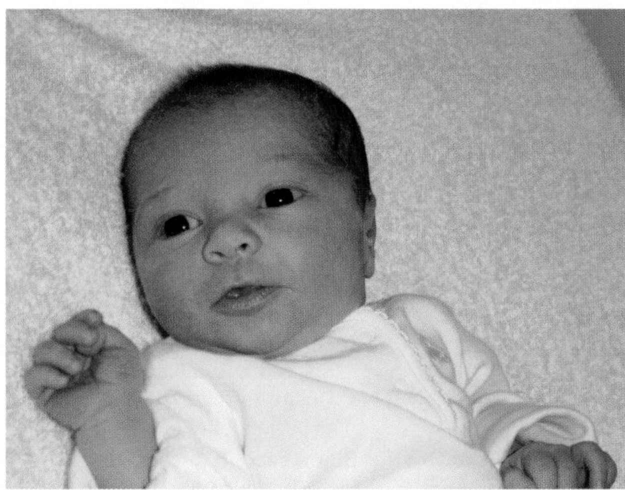

Fig. 15-5 Infant in alert state. (Courtesy Kathryn Alden, Chapel Hill, NC.)

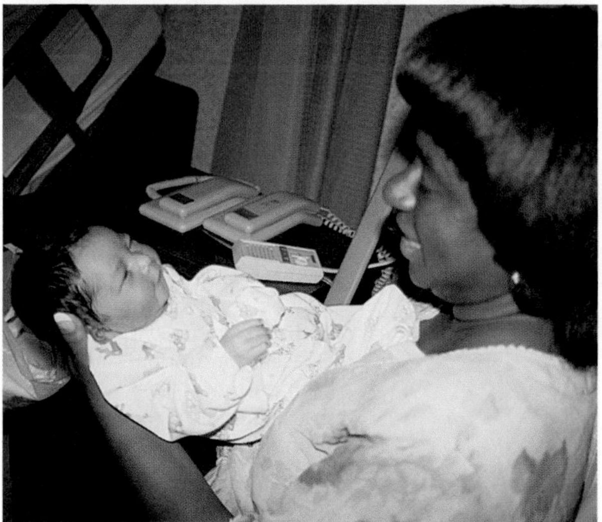

Fig. 15-6 Sharing a smile: example of synchrony. (Courtesy Marjorie Pyle, RNC, Lifecircle, Costa Mesa, CA.)

The term *synchrony* refers to the "fit" between the infant's cues and the parent's response. When parent and infant experience a synchronous interaction, it is mutually rewarding (Fig. 15-6). Parents need time to interpret the infant's cues correctly. For example, after a certain time the infant develops a specific cry in response to different situations such as boredom, loneliness, hunger, and discomfort. The parent may need assistance in interpreting these cries, along with trial and error interventions, before synchrony develops.

PARENTAL ROLE AFTER CHILDBIRTH

Adaptation involves a stabilizing of tasks, a coming to terms with commitments. Parents demonstrate growing competence in child care activities and become increasingly more attuned to their infant's behavior. Typically, the period from the decision to conceive through the first months of having a child is termed the **transition to parenthood.**

Transition to Parenthood

Historically, the transition to parenthood was viewed as a crisis. The current perspective is that parenthood is a developmental transition rather than a major life crisis. The transition to parenthood is a time of disorder and disequilibrium, as well as satisfaction, for mothers and their partners. Usual methods of coping often seem ineffective during this time. Some parents are so distressed that they are unable to be supportive of each other. Because men typically identify their spouses as their primary or only source of support, the transition can be comparatively harder for the fathers. They often feel deprived when the mothers, who are also experiencing stress, cannot provide their usual level of support. Many parents are unprepared for the strong emotions such as helplessness, inadequacy, and anger that arise when dealing with a crying infant. On the other hand, parenthood allows adults to develop and display a selfless, warm, and caring side of themselves that may not be expressed in other adult roles.

For the majority of mothers and their partners the transition to parenthood is an opportunity rather than a time of danger. Parents try new coping strategies as they work to master their new roles and reach new developmental levels. As they work through the transition, they often find personal strength and resourcefulness.

Parental Tasks and Responsibilities

Parents need to reconcile the actual child with the fantasy and dream child. This process means coming to terms with the infant's physical appearance, sex, innate temperament, and physical status. If the real child differs greatly from the fantasy child, some parents delay acceptance of the child. In some instances, they never accept the child.

Many parents know the sex of the infant before birth because of the use of ultrasound assessments. For those who do not have this information, disappointment over the baby's sex can take time to resolve. The parents may provide adequate physical care but have difficulty in being sincerely involved with the infant until this internal conflict has been resolved. As one mother remarked, "I really wanted a boy. I know it is silly and irrational, but when they said, 'She's a lovely little girl,' I was so disappointed and angry–yes, angry–I could hardly look at her. Oh, I looked after her okay, her feedings and baths and things, but I couldn't feel excited. To tell the truth, I felt like a monster not liking my child. Then one day, she was lying there and she turned her head and looked right at me. I felt a flooding of love for her come over me, and we looked at each other a long time. It's okay now. I wouldn't change her for all the boys in the world."

The normal appearance of the neonate–size, color, molding of the head, or bowed appearance of the legs–is startling for some parents. Nurses can encourage parents to examine their babies and to ask questions about newborn characteristics.

Parents need to become adept in the care of the infant, including caregiving activities, noting the communication cues given by the infant to indicate needs, and responding appropriately to the infant's needs. Self-esteem grows with competence. Breastfeeding makes mothers believe that they are contributing in a unique way to the welfare of the infant. The parent may interpret the infant's response to the parental care and attention as a comment on the quality of that care. Infant behaviors that parents interpret as positive responses to their care include being consoled easily, enjoying being cuddled, and making eye contact. Spitting up frequently after feedings, crying, and being unpredictable are often perceived as negative responses to parental care. Continuation of these infant responses that parents view as negative can result in alienation of parent and infant, which will not benefit the infant.

Some people view assistance, including advice by husbands, partners, wives, mothers, mothers-in-law, and health care professionals, as supportive. Others view advice as criticism or an indication of how inept these people judge the new parents to be. Criticism, real or imagined, of the new parents' ability to provide adequate physical care, nutrition, or social stimulation for the infant can be devastating. By providing encouragement and praise for parenting efforts, nurses can bolster the new parents' confidence.

Parents must establish a place for the newborn within the family group. Whether the infant is the firstborn or the last born, all family members must adjust their roles to accommodate the newcomer.

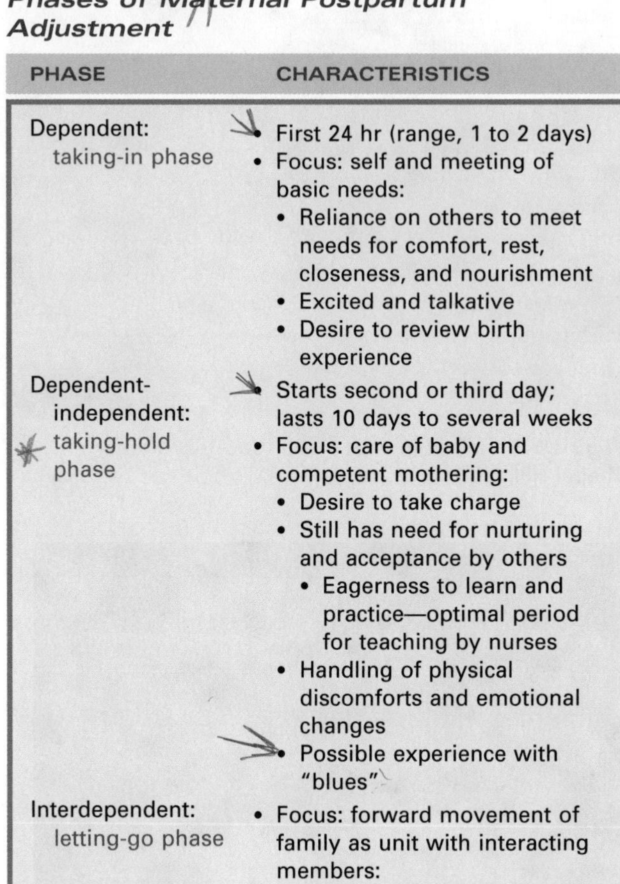

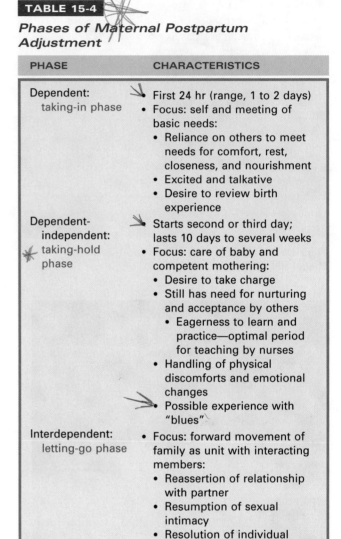

TABLE 15-4
Phases of Maternal Postpartum Adjustment

PHASE	CHARACTERISTICS

Dependent: taking-in phase	• First 24 hr (range, 1 to 2 days)
	• Focus: self and meeting of basic needs:
	  • Reliance on others to meet needs for comfort, rest, closeness, and nourishment
	  • Excited and talkative
	  • Desire to review birth experience

Dependent-independent: taking-hold phase	• Starts second or third day; lasts 10 days to several weeks
	• Focus: care of baby and competent mothering:
	  • Desire to take charge
	  • Still has need for nurturing and acceptance by others
	    • Eagerness to learn and practice—optimal period for teaching by nurses
	  • Handling of physical discomforts and emotional changes
	  • Possible experience with "blues"

Interdependent: letting-go phase	• Focus: forward movement of family as unit with interacting members:
	  • Reassertion of relationship with partner
	  • Resumption of sexual intimacy
	  • Resolution of individual roles

Source: Rubin, R. (1961). Basic maternal behavior. *Nursing Outlook, 9,* 683-686.

Becoming a Mother

Rubin (1961) identified three phases of maternal role attainment in which the mother adjusts to her parental role. These phases are characterized by dependent behavior, dependent-independent behavior, and interdependent behavior. The phases extend over the first several weeks (Table 15-4). Rubin's research was conducted when the length of stay in the hospital was for a longer period (3 to 5 or more days). With today's early discharge, women seem to move through the phases faster than before.

Mercer (2004) suggested that the concept of *maternal role attainment,* introduced by Rubin in 1961, be replaced with **becoming a mother** to signify the transformation and growth of the mother identity. Becoming a mother implies more than attaining a role. It includes learning new skills and increasing her confidence in herself as she meets new challenges in caring for her child or children.

Mercer (2004) identified four stages in the process of becoming a mother. These stages include "(a) commitment, attachment to the unborn baby, and preparation for delivery and motherhood during pregnancy; (b) acquaintance/attachment to the infant, learning to care for the infant, and physical restoration during the first 2 to 6 weeks following birth; (c) moving toward a new normal; and (d) achievement of a maternal identity through redefining self to incorporate motherhood (around 4 months)" (Mercer & Walker, 2006, pp. 568-569). The time of achievement of the stages is variable and the stages may overlap. Achievement is influenced by mother and infant variables and the social environment.

Maternal sensitivity or maternal responsiveness is an important determinant of the maternal-infant relationship. It can be defined as the quality of a mother's sensitive behaviors that are based on her awareness, perception, and responsiveness to infant cues and behaviors. Maternal sensitivity significantly influences the infant's physical, psychologic, and cognitive development. Maternal qualities inherent to this sensitivity include awareness and responsiveness to infant cues, affect, timing, flexibility, acceptance, and conflict negotiation. Maternal sensitivity is dynamic and develops over time in a reciprocal give-and-take with the infant (Shin, Park, Ryu, & Seomun, 2008).

The transition to motherhood requires adjustment for the mother and her family. Disruption is inherent in that adjustment. Circumstances such as problems in postpartum recovery or giving birth to a high risk infant add to the disruption (Lutz & May, 2007).

Nelson (2003) identified two social processes in maternal transition. The primary process is engagement, that is, making a commitment to being a mother, actively caring for her child, and experiencing his or her presence. The secondary process is experiencing herself as a mother, which leads to growth and transformation. During this process, she must learn how to mother and adapt to a changed relationship with her partner, family, and friends. The woman must examine herself in relation to the past and her present and come to view herself as a mother. She must make important decisions such as whether to return to work and, if so, when.

Not all mothers experience the transition to motherhood in the same way. For some women, becoming a mother entails multiple losses. For example, for some single women, a loss of the family of origin may occur when they do not accept her decision to have the child. There may be loss of a relationship with the father of the baby, with friends, and with their own sense of self. Women describe a loss of dreams that includes loss of job, financial security, and a future profession. Accompanying these losses is a loss of support.

Nurses must individualize their assessments and interventions. More reality-based perinatal education programs are necessary to prepare mothers better and decrease their anxiety. Live classes allow time for questions to be answered and for mothers to lend support to one another. Mothers need to know that during the first months of parenthood it is common to feel overwhelmed and insecure and to experience physical and mental fatigue. They need to be assured that this situation is temporary and that 3 to 6 months may be needed to become comfortable in caregiving and in being a mother. Maternal support by professionals should not end with hospital discharge but extend over the next 4 to 6 months; long-term interventions tend to be more successful than one-time encounters. Nurses can advocate for the extension of such support services well into the postpartum period (Mercer & Walker, 2006).

During pregnancy and after birth nurses can discuss the usual postpartum concerns that mothers experience. They can provide anticipatory guidance on coping strategies, such as resting when the infant sleeps and planning with an extended family member or friend to do the housework for the first week or two after the baby is born. Once a mother is home, periodic telephone calls from the nurse who cared for her in the birth setting can provide the mother with an opportunity to vent her concerns and get support and advice from "her nurse." Nurses should plan additional supportive counseling for first-time mothers inexperienced in child care, women whose careers had provided outside stimulation, women who lack friends or family members with whom to share delights and concerns, and adolescent mothers. When possible, postpartum home visits are included in the plan of care.

Postpartum "blues"

Critical Thinking Exercise: Postpartum Home Care

The "pink" period surrounding the first day or two after birth, characterized by heightened joy and feelings of well-being, is often followed by a "blue" period. Up to 80% of women of all ethnic and racial groups experience the **postpartum blues** or "baby blues." During the blues, women are emotionally labile and often cry easily for no apparent reason. This lability seems to peak around the fifth day and subside by the tenth day. Other symptoms of postpartum blues include depression, a let-down feeling, restlessness, fatigue, insomnia, headache, anxiety, sadness, and anger. Biochemical, psychologic, social, and cultural factors have been explored as possible causes of postpartum blues; however, the cause remains unknown.

Whatever the cause, the early postpartum period appears to be one of emotional and physical vulnerability for new mothers, who are often psychologically overwhelmed by the reality of parental responsibilities. Mothers feel deprived of the supportive care they received from family members and friends during pregnancy. Some mothers regret the loss of the mother–unborn child relationship and mourn its passing. Still others experience a let-down feeling when labor and birth are complete. The majority of women experience fatigue after childbirth, which is compounded by the around-the-clock demands of the new baby and can accentuate the feelings of depression. Postpartum fatigue increases the risk of postpartum depressive symptoms and can have a negative effect on maternal role attainment (Corwin & Arbour, 2007; Kurth, Kennedy, Spichiger, et al., 2011). To help mothers cope with postpartum blues, nurses can suggest various strategies (Patient Instructions for Self-Management box).

A few questions on a discharge checklist can help mothers to assess their level of "blues" and to decide when to seek advice from their nurse, nurse-midwife, or physician. Home visits and telephone follow-up calls by a nurse are important to assess the mother's pattern of "blue" feelings and behavior over time.

Although the postpartum blues are usually mild and short lived, approximately 10% to 15% of women experience a more severe syndrome termed *postpartum depression* (PPD). Symptoms of PPD can range from mild to severe, with women having "good days" and "bad days." Fathers can also experience PPD. Screening for PPD should be performed with both mothers and fathers. PPD can go

NURSING CARE PLAN *Home Care Follow-Up: Transition to Parenthood*

NURSING DIAGNOSIS Deficient knowledge of infant care related to lack of experience or lack of support

Expected Outcomes *The parents provide safe and adequate care and the infant appears healthy.*

Nursing Interventions/*Rationales*

- Observe infant care routines (bathing, diapering, feeding, play) *to evaluate parental ease with care and adequacy of techniques.*
- Observe the infant's appearance (height-weight ratio, head circumference, fontanels, skin tone and turgor), and assess the infant's vital signs, overall tone, reflexes, and age-appropriate developmental skills *to evaluate for signs indicative of inadequate care.*
- Explore available support systems for infant care *to determine the adequacy of existing system.*
- Demonstrate troublesome care routines, and have involved family members return the demonstration *to facilitate improvements in care.*
- Provide ongoing follow-up and referrals as needed *to ensure that identified potential and actual care deficits are addressed and resolved.*

NURSING DIAGNOSIS Disturbed sleep pattern related to infant demands and environmental interruptions

Expected Outcomes *Woman sleeps for uninterrupted periods and states that she feels rested on waking.*

Nursing Interventions/*Rationales*

- Discuss the woman's routine, and specify factors that interfere with sleep *to determine the scope of the problem and direct interventions.*
- Explore ways the woman and significant others can make the environment more conducive to sleep (e.g., privacy, darkness, quiet, back rubs, soothing music, warm milk), and teach the use of guided imagery and relaxation techniques *to promote optimal conditions for sleep.*
- Eliminate factors or routines (e.g., caffeine, foods that induce heartburn, strenuous mental or physical activity) *that may interfere with sleep.*
- Advise the family to limit visitors and activities *to prevent further stress and fatigue.*
- Have the family plan specific times to care for the newborn *to allow mother time to sleep;* have the mother learn to use infant nap time as a time for her to nap as well *to replenish energy and decrease fatigue.*
- Assist the family to identify persons such as family members or friends who can provide help with household tasks, infant care, and care of other children *to allow the mother more time to rest.*

NURSING DIAGNOSIS Risk for impaired home maintenance related to addition of new family member, inadequate resources, or inadequate support systems

Expected Outcome *Home exhibits signs of safe and functional environment.*

Nursing Interventions/*Rationales*

- Observe the home environment (e.g., available living space and sleeping arrangements; adequacy of facilities for food preparation and storage, hygiene, and toileting; overall state of repair; cleanliness; presence of safety hazards) *to determine the adequacy and effective use of resources.*
- Observe arrangements for the newborn, such as sleeping space, care equipment, and supplies (bathing, changing, feeding, transportation) *to determine the adequacy of resources.*
- Explore who is responsible for cooking, cleaning, child care, and newborn care, and determine whether the mother seems adequately rested *to determine the adequacy of support systems.*
- Identify and arrange referrals to needed social agencies (e.g., Temporary Assistance for Needy Families [TANF]; Special Supplemental Nutrition Program for Women, Infants, and Children [WIC] program; food pantries) *to address resource deficits (finances, supplies, equipment).*

NURSING DIAGNOSIS Risk for interrupted family processes related to inclusion of the new family member

Expected Outcome *Infant is successfully incorporated into the family structure.*

Nursing Interventions/*Rationales*

- Explore with the family the ways that the birth and neonate have changed the family structure and function *to evaluate functional and role adjustment.*
- Observe the family's interaction with the newborn, and note degree of bonding, evidence of sibling rivalry, and involvement in newborn care *to evaluate the acceptance of the newest family member.*
- Clarify identified misinformation and misperceptions *to promote clear communication.*
- Assist the family in exploring options for solutions to identified problems *to promote effective problem resolution.*
- Support the family's efforts as they move toward adjusting and incorporating the new member *to reinforce new functions and roles.*
- If needed, make referrals to appropriate social services or community agencies *to ensure ongoing support and care.*

undetected because new parents generally do not voluntarily admit to this kind of emotional distress out of embarrassment, guilt, or fear. Nurses need to include teaching about how to differentiate symptoms of the "blues" and PPD and urge parents to report depressive symptoms promptly if they occur (see Chapter 23).

Becoming a Father

Research on paternal adjustment to parenthood indicates that men go through predictable phases during their transition to parenthood as they seek to become involved fathers (Goodman, 2005). In the first phase, men enter parenthood with intentions of being an emotionally

PATIENT INSTRUCTIONS FOR SELF-MANAGEMENT

Coping with Postpartum Blues

- Remember that the "blues" are normal and that both the mother and the father or partner may experience them.
- Get plenty of rest; nap when the baby does if possible. Go to bed early, and let friends and family know when to visit and how they can help. (Remember, you are not "Supermom.")
- Use relaxation techniques learned in childbirth classes (or ask the nurse to teach you and your partner some techniques).
- Do something for yourself. Take advantage of the time your partner or family members care for the baby—soak in the tub (a 20-minute soak can be the equivalent of a 2-hour nap), or go for a walk.
- Plan a day out of the house—go to the mall with the baby, being sure to take a stroller or carriage, or go out to eat with friends without the baby. Many communities have churches or other agencies that provide child care programs such as Mothers' Morning Out.
- Talk to your partner about the way you feel—for example, about feeling tied down, how the birth met your expectations, and things that will help you (do not be afraid to ask for specifics).
- If you are breastfeeding, give yourself and your baby time to learn.
- Seek out and use community resources such as La Leche League or community mental health centers. One nationally recognized resource is:

  Postpartum Support International
  927 North Kellogg Ave.
  Santa Barbara, CA 93111
  (805) 967-7636

involved father with deep connections to the infant. Many men desire to parent differently than their own fathers. The second phase is a time of confronting reality, when men realize that their expectations were inconsistent with the realities of life with a newborn during the first few weeks. During this period, fathers experience intense emotions. Many fathers acknowledge that their expectations were of limited value once they were immersed in the reality of parenthood. Feelings that often accompany this reality are sadness, ambivalence, jealousy, frustration at not being able to participate in breastfeeding, and an overwhelming desire to be more involved. Some men are surprised that establishing a relationship with the infant is more gradual than expected. Fathers often feel alone, having no one with whom to discuss their feelings during this time. Mothers are preoccupied with infant care and their own transition to parenting. On the other hand, some fathers are pleasantly surprised at the ease and fun of parenting and take an active role. Many fathers of breastfeeding infants find ways to be involved in infant care other than feeding. The third phase is working to create the role of involved father. The realities of the first few weeks at home with a newborn cause fathers to change their expectations, set new priorities, and redefine their role. They develop strategies for balancing work, their own needs, and the needs of their partner and infant. Men become increasingly more comfortable with infant care. During this time, they may struggle for recognition and positive feedback from their partner, the infant, and others. They may feel excluded from support and attention by health care providers. The final phase of becoming an involved father is one of reaping rewards, the most significant one being reciprocity from the infant, such as a smile. This phase typically occurs around 6 weeks to 2 months. Increased sociability of the infant enhances the father-infant relationship (Goodman, 2005) (Table 15-5).

TABLE 15-5

Early Development of the Involved Father Role

PHASES	CHARACTERISTICS
Expectations and intentions	Desire for emotional involvement and deep connection with infant
Confronting reality	Dealing with unrealistic expectations, frustration, disappointment, feelings of guilt, helplessness, and inadequacy
Creating the role of involved father	Altering expectations, establishing new priorities, redefining role, negotiating changes with partner, learning to care for infant, increasing interaction with infant, struggling for recognition
Reaping rewards	Infant smile, sense of meaning, completeness and immortality

Source: Goodman, J. (2005). Becoming an involved father of an infant. *Journal of Obstetric, Gynecologic, and Neonatal Nursing, 34*(2), 190-200.

First-time fathers perceive the first 4 to 10 weeks of parenthood in much the same way that mothers do. It is a period characterized by uncertainty, increased responsibility, disruption of sleep, and inability to control time needed to care for the infant and reestablish the marital dyad. Fathers express concerns about decreased attention from their partners relative to their personal relationship, the mother's lack of recognition of the father's desire to participate in decision making for the infant, and limited time available to establish a relationship with the infant. These concerns can precipitate feelings of jealousy of the infant. The father should discuss his individual concerns and needs with the mother and become more involved with the infant. This effort can help alleviate feelings of jealousy.

In North American culture, neonates have a powerful impact on their fathers who become intensely involved with their babies. The term used for the father's absorption, preoccupation, and interest in the infant is **engrossment**. Characteristics of engrossment include some of the sensual responses relating to touch and eye-to-eye contact that were discussed earlier and the father's keen awareness of features both unique and similar to himself that validate his claim to the infant. An outstanding response is one of strong attraction to the newborn. Fathers spend considerable time "communicating" with the infant and taking delight in the infant's response to them (Fig. 15-7). Fathers experience increased self-esteem and a sense of being proud, bigger, more mature, and older after seeing their baby for the first time.

Fathers spend less time than mothers with infants, and their interactions with infants tend to be characterized by stimulating social play rather than caretaking. The variations in infant stimulation from both parents provide a wider social experience for the infant.

Fathers lack interpersonal and professional support compared with mothers and may feel excluded from antenatal appointments and antenatal classes. They need information and encouragement during pregnancy and in the postnatal period related to infant care, parenting, and relationship changes. During the postpartum hospital stay, nurses can arrange to teach infant care when the father is present and provide anticipatory guidance for fathers about the transition to parenthood. Separate prenatal and parenting classes and parenting support groups for fathers can provide them with an opportunity to discuss their concerns and have some of their needs met. Postpartum telephone calls and home visits by the nurse should include time for assessment of the father's adjustment and needs (Deave, Johnson, & Ingram, 2008; Fletcher, Vimpani, Russell, & Sibbritt, 2008; Halle et al., 2008; St. John, Cameron, & McVeigh, 2005).

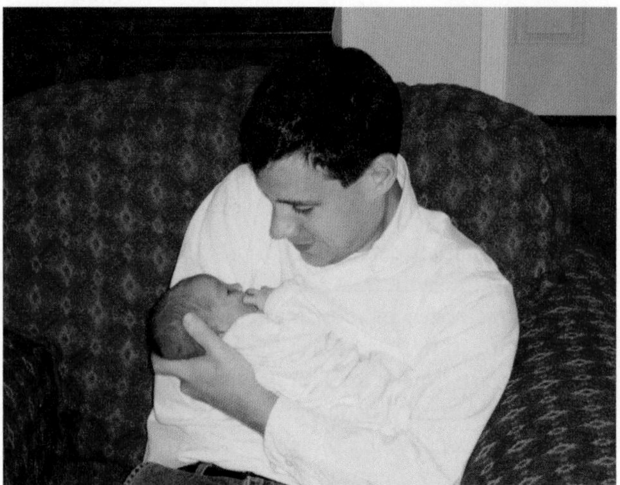

Fig. 15-7 Engrossment. Father is absorbed in looking at his newborn. (Courtesy Kathryn Alden, Chapel Hill, NC.)

Adjustment for the Couple

The transition to parenthood brings about changes in the relationship between the mother and her partner. A strong, healthy marriage or couple relationship is the best foundation for parenthood, although even the best relationships are often shaken with the addition of a new baby. During the first few weeks after birth, parents experience a plethora of emotions. Even though they may feel an overwhelming love and a sense of amazement toward their newborn, they also feel a great responsibility. Even if the mother and her partner have been to prenatal classes, read books, or sought advice from family or friends, they are usually surprised by the realities of life with a new baby and the changes in their relationship (Deave et al., 2008). Because men and women experience pregnancy and birth differently, the expectation is that they will also vary in their adjustment to parenthood.

Common issues that couples face as they become parents include changes in their relationship with one another, division of household and infant care responsibilities, financial concerns, balancing work and parental responsibilities, and social activities. To assist new parents in their transition, nurses can encourage them during pregnancy and in the postpartum period to share personal expectations with each other and to assess their relationship periodically. Couples need to schedule time into their busy lives for one-on-one conversation and try to have regular "dates" or time apart from the infant. The mother and her partner need to express appreciation for one another and for their baby. Support from family, friends, and community health professionals should be identified early and used as needed during pregnancy and in the postpartum period and beyond. The couple who is willing to experiment with new approaches to their lifestyle and habits may find the transition to parenthood less difficult (Brotherson, 2007).

Resuming sexual intimacy

Nurses need to remind new parents to resume intimacy and their sexual relationship. The couple may begin to engage in sexual intercourse during the second to fourth week after the baby is born. Some couples begin earlier, as soon as it can be accomplished without discomfort, depending on factors such as timing, amount of vaginal dryness, and breastfeeding status. Sexual intimacy enhances the adult aspect of the family, and the adult pair shares a closeness denied to other family members. Changes in a woman's sexuality after childbirth are related to hormonal shifts, increased breast size, uneasiness with a body that has yet to return to a prepregnant size, chronic fatigue related to sleep deprivation, and physical exhaustion. Many new fathers speak of feeling alienated when they observe the intimate mother-infant relationship, and some are frank in expressing feelings of jealousy toward the infant. The resumption of sexual intimacy seems to bring the parents' relationship back into focus. Before and after birth, nurses should review with new parents their plans for other pregnancies and their preferences for contraception.

Postpartum adjustment in the lesbian couple

Little is known about postpartum maternal adjustment in the lesbian couple. Relationship satisfaction in first-time lesbian parent couples appears related to egalitarianism, commitment, sexual compatibility, and communication skills, as well as to the birth mother's decision for insemination by an anonymous sperm donor. Similar to heterosexual parent couples, most lesbian parent couples voice concern about less time and energy for their relationship after the arrival of the baby. Both partners consider themselves to be equal parents of the baby who share actively in childrearing. A primary concern of co-mothers is the legal vulnerability of lesbian families confounded by their social invisibility.

Lesbian couples face strong social sanctions regarding pregnancy and parenting. Their families may not have resolved the initial dismay and guilt over learning of their daughters' homosexuality, or they may disagree with the lesbian couple's decision to conceive and be parents. Lesbian parents deal with public ignorance, social and legal invisibility, and the lack of biologic connection to the child by using various techniques. These techniques include carefully planning and accomplishing their transition to parenthood, displaying public acts of equal mothering, sharing parenting at home, establishing a distinct parenting role within the family, and supporting each partner's sense of identity as a mother. In situations in which family support is limited or absent the nurse can help lesbian couples locate supportive social groups, lesbian or heterosexual.

DIVERSITY IN TRANSITIONS TO PARENTHOOD

Various factors, including age, social networks, socioeconomic conditions, and personal aspirations for the future, influence how parents respond to the birth of a child. Cultural beliefs and practices also affect parenting behaviors. Factors that are recognized to increase the risk of parenting problems include poverty, low education level, single parenting, adolescent pregnancy and advanced maternal age.

Age

Maternal age has a definite effect on the transition to parenting. The mother, fetus, and newborn are at highest risk when the mother is an adolescent or is older than 35 years.

Adolescent mother

Although becoming a parent is biologically possible for the adolescent female, her egocentricity and concrete thinking often interfere with the ability to parent effectively. Higher mortality rates among infants of adolescent mothers are attributed to inexperience, lack of knowledge, and immaturity of the mothers, causing them to be unable to recognize a problem and obtain the necessary resources to rectify the situation. Nevertheless, in most instances, with adequate support and developmentally appropriate teaching, adolescents can learn effective parenting skills.

The transition to parenthood may be difficult for adolescent parents. Because many adolescents have their own unmet developmental needs, coping with the developmental tasks of parenthood is often difficult. Some young parents experience difficulty accepting a changing self-image and adjusting to new roles related to the responsibilities of infant care. Other adolescent parents, however, may have higher self-concepts than their nonparenting peers.

Critical Thinking/Clinical Decision Making

Transition to Parenthood for the Adolescent Couple

As a mother-baby nurse, you are assigned the care of Tamika, a 16 year old, who is being discharged from the hospital 72 hours after giving birth by cesarean to a 5-pound baby girl. Tamika has been trying to breastfeed, but the baby has lost 8% of her birth weight, and the pediatrician ordered formula supplementation after breastfeeding. Her breasts are engorged, and painful. Tamika says she slept very little last night because she was trying to feed the baby. She is tearful and says it hurts too much to breastfeed. She asks you to take the baby back to the nursery and give her a bottle. Her mother is staying with her. The baby's father, Thomas, 16 years of age, is in the room with Tamika. He has come to take Tamika and the baby home. Thomas has been to visit a few times but is trying to go to school and work his evening job at the local grocery store.

1. Evidence—Is evidence sufficient to draw conclusions about the education and care these new parents need?
2. Assumptions—What assumptions can be made about the following factors?
   a. The relationship of maternal age and postpartum adjustment
   b. The need for social support in the postnatal period
   c. The need for perinatal education
   d. Long-term prognosis for positive outcomes
3. What implications and priorities for nursing care can be drawn at this time?
4. Does the evidence objectively support your conclusion?
5. Do alternative perspectives to your conclusion exist?

As adolescent parents move through the transition to parenthood, they may feel "different" from their peers, excluded from "fun" activities, and prematurely forced to enter an adult social role. The conflict between their own desires and the infant's demands, in addition to the low tolerance for frustration that is typical of adolescence, further contribute to the normal psychosocial stress of childbirth and parenting. Maintaining a relationship with the baby's father is beneficial for the teen mother and her infant, although adolescent pregnancy often heralds the departure of the young father from the relationship (Herrman, 2008).

Adolescent mothers provide warm and attentive physical care; however, they use less verbal interaction than older parents, and adolescents tend to be less responsive and to interact less positively with their infants than older mothers. Interventions emphasizing verbal and nonverbal communication skills between mother and infant are important. Such intervention strategies must be concrete and specific because of the cognitive level of adolescents. Although some observers suggest that some adolescents may use more aggressive behaviors, a higher-than-normal incidence of child abuse has not been documented. In comparison to older mothers, teenage mothers have a limited knowledge of child development. They tend to expect too much of their infants too soon and often characterize their infants as being fussy. This limited knowledge may cause teenagers to respond to their infants inappropriately.

Many young mothers pattern their maternal role on what they themselves experienced. Therefore nurses need to determine the type of support that people close to the young mother are able and prepared to give, as well as the kinds of community assistance available to supplement this support. Many teen mothers can identify a source of social support, with the predominant source being their own mothers. Community-based programs for pregnant adolescents and adolescent parents improve access to health care, education, and other support services.

The need for continued assessment of the new mother's parenting abilities during this postbirth period is essential. Continued support is facilitated by involving the grandparents and other family members, as well as through home visits and group sessions for discussion of infant care and parenting problems. Serious problems can be prevented through outreach programs concerned with self-management, parent-child interactions, infant development, child injuries, and failure to thrive. As the adolescent performs her mothering role within the framework of her family, she may need to address dependency versus independency issues. The adolescent's family members also may need help adapting to their new roles. Some mothers and fathers of adolescents feel they are too young and unprepared to be grandparents.

Adolescent father

The adolescent father and mother face immediate developmental crises, which include completing the developmental tasks of adolescence, making a transition to parenthood, and sometimes adapting to marriage. These transitions are often stressful. The nurse may initiate interaction with the adolescent father if he is present during prenatal visits or if he is with his partner during labor and birth. During the hospital stay the nurse can include the adolescent father in teaching sessions about infant care and parenting. The nurse can ask him to be present during postpartum home visits and to accompany the mother and the baby to well-baby checkups at the clinic or pediatrician's office. With the adolescent mother's agreement the nurse may contact the father directly. Adolescent fathers need support to discuss their emotional responses to the pregnancy, birth, and fatherhood. The nurse needs to be aware of the father's feelings of guilt, powerlessness, or bravado because these feelings may have negative consequences for both the parents and the child. Counseling of adolescent fathers needs to be reality oriented and should include topics such as finances, child care, parenting skills, and the father's role in the parenting experience. Teenage fathers also need to know about reproductive physiology and birth control options, as well as sex practices that lower the risk of pregnancy and sexually transmitted infections.

The adolescent father may continue to be involved in an ongoing relationship with the young mother and his baby. In many instances, he also plays an important role in the decisions about child care and raising the child. He may need help to develop realistic perceptions of his role as "father to a child" and is encouraged to use coping mechanisms that are not harmful to his own, his partner's, or his child's well-being. The nurse enlists support systems, parents, and professional agencies on his behalf.

Maternal age older than 35 years

Women older than 35 years have always continued their childbearing either by choice or because of a lack of or a failure of contraception during the perimenopausal years. Added to this group are women who have postponed pregnancy because of careers or other reasons, as well as women of infertile couples who finally become pregnant with the aid of technologic advances.

Support from partners aids in the adjustment of older mothers to changes involved in becoming a parent and seeing themselves as competent. Support from other family members and friends is also important for positive self-evaluation of parenting, a sense of well-being and satisfaction, and help in dealing with stress. Women of advanced maternal age may experience social isolation. Older mothers may have less family and social support than younger mothers. They are less likely to live near family, and their own parents, if still living, may be unable to provide assistance or support because of age or health issues. Mothers of advanced maternal age are often caught in the "sandwich generation," taking on responsibility for care of aging parents. Social support may be lacking because their peers are probably busy with their careers and have limited time to help. Their friends are likely to have older children and have less in common with the new mother (Suplee, Dawley, & Bloch, 2007).

Changes in the sexual aspect of a relationship can create stress for new midlife parents. Mothers report that finding time and energy for a romantic rendezvous is difficult. They attribute much of this difficulty to the reality of caring for an infant, but the decreasing libido that normally accompanies getting older also contributes.

Work and career issues are sources of conflict for older mothers. Conflicts emerge over being disinterested in work, worrying about giving enough attention to work with the distractions of a new baby, and anticipating what returning to work will entail. Child care is a major factor causing stress about work.

Another major issue for older mothers with careers is the perception of loss of control. Mothers older than 35 years, when compared with younger mothers, are at a different stage in their careers, having attained high levels of education, career, and income. The loss of control experienced when going from the consistency of a work role to the inconsistency of the parent role comes as a surprise to many older women. Helping the older mother have realistic expectations of herself and of parenthood is essential.

New mothers who are also perimenopausal may have difficulty distinguishing fatigue, loss of sleep, decreased libido, or other physiologic symptoms as the causes of the change in their sex lives. Although many women view menopause as a natural stage of life, for midlife mothers, this cessation of menstruation coincides with the state of parenthood. The changes of midlife and menopause can add more emotional and physical stress to older mothers' lives because of the time- and energy-consuming aspects of raising a young child.

Paternal age older than 35 years

Although many older fathers describe their experience of midlife parenting as wonderful, they also recognize drawbacks. Positive aspects of fatherhood in older years include increased love and commitment between the two parents, a reinforcement of why one married in the first place, a feeling of being complete, experiencing of "the child" again in oneself, more financial stability than in younger years, and more freedom to focus on parenting rather than on career. A common drawback of midlife parenting is the change that it brings about in the relationships with their partners.

Social Support

Social support is strongly related to positive adaptation by new parents, including adolescent parents, during the transition to parenthood. Social support is multidimensional and includes the number of members in a person's social network, types of support, perceived general support, actual support received, and satisfaction with support available and received. The type and satisfaction of support seems to be more important than the total number of support network members.

Across cultural groups, families and friends of new parents form an important dimension of the parent's social network. Through seeking help within the social network, new mothers learn culturally valued practices and develop role competency.

Social networks provide a support system on which parents can rely for assistance, but they also can be a source of conflict. Sometimes a large network can cause problems because it results in conflicting advice that comes from numerous people. Grandparents or in-laws are most appreciated when they assist with household responsibilities and do not intrude into the parents' privacy or judge them critically.

Because of the extent of restructuring and reorganization that occurs in a family with the birth of another child, the mothers' moods and fatigue in the postpartum period can be helped more by situation-specific support from family and friends than by general support. General support addresses feeling loved, respected, and valued. Situation-specific support relates to practical concerns such as physical needs and child care. For example, the practical support of a grandparent bathing the infant can help lessen a second-time mother's feelings of loss by providing her time to be with her firstborn child.

Culture

Cultural beliefs and practices are important determinants of parenting behaviors. Culture influences the interactions with the baby, as well as the parents' or the family's caregiving style. For example, the provision for a period of rest and recuperation for the mother after birth is prominent in several cultures. Asian mothers must remain at home with the baby at least 30 days after birth and are not supposed to engage in household chores, including care of the baby. Many times the grandmother takes over the baby's care immediately, even before discharge from the hospital. Jordanian mothers have a 40-day lying-in after birth during which their mothers or sisters care for the baby. Japanese mothers rest for the first 2 months after childbirth. Latinas practice an intergenerational family ritual, *la cuarentena.* For 40 days after birth the mother is expected to recuperate and get acquainted with her infant. Traditionally, this process involves many restrictions concerning food (spicy or cold foods, fish, pork, and citrus are avoided; tortillas and chicken soup are encouraged), exercise, and activities, including sexual intercourse. Many women avoid bathing and washing their hair. Traditional Latino husbands do not expect to see their wives or infants until both have been cleaned and dressed after birth. *La cuarentena* incorporates individuals into the family, instills parental responsibility, and integrates the family during a critical life event (D'Avanzo, 2008).

All cultures place importance on desiring and valuing children. In Asian families, children are a source of family strength and stability, are perceived as wealth, and are objects of parental love and affection. Infants are almost always given an affectionate "cradle" name that is used during the first years of life; for example, a Filipino girl might be called "Ling-Ling" and a boy "Bong-Bong."

Differing cultural values can influence parents' interactions with health care professionals. For example, Asians are taught to be humble and obedient; to be outspoken is frowned on. They are brought up to refrain from questioning authority figures (e.g., a nurse), to avoid confrontation, and to respect the yin/yang balance in nature. Because of these learned values, an Asian mother might not confront the nurse about the length of time taken to receive the medication requested for her episiotomy pain. A mother may nod and say, "Yes," in response to the nurse's directions for using an iced sitz bath but then will not use the sitz bath. The "yes," in this case, is a gesture of courtesy, meaning, "I'm listening"; it is not an indication of agreement to comply. The mother does not use the iced sitz bath because of her traditional avoidance of bathing and cold after birth. Because not all members of a cultural group adhere to traditional practices, it is necessary to validate which cultural practices are important to individual parents.

Knowledge of cultural beliefs can help the nurse make more accurate assessments and diagnoses of observed parenting behaviors. For example, nurses may become concerned when they observe cultural practices that appear to reflect poor maternal-infant bonding. Algerian mothers may not unwrap and explore their infants as part of the acquaintance process because, in Algeria, babies are wrapped tightly in swaddling clothes to protect them physically and psychologically (D'Avanzo, 2008). The nurse may observe a Vietnamese woman who gives minimal care to her infant but refuses to cuddle or further interact with her baby. This apparent lack of interest in the newborn is this cultural group's attempt to ward off "evil spirits" and actually reflects an intense love and concern for the infant. An Asian mother might be criticized for almost immediately relinquishing the care of the infant to the grandmother and not even attempting to hold her baby when it is brought to her room. However, in Asian extended families, members show their support for a new mother's rest and recuperation by assisting with the care of the baby. Contrary to the guidance that is sometimes given to mothers in the United States about "nipple confusion," a mix of breastfeeding and bottle-feeding is standard practice for Japanese mothers. This tradition is related to concern for the mother's rest during the first 2 to 3 months and does not usually lead to problems with lactation; breastfeeding is widespread and successful among Japanese women.

Cultural beliefs and values give perspective to the meaning of childbirth for a new mother. Nurses can provide an opportunity for a new mother to talk about her perception of the meaning of childbearing. In helping new families adjust to parenthood, nurses must provide culturally sensitive care by following principles that facilitate nursing practice within transcultural situations.

Socioeconomic Conditions

Socioeconomic conditions often determine access to available resources. Parents whose economic condition is made worse with the birth of each child and who are unable to use an effective method of fertility management may find childbirth complicated by concern for their own health and a sense of helplessness. Mothers who are single, separated, or divorced from their husbands or without a partner, family, and friends may view the birth of a child with dread. Serious financial problems may negatively affect mothering behaviors. Similarly, fathers who are overwhelmed with financial stresses may lack effective parenting skills and behaviors.

Personal Aspirations

For some women, parenthood interferes with or blocks plans for personal freedom or career advancement. Unresolved resentment will affect caregiving activities and adjustment to parenting. This situation may result in indifference and neglect of the infant or in excessive concerns; the mother may set impossibly high standards for her own behavior or the child's performance.

Nursing interventions include providing opportunities for mothers to express their feelings freely to an objective listener, to discuss measures to permit personal growth, and to learn about the care of their infant. Referring the woman to a support group of other mothers "in the same situation" may also be helpful.

Nurses can be proactive in influencing changes in work policies related to maternity and paternity leaves, varying models of work sharing and "family-friendly" work environments. Some corporations already structure their work sites to support new mothers (e.g., by providing on-site day care facilities and lactation rooms).

COMMUNITY ACTIVITY

Visit an obstetric or pediatric office or clinic in your community. Interview a member of the health team or a new mother. Identify issues related to postpartum adaptation for new mothers and families. Include concerns related to parental expectations, social support, lack of experience, inadequate resources, age, and culture. Include the role of siblings and grandparents in the adaptation process.

PARENTAL SENSORY IMPAIRMENT

In early interactions between the parent and child, all senses–sight, hearing, touch, taste, and smell–are used by each individual to initiate and sustain the attachment process. A parent who has an impairment of one of the senses needs to maximize use of the remaining senses.

Visually Impaired Parent

Visual impairment alone does not seem to have a negative effect on mothers' early parenting experiences. These mothers, just as sighted mothers, express the wonders of parenthood and encourage other visually impaired persons to become parents. Mothers with disabilities tend to value the importance of performing parenting tasks in the perceived culturally usual way.

Although visually impaired mothers initially feel a pressure to conform to traditional, sighted ways of parenting, they soon adapt these ways and develop methods better suited to themselves. Examples of activities that visually impaired mothers perform differently include preparation of the infant's nursery, clothes, and supplies. Some mothers put an entire clothing outfit together and hang it in the closet rather than keeping items separate in drawers. Some develop a labeling system for the infant's clothing and put diapering, bathing, and other care supplies where they will be easy to locate. A strength that visually impaired parents have is a heightened sensitivity to other sensory outputs. A visually impaired mother can tell when her infant is facing her because she notices the baby's breath on her face.

One of the major difficulties that visually impaired parents experience is the skepticism, open or hidden, of health care professionals. Visually impaired people sense reluctance on the part of others to acknowledge that they have a right to be parents. All too often, nurses and physicians lack the experience to deal with the childbearing and childrearing needs of visually impaired mothers, as well as mothers with other disabilities, such as the hearing impaired, physically impaired, and mentally challenged. The nurse's best approach is to assess the mother's capabilities and to use that information as a basis for making plans to assist the woman, often in much the same way as for a mother without impairments. Visually impaired mothers have made suggestions for providing care for women such as themselves during childbearing (Box 15-2). Such approaches can help avoid a sense of increased vulnerability on the mother's part.

Eye contact is important in U.S. culture. With a parent who is visually impaired, this critical factor in the parent-child attachment process is obviously missing. However, the blind parent, who may never have experienced this method of strengthening relationships, does not miss it. The infant will need other sensory input from that parent. An infant looking into the eyes of a mother who is blind may be unaware that the eyes are unseeing. Other people in the newborn's environment can also participate in active eye-to-eye contact to supply this need. A problem may arise, however, if the visually impaired parent has little facial expression. Her infant, after making repeated unsuccessful attempts to engage in face play with the mother, will abandon the behavior with her and intensify it with the father or other people in the household. Nurses can provide anticipatory guidance regarding this situation and help the mother learn to nod and smile while talking and cooing to the infant.

BOX 15-2

Nursing Approaches for Working with Visually Impaired Parents

- Parents who are blind need verbal teaching by health care providers because pregnancy and childbirth information is usually not accessible to blind people.
- A visually impaired parent needs an orientation to the hospital room that allows the parent to move about the room independently. For example, "Go to the left of the bed and trail the wall until you feel the first door. That is the bathroom."
- Parents who are blind need explanations of routines.
- Parents who are blind need to feel devices (e.g., monitors, pelvic models) and to hear descriptions of the devices.
- Visually impaired parents need a chance to ask questions.
- Visually impaired parents need the opportunity to hold and touch the baby after birth.
- Nurses need to demonstrate baby care by touch and to follow with, "Now show me how you would do it."
- Nurses need to give instructions such as, "I'm going to give you the baby. The head is to your left side."

Hearing-Impaired Parent

The parent who has a hearing impairment faces challenges in caregiving and parenting, particularly if the deafness dates from birth or early childhood. The mother and her partner are likely to have established an independent household. Devices that transform sound into light flashes can be fitted into the infant's room to permit immediate detection of crying. Even if the parent is not speech trained, vocalizing can serve as both a stimulus and a response to the infant's early vocalizing. Deaf parents can provide additional vocal training by use of recordings and television so that from birth the child is aware of the full range of the human voice. Young children acquire sign language readily, and the first sign used is as varied as the first word.

Section 504 of the Rehabilitation Act of 1973 requires that hospitals and other institutions receiving funds from the U.S. Department of Health and Human Services use various communication techniques and resources with the deaf, including having staff members or certified interpreters who are proficient in sign language. For example, provision of written materials with demonstrations and having nurses stand where the parent can read their lips (if the parent practices lip reading) are two techniques that can be used. A creative approach is for the nursing unit to develop videos in which information on postpartum care, infant care, and parenting issues is signed by an interpreter and spoken by a nurse. A videotape in which a nurse signs while speaking would be ideal. With the advent of the Internet, many resources are available to the deaf parent.

SIBLING ADAPTATION

Because the family is an interactive, open unit, the addition of a new family member affects everyone in the family. Siblings have to assume new positions within the family hierarchy. Parents often face the task of caring for a new child while not neglecting the others. Parents need to distribute their attention in an equitable manner. When the newborn was born prematurely or has special needs, this task can be difficult.

Reactions of siblings result from temporary separation from the mother, changes in the mother's or father's behavior, or the siblings' response to the infant's coming home. Positive behavioral changes of siblings include interest in and concern for the baby (Fig. 15-8) and increased independence. Regression in toileting and sleep habits, aggression toward the baby, and increased seeking of attention and whining are examples of negative behaviors.

The parents' attitudes toward the arrival of the baby can set the stage for the other children's reactions. Because the baby absorbs the time and attention of the important people in the other children's lives, jealousy (**sibling rivalry**) is common once the initial excitement of having a new baby in the home is over. However, sibling rivalry, or negative behaviors in siblings, may have been overemphasized in the past and exists for a comparatively short time. Developmentally appropriate behaviors in siblings are similar before and after the baby arrives. Firstborn children seem to continue their usual routines and are more pleased with newborns and more understanding of the baby's need for care than the parents predict.

Parents, especially mothers, spend much time and energy promoting sibling acceptance of a new baby. Participating in sibling preparation classes makes a difference in the ability of mothers to cope with sibling behavior. Older children are actively involved in preparing for the infant, and this involvement intensifies after the birth of the child. Parents have to manage the feeling of guilt that the older children are being deprived of parental time and attention. Parents have to monitor the behavior of older children toward the more vulnerable infant and divert aggressive behavior. Box 15-3 presents strategies that parents have used to facilitate acceptance of a new baby by siblings.

Siblings demonstrate acquaintance behaviors with the newborn. The acquaintance process depends on the information given to the child before the baby is born and on the child's cognitive development level. The initial behaviors of siblings with the newborn include looking at the infant and touching the head (see Fig. 15-8). The initial adjustment of older children to a newborn takes time, and parents should allow children to interact at their own pace rather than forcing them to interact. To expect a young child to accept and love a rival for the parents' affection assumes an unrealistic level of maturity. Sibling love grows as does other love, that is, by being with another person and sharing experiences. The bond between siblings involves a secure base in which one child provides support for the other, is missed when absent, and is looked to for comfort and security.

BOX 15-3

Strategies for Facilitating Sibling Acceptance of a New Baby

- Take your older child (or children) on a tour of your hospital room and point out similarities between this birth and his or her birth. "This is like the room I was in with you, and the baby is in the same kind of bassinet that you were in."
- Have a small gift from the baby to give to your older child each day he or she visits in the hospital.
- Give the older child a T-shirt that says "I'm a big brother" [or "sister"].
- Arrange for your children to be among the first to see the newborn. Let them hold the baby in the hospital. One mother and father arranged for their firstborn son to be present at the births of his three brothers and to be the first one to hold them.
- When the older child visits for the first time, make sure you are not holding the new baby. Your arms need to be open and available for the older child. Instruct the person accompanying the older child to call ahead or give a warning knock to give you time to lay the baby down or have someone else hold the baby.
- Plan individual time with each child. The father or partner can spend time with the older siblings while the mother is taking care of the baby and vice versa. Siblings like to have time and attention from both parents.
- Give preschool and early school-age siblings a newborn doll as "their baby." Give the sibling a photograph of the new baby to take to school to show off "his" or "her" baby. Older siblings may enjoy the responsibility of helping care for the newborn, such as learning how to give the baby a bottle or change a diaper. Remember to supervise interactions between the siblings and new baby.

GRANDPARENT ADAPTATION

Grandparents experience a transition to grandparenthood. Intergenerational relationships shift, and grandparents must deal with changes in practices and attitudes toward

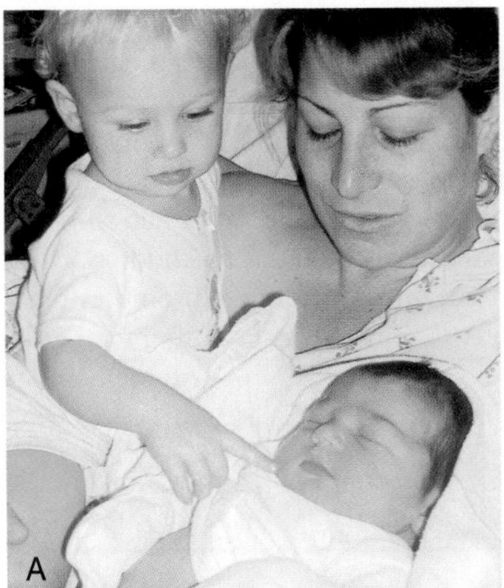

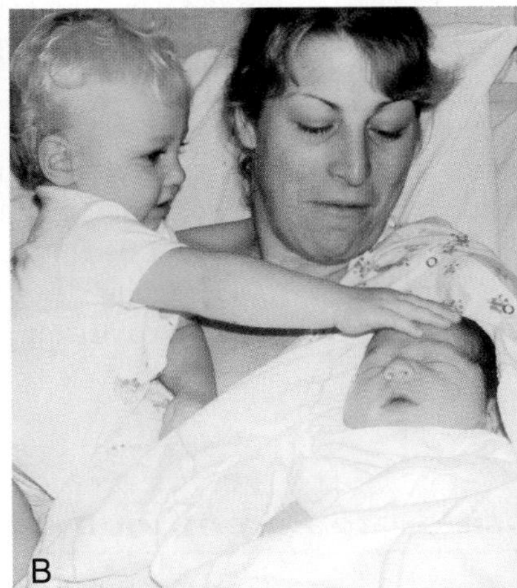

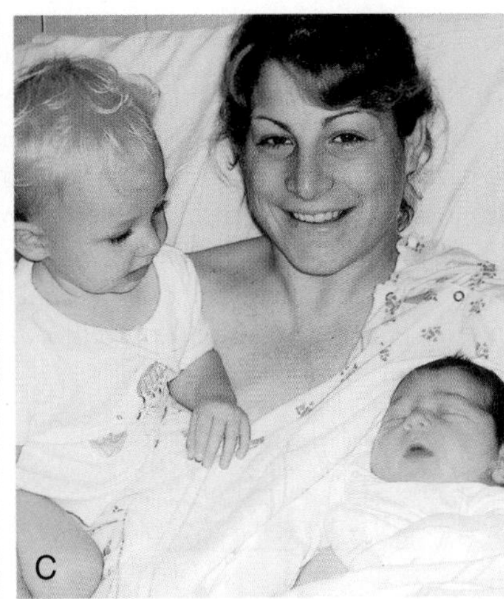

Fig. 15-8 First meeting. Sister with mother during first meeting with new sibling. **A**, First tentative touch with fingertip. **B**, Relationship is more secure; touching with whole hand is now okay. **C**, Smiles indicate acceptance. (Courtesy Sara Kossuth, Los Angeles, CA.)

childbirth, childrearing, and men's and women's roles at home and in the workplace. The degree to which grandparents understand and accept current practices can influence how supportive they are to their adult children.

At the same time that they are adjusting to grandparenthood the majority of grandparents are experiencing normative middle- and old-age life-transition issues, such as retirement and a move to smaller housing, and need support from their adult children. Some may feel regret about their limited involvement because of poor health or geographic distance.

The extent of grandparent involvement in the care of the newborn depends on many factors such as the willingness of the grandparents to become involved, the proximity of the grandparents, and ethnic and cultural expectations of the grandparents' role. For example, if the new parents live in the United States, Asian grandparents typically come to the United States to care for the baby and the mother after birth and to care for the children once the parents return to work. In the United States, paternal grandparents, in contrast to those in other cultures, frequently consider themselves secondary to the maternal grandparents. Less seems expected of them, and they are initially less involved. Nevertheless, these grandparents are eager to help and express great pleasure in their son's fatherhood and his involvement with the baby (Fig. 15-9).

For first-time parents, pregnancy and parenthood can reawaken old issues related to dependence versus independence. Couples often do not plan on their parents' help immediately after the baby arrives. They want time "to be a family," implying a couple-baby unit, not the intergenerational family network. Contrary to their expectations, however, new parents do call on their parents for help, especially the maternal grandmother. Many grandparents are aware of their adult children's wishes for autonomy, respect these wishes, and remain available to help when asked.

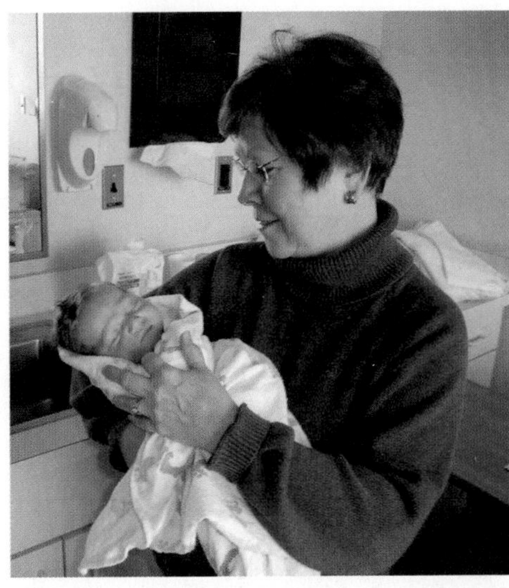

Fig. 15-9 Grandmother and new grandson get acquainted. (Courtesy Nicole Larson, Eden Prairie, MN.)

Grandparents' classes can be used to bridge the generation gap and to help the grandparents understand their adult children's parenting concepts. The classes include information on up-to-date childbearing practices; family-centered care; infant care, feeding, and safety (car seats); and exploration of roles that grandparents play in the family unit.

Increasing numbers of grandparents are providing permanent care to their grandchildren as a result of divorce, substance abuse, child abuse or neglect, abandonment, teenage pregnancy, death, human immunodeficiency virus and acquired immunodeficiency syndrome, unemployment, incarceration, and mental health problems. This emerging trend requires the nurse to evaluate the role of the grandparent in parenting the infant. Educational and financial considerations must be addressed and available support systems identified for these families.

Nursing Care Plan: The Multiparous Woman and Family

CARE MANAGEMENT

Numerous changes occur during the first weeks of parenthood. Nursing care management should be directed toward helping parents cope with infant care, role changes, altered lifestyle, and change in family structure resulting from the addition of a new baby. Developing skill and confidence in caring for an infant can be anxiety provoking. Anticipatory guidance can help prevent a shock of reality in the transition from hospital or birthing center to home that might negate the parents' joy or cause them undue stress.

Through education, support, and encouragement, nurses are instrumental in assisting mothers and their partners in the transition to parenthood, whether they are first-time parents or parents of several other children. Early and ongoing assessment and intervention promotes positive outcomes for parents, infants, and family members.

NURSING PROCESS *Transition to Parenthood*

ASSESSMENT

- Assessment should include a psychosocial assessment focusing on:
  - Parent-infant attachment
  - Adjustment to the parental role
  - Sibling adjustment
  - Social support
  - Education needs
  - Mother's and baby's physical adaptation
- Early home visits are an excellent opportunity for the nurse to assess beginnings of positive or negative parenting behaviors and to provide positive reinforcement for loving and nurturing behaviors with the infant.
- Parents who interact in inappropriate or abusive ways with their infants should be monitored closely, and an appropriate mental health practitioner or professional social worker should be notified.

NURSING DIAGNOSES

Examples of nursing diagnoses related to transition to parenthood include:

- *Readiness for enhanced family coping* related to
  - Positive attitude and realistic expectations for newborn and adapting to parenthood
  - Nurturing behaviors with newborn
  - Verbalizing positive factors in lifestyle change
- *Risk for impaired parenting* related to
  - Lack of knowledge of infant care
  - Feelings of incompetence or lack of confidence
  - Unrealistic expectations of newborn or infant
  - Fatigue from interrupted sleep
- *Parental role conflict* related to
  - Role transition and role attainment
  - Unwanted pregnancy
  - Lack of resources to support parenting (e.g., no paid leave)
- *Risk for impaired parent-child attachment* related to
  - Difficult labor and birth
  - Postpartum complications
  - Neonatal complications or anomalies

EXPECTED OUTCOMES

Expected outcomes for effective transition to parenthood include that the parents will:

- Demonstrate behaviors that reflect appreciation of sensory and behavioral capacities of the infant.
- Verbalize increasing confidence and competence in feeding, diapering, dressing, and sensory stimulation of the infant.
- Identify deviations from normal in the infant that should be brought to the immediate attention of the primary health care provider.
- Relate effectively to the newborn's siblings and grandparents.

PLAN OF CARE AND INTERVENTIONS

A plan of care is formulated in collaboration with the family, incorporating their priorities and preferences, to meet their specific needs.

- Provide practical suggestions for infant care (see Chapter 17).
- Provide anticipatory guidance on what to expect as newborn grows and develops:
  - Sleep-wake cycles
  - Interpretation of crying and quieting techniques
  - Infant developmental milestones
  - Sensory enrichment/infant stimulation
  - Recognizing signs of illness
  - Well-baby follow-up and immunizations

EVALUATION

Evaluation is based on the expected outcomes of care. The plan is revised as needed based on the evaluation findings.

KEY POINTS

- The birth of a child necessitates changes in the existing interactional structure of a family.
- Attachment is the process by which the parent and infant come to love and accept each other.
- Attachment is strengthened through the use of sensual responses or interactions by both partners in the parent-infant interaction.
- In adjusting to the parental role the mother moves from a dependent state (taking in) to an interdependent state (letting go).
- Many mothers exhibit signs of postpartum blues (baby blues).
- Fathers experience emotions and adjustments during the transition to parenthood that are similar to, and also distinctly different from, those of mothers.
- Modulation of rhythm, modification of behavioral repertoires, and mutual responsivity facilitate infant-parent adjustment.
- Many factors influence adaptation to parenthood (e.g., age, culture, socioeconomic level, expectations of what the child will be like).
- Sibling adjustment to a new baby requires creative parental interventions.
- Grandparents can have a positive influence on the postpartum family.

Audio Chapter Summaries Access an audio summary of these Key Points on evolve

References

Brotherson, S. (2007). From partners to parents: Couples and the transition to parenthood. *International Journal of Childbirth Education*, *22*(2), 7-12.

Corwin, E. J., & Arbour, M. (2007). Postpartum fatigue and evidence-based interventions. *MCN American Journal of Maternal/Child Nursing*, *32*(4), 215-220.

Deave, T., Johnson, D., & Ingram, J. (2008). Transition to parenthood: The needs of parents in pregnancy and early parenthood. *BMC Pregnancy and Childbirth*, *8*(30), 1-11. Retrieved June 5, 2009 from www.biomedcentral.com/1471-2393/8/30.

D'Avanzo, C. (2008). *Mosby's pocket guide to cultural health assessment* (4th ed.). St. Louis: Mosby.

Flacking, A., Lehtonen, L., Thomson, G., et al. (2012). Closeness and separation in neonatal intensive care. *Acta Paediatrica*, *101*(10), 1032-1037.

Fletcher, R., Vimpani, G., Russell, G., & Sibbritt, D. (2008). Psychosocial assessment of expectant fathers. *Archives of Women's Mental Health*, *11*(1), 27-32.

Giger, J. N. (2012). *Transcultural nursing: Assessment and intervention* (6th ed.). St. Louis: Mosby.

Goodman, J. (2005). Becoming an involved father of an infant. *Journal of Obstetric, Gynecologic, and Neonatal Nursing*, *34*(2), 190-200.

Halle, C., Dowd, T., Fowler, C., Rissel, K., Hennessy, K., MacNevin, R., et al. (2008). Supporting fathers in the transition to parenthood. *Contemporary Nurse*, *31*(1), 57-70.

Herrman, J. (2008). Adolescent perceptions of teen births. *Journal of Obstetric, Gynecologic, and Neonatal Nursing*, *37*(1), 42-50.

Hung, K. J., Berg, O. (2011). Early skin-to-skin after cesarean to improve breastfeeding. *MCN American Journal of Maternal Child Nursing*, *36*(5), 318-324.

Klaus, M., & Kennell, J. (1976). *Maternal-infant bonding*. St. Louis: Mosby.

Klaus, M., & Kennell, J. (1982). *Parent-infant bonding* (2nd ed.). St. Louis: Mosby.

Kurth, E., Kennedy, H. P., Spichiger, E., et al. (2011). Crying babies, tired mothers: What do we know? A systematic review. *Midwifery*, *27*(2), 187-194.

Lutz, K., & May, K. A. (2007). The impact of high-risk pregnancy on the transition to parenthood. *International Journal of Childbirth Education*, *22*(3), 20-22.

Mercer, R. (2004). Becoming a mother versus maternal role attainment. *Journal of Nursing Scholarship*, *36*(3), 226-232.

Mercer, R., & Walker, L. (2006). A review of nursing interventions to foster becoming a mother. *Journal of Obstetric, Gynecologic, and Neonatal Nursing*, *35*(5), 568-582.

Moore, E., Anderson, G., Bergman, N., et al. (2012). Early skin-to-skin contact for mothers and their healthy newborn infants. *Cochrane Database of Systematic Reviews*, May 15(5), CD003519. pub 3. DOI: 10.1002/14651858.

Nelson, A. (2003). Transition to motherhood. *Journal of Obstetric, Gynecologic, and Neonatal Nursing*, *32*(4), 465-477.

Rubin, R. (1961). Basic maternal behavior. *Nursing Outlook*, *9*, 683-686.

Shin, H., Park, Y., Ryu, H., & Seomun, G. (2008). Maternal sensitivity: a concept analysis. *Journal of Advanced Nursing*, *64*(3), 304-314.

St. John, W., Cameron, C., & McVeigh, C. (2005). Meeting the challenge of new fatherhood during the early weeks. *Journal of Obstetric, Gynecologic, and Neonatal Nursing*, *34*(2), 180-189.

Suplee, P., Dawley, K., & Bloch, J. (2007). Tailoring peripartum nursing care for women of advanced maternal age. *Journal of Obstetric, Gynecologic, and Neonatal Nursing*, *36*(6), 616-623.

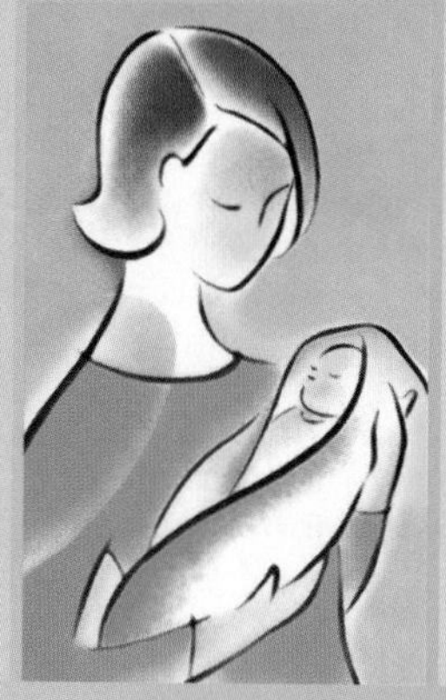

CHAPTER 16

Physiologic and Behavioral Adaptations of the Newborn

SHANNON E. PERRY

LEARNING OBJECTIVES

- *Discuss the physiologic adaptations of the neonate during the transition to extrauterine life.*
- *Describe the sequence to follow in assessing the newborn.*
- *Recognize deviations from normal physiologic findings during the examination of the newborn.*
- *Explain thermoregulation in the neonate and the types of heat loss.*
- *Describe the behavioral adaptations of the newborn, including periods of reactivity and sleep-wake states.*
- *Discuss the sensory and perceptual functioning of the neonate.*

KEY TERMS AND DEFINITIONS

acrocyanosis Peripheral cyanosis; blue color of hands and feet in most infants at birth that may persist for 7 to 10 days

brown fat Source of heat unique to neonates that is capable of greater thermogenic activity than ordinary fat; deposits are found around the adrenals, kidneys, and neck; between the scapulae; and behind the sternum for several weeks after birth

caput succedaneum Swelling of the tissue over the presenting part of the fetal head caused by pressure during labor

cephalhematoma Extravasation of blood from ruptured vessels between a skull bone and its external covering, the periosteum; swelling is limited by the margins of the cranial bone affected (usually parietals)

cold stress Excessive loss of heat that results in increased respirations and nonshivering thermogenesis to maintain core body temperature

erythema toxicum Innocuous pink papular neonatal rash of unknown cause, with superimposed vesicles appearing within 24 to 48 hours after birth and resolving spontaneously within a few days

habituation Psychologic and physiologic phenomenon whereby the response to a constant or repetitive stimulus is decreased

jaundice Yellow color of skin due to increased level of bilirubin in body tissues

meconium Greenish black, viscous first stool formed during fetal life from the amniotic fluid and its constituents, intestinal secretions (including bilirubin), and cells (shed from the mucosa)

milia Small, white sebaceous glands, appearing as tiny, white, pinpoint papules on the forehead, nose, cheeks, and chin of the neonate

mongolian spots Bluish gray or dark nonelevated pigmented areas usually found over the lower back and buttocks that are present at birth in some infants, primarily nonwhite, usually fading by school age

sleep-wake states Variation in states of newborn consciousness from deep sleep to extreme irritability

surfactant Phosphoprotein necessary for normal respiratory function that prevents alveolar collapse (atelectasis)

thermogenesis Creation or production of heat, especially in the body

thermoregulation Control of temperature; a balance between heat loss and heat production

transition period Period from birth to 4 to 6 hours later in which the infant passes through a period of reactivity, sleep, and a second period of reactivity

vernix caseosa Protective gray-white fatty substance of cheesy consistency covering the fetal skin

WEB RESOURCES

Additional related content can be found on the companion website at evolve

http://evolve.elsevier.com/Lowdermilk/Maternity/

- NCLEX Review Questions
- Anatomy Review: Sutures and Fontanels
- Assessment Videos: Buttocks, Cremasteric Reflex, Legs (Symmetry, Length), Male Breasts (Supine Position), Moro Reflex, Neck (Posterior), Plantar Grasp, Rooting and Sucking, Upper Extremities
- Case Study: Newborn Health Problems
- Skill: Thermoregulation

The neonatal period includes the time from birth through day 28 of life. By term gestation, the various anatomic and physiologic systems of the fetus have reached a level of development and functioning that permits a separate existence from the mother. At birth the newborn infant exhibits behavioral competencies and a readiness for social interaction. These adaptations set the stage for future growth and development.

TRANSITION TO EXTRAUTERINE LIFE

Newborns undergo phases of instability during the first 6 to 8 hours after birth. These phases are collectively called the **transition period** between intrauterine and extrauterine existence. The first phase of the transition period lasts up to 30 minutes after birth and is called the *first period of reactivity*. The newborn's heart rate increases rapidly to 160 to 180 beats/minute but gradually falls after 30 minutes or so to a baseline rate of between 100 and 120 beats/minute. Respirations are irregular, with a rate between 60 and 80 breaths/minute. Fine crackles may be present on auscultation; audible grunting, nasal flaring, and retractions of the chest also may be noted, but these should cease within the first hour of birth. The infant is alert and may have spontaneous startles, tremors, crying, and movement of the head from side to side. Bowel sounds are audible, and meconium may be passed.

After the first period of reactivity the newborn either sleeps or has a marked decrease in motor activity. This period of unresponsiveness, often accompanied by sleep, lasts from 60 to 100 minutes and is followed by a second period of reactivity.

The second period of reactivity occurs roughly between 4 and 8 hours after birth and lasts from 10 minutes to several hours. Brief periods of tachycardia and tachypnea occur, associated with increased muscle tone, skin color, and mucous production. Meconium is commonly passed at this time. Most healthy newborns experience this transition regardless of gestational age or type of birth; extremely and very preterm infants do not because of physiologic immaturity.

PHYSIOLOGIC ADAPTATIONS

Respiratory System

With the cutting of the umbilical cord the infant undergoes rapid and complex physiologic changes. The most critical and immediate adjustment a newborn makes at birth is the establishment of respirations. With a vaginal birth some lung fluid is squeezed from the newborn's trachea and lungs; in infants who are born by cesarean birth some lung fluid may be retained within the alveoli. With the first breath of air the newborn begins a sequence of cardiopulmonary changes (Table 16-1).

Initial breathing is probably the result of a reflex triggered by pressure changes, exposure to cool air temperature, noise, light, and other sensations related to the birth process. In addition, the chemoreceptors in the aorta and carotid bodies initiate neurologic reflexes when arterial oxygen pressure (PO_2) falls, arterial carbon dioxide pressure (PCO_2) rises, and arterial pH falls. In most cases an exaggerated respiratory reaction follows within 1 minute of birth, and the infant takes a first gasping breath and cries.

Once respirations are established, breaths are shallow and irregular, ranging from 30 to 60 breaths/minute, with periods of periodic breathing that include pauses in respirations lasting less than 20 seconds. These episodes of periodic breathing occur most often during the active (rapid eye movement [REM]) sleep cycle and decrease in frequency and duration with age. Apneic periods longer than 20 seconds are an indication of a pathologic process and should be thoroughly evaluated.

Signs of Respiratory Distress

Most term infants breathe spontaneously and continue to have normal respirations. Signs of respiratory distress may include nasal flaring, intercostal or subcostal retractions (in-drawing of tissue between the ribs or below the rib cage), or grunting with respirations. Suprasternal or subclavicular retractions with stridor or gasping most often represent an upper airway obstruction. Seesaw or paradoxical respirations (exaggerated rise in abdomen, with respiration, as the chest falls) instead of abdominal respirations are abnormal and should be reported. A respiratory rate of less than 30 or greater than 60 breaths/minute with

TABLE 16-1

Characteristics of the Respiratory System of the Neonate

CHARACTERISTIC	EFFECT ON FUNCTION
Decreased lung elastic tissue and recoil	Decreased lung compliance requiring higher pressures and more work to expand; increased risk of atelectasis
Reduced diaphragm movement and maximal force potential	Less effective respiratory movement; difficulty generating negative intrathoracic pressures; risk of atelectasis
Tendency to nose breathe; altered position of larynx and epiglottis	Enhanced ability to synchronize swallowing and breathing; risk of airway obstruction; possibly more difficult to intubate
Small compliant airway passages with higher airway resistance; immature reflexes	Risk of airway obstruction and apnea
Increased pulmonary vascular resistance with sensitive pulmonary arterioles	Risk of ductal shunting and hypoxemia with events such as hypoxia, acidosis, hypothermia, hypoglycemia, and hypercarbia
Increased oxygen consumption	Increased respiratory rate and work of breathing; risk of hypoxia
Increased intrapulmonary right-left shunting	Increased risk of atelectasis with wasted ventilation; lower Pco_2
Immaturity of pulmonary surfactant system in immature infants	Increased risk of atelectasis and respiratory distress syndrome; increased work of breathing
Immature respiratory control	Irregular respirations with periodic breathing; risk of apnea; inability to rapidly alter depth of respirations

From Blackburn, S. (2007). *Maternal, fetal, & neonatal physiology: A clinical perspective* (3rd ed.). St. Louis: Saunders.
Pco_2: Partial pressure of carbon dioxide.

the infant at rest must be thoroughly evaluated. The respiratory rate of the infant can be slowed, depressed, or absent due to the effects of analgesics or anesthetics administered to the mother during labor and birth. Apneic episodes can be related to several events (rapid increase in body temperature; hypothermia, hypoglycemia, and sepsis) that require thorough evaluation. Tachypnea may result from inadequate clearance of lung fluid, or it may be an indication of newborn respiratory distress syndrome.

Maintaining adequate oxygen supply

During the first hour of life the pulmonary lymphatics continue to remove large amounts of fluid. Removal of fluid is also a result of the pressure gradient from alveoli to interstitial tissue to blood capillary. Reduced vascular resistance accommodates this flow of lung fluid. Retention of lung fluid may interfere with the infant's ability to maintain adequate oxygenation, especially if other factors that compromise respirations are present (meconium aspiration, congenital diaphragmatic hernia, esophageal atresia with fistula, choanal atresia, congenital cardiac defect, immature alveoli [absent or decreased]).

The term newborn's chest circumference is approximately 30 to 33 cm at birth. Auscultation of the chest of a newborn reveals loud, clear breath sounds that seem very near because the infant has little chest wall musculature. The ribs of the infant articulate with the spine at a horizontal rather than a downward slope; consequently, the rib cage cannot expand with inspiration as readily as that of an adult. Because neonatal respiratory function is largely a matter of diaphragmatic contraction, abdominal breathing is characteristic of newborns. That is, the newborn infant's chest and abdomen rise simultaneously with inspiration, but because of the large size of the abdomen, chest movement is not as visible.

The outer walls of the alveoli are lined with **surfactant**, a protein manufactured in type II cells of the lungs. Lung expansion is largely dependent on chest wall contraction and adequate presence and secretion of surfactant. Surfactant lowers surface tension, therefore reducing the pressure required to keep the alveoli open with inspiration, and prevents total alveolar collapse on exhalation, thereby maintaining alveolar stability. With absent or decreased surfactant, more pressure must be generated for inspiration, which may soon tire or exhaust preterm or sick term infants. Surfactant may be compared with soapy water on the inside of a balloon. Sometimes the sides of an uninflated balloon stick together and cannot expand. If some soapy water is poured into the balloon, the surfaces are slippery and prevent the sides from sticking; this allows the balloon to expand.

Cardiovascular System

The cardiovascular system changes significantly after birth. The infant's first breaths, combined with increased alveolar capillary distention, inflate the lungs and reduce pulmonary vascular resistance to the pulmonary blood flow from the pulmonary arteries. Pulmonary artery pressure drops, and pressure in the right atrium declines. Increased pulmonary blood flow to the left side of the heart increases pressure in the left atrium, which causes a functional closure of the foramen ovale. During the first few days of life, crying may reverse the flow through the foramen ovale temporarily and lead to mild cyanosis (Table 16-2).

TABLE 16-2

Cardiovascular Changes at Birth

PRENATAL STATUS	POSTBIRTH STATUS	ASSOCIATED FACTORS
PRIMARY CHANGES		
Pulmonary circulation: high pulmonary vascular resistance, increased pressure in right ventricle and pulmonary arteries	Low pulmonary vascular resistance; decreased pressure in right atrium, ventricle, and pulmonary arteries	Expansion of collapsed fetal lung with air
Systemic circulation: low pressures in left atrium, ventricle, and aorta	High systemic vascular resistance; increased pressure in left atrium, ventricle, and aorta	Loss of placental blood flow
SECONDARY CHANGES		
Umbilical arteries: patent, carrying of blood from hypogastric arteries to placenta	Functionally closed at birth; obliteration by fibrous proliferation possibly taking 2-3 mo, distal portions becoming lateral vesicoumbilical ligaments, proximal portions remaining open as superior vesicle arteries	Closure preceding that of umbilical vein, probably accomplished by smooth muscle contraction in response to thermal and mechanical stimuli and alteration in oxygen tension, mechanically severed with cord at birth
Umbilical vein: patent, carrying of blood from placenta to ductus venosus and liver	Closed, becoming ligamentum teres hepatis after obliteration	Closure shortly after umbilical arteries, hence blood from placenta possibly entering neonate for short period after birth, mechanically severed with cord at birth
Ductus venosus: patent, connection of umbilical vein to inferior vena cava	Closed, becoming ligamentum venosum after obliteration	Loss of blood flow from umbilical vein
Ductus arteriosus: patent, shunting of blood from pulmonary artery to descending aorta	Functionally closed almost immediately after birth, anatomic obliteration of lumen by fibrous proliferation requiring 1-3 mo, becoming ligamentum arteriosum	Increased oxygen content of blood in ductus arteriosus creating vasospasm of its muscular wall High systemic resistance increasing aortic pressure; low pulmonary resistance reducing pulmonary arterial pressure
Foramen ovale: formation of a valve opening that allows blood to flow directly to left atrium (shunting of blood from right to left atrium)	Functionally closed at birth, constant apposition gradually leading to fusion and permanent closure within a few months or years in majority of persons	Increased pressure in left atrium and decreased pressure in right atrium causing closure of valve over foramen

In utero, fetal PO_2 is 27 mm Hg. After birth, when the PO_2 level in the arterial blood approximates 50 mm Hg, the ductus arteriosus constricts in response to increased oxygenation. Circulating levels of the hormone prostaglandin E (PGE_2) also have an important role in closure of the ductus arteriosus. Later, the ductus arteriosus closes completely and becomes a ligament. With the clamping of the cord, the umbilical arteries, umbilical vein, and ductus venosus close and are converted into ligaments. The hypogastric arteries also occlude and become ligaments.

Heart rate and sounds

The heart rate averages 100 to 160 beats/minute, with variations noted during sleeping and waking states. Shortly after the first cry the infant's heart rate may accelerate as high as 175 to 180 beats/minute. The range of the heart rate in the term infant is approximately 85 to 90 beats/minute during deep sleep and up to 170 or more beats/minute while the infant is awake. A heart rate of 180 beats/minute is not unusual when the infant cries. A heart rate that is either consistently high (>170 beats/min) or low (<80 beats/min) with the newborn at rest should be reevaluated within an hour or when the activity of the infant changes.

The apical impulse (point of maximal impulse [PMI]) in the newborn is located at the fourth intercostal space and to the left of the midclavicular line. The PMI is often visible and easily palpable because of the thin chest wall; this is also called precordial activity.

Apical pulse rates should be assessed on all infants. Auscultation should be for a full minute, preferably when the infant is asleep. An irregular heart rate is not uncommon in the first few hours of life. After this time an irregular heart rate not attributed to changes in activity or respiratory pattern should be further evaluated.

Heart sounds during the neonatal period are of higher pitch, shorter duration, and greater intensity than those during adult life. The first sound (S_1) is typically louder and duller than the second sound (S_2), which is sharp. The third and fourth heart sounds are not auscultated in newborns. Most heart murmurs heard during the first few days of life have no pathologic significance, and more than one half of the murmurs disappear by 6 months. However, the presence of a murmur and accompanying signs such as poor feeding, apnea, cyanosis, or pallor are considered abnormal and should be further investigated.

Blood pressure

The newborn infant's average systolic blood pressure (BP) is 60 to 80 mm Hg, and the average diastolic pressure is 40 to 50 mm Hg. The BP increases by the second day of life, with minor variations noted during the first month of life. A drop in systolic BP (approximately 15 mm Hg) in the first hour of life is common. Crying and movement usually cause increases in the systolic pressure. The measurement of BP is best accomplished with an oscillometric device while the infant is at rest. A correctly sized cuff must be used for accurate measurement of an infant's BP.

Unless a specific indication exists, BP is not usually measured in the newborn on a routine basis except as a baseline. The practice of obtaining four extremity BPs in the early newborn period to detect coarctation of the aorta (COA) has been recently questioned (Razmus & Lewis, 2006). This is based on evidence that COA defects do not occur in the immediate postbirth period but more typically at approximately 12 to 14 days of age, a time when the ductus arteriosus closes (Taylor, 2005).

Blood volume

The blood volume of the newborn is approximately 80 to 85 ml/kg of body weight. Immediately after birth the total blood volume averages 300 ml, but this volume can increase by as much as 100 ml, depending on the length of time before the cord is clamped and cut. The preterm infant has a relatively greater blood volume than the term newborn because the preterm infant has a proportionately greater plasma volume, not a greater red blood cell (RBC) mass.

Early or late clamping of the umbilical cord changes the circulatory dynamics of the newborn. Late clamping expands the blood volume from the so-called placental transfusion of blood to the newborn. Delayed cord clamping (≥2 minutes after birth) has been reported to result in polycythemia with subsequent clinical signs of hyperviscosity (hematocrit ≥65%, plethoric or ruddy red appearance, sluggish circulation leading to possible emboli in the microvasculature and organ damage, respiratory distress, and possibly hyperbilirubinemia as a result of red cell breakdown) (Armentrout & Huseby, 2003). However, recent data showed delayed cord clamping (no longer than 2 minutes after birth) in full-term neonates was found to be beneficial in improving hematocrit and iron status and in decreasing anemia; such benefits were observed over ages 2 to 6 months. Polycythemia occurred with delayed clamping but was not harmful (Hutton & Hassan, 2007).

Hematopoietic System

The hematopoietic system of the newborn exhibits certain variations from that of the adult. Levels of RBCs and leukocytes differ, but platelet levels are relatively the same.

Red blood cells and hemoglobin

At birth the average levels of RBCs and hemoglobin (fetal hemoglobin is predominant) are higher than those in the adult. Cord blood of the term newborn may have a hemoglobin concentration of 14 to 24 g/dl (mean, 17 g/dl). The hematocrit ranges from 44% to 64% (mean, 55%). The RBC count is correspondingly elevated, ranging from 4.8 to 7.1 million/mm^3 (mean, 5.14 million/mm^3). By the end of the first month, these values fall and reach the average levels of 11 to 17 g/dl and 4.2 to 5.2 million/mm^3, respectively.

The blood values may be affected by delayed clamping of the cord, which results in a rise in hemoglobin, RBCs, and hematocrit. The source of the sample is a significant factor because capillary blood yields higher values than venous blood. The timing of blood sampling is also significant; the slight rise in RBCs after birth is followed by a substantial drop. At birth the infant's blood contains an average of 70% fetal hemoglobin, but because of the shorter life span of the cells containing fetal hemoglobin, the percentage falls to 55% by 5 weeks and to 5% by 20 weeks. Iron stores generally are sufficient to sustain normal RBC production for 4 to 5 months in the term infant, at which time a physiologic anemia that is usually transient can occur.

Leukocytes

Leukocytosis, with a white blood cell (WBC) count of approximately 18,000 cells/mm^3 (range, 9000 to 30,000 cells/mm^3), is normal at birth. The number of WBCs increases to 23,000 to 24,000 cells/mm^3 during the first day after birth. This initial high WBC count of the newborn decreases rapidly, and a resting level of 11,500 cells/mm^3 is normally maintained during the neonatal period. Serious infection is not well tolerated by the newborn; leukocytes are slow to recognize foreign protein and to localize and fight infection early in life. Sepsis may be accompanied by a concomitant rise in WBCs (neutrophilia); however, some infants may exhibit clinical signs of sepsis without a significant elevation in WBCs. In addition, events other than infection may cause neutrophilia in the newborn. These events include prolonged crying, maternal hypertension, asymptomatic hypoglycemia, hemolytic disease, meconium aspiration syndrome, labor induction with oxytocin, surgery, difficult labor, high altitude, and maternal fever.

Platelets

The platelet count ranges between 200,000 and 300,000 cells/mm^3 and is essentially the same in newborns as in adults. The levels of factors II, VII, IX, and X, found in the liver, are decreased during the first few days of life because the newborn cannot synthesize vitamin K. However, bleeding tendencies in the newborn are uncommon, and unless the vitamin K deficiency is great, clotting is sufficient to prevent hemorrhage.

Blood groups

The infant's blood group is genetically determined and established early in fetal life. However, during the neonatal period the strength of the agglutinogens present in the RBC membrane gradually increases. Cord blood samples may be used to identify the infant's blood type and Rh status.

Thermogenic System

Next to establishing respirations and adequate circulation, heat regulation is most critical to the newborn's survival. **Thermoregulation** is the maintenance of balance between heat loss and heat production. Newborns attempt to stabilize their core body temperatures within a narrow range. Hypothermia from excessive heat loss is a common and dangerous problem in neonates. The newborn infant's ability to produce heat (**thermogenesis**) often approaches that of the adult; however, the tendency toward rapid heat loss in a cold environment is increased in the newborn and poses a hazard.

Thermogenesis

The shivering mechanism of heat production is rarely operable in the newborn. Nonshivering thermogenesis is accomplished primarily by metabolism of **brown fat,** which is unique to the newborn, and secondarily by increased metabolic activity in the brain, heart, and liver. Brown fat is located in superficial deposits in the interscapular region and axillae, as well as in deep deposits at the thoracic inlet, along the vertebral column, and around the kidneys. Brown fat has a richer vascular and nerve supply than ordinary fat. Heat produced by intense lipid metabolic activity in brown fat can warm the newborn by increasing heat production as much as 100%. Reserves of brown fat, usually present for several weeks after birth, are rapidly depleted with cold stress. The amount of brown fat reserve increases with the weeks of gestation. A full-term newborn has greater stores than a preterm infant.

Heat loss

Heat loss in the newborn occurs by four modes:

- *Convection* is the flow of heat from the body surface to cooler ambient air. Because of heat loss by convection the ambient temperature in the nursery is kept at approximately 24° C, and newborns in open bassinets are wrapped to protect them from the cold.
- *Radiation* is the loss of heat from the body surface to a cooler solid surface not in direct contact but in relative proximity. To prevent this type of loss, nursery cribs and examining tables are placed away from outside windows, and care is taken to avoid direct air drafts.
- *Evaporation* is the loss of heat that occurs when a liquid is converted to a vapor. In the newborn, heat loss by evaporation occurs as a result of vaporization of moisture from the skin. This heat loss can be intensified by failure to dry the newborn directly after birth or by drying the infant too slowly after a bath. The less mature the newborn is, the more severe the evaporative heat loss will be. Evaporative heat loss, as a component of insensible water loss, is the most significant cause of heat loss in the first few days of life.
- *Conduction* is the loss of heat from the body surface to cooler surfaces in direct contact. When admitted to the nursery the newborn is placed in a warmed crib to minimize heat loss. The scales used for weighing the newborn should have a protective cover to minimize conductive heat losses as well.

Skill: Thermoregulation

Loss of heat must be controlled to protect the infant. Control of such modes of heat loss is the basis of caregiving policies and techniques. One method for promoting maternal-newborn interaction is to place the naked healthy newborn next to the mother's skin and cover both with a blanket. This skin-to-skin contact enhances newborn temperature control and interaction (Fig. 16-1).

Temperature regulation

Anatomic and physiologic differences among the newborn, child, and adult are notable. The newborn's ability to produce heat is initially less than that of an adult. Newborns have larger body surface-body weight (mass) ratios than children and adults. The flexed position of the newborn helps guard against heat loss because it diminishes the amount of body surface exposed to the environment. Infants can also reduce the loss of internal heat through the body surface by constricting peripheral blood vessels.

Cold stress imposes metabolic and physiologic demands on all infants, regardless of gestational age and condition. The respiratory rate increases in response to the increased need for oxygen. In the cold-stressed infant, oxygen consumption and energy are diverted from maintaining normal brain and cardiac function and growth to thermogenesis for survival. If the infant cannot maintain an adequate oxygen tension, vasoconstriction follows and jeopardizes pulmonary perfusion. As a consequence, the

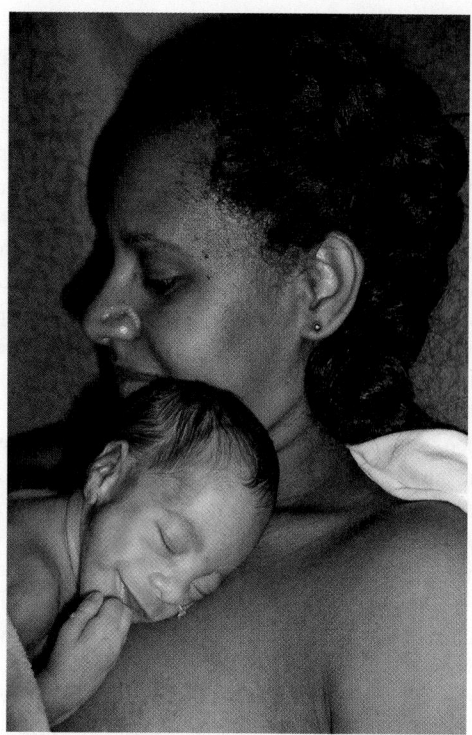

Fig. 16-1 Infant in skin-to-skin contact with mother. (Courtesy Cheryl Briggs, RN, Annapolis, MD.)

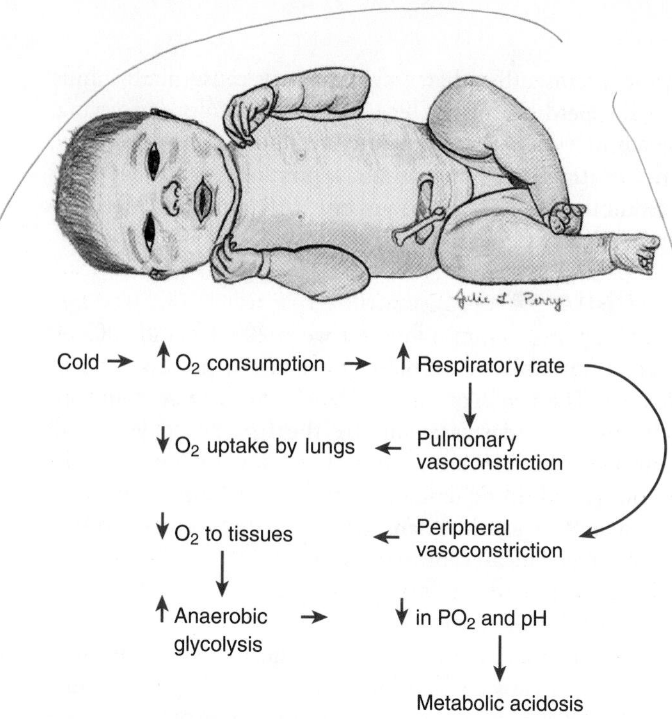

Fig. 16-2 Effects of cold stress. When an infant is stressed by cold, oxygen consumption increases, and pulmonary and peripheral vasoconstriction occur, thereby decreasing oxygen uptake by the lungs and oxygen to the tissues; anaerobic glycolysis increases; and the Po_2 and pH decrease, leading to metabolic acidosis.

Po_2 is decreased, and the blood pH drops. These changes may prompt a transient respiratory distress or may aggravate existing respiratory distress syndrome. Moreover, decreased pulmonary perfusion and oxygen tension may maintain or reopen the right-to-left shunt across the patent ductus arteriosus.

The basal metabolic rate increases with cold stress (Fig. 16-2). If cold stress is protracted, anaerobic glycolysis occurs, resulting in increased production of acids. Metabolic acidosis develops, and if a defect in respiratory function is present, respiratory acidosis also develops. Excessive fatty acids may displace the bilirubin from the albumin-binding sites and exacerbate hyperbilirubinemia.

Hypoglycemia is another metabolic consequence of cold stress. The process of anaerobic glycolysis uses approximately three to four times the amount of blood glucose, thereby depleting existing stores. If the infant is sufficiently stressed and low glucose stores are not replaced, hypoglycemia, which can be asymptomatic in the newborn, may develop.

Hyperthermia develops more rapidly in the newborn than in the adult because of the decreased ability to increase evaporative skin water losses. Although newborn infants have six times as many sweat glands per unit area as adults, in most newborns these glands do not function sufficiently to allow the infant to sweat. Serious overheating of the newborn can cause cerebral damage from dehydration or heat stroke and death.

Renal System

At term gestation the kidneys occupy a large portion of the posterior abdominal wall. The bladder lies close to the anterior abdominal wall and is an abdominal organ and a pelvic organ. In the newborn almost all palpable masses in the abdomen are renal in origin.

A small quantity (approximately 40 ml) of urine is usually present in the bladder of a full-term infant at birth. The frequency of voiding varies from two to six times per day during the first and second days of life and from 5 to 25 times per day thereafter. Approximately six to eight voidings per day of pale straw-colored urine are indicative of adequate fluid intake after the first 3-4 days. Generally, term infants void 15 to 60 ml of urine/kg/day.

Full-term infants have limited capacity to concentrate urine; therefore the specific gravity of the urine may range from 1.001 to 1.020. The ability to concentrate urine fully is attained by approximately 3 months of age. After the first voiding the infant's urine may appear cloudy (because of mucous content) and have a much higher specific gravity. This level decreases as fluid intake increases. Normal urine during early infancy is usually straw colored and almost odorless. During the first week after birth, urine contains an abundance of uric acid crystals that may appear as pink or orange stains ("brick dust") on the diaper. If this occurs after the first week, it can be an indication of insufficient intake.

It is common for newborns to lose 5% to 7% of their birth weight during the first 3 to 5 days of life. This is the result of fluid loss through urine, feces, and lungs, as well as an increased metabolic rate and limited fluid intake. If the mother is breastfeeding and her milk supply has not yet transitioned to the higher volume mature milk by the third or fourth day, the neonate is somewhat protected from dehydration by the increased extracellular fluid volume that is present at birth. Weight loss in excess of 7% of birth weight can indicate feeding problems, especially in the breastfeeding infant. This warrants further assessment of feedings. If the weight loss reaches 10% of birth weight during the first week of life, there is cause for concern. The neonate should regain the birth weight within 10 to 14 days, depending on the feeding method (breast or bottle).

Because renal thresholds are low in the infant, bicarbonate concentration and buffering capacity are decreased. This reduction may lead to acidosis and electrolyte imbalance.

Fluid and electrolyte balance

Approximately 40% of the body weight of the newborn is extracellular fluid. Each day the newborn takes in and excretes roughly 600 to 700 ml of fluid, which is 20% of the total body fluid or 50% of the extracellular fluid. The glomerular filtration rate of a newborn is approximately 30% to 50% that of the adult. This lower filtration rate results in a decreased ability to remove nitrogenous and other waste products from the blood. However, the newborn's ingested protein is almost totally metabolized for growth.

Sodium reabsorption is decreased as a result of a lowered sodium- or potassium-activated adenosine triphosphatase activity. The decreased ability to excrete excessive sodium results in hypotonic urine compared with plasma, leading to a higher concentration of sodium, phosphates, chloride, and organic acids and a lower concentration of bicarbonate ions. The infant has a higher renal threshold for glucose than adults.

Gastrointestinal System

The term newborn is capable of swallowing, digesting, metabolizing, and absorbing proteins and simple carbohydrates and emulsifying fats. With the exception of pancreatic amylase the characteristic enzymes and digestive juices are present even in low-birth-weight neonates.

In the adequately hydrated infant the mucous membrane of the mouth is moist and pink. The hard and soft palates are intact. The presence of moderate to large amounts of mucus is common in the first few hours after birth. Small whitish areas (Epstein pearls) may be found on the gum margins and at the juncture of the hard and soft palate. The cheeks are full because of well-developed sucking pads. These pads, like the labial tubercles (sucking calluses) on the upper lip, disappear around the age of 12 months, when the sucking period is over.

Even though sucking motions in utero have been recorded by ultrasound, these motions are not coordinated with swallowing in any infant born before 32 to 33 weeks of gestation. Sucking behavior is influenced by neuromuscular maturity, maternal medications received during labor and birth, and the type of initial feeding.

A special mechanism present in healthy term newborns coordinates the breathing, sucking, and swallowing reflexes necessary for oral feeding. Sucking in the newborn takes place in small bursts of three or four and up to eight to ten sucks at a time, with a brief pause in between bursts. The infant is unable to move food from the lips to the pharynx; therefore placing the nipple (breast or bottle) well inside the baby's mouth is necessary. Peristaltic activity in the esophagus is uncoordinated in the first few days of life. It quickly becomes a coordinated pattern in healthy full-infants and they swallow easily.

Teeth begin developing in utero, with enamel formation continuing until approximately age 10 years. Tooth development is influenced by neonatal or infant illnesses, medications, and illnesses of or medications taken by the mother during pregnancy. The fluoride level in the water supply also influences tooth development. Occasionally an infant may be born with one or more teeth.

Bacteria are not present in the infant's gastrointestinal tract at birth. Soon after birth, oral and anal orifices permit entry of bacteria and air. Generally, the highest bacterial concentration is found in the lower portion of the intestine, particularly in the large intestine. Normal colonic bacteria are established within the first week after birth, and normal intestinal flora help synthesize vitamin K, folate, and biotin. Bowel sounds can usually be heard shortly after birth.

The capacity of the stomach varies from 30 to 90 ml, depending on the size of the infant. Emptying time for the stomach is highly variable. Several factors, such as time and volume of feedings or type and temperature of food, may affect the emptying time. The cardiac sphincter and nervous control of the stomach are immature, thus some regurgitation may occur. Regurgitation during the first day or two of life can be decreased by avoiding overfeeding, by burping the infant, and by positioning the infant with the head slightly elevated.

Digestion

The infant's ability to digest carbohydrates, fats, and proteins is regulated by the presence of certain enzymes. Most of these enzymes are functional at birth. One exception is amylase, produced by the salivary glands after approximately 3 months and by the pancreas at approximately 6 months of age. This enzyme is necessary to convert starch into maltose and occurs in high amounts in colostrum. The other exception is lipase, also secreted by the pancreas; it is necessary for the digestion of fat. Therefore the normal newborn is capable of digesting simple carbohydrates and proteins but has a limited ability to digest fats.

BOX 16-1

Change in Stooling Patterns of Newborns

MECONIUM
- Infant's first stool is composed of amniotic fluid and its constituents, intestinal secretions, shed mucosal cells, and possibly blood (ingested maternal blood or minor bleeding of alimentary tract vessels).
- Passage of meconium should occur within the first 24 to 48 hours, although it may be delayed up to 7 days in very low-birth-weight infants.

TRANSITIONAL STOOLS
- Usually appear by third day after initiation of feeding; greenish brown to yellowish brown, thin, and less sticky than meconium; may contain some milk curds

MILK STOOL
- Usually appears by fourth day
- Breastfed infants: stools yellow to golden, pasty in consistency, with an odor similar to that of sour milk
- Formula-fed infants: stools pale yellow to light brown, firmer in consistency, with a more offensive odor

Further digestion and absorption of nutrients occur in the small intestine in the presence of pancreatic secretions, secretions from the liver through the common bile duct, and secretions from the duodenal portion of the small intestine.

Stools

At birth the lower intestine is filled with meconium. **Meconium** is formed during fetal life from the amniotic fluid and its constituents, intestinal secretions (including bilirubin), and cells (shed from the mucosa). Meconium is greenish black and viscous and contains occult blood. The first meconium passed is usually sterile, but within hours, all meconium passed contains bacteria. The majority of healthy term infants pass meconium within the first 12 to 24 hours of life, and almost all do so by 48 hours (Blackburn, 2007). The number of stools passed varies during the first week, being most numerous between the third and sixth days. Newborns fed early pass stools sooner. Progressive changes in the stooling pattern indicate a properly functioning gastrointestinal tract (Box 16-1).

Hepatic System

The liver and gallbladder are formed by the fourth week of gestation. In the newborn the liver can be palpated approximately 1 cm below the right costal margin because it is enlarged and occupies approximately 40% of the abdominal cavity. The infant's liver plays an important role in iron storage, carbohydrate metabolism, conjugation of bilirubin, and coagulation.

Iron storage

The fetal liver, which serves as the site for production of hemoglobin after birth, begins storing iron in utero. The infant's iron store is proportional to total body hemoglobin content and length of gestation. At birth the term infant has an iron store sufficient to last 4 to 6 months. Iron stores of preterm and small-for-gestational age infants are often lower and are depleted sooner than in healthy infants.

Carbohydrate metabolism

At birth the newborn is cut off from its maternal glucose supply and, as a result, has an initial decrease in serum glucose levels. The newborn's increased energy needs, decreased hepatic release of glucose from glycogen stores, increased RBC volume, and increased brain size may initially contribute to the rapid depletion of stored glycogen within the first 24 hours after birth. In most healthy term newborns, blood glucose levels stabilize at 50 to 60 mg/dl during the first several hours after birth; by the third day of life the blood glucose levels should be approximately 60 to 70 mg/dl. The initiation of feedings assists in the stabilization of the newborn's blood glucose levels. Colostrum contains high amounts of glucose thus also assisting in the stabilization of blood glucose levels in breastfed neonates (colostrum is higher in protein, but lower in glucose, than mature milk) (see Evidence-Based Practice box in Chapter 17).

Jaundice

Jaundice is the manifestation of the pigment bilirubin in the tissues of the body. Jaundice does not usually appear until the bilirubin level reaches 5 mg/dl. Any visible jaundice within the first 24 hours of life or persistence of jaundice beyond 7 to 10 days requires further investigation into the cause as this represents an underlying pathologic process (Fig. 16-3). See Chapter 17 for a further discussion of bilirubin metabolism and hyperbilirubinemia.

Coagulation

Coagulation factors, which are synthesized in the liver, are activated by vitamin K. The lack of intestinal bacteria needed to synthesize vitamin K results in transient blood coagulation deficiency between the second and fifth days of life. The administration of intramuscular vitamin K shortly after birth helps prevent clotting problems.

Immune System

The cells that provide the infant with immunity are developed early in fetal life; however, they are not activated for weeks to months after birth. For the first 3 months of life the healthy term infant is somewhat protected by passive immunity received from the mother; however, this status is dependent on the mother's previous exposure to antigens and her immunologic response. The membrane-protective immunoglobulin A (IgA) is missing from the

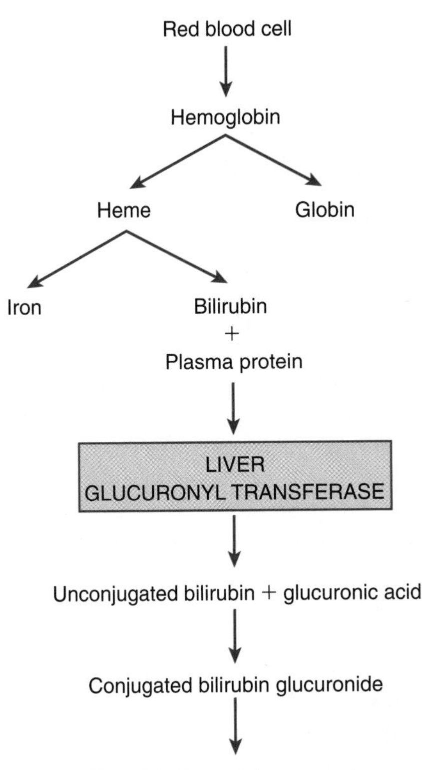

Fig. 16-3 Formation and excretion of bilirubin.

Critical Thinking/Clinical Decision Making

Near Term Infant with Physiologic Jaundice

Veronica gave birth vaginally with the assistance of vacuum extraction to a 7-lb baby boy 36 hours ago. The baby was estimated to be at 35 to 36 weeks of gestation. As a result of the vacuum extraction the baby's occiput is bruised and slightly edematous (his condition appeared much worse yesterday). For the first 24 hours, he was very sleepy and difficult to arouse for feedings, but for the last 12 hours, he has breastfed every 2 to 3 hours for approximately 15 minutes. He has voided twice and passed only one small meconium stool since birth. Randy was holding his baby this morning and stated, "Look at his handsome skin tones! Why, he looks like he has been on vacation and started to get his suntan."

1. Evidence—Is evidence sufficient to draw conclusions about the baby's skin color?
2. Assumptions—What assumptions can be made about the following?
   a. The baby's skin color
   b. Baby's intake and output since birth
   c. The parents' understanding of physiologic jaundice
3. What implications and priorities for nursing care can be drawn at this time?
4. Does the evidence objectively support your conclusion?
5. Do alternative perspectives to your conclusion exist?

respiratory and urinary tracts, and unless the newborn is breastfed, is also absent from the gastrointestinal tract. The infant begins to synthesize IgG, and approximately 40% of adult levels are reached by age 1 year. Significant amounts of IgM are produced at birth, and adult levels are reached by 9 months of age. The production of IgA, IgD, and IgE is much more gradual, and maximal levels are not attained until early childhood. The infant who is breastfed receives significant passive immunity through the colostrum and breast milk.

Integumentary System

All skin structures are present at birth. The epidermis and dermis are loosely bound and extremely thin. **Vernix caseosa** (a cheeselike, whitish substance) is fused with the epidermis and serves as a protective covering. The infant's skin is very sensitive and can be easily damaged. The term infant has an erythematous (red) skin color for a few hours after birth, after which it fades to its normal color. The skin often appears blotchy or mottled, especially over the extremities. The hands and feet appear slightly cyanotic **(acrocyanosis)**, which is caused by vasomotor instability and capillary stasis. Acrocyanosis is normal and appears intermittently over the first 7 to 10 days, especially with exposure to cold.

The healthy term newborn has a plump appearance because of large amounts of subcutaneous tissue and extracellular water content. Fine lanugo hair may be noted over the face, shoulders, and back. Edema of the face and ecchymosis (bruising) or petechiae may be present as a result of face presentation, forceps-assisted birth, or vacuum extraction (see Fig. 17-6).

Creases can be found on the palms of the hands. The simian line, a single palmar crease, is often found in Asian infants or in infants with Down syndrome.

Caput succedaneum

Caput succedaneum is a generalized, easily identifiable edematous area of the scalp, most commonly found on the occiput (Fig. 16-4, *A*). The sustained pressure of the presenting vertex against the cervix results in compression of local vessels, thereby slowing venous return. The slower venous return causes an increase in tissue fluids within the skin of the scalp, and an edematous swelling develops. This edematous swelling, present at birth, extends across suture lines of the skull and disappears spontaneously within 3 to 4 days. Infants who are born with the assistance of vacuum extraction usually have a caput in the area where the cup was applied.

Case Study: Newborn Health Problems

Cephalhematoma

Cephalhematoma is a collection of blood between a skull bone and its periosteum; therefore a cephalhematoma does not cross a cranial suture line (Fig. 16-4, *B*). Caput succedaneum and cephalhematoma often occur simultaneously.

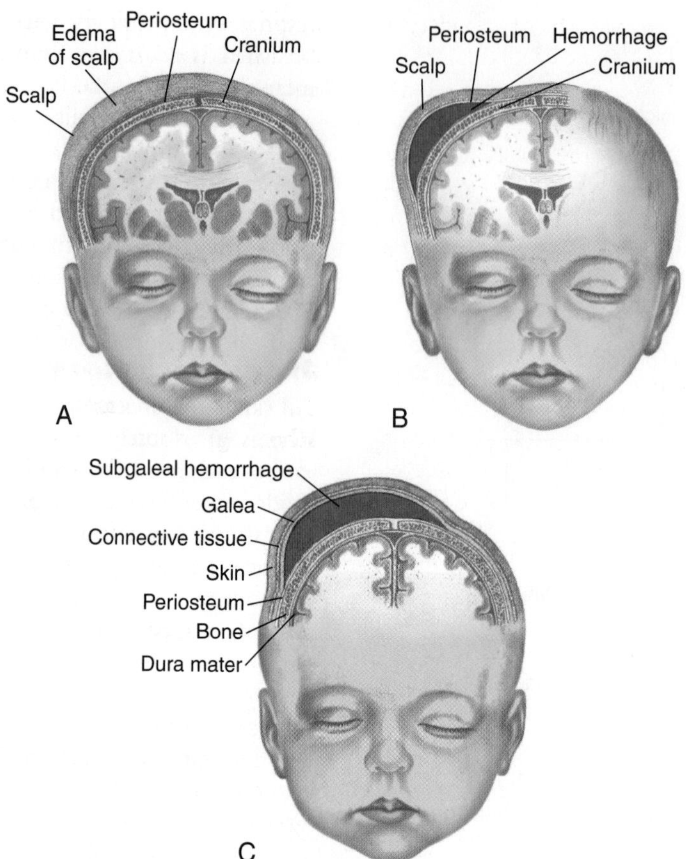

Fig. 16-4 **A,** Caput succedaneum. **B,** Cephalhematoma. **C,** Subgaleal hemorrhage. (**A** and **C** From Seidel, H. M., Ball J. W., Dains, J. E., & Benedict, G. W. [2006]. *Mosby's guide to physical examination* [6th ed.]. St. Louis: Mosby.)

Bleeding may occur with spontaneous birth from pressure against the maternal bony pelvis. Low forceps birth and difficult forceps rotation and extraction may also cause bleeding. This soft, fluctuating, irreducible fullness does not pulsate or bulge when the infant cries. It appears several hours or the day after birth and may not become apparent until a caput succedaneum is absorbed. A cephalhematoma is usually largest on the second or third day, by which time the bleeding stops. The fullness of a cephalhematoma spontaneously resolves in 3 to 6 weeks. It is not aspirated because infection may develop if the skin is punctured. As the hematoma resolves, hemolysis of RBCs occurs, and jaundice may result. Hyperbilirubinemia and jaundice may occur after the newborn is discharged home.

Subgaleal hemorrhage

Subgaleal hemorrhage is bleeding into the subgaleal compartment (Fig. 16-4, *C*). The subgaleal compartment is a potential space that contains loosely arranged connective tissue; it is located beneath the galea aponeurosis, the tendinous sheath that connects the frontal and occipital muscles and forms the inner surface of the scalp. The injury occurs as a result of forces that compress and then drag the head through the pelvic outlet (Paige & Moe, 2006). Researchers have reported concern regarding the increased use of the vacuum extractor at birth and an association with cases of subgaleal hemorrhage, neonatal morbidity, and deaths (Boo, Foong, Mahdy, Yong, & Jaafar, 2005: Uchil & Arulkumaran, 2003). The bleeding extends beyond bone, often posteriorly into the neck, and continues after birth, with the potential for serious complications such as anemia or hypovolemic shock.

Early detection of the hemorrhage is vital; serial head circumference measurements and inspection of the back of the neck for increasing edema and a firm mass are essential. A boggy scalp, pallor, tachycardia, and increasing head circumference may also be early signs of a subgaleal hemorrhage (Doumouchtsis & Arulkumaran, 2006). Computed tomography or magnetic resonance imaging is useful in confirming the diagnosis. Replacement of lost blood and clotting factors is required in acute cases of hemorrhage. Another possible early sign of subgaleal hemorrhage is a forward and lateral positioning of the infant's ears because the hematoma extends posteriorly. Monitoring the infant for changes in level of consciousness and a decrease in the hematocrit are also key to early recognition and management. An increase in serum bilirubin levels may be seen as a result of the breakdown of blood cells within the hematoma.

Sweat glands

Sweat glands are present at birth but do not respond to increases in ambient or body temperature. Some fetal sebaceous gland hyperplasia and secretion of sebum result from the hormonal influences of pregnancy. Vernix caseosa is a product of the sebaceous glands. Removal of the vernix is followed by desquamation of the epidermis in most infants. Vernix has been shown to be an epidermal barrier with positive benefits for neonatal skin such as decreasing the skin pH, decreased skin erythema, and improved skin hydration (Visscher et al., 2005). Distended, small, white sebaceous glands (**milia**) may be noticeable on the newborn face.

Desquamation

Desquamation (peeling) of the skin of the term infant does not occur until a few days after birth. Large generalized areas of skin desquamation present at birth may be an indication of postmaturity.

Mongolian spots

Mongolian spots, bluish-black areas of pigmentation, may appear over any part of the exterior surface of the body, including the extremities. They are more commonly noted on the back and buttocks (Fig. 16-5). These pigmented areas are most frequently noted in newborns whose ethnic origins are in the Mediterranean area, Latin America, Asia, or Africa. They are more common in dark-skinned individuals but may occur in 5% to 13% of Caucasians as well (Blackburn, 2007). They fade gradually over months or years.

Nevi

Telangiectatic nevi, known as "stork bites," are pink and easily blanched (Fig. 16-6, *A*). They appear on the upper eyelids, nose, upper lip, lower occipital area, and nape of the neck. They have no clinical significance and fade by the second year of life.

The nevus vasculosus is a common type of capillary hemangioma. It consists of dilated, newly formed capillaries occupying the entire dermal and subdermal layers, with associated connective tissue hypertrophy. The typical lesion is a raised, sharply demarcated, bright- or dark-red, rough-surfaced swelling. As the infant grows the hemangioma may proliferate and become more vascular, thereby often being called a *strawberry hemangioma.* Lesions are usually single but may be multiple, with 75% occurring on the head. These lesions can remain until the child is of school age or sometimes even longer but can be removed successfully with pulsed dye laser therapy, interferon therapy, and prednisone administration. In some cases, subcutaneous injections of interferon alfa-2a or interferon alfa-2b may be required if prednisone therapy and the pulsed dye laser fail to control a problematic hemangioma.

A port-wine stain, or nevus flammeus, is usually observed at birth and is composed of a plexus of newly formed capillaries in the papillary layer of the corium. It is red to purple; varies in size, shape, and location; and is not elevated. True port-wine stains do not blanch on pressure or disappear. They are most commonly found on the face and neck.

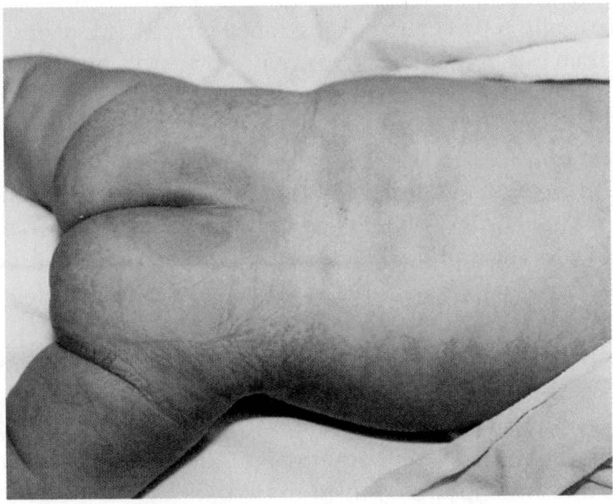

Fig. 16-5 Mongolian spot.

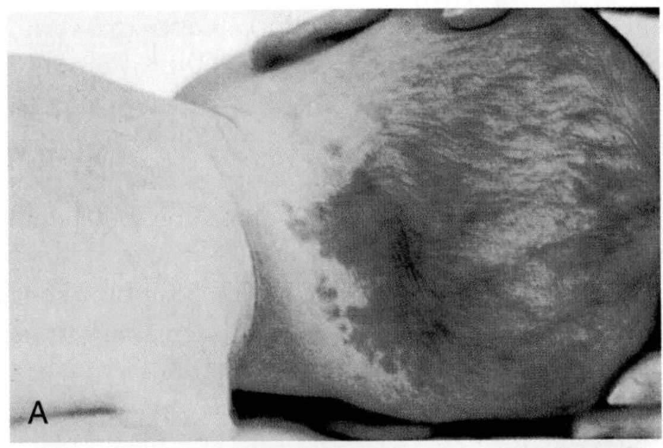

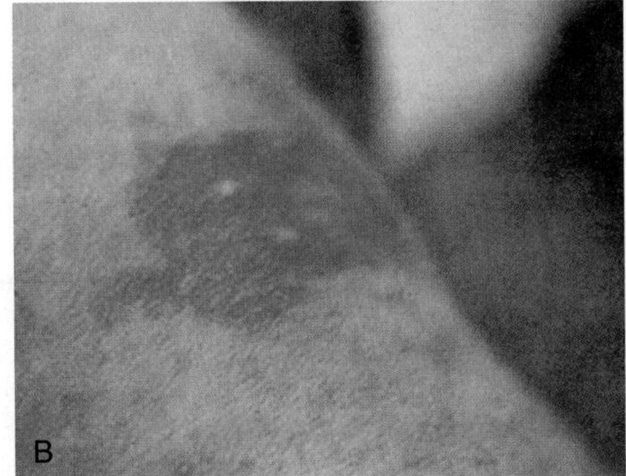

Fig. 16-6 **A,** Telangiectatic nevi (stork bite). **B,** Erythema toxicum (flea bite). (Courtesy Mead Johnson & Co., Evansville, IN.)

Erythema toxicum

A transient rash, **erythema toxicum,** is also called *erythema neonatorum, newborn rash,* or *flea bite dermatitis.* It is found in term neonates during the first 3 weeks of life. Erythema toxicum produces lesions in different stages: erythematous macules, papules, and small vesicles (Fig. 16-6, *B*). The lesions may appear suddenly anywhere on the body. The rash is thought to be an inflammatory response. Eosinophils, which help decrease inflammation, are found in the vesicles. Although the appearance is alarming, the rash has no clinical significance and requires no treatment.

Reproductive System

Female

At birth the ovaries contain thousands of primitive germ cells. These cells represent the full complement of potential ova; no oogonia form after birth in term infants. The ovarian cortex, which is made up primarily of primordial follicles, occupies a larger portion of the ovary in the newborn female than in the adult female. From birth to sexual maturity the number of ova decreases by approximately 90%.

An increase of estrogen during pregnancy followed by a decrease after birth results in a mucoid vaginal discharge and even some slight bloody spotting (pseudomenstruation). External genitals (i.e., labia majora and minora) are usually edematous with increased pigmentation. In term infants the labia majora and minora cover the vestibule (Fig. 16-7, *A*). In preterm infants, the clitoris is prominent, and the labia majora are small and widely separated. Vaginal or hymenal tags are common findings and have no clinical significance. Vernix caseosa may be present between the labia and should not be forcibly removed during bathing.

If the infant was born in the breech position, the labia may be edematous and bruised. The edema and bruising resolve in a few days; no treatment is necessary.

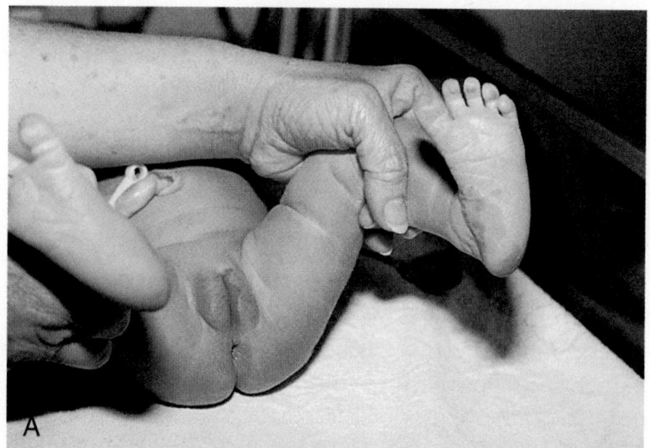

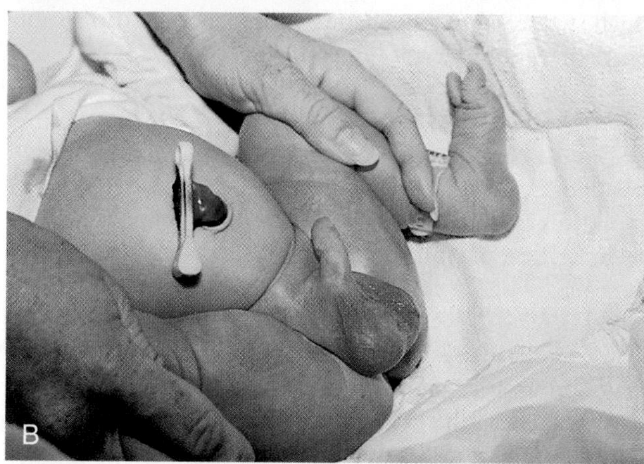

Fig. 16-7 External genitalia. **A,** Genitals in female term infant. Note mucoid vaginal discharge. **B,** Genitals in male infant. Uncircumcised penis. Rugae cover scrotum, indicating term gestation. Cord has been swabbed with ethylene blue to prevent infection. (Courtesy Marjorie Pyle, RNC, Lifecircle, Costa Mesa, CA.)

Male

The testes descend into the scrotum by birth in 90% of newborn boys. Although this percentage decreases with premature birth, by 1 year of age the incidence of undescended testes in all boys is less than 1%.

A tight prepuce (foreskin) is common in newborns. The urethral opening may be completely covered by the prepuce, which may not be retractable for 3 to 4 years. Smegma, a white, cheesy substance, is commonly found under the foreskin. Small, white, firm lesions called *epithelial pearls* may be seen at the tip of the prepuce. In the preterm male infant of less than 28 weeks of gestation the testes remain within the abdominal cavity and the scrotum appears high and close to the body. By 28 to 36 weeks of gestation the testes can be palpated in the inguinal canal, and a few rugae appear on the scrotum. At 36 to 40 weeks of gestation the testes are palpable in the upper scrotum, and rugae appear on the anterior portion. After 40 weeks the testes can be palpated in the scrotum, and rugae cover the scrotal sac. The postterm neonate has deep rugae and a pendulous scrotum. The scrotum is usually more deeply pigmented than the rest of the skin (Fig. 16-7, *B*) and is especially apparent in darker-skinned infants. This pigmentation is a response to maternal estrogen. A hydrocele, caused by an accumulation of fluid around the testes, may be present. It can be transilluminated with a light and usually decreases in size without treatment.

If the male infant is born in a breech presentation, the scrotum can be very edematous and bruised (Fig. 16-8). The swelling and discoloration subside within a few days.

Swelling of breast tissue

Swelling of the breast tissue in term infants of both sexes is caused by the hyperestrogenism of pregnancy. In a few infants a thin discharge (witch's milk) can be seen. This finding has no clinical significance, requires no treatment, and subsides within a few days as the maternal hormones are eliminated from the infant's body.

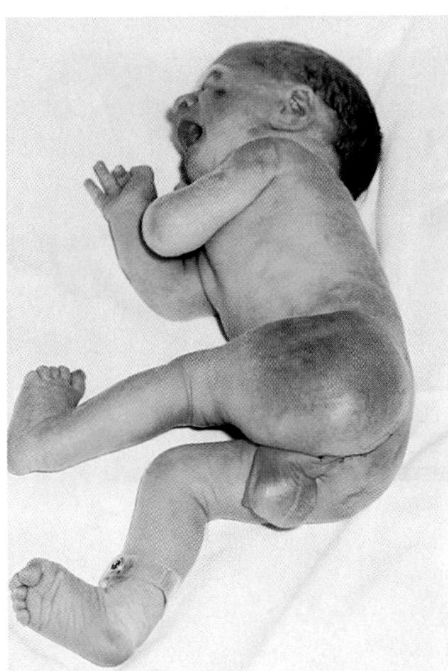

Fig. 16-8 Swelling of the genitals and bruising of the buttocks after a breech birth. (From O'Doherty, N. [1986]. *Neonatology: Micro atlas of the newborn.* Nutley, NJ: Hoffman-LaRoche.)

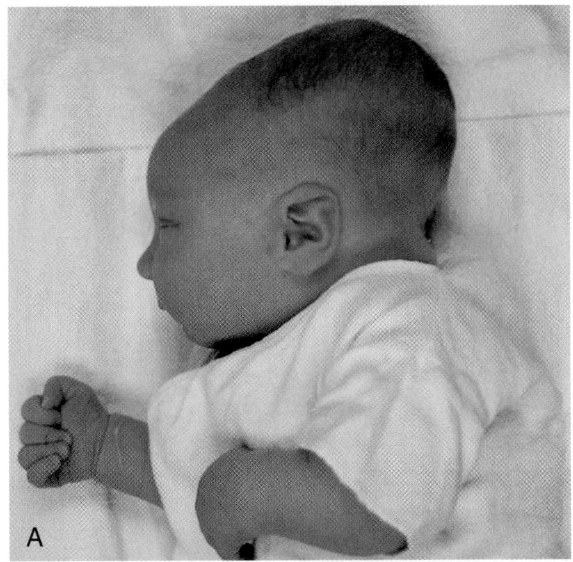

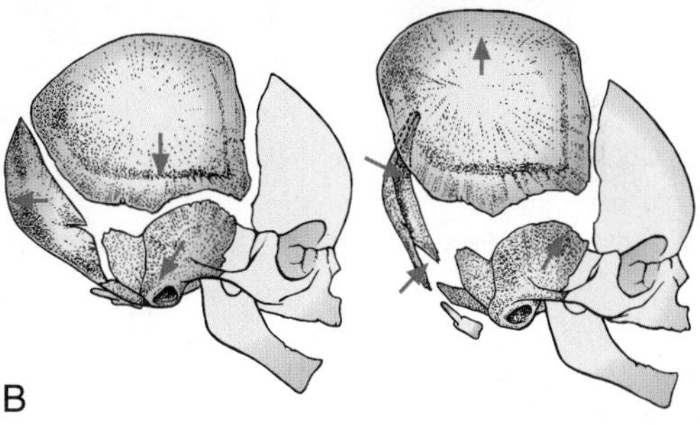

Fig. 16-9 Molding. **A**, Significant molding, soon after birth. **B**, Schematic of bones of skull when molding is present. (**A**, Courtesy Kim Molloy, Knoxville, IA.)

The nipples should be symmetric on the chest. Breast tissue and areola size increase with gestation. The areola appears slightly elevated at 34 weeks of gestation. By 36 weeks a breast bud of 1 to 2 mm is palpable and increases to 12 mm by 42 weeks.

Skeletal System

The infant's skeletal system undergoes rapid development during the first year of life. At birth, more cartilage is present than ossified bone. Because of cephalocaudal (head-to-rump) development the newborn appears somewhat out of proportion.

At term the head is one fourth of the total body length. The arms are slightly longer than the legs. In the newborn the legs are one third of the total body length but only 15% of the total body weight. As growth proceeds the midpoint in head-to-toe measurements gradually descends from the level of the umbilicus at birth to the level of the symphysis pubis at maturity.

The face appears small in relation to the skull, which appears large and heavy. Cranial size and shape can be distorted by molding (the shaping of the fetal head by the overlapping of cranial bones to facilitate movement through the birth canal during labor) (Fig. 16-9).

The bones in the vertebral column of the newborn form two primary curvatures–one in the thoracic region and one in the sacral region. Both are forward, concave curvatures. As the infant gains head control at approximately age 3 months, a secondary curvature appears in the cervical region.

Some newborns exhibit a significant separation of the knees when the ankles are held together, resulting in an appearance of bowlegs. At birth, no apparent arch to the foot is seen. The extremities should be symmetric and of equal length. Skin folds should be equal and symmetric. The hips are checked for dysplasia by a trained clinician using the Ortolani maneuver (Fig. 16-10). Fingers and toes should be equal in number and have nails. Extra digits (polydactyly) are sometimes found on the hands and feet. Fingers or toes may be fused (syndactyly). Creases can be found on the palms of the hands and cover the soles of the term newborn's feet. If the infant's presentation was breech, the knees may remain extended and the infant will maintain the in utero position for several weeks (Fig. 16-11).

Two reflexes are elicited, the grasp reflex and the Babinski reflex. To assess the grasp reflex, the palms of the hands or soles of the feet are touched near the base of the digits; this causes flexion or grasping (Fig. 16-12). To assess the *Babinski reflex,* the outer sole of the foot is stroked upward from the heel across the ball of the foot; this causes the big toe to dorsiflex and the other toes to hyperextend (Table 16-3).

The newborn's spine appears straight and can be flexed easily. The vertebrae should appear straight and flat. The base of the spine should be free from a dimple. If a dimple

Text continued on p. 457.

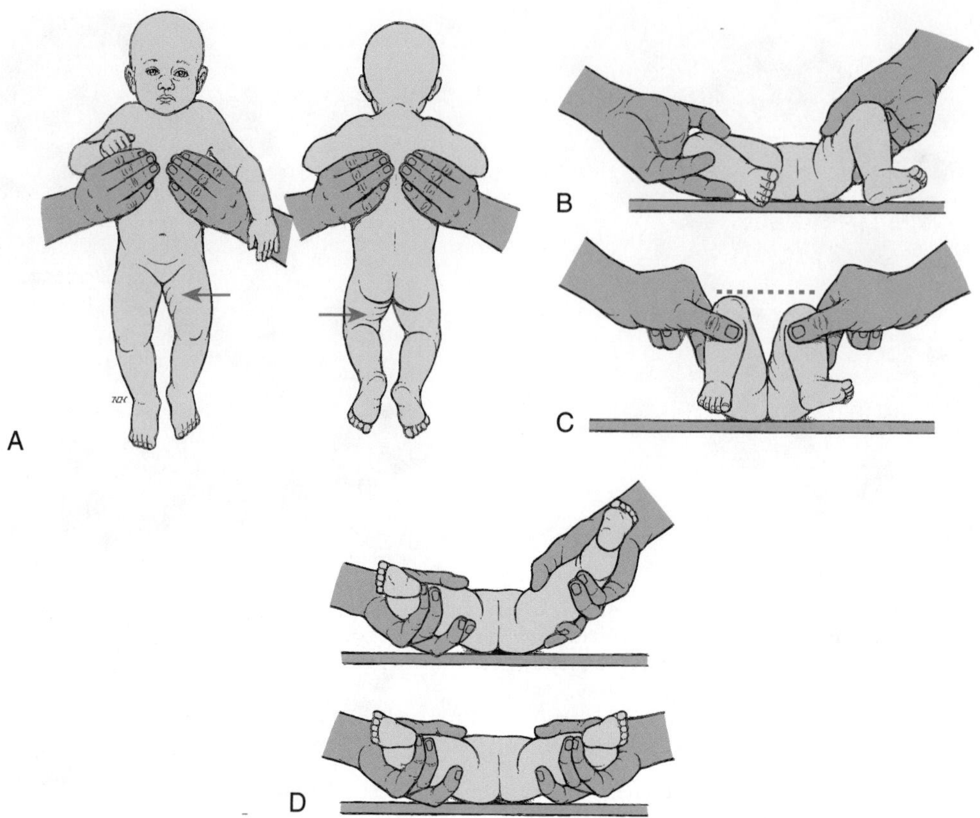

Fig. 16-10 Signs of developmental dysplasia of the hip. **A,** Asymmetry of gluteal and thigh folds with shortening of the thigh (Galeazzi sign). **B,** Limited hip abduction, as seen in flexion (Ortolani test). **C,** Apparent shortening of the femur, as indicated by the level of the knees in flexion (Allis sign). **D,** Ortolani test with femoral head moving in and out of acetabulum (in infants 1 to 2 months of age). (From Hockenberry, M. J. & Wilson, D. [2009]. *Wong's essentials of pediatric nursing* [8th ed.]. St. Louis: Mosby.)

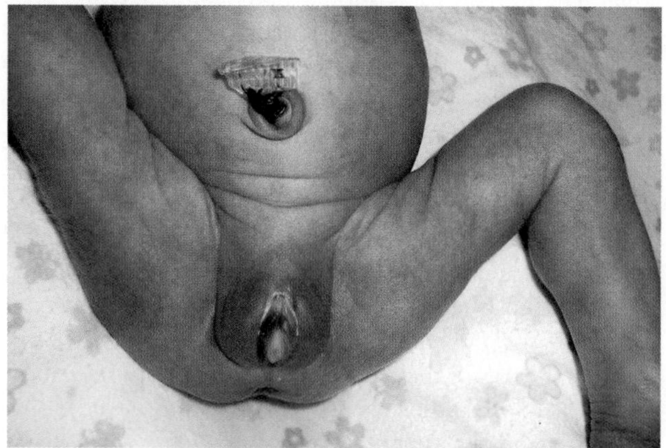

Fig. 16-11 Position of infant's legs after breech birth. (Courtesy Cheryl Briggs, RN, Annapolis, MD.)

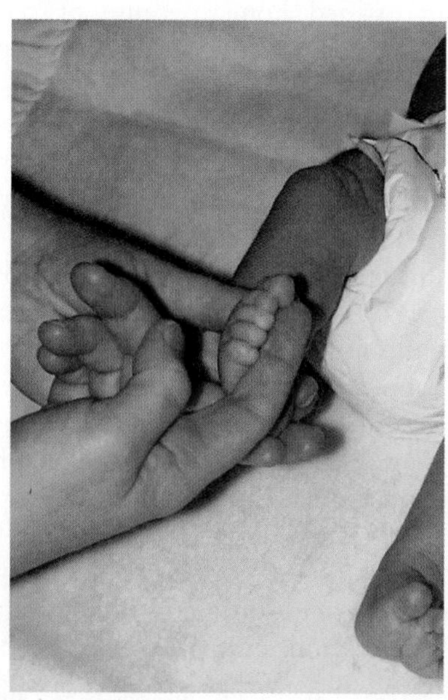

Fig. 16-12 Plantar grasp reflex. (From Zitelli, B. J. & Davis, H. W. [2007]. *Atlas of pediatric physical diagnosis* [6th ed.]. St. Louis: Mosby.)

TABLE 16-3

Assessment of Newborn's Reflexes

REFLEX	ELICITING THE REFLEX	CHARACTERISTIC RESPONSE	COMMENTS
Sucking and rooting	Touch infant's lip, cheek, or corner of mouth with nipple	Infant turns head toward stimulus, opens mouth, takes hold, and sucks	Response is difficult if not impossible to elicit after infant has been fed; if response is weak or absent, consider prematurity or neurologic defect Parental guidance: Avoid trying to turn head toward breast or nipple, allow infant to root; response disappears after 3 to 4* mo but may persist up to 1 yr If response is weak or absent, may indicate prematurity or neurologic defect
Swallowing	Feed infant; swallowing usually follows sucking and obtaining fluids	Swallowing is usually coordinated with sucking and usually occurs without gagging, coughing, or vomiting	Sucking and swallowing are often uncoordinated in preterm infant
Grasp:			
Palmar	Place finger in palm of hand	Infant's fingers curl around examiner's fingers	Palmar response lessens by 3 to 4 mo; parents enjoy this contact with infant. Plantar response lessens by 8 mo
Plantar	Place finger at base of toes	Toes curl downward (see Fig. 16-12)	
Extrusion	Touch or depress tip of tongue	Newborn forces tongue outward	Response disappears about fourth month of life
Glabellar (Myerson sign)	Tap over forehead, bridge of nose, or maxilla of newborn whose eyes are open	Newborn blinks for first four or five taps	Continued blinking with repeated taps is consistent with extrapyramidal disorder
Tonic neck or "fencing"	With infant falling asleep or sleeping, turn head quickly to one side	With infant facing left side, arm and leg on that side extend; opposite arm and leg flex (turn head to right, and extremities assume opposite postures)	Responses in leg are more consistent Complete response disappears by 3 to 4 mo, incomplete response may be seen until third or fourth year After 6 wk, persistent response is sign of possible cerebral palsy

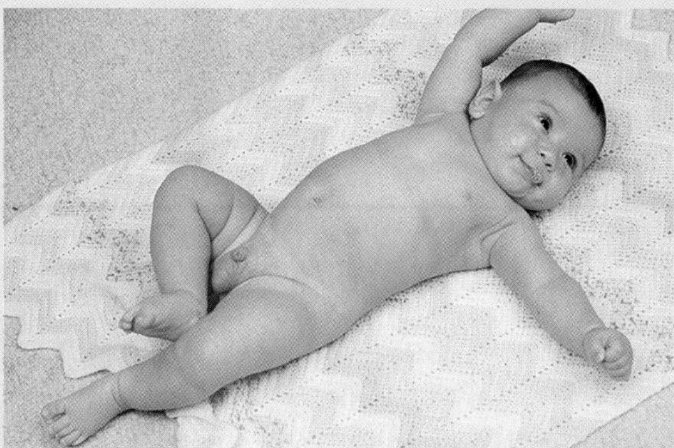

Classic pose in spontaneous tonic neck reflex. (Courtesy Marjorie Pyle, RNC, Lifecircle, Costa Mesa, CA.)

*All durations for persistence of reflexes are based on time elapsed after 40 weeks of gestation; that is, if this newborn was born at 36 weeks of gestation, add 1 month to all time limits given.

Continued

Assessment Video: Rooting and Sucking

Assessment Video: Plantar Grasp

Assessment Video: Moro Reflex

TABLE 16-3

Assessment of Newborn's Reflexes—cont'd

REFLEX	ELICITING THE REFLEX	CHARACTERISTIC RESPONSE	COMMENTS
Moro	Hold infant in semisitting position, allow head and trunk to fall backward to an angle of at least 30 degrees Place infant on flat surface, strike surface to startle infant	Symmetric abduction and extension of arms are seen; fingers fan out and form a C with thumb and forefinger; slight tremor may be noted; arms are adducted in embracing motion and return to relaxed flexion and movement Legs may follow similar pattern of response Preterm infant does not complete "embrace"; instead, arms fall backward because of weakness	Response is present at birth; complete response may be seen until 8 wk; body jerk is seen only between 8 and 18 wk; response is absent by 6 mo if neurologic maturation is not delayed; response may be incomplete if infant is deeply asleep; give parental guidance about normal response Asymmetric response may connote injury to brachial plexus, clavicle, or humerus Persistent response after 6 mo indicates possible brain damage
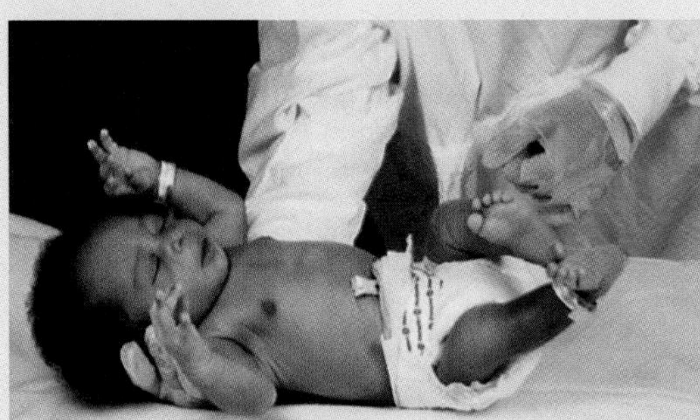 Moro reflex. (From Dickason, E., Silverman, B., & Kaplan, J. [1998]. *Maternal-infant nursing care* [3rd ed.]. St. Louis; Mosby.)			
Stepping or "walking"	Hold infant vertically, allowing one foot to touch table surface	Infant will simulate walking, alternating flexion and extension of feet; term infants walk on soles of their feet, and preterm infants walk on their toes	Response is normally present for 3 to 4 wk
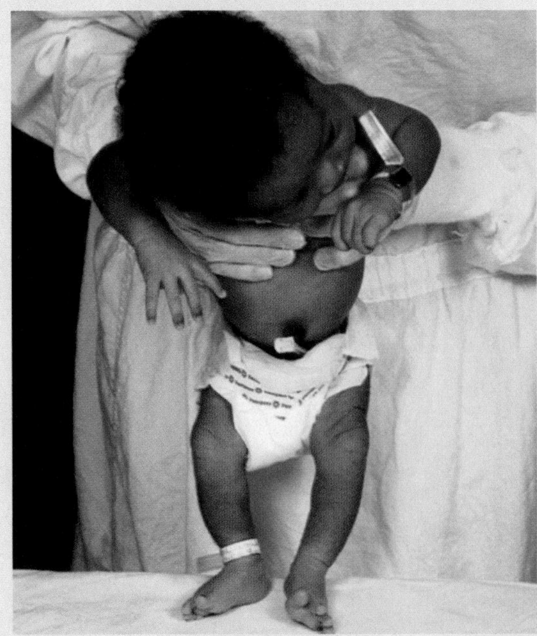 Stepping reflex. (From Dickason, E., Silverman, B., & Kaplan, J. [1998]. *Maternal-infant nursing care* [3rd ed.]. St. Louis: Mosby.)			

TABLE 16-3

Assessment of Newborn's Reflexes—cont'd

REFLEX	ELICITING THE REFLEX	CHARACTERISTIC RESPONSE	COMMENTS
Crawling	Place newborn on abdomen	Newborn makes crawling movements with arms and legs	Response should disappear about 6 wk of age
Deep tendon	Use finger instead of percussion hammer to elicit patellar, or knee jerk, reflex; newborn must be relaxed	Reflex jerk is present; even with newborn relaxed, nonselective overall reaction may occur	
Crossed extension	Infant should be supine; extend one leg, press knee downward, stimulate bottom of foot; observe opposite leg	Opposite leg flexes, adducts, and then extends	This reflex should be present during newborn period.

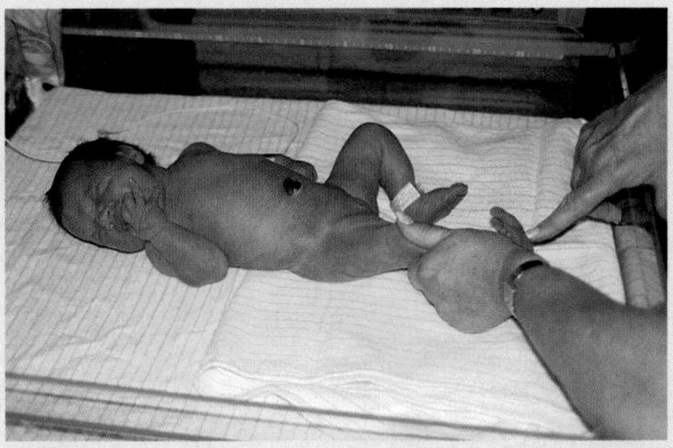

Crossed extension reflex. (Courtesy Marjorie Pyle, RNC, Lifecircle, Costa Mesa, CA.)

REFLEX	ELICITING THE REFLEX	CHARACTERISTIC RESPONSE	COMMENTS
Startle	Perform sharp hand clap; best elicited if newborn is 24 to 36 hr old or older	Arms abduct with flexion of elbows, hands stay clenched	Response should disappear by 4 mo of age Response is elicited more readily in preterm newborn (inform parents of this characteristic)
Babinski sign (plantar)	On sole of foot, beginning at heel, stroke upward along lateral aspect of sole, then move finger across ball of foot	All toes hyperextend, with dorsiflexion of big toe; recorded as a positive sign	Absence requires neurologic evaluation, should disappear after 1 yr of age

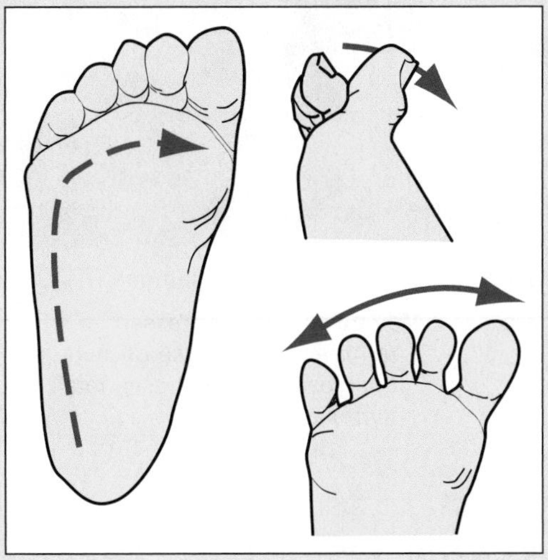

Babinski reflex. (From Hockenberry, M., et al. [2007]. *Wong's nursing care of infants and children* [8th ed.]. St. Louis: Mosby.)

Continued

TABLE 16-3

Assessment of Newborn's Reflexes—cont'd

REFLEX	ELICITING THE REFLEX	CHARACTERISTIC RESPONSE	COMMENTS
Pull-to-sit (traction)	Pull infant up by wrists from supine position with head in midline	Head will lag until infant is in upright position, then head will be held in same plane with chest and shoulder momentarily before falling forward; infant will attempt to right head	Response depends on general muscle tone and maturity and condition of infant
Trunk incurvation (Galant)	Place infant prone on flat surface, run finger down back about 4 to 5 cm lateral to spine, first on one side and then down other	Trunk is flexed, and pelvis is swung toward stimulated side	Response disappears by fourth week Response may vary but should be obtainable in all infants, including preterm ones. Absence suggests general depression of nervous system With transverse lesions of cord, no response below the level of the lesion is present.
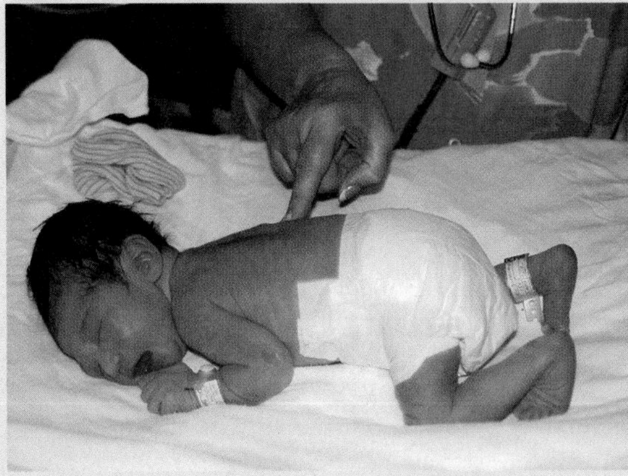 Trunk incurvation reflex. (Courtesy Marjorie Pyle, RNC, Lifecircle, Costa Mesa, CA.)			
Magnet	Place infant in supine position, partially flex both lower extremities, and apply pressure to soles of feet	Both lower limbs should extend against examiner's pressure	Absence suggests damage to spinal cord or malformation Reflex may be weak or exaggerated after breech birth
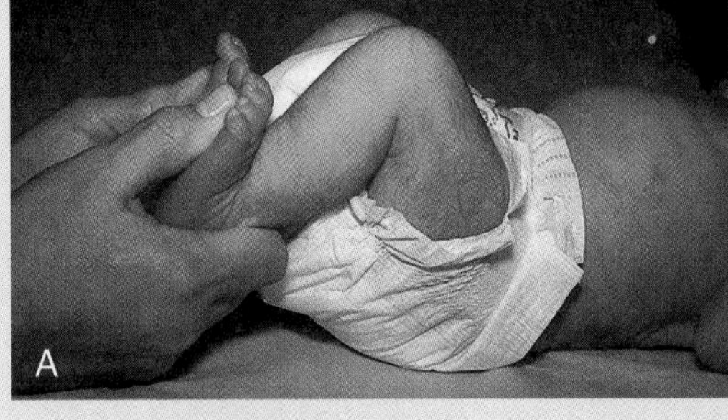 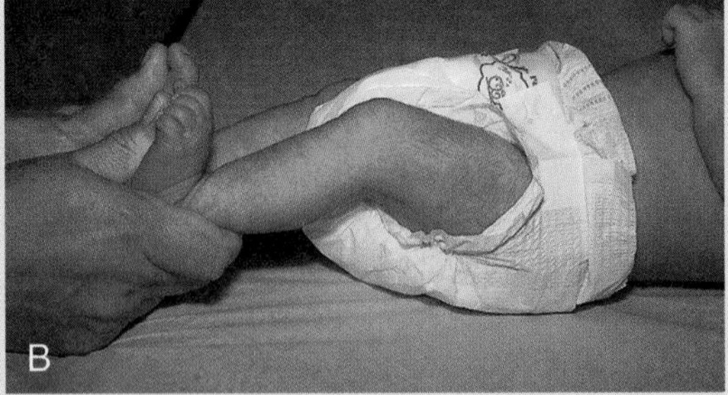 Magnet reflex. (Courtesy Michael S. Clement, M.D., Mesa, AZ.)			
Additional newborn responses: yawn, stretch, burp, hiccup, sneeze	These responses are spontaneous behaviors	May be slightly depressed temporarily because of maternal analgesia or anesthesia, fetal hypoxia, or infection	Parental guidance: most of these behaviors are pleasurable to parents Parents need to be assured that behaviors are normal Sneeze is usually response to lint, etc., in nose and not an indicator of a cold No treatment is needed for hiccups; sucking may help

is noted, further inspection is required to determine whether a sinus is present. A pilonidal dimple, especially with a sinus and nevus pilosis (hairy nevus), can be associated with spina bifida.

Neuromuscular System

The neuromuscular system is almost completely developed at birth. The term newborn is a responsive and reactive being with remarkable capacity for social interaction and self-organization.

Growth of the brain after birth follows a predictable pattern of rapid growth during infancy and early childhood, and growth becomes more gradual during the remainder of the first decade and minimal during adolescence. By the end of the first year, the cerebellum ends its growth spurt which began at approximately 30 gestational weeks.

The brain requires glucose as a source of energy and a relatively large supply of oxygen for adequate metabolism. Such requirements signal a need for careful assessment of the infant's respiratory status. The necessity for glucose requires attentiveness to those neonates who are at risk for hypoglycemia (e.g., infants of diabetic mothers, infants who are macrosomic or small for gestational age, and newborns experiencing prolonged birth, hypoxia, or preterm birth).

Spontaneous motor activity can be seen as transient tremors of the mouth and chin, especially during crying episodes, and of the extremities, notably the arms and hands. Transient tremors are normal and can be observed in nearly every newborn. These tremors should not be present when the infant is quiet and should not persist beyond 1 month of age. Persistent tremors or tremors involving the total body can indicate pathologic conditions. Normal tremors, tremors of hypoglycemia, and central nervous system (CNS) disorders must be differentiated so corrective care can be instituted as necessary.

Neuromuscular control, although very limited, can be noted. If newborns are placed face down on a firm surface, they will turn their heads to the side. They attempt to hold their heads in line with their bodies if they are raised by their arms. Various reflexes serve to promote safety and adequate food intake.

Newborn reflexes

The newborn has many primitive reflexes. The times at which these reflexes appear and disappear reflect the maturity and intactness of the developing nervous system. The most common reflexes found in the normal newborn are described in Table 16-3 (pp. 453-456).

PHYSICAL ASSESSMENT

The assessment of the newborn should progress in a systematic manner, with evaluation and assessment of each system (e.g., respiratory, cardiovascular). Experts recommend that assessment of features (e.g., observing general color and posture, auscultating heart tones and breath sounds) that least disturb the newborn be conducted first and then proceed in a head-to-toe manner once the newborn is awake and active. The findings provide a database for implementing the nursing process with newborns and for providing anticipatory guidance for the parents. An immediate assessment of the newborn is carried out to evaluate the infant's transition to extrauterine life. The Apgar score (see Chapter 17), determined at 1 and 5 minutes, provides information that must be considered in the context of data from the total assessment.

A complete physical examination should be performed within 24 hours after birth, after the newborn's temperature stabilizes or while under a radiant warmer. The area used for examination should be well-lighted, warm, and free from drafts. The infant is undressed as needed and placed on a firm, warmed, flat surface. The physical assessment should begin with a review of the maternal history and prenatal and intrapartal records, providing a background for the recognition of any potential problems. This assessment also includes general appearance, behavior, vital signs measurements, and maternal-infant interactions. Descriptions of any variations from normal and all abnormal findings are included (Table 16-4). Ongoing assessments of the newborn are made and an evaluation is performed before discharge.

General Appearance

The neonate's maturity level can be gauged by assessment of general appearance. Features to assess in the general survey include posture, activity, any overt signs of anomalies that may cause initial distress, presence of bruising or other consequences of delivery, and state of alertness. The normal resting position of the neonate is one of general flexion (Fig. 16-13).

Vital Signs

The temperature, heart rate, and respiratory rate are always obtained. BP is not assessed unless cardiac problems are

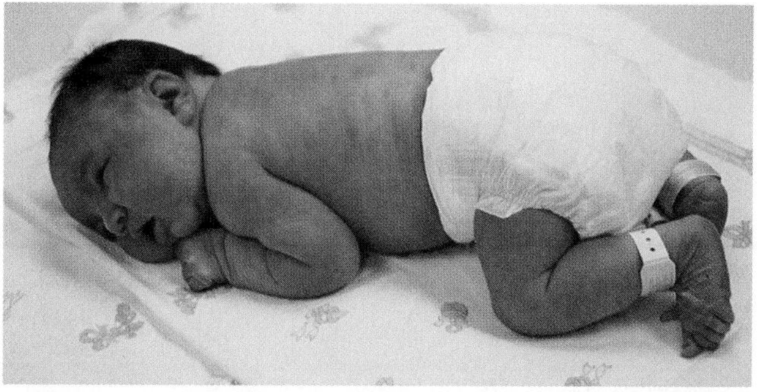

Fig. 16-13 Newborn in position of flexion in prone position while awake. (From Hockenberry, M. J. & Wilson, D. [2007]. *Wong's nursing care of infants and children,* [8th ed.]. St. Louis: Mosby.)

Text continued on p. 472.

TABLE 16-4

Physical Assessment of Newborn

AREA ASSESSED AND APPRAISAL PROCEDURE	NORMAL FINDINGS: AVERAGE FINDINGS	NORMAL FINDINGS: NORMAL VARIATIONS	DEVIATIONS FROM NORMAL RANGE: POSSIBLE PROBLEMS (ETIOLOGY)
POSTURE			
Inspect newborn before disturbing for assessment. Refer to maternal chart for fetal presentation, position, and type of birth (vaginal, surgical), given that newborn readily assumes in utero position.	Vertex: arms, legs in moderate flexion; fists clenched Resistance to having extremities extended for examination or measurement, crying possible when attempted Cessation of crying when allowed to resume curled-up fetal position (lateral) Normal spontaneous movement bilaterally asynchronous (legs moving in bicycle fashion) but equal extension in all extremities	Frank breech: legs straighter and stiff, newborn assuming intrauterine position in repose for a few days Prenatal pressure on limb or shoulder possibly causing temporary facial asymmetry or resistance to extension of extremities	Hypotonia, relaxed posture while awake (preterm or hypoxia in utero, maternal medications, neuromuscular disorder such as spinal muscular atrophy) Hypertonia (chemical dependence, central nervous system [CNS] disorder) Limitation of motion in any of extremities (see Skeletal System, p. 451 and Extremities, pp. 470-472)
VITAL SIGNS			
Check heart rate and pulses: Thorax (chest) Inspection Palpation Auscultation Apex: mitral valve Second interspace, left of sternum: pulmonic valve Second interspace, right of sternum: aortic valve Junction of xiphoid process and sternum: tricuspid valve	Visible pulsations in left midclavicular line, fifth intercostal space Apical pulse, fourth intercostal space 100-160 beats/min Quality: *first sound* (closure of mitral and tricuspid valves) and *second sound* (closure of aortic and pulmonic valves) sharp and clear	80-100 beats/min (sleeping) to 180 beats/min (crying); possibly irregular for brief periods, especially after crying Murmur, especially over base or at left sternal border in interspace 3 or 4 (foramen ovale anatomically closing at approximately 1 yr)	Tachycardia: persistent, ≥180 beats/min (respiratory distress syndrome [RDS]; pneumonia) Bradycardia: persistent, ≤80 beats/min (congenital heart block, maternal lupus) Murmur (possibly functional) Arrhythmias: irregular rate Sounds: Distant (pneumopericardium) Poor quality Extra Heart on right side of chest (dextrocardia, often accompanied by reversal of intestines)
Peripheral pulses: femoral, brachial, popliteal, posterior tibial	Peripheral pulses equal and strong		Weak or absent peripheral (decreased cardiac output, thrombus, possible coarctation of aorta if weak on left and strong on right) Bounding

TABLE 16-4

Physical Assessment of Newborn—cont'd

AREA ASSESSED AND APPRAISAL PROCEDURE	NORMAL FINDINGS		DEVIATIONS FROM NORMAL RANGE: POSSIBLE PROBLEMS (ETIOLOGY)
	AVERAGE FINDINGS	NORMAL VARIATIONS	
Obtain temperature: Axillary: method of choice Temporal and intraauricular thermometers are not effective in measuring newborn temperature.	Axillary: 37° C Temperature stabilized by 8-10 hr of age	36.5°-37.5° C Heat loss: from evaporation, conduction, convection, radiation	Subnormal (preterm birth, infection, low environmental temperature, inadequate clothing, dehydration) Increased (infection, high environmental temperature, excessive clothing, proximity to heating unit or in direct sunshine, chemical dependence, diarrhea and dehydration) Temperature not stabilized by 6-8 hr after birth (if mother received magnesium sulfate, newborn less able to conserve heat by vasoconstriction; maternal analgesics possibly reducing thermal stability in newborn)
Observe and monitor respiratory rate and effort:			
Observe respirations when infant is at rest Count respirations for full minute Listen for sounds audible without stethoscope Observe respiratory effort	40/min Tendency to be shallow and irregular in rate, rhythm, and depth when infant is awake Crackles may be heard after birth No adventitious sounds audible on inspiration and expiration Breath sounds: bronchial: loud, clear	30-60/min Short periodic breathing episodes and no evidence of respiratory distress or apnea (>20 seconds); periodic breathing, First period (reactivity): 50-60/min Second period: 50-70/min Stabilization (1-2 days): 30-40/min Crackles (fine)	Apneic episodes: >20 sec (preterm infant: rapid warming or cooling of infant; CNS or blood glucose instability) Bradypnea: <25/min (maternal narcosis from analgesics or anesthetics, birth trauma) Tachypnea: >60/min (RDS, transient tachypnea of the newborn, congenital diaphragmatic hernia) Breath Sounds: Crackles (coarse), rhonchi, wheezing Expiratory grunt (narrowing of bronchi) Distress evidenced by nasal flaring, grunting, retractions, labored breathing Stridor (upper airway occlusion)

Continued

TABLE 16-4

Physical Assessment of Newborn—cont'd

AREA ASSESSED AND APPRAISAL PROCEDURE	NORMAL FINDINGS: AVERAGE FINDINGS	NORMAL FINDINGS: NORMAL VARIATIONS	DEVIATIONS FROM NORMAL RANGE: POSSIBLE PROBLEMS (ETIOLOGY)
Obtain blood pressure (BP) (usually not done in normal term infand) Check oscillometric monitor BP cuff: BP cuff width affects readings, use appropriately sized cuff and palpate brachial, popliteal, or posterior tibial pulse (depending on measurement site)	80s-90s/40s-50s (approximate ranges) At birth Systolic: 60-80 mm Hg Diastolic: 40-50 mm Hg At 10 days Systolic: 95-100 mm Hg Diastolic: 45-75 mm Hg	Variation with change in activity level: awake, crying, sleeping	Difference between upper and lower extremity pressures (coarctation of aorta) Hypotension (sepsis, hypovolemia) Hypertension (coarctation of aorta, renal involvement, thrombus)
WEIGHT*			
Put protective liner cloth or paper in place and adjust scale to 0 grams or pounds and ounces Weigh at same time each day Protect newborn from heat loss	Female 3400 g Male 3500 g Regaining of birth weight within first 2 weeks	2500-4000 g Acceptable weight loss: 10% or less in first 3-5 days Second baby weighing more than first (on average)	Weight ≤2500 g (preterm, small for gestational age, rubella syndrome) Weight ≥4000 g (large for gestational age, maternal diabetes, heredity—normal for these parents) Weight loss over 10% to 15% (growth failure, dehydration); assess breastfeeding success
Weighing the infant. Note that a hand is held over infant as a safety measure. The scale is covered to protect against cross-infection. (Courtesy Kim Molloy, Knoxville, IA.)			
LENGTH			
Measure length from top of head to heel; measuring is difficult in term infant because of presence of molding, incomplete extension of knees	50 cm	45-55 cm	<45 cm or >55 cm (chromosomal abnormality, heredity—normal for these parents); some syndromes present shorter than average limb length (skeletal dysplasias, achondroplasia)

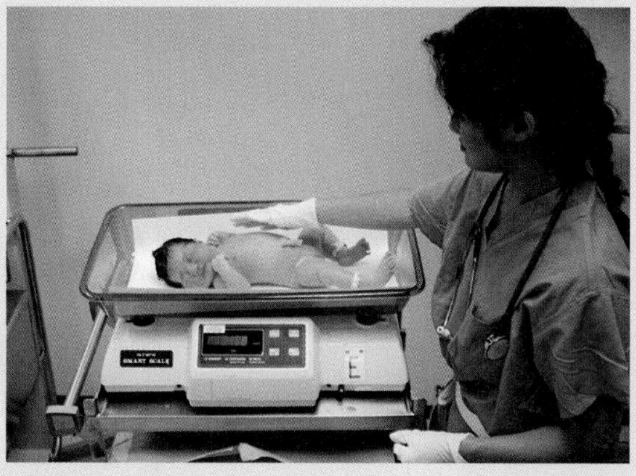

NOTE: Weight, length, and head circumference should all be close to the same percentile for any child.

TABLE 16-4

Physical Assessment of Newborn—cont'd

AREA ASSESSED AND APPRAISAL PROCEDURE	NORMAL FINDINGS: AVERAGE FINDINGS	NORMAL FINDINGS: NORMAL VARIATIONS	DEVIATIONS FROM NORMAL RANGE: POSSIBLE PROBLEMS (ETIOLOGY)
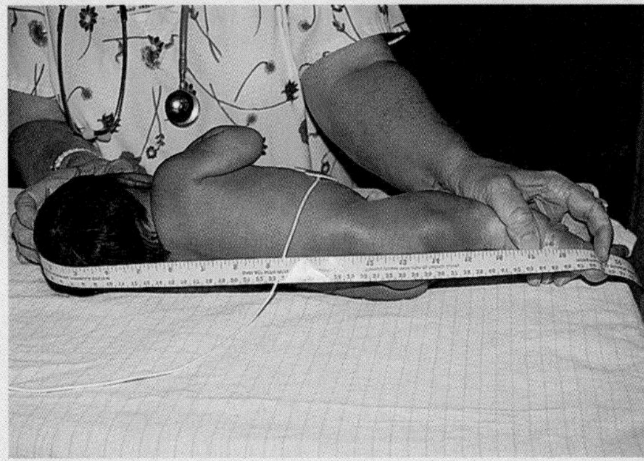 Measuring length, crown to heel. To determine total length, include length of legs. If measurements are taken before the infant's initial bath, wear gloves. (Courtesy Marjorie Pyle, RNC, Lifecircle, Costa Mesa, CA.)			
HEAD CIRCUMFERENCE			
Measure head at greatest diameter: occipitofrontal circumference May need to remeasure on second or third day after resolution of molding and caput succedaneum	33-35 cm Circumference of head and chest approximately the same for first 1 or 2 days after birth; chest rarely measured on routine basis	32-36.8 cm	Microcephaly, head ≤32 cm: (maternal rubella, toxoplasmosis, cytomegalovirus, fused cranial sutures [craniosynostosis]) Hydrocephaly: sutures widely separated, circumference ≥4 cm more than chest circumference (infection) Increased intracranial pressure (hemorrhage, space-occupying lesion)
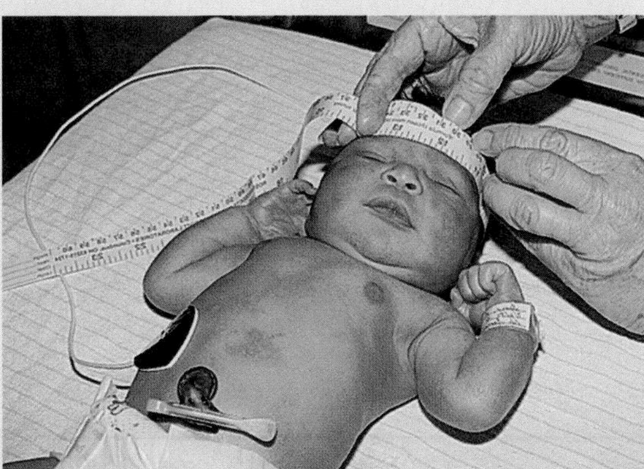 Measuring circumference of head. (Courtesy Marjorie Pyle, RNC, Lifecircle, Costa Mesa, CA.)			

Continued

TABLE 16-4

Physical Assessment of Newborn—cont'd

AREA ASSESSED AND APPRAISAL PROCEDURE	NORMAL FINDINGS		DEVIATIONS FROM NORMAL RANGE: POSSIBLE PROBLEMS (ETIOLOGY)
	AVERAGE FINDINGS	NORMAL VARIATIONS	
CHEST CIRCUMFERENCE			
Measure at nipple line	2-3 cm less than head circumference; averages between 30 and 33 cm	≤30 cm	Prematurity

Measuring circumference of chest. (Courtesy Marjorie Pyle, RNC, Lifecircle, Costa Mesa, CA.)

AREA ASSESSED AND APPRAISAL PROCEDURE	AVERAGE FINDINGS	NORMAL VARIATIONS	DEVIATIONS FROM NORMAL RANGE: POSSIBLE PROBLEMS (ETIOLOGY)
SKIN			
Check color Inspect and palpate Inspect semi-naked newborn in well-lighted, warm area without drafts; natural daylight best Inspect newborn when quiet and alert	Generally pink Varying with ethnic origin, skin pigmentation beginning to deepen right after birth in basal layer of epidermis Acrocyanosis common after birth	Mottling Harlequin sign Plethora Telangiectases ("stork bites" or capillary hemangiomas) (see Fig. 16-6, *A*) Erythema toxicum/neonatorum ("newborn rash") (see Fig. 16-6, *B*) Milia Petechiae over presenting part Ecchymoses from forceps in vertex births or over buttocks, genitalia, and legs in breech births	Dark red (preterm, polycythemia) Gray (hypotension, poor perfusion) Pallor (cardiovascular problem, CNS damage, blood dyscrasia, blood loss, twin-to-twin transfusion, infection) Cyanosis (hypothermia, infection, hypoglycemia, cardiopulmonary diseases, neurologic, or respiratory malformations) Generalized petechiae (clotting factor deficiency, infection) Generalized ecchymoses (hemorrhagic disease)
Observe for jaundice	None at birth	Physiologic jaundice in up to 60% of term infants in first week of life	Jaundice within first 24 hr (increased hemolysis, Rh isoimmunization, ABO incompatibility)
Observe for birthmarks or bruises: Inspect and palpate for location, size, distribution, characteristics, color, if obstructing airway or oral cavity		Mongolian spot (see Fig. 16-5) in infants of African-American, Asian, and Native-American origin	Hemangiomas Nevus flammeus: port-wine stain Nevus vasculosus: strawberry mark Cavernous hemangioma

TABLE 16-4

Physical Assessment of Newborn—cont'd

AREA ASSESSED AND APPRAISAL PROCEDURE	NORMAL FINDINGS: AVERAGE FINDINGS	NORMAL FINDINGS: NORMAL VARIATIONS	DEVIATIONS FROM NORMAL RANGE: POSSIBLE PROBLEMS (ETIOLOGY)
Check skin condition: Inspect and palpate for intactness, smoothness, texture, edema, pressure points if ill or immobilized	Confined to eyelid edema (result of eye prophylaxis) Opacity: few large blood vessels visible indistinctly over abdomen	Slightly thick; superficial cracking, peeling, especially of hands, feet No visible blood vessels, a few large vessels clearly visible over abdomen Some fingernail scratches	Edema on hands, feet; pitting over tibia; periorbital (over hydration; hydrops) Texture thin, smooth, or of medium thickness; rash or superficial peeling visible (preterm, postterm) Numerous vessels very visible over abdomen (preterm) Texture thick, parchment-like; cracking, peeling (postterm) Skin tags, webbing Papules, pustules, vesicles, ulcers, maceration (impetigo, candidiasis, herpes, diaper rash)
Weigh infant routinely Inspect and palpate Gently pinch skin between thumb and forefinger over abdomen and inner thigh to check for turgor Note presence of subcutaneous fat deposits (adipose pads) over cheeks, buttocks	Dehydration: loss of weight best indicator After pinch released, skin returns to original state immediately	Normal weight loss after birth: up to 10% of birth weight Possibly puffy Variation in amount of subcutaneous fat	Loose, wrinkled skin (prematurity, postmaturity, dehydration: fold of skin persisting after release of pinch) Tense, tight, shiny skin (edema, extreme cold, shock, infection) Lack of subcutaneous fat, prominence of clavicle or ribs (preterm, malnutrition)
Check vernix caseosa: Observe color and odor before bath or removing	Whitish, cheesy, odourless	Usually more found in creases, folds	Absent or minimal (postmature infant) Abundant (preterm) Green color (possible in utero release of meconium or presence of bilirubin) Odor (possible intrauterine infection)
Assess lanugo: Inspect for this fine, downy hair, amount and distribution	Over shoulders, pinnas of ears, forehead	Variation in amount	Absent (postmature) Abundant (preterm, especially if lanugo abundant, long and thick over back)
HEAD			
Palpate skin	(See Skin)	Caput succedaneum, possibly showing some ecchymosis (see Fig. 16-4, *A*)	Cephalhematoma (see Fig. 16-4, *B*)
Inspect shape, size	Making up one fourth of body length Molding (see Fig. 16-9)	Slight asymmetry from intrauterine position Lack of molding (preterm, breech presentation, cesarean birth)	Severe molding (birth trauma) Indentation (fracture from trauma)

Continued

Assessment Video: Sutures and Fontanels

TABLE 16-4

Physical Assessment of Newborn—cont'd

AREA ASSESSED AND APPRAISAL PROCEDURE	NORMAL FINDINGS: AVERAGE FINDINGS	NORMAL FINDINGS: NORMAL VARIATIONS	DEVIATIONS FROM NORMAL RANGE: POSSIBLE PROBLEMS (ETIOLOGY)
Palpate, inspect, and note size and status of fontanels (open vs. closed)	Anterior fontanel 5-cm diamond, increasing as molding resolves Posterior fontanel triangle, smaller than anterior	Variation in fontanel size with degree of molding Difficulty in feeling fontanels possible because of molding	Fontanels: Full, bulging (tumor, hemorrhage, infection) Large, flat, soft (malnutrition, hydrocephaly, delayed bone age, hypothyroidism) Depressed (dehydration)
Palpate sutures	Palpable and separated sutures	Possible overlap of sutures with molding	Sutures: Widely spaced (hydrocephaly) Premature closure (fused) (craniosynostosis)
Inspect pattern, distribution, amount of hair; feel texture	Silky, single strands lying flat; growth pattern toward face and neck	Variation in amount	Fine, wooly (preterm) Unusual swirls, patterns, or hairline; or coarse, brittle (endocrine or genetic disorders)
EYES			
Check placement on face	Eyes and space between eyes each one third the distance from outer-to-outer canthus	Epicanthal folds: characteristic in some ethnicities	Epicanthal folds when present with other signs (chromosomal disorders such as Down, cri-du-chat syndromes)

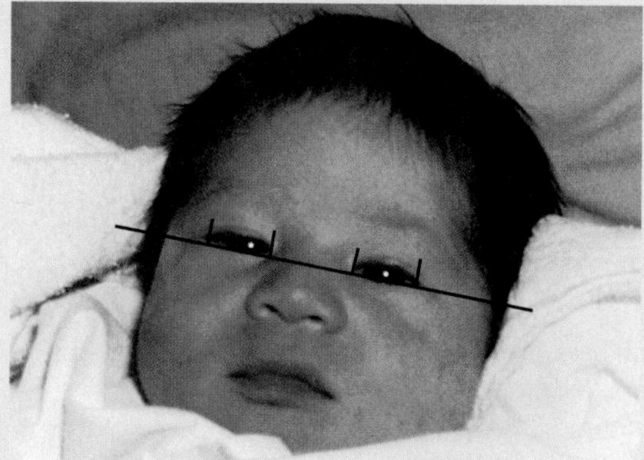

Eyes. In pseudostrabismus, inner epicanthal folds cause the eyes to appear misaligned; however, corneal light reflexes are perfectly symmetric. Eyes are symmetric in size and shape and are well placed.

AREA ASSESSED AND APPRAISAL PROCEDURE	AVERAGE FINDINGS	NORMAL VARIATIONS	DEVIATIONS FROM NORMAL RANGE
Check for symmetry in size, shape	Symmetric in size, shape		
Check eyelids for size, movement, blink	Blink reflex	Edema if eye prophylaxis drops or ointment instilled	

TABLE 16-4

Physical Assessment of Newborn—cont'd

AREA ASSESSED AND APPRAISAL PROCEDURE	NORMAL FINDINGS: AVERAGE FINDINGS	NORMAL FINDINGS: NORMAL VARIATIONS	DEVIATIONS FROM NORMAL RANGE: POSSIBLE PROBLEMS (ETIOLOGY)
Assess for discharge	None No tears	Some discharge if silver nitrate used Occasional presence of some tears	Discharge: purulent (infection) Chemical conjunctivitis from eye medication is common—requires no treatment
Evaluate eyeballs for presence, size, shape	Both present and of equal size, both round, firm	Subconjunctival hemorrhage	Agenesis or absence of one or both eyeballs Lens opacity or absence of red reflex (congenital cataracts, possibly from rubella, retinoblastoma [cat's eye reflex]) Lesions: coloboma, absence of part of iris (congenital) Pink color of iris (albinism) Jaundiced sclera (hyperbilirubinemia)
Check pupils	Present, equal in size, reactive to light		Pupils: unequal, constricted, dilated, fixed (intracranial pressure, medications, tumor)
Evaluate eyeball movement	Random, jerky, uneven, focus possible briefly, following to midline	Transient strabismus or nystagmus until third or fourth month	Persistent strabismus Doll's eyes (increased intracranial pressure) Sunset (increased intracranial pressure)
Assess eyebrows: amount of hair, pattern	Distinct (not connected in midline)		Connection in midline (Cornelia de Lange syndrome)
NOSE			
Observe shape, placement, patency, configuration	Midline Some mucus but no drainage Preferential nose breather Sneezing to clear nose	Slight deformity (flat or deviated to one side) from passage through birth canal	Copious drainage (rarely congenital syphilis); blockage-membranous or bone with cyanosis at rest and return of pink color with crying (choanal atresia) Malformed (congenital syphilis, chromosomal disorder) Flaring of nares (respiratory distress)
EARS			
Observe size, placement on head, amount of cartilage, open auditory canal	Correct placement line drawn through inner and outer canthi of eyes reaching to top notch of ears (at junction with scalp) Well-formed, firm cartilage	Size: small, large, floppy Darwin's tubercle (nodule on posterior helix)	Agenesis Lack of cartilage (preterm) Low placement (chromosomal disorder, mental retardation, kidney disorder) Preauricular tag or sinus Size: possibly overly prominent or protruding ears

Continued

TABLE 16-4

Physical Assessment of Newborn—cont'd

AREA ASSESSED AND APPRAISAL PROCEDURE	NORMAL FINDINGS: AVERAGE FINDINGS	NORMAL FINDINGS: NORMAL VARIATIONS	DEVIATIONS FROM NORMAL RANGE: POSSIBLE PROBLEMS (ETIOLOGY)
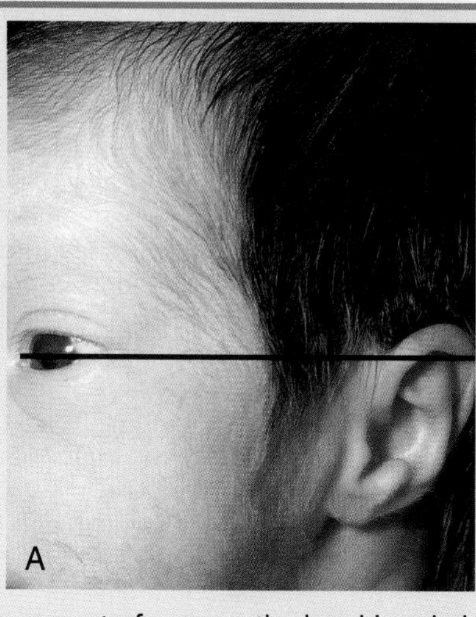 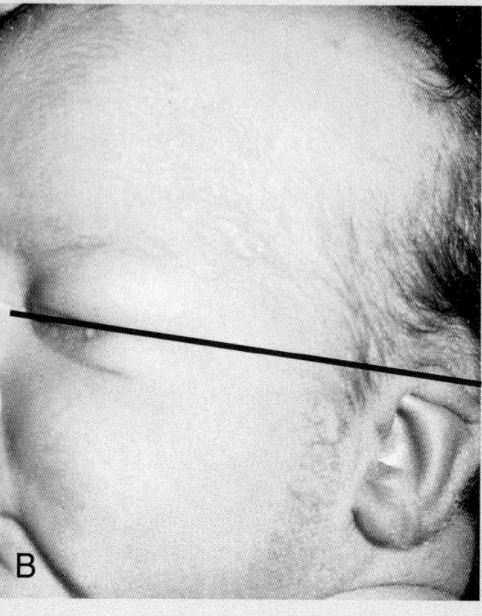 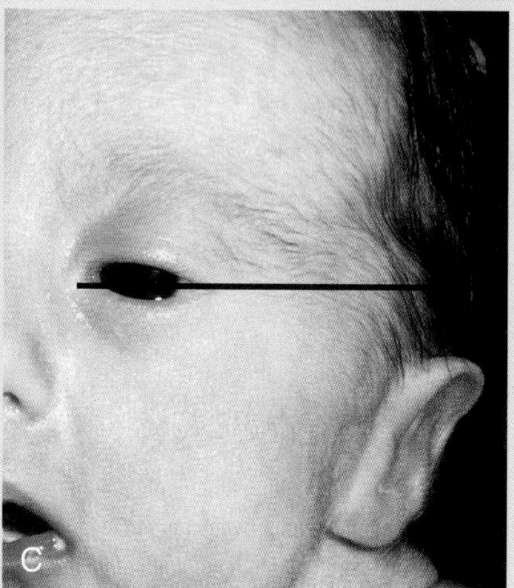 Placement of ears on the head in relation to a line drawn from the inner to the outer canthus of the eye. **A,** Normal position. **B,** Abnormally angled ear. **C,** True low-set ear. (Courtesy Mead Johnson Nutritionals, Evansville, IN.)			
Assess hearing Perform universal newborn hearing screening to identify deficits (Fig. 16-15).	Responds to voice and other sounds	State (e.g., alert, asleep) influencing response	Lack of response to loud noise *should not* imply deafness
FACIES			
Observe overall appearance and symmetry of face	Rounded and symmetric; influenced by birth type, molding, or both	Positional deformities	Usually accompanied by other features such as low-set ears, other structural disorders (hereditary, chromosomal aberration)
MOUTH			
Inspect and palpate Assess buccal mucosa Dry or moist Pink Status intact Assess lips for color, configuration, movement	Symmetry of lip movement	Transient circumoral cyanosis	Gross anomalies in placement, size, shape (cleft lip or palate [or both], gums) Cyanosis, circumoral pallor (respiratory distress, hypothermia) Asymmetry in movement of lips (seventh cranial nerve paralysis)
Check gums	Pink gums	Inclusion cysts (Epstein pearls—Bohn nodules, whitish, hard nodules on gums or roof of mouth)	Teeth: predeciduous or deciduous (hereditary)
Assess tongue for color, mobility, movement, size	Tongue not protruding, freely movable, symmetric in shape, movement Sucking pads inside cheeks	Short lingual frenulum	Macroglossia (preterm, chromosomal disorder) Thrush: white plaques on cheeks or tongue that bleed if touched *(Candida albicans)*

TABLE 16-4

Physical Assessment of Newborn—cont'd

AREA ASSESSED AND APPRAISAL PROCEDURE	NORMAL FINDINGS		DEVIATIONS FROM NORMAL RANGE: POSSIBLE PROBLEMS (ETIOLOGY)
	AVERAGE FINDINGS	NORMAL VARIATIONS	
Assess palate (soft, hard): Arch Uvula	Soft and hard palates intact Uvula in midline	Anatomic groove in palate to accommodate nipple, disappearance by 3 to 4 yr of age Epstein pearls	Cleft hard or soft palate
Assess chin	Distinct chin		Micrognathia—recessed chin with prominent overbite (Pierre Robin sequence or other syndrome)
Evaluate saliva for amount, character	Mouth moist, pink		Excessive salivation and choking or turning blue (esophageal atresia, tracheoesophageal fistula)
Check reflexes: Rooting Sucking Extrusion	Reflexes present	Reflex response dependent on state of wakefulness and hunger	Absent (preterm)
NECK			
Inspect and palpate for movement, flexibility, masses, bruising	Short, thick, surrounded by skin folds; no webbing		Webbing (Turner syndrome)
Check sternocleidomastoid muscles, movement and position of head	Head held in midline (sternocleidomastoid muscles equal), no masses Freedom of movement from side to side and flexion and extension, no movement of chin past shoulder	Transient positional deformity apparent when newborn is at rest: passive movement of head possible	Restricted movement, holding of head at angle (torticollis [wryneck], opisthotonos) Absence of head control (preterm birth, Down syndrome, hypotonia [spinal muscular atrophy])
Assess trachea for position and thyroid gland	Thyroid not palpable		Masses (enlarged thyroid) Distended veins (cardiopulmonary disorder) Skin tags
CHEST			
Inspect and palpate Shape	Almost circular, barrel shaped	Tip of sternum possibly prominent	Bulging of chest, unequal movement (pneumothorax, pneumomediastinum) Malformation (funnel chest—pectus excavatum)
Observe respiratory movements	Symmetric chest movements, chest and abdominal movements synchronized during respirations	Occasional retractions, especially when crying	Retractions with or without respiratory distress (preterm, RDS) Paradoxical breathing
Evaluate clavicles	Clavicles intact		Fracture of clavicle (trauma); crepitus
Assess ribs	Rib cage symmetrical, intact; moves with respirations		Poor development of rib cage and musculature (preterm)

Assessment Video: Neck (Posterior)

Continued

TABLE 16-4

Physical Assessment of Newborn—cont'd

AREA ASSESSED AND APPRAISAL PROCEDURE	NORMAL FINDINGS		DEVIATIONS FROM NORMAL RANGE: POSSIBLE PROBLEMS (ETIOLOGY)
	AVERAGE FINDINGS	NORMAL VARIATIONS	
Assess nipples for size, placement, number	Nipples prominent, well formed; symmetrically placed		Nipples Supernumerary, along nipple line Malpositioned or widely spaced
Check breast tissue	Breast nodule: approximately 6 mm in term infant	Breast nodule: 3-10 mm Secretion of witch's milk	Lack of breast tissue (preterm) Sounds: bowel sounds may be heard in diaphragmatic hernia (see Abdomen)
Auscultate: Heart sounds and rate and breath sounds (see Vital Signs)			
ABDOMEN			
Inspect and palpate umbilical cord	Two arteries, one vein Whitish gray Definite demarcation between cord and skin, no intestinal structures within cord Dry around base, drying Odorless Cord clamp in place for 24 hr		One artery (renal anomaly) Meconium stained (intrauterine distress) Bleeding or oozing around cord (hemorrhagic disease) Redness or drainage around cord (infection, possible persistence of urachus)
		Reducible umbilical hernia	Hernia: herniation of abdominal contents through cord opening (e.g., omphalocele); defect covered with thin, friable membrane, possibly extensive
Inspect size of abdomen and palpate contour	Rounded, prominent, dome shaped because abdominal musculature not fully developed Liver possibly palpable 1-2 cm below right costal margin No other masses palpable No distention Few visible veins on abdominal surface	Some diastasis recti (separation) of abdominal musculature	Gastroschisis: herniation of abdominal contents to the side or above the cord, contents not covered by membranous tissue and may include liver Distention at birth: Ruptured viscus, genitourinary masses or malformations: hydronephrosis, teratomas, abdominal tumors Mild (overfeeding, high gastrointestinal tract obstruction) Marked (lower gastrointestinal tract obstruction, anorectal malformation, anal stenosis), often with bilious emesis Intermittent or transient (overfeeding) Partial intestinal obstruction (stenosis of bowel) Visible peristalsis (obstruction) Malrotation of bowel or adhesions Sepsis (infection)

Assessment Video: Male Breasts (Supine Position)

TABLE 16-4

Physical Assessment of Newborn—cont'd

AREA ASSESSED AND APPRAISAL PROCEDURE	NORMAL FINDINGS: AVERAGE FINDINGS	NORMAL FINDINGS: NORMAL VARIATIONS	DEVIATIONS FROM NORMAL RANGE: POSSIBLE PROBLEMS (ETIOLOGY)
Auscultate bowel sounds and note number, amount, and character of stools	Sounds present within minutes after birth in healthy term infant Meconium stool passing within 24-48 hr after birth		Scaphoid, with bowel sounds in chest and severe respiratory distress (congenital diaphragmatic hernia)
Assess color		Linea nigra possibly apparent and caused by hormone influence during pregnancy	
Observe movement with respiration	Respirations primarily diaphragmatic, abdominal and chest movement synchronous		Decreased or absent abdominal movement with breathing (phrenic nerve palsy, congenital diaphragmatic hernia)
GENITALIA			
Female (see Fig. 16-7, *A*)			
Inspect and palpate General appearance Clitoris Labia majora	Female genitals: Usually edematous Usually edematous, covering labia minora in term newborns	Increased pigmentation caused by pregnancy hormones Edema and ecchymosis after breech birth Some vernix caseosa between labia possible	Ambiguous genitalia—wide variation (small phallus not well distinguished from enlarged clitoris) Virilized female—extremely large clitoris (congenital adrenal hyperplasia)
Labia minora	Possible protrusion over labia majora		Enlarged clitoris with urinary meatus on tip, absent scrotum, micropenis, fused labia
Discharge Vagina	Smegma Open orifice Mucoid discharge Hymenal/vaginal tag	Blood-tinged discharge from pseudomenstruation caused by pregnancy hormones	Stenosed meatus Labia majora widely separated and labia minora prominent (preterm) Absence of vaginal orifice Fecal discharge (fistula)
Urinary meatus	Beneath clitoris, difficult to see	Rust-stained urine (uric acid crystals)	Bladder exstrophy (bladder outside abdominal cavity and turned inside out)
Check urination	Voiding 2-6 times per day for first 1-2 days; voiding 6-10 times per day by day 5 or 6	Rust-stained urine (uric acid crystals)	No void within first 24 hours (renal agenesis; Potter syndrome)
Male (see Fig. 16-7, *B*)			
Inspect and palpate General appearance Penis Urinary meatus appearance—should be at tip of penile shaft	Male genitals: Foreskin covers glans (if uncircumcised), meatus at tip of penis	Increased size and pigmentation caused by pregnancy hormones	Ambiguous genitalia Micropenis Urinary meatus not on tip of glans penis (hypospadias, epispadias, foreskin may be retracted or absent)
Prepuce (foreskin)—do not forcibly retract foreskin if uncircumcised	Prepuce covering glans penis and not retractable	Prepuce removed if circumcised Wide variation in size of genitals	Round meatal opening

Continued

TABLE 16-4

Physical Assessment of Newborn—cont'd

AREA ASSESSED AND APPRAISAL PROCEDURE	NORMAL FINDINGS: AVERAGE FINDINGS	NORMAL FINDINGS: NORMAL VARIATIONS	DEVIATIONS FROM NORMAL RANGE: POSSIBLE PROBLEMS (ETIOLOGY)
Scrotum: Rugae (wrinkles)	Large, edematous, pendulous in term infant; covered with rugae	Scrotal edema and ecchymosis if breech birth Hydrocele, small, noncommunicating	Scrotum smooth and testes undescended (preterm, cryptorchidism) Bifid scrotum Hydrocele Inguinal hernia
Testes	Palpable on each side	Bulge palpable in inguinal canal	Undescended (preterm)
Check urination	Voiding within 24 hr, stream adequate	Rust-stained urine (uric acid crystals)	No void in first 24 hours (renal agenesis; Potter syndrome)
Check reflexes: Cremasteric	Testes retracted, especially when newborn is chilled		
EXTREMITIES			
Make a general check: Inspect and palpate Degree of flexion Range of motion Symmetry of motion Muscle tone	Assuming of position maintained in utero Attitude of general flexion Full range of motion, spontaneous movements	Transient positional deformities	Limited motion (malformations) Poor muscle tone (preterm, maternal medications, CNS anomalies)
Check arms and hands: Inspect and palpate Color Intactness Appropriate placement	Longer than legs in newborn period Contours and movements symmetric	Slight tremors sometimes apparent Some acrocyanosis	Asymmetry of movement (fracture/crepitus, brachial nerve trauma, malformations) Asymmetry of contour (malformations, fracture) Amelia or phocomelia (teratogens) Palmar creases Simian line with short, incurved little fingers (Down syndrome)
Count number of fingers	Five on each hand Fist often clenched with thumb under fingers		Webbing of fingers: syndactyly Absence or excess of fingers Strong, rigid flexion; persistent fists; positioning of fists in front of mouth constantly (CNS disorder) Yellowed nail beds (meconium staining)
Evaluate joints Shoulder Elbow Wrist Fingers	Full range of motion, symmetric contour		Increased tonicity, clonus, prolonged tremors (CNS disorder)

Ⓔ Assessment Video: Cremasteric Reflex

Ⓔ Assessment Video: Upper Extremities

TABLE 16-4

Physical Assessment of Newborn—cont'd

AREA ASSESSED AND APPRAISAL PROCEDURE	NORMAL FINDINGS: AVERAGE FINDINGS	NORMAL FINDINGS: NORMAL VARIATIONS	DEVIATIONS FROM NORMAL RANGE: POSSIBLE PROBLEMS (ETIOLOGY)
Check reflex: grasp (palmar and plantar)			
Check legs and feet: Inspect and palpate Color Intactness Length in relation to arms and body and to each other	Appearance of bowing because lateral muscles more developed than medial muscles	Feet appearing to turn in but can be easily rotated externally, positional defects tending to correct while infant is crying Acrocyanosis	Amelia, phocomelia (chromosomal defect, teratogenic effect) Temperature of one leg differing from that of the other (circulatory deficiency, CNS disorder)
Number of toes	Five on each foot		Webbing, syndactyly (chromosomal defect) Absence or excess of digits (chromosomal defect, familial trait)
Femur Head of femur as legs are flexed and abducted, placement in acetabulum (see Fig. 16-10)	Intact femur		Femoral fracture (difficult breech birth) Developmental dysplasia of the hip
Major gluteal folds Soles of feet	Major gluteal folds even Soles well lined (or wrinkled) over two thirds of foot in term infants Plantar fat pad giving flat-footed effect		Hip dysplasia Soles of feet: Few creases (preterm) Covered with creases (postmature) Congenital clubfoot
Evaluate joints Hip Knee Ankle Toes	Full range of motion, symmetric contour		Hypermobility of joints (Down syndrome)
Check reflexes (see Table 16-3)			Asymmetric movement (trauma, CNS disorder)
BACK			
Assess anatomy: Inspect and palpate Spine Shoulders Scapulae Iliac crests Base of spine—pilonidal dimple or sinus	Spine straight and easily flexed Infant able to raise and support head momentarily when prone Shoulders, scapulae, and iliac crests lining up in same plane	Temporary minor positional deformities, correction with passive manipulation	Limitation of movement (fusion or deformity of vertebra) Spina bifida cystica (meningocele, myelomeningocele) Pigmented nevus with tuft of hair, location anywhere along the spine, often associated with spina bifida occulta Sinus (opening to spinal cord)
Check reflexes (spinal related)			
Test trunk incurvation reflex	Trunk flexed and pelvis swings to stimulated side	May not be apparent in first few days but is usually present in 5-6 days	If transverse lesion is present, no response below lesion; absence of response: central nervous system abnormality or CNS depression

Assessment Video: Legs (Symmetry, Length)

Continued

TABLE 16-4

Physical Assessment of Newborn—cont'd

AREA ASSESSED AND APPRAISAL PROCEDURE	NORMAL FINDINGS		DEVIATIONS FROM NORMAL RANGE: POSSIBLE PROBLEMS (ETIOLOGY)
	AVERAGE FINDINGS	NORMAL VARIATIONS	
Test magnet reflex	Lower limbs extend as pressure applied to feet with legs in semiflexed position	Weak or exaggerated response with breech presentation	Absence: suggestive of CNS damage or malformation
ANUS			
Inspect and palpate Placement Patency Test for sphincter response (active "wink" reflex)	One anus with good sphincter tone Passage of meconium within 24 hr after birth Anal "wink" present, anal opening patent	Passage of meconium within 48 hr of birth	Imperforate anus without fistula Rectal atresia and stenosis Absence of anal opening; drainage of fecal material from vagina in female or urinary meatus in male (rectal fistula) or along perineal raphe (midline area between base of penis and anus)—anorectal malformation
Observe for the following: Abdominal distention Passage of meconium from anal opening Fecal drainage from perineum, penis, vagina			
STOOLS			
Observe frequency, color, consistency	Meconium followed by transitional and soft yellow stool		No stool (obstruction) Frequent watery stools (infection, phototherapy)

Assessment Video: Buttocks

suspected. An irregular, very slow, or very fast heart rate may indicate a need for further evaluation of circulatory status including BP measurement.

The axillary temperature is a safe, accurate measurement of temperature. Electronic thermometers have expedited this task and provide a reading within 1 minute. Temporal artery, tympanic, and oral routes for measuring temperature in the newborn are not considered accurate (Asher & Northington, 2008). Taking an infant's temperature may cause the infant to cry and struggle against the placement of the thermometer in the axilla. Before taking the temperature the examiner can determine the apical heart rate and respiratory rate while the infant is quiet and at rest. The normal axillary temperature averages 37° C with a range from 36.5° to 37.5° C.

The respiratory rate varies with the state of alertness and activity after birth. Respirations are abdominal in nature and can be counted by observing or by lightly feeling the rise and fall of the abdomen. Neonatal respirations are shallow and irregular. The respirations should be counted for a full minute to obtain an accurate count because of periods of periodic breathing wherein respirations may cease for seconds (≤20) and resume again. The examiner should also observe for symmetry of chest movement. The average respiratory rate is 40 breaths/minute but will vary between 30 and 60 breaths/minute or may be higher than 60 breaths/minute if the newborn is very active or crying (see Table 16-1).

An apical pulse rate should be obtained on all newborns. Auscultation should be for a full minute, preferably when the infant is asleep or in a quiet alert state. The infant may need to be held and comforted during assessment. Heart rate may range from 80 to 170 or more beats/minute shortly after birth and, when the infant's condition has stabilized, from 120 to 140 beats/minute. Brachial and femoral pulses are assessed for equality and strength.

If BP is measured, an oscillometric monitor calibrated for neonatal pressures is preferred. An appropriate sized cuff (width-to-arm or calf ratio of 0.45 to 0.70 or approximately ½ to ¾) is essential for accuracy. Neonatal BP is usually highest immediately after birth and falls to a minimum by 3 hours after birth. It then begins to rise steadily and reaches a plateau between 4 and 6 days after birth. This measurement is usually equal to that of the immediate postbirth BP. The BP varies with the neonate's activity; accurate measurement is best obtained while the newborn is at rest.

A baseline pulse oximetry measurement may be obtained as well as palpation of peripheral pulses (brachial, femoral, pedal), before the infant's discharge from the birth institution, especially if a congenital cardiac defect is suspected.

Baseline Measurements of Physical Growth

Baseline measurements are taken and recorded to help assess the progress and determine the growth patterns of the neonate. These measurements may be recorded on growth charts. The following measurements are made when the neonate is assessed.

Weight

The newborn is usually weighed shortly after birth. This assessment may be performed in the labor and birthing area, the mother's room, or on admission to the nursery. Care must be taken to ensure that the scales are balanced. The totally unclothed neonate is placed in the center of the scale, which is usually covered with a disposable pad or cloth to prevent heat loss via conduction to prevent cross-infection. The nurse should place one hand over (but not touching) the neonate to prevent the infant from falling off the scales (p. 460). Weighing the infant at the same time every day is common during the hospital stay. Birth weight of a term infant typically ranges from 2500 to 4000 g.

Head circumference and body length

The head is measured at the widest part, which is the occipitofrontal diameter (p. 461). The tape measure is placed around the head just above the infant's eyebrows. The term neonate's head circumference ranges from 32 to 36.8 cm.

The length may be difficult to obtain because of the flexed posture of the newborn (p. 461). The examiner places the newborn on a flat surface and extends the leg until the knee is flat against the surface. Placing the head against a perpendicular surface and extending the leg may assist with obtaining this measurement. In the term neonate, head-to-heel length ranges from 45 to 55 cm.

Neurologic Assessment

The physical examination includes a neurologic assessment of newborn reflexes (see Table 16-3). This assessment provides useful information about the infant's nervous system and state of neurologic maturation. Many reflex behaviors (e.g., sucking, rooting) are important for proper development. Other reflexes such as gagging and sneezing act as primitive safety mechanisms. The assessment needs to be carried out as early as possible because abnormal signs present in the early neonatal period may require further investigation before the newborn is discharged home.

BEHAVIORAL CHARACTERISTICS

The healthy infant must accomplish behavioral and biologic tasks to develop normally. Behavioral characteristics form the basis of the social capabilities of the infant. Healthy newborns differ in their activity levels, feeding patterns, sleeping patterns, and responsiveness. Parents' reactions to their newborns are often determined by these differences. Showing parents the unique characteristics of their infant assists parents to develop a more positive perception of the infant with increased interaction between infant and parent.

Behavioral responses, as well as physical characteristics, change during the period of transition. The Brazelton Neonatal Behavioral Assessment Scale (BNBAS) can be used to assess the infant's behavior systematically (Brazelton, 1999; Brazelton & Nugent, 1996). The BNBAS is an interactive examination that assesses the infant's response to 28 areas organized according to the clusters in Box 16-2. It is generally used as a research or diagnostic tool and requires special training.

In addition to use as initial and ongoing tools to assess neurologic and behavioral responses, the scales can be used to assess initial parent-infant relationships and as a

BOX 16-2

Clusters of Neonatal Behaviors in the Brazelton Neonatal Behavioral Assessment Scale (BNBAS)

Habituation: ability to respond to and then inhibit responding to discrete stimuli (light, rattle, bell, pinprick) while asleep
Orientation: quality of alert states and ability to attend to visual and auditory stimuli while alert
Motor performance: quality of movement and tone
Range of state: measure of general arousal level or arousability of infant
Regulation of state: how infant responds when aroused
Autonomic stability: signs of stress (tremors, startles, skin color) related to homeostatic (self-regulator) adjustment of the nervous system
Reflexes: assessment of several neonatal reflexes

guide for parents to help them focus on their infant's individuality and to develop a deeper attachment to their child. See Chapter 15 for further discussion of attachment.

Sleep-Wake States

Variations in the state of consciousness of infants are called **sleep-wake states**. The six states form a continuum from deep sleep to extreme irritability (Fig. 16-14): two sleep states (deep sleep and light sleep) and four wake states (drowsy, quiet alert, active alert, and crying) (Blackburn 2007). Each state has specific characteristics and state-related behaviors. The optimal state of arousal is the quiet alert state. During this state, infants smile, vocalize, move in synchrony with speech, watch their parents' faces, and respond to people talking to them. Infants respond to internal and external environmental factors by controlling sensory input and regulating the sleep-wake states; the ability to make smooth transitions between states is called *state modulation*. The ability to regulate sleep-wake states is essential in the infant's neurobehavioral development. As infants approach term gestation, they are better able to cope with external or internal factors that affect the sleep-wake patterns.

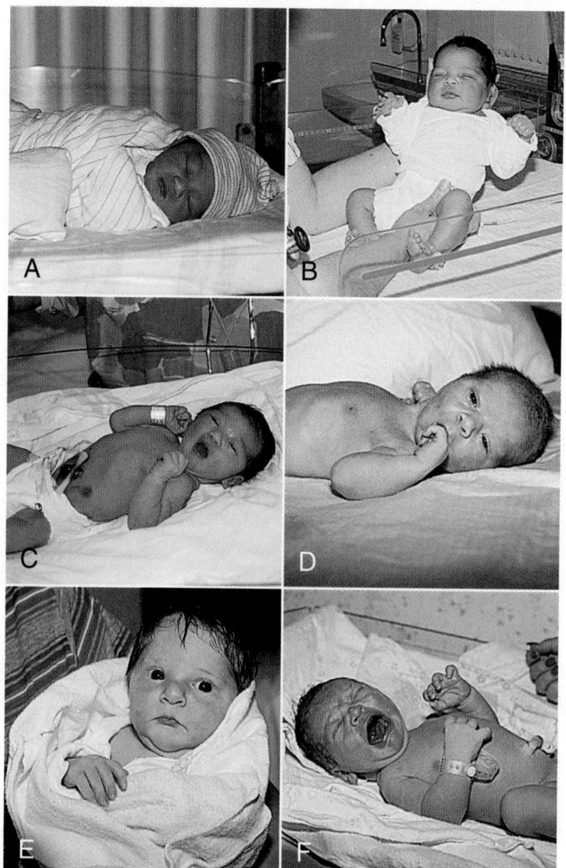

Fig. 16-14 Summary of newborn sleep-wake states. States of consciousness: **A**, Deep sleep. **B**, Light sleep. **C**, Drowsy. **D**, Quiet alert. **E**, Active alert. **F**, Crying. (Courtesy Marjorie Pyle, RNC, Lifecircle, Costa Mesa, CA.)

Infants use purposeful behavior to maintain the optimal arousal state as follows: (1) actively withdrawing by increasing physical distance, (2) rejecting by pushing away with hands and feet, (3) decreasing sensitivity by falling asleep or breaking eye contact by turning head, or (4) using signaling behaviors, such as fussing and crying. These behaviors permit infants to quiet themselves and reinstate readiness to interact.

The first 6 weeks of life involve a steady decrease in the proportion of active REM sleep to total sleep. A steady increase in the proportion of quiet sleep to total sleep also occurs. Periods of wakefulness increase. For the first few weeks the wakeful periods seem dictated by hunger but soon a need for socializing appears as well. The newborn sleeps on average approximately 17 hours a day, with periods of wakefulness gradually increasing. By the fourth week of life, some infants stay awake from one feeding to the next.

Other Factors Influencing Newborn Behavior

Gestational age

The gestational age of the infant and level of CNS maturity affect the observed behavior. In an infant with an immature CNS (preterm) the entire body responds to a pinprick of the foot although the response may not be observed by an untrained observer. The more mature infant withdraws only the foot. CNS immaturity is reflected in reflex development, sleep-wake states, and ability (or lack thereof) to regulate or modulate a smooth transition between different states. Preterm infants have brief periods of alertness but have difficulty maintaining alertness without becoming overstimulated, which leads to autonomic instability unless intervention is implemented. Premature or sick infants show signs of fatigue or physiologic stress sooner than full-term healthy infants.

Time

The time elapsed since birth affects the behavior of infants as they attempt to become organized initially. Time elapsed since the previous feeding and time of day also may influence infants' responses.

Stimuli

Environmental events and stimuli affect the behavioral responses of infants. The newborn responds to animate and inanimate stimuli. Nurses in intensive care nurseries observe that infants respond to loud noises, bright lights, monitor alarms, and tension in the unit. If a mother is tense, nervous, or uncomfortable while feeding her infant, the infant may sense her tension and demonstrate difficulty feeding.

Medication

Controversy surrounds the effects on infant behavior of maternal medication (e.g., analgesia and anesthesia) during labor. Some researchers note that infants of mothers given certain analgesic medications may have disturbances in newborn behavior, that is, more crying, an increase in temperature, and some difficulty in breastfeeding (Ransjö-Arvidson, Matthiesen, Lilja, Nissen, Widström, & Uvnäs-Moberg, 2001). Other researchers maintain that the effect on infant behavior is nonexistent (Chang & Heaman, 2006).

Sensory Behaviors

From birth, infants possess sensory capabilities that indicate a state of readiness for social interaction. Infants effectively use behavioral responses in establishing their first dialogues. These responses, coupled with the newborns' "baby appearance" (e.g., facial proportions of forehead, eyes larger than the lower portion of the face) and their small size and helplessness, rouse feelings of wanting to hold, protect, and interact with them.

Vision

At birth the eye is structurally incomplete and the muscles are immature. The process of accommodation is not present at birth but improves over the first 3 months of life. The pupils react to light, the blink reflex is easily stimulated, and the corneal reflex is activated by light touch. Term newborns can see objects as far away as 50 cm (2.5 feet). The clearest visual distance is 17 to 20 cm (8-12 inches), which is approximately the distance between the mother's face and the infant's face during breastfeeding or cuddling. Infants are sensitive to light; they will frown if a bright light is flashed in their eyes, and will turn toward a soft, red light. If the room is darkened, they will open their eyes wide and look about. By 2 months of age, they can detect color; but at 5 days of age and younger, they seem more attracted by black-and-white patterns.

Response to movement is noticeable. If a bright light is shown to newborns (even at 15 minutes of age), they will follow it visually; some will even turn their heads to do so. Because human eyes are bright, shiny objects, newborns will track their parents' eyes. Parents often comment on their excitement in observing this behavior. The development of eye-to-eye contact is very important for parent-infant attachment. Children of blind parents, and parents who have blind children, must circumvent this obstacle for the formation of a relationship.

Visual acuity is surprising; even at 2 weeks of age, infants can distinguish patterns with stripes 3 mm apart. By 6 months their vision is as acute as that of an adult. They prefer to look at patterns rather than plain surfaces, even if the latter are brightly colored. Infants prefer more complex patterns to simple ones. They prefer novelty (changes in pattern) by 2 months of age. The infant of a few weeks of age is therefore capable of responding actively to an enriched environment.

Hearing

As soon as the amniotic fluid drains from the ears the infant's hearing is similar to that of an adult. Loud sounds of approximately 90 db cause the infant to respond with a startle reflex. The newborn responds to low-frequency sounds such as a heartbeat or lullaby by decreasing motor activity or stopping crying. High-frequency sound elicits an alerting reaction.

The infant responds readily to the mother's voice. Studies indicate a selective listening to maternal voice sounds and rhythms during intrauterine life that prepares newborns for recognition and interaction with their primary caregivers–their mothers. Newborns are accustomed in the uterus to hearing the regular rhythm of the mother's heartbeat. As a result, they respond by relaxing and ceasing to fuss and cry if a regular heartbeat simulator is placed in their cribs.

Hearing loss is a common major abnormality at birth; approximately 1 to 3 in 1000 term infants have bilateral hearing loss (American Academy of Pediatrics, 1999). To identify affected infants the hearing of all infants is screened before discharge from the birth institution (Fig. 16-15).

Smell

Newborns react to strong odors such as alcohol or vinegar by turning their heads away. Breastfed infants are able to smell breast milk and can differentiate their mothers from other lactating women by the smell (Lawrence & Lawrence, 2005).

Taste

The newborn can distinguish among tastes, and various types of solutions elicit differing facial expressions. A tasteless solution produces no response; a sweet solution elicits eager sucking. A sour solution causes a puckering of the lips, and a bitter liquid produces a grimace.

COMMUNITY ACTIVITY

Locate a newborn class in your community. Is the class given during pregnancy or in the early postnatal period? If in the postnatal period, do parents bring their infants to the class? Are the classes available in more than one language? Interview the instructor to determine what is included in the class content. Are deviations from the norm included as well as normal physical characteristics of the neonate? What information do parents receive related to newborn behaviors? Are feeding and sleeping behaviors addressed? What suggestions would you make to include content related to physiologic and behavioral adaptations of the newborn? Are cultural variations addressed? What is the value of providing expectant parents with this information?

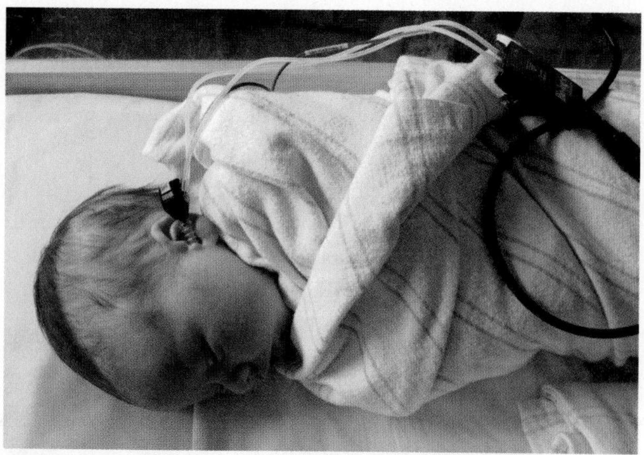

Fig. 16-15 Hearing screening in the newborn nursery. (Courtesy Julie and Darren Nelson, Loveland, CO.)

Young infants are particularly oriented toward the use of their mouths, both for meeting their nutritional needs for rapid growth and for releasing tension through sucking. The early development of circumoral sensation, muscle activity, and taste would seem to be preparation for survival in the extrauterine environment.

Touch

The infant is responsive to touch on all parts of the body. The face (especially the mouth), the hands, and the soles of the feet seem to be the most sensitive. Reflexes can be elicited by stroking the infant. The newborn's responses to touch suggest that this sensory system is well prepared to receive and process tactile messages. Touch and motion are essential to normal growth and development. However, each infant is unique, and variations can be seen in newborns' responses to touch. Birth trauma or stress and depressant drugs taken by the mother decrease the infant's sensitivity to touch or painful stimuli.

Response to Environmental Stimuli

Temperament

Classic studies (e.g., Thomas, Birch, Chess, & Robbins, 1961; Thomas, Chess, & Birch, 1970) identified individual variations in the primary reaction pattern of newborns and described them as temperament. Their style of behavioral response to stimuli is guided by the temperament affecting the newborn's sensory threshold, ability to habituate, and response to maternal behaviors. The newborn possesses individual characteristics that affect selective responses to various stimuli present in the internal and external environment.

Habituation

Habituation is a protective mechanism that allows the infant to become accustomed to environmental stimuli. Habituation is a psychologic and physiologic phenomenon in which the response to a constant or repetitive stimulus is decreased. In the term newborn, habituation can be demonstrated in several ways. Shining a bright light into a newborn's eyes will cause a startle or squinting the first two or three times. The third or fourth flash will elicit a diminished response, and by the fifth or sixth flash the infant ceases to respond (Brazelton, 1999; Brazelton & Nugent, 1996). The same response pattern holds true for the sounds of a rattle or a pinprick to the heel.

The ability to habituate also allows the newborn to select stimuli that promote continued learning about the social world, thus preventing overload. The intrauterine experience seems to have programmed the newborn to be especially responsive to human voices, soft lights, soft sounds, and sweet tastes.

The newborn quickly learns the sounds in the home environment and is able to sleep in their midst. The selective responses of the newborn indicate cerebral organization capable of memory and making choices. The ability to habituate depends on state of consciousness, hunger, fatigue, and temperament. These factors also affect consolability, cuddliness, irritability, and crying.

Consolability

Newborns vary in their ability to console themselves or to be consoled. In the crying state, most newborns initiate one of several methods for reducing their distress. Hand-to-mouth movements are common, with or without sucking, as well as alerting to voices, noises, or visual stimuli.

Cuddliness

Cuddliness is especially important to parents because they often gauge their ability to care for the child by the child's responses to their actions. Variability is noted in the degree to which newborns will mold into the contours of the persons holding them. Babies are soothed and become alert with the vestibular stimulation of being picked up and moved.

Irritability

Some newborns cry longer and harder than others. For some infants the sensory threshold seems low. They are readily upset by unusual noises, hunger, wetness, or new experiences and respond intensely to these stimuli. Others with a high sensory threshold require a great deal more stimulation and variation to reach the active, alert state.

Crying

Crying in an infant may signal hunger, pain, desire for attention, or fussiness. Most mothers learn to distinguish among the cries. The duration of crying is highly variable in each infant; newborns may cry for as little as 5 minutes or as much as 2 hours or more per day. The amount of crying peaks in the second month and then decreases. A diurnal rhythm of crying can be noted, with more crying in the evening hours. Crying does not seem to differ with different caregivers.

KEY POINTS

- By full term the infant's various anatomic and physiologic systems have reached a level of development and functioning that permits a physical existence apart from the mother.
- The healthy term infant has sensory capabilities that indicate a state of readiness for social interaction.
- Several significant differences exist among the respiratory, renal, and thermogenic systems of the newborn and those of an adult.
- Heat loss in the healthy term newborn may exceed the capacity to produce heat, which can lead to metabolic and respiratory complications that threaten the newborn's well-being.
- Assessment of the newborn requires data from the prenatal, intrapartal, and postpartal periods.
- The newborn assessment should proceed systematically so that each system is thoroughly evaluated.
- Some reflex behaviors are important for the newborn's survival.
- Individual personalities and behavioral characteristics of infants play major roles in their ultimate relationships with their parents.
- Sleep-wake states and other factors influence the newborn's behavior.
- Each full-term newborn has a predisposed capacity to handle the multitude of stimuli in the external world.

Audio Chapter Summaries: Access an audio summary of these Key Points on evolve

References

American Academy of Pediatrics (AAP) Task Force on Newborn and Infant Hearing. (1999). Newborn and infant hearing loss: Detection and intervention. *Pediatrics, 103*(2), 527-530.

Armentrout, D. C. & Huseby, V. (2003). Polycythemia in the newborn. *MCN: The American Journal of Maternal/Child Nursing, 28*(4), 234-239.

Asher, C. & Northington, L. K. (2008). Position statement for measurement of temperature/fever in children. *Journal of Pediatric Nursing, 23*(3), 234-235.

Blackburn, S. (2007). *Maternal, fetal, & neonatal physiology: A clinical perspective* (3rd ed.). St. Louis: Saunders.

Boo, N. Y., Foong, K. W., Mahdy, Z. A., Yong, S. C., & Jaafer, R. (2005). Risk factors associated with subaponeurotic haemorrhage in full-term infants exposed to vacuum extraction. *British Journal of Obstetrics and Gynaecology, 112*, 1516-1521.

Brazelton, T. (1999). Behavioral competence. In G. Avery, M. Fletcher, & M. MacDonald (Eds.), *Neonatology: Pathophysiology and management of the newborn* (5th ed.). Philadelphia: Lippincott Williams & Wilkins.

Brazelton, T. & Nugent, K. (1996). *Neonatal behavioural assessment scale* (3rd ed.). London: MacKeith.

Chang, Z. M., & Heaman, M. I. (2006). Epidural analgesia during labor and delivery: Effects on the initiation and continuation of effective breastfeeding. *Journal of Human Lactation, 21*(3), 305-314.

Doumouchtsis, S. K., & Arulkumaran, S. (2006). Head injuries after instrumental vaginal deliveries, *Current Opinion in Obstetrics and Gynecology, 18*(2), 129-134.

Hutton, E. K. & Hassan, E. S. (2007). Late vs early clamping of the umbilical cord in full-term neonates: Systematic review and meta-analysis of controlled trials. *Journal of the American Medical Association, 297*(11), 1241-1252.

Kent, A. L., Kecskes, Z., Shadbolt, B., & Falk, M. C. (2007). Blood pressure in the first year of life in healthy infants born at term. *Pediatric Nephrology, 22*(10), 1743-1749.

Lawrence, R. & Lawrence R. (2005). *Breastfeeding: A guide for the medical profession* (6th ed.). Philadelphia: Mosby.

Paige, P. & Moe, P. C. (2006). Neurologic disorders. In G. Merenstein & S. Gardner (Eds.), *Handbook of neonatal intensive care* (6th ed.). St. Louis: Mosby.

Ransjö-Arvidson, A. B., Matthiesen, A. S., Lilja, G., Nissen, E., Widström, A. M., & Uvnäs-Moberg, K. (2001). Maternal analgesia during labor disturbs newborn behavior: Effects on breastfeeding temperature, and crying. *Birth, 28*(1), 5-12.

Razmus, I. J. & Lewis, L. (2006). Using four limb blood pressures as a screening tool in normal newborns. *Society of Pediatric Nursing News, 15*(6), 5-7.

Taylor, M. L. (2005). Coarctation of the aorta: Critical catch for newborn well-being. *The Nurse Practitioner, 30*(12), 34-43.

Thomas, A., Birch, H.G., Chess, S., & Robbins, L.C. (1961). Individuality in responses of children to similar environmental situations. *American Journal of Psychiatry, 117*, 798-803.

Thomas, A., Chess, S., & Birch, H. G. (1970). The origin of personality. *Scientific American, 223*(2), 102-109.

Uchil, D. & Arulkumaran, S. (2003). Neonatal subgaleal hemorrhage and its relationship to delivery by vacuum extraction. *Obstetric and Gynecology Survey, 58*(10), 687-693.

Visscher, M. O., Narendran, V., Pickens, W. L., LaRuffa, A. A., Meinzen-Derr, J., Allen, K., et al. (2005). Vernix caseosa in neonatal adaptation. *Journal of Perinatology, 25*(7), 440-446.

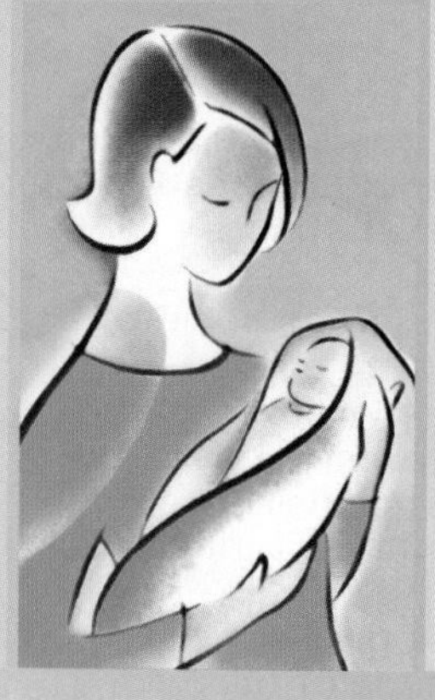

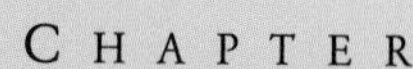

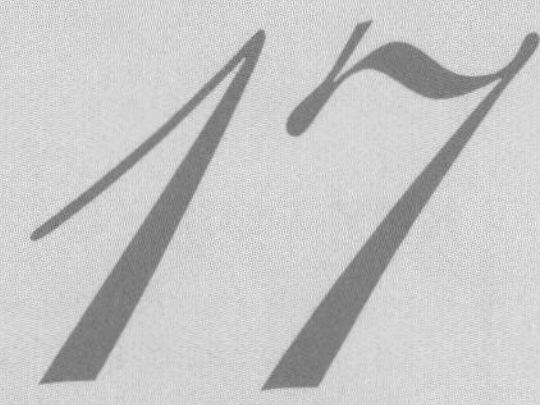

Assessment and Care of the Newborn and Family

SHANNON E. PERRY

LEARNING OBJECTIVES

- *Explain the purpose and components of the Apgar score.*
- *Compare and contrast the characteristics of the preterm, late preterm, term, and postterm neonate.*
- *Perform a gestational age assessment of a newborn.*
- *Explain the elements of a safe environment.*
- *Discuss phototherapy and the guidelines for teaching parents about this treatment.*
- *Explain the purposes for and methods of circumcision, the postoperative care of the circumcised infant, and parent teaching regarding circumcision.*
- *Review the procedures for performing a heel stick, collecting urine specimens, and assisting with venipuncture.*
- *Evaluate pain in the newborn based on physiologic changes and behavioral observations.*
- *Review anticipatory guidance nurses provide to parents before discharge.*

KEY TERMS AND DEFINITIONS

Apgar score Numeric expression of the condition of a newborn obtained by rapid assessment at 1 and 5 minutes of age; developed by Dr. Virginia Apgar

circumcision Excision of the prepuce (foreskin) of the penis, exposing the glans

hyperbilirubinemia Elevation of unconjugated serum bilirubin concentrations

hypothermia Temperature that falls below the normal range, that is, below 35° C, usually caused by exposure to cold

kernicterus Pathologic process characterized by deposition of bilirubin in the brain

late preterm infant Infants born at 34 0/7 to 36 6/7 weeks of gestation

ophthalmia neonatorum Infection in the neonate's eyes usually resulting from gonorrheal, chlamydial, or other infection contracted when the fetus passes through the birth canal (vagina)

phototherapy Use of lights to reduce serum bilirubin levels by oxidation of bilirubin into water-soluble compounds that are processed in the liver and excreted in bile and urine

physiologic jaundice Yellow tinge to skin and mucous membranes in response to increased serum levels of unconjugated bilirubin; not usually apparent until after 24 hours; also called *neonatal jaundice, physiologic hyperbilirubinemia*

WEB RESOURCES

Additional related content can be found on the companion website at evolve

http://evolve.elsevier.com/Lowdermilk/Maternity/

- NCLEX Review Questions
- Assessment Videos: Circumcision, Crying Female Neonate
- Case Study: The Normal Newborn
- Critical Thinking Exercise: Circumcision
- Critical Thinking Exercise: Jaundice
- Nursing Care Plan: Immediate Care of the Newborn
- Nursing Care Plan: The Normal Newborn and Family
- Skill: Changing a Diaper
- Skill: Infant Bathing
- Skill: Pain Assessment
- Skill: Swaddling
- Spanish Guidelines: Daily Care
- Spanish Guidelines: General Advice
- Spanish Guidelines: Infant Quieting Techniques

Although most infants make the necessary biopsychosocial adjustments to extrauterine existence without undue difficulty, their well-being depends on the care they receive from others. This chapter describes the assessment and care of the infant immediately after birth until discharge, as well as important anticipatory guidance related to ongoing infant care. A discussion of pain in the neonate and its management is included.

BIRTH THROUGH THE FIRST 2 HOURS

NURSING CARE MANAGEMENT

Care begins immediately after birth and focuses on assessing and stabilizing the newborn's condition. The nurse has the primary responsibility for the infant during this period because the physician or midwife is involved with care of the mother. The nurse must be alert for any signs of distress and initiate appropriate interventions.

With the possibility of transmission of viruses such as hepatitis B virus (HBV) and human immunodeficiency virus (HIV) through maternal blood and blood-stained amniotic fluid, the newborn must be considered a potential contamination source until proved otherwise. As part of Standard Precautions, nurses should wear gloves when handling the newborn until blood and amniotic fluid are removed by bathing.

Assessment

Initial Assessment and Apgar Scoring

The initial assessment of the neonate is performed immediately after birth using the Apgar score (Table 17-1) and a brief physical examination (Box 17-1). A gestational age assessment is completed within the first hours of birth in a stable newborn. A more comprehensive physical assessment is completed within 24 hours of birth (see Table 16-4).

BOX 17-1

Initial Physical Assessment by Body System

Central nervous system	[ ] Moves extremities, muscle tone good [ ] Symmetric features, movement [ ] Suck, rooting, Moro response, grasp reflexes good [ ] Anterior fontanel soft and flat
Cardiovascular system	[ ] Heart rate strong and regular [ ] No murmurs heard [ ] Pulses strong and equal bilaterally
Respiratory system	[ ] Lungs clear to auscultation bilaterally [ ] No retractions or nasal flaring [ ] Respiratory rate, 30-60 breaths/min [ ] Chest expansion symmetric [ ] No upper airway congestion
Genitourinary system	[ ] Male: urethral opening at tip of penis; testes descended bilaterally [ ] Female: vaginal opening apparent
Gastrointestinal system	[ ] Abdomen soft, no distention [ ] Cord attached and clamped [ ] Anus appears patent
Ear, nose, throat	[ ] Eyes clear [ ] Palates intact [ ] Nares patent
Skin	Color [ ] pink [ ] acrocyanotic [ ] No lesions or abrasions [ ] No peeling [ ] Birthmarks [ ] Caput and molding [ ] Vacuum "cap" [ ] Forceps marks [ ] Other

Comments:

____

____

____

TABLE 17-1

Apgar Score

	SCORE		
SIGN	0	1	2
Heart rate	Absent	Slow (<100)	>100
Respiratory rate	Absent	Slow, weak cry	Good cry
Muscle tone	Flaccid	Some flexion of extremities	Well flexed
Reflex irritability	No response	Grimace	Cry
Color	Blue, pale	Body pink, extremities blue	Completely pink

Apgar score

The **Apgar score** permits a rapid assessment of the newborn's transition to extrauterine existence based on five signs that indicate the physiologic state of the neonate: (1) heart rate, based on auscultation with a stethoscope or palpation of the umbilical cord; (2) respiratory rate, based on observed movement of respiratory efforts; (3) muscle tone, based on degree of flexion and movement of the extremities; (4) reflex irritability, based on response to bulb syringe or catheter inserted in the nasopharynx; and (5) generalized skin color, described as pallid, cyanotic, or pink (see Table 17-1). Evaluations are made at 1 and 5 minutes after birth and can be completed by the nurse or birth attendant. Scores of 0 to 3 indicate severe distress, scores of 4 to 6 indicate moderate difficulty, and scores of 7 to 10 indicate that the infant is having minimal or no difficulty adjusting to extrauterine life. Apgar scores do not predict future neurologic outcome but are useful for describing the newborn's transition to extrauterine environment (Box 17-2). If resuscitation is required, it should be initiated before the 1-minute Apgar score (American Academy of Pediatrics [AAP] and American College of Obstetricians and Gynecologists [ACOG], 2007).

BOX 17-2

Significance of the Apgar Score

The Apgar score was developed to provide a systematic method of assessing an infant's condition at birth. Researchers have tried to correlate Apgar scores with various outcomes such as development, intelligence, and neurologic development. In some instances, researchers have attempted to attribute causality to the Apgar score, that is, to suggest that the low Apgar score caused or predicted later problems. This use of the Apgar score is inappropriate. Instead the score should be used to ensure that infants are systematically observed at birth to ascertain the need for immediate care. Either a physician or a nurse may assign the score; however, to avoid the real or perceived appearance of bias, the person assisting with the birth should not assign the score. Lack of consistency in the assigned scores limits studies of the Apgar's long-term predictive value. Prospective parents and the public need education on the significance of the Apgar score, as well as its limits. Because infants often do not receive the maximal score of 10, parents need to know that scores of 7 to 10 are within normal limits. Attorneys involved in litigation related to injury of an infant at birth or negative outcomes, either short term or long term, also need education about the Apgar score, its significance, and its limits. This useful tool needs to be used appropriately; health care providers, parents, and the public may need education to ensure appropriate use of the score.

Source: Montgomery, K. (2000). Apgar scores: Examining the long-term significance. *Journal of Perinatal Education, 9*(3), 5-9.

Initial physical assessment

The initial physical assessment includes a brief review of systems (see Box 17-1):

1. *External:* Note skin color, general activity, position; assess nasal patency by closing one nostril at a time while observing respirations; skin: peeling, or lack of subcutaneous fat (preterm or postterm); temperature; note meconium staining of cord, skin, fingernails, or amniotic fluid (staining may indicate fetal release of meconium); note length of nails and development of creases on soles of feet.
2. *Chest:* Auscultate apical heart for rate and rhythm, heart tones, and presence of abnormal sounds; assess rate and character of respirations and presence of crackles or other adventitious sounds; note equality of breath sounds by auscultation and observation.
3. *Abdomen:* Verify characteristics of the abdomen (rounded, flat, concave) and absence of anomalies; auscultate bowel sounds; note number of vessels in the cord and general status of the cord (e.g., thin, emaciated; thick, tortuous; presence of hematoma).
4. *Neurologic:* Check muscle tone, and assess Moro and suck reflexes; palpate anterior fontanel; note by palpation the presence and size of the fontanels and sutures; note bulging or depression of the anterior fontanel.
5. *Genitourinary:* Note external sex characteristics and any abnormality of genitalia; check anal patency (presence of meconium); note passage of urine.
6. *Other observations:* Note gross structural malformations obvious at birth that may require immediate medical attention (e.g., omphalocele, meningocele).

The nurse responsible for the care of the newborn immediately after birth verifies that respirations have been established, dries the infant thoroughly, assesses temperature, and places identical identification bracelets on the infant and the mother. In some settings the father or partner also wears an identification bracelet. In many settings, immediately after birth the infant is placed on the mother's abdomen to allow skin-to-skin contact. This action contributes to stabilizing and maintaining the newborn's body temperature and promotes parental bonding. In other settings, the neonate may be wrapped in a warm blanket and placed in the mother's arms, given to the partner to hold, or kept partially undressed under a radiant warmer. The infant may be admitted to a nursery or may remain with the parents throughout the hospital stay.

The initial examination of the newborn can occur while the nurse is drying and wrapping the infant, or observations can be made while the infant is lying on the mother's abdomen or in her arms immediately after birth. Efforts should be directed toward minimizing interference in the initial parent-infant acquaintance process. If the infant is breathing effectively, is pink in color, and has no apparent life-threatening anomalies or risk factors requiring immediate attention (e.g., infant of a diabetic mother), further examination can be delayed until after the parents have had an opportunity to interact with the infant. Routine procedures and the admission process can be carried out in the mother's room or in a separate nursery.

The nursing process in the immediate care of the newborn and family is outlined in the Nursing Process box.

Interventions

Changes can occur rapidly in newborns immediately after birth. Assessment must be followed quickly by the implementation of appropriate care.

Airway maintenance

Generally, the healthy term infant born vaginally has little difficulty clearing the airway. Most secretions are moved by gravity and brought by the cough reflex to the oropharynx to be drained or swallowed. The infant is often maintained in a side-lying position (head stabilized, not in the Trendelenburg position) with a rolled blanket at the back to facilitate drainage.

If the infant has excess mucus in the respiratory tract, the mouth and nasal passages can be gently suctioned with a bulb syringe (Fig. 17-1). Routine chest percussion and suctioning of healthy term or late preterm infants is avoided; evidence is insufficient to support anything other than gentle nasopharyngeal and oropharyngeal suctioning to clear secretions (Hagedorn, 2006). The infant who is choking on secretions should be supported with the head to the side. The mouth is suctioned first to prevent the infant from inhaling pharyngeal secretions by gasping as the nares are touched. The bulb is compressed and inserted into one side of the mouth. The center of the mouth is avoided because the gag reflex could be stimulated. The nasal passages are suctioned one nostril at a time. The

NURSING PROCESS *Care of the Newborn and Family*

ⓔ Nursing Care Plan: Immediate Care of the Newborn

ASSESSMENT

A brief initial assessment is performed to detect problems that can interfere with effective newborn transition. After the infant is stabilized and mother-infant contact has occurred, a gestational assessment and a complete examination can be performed (see Box 17-1, Fig. 17-1, and Table 16-4).

Assessment should include a psychosocial assessment focusing on parent-infant attachment, adjustment to the parental role, sibling adjustment, social support, and education needs, as well as the mother's and the baby's physical adaptation (see Chapter 15).

NURSING DIAGNOSES

Nursing diagnoses for the newborn are established after analyzing the findings of the physical assessment and may include the following:

- *Ineffective airway clearance* related to:
  - Airway obstruction with mucus, blood, and amniotic fluid
  - Inability to clear mucus by cough or expectoration
- *Impaired gas exchange* related to:
  - Airway obstruction
  - Ineffective breathing pattern
- *Risk for imbalanced body temperature* related to:
  - Imbalance between body heat loss and heat production
- *Pain* related to:
  - Heel stick, circumcision, venipuncture

Possible nursing diagnoses for the parents are as follows:

- *Readiness for enhanced parenting* related to:
  - Knowledge of newborn's social capabilities and dependency needs
  - Knowledge of newborn's biologic characteristics
- *Readiness for enhanced family coping* related to:
  - Positive attitude and realistic expectations for newborn and adapting to parenthood
  - Nurturing behaviors with newborn
  - Verbalizing positive factors in lifestyle change
- *Risk for impaired parent-infant* attachment related to:
  - Difficult labor and birth
  - Postpartum complications
  - Neonatal complications or anomalies
- *Situational low self-esteem* related to:
  - Misinterpretation of newborn's behavioral cues

EXPECTED OUTCOMES OF CARE

Expected outcomes can apply to both the infant and the caregiver. Expected outcomes for the newborn during the immediate recovery period include that the infant will achieve the following:

- Maintain an effective breathing pattern
- Maintain effective thermoregulation
- Remain free from infection
- Receive necessary nutrition for growth
- Establish adequate elimination patterns
- Experience minimal pain
- Remain injury free

Expected outcomes for the parents include that they will accomplish the following:

- Attain knowledge, skill, and confidence relevant to infant care activities.
- State understanding of biologic and behavioral characteristics of the newborn.
- Identify deviations from normal that should be brought to the attention of the primary health care provider.
- Have opportunities to intensify their relationship with the infant.
- Begin to integrate the infant into the family.

PLAN OF CARE AND INTERVENTIONS

Several intervention strategies for the newborn infant and family are discussed on pp. 482-488.

EVALUATION

Evaluation is based on the expected outcomes of care. The plan is revised as needed based on the evaluation findings.

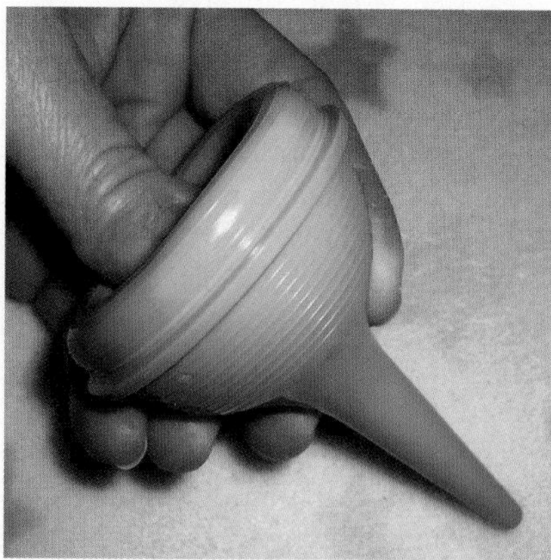

Fig. 17-1 Bulb syringe. Bulb must be compressed before insertion. (Courtesy Cheryl Briggs, RN, Annapolis, MD.)

nurse should listen to the infant's respirations and lung sounds with a stethoscope to determine whether crackles, rhonchi, or inspiratory stridor are present. Fine crackles may be auscultated for several hours after birth. If the bulb syringe does not clear mucus interfering with respiratory effort, mechanical suction can be used.

The bulb syringe should always be kept in the infant's crib. The parents should be given a demonstration of how to use the bulb syringe and asked to perform a return demonstration.

If the newborn has an obstruction that is not cleared with suctioning, further investigation must occur to determine if a mechanical defect (e.g., tracheoesophageal fistula, choanal atresia [see Chapter 24]) is causing the obstruction.

Deeper suctioning may be needed to remove mucus from the newborn's nasopharynx or posterior oropharynx. However, this type of suctioning should be performed only after an assessment of the risks involved. Proper tube insertion and suctioning for 5 seconds or less per tube insertion helps prevent vagal stimulation and hypoxia. If wall suction is used, the pressure should be adjusted to less than 80 mm Hg. After the catheter is properly placed, suction is created by intermittently placing one's thumb over the control as the catheter is carefully rotated and gently withdrawn. This procedure may need to be repeated until the infant has a clear airway (see Procedure box).

Maintaining an adequate oxygen supply. Four conditions are essential for maintaining an adequate oxygen supply:

- A clear airway
- Effective establishment of respirations
- Adequate circulation, adequate perfusion, and effective cardiac function
- Adequate thermoregulation (Exposure to cold stress increases oxygen and glucose needs.)

Signs of potential complications related to abnormal breathing are listed in the Signs of Potential Complications box.

Procedure

Suctioning with a Bulb Syringe

- The bulb syringe should always be kept in the infant's crib.
- The mouth is suctioned first to prevent the infant from inhaling pharyngeal secretions by gasping as the nares are touched.
- The bulb is compressed (see Fig. 17-1) and inserted into one side of the mouth. The center of the infant's mouth is avoided because the gag reflex could be stimulated.
- The nasal passages are suctioned one nostril at a time.
- When the infant's cry does not sound as though it is through mucus or a bubble, suctioning can be stopped.
- The parents should be given demonstrations on how to use the bulb syringe and asked to perform a return demonstration.

Maintaining body temperature

Effective neonatal care includes maintenance of an optimal thermal environment (see Chapter 16). Cold stress increases the need for oxygen and may deplete glucose stores. The infant may react to exposure to cold by increasing the respiratory rate and may become cyanotic. Ways to stabilize the newborn's body temperature include placing the infant directly on the mother's abdomen and covering with a warm blanket (skin-to-skin contact), drying and wrapping the newborn in warmed blankets immediately after birth, keeping the head well covered, and keeping the ambient temperature of the nursery at 22° to 26° C (AAP & ACOG, 2012). Allowing vernix caseosa to remain on the infant's skin has not been associated with a decrease in axillary temperature in the first hour after birth (Visscher et al., 2005).

If the infant does not remain with the mother during the first 1 to 2 hours after birth, the nurse places the thoroughly dried infant under a radiant warmer or in a warm incubator until the body temperature stabilizes. The infant's skin temperature is used as the point of control in a warmer with a servo-controlled mechanism. The control panel is usually maintained between 36° and 37° C. This setting should maintain the healthy term newborn's skin temperature at approximately 36.5° to 37° C. A thermistor probe (automatic sensor) is usually placed on the upper quadrant of the abdomen immediately below the right or left costal margin (never over a bone). A reflector adhesive patch may be used over the probe to provide adequate warming. This probe will ensure detection of minor temperature changes resulting from external environmental factors or neonatal factors (peripheral vasoconstriction, vasodilation, or increased metabolism) before a dramatic change in core body temperature develops. The servo-controller adjusts the temperature of the warmer to main-

NURSING CARE PLAN Normal Newborn

NURSING DIAGNOSIS Risk for ineffective airway clearance related to excess mucus production or improper positioning

Expected Outcomes *Neonate's airway remains patent; breath sounds are clear, and no respiratory distress is evident.*

Nursing Interventions/*Rationales*

- Teach the parents that gagging, coughing, and sneezing are normal neonatal responses *that assist the neonate in clearing the airways.*
- Teach the parents feeding techniques that prevent overfeeding and distention of the abdomen and to burp the neonate frequently *to prevent regurgitation and aspiration.*
- Position the neonate on the back when sleeping *to prevent suffocation.*
- Suction the mouth and nasopharynx with a bulb syringe as needed; clean the nares of crusted secretions *to clear the airway and prevent aspiration and airway obstruction.*

NURSING DIAGNOSIS Risk for imbalanced body temperature related to larger body surfaces relative to mass

Expected Outcome *Neonate temperature remains in range of 36.5° to 37.5° C.*

Nursing Interventions/*Rationales*

- Maintain a neutral thermal environment *to identify any changes in the neonate's temperature that may be related to other causes.*
- Monitor the neonate's axillary temperature frequently *to identify any changes promptly and ensure early interventions.*
- Bathe the neonate efficiently when temperature is stable, using warm water, drying carefully, and avoiding exposing neonate to drafts *to avoid heat losses from evaporation and convection.*
- Report any alterations in temperature findings promptly *to assess and treat for possible infection.*

NURSING DIAGNOSIS Risk for infection related to immature immunologic defenses and environmental exposure

Expected Outcome *The neonate will be free from signs of infection.*

Nursing Interventions/*Rationales*

- Review the maternal record for evidence of any risk factors *to ascertain whether the neonate may be predisposed to infection.*
- Monitor vital signs *to identify early possible evidence of infection, especially temperature instability.*
- Have all care providers, including parents, practice good handwashing techniques before handling the newborn *to prevent the spread of infection.*
- Provide the prescribed eye prophylaxis *to prevent infection.*
- Keep the genital area clean and dry using proper cleansing techniques *to prevent skin irritation, cross-contamination, and infection.*
- Keep the umbilical stump clean and dry, and keep it exposed to the air *to allow to dry and minimize the chance of infection.*
- If the infant is circumcised, keep the site clean, and apply the diaper loosely *to prevent trauma and infection.*
- Teach the parents to keep the neonate away from crowds and environmental irritants *to reduce potential sources of infection.*

NURSING DIAGNOSIS Risk for injury related to sole dependence on caregiver

Expected Outcome *Neonate remains free of injury.*

Nursing Interventions/*Rationales*

- Monitor the environment for hazards such as sharp objects, long fingernails of the caretaker and neonate, and jewelry of the caretaker that may be sharp *to prevent injury.*
- Handle the neonate gently and support the head, ensure the use of a car seat by parents, teach parents to avoid placing the neonate on a high surface unsupervised and to supervise pet and sibling interactions *to prevent injury.*
- Assess the neonate frequently for any evidence of jaundice *to identify rising bilirubin levels, treat promptly, and prevent kernicterus.*

NURSING DIAGNOSIS Readiness for enhanced family coping related to anticipatory guidance regarding responses to the neonate's crying

Expected Outcome *Parents will verbalize their understanding of the methods of coping with the neonate's crying, and describe increased success in interpreting the neonate's cries.*

Nursing Interventions/*Rationales*

- Alert the parents to crying as the neonate's form of communication and that cries can be differentiated to indicate hunger, wetness, pain, and loneliness *to provide reassurance that crying is not indicative of the neonate's rejection of parents and that parents will learn to interpret the different cries of their child.*
- Differentiate self-consoling behaviors from fussing or crying *to give parents concrete examples of interventions.*
- Discuss methods of consoling a neonate who has been crying, such as checking and changing diapers, talking softly to the neonate, holding the neonate's arms close to the body, swaddling, picking the neonate up, rocking, using a pacifier, feeding, or burping *to provide anticipatory guidance.*

Procedure

Suctioning with a Nasopharyngeal Catheter with Mechanical Suction Apparatus

To remove excessive or tenacious mucus from the infant's nasopharynx:

- If wall suction is used, adjust the pressure to under 80 mm Hg. Proper tube insertion and suctioning for 5 seconds per tube insertion help prevent laryngospasms and oxygen depletion.
- Lubricate the catheter in sterile water and then insert either orally along the base of the tongue or up and back into the nares.
- After the catheter is properly placed, create suction by intermittently placing your thumb over the control as the catheter is carefully rotated and gently withdrawn.
- Repeat the procedure until the infant's cry sounds clear and air entry into the lungs is heard by stethoscope.

tain the infant's skin temperature within the preset range. The sensor needs to be checked periodically to make sure it is securely attached to the infant's skin. The axillary temperature of the newborn is checked every hour (or more often as needed) until the newborn's temperature stabilizes. The length of time to stabilize and maintain body temperature varies; each newborn should therefore be allowed to achieve thermal regulation as necessary, and care should be individualized.

During all procedures, heat loss must be avoided or minimized for the newborn; therefore examinations and activities are performed with the newborn under a heat panel. The initial bath is postponed until the newborn's skin temperature is stable and can adjust to heat loss from a bath. The exact and optimal timing of the bath for each newborn remains unknown.

Even a healthy term infant can become hypothermic. Birth in a car on the way to the hospital, a cold birthing room, or inadequate drying and wrapping immediately after birth may cause the newborn's temperature to fall below the normal range (hypothermia). Warming the hypothermic infant is accomplished with care. Rapid warming may cause apneic spells and acidosis in an infant. Therefore the warming process is monitored to progress slowly over a period of 2 to 4 hours.

Immediate interventions

One of the nurse's responsibilities is to perform certain interventions soon after birth to provide for the safety of the newborn. Such interventions can be delayed for an hour or two so that uninterrupted maternal-infant bonding can occur.

Eye prophylaxis. The instillation of a prophylactic agent in the eyes of all neonates (Fig. 17-2) is mandatory in the United States. This is a precautionary measure against **ophthalmia neonatorum,** which is an inflammation of the eyes resulting from gonorrheal or chlamydial infection contracted by the newborn during passage through the mother's birth canal. In the United States, if parents object to this treatment, they may be asked to sign an informed refusal form, and their refusal will be noted in the neonate's record. The agent used for prophylaxis varies according to hospital protocols, but usual agents include forms of erythromycin, tetracycline, or silver nitrate (Medication Guide). Canadian hospitals have not recommended the use of silver nitrate since 1986. Its use in the United States is minimal because silver nitrate does not protect against chlamydial infection and can cause chemical conjunctivitis. Instillation of eye prophylaxis may be delayed until an hour or so (up to 2 hours in Canada) after birth so that eye contact and parent-infant attachment and bonding are facilitated.

Topical antibiotics such as tetracycline and erythromycin, silver nitrate, and a 2.5% povidone-iodine solution

signs of POTENTIAL COMPLICATIONS

Abnormal Newborn Breathing

- Bradypnea (≤25 respirations/min)
- Tachypnea (≥60 respirations/min)
- Abnormal breath sounds: crackles, rhonchi, wheezes, expiratory grunt
- Respiratory distress: nasal flaring, retractions, chin tug
- Skin color: cyanosis, mottling
- Pulse oximetry value: <95%

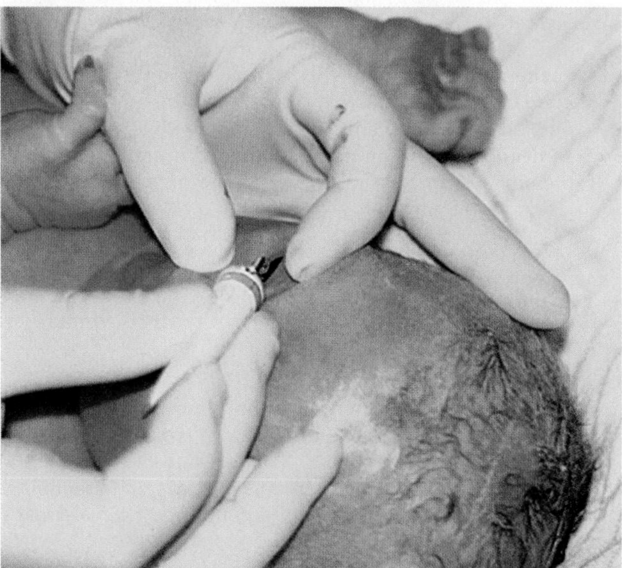

Fig. 17-2 Instillation of medication into eye of newborn. Thumb and forefinger are used to open the eye; medication is placed in the lower conjunctiva from the inner to the outer canthus. (Courtesy Marjorie Pyle, RNC, Lifecircle, Costa Mesa, CA.)

Medication Guide

Eye Prophylaxis: Erythromycin Ophthalmic Ointment, 0.5%, and Tetracycline Ophthalmic Ointment, 1%

ACTION

- These antibiotic ointments are both bacteriostatic and bactericidal. They provide prophylaxis against ophthalmia neonatorum.

INDICATION

- These medications are applied to prevent ophthalmia neonatorum in newborns of mothers who are infected with gonorrhea, conjunctivitis, and chlamydia.

NEONATAL DOSAGE

- Apply a 1- to 2-cm ribbon of ointment to the lower conjunctival sac of each eye; may also be used in drop form.

ADVERSE REACTIONS

- May cause chemical conjunctivitis that lasts 24 to 48 hours; vision may be blurred temporarily.

NURSING CONSIDERATIONS

- Administer within 1 to 2 hours of birth. Wear gloves. Cleanse the eyes if necessary before administration. Open the eyes by putting a thumb and finger at the corner of each lid and gently pressing on the periorbital ridges. Squeeze the tube and spread the ointment from the inner canthus of the eye to the outer canthus. Do not touch the tube to the eye. After 1 minute, excess ointment may be wiped off. Observe eyes for irritation. Explain the treatment to the parents.
- Eye prophylaxis for ophthalmia neonatorum is required by law in all states of the United States.

(currently unavailable in commercial form in the United States) are not effective in the treatment of chlamydial conjunctivitis. A 14-day course of oral erythromycin or an oral sulfonamide may be given for chlamydial conjunctivitis (AAP, 2006).

Vitamin K prophylaxis. Administering vitamin K intramuscularly is routine in the newborn period in the United States. A single intramuscular injection of 0.5 to 1 mg of vitamin K is given soon after birth to prevent hemorrhagic disease of the newborn. Administration can be delayed until after the first breastfeeding in the birthing room (AAP & ACOG, 2012). Vitamin K is produced in the gastrointestinal tract by bacteria starting soon after microorganisms are introduced. By day 8, healthy newborns are able to produce their own vitamin K (Medication Guide).

NURSING ALERT Vitamin K is never administered by the intravenous route for the prevention of hemorrhagic disease of the newborn except in some cases of a preterm infant who has no muscle mass. In such cases the medication should be diluted and given over 10 to 15 minutes, with the infant being closely monitored with a cardiorespiratory monitor. Rapid bolus administration of vitamin K can cause cardiac arrest.

Umbilical cord care. The cord is clamped immediately after birth. The goal of cord care is to prevent or decrease the risk of hemorrhage and infection. The umbilical cord stump is an excellent medium for bacterial growth and can easily become infected. The cord clamp is removed once the stump has started drying and is no longer bleeding (Fig. 17-3), typically in 24 hours.

Hospital protocol determines the technique for routine cord care. Common methods include the use of an antimicrobial agent such as bacitracin or triple dye, although some experts advocate the use of alcohol alone, soap and water, sterile water, povidone-iodine, or no treatment (natural healing). Current recommendations for cord

Medication Guide

Vitamin K: Phytonadione (AquaMEPHYTON, Konakion)

ACTION

- This intervention provides vitamin K because the newborn does not have the intestinal flora to produce this vitamin in the first week after birth. It also promotes formation of clotting factors (II, VII, IX, X) in the liver.

INDICATION

- Vitamin K is used for the prevention and treatment of hemorrhagic disease in the newborn.

NEONATAL DOSAGE

- Administer a 0.5- to 1-mg (0.25- to 0.5-ml) dose intramuscularly (IM) within 2 hours of birth; can be repeated if the newborn shows bleeding tendencies. Vitamin K is never administered by the intravenous route for the prevention of hemorrhagic disease of the newborn except in some cases of a preterm infant who has no muscle mass. In such instances, the medication is diluted and given over 10 to 15 minutes while closely monitoring the infant with a cardiorespiratory monitor. Rapid IV administration of vitamin K can cause cardiac arrest.

ADVERSE REACTIONS

- Edema, erythema, and pain at the injection site may occur rarely; hemolysis, jaundice, and hyperbilirubinemia have been reported, particularly in preterm infants.

NURSING CONSIDERATIONS

- Follow procedure for IM injections on pp. 503-504 and Fig. 17-16.

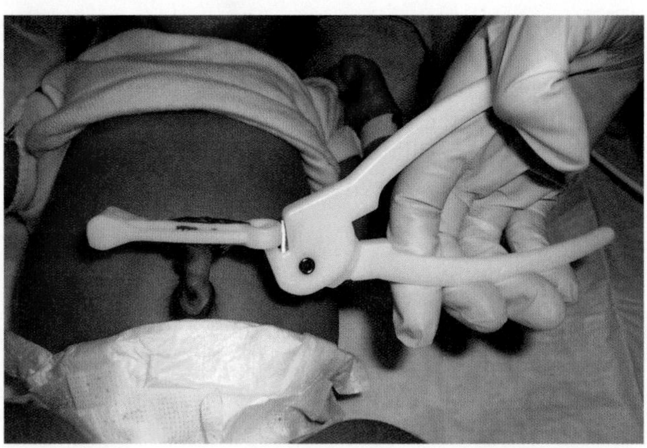

Fig. 17-3 With special scissors, remove clamp after cord dries (approximately 24 hours). (Courtesy Cheryl Briggs, RN, Annapolis, MD.)

care by the Association of Women's Health, Obstetric and Neonatal Nurses (AWHONN, 2007) include cleaning the cord with sterile water initially and subsequently with plain water. A one-time application of triple dye has been shown to be superior to alcohol, povidone-iodine, or topical antibiotics in reducing colonization or infection; the use of alcohol is associated with prolonged cord drying and separation (McConnell, Lee, Couillard, & Sherrill, 2004; Zupan, Garner, & Omari, 2004).

The stump and base of the cord should be assessed for edema, redness, and purulent drainage with each diaper change. The nurse cleanses the cord and skin area around the base of the cord with the prescribed preparation (e.g., sterile water, erythromycin solution, or triple-blue dye). The stump deteriorates through the process of dry gangrene; therefore odor alone is not a positive indicator of omphalitis (infection of the umbilical stump). Cord separation time is influenced by several factors, including type of cord care, type of birth, and other perinatal events. The average cord separation time is 10 to 14 days. Some dried blood may be seen in the umbilicus at separation (Fig. 17-4).

Promoting parent-infant interaction

Today's childbirth practices strive to promote the family as the focus of care. Parents generally desire to share in the birth process and to have early contact with their infants (see Fig. 1-2). The infant can be put to breast soon after birth. Early contact between mother and newborn can be important in developing future relationships; it also has a positive effect on the duration of breastfeeding. Early mother-infant contact produces physiologic benefits. Oxytocin and prolactin levels rise in the mother and infant suckling is activated. The process of developing active immunity begins as the infant ingests antibodies from the mother's colostrum.

Case Study: The Normal Newborn

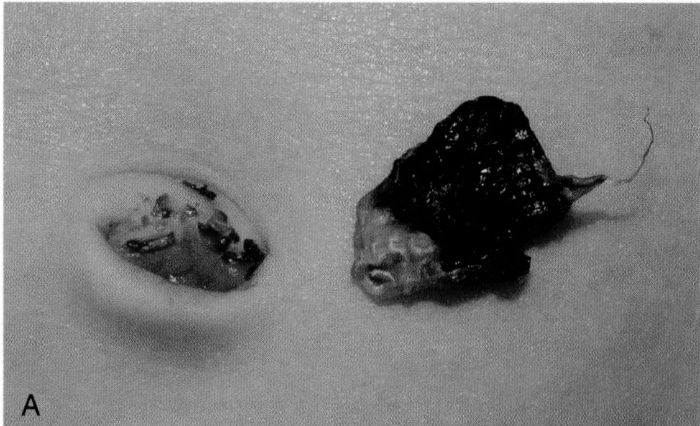

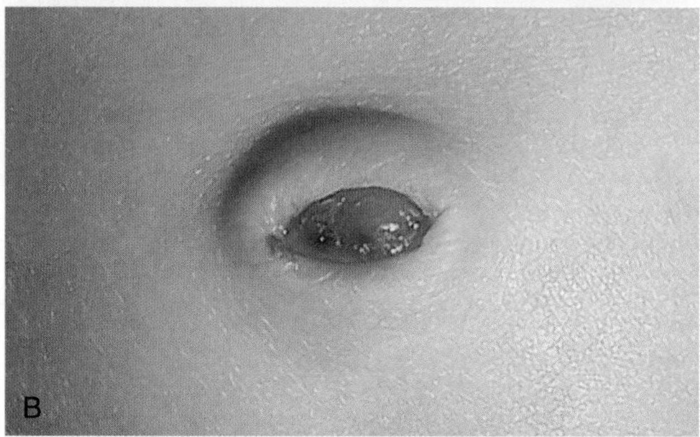

Fig. 17-4 Cord separation. **A,** Cord separated with some dried blood still in the umbilicus. **B,** Umbilicus cleansed and beginning to heal. (Courtesy Cheryl Briggs, RN, Annapolis, MD.)

FROM 2 HOURS AFTER BIRTH UNTIL DISCHARGE

NURSING CARE MANAGEMENT

In an effort to provide more family-centered care, many hospitals have adopted variations of single-room maternity care (SRMC) or mother-baby (couplet) care in which one nurse provides care for the mother and newborn. SRMC allows the infant to remain with the parents after the birth. Many of the procedures, such as assessment of weight and measurement (i.e., circumference of head and length), instillation of eye medication, administration of vitamin K, and physical assessment, are carried out in the labor and birth unit. Nurses who work in an SRMC unit; the labor, delivery, and recovery (LDR) room; or the labor, delivery, recovery, and postpartum (LDRP) room must be educated and competent in providing intrapartal, neonatal, and postpartum nursing care. If an infant is transferred to the nursery, the nurse receiving the newborn verifies the infant's identification, places the baby in a warm environment, and begins the admission process.

Assessment

Physical assessment

A complete physical examination is performed within 24 hours, after the infant's condition has stabilized (Box

17-3). See Chapter 16 for a detailed description of this examination.

Gestational age assessment

Assessment of gestational age is important because perinatal morbidity and mortality rates are related to gestational age and birth weight. A frequently used method of determining gestational age is the simplified Assessment of Gestational Age scale (Ballard, Novak, & Driver, 1979) (see Fig. 17-5, *A*). This scale, an abbreviated version of the Dubowitz scale, can be used to measure gestational ages of infants between 35 and 42 weeks. It assesses six external physical and six neuromuscular signs. Each sign has a numerical score, and the cumulative score correlates with a maturity rating of 26 to 44 weeks of gestation.

The New Ballard Score, a revision of the original scale, can be used with newborns as young as 20 weeks of gestation. The tool has the same physical and neuromuscular sections but includes –1 to –2 scores that reflect signs of extremely premature infants, such as fused eyelids; imperceptible breast tissue; sticky, friable, transparent skin; no lanugo; and square-window (flexion of wrist) angle greater than 90 degrees (see Fig. 17-5, *A*). The examination of infants with a gestational age of 26 weeks or less should be performed at a postnatal age of less than 12 hours. For infants with a gestational age of at least 26 weeks the examination can be performed up to 96 hours after birth. To ensure accuracy, experts recommend that the initial examination be performed within the first 48 hours of life. Neuromuscular adjustments after birth in extremely immature neonates require that a follow-up examination be performed to further validate neuromuscular criteria. The New Ballard Scale overestimates gestational age by 2 to 4 days in infants younger than 37 weeks of gestation, especially at gestational ages of 32 to 37 weeks (Ballard, Khoury, Wedig, Wang, Eilers-Walsman, & Lipp, 1991). Box 17-4 highlights specific maneuvers used in gestational age assessment.

Classification of newborns by gestational age and birth weight

Classification of infants at birth by both birth weight and gestational age provides a more satisfactory method

BOX 17-3

Physical Examination of the Newborn

- Provide a normothermic and nonstimulating examination area.
- Check that equipment and supplies are working properly and are accessible.
- Undress only the body area to be examined to prevent heat loss.
- Proceed in an orderly sequence (usually head to toe) with the following exceptions:
  - Perform all procedures that require quiet first, such as observing respirations, position, skin color, tone, and condition.
  - Next, auscultate the lungs, heart, and abdomen.
  - Perform more disturbing procedures, such as testing reflexes, last.
  - Measure head and length at same time to compare results.
- Proceed quickly to prevent stressing the infant.
- Comfort the infant during and after the examination; involve the parent in the following:
  - Talk softly.
  - Hold the infant's hands against his or her chest.
  - Swaddle and hold.
  - Give a pacifier or gloved finger to suck.

BOX 17-4

Maneuvers Used in Assessing Gestational Age

POSTURE

With infant quiet and in a supine position, observe degree of flexion in arms and legs. Muscle tone and degree of flexion increase with maturity. Full flexion of the arms and legs = score 4.*

SQUARE WINDOW

With thumb supporting back of arm below wrist, apply gentle pressure with index and third fingers on dorsum of hand without rotating infant's wrist. Measure angle between base of thumb and forearm. Full flexion (hand lies flat on ventral surface of forearm) = score 4.*

ARM RECOIL

With infant supine, fully flex both forearms on upper arms and hold for 5 seconds; pull down on hands to extend fully, and rapidly release arms. Observe rapidity and intensity of recoil to a state of flexion. A brisk return to full flexion = score 4.*

POPLITEAL ANGLE

With infant supine and pelvis flat on a firm surface, flex lower leg on thigh and then flex thigh on abdomen. While holding knee with thumb and index finger, extend lower leg with index finger of other hand. Measure degree of angle behind knee (popliteal angle). An angle of less than 90 degrees = score 5.*

SCARF SIGN

With infant supine, support head in midline with one hand; use other hand to pull infant's arm across the shoulder so that infant's hand touches shoulder. Determine location of elbow in relation to midline. Elbow does not reach midline = score 4.*

HEEL TO EAR

With infant supine and pelvis flat on a firm surface, pull foot as far as possible up toward ear on same side. Measure distance of foot from ear and degree of knee flexion (same as popliteal angle). Knees flexed with a popliteal angle of less than 10 degrees = score 4.*

Source: Hockenberry, M. J. & Wilson, D. (2011). *Wong's nursing care of infants and children* (9th ed.). St Louis: Mosby.

*See Fig. 17-5 for scale and interpretation of scores.

NEUROMUSCULAR MATURITY

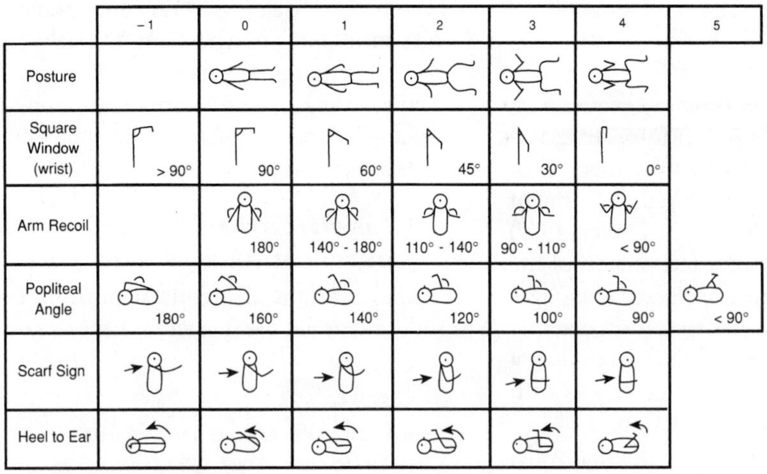

	−1	0	1	2	3	4	5
Posture							
Square Window (wrist)	> 90°	90°	60°	45°	30°	0°	
Arm Recoil		180°	140° - 180°	110° - 140°	90° - 110°	< 90°	
Popliteal Angle	180°	160°	140°	120°	100°	90°	< 90°
Scarf Sign							
Heel to Ear							

PHYSICAL MATURITY

Skin	sticky friable transparent	gelatinous red, translucent	smooth pink, visible veins	superficial peeling or rash, few veins	cracking pale areas rare veins	parchment deep cracking no vessels	leathery cracked wrinkled
Lanugo	none	sparse	abundant	thinning	bald areas	mostly bald	
Plantar Surface	heel-toe 40-50 mm: -1 <40 mm: -2	>50 mm no crease	faint red marks	anterior transverse crease only	creases ant. 2/3	creases over entire sole	
Breast	imperceptible	barely perceptible	flat areola no bud	stippled areola 1-2 mm bud	raised areola 3-4 mm bud	full areola 5-10 mm bud	
Eye/Ear	lids fused loosely: -1 tightly: -2	lids open pinna flat stays folded	sl. curved pinna; soft; slow recoil	well-curved pinna; soft but ready recoil	formed & firm instant recoil	thick cartilage ear stiff	
Genitals (male)	scrotum flat, smooth	scrotum empty faint rugae	testes in upper canal rare rugae	testes descending few rugae	testes down good rugae	testes pendulous deep rugae	
Genitals (female)	clitoris prominent labia flat	prominent clitoris small labia minora	prominent clitoris enlarging minora	majora & minora equally prominent	majora large minora small	majora cover clitoris & minora	

MATURITY RATING

score	weeks
-10	20
-5	22
0	24
5	26
10	28
15	30
20	32
25	34
30	36
35	38
40	40
45	42
50	44

A

Fig. 17-5 Estimation of gestational age. **A,** New Ballard scale for newborn maturity rating. Expanded scale includes extremely premature infants and has been refined to improve accuracy in more mature infants. (From Ballard, J., Khoury, J. K., Wang, L., Eilers-Walsman, B., & Lipp, R. [1991]. New Ballard score, expanded to include extremely premature infants, *Journal of Pediatrics, 119*[3], 417.)

for predicting mortality risks and providing guidelines for management of the neonate than estimating gestational age or birth weight alone. The infant's birth weight, length, and head circumference are plotted on standardized graphs that identify normal values for gestational age. A normal range of birth weights exists for each gestational week (see Fig. 17-5, *B*).

Intrauterine growth curves developed by Battaglia and Lubchenco (1967) have been used to classify infants according to birth weight and gestational age. Since that time, other intrauterine growth charts have emerged to reflect a more heterogeneous sample population than previously described. The primary intrauterine growth charts that provide national reference data include the work of Alexander, Himes, Kaufman, Mor, and Kogan (1996), which is representative of more than 3.1 million live births in the United States; the work of Thomas, Peabody, Turnier, and Clark (2000); Arbuckle, Wilkins, and Sherman (1993); and Kramer and colleagues (2001), which are representative of intrauterine growth among the Canadian population. Thomas and colleagues concluded that intrauterine growth measured by head circumference, birth weight, and length varies according to race and gender. These researchers also found that altitude did not seem to affect birth weight significantly, as has been suggested by other authors. In one study, Asian and Hispanic newborns had lower

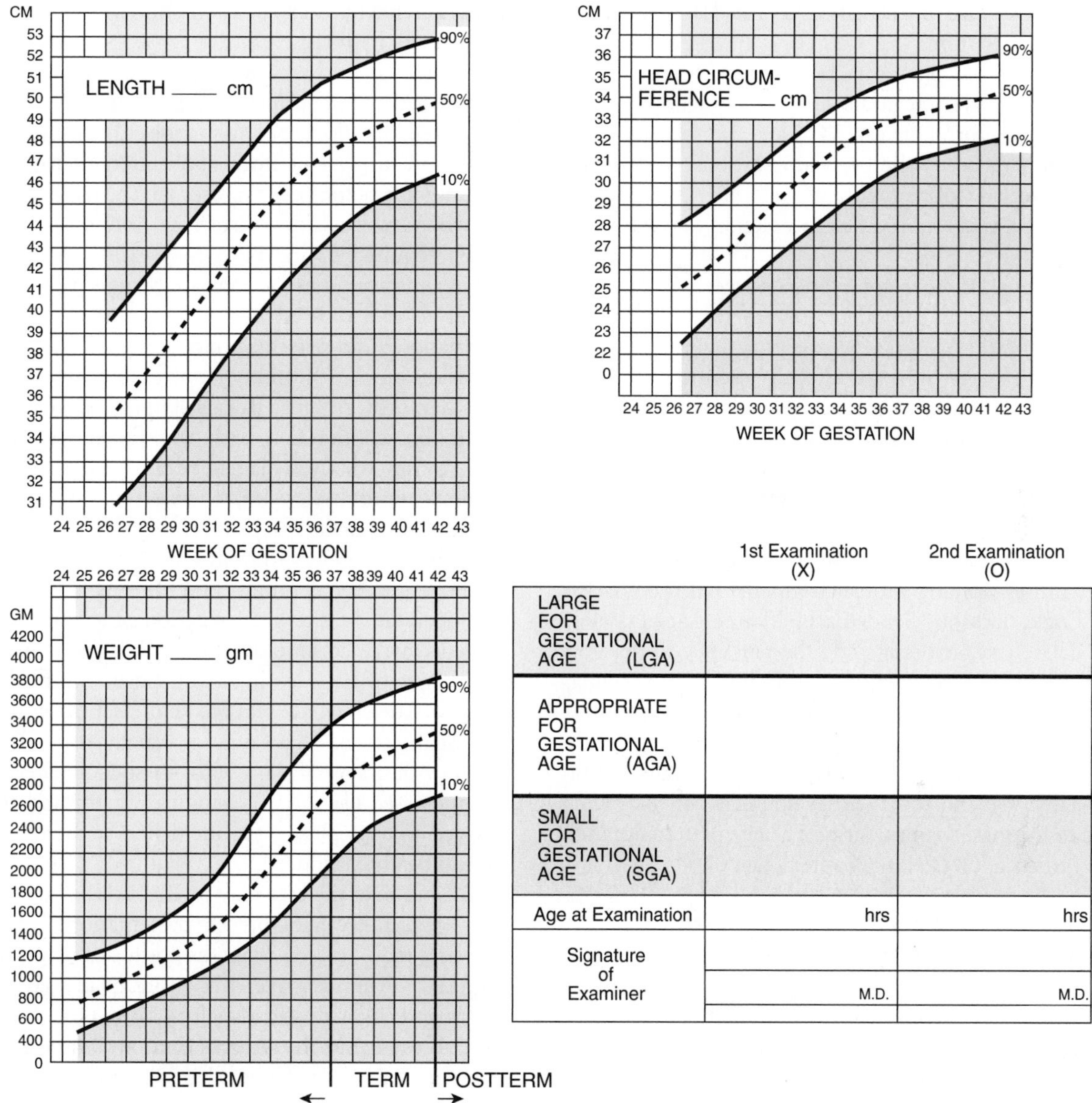

Fig. 17-5, cont'd B, Intrauterine growth: birth weight percentiles based on live single births at gestational ages 20 to 44 weeks. (Data from Alexander, G., Himes, J., Kaufman, R., Mor, J., & Kogan, M. [1996]. A United States national reference for fetal growth. *Obstetrics & Gynecology, 87*[2], 163-168.)

mean birthweights, shorter mean lengths, and smaller mean head circumferences than Caucasian newborns (Madan, Holland, Humbert, & Benitz, 2002). The reader should access and use the most current intrauterine growth chart specific to the referent population being evaluated, especially when considering multiples such as twins.

The infant whose weight is appropriate for gestational age (AGA) (between the 10th and 90th percentiles) can be presumed to have grown at a normal rate regardless of the length of gestation–preterm, term, or postterm. The infant who is large for gestational age (LGA) (above the 90th percentile) can be presumed to have grown at an accelerated rate during fetal life; the small-for-gestational-age (SGA) infant (below the 10th percentile) can be presumed to have grown at a restricted rate during intrauterine life. When gestational age is determined according to the Ballard Scale, the newborn will fall into one of the following nine possible categories for birth weight and gestational age: AGA–term, preterm, postterm; SGA–term, preterm, postterm; or LGA–term, preterm, postterm. Birth weight influences mortality: the lower the birth weight, the higher the mortality. The same is true for gestational age: The lower the gestational age, the higher the mortality (Stoll, 2007).

Infants may also be classified in the following ways according to gestation:

- *Preterm or premature*–born before completion of 37 weeks of gestation, regardless of birth weight
- *Late preterm*–born between $34\frac{0}{7}$ and $36\frac{6}{7}$ weeks
- *Term*–born between the beginning of week 38 and the end of week 42 of gestation
- *Postterm (postdate)*–born after completion of week 42 of gestation
- *Postmature*–born after completion of week 42 of gestation and showing the effects of progressive placental insufficiency

Late preterm infant. Recent attention has been focused on infants who are considered "late preterm." These infants are often the size and weight of term infants and may be admitted to the healthy newborn nursery and treated as healthy newborns. **Late preterm infants**, born at $34\frac{0}{7}$ to $36\frac{6}{7}$ weeks of gestation, have risk factors resulting from their physiologic immaturity that require close attention by nurses working with such infants (Bakewell-Sachs, 2007; Engle, Jackson, Sendelbach, Manning, & Frawley, 2007). These risk factors include the tendency to develop respiratory distress, temperature instability, hypoglycemia, apnea, feeding difficulties, and jaundice and hyperbilirubinemia. Nurses working with healthy term infants must be cognizant of the risk factors for late preterm infants and be continually vigilant for the development of problems related to the infant's immaturity. The late preterm infant's care is further addressed in Chapter 24.

Common Newborn Problems

Physical injuries

Birth trauma includes any physical injury sustained by a newborn during labor and birth. Although most injuries are minor and resolve during the neonatal period without treatment, some types of trauma require intervention; a few are serious enough to be fatal.

Several factors predispose an infant to birth trauma. Maternal factors include uterine dysfunction that leads to prolonged or precipitous labor, preterm or postterm labor, and cephalopelvic disproportion. Injury may result from dystocia caused by fetal macrosomia, multifetal gestation, abnormal or difficult presentation, and congenital anomalies. Intrapartum events that can result in scalp injury include the use of intrapartum monitoring of the fetal heart rate and fetal scalp blood sampling. Obstetric birth techniques can also cause injury. These techniques include forceps birth, vacuum extraction, external version and extraction, and cesarean birth (see Skeletal Injuries and Peripheral Nervous System Injuries in Chapter 24). Caput succedaneum and cephalhematoma are discussed in Chapter 16 (see Fig. 16-4).

Soft-tissue injuries. Subconjunctival and retinal hemorrhages result from rupture of capillaries caused by increased pressure during birth. These hemorrhages usually clear within 5 days after birth and present no further problems. Parents need explanation and reassurance that these injuries are harmless.

Erythema, ecchymoses, petechiae, abrasions, lacerations, or edema of buttocks and extremities may be present. Localized discoloration may appear over the presenting parts and may result from application of forceps or the vacuum extractor. Ecchymoses and edema may appear anywhere on the body. Petechiae (pinpoint hemorrhagic areas) acquired during birth may extend over the upper trunk and face. These lesions are benign if they disappear within 2 or 3 days of birth and no new lesions appear. Ecchymoses and petechiae may be signs of a more serious disorder, such as thrombocytopenic purpura. To differentiate hemorrhagic areas from a skin rash or discolorations, try to blanch the skin with two fingers. Petechiae and ecchymoses will not blanch because extravasated blood remains within the tissues, whereas skin rashes and discolorations do blanch.

Trauma secondary to dystocia can occur to the presenting fetal part. Forceps injury and bruising from the vacuum cup occur at the site of application of the instruments. A forceps injury commonly produces a linear mark across both sides of the face in the shape of the blades of the forceps. The affected areas are kept clean to minimize the risk of infection. These injuries usually resolve spontaneously within several days with no specific therapy. With the increased use of the vacuum extractor and the use of padded forceps blades, the incidence of these lesions can be significantly reduced.

Bruises over the face may be the result of face presentation (Fig. 17-6). In a breech presentation, bruising and swelling may be seen over the buttocks or genitalia (see Fig. 16-8). The skin over the entire head may be ecchymotic and covered with petechiae caused by a tight nuchal cord. If the hemorrhagic areas do not disappear spontaneously in 2 days, or if the infant's condition changes, the physician is notified.

Accidental lacerations may be inflicted with a scalpel during a cesarean birth. These cuts may occur on any part of the body but are most often found on the scalp, buttocks, and thighs. They are usually superficial and need only to be kept clean. Butterfly adhesive strips will hold together the edges of more serious lacerations. Rarely are sutures needed.

Physiologic problems

Conjugation of bilirubin. Bilirubin is one of the products derived from the hemoglobin released with the breakdown of red blood cells (RBCs) and the myoglobin in muscle cells. The hemoglobin is broken down by the reticuloendothelial cells, converted to bilirubin, and released in an unconjugated form. Unconjugated (indirect)

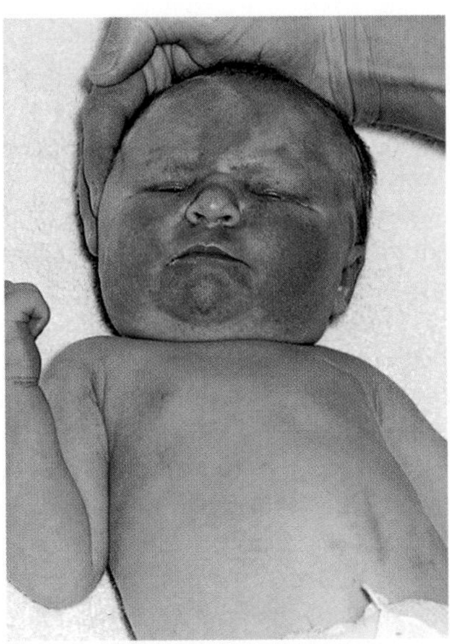

Fig. 17-6 Marked bruising on the entire face of an infant born vaginally after face presentation. Less severe ecchymoses were present on the extremities. Phototherapy was required for treatment of jaundice resulting from the breakdown of accumulated blood. (From O'Doherty, N. [1986]. *Neonatology: Micro atlas of the newborn.* Nutley, NJ: Hoffman-LaRoche.)

bilirubin is relatively insoluble and almost entirely bound to circulating albumin, a plasma protein. The unbound bilirubin can leave the vascular system and permeate other extravascular tissues (e.g., skin, sclera, oral mucous membranes). The resulting yellow coloring is termed *jaundice.*

In the liver the unbound bilirubin is conjugated with glucuronide in the presence of the enzyme glucuronyl transferase. The conjugated form of bilirubin (direct bilirubin) is soluble and is excreted from liver cells as a constituent of bile. Along with other components of bile, direct bilirubin is excreted into the biliary tract system that carries the bile into the duodenum. Bilirubin is converted to urobilinogen and stercobilinogen within the duodenum through the action of the bacterial flora. Urobilinogen is excreted in urine and feces; stercobilinogen is excreted in the feces (see Fig. 16-3). The total serum bilirubin level is the sum of the levels of both conjugated and unconjugated bilirubin.

Physiologic jaundice

Approximately 50% to 60% of all full-term newborns are visibly jaundiced (yellow) during the first 3 days of life. Serum bilirubin levels less than 5 mg/dl are not usually reflected in visible skin jaundice. Although the neonate has the functional capacity to convert bilirubin, physiologic hyperbilirubinemia commonly occurs in infants. **Physiologic jaundice** or **neonatal hyperbilirubinemia** occurs in 80% of preterm newborns. The incidence of physiologic jaundice is increased in Asian, Native American, and Eskimo infants. Although neonatal jaundice is considered benign, bilirubin may accumulate to hazardous levels and lead to a pathologic condition. Neonatal jaundice occurs because the newborn has a higher rate of bilirubin production than does an adult, and considerable reabsorption of bilirubin occurs from the neonatal small intestine.

Two phases of physiologic jaundice have been identified in full-term infants. In the first phase, bilirubin levels of formula-fed Caucasian and African-American infants gradually increase to approximately 5 to 6 mg/dl by 60 to 72 hours of life then decrease to a plateau of 2 to 3 mg/dl by the fifth day (Blackburn, 2007). In Asian and Asian-American infants, levels reach a peak of 10 to 14 mg/dl around the third to fifth day of life; the levels gradually fall to 2 to 3 mg/dl by the seventh to tenth day. Bilirubin levels maintain a steady plateau state in the second phase without increasing or decreasing until approximately 12 to 14 days, at which time levels fall to the normal value of 1 mg/dl (Blackburn). This pattern varies according to racial group, method of feeding (breast versus bottle), and gestational age. In preterm formula-fed infants, serum bilirubin levels may peak as high as 10 to 12 mg/dl at 5 to 6 days of life and decrease slowly over a period of 2 to 4 weeks.

Some characteristics of physiologic jaundice include the following:

- The infant is otherwise well relative to cardiorespiratory status, neurologic status, carbohydrate metabolism, feeding pattern, and elimination.
- In term infants, jaundice first appears *after* 24 hours and disappears by the end of the seventh day.
- In preterm infants, jaundice is first evident after 48 hours and disappears by the ninth or tenth day.
- The infant's predischarge total serum bilirubin falls below the high risk category (<95th percentile) on the hour-specific nomogram (see Fig. 17-8).
- The serum concentration of unconjugated bilirubin usually does not exceed 12 mg/dl in term infants and 15 mg/dl in preterm infants.
- Direct bilirubin does not exceed 1 to 1.5 mg/dl.
- Indirect or unconjugated bilirubin concentration does not increase by more than 5 mg/dl per day.

See Table 17-2 for the varying causes of neonatal indirect hyperbilirubinemia.

NURSING ALERT The appearance of jaundice during the first 24 hours of life or persistence beyond the ages previously delineated usually indicates a potential pathologic process that requires further investigation.

Critical Thinking Exercise: Jaundice

In the newborn intestine the enzyme β-glucuronidase is able to convert conjugated bilirubin into the unconjugated form, which is subsequently reabsorbed by the intestinal mucosa and transported to the liver. This process, known as *enterohepatic circulation*, or *enterohepatic shunting*, is accentuated in the newborn and is thought to be a primary mechanism in physiologic jaundice (Maisels, 2005). Feeding is important in reducing serum bilirubin levels because it stimulates peristalsis and produces more

TABLE 17-2

Causes of Neonatal Indirect Hyperbilirubinemia

BASIS	CAUSES
INCREASED PRODUCTION OF BILIRUBIN	
Increased hemoglobin destruction	Fetomaternal blood group incompatibility (Rh, ABO) Congenital red blood cell abnormalities Congenital enzyme deficiencies (G6PD, galactosemia) Sepsis Enclosed hemorrhage (cephalhematoma, bruising)
Increased amount of hemoglobin	Polycythemia (maternal-fetal or twin-twin transfusion, SGA) Delayed cord clamping
Increased enterohepatic circulation	Delayed passage of meconium, meconium ileus, or plug Fasting or delayed initiation of feeding Intestinal atresia or stenosis
ALTERED HEPATIC CLEARANCE OF BILIRUBIN	
Alteration in uridine diphosphoglucuronyl transferase production or activity	Immaturity Metabolic/endocrine disorders (e.g., Crigler-Najjar disease, hypothyroidism, disorders of amino acid metabolism)
Alteration in hepatic function and perfusion (and thus conjugating ability)	Sepsis (also causes inflammation) Asphyxia, hypoxia, hypothermia, hypoglycemia Drugs and hormones (e.g., novobiocin, pregnanediol)
Hepatic obstruction (associated with direct hyperbilirubinemia)	Congenital anomalies (biliary atresia, cystic fibrosis) Biliary stasis (hepatitis, sepsis) Excessive bilirubin load (often seen with severe hemolysis)

Source: Blackburn, S. T. (2007). *Maternal, fetal, and neonatal physiology: A clinical perspective* (3rd ed.). St. Louis: Saunders.
G6PD, Glucose-6-phosphate dehydrogenase; *SGA,* small for gestational age.

rapid passage of meconium, thus diminishing the amount of reabsorption of unconjugated bilirubin. Feeding also introduces bacteria to aid in the reduction of bilirubin to urobilinogen. Colostrum, a natural laxative, facilitates meconium evacuation.

Every newborn is assessed for jaundice. To differentiate cutaneous jaundice from normal skin color, apply pressure with a finger over a bony area (e.g., the nose, forehead, sternum) for several seconds to empty all the capillaries in that spot. If jaundice is present, the blanched area will look yellow before the capillaries refill. The conjunctival sacs and buccal mucosa also are assessed, especially in darker-skinned infants. Assessing for jaundice in natural light is recommended because artificial lighting and reflection from nursery walls can distort the actual skin color. Visual assessment of jaundice does not, however, provide an accurate assessment of the level of serum bilirubin.

Jaundice is generally noticeable first in the head, especially in the sclera and mucous membranes, and then progresses gradually to the thorax, abdomen, and extremities. The degree of jaundice is determined by serum bilirubin measurements. Normal values of unconjugated bilirubin are 0.2 to 1.4 mg/dl.

An important point to remember is that the evaluation of jaundice is not based solely on serum bilirubin and transcutaneous bilirubin levels; it is also based on the timing of the appearance of clinical jaundice, gestational age at birth, age in hours since birth, family history that includes maternal blood type and Rh status and history of hyperbilirubinemia in a sibling, evidence of hemolysis, feeding method, the infant's physiologic status, and the progression of serial serum bilirubin levels.

Pathologic jaundice is that level of serum bilirubin which, if left untreated, can result in sensorineural hearing loss, mild cognitive delays, and **kernicterus,** which is the deposition of bilirubin in the brain. With ever-changing medical terminology in the literature, less emphasis is placed on pathologic jaundice more by omission than anything else. Nonetheless, one might consider any newborn jaundice as being physiologic (see preceding discussion) unless proven otherwise, in which case the condition may be considered pathologic.

Kernicterus describes the yellow staining of the brain cells that may result in bilirubin encephalopathy. The damage occurs when the serum concentration reaches toxic levels, regardless of cause. There is evidence that a fraction of unconjugated bilirubin crosses the blood-brain barrier in neonates with physiologic hyperbilirubinemia. When certain pathologic conditions exist in addition to elevated bilirubin levels, the permeability of the blood-brain barrier to unconjugated bilirubin is increased, which creates the potential for irreversible damage. The exact level of serum bilirubin required to cause damage is not known. The signs of bilirubin encephalopathy are those of central nervous system depression or excitation. Prodromal symptoms consist of decreased activity, lethargy, irritability, hypotonia, and seizures. Later, these subtle findings are followed by development of athetoid cerebral palsy, mental retardation, and deafness. Neonates who survive may eventually show evidence of neurologic damage, such as mental retardation, attention-deficit/hyperactivity disorder, delayed or abnormal motor movement (especially ataxia or athetosis), behavior disorders, perceptual problems, or sensorineural hearing loss.

Noninvasive monitoring of bilirubin using cutaneous reflectance measurements (transcutaneous bilirubinometry [TcB]) allows for repetitive estimations of bilirubin (Fig. 17-7). These devices work well on both dark- and light-skinned infants and demonstrate linear correlation with serum determinations of bilirubin levels in full-term infants. TcB monitors may be used to screen clinically significant jaundice and decrease the need for serum bilirubin measurements. With shorter maternity stays the value of transcutaneous bilirubin measurements as an assessment tool in follow-up home care has been demonstrated in a homogeneous population. However, because transcutaneous bilirubin measurements are affected by race, gestational age, and birth weight, their use in heterogeneous populations remains limited for diagnostic purposes. In addition, the intensity of jaundice is not always related to the degree of hyperbilirubinemia. The new TcB monitors provide accurate measurements within 2 to 3 mg/dl in most neonatal populations at serum levels below 15 mg/dl (AAP Subcommittee on Hyperbilirubinemia, 2004). After phototherapy has been initiated, TcB is no longer useful as a screening tool.

The use of hour-specific serum bilirubin levels to predict term newborns at risk for rapidly rising levels has now become an official recommendation by the AAP Subcommittee on Hyperbilirubinemia (2004) for the monitoring of healthy neonates at 35 weeks of gestation or greater before discharge from the hospital. Using a nomogram (Fig. 17-8) with three levels (high, intermediate, or low risk) of rising total serum bilirubin values assists in the determination of which newborns might need further evaluation after discharge. Universal bilirubin screening based on hour-specific total serum bilirubin can be performed at the same time as the routine newborn profile (phenylketonuria [PKU], galactosemia, and others) (AAP Subcommittee on Hyperbilirubinemia). The hour-specific bilirubin risk nomogram is used to determine the infant's risk for development of hyperbilirubinemia requiring medical treatment or closer screening. Studies have demonstrated the accuracy of the nomogram in predicting infants with rapidly rising bilirubin levels requiring evaluation or treatment (Keren, Luan, Friedman, Sadlemire, Cnaan, Bhutani, 2008).

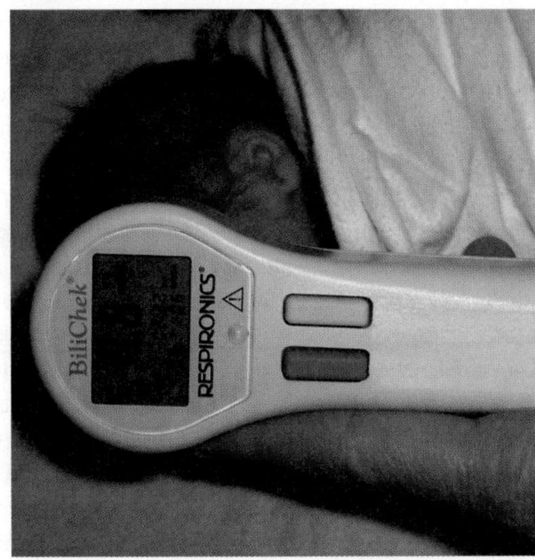

Fig. 17-7 Transcutaneous monitoring of bilirubin with a TcB monitor. (Courtesy Cheryl Briggs, RN, Annapolis, MD.)

Risk factors recognized to place infants in the high risk category include gestational age less than 38 weeks, breastfeeding, previous sibling with significant jaundice, and jaundice appearing before discharge (APA Subcommittee on Hyperbilirubinemia, 2004). Experts recommend that healthy infants (35 weeks or greater) receive follow-up care and assessment of bilirubin within 3 days of discharge if discharged at less than 24 hours and a risk assessment with tools such as the hour-specific nomogram. Newborns discharged at 24 to 47.9 hours should receive follow-up evaluation within 4 days (96 hours), and those discharged between 48 and 72 hours should receive follow-up within 5 days (APA Subcommittee on Hyperbilirubinemia). The guidelines for monitoring and treating neonatal hyperbilirubinemia are published extensively elsewhere (see Resources on this book's website).

One technology that is being investigated for noninvasive bilirubin monitoring includes measuring carbon monoxide indices (end-tidal carbon monoxide concentration [ETCOc]) in exhaled breath (carbon monoxide is produced when RBCs are broken down, thus the extent of hemolysis may be assessed). This technology is currently not being used significantly in the clinical setting because of its expense and lack of predictability in determining neonatal hemolysis (Mincey & Gonzaba, 2007).

Jaundice associated with breastfeeding

Breastfeeding is associated with an increased incidence of jaundice. Two types have been identified; however, the nomenclature may vary among experts. In addition, these types may overlap and may not be easily differentiated from each other (Blackburn, 2007). Breastfeeding-associated jaundice (early-onset jaundice) begins at 2 to 4 days of age and occurs in approximately 10% to 25% of breastfed newborns. The jaundice is related to the process of breastfeeding and probably results from decreased caloric and fluid intake by breastfed infants before the milk supply is well established because lack of sufficient intake is associated with decreased hepatic clearance of bilirubin (Blackburn).

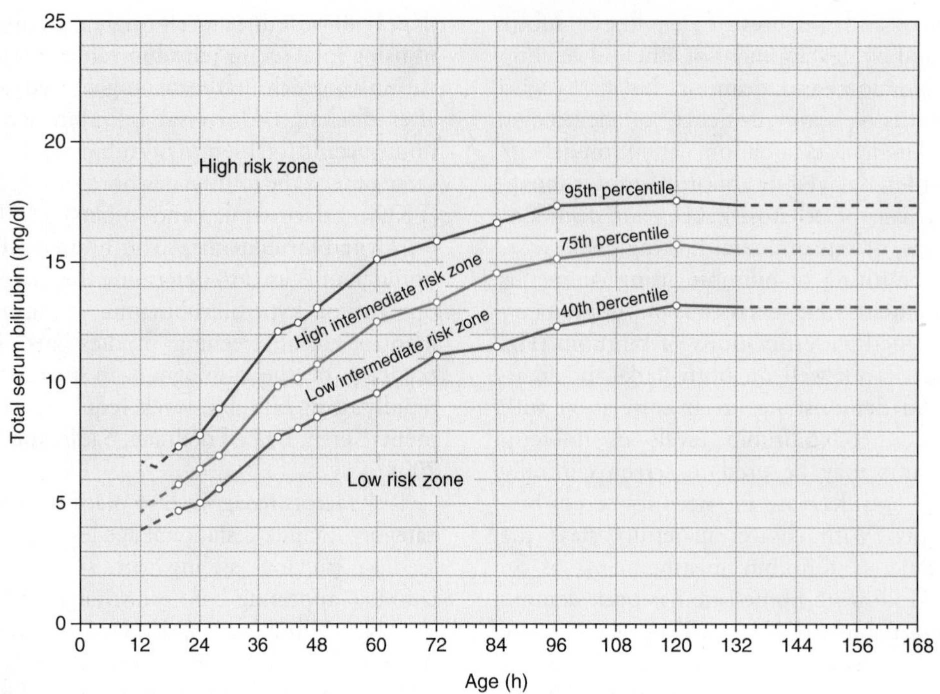

Fig. 17-8 Nomogram for designation of risk in 2840 well newborns at 36 or more weeks of gestational age with birth weight of 2000 g or more or 35 or more weeks of gestational age and birth weight of 2500 g or more based on the hour-specific serum bilirubin values. (This nomogram should not be used to represent the natural history of neonatal hyperbilirubinemia.) (From Bhutani, V. K., Johnson, L., & Sivieri, E. M. [1999]. Predictive ability of a predischarge hour-specific serum bilirubin for subsequent significant hyperbilirubinemia in healthy term and near-term newborns. *Pediatrics, 103*[1], 6-14.)

The presence of decreased caloric intake (less milk), weight loss of more than 5% to 7% in the first 5 days of life, increasing serum bilirubin (unconjugated) levels, decreased stooling, and increased jaundice is also sometimes called *starvation jaundice* or *nonbreastfeeding jaundice*. To prevent this pattern the following measures are suggested: initiation of breastfeeding within the first few hours of life, continuous rooming-in with the mother, breastfeeding 10 to 12 times per day, no supplements, and recognition of and response to hunger cues.

Breast-milk jaundice (late-onset jaundice) may initially begin as the early-onset variety or may begin at age 4 to 6 days and occurs in 2% to 3% of breastfed infants. Rising levels of bilirubin peak during the second week and gradually diminish. Despite high levels of bilirubin that may persist for 3 to 12 weeks, these infants are well and have no signs of hemolysis or liver dysfunction. The jaundice may be caused by factors in the breast milk (pregnanediol, fatty acids, and β-glucuronidase) that either inhibit the conjugation or decrease the excretion of bilirubin. Less-frequent stooling by breastfed infants may allow for extended time for reabsorption of bilirubin from stools (Blackburn, 2007) (see Chapter 18 for a discussion of these conditions in relation to nutrition).

Hypoglycemia. Hypoglycemia during the early newborn period of a term infant is defined as a blood glucose concentration less than adequate to support neurologic, organ, and tissue function; however, the precise level at which this concentration occurs in every neonate is not known. At birth the maternal source of glucose is cut off with the clamping of the umbilical cord. Most healthy term newborns experience a transient decrease in glucose levels, with a subsequent mobilization of free fatty acids and ketones to help maintain adequate glucose levels (Blackburn, 2007). Insulin does not cross the placental barrier, thus predisposing some infants to low glucose levels as a result of increased insulin activity. Infants who are asphyxiated or have other physiologic stress may experience hypoglycemia as a result of a decreased glycogen supply, inadequate gluconeogenesis, or overutilization of glycogen stored during fetal life.

For the healthy full-term infant born after an uneventful pregnancy and birth, recommendations are to monitor glucose levels only in the presence of risk factors, which may be transient but recurrent (e.g., jitteriness, an irregular respiratory effort, cyanosis, apnea, a weak and high-pitched cry, feeding difficulty, hunger, lethargy, twitching, eye rolling, seizures) or clinical manifestations of hypoglycemia; in these infants a plasma glucose of less than 45 mg/dl (2.5 mmol/L) requires intervention. Healthy full-term, breastfed newborns may not fit into this category because human milk appears to provide adequate substrate (Cornblath et al., 2000). Hoseth, Joergensen, Ebbesen, and Moeller (2000) evaluated blood glucose levels in healthy, full-term, breastfed infants and found significant hypoglycemia in only two of the 223 infants during the first 4 days of life.

Close observation and monitoring of blood glucose levels within 2 to 3 hours of birth are recommended for infants who are at risk for altered metabolism as a result of maternal illness factors (diabetes, gestational hypertension, terbutaline administration) or newborn factors (perinatal hypoxia, infection, hypothermia, polycythemia, congenital malformations, hyperinsulinism, small for gestational age, fetal hydrops). If the newborn has a blood glucose level below 36 mg/dl (2.0 mmol/L), intervention such as breastfeeding or bottle-feeding should be instituted. If levels remain low despite feeding, intravenous dextrose is warranted. In such infants the treatment should be aimed at maintaining the blood glucose levels above 45 mg/dl (2.5 mmol/L) (Cornblath et al., 2000). Blood glucose levels for infants with severe hyperinsulinism may need to be higher (60 mg/dl; 3.3 mmol/L) to prevent serious effects. Hypoglycemia in preterm infants requires further studies, but experts have suggested that values be maintained above 47 mg/dl (2.6 mmol/L) (Cornblath et al.).

Experts further recommend that emphasis be placed less on an absolute glucose value but rather on promoting normoglycemia with interventions for less optimal values (Blackburn, 2007). Monitoring blood glucose in the asymptomatic healthy term neonate (not at risk) on a routine basis is not recommended.

Hypoglycemia in the low risk term infant is usually eliminated by feeding the infant a source of carbohydrate (i.e., human milk or formula). Occasionally the intravenous administration of glucose is required for infants with persistently high insulin levels or in those with depleted glycogen stores (Evidence-Based Practice).

Hypocalcemia. Hypocalcemia is defined as serum calcium levels of less than 7.8 to 8 mg/dl in term infants and slightly lower (7 mg/dl) in preterm infants; ideally, ionized fraction levels reflect the biologically active form and levels range from 3 to 4.4 mg/dl depending on the measurement method (Blackburn, 2007). Hypocalcemia may occur in infants of diabetic mothers or in those who had perinatal asphyxia or trauma, and in low-birth-weight and preterm infants. Early-onset hypocalcemia usually occurs within the first 24 to 48 hours after birth. Signs of hypocalcemia include jitteriness, high-pitched cry, irritability, apnea, intermittent cyanosis, abdominal distention, and laryngospasm, although some hypocalcemic infants are asymptomatic (Blackburn).

In most instances, early-onset hypocalcemia is self-limiting and resolves within 1 to 3 days. Treatment includes early feeding of an appropriate source of calcium such as fortified human milk or a preterm infant formula. In some cases (e.g., the medically unstable extremely low-birth-weight-infant) the administration of intravenous elemental calcium and phosphorus may be necessary.

Jitteriness is a symptom of both hypoglycemia and hypocalcemia; therefore hypocalcemia must be considered if the therapy for hypoglycemia proves ineffective.

LABORATORY AND DIAGNOSTIC TESTS

Because newborns experience many transitional events in the first 28 days of life, laboratory samples are often collected to determine adequate physiologic adaptation and to identify disorders that can adversely affect the child's life beyond the neonatal period. Blood samples for most laboratory tests can be obtained from the neonate with a heel puncture. Tests commonly performed include blood glucose levels, bilirubin levels, newborn screening tests (e.g., PKU, thyroxine [T_4], sickle cell disease, galactosemia) and drug serum levels. Standard laboratory values for a term newborn are given in Box 17-5.

Mandated by U.S. law, newborn genetic screening is an important public health program that is aimed at early detection of genetic diseases that result in severe health problems if not treated early. All states screen for PKU and hypothyroidism, but each state determines whether other tests are performed. Other genetic defects that are included in some screening programs include galactosemia, cystic fibrosis, maple syrup urine disease, and sickle cell disease. Experts recommend that the screening test be repeated at age 1 to 2 weeks if the initial specimen was obtained when the infant was younger than 24 hours (Albers & Levy, 2005).

With the increased mobility of the population, newborns at high risk for certain metabolic diseases may not be appropriately screened. Therefore families need to be educated regarding the availability of metabolic tests routinely screened in their state of residence. Tandem mass spectrometry has the potential for identifying more than 30 disorders in addition to the standard inborn errors of metabolism (IEMs). With tandem mass spectrometry, earlier identification of IEMs may prevent further developmental delays and morbidities in affected children.

Information about which tests are required in a state can be obtained from state health departments (see Resources on this book's website). Some of the major disorders for which infants are screened are described in Table 17-3.

Collection of Specimens

Ongoing evaluation and screening of a newborn often requires obtaining blood by the heel-stick or venipuncture or the collection of a urine specimen.

Heel stick

Most blood specimens are drawn by laboratory technicians. Nurses, however, may be required to perform heel sticks to obtain blood for glucose monitoring or newborn

EVIDENCE-BASED PRACTICE

Monitoring for Hypoglycemia

Pat Gingrich

ASK THE QUESTION

What are the current recommendations for monitoring and treating neonatal hypoglycemia?

SEARCH FOR EVIDENCE

Search Strategies: Professional organization guidelines, meta-analyses, systematic reviews, randomized controlled trials, nonrandomized prospective studies, and retrospective studies since 2006.

Search Databases: Cumulative Index to Nursing and Allied Health Literature, Cochrane, Medline, National Guideline Clearinghouse, TRIP Database Plus, and the websites for the American Academy of Pediatrics, the Association of Women's Health, Obstetric and Neonatal Nurses, the Centers for Disease Control and Prevention, and the World Health Organization.

CRITICALLY ANALYZE THE EVIDENCE

Hypoglycemia affects less than 1% of healthy newborns. Risk factors for hypoglycemia included weight below 2 kilograms or above 4 kilograms, small or large for gestational age, intrauterine growth-restricted infants, less than 37 weeks of gestation, maternal diabetes or glucose imbalance, and sepsis. Hypoglycemia of the newborn is infrequently a symptom of underlying disease. Signs of hypoglycemia include irritability, jitteriness, high-pitched cry, pallor, sweating, lethargy, poor feeding, seizures, and respiratory difficulties. A Best Practice Guideline from the Joanna Briggs Institute concluded that breastfeeding early and often, with thermoregulation through skin-to-skin contact, will normalize the glucose levels of most term, normal-weight infants during their first 48 hours (Joanna Briggs Institute, 2006). The guidelines recommended against any supplemental glucose or water feedings or routine glucose monitoring, except in the case of obvious physical signs of hypoglycemia.

This emphasis on breastfeeding early (first hour) and often (10-12 feedings in first 24 hours) concurs with the guidelines for breastfeeding by the Association of Women's Health, Obstetric and Neonatal Nurses (2007) and the Academy of Breastfeeding Medicine (ABM) (2006). The ABM guidelines recommend breastfeeding every 1 to 2 hours and monitoring blood glucose (BG) level. If the BG does not reach the goal of more than 45 mg/dL, consider administering glucose intravenously.

IMPLICATIONS FOR PRACTICE

As noted in the Evidence-Based Practice box in Chapter 24 skin-to-skin contact and early breastfeeding have proven benefits for early temperature and glucose stabilization of the newborn, as well as bonding during the newborn's first awake, interactive period. All nonessential tasks, such as administration of eye medications and vitamin K, should be delayed so as to facilitate this enriching time together. The nurse should be alert to the signs of hypoglycemia, which can appear very late. For most cases without underlying pathology, monitoring the glucose levels and encouraging breastfeeding, rather than supplemental formula or glucose, and skin-to-skin contact will correct the hypoglycemia within minutes or hours. Finally, the nurse should remember that every baby has its own normal range of glucose, which may run high or low in the normal range.

References:

Association of Women's Health Obstetric and Neonatal Nurses (AWHONN). (2007). *Breastfeeding support: Prenatal care through the first year* (2nd ed.). Evidence–Based Clinical Practice Guideline. Washington, DC: AWHONN.

Joanna Briggs Institute of Evidence Based Nursing. (2006). Management of asymptomatic hypoglycemia in healthy term neonates for nurses and midwives. *Best Practice, 10*(1), 1-4.

Wight, N. & Marinelli, K. A. (2006). Academy of Breastfeeding Medicine Protocol Committee: ABM Clinical Protocol No. 1: Guidelines for glucose monitoring and treatment of hypoglycemia in breastfed neonates. *Breastfeeding Medicine, 1*, 178-184.

screening. The same technique is used to obtain a blood sample for a PKU or to test for galactosemia and hypothyroidism or other IEMS (see Table 17-3).

Warming the heel before the sample is taken is often helpful; application of heat for 5 to 10 minutes helps dilate the vessels in the area. A cloth soaked with warm water and wrapped loosely around the foot provides effective warming. Disposable heel warmers also are available from a variety of companies but should be used with care to prevent burns. Nurses should wear gloves when collecting any specimen. The nurse cleanses the area with an appropriate skin antiseptic, restrains the infant's foot with a free hand, and then punctures the site. A spring-loaded automatic puncture device causes less pain and requires fewer punctures than a manual lance blade.

The most serious complication of an infant heel stick is necrotizing osteochondritis resulting from lancet penetration of the bone. To prevent this problem the stick should be made at the outer aspect of the heel and should penetrate no deeper than 2.4 mm. To identify the appropriate puncture site the nurse should draw an imaginary line from between the fourth and fifth toes and parallel to the lateral aspect of the foot to the heel where the stick should be made; a second line can be drawn from the great toe to the medial aspect of the heel (Fig. 17-9, *A*). Repeated trauma to the walking surface of the heel can cause fibrosis and scarring that may lead to problems with walking later in life.

After the specimen has been collected, pressure should be applied with a dry gauze square. No further skin cleanser should be applied because it will cause the site to continue to bleed. The site is then covered with an adhesive bandage. The nurse ensures proper disposal of equipment used, reviews the laboratory requisition for correct

BOX 17-5

Standard Laboratory Values in the Neonatal Period

			NEONATAL
1. HEMATOLOGIC VALUES			
Clotting factors			
Activated clotting time (ACT)			2 min
Bleeding time (Ivy)			2 to 7 min
Clot retraction			Complete 1 to 4 hr
Fibrinogen			125 to 300 mg/dl*

	TERM	PRETERM
Hemoglobin (g/dl)	14 to 24	15 to 17
Hematocrit (%)	44 to 64	45 to 55
Reticulocytes (%)	0.4 to 6	Up to 10
Fetal hemoglobin (% of total)	40 to 70	80 to 90
Red blood cells (RBCs)/mcl†	4.8×10^6 to 7.1×10^6	
Platelet count/mm³	150,000 to 300,000	120,000 to 180,000
White blood cells (WBCs)/mcl	9000 to 30,000	10,000 to 20,000
Neutrophils (%)	54 to 62	47
Eosinophils and basophils (%)	1 to 3	
Lymphocytes (%)	25 to 33	33
Monocytes (%)	3 to 7	4
Immature WBCs (%)	10	16

			NEONATAL
2. BIOCHEMICAL VALUES			
Bilirubin, direct			0 to 1 mg/dl
Bilirubin, total	Cord:		<2 mg/dl
	Peripheral blood:	0 to 1 day	6 mg/dl
		1 to 2 days	8 mg/dl
		2 to 5 days	12 mg/dl
Blood gases		Arterial:	pH 7.31 to 7.49
			P_{CO_2} 26 to 41 mm Hg
			P_{O_2} 60 to 70 mm Hg
		Venous:	pH 7.31 to 7.41
			P_{CO_2} 40 to 50 mm Hg
			P_{O_2} 40 to 50 mm Hg
Serum glucose			40 to 60 mg/dl
3. URINALYSIS			
Color			Clear, straw
Specific gravity			1.001 to 1.020
pH			5 to 7
Protein			Negative
Glucose			Negative
Ketones			Negative
RBCs			0 to 2
WBCs			0 to 4
Casts			None

Sources: Hockenberry, M. & Wilson, D. (2011). *Wong's nursing care of infants and children* (9th ed.). St. Louis: Mosby; Pagana, K. & Pagana, T. (2006). *Mosby's manual of diagnostic and laboratory tests* (3rd ed.). St. Louis: Mosby.

**dl* refers to deciliter (1 dl=100 ml); this conforms to the SI system (standardized international measurements).

†*mcl* refers to microliter.

Volume: 24 to 72 ml/kg excreted daily in the first few days; by week 1, 24-hr urine volume close to 200 ml.

Protein: may be present in first 2 to 4 days.

Osmolarity (mOsm/L): 100 to 600.

P_{CO_2}, partial pressure of carbon dioxide; P_{O_2}, partial pressure of oxygen; *RBCs*, red blood cells; *WBCs*, white blood cells.

TABLE 17-3

Newborn Screening Summary

DISORDER/EVIDENCE	SYMPTOMS	SCREENING INCIDENCE	TREATMENT
PKU (classic) Elevated phenylalanine (plasma concentrations >20 mg/dl)	Severe mental retardation if early detection and treatment not started eczema, seizures, behavior disorders, decreased pigmentation, distinctive musty or mouse-like odor	1:13,500 to 1:20,000 More common in Caucasians and Native Americans	Lifelong dietary management with low-phenylalanine diet; possible tyrosine supplementation
Congenital hypothyroidism (primary) Low T_4, elevated TSH	Asymptomatic at birth; mental and motor delays (although neonatal detection and treatment has decreased incidence of mental retardation), short stature, coarse, dry skin and hair, hoarse cry, constipation	1:3600 to 1 in 5000 live births with some ethnic variation 1:32,000 African-American 1:2000 Hispanic and Native American	Maintain L-thyroxine levels in upper half of normal range; periodic bone age to monitor growth
Galactosemia (transferase deficiency) Elevated galactose; low or absent fluorescence	Hypotonia, lethargy, vomiting, diarrhea, metabolic acidosis, *Escherichia coli* sepsis, or liver dysfunction; mental retardation, jaundice, blindness, cataracts, long-term behavioral problems, and neurologic impairment	1:60,000 to 1:250,000	Eliminate galactose and lactose from the diet; soy formulas in infancy; lactose-free solid foods
Maple syrup urine disease (MSUD) Elevated leucine	Poor feeding, lethargy, hypotonia, vomiting, ketoacidosis, and seizures; sweet maple syrup odor may occur in urine, cerumen, or sweat	1:90,000 to 1:100,000; higher in certain Mennonite (Older Order) populations, 1 in 176 to 1 in 358	Branched-chain amino acid–free formula with added protein-based formula; thiamine supplement in some individuals; lifelong treatment and monitoring necessary
Homocystinuria Elevated methionine and homocysteine	Infancy: nonspecific growth failure; developmental delay; more commonly diagnosed around 3 yrs—mental retardation, seizures, behavioral disorders, early-onset thromboses, dislocated lenses, tall lanky body habitus	1:150,000 to 1:200,000; more prevalent in Ireland and New South Wales, Australia (1 in 60,000)	Methionine-restricted diet; cystine supplement; vitamin B_6 supplement if responsive
Congenital adrenal hyperplasia (CAH) Elevated 17-hydroxyprogesterone; abnormal electrolytes	Hyponatremia, hyperkalemia, hypoglycemia, dehydration; weight loss; hypotension; shock in "salt wasting" type; female virilization; progressive virilization in both sexes	1:10,000 to 1:20,000; higher in Native Alaskans, 1 in 300	Reduce excessive corticotrophins; replace glucocorticoids and mineral corticoids; corrective surgery for ambiguous genitalia (intersex assignment is controversial)
Sickle cell/hemoglobin SC (thalassemias)	Repeated infections, growth failure , pallor, hemolytic anemia; sickle cell crisis	Sickle cell anemia (SCA), 1 in 2,647 in non–African-Americans; 1 in 375 African-Americans; 1 in 36,000 Hispanics	Preventive care: treatment of meningococcal and pneumococcal infections; hydroxyurea (antisickling agent); prevent human parvovirus B19 infection (limits production of reticulocytes)
Biotinidase deficiency Deficient or absent activity of biotinidase on colorimetric assay	Myoclonic seizures, hypotonia, feeding difficulties, organic aciduria, fungal infections, ataxia, skin rash, hearing loss, alopecia, optic nerve atrophy, developmental delay, coma, and death	1:60,000 to 1:137,000	5-20 mg biotin daily; less with partial deficiency

Sources: DeBaun, M. R. & Vichinsky, E. (2007). Hemoglobinopathies. In R. M. Kliegman R. E. Behrman, H. B. Jenson, & B. F. Stanton (Eds.), *Nelson textbook of pediatrics* (18th ed.). Philadelphia: Saunders; LaFranchini, S. (2007). Disorders of the thyroid gland. In R. M. Kliegman, R. E. Behrman, H. B. Jenson, & B. F. Stanton (Eds.), *Nelson textbook of pediatrics* (18th ed.). Philadelphia: Saunders; Lashley, F. R. (2002). Newborn screening: New opportunities and new challenges. *Newborn & Infant Nursing Reviews, 2*(4), 228-242; Rezvani, I. (2007). Metabolic diseases. In R. M. Kliegman R. E. Behrman, H. B. Jenson, & B. F. Stanton (Eds.), *Nelson textbook of pediatrics* (18th ed.). Philadelphia: Saunders.
PKU, phenylketonuria; T_4, thyroxine, *TSH*, thyroid-stimulating hormone.

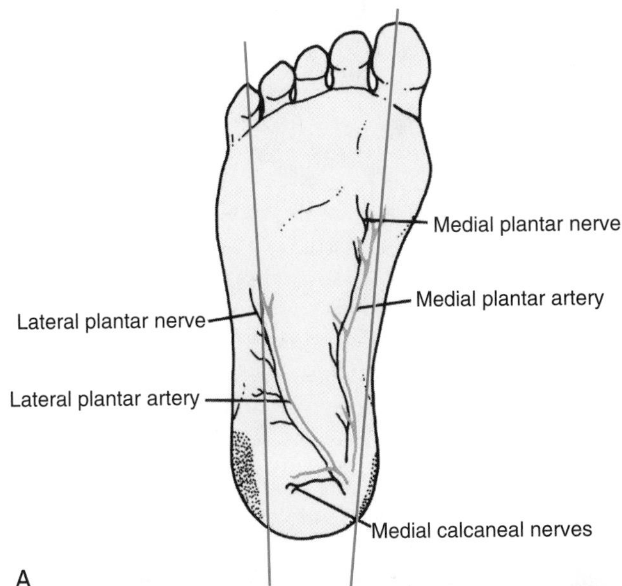

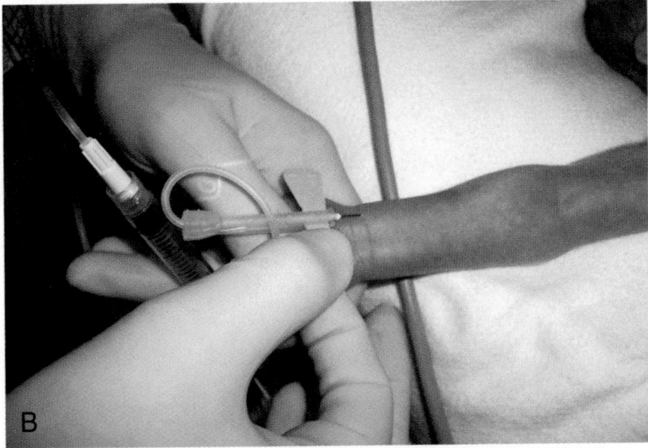

Fig. 17-9 Heel stick and venipuncture. **A,** Heel-stick sites (*shaded areas*) on infant's foot for obtaining samples of capillary blood. **B,** Venipuncture using a butterfly needle. (**B,** Courtesy Cheryl Briggs, RN, Annapolis, MD.)

identification, and checks the specimen for accurate labeling and routing.

A heel stick is traumatic for the infant and causes pain. After several heel sticks, infants have been observed to withdraw their feet when they are touched. To reassure the infant and promote feelings of safety the neonate should be cuddled and comforted when the procedure is complete and appropriate pain management measures taken to minimize the pain.

Venipuncture

Venous blood samples can be drawn from antecubital, saphenous, superficial wrist, and rarely, scalp veins. If an existing intravenous site is used to obtain a blood specimen, the type of infusion fluid is an important consideration; contamination of the blood sample with the fluid can alter the results.

When venipuncture is required, positioning of the needle is extremely important. Although regular venipuncture needles can be used, butterfly needles are sometimes preferred (Fig. 17-9, *B*). A 25-gauge needle is adequate for blood sampling in neonates, with minimal hemolysis occurring when the proper procedure is followed. Patience is required during the procedure because the blood return in small veins is slow, and consequently the small needle must remain in place longer than larger needles. A tourniquet is optional but can help increase blood flow with venipuncture. The mummy restraint is commonly used to help secure the infant (Fig. 17-10). Other methods of restraint are in Fig. 17-11.

For blood gas studies the blood sample container is packed in ice (to reduce blood cell metabolism) and taken immediately to the laboratory for analysis.

Pressure must be maintained over an arterial or femoral vein puncture with a dry gauze square for at least 3 to 5 minutes to prevent bleeding from the site. For an hour after any venipuncture the nurse should observe the infant frequently for evidence of bleeding or hematoma formation at the puncture site. The infant's tolerance of the procedure should be noted and recorded. The infant should be cuddled and comforted (e.g., rocked, given a pacifier) when the procedure is completed and appropriate pain management measures taken to minimize pain associated with the procedure.

NURSING ALERT Only venous or capillary blood samples can be used for newborn screening and genetic studies; cord blood is not used for such samples.

Obtaining a urine specimen

Examination of urine is a valuable laboratory tool for infant assessment; the way in which the specimen is collected may influence the results. The urine sample should be fresh and analyzed within 1 hour of collection.

A variety of urine collection bags are available (Fig. 17-12). These containers are clear plastic, single-use bags with an adhesive material around the opening at the point of attachment.

To prepare the infant the nurse removes the diaper and places the infant in a supine position. The genitalia, perineum, and surrounding skin are washed and thoroughly dried because the adhesive on the bag will not stick to moist, powdered, or oily skin surfaces. The protective paper is removed to expose the adhesive (Fig. 17-12, *A*). In female infants the perineum is stretched to flatten skin folds; then the adhesive area on the bag is pressed firmly to the skin all around the urinary meatus and vagina. (NOTE: Start with the narrow portion of the butterfly-shaped adhesive patch.) Starting the application at the bridge of skin separating the rectum from the vagina and working upward is most effective (Fig. 17-12, *B*). In male infants the penis (and scrotum, depending on the size of the collection device) is tucked through the opening into the collector before the protective paper is removed

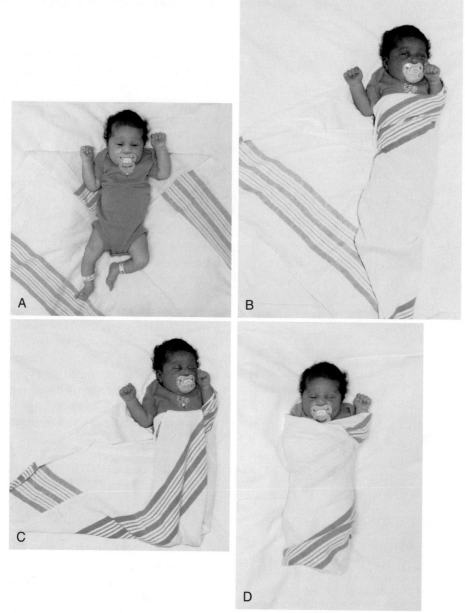

Fig. 17-10 Application of mummy restraint (swaddling). **A,** Infant is placed on folded corner of blanket. **B,** One corner of blanket is brought across body and secured beneath the body. **C,** Lower corner is folded and tucked and second corner is brought across body and secured. **D,** Modified mummy restraint with one hand uncovered. (Courtesy Cheryl Briggs, RN, Annapolis, MD.)

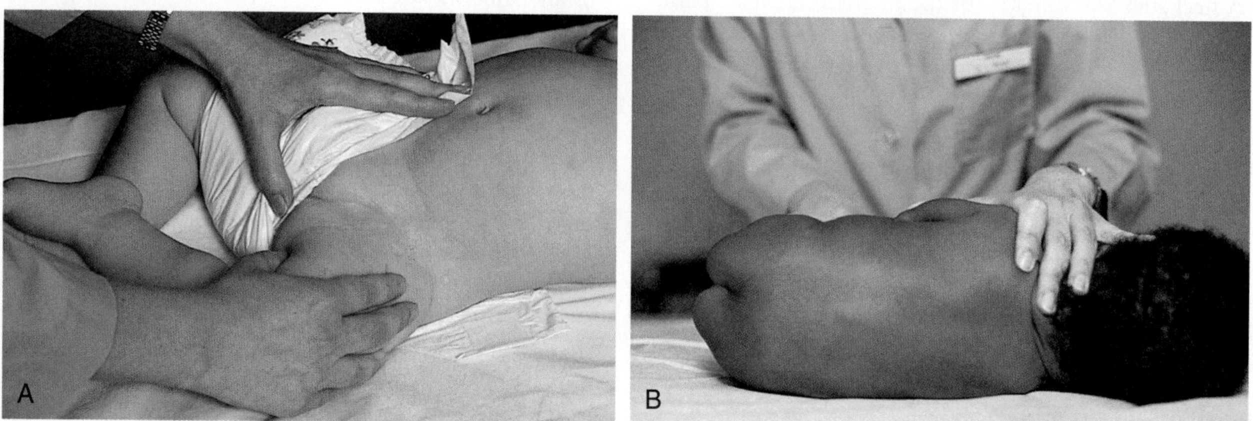

Fig. 17-11 Alternate methods of infant restraint. **A,** Restraining infant for femoral vein puncture. **B,** Modified side-lying position for lumbar puncture. (From Hockenberry, M. & Wilson, D. [2007]. *Wong's nursing care of infants and children* [8th ed.]. St. Louis: Mosby.)

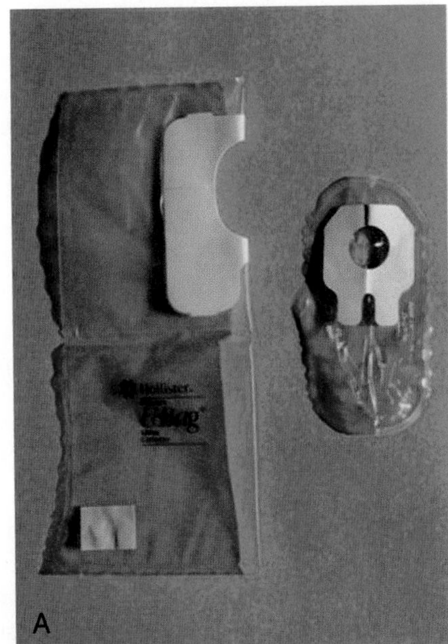

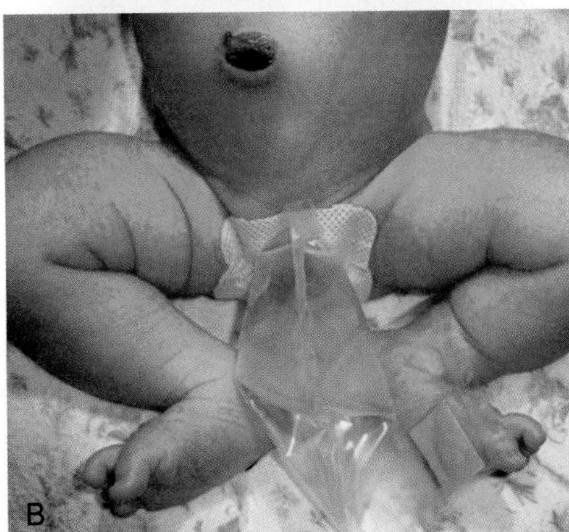

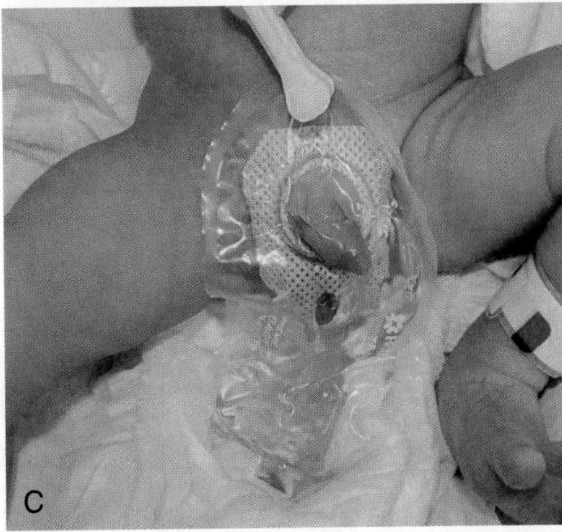

Fig. 17-12 Collection of urine specimen. **A,** Protective paper is removed from the adhesive surface. **B,** Applied to female infants. **C,** Applied to male infants. (Courtesy Cheryl Briggs, RN, Annapolis, MD.)

from the adhesive; the protective paper is then removed, and the flaps are pressed firmly onto the perineum, making sure the entire adhesive is firmly attached to skin and the edges of the opening do not pucker (Fig. 17-12, *C*). This method helps ensure a leak-proof seal and decreases the chance of contamination from stool. Cutting a slit in the diaper and pulling the bag through the slit can also help prevent leaking.

The diaper is carefully replaced, and the bag is checked frequently. When a sufficient amount of urine (this amount varies according to the test done) appears, the bag is removed. The infant's skin is observed for signs of irritation while the bag is in place. The specimen can be aspirated with a syringe or drained directly from the bag. For draining the bag is held in one hand and tilted to keep urine away from the tab. The tab is then removed and the urine is drained into a clean receptacle.

Collection of a 24-hour specimen from an infant can be a challenge; the infant may need light restraint with elbow restraints for appropriate collection of the specimen. The 24-hour urine bag is applied in the manner just described, and the urine is drained into a receptacle. During the collection the infant's skin is observed closely for signs of irritation and for lack of a proper seal.

For some types of urine tests, urine can be aspirated directly from the diaper by means of a syringe without a needle. If the diaper has absorbent gelling material that traps urine, a small gauze dressing or cotton balls can be placed inside the diaper and the urine aspirated from the cotton or gauze.

Restraining the infant

Infants may need to be restrained to (1) protect them from injury, (2) facilitate examinations, and (3) limit discomfort during tests, procedures, and specimen collections (see Figs. 17-10 and 17-11). The following special considerations must be kept in mind when restraining an infant:

- Apply restraints and check them to make sure they are not irritating the skin or impairing circulation.
- Maintain proper body alignment.
- Apply restraints without using knots or pins if possible. If knots are necessary, make the kind that can be released quickly. Use pins with care to eliminate the danger of their puncturing or pressing against the infant's skin.
- Check the infant hourly, or more frequently if indicated.

Restraint without appliance. The nurse may restrain the infant by using the hands and body. Fig. 17-11, *A* illustrates ways to restrain an infant in this manner.

Interventions

Protective environment

The provision of a protective environment is basic to the care of the newborn. The construction, maintenance, and operation of nurseries in accredited hospitals is monitored by national professional organizations such as the AAP, Joint Commission, Occupational Safety and Health Administration, and local or state governing bodies. In addition, hospital personnel develop their own policies and procedures for protecting the newborns under their care. Prescribed standards cover areas such as environmental factors, measures to control infection, and safety factors.

Environmental factors. Environmental factors include provision of adequate lighting, elimination of potential fire hazards, safety of electrical appliances, adequate ventilation, and controlled temperature (i.e., warm and free of drafts) and humidity (i.e., 40% to 60%) (AAP & ACOG, 2012).

Measures to control infection. Measures to control infection include adequate floor space to permit the positioning of bassinets at least 3 feet apart in all directions, handwashing facilities, and areas for cleaning and storing equipment and supplies. Only specified personnel directly involved in the care of mothers and infants are allowed in these areas, thereby reducing the opportunities for the transmission of pathogenic organisms.

NURSING ALERT Personnel are instructed to use good handwashing techniques. The most important single measure in the prevention of neonatal infection is handwashing between handling different infants and after contact with potentially contaminated objects (e.g., computer keyboards, telephone, countertop surfaces).

Health care workers must wear gloves when handling infants until blood and amniotic fluid have been removed from the skin, when drawing blood (e.g., heel stick), when caring for a fresh wound (e.g., circumcision), and during diaper changes.

Visitors and health care providers such as nurses, physicians, parents, siblings, grandparents are expected to wash their hands before having contact with infants or equipment. Individuals with infectious conditions are excluded from contact with newborns or must take special precautions when working with infants. This group includes persons with upper respiratory tract infections, gastrointestinal tract infections, and infectious skin conditions.

Safety: Preventing infant abduction. Health care institutions must be proactive in protecting newborns from abductions. Examples of measures taken include placing matching identification bracelets on infants and their parents, using identification bands with radiofrequency transmitters (Fig. 17-13) that set off an alarm if the bracelet is removed or if a certain threshold is crossed (doorway to exit the unit or building), and footprinting or taking identification pictures immediately after birth, before the infant leaves the mother's side. In addition, agencies must conduct periodic unit- and hospital-wide drills aimed at preventing newborn abductions. Personnel caring for newborns must be clearly identified by photo identification, and parents must be educated regarding measures to prevent abduction from the mother's room (i.e., be certain they know the identity of anyone who cares for the infant and never to release the infant to anyone who is not wearing the appropriate identification). Parents are educated before discharge regarding measures to minimize the risk for abduction from the home setting.

Supporting parents in the care of their infant

The sensitivity of the caregiver to the social responses of the infant is basic to the development of a mutually satisfying parent-child relationship. Sensitivity increases over time as parents become more aware of their infant's social capabilities (Cultural Considerations box).

Social interaction. The activities of daily care during the neonatal period are the best times for infant and family interactions. While caring for their newborn the mother and father can talk to the infant, play baby games, caress and cuddle the child, and perhaps use infant massage. In Fig. 17-14 a great-grandmother and infant are shown engaging in arousal, imitation of facial expression,

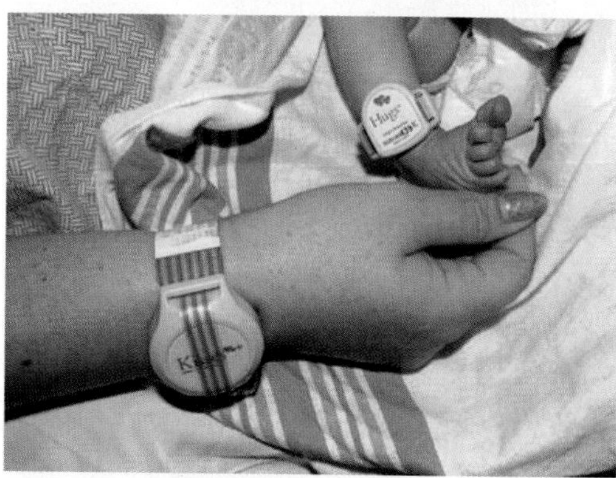

Fig. 17-13 Neonatal safety device. (Courtesy Shannon Perry, Phoenix, AZ.)

Cultural Considerations

Cultural Beliefs and Practices Related to Infant Care

Nurses working with childbearing families from other cultures and ethnic groups must be aware of cultural beliefs and practices that are important to individual families. People with a strong sense of heritage may hold on to traditional health beliefs long after adopting other U.S. lifestyle practices. These health beliefs may involve practices regarding the newborn. For example, some Asians, Latinas, eastern Europeans, and Native Americans delay breastfeeding because they believe that colostrum is "bad." Some Hispanics and African-Americans place a belly band over the infant's umbilicus. The birth of a male child is generally preferred by Asians and Indians, and some Asians and Haitians delay naming their infants (D'Avanzo, 2008).

and smiling. Too much stimulation should be avoided after feeding and before a sleep period. Older children's contact with a newborn is encouraged and supervised based on the developmental level of the child (Fig. 17-15). Parents often keep memento books that record the birth, the hospital stay, and their infant's progress. Other parents create blogs (e.g., www.wordpress.com) to share their development as a family.

Infant feeding. The infant is put to breast as soon as possible after birth or at least within 4 hours. Newborns are allowed to feed when they awaken and demonstrate typical hunger cues regardless of the time lapsed from the previous feeding. Ordinarily, mothers are encouraged to breastfeed their infants every 2 to 3 hours (bottle-feed every 3 to 4 hours, or as the bady exhibits hunger cues) during the day and only when the infant awakens during the night in the first few days after birth. Breastfed babies nurse more often than bottle-fed babies because breast milk is digested faster than formulas made from cow's milk, and the stomach empties sooner as a result. Water and dextrose water supplements are not recommended because they have a tendency to decrease breastfeeding. No evidence has been found to support dextrose or water feedings in newborns (see Evidence-Based Practice). For a thorough discussion of infant feeding, see Chapter 18.

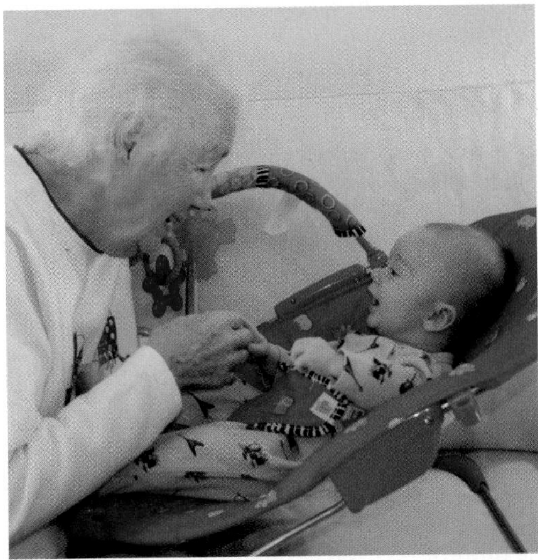

Fig. 17-14 Great-grandmother and infant enjoying social interaction. (Courtesy Freida Belding, Bird City, KS.)

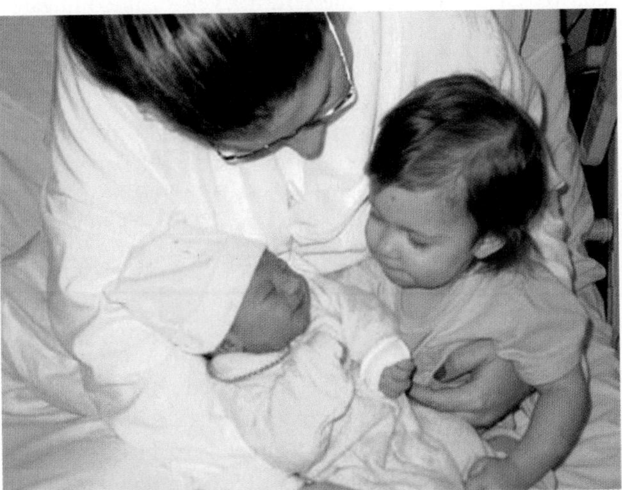

Fig. 17-15 Mother supervising contact of older sibling with newborn. (Courtesy Rebekah Vogel, Fort Collins, CO.)

THERAPEUTIC AND SURGICAL PROCEDURES

Intramuscular Injection

As discussed previously, administering a single dose of 0.5 to 1 mg of vitamin K intramuscularly to an infant is routine soon after birth (see Medication Guide box on p. 487).

Hepatitis B (HB) vaccination is recommended for all infants. Infants at highest risk for contracting HB are those born to women who have hepatitis or whose HB status is unknown. If the infant is born to an infected mother or to a mother who is a chronic carrier, HB vaccine and HB immune globulin (HBIG) should be administered within 12 hours of birth (Medication Guides). The HB vaccine is given in one site and the HBIG in another. For infants born to HB-negative women the first dose of the vaccine may be given at birth or at 1 month of age. Parental consent should be obtained before administering these vaccines.

Selection of the appropriate equipment and site for injection is important. In most cases a 25-gauge, ⅝-inch needle should be used for the vitamin K and HB vaccine injections. Injections must be given in muscles large enough to accommodate the medication, and major nerves and blood vessels must be avoided. The muscles of newborns may not tolerate more than a 0.5 ml per intramuscular injection. The preferred injection site for newborns is the vastus lateralis (Fig. 17-16). The dorsogluteal muscle is very small, poorly developed, and dangerously close to the sciatic nerve, which occupies a proportionately larger area in infants than in older children. Therefore it is not recommended as an injection site in small children. The newborn's deltoid muscle has an inadequate amount of muscle for intramuscular administration. A key factor in preventing and minimizing local reaction to intramuscular injections is adequate deposition of the medication deep within the muscle; therefore muscle size, needle length, and amount of medication injected should be carefully considered.

For an injection the neonate's leg should be stabilized. Gloves are worn. The nurse cleanses the injection site with an appropriate skin antiseptic, then stabilizes the infant's muscle between the thumb and forefinger. The needle is inserted into the vastus lateralis at a 90-degree angle. The

Medication Guide

Hepatitis B Vaccine (Recombivax HB, Engerix-B)

ACTION

- Hepatitis B vaccine induces protective antihepatitis B antibodies in 95% to 99% of healthy infants who receive the recommended three doses. The duration of protection of the vaccine is unknown.

INDICATION

- Hepatitis B vaccine is for immunization against infection caused by all known subtypes of hepatitis B virus (HBV).

NEONATAL DOSAGE

- The usual dosage is Recombivax HB, 5 mg/0.5 ml, or Engerix-B, 10 mg/0.5 ml, at 0, 1, and 6 months.

ADVERSE REACTIONS

- Common adverse reactions are rash, fever, erythema, swelling, and pain at injection site.

NURSING CONSIDERATIONS

- Parental consent must be obtained before administration. Follow proper procedure for administration of intramuscular (IM) injection. If infant also needs hepatitis B immune globulin (HBIG), use separate sites for the two injections.
- For infants of mothers with negative hepatitis B status: administer hepatitis B (HepB) vaccine before discharge from hospital.
- For infants born to hepatitis B surface antigen (HBsAg)–positive mothers: administer HepB vaccine and HBIG within 12 hours after birth.
- For infants born to mothers whose hepatitis B status is unknown:
  - ≤2000 g: administer HepB vaccine and HBIG within 12 hours after birth
  - ≥2000 g: administer HepB vaccine as soon as possible; if mother's HepB results are positive, give HBIG by 1 week of age

Medication Guide

Hepatitis B Immune Globulin

ACTION

- Hepatitis B immune globulin (HBIG) provides a high titer of antibody to hepatitis B surface antigen (HBsAg).

INDICATION

- The HBIG vaccine provides prophylaxis against infection in infants born of HBsAg-positive mothers.

NEONATAL DOSAGE

- Administer one 0.5-ml dose intramuscularly within 12 hours of birth.

ADVERSE REACTIONS

- Hypersensitivity may occur.

NURSING CONSIDERATIONS

- The HBIG vaccine must be given within 12 hours of birth. Follow proper procedure for administration of IM injection. (See guidelines for administration in Medication Guide: Hepatitis B Vaccine, at left.) The HBIG vaccine can be given at the same time as the hepatitis B vaccine but at a different site. Document the date, time, and site of injection, as well as the lot number and expiration date of the vaccine, according to agency policy.

plunger of the syringe is gently withdrawn, and if no blood is aspirated, the medication is injected. If blood is aspirated, the needle is withdrawn, and the injection is given in another site. The needle is withdrawn quickly and pressure is maintained at the site to minimize pain.

The nurse should always remember to comfort the infant after an injection and to discard equipment properly. Needles should never be recapped but should be properly discarded in an appropriate safety container. The name of the medication, date and time, amount, route, and site of injection must be recorded on the newborn's record.

Therapy for Hyperbilirubinemia

The best therapy for hyperbilirubinemia is prevention. Because bilirubin is excreted in meconium, prevention can be facilitated by early feeding, which stimulates the passage of meconium. However, despite early passage of meconium, the term infant may have trouble conjugating the increased amount of bilirubin derived from disintegrating fetal RBCs. As a result, the serum levels of unconjugated bilirubin can rise beyond normal limits, causing hyperbilirubinemia. The goal of treatment of hyperbilirubinemia is to help reduce the newborn's serum levels of unconjugated bilirubin. The two principal ways of reaching this goal are phototherapy and, rarely, exchange blood transfusion. Exchange transfusion is used to treat infants whose levels of serum bilirubin are rising rapidly despite the use of intensive phototherapy (see discussion on p. 507).

Phototherapy

During **phototherapy** the unclothed infant is placed under a bank of lights approximately 45 to 50 cm from the light source. The distance may vary based on unit protocol and type of light used. A Plexiglas panel or shield should always be placed between the lights and the infant when conventional lighting is used. The most effective

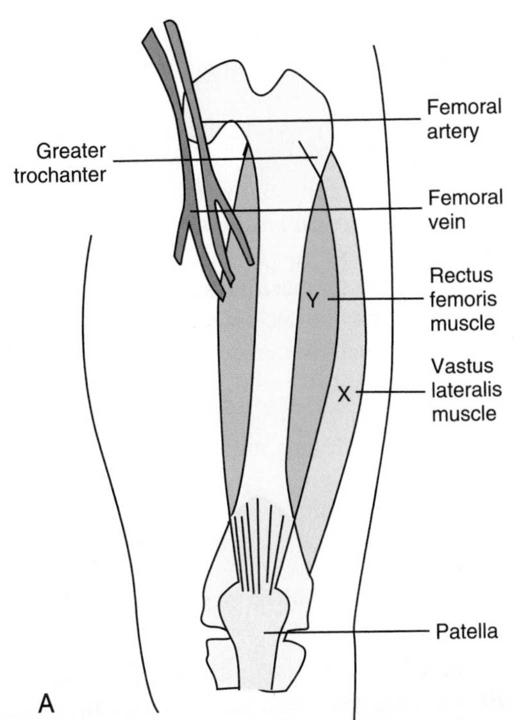

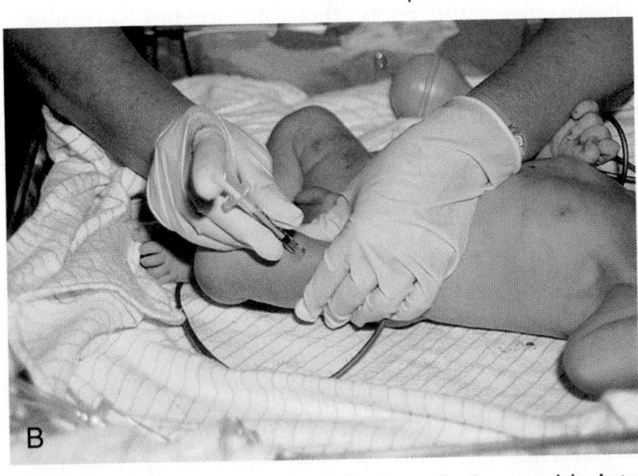

Fig. 17-16 Intramuscular injection. **A,** Acceptable intramuscular injection site for newborn infant. *X,* Injection site. **B,** Infant's leg stabilized for intramuscular injection. Nurse is wearing gloves to give injection. (**B,** Courtesy Marjorie Pyle, RNC, Lifecircle, Costa Mesa, CA.)

therapy is achieved with lights at 400 to 500 manometers, and a blue-green light spectrum is the most efficient (Steffensrud, 2004). The lamp's energy output should be monitored routinely with a photometer during treatment to ensure efficacy of therapy. Phototherapy is carried out until the infant's serum bilirubin level decreases to within an acceptable range. The decision to discontinue therapy is based on the observation of a definite downward trend in the bilirubin values.

Several precautions must be taken while the infant is undergoing phototherapy. The infant's eyes must be protected by an opaque mask to prevent overexposure to the light. The eye shield should cover the eyes completely but not occlude the nares. Before the mask is applied the infant's eyes should be closed gently to prevent excoriation of the corneas. The mask should be removed periodically and during infant feedings so that the eyes can be checked and cleansed with water and the parents can have visual contact with the infant (Fig. 17-17).

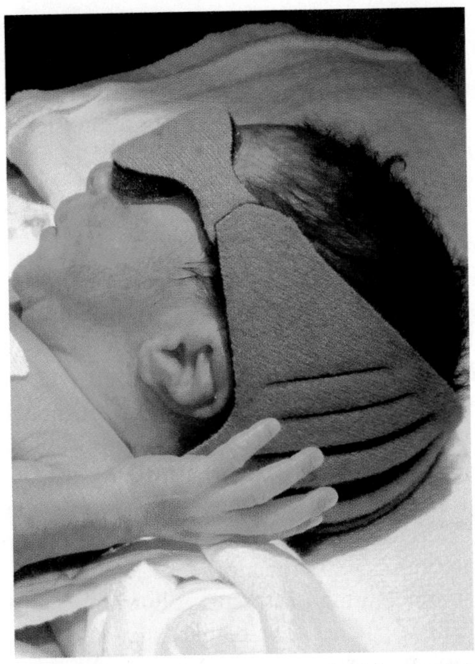

Fig 17-17 Infant with eyes covered while receiving phototherapy. (Courtesy Cheryl Briggs, RN, Annapolis, MD.)

To promote optimal skin exposure during phototherapy a "string bikini" made from a disposable facemask is often used instead of a diaper, which allows optimal skin exposure and provides protection for the genitals and the bedding. Before use the metal strip must be removed from the mask to prevent burning the infant. Lotions and ointments should not be used during phototherapy because they absorb heat and can cause burns.

Phototherapy can cause changes in the infant's temperature, depending partially on the bed used: bassinet, incubator, or radiant warmer. The infant's temperature should be closely monitored. Phototherapy lights can increase the rate of insensible water loss, which contributes to fluid loss and dehydration. Therefore the infant must be adequately hydrated. Hydration maintenance in the healthy newborn is accomplished with human milk or infant formula; administering glucose water or plain water has no advantage or benefit because these liquids do not promote excretion of bilirubin in the stools and may actually perpetuate enterohepatic circulation, thus delaying bilirubin excretion.

It is important to closely monitor urinary output while the infant is receiving phototherapy. Urine output may be decreased or unaltered; the urine may have a dark-gold or brown appearance.

The number and consistency of stools are monitored. Bilirubin breakdown increases gastric motility, which results in loose stools that can cause skin excoriation and breakdown. The infant's buttocks must be cleaned after each stool to help maintain skin integrity. A fine maculopapular rash may appear during phototherapy, but this condition is transient. Because visualization of the infant's skin color is difficult with blue light, appropriate cardiorespiratory monitoring should be implemented based on the infant's overall condition.

Critical Thinking Exercise: Circumcision

Alternative devices for phototherapy that are safe and effective are a fiberoptic panel attached to an illuminator and a Bilibed. The fiberoptic blanket is flexible and can be placed around the infant's torso or flat in the bed, thus delivering continuous phototherapy. Although fiberoptic lights do not produce heat as do conventional lights, staff should ensure that a covering pad is placed between the infant's skin and the fiberoptic device to prevent skin burns, especially in preterm infants. The newborn can remain in the mother's room in an open crib or in her arms during treatment. Follow unit protocol for the use of eye patches. The blanket may also be used for home phototherapy. In certain instances the infant's bilirubin levels may be increasing rapidly, and intensive phototherapy is required; this situation involves the use of a combination of conventional lights and fiberoptic blankets to maximize bilirubin reduction. All aspects of phototherapy should be accurately recorded in the infant's medical record.

The Bilibed uses a LED based phototherapy system. The baby is placed directly in the cradle above the light source. There is no need to adjust the distance between the baby and the light source. Follow unit protocol for the use of eye patches. The LEDs do not produce heat and can be used with radiant warmers.

Parent education. Serum levels of bilirubin in the newborn continue to rise until the fifth day of life. Many parents leave the hospital within 24 hours of birth, and some as early as 6 hours after birth. Therefore parents must receive education regarding jaundice and its treatment. They should have written instructions for assessing the infant's condition and the name of a contact person for reporting their findings and raising their concerns. Some institutions or third-party providers pay for a home visit to evaluate the infant's condition and to monitor the mother's health. If measuring serum bilirubin levels proves necessary after discharge from the hospital, a health care technician or nurse may draw the blood for the specimen, or the parents may take the baby to a laboratory to have blood drawn for a serum bilirubin. In some cases, parents may take the newborn to an outpatient clinic or physician's office to be evaluated.

Home phototherapy. Healthy term infants may at times be discharged home and need phototherapy for hyperbilirubinemia. Candidates for home phototherapy include infants who are healthy and active with no signs and symptoms of other complications. The parents or other caregivers must be willing and able to assume the responsibility for therapy maintenance and monitoring, and the home environment should be adequate with a telephone, heat, and electricity.

The company that provides the home therapy equipment is responsible for setting up the phototherapy unit and teaching the parents or caregivers how to use the equipment. The home care nurse schedules home visits to assess the infant's response to therapy, including weight, feeding, output, and temperature stability. Additional education of parents may be necessary; their understanding of the therapy and their responsibilities is assessed. Blood may be drawn for laboratory work and results reported to the primary health care provider. When therapy is discontinued, follow-up visits for monitoring may be ordered. The equipment company is called to arrange for pick-up of the phototherapy unit.

Circumcision

Circumcision of male newborns is commonly performed in the United States, although its value is controversial. The AAP Task Force on Circumcision (1999) noted that, although scientific evidence exists of potential medical benefits of circumcision, the data are not sufficient to recommend routine circumcision. The Task Force further recommended that if circumcision is performed, analgesia should be used; this policy statement was reaffirmed in 2005 (AAP, 2005a). ACOG (2001) and the American Medical Association Council on Scientific Affairs (2005) have issued similar recommendations regarding newborn circumcision.

Circumcision is a matter of personal parental choice. Parents usually decide to have their newborn circumcised for one or more of the following reasons: hygiene, religious conviction, tradition, culture, or social norms. Regardless of the reason for the decision, parents should be given unbiased information and the opportunity to discuss the benefits and risks of the procedure.

Suggested medical benefits of circumcision for the infant include decreased incidence of urinary tract infection and decreased risk for sexually transmitted infection, penile cancer, and human papillomavirus infection. The risk of cervical cancer among female partners of circumcised men may be reduced. In 2012, the AAP issued a policy stating that the health benefits outweigh the risks and that circumcision should be available for families who choose it (AAP Task Force on Circumcision, 2012). Risks and potential complications associated with circumcision include hemorrhage, infection, and penile injury (removal of excessive skin, damage to the meatus or glans).

Expectant parents should begin learning about circumcision during the prenatal period, but circumcision is not often discussed with parents before labor. In many instances, parents are first confronted with the decision regarding circumcision as the mother is being admitted to the hospital or birth unit. The stress of the intrapartal period makes this time difficult for parental decision making and is not an ideal time to broach the topic of circumcision and expect a well-thought-out decision.

Procedure

Circumcision involves removing the prepuce (foreskin) of the glans. The procedure is not usually performed immediately after birth because of the danger of cold stress and decreased clotting factors, but it is often performed in the hospital before the infant's discharge. The circumcision of a Jewish male infant is commonly performed on the eighth day after birth and is performed at home in a ceremony called a *bris* (unless the infant is ill). This timing is logical from a physiologic standpoint because clotting factors decrease somewhat immediately after birth and do not return to prebirth levels until the end of the first week.

Feedings are usually withheld up to 2 to 3 hours before the circumcision to prevent vomiting and aspiration. To prepare the infant for the circumcision, he is positioned on a plastic restraint form (Fig. 17-18), and the penis is cleansed with soap and water or a preparatory solution such as povidone-iodine. The infant is draped to provide warmth and a sterile field, and the sterile equipment is readied for use.

Although some circumcision procedures require no special equipment or appliances, numerous instruments have been designed for this purpose. Use of the Yellen (Gomco) (Fig. 17-19) or Mogen clamp may make this operation almost bloodless. The procedure itself takes only a few minutes. After completion, a small petrolatum gauze dressing or a generous amount of petrolatum or A & D ointment may be applied to the penis for the first few days to prevent the diaper from adhering to the site. A PlastiBell is another device used for circumcision. The advantages to its use are that it applies constant direct pressure to prevent hemorrhage during the procedure and afterward protects against infection, keeps the site from sticking to the diaper, and prevents pain with urination. When used for circumcision the PlastiBell is first fitted over the glans, the suture is tied around the rim of the bell, and excess prepuce is cut away. The plastic rim remains in place for approximately a week. It falls off after healing has taken place, usually within 5 to 7 days (Fig. 17-20). Petrolatum is not usually needed when the PlastiBell is used.

Assessment Video: Circumcision

Procedural pain management

Circumcision is painful. The pain is characterized by both physiologic and behavioral changes in the infant (see discussion that follows). Four types of anesthesia and analgesia are used in newborns who undergo circumcisions: ring block, dorsal penile nerve block (DPNB), topical anesthetic such as eutectic mixture of local anesthetic (EMLA) (prilocaine-lidocaine) or LMX4 (4% lidocaine), and concentrated oral sucrose. Nonpharmacologic methods such as nonnutritive sucking, containment, and swaddling may be used to enhance pain management. The Cochrane group exploring pain relief for neonatal circumcision (Brady-Fryer, Wiebe, & Lander, 2004) found that DPNB was the most effective intervention for decreasing the pain of circumcision. Studies exploring the use of several strategies concurrently, such as that conducted by Razmus, Dalton, and Wilson (2004), which included groups receiving both concentrated oral sucrose and ring block compared with ring block alone, have the most potential to clarify optimal strategies.

A ring block is the injection of buffered lidocaine administered subcutaneously on each side of the penile shaft. A DPNB includes subcutaneous injections of buffered lidocaine at the 2 o'clock and 10 o'clock positions at the base of the penis. The circumcision should not be performed for at least 5 minutes after these injections.

A topical cream containing prilocaine-lidocaine such as EMLA can be applied to the base of the penis at least 1

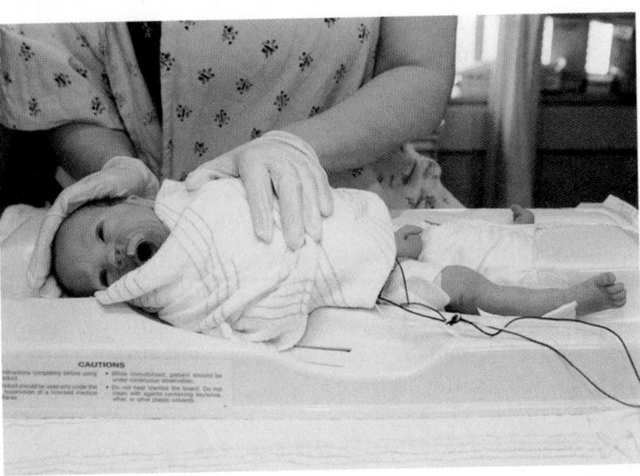

Fig. 17-18 Proper positioning of infant in Circumstraint. (Photo by Paul Vincent Kuntz, Texas Children's Hospital, Houston, TX.)

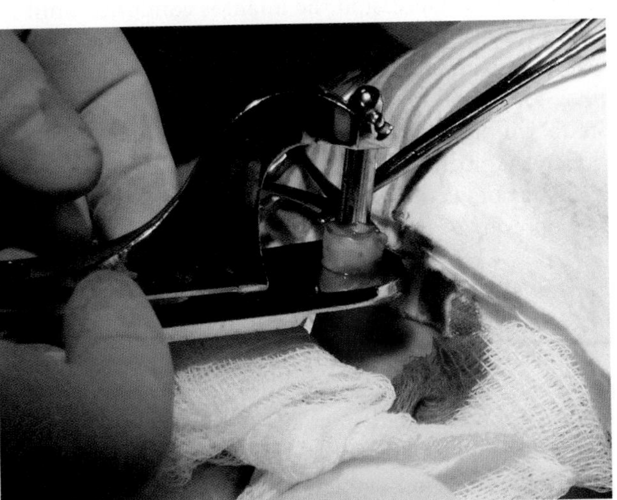

Fig. 17-19 Circumcision with Yellen clamp. After hemostasis occurs, the prepuce (over cone) will be cut away. (Courtesy Cheryl Briggs, RN, Annapolis, MD.)

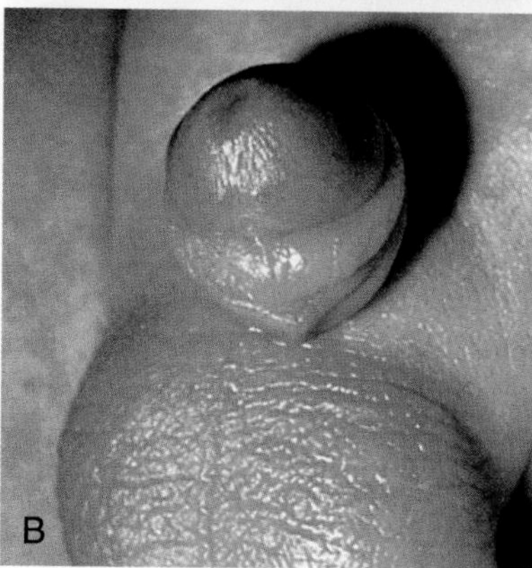

Fig. 17-20 Circumcision by using Hollister PlastiBell. **A,** Suture around rim of PlastiBell controls bleeding. **B,** Plastic rim and suture drop off in 7 to 10 days. (Permission to use or reproduce this copyrighted material has been granted by the owner, Hollister, Inc., Libertyville, IL.)

Skill: Pain Assessment

hour before the circumcision. The area where the prepuce attaches to the glans is well coated with 1 g of the cream and then covered with a transparent occlusive dressing or finger cot. Just before the procedure the cream is removed. Blanching or redness of the skin may occur.

After the circumcision the infant is comforted until he is quieted. If the parents were not present during the procedure, the infant is returned to them. The infant can be fussy for several hours and can have disturbed sleep-wake states and disorganized feeding behaviors. Oral acetaminophen may be administered after the procedure every 4 hours (as ordered by the practitioner) for a maximum of five doses in 24 hours or a maximum of 75 mg/kg/day.

Care of the newly circumcised infant

Post-circumcision protocols vary. In many settings, the circumcision site is assessed for bleeding every 30 minutes for the first hour and then hourly for the next 4 to 6 hours. The nurse monitors the infant's urinary output, noting the time and amount of the first voiding after the circumcision. If bleeding is noted from the circumcision, the nurse applies gentle pressure to the site of bleeding with a folded sterile gauze square. A hemostatic agent such as Gelfoam® powder or sponge may be applied to the circumcision site to help control the bleeding. If bleeding is not easily controlled, a blood vessel may need to be ligated. In this event, one nurse notifies the physician and prepares the necessary equipment (i.e., circumcision tray and suture material), while another nurse maintains intermittent pressure until the physician arrives. If the parents take the baby home before the end of the observation period, they must be taught proper home care (Teaching Guidelines box).

Nursing actions are planned and implemented to prevent infection. Prepackaged commercial wipes for cleaning the diaper area should not be used because they contain alcohol, which delays healing and causes discomfort. Instead, the nurse washes the penis gently with water to remove urine and feces and, if necessary, applies fresh petrolatum around the glans after each diaper change. The glans penis, normally dark red during healing, becomes covered with a yellow exudate in 24 hours, which is part of normal healing, not an infective process. No attempt should be made to remove the exudate, which persists for 2 to 3 days. Parents should be taught to apply the diaper so that it does not press on the circumcised area. They should be encouraged to change the diaper at least every 4 hours to prevent it from sticking to the penis.

NEONATAL PAIN

Pain has physiologic and psychologic components. The psychologic component of pain and the diffuse total body response to pain exhibited by the neonate led many health care providers to believe that infants, especially preterm infants, do not experience pain. The central nervous system is well developed, however, as early as 24 weeks of gestation. The peripheral and spinal structures that transmit pain information are present and functional between the first and second trimester. The pituitary-adrenal axis is also well developed at this time, and a fight-or-flight reaction is observed in response to the catecholamines released in response to stress.

The physiologic response to pain in neonates can be life threatening. Pain response can decrease tidal volume, increase demands on the cardiovascular system, increase metabolism, and cause neuroendocrine imbalance. The hormonal-metabolic response to pain in a term infant has greater magnitude and shorter duration than that in adults. The newborn's sympathetic response to pain is less mature and therefore less predictable than an adult's.

Newborns react to painful stimuli in a variety of ways. Pain responses can be categorized as behavioral, physiologic or autonomic, and metabolic.

Neonatal Responses to Pain

The most common behavioral sign of pain is a vocalization or crying, ranging from a whimper to a distinctive high-pitched, shrill cry. Facial expressions of pain include

TEACHING GUIDELINES

Care of the Circumcised Newborn at Home

- Wash hands before touching the newly circumcised penis.

CHECK FOR BLEEDING

- Check circumcision for bleeding with each diaper change.
- If bleeding occurs, apply gentle pressure with a folded sterile gauze square. If bleeding does not stop with pressure, notify primary health care provider.

OBSERVE FOR URINATION

- Check to see that the infant urinates after being circumcised.
- Infant should have a wet diaper 2 to 6 times per 24 hours the first 1 to 2 days after birth, then 6 to 10 times per 24 hours after 3 to 4 days.

KEEP AREA CLEAN

- Change the diaper and inspect the circumcision at least every 4 hours.
- Wash the penis gently with warm water to remove urine and feces. Apply petrolatum to the glans with each diaper change (omit petrolatum if a PlastiBell was used).
- Use soap only after the circumcision is healed (5 to 6 days).
- Apply the diaper to prevent pressure on the circumcised area.

CHECK FOR INFECTION

- Glans penis is dark red after circumcision then becomes covered with yellow exudate in 24 hours, which is normal and will persist for 2 to 3 days. Do not attempt to remove it.
- Redness, swelling, discharge, or odor indicates infection. Notify the primary health care provider if you think the circumcision area is infected.

PROVIDE COMFORT

- Circumcision is painful. Handle the area gently.
- Provide extra holding, feeding, and opportunities for nonnutritive sucking for a day or two.

grimacing, eye squeeze, brow contraction, deepened nasolabial furrows, a taut and quivering tongue, and an open mouth. The infant will flex and adduct the upper body and lower limbs in an attempt to withdraw from the painful stimulus. The preterm infant has a lower-than-normal threshold for initiation of this flex response. An infant who receives a muscle-paralyzing agent such as vecuronium will be unable to mount a behavioral or visible pain response.

Significant changes in heart rate, blood pressure (increased or decreased), intracranial pressure, vagal tone, respiratory rate, and oxygen saturation occur during noxious stimulation (Walden & Franck, 2003). Infants release epinephrine, norepinephrine, glucagon, corticosterone, cortisol, 11-deoxycorticosterone, lactate, pyruvate, and glucose (Walden & Franck, 2003).

Assessment of Neonatal Pain

In assessing pain the care provider needs to consider the health of the neonate, the type and duration of the painful stimulus, environmental factors, and the infant's state of alertness. For example, severely compromised neonates may be unable to generate a pain response, although they are, in fact, experiencing pain.

Every patient should have an initial pain assessment, as well as a pain management plan; this mandate includes newborns. The National Association of Neonatal Nurses (NANN) developed practice guidelines stating that all nurses who care for newborns should have education and competency validation in pain assessment. Pain should be assessed and documented on a regular basis (Walden & Gibbins, 2008).

Several pain assessment tools have been developed for use with neonates. A combination of behavioral and physiologic indicators of pain is used to diagnose and differentiate infant pain levels. Tools that have been shown to have validity and reliability include the Neonatal Infant Pain Scale (NIPS) (Lawrence, Alcock, McGrath, Kay, MacMurray, & Dulberg, 1993) and the Premature Infant Pain Profile (PIPP) (Stevens, Johnston, Petryshen, & Taddio, 1996). A pain assessment tool used by nurses in the neonatal intensive care unit is the CRIES (Krechel & Bildner, 1995) (Table 17-4). This tool was developed for use by nurses who work with preterm and term infants. CRIES is an acronym for the physiologic and behavioral indicators of pain used in the tool: *c*rying, *r*equiring increased oxygen, *i*ncreased vital signs, *e*xpression, and *s*leeplessness. Each indicator is scored from 0 to 2. The total possible pain score, which represents the worst pain, is 10. A pain score greater than 4 should be considered significant. This tool can be used on infants between 32 weeks of gestation and 20 weeks after birth (Pasero, 2002).

Management of Neonatal Pain

The goals of the management of neonatal pain are to (1) minimize the intensity, duration, and physiologic cost of the pain and (2) maximize the neonate's ability to cope with and recover from the pain. Nonpharmacologic and pharmacologic strategies are used.

Nonpharmacologic management

Containment, also known as *swaddling*, is effective in reducing excessive immature motor responses. Containment may provide comfort through other senses, such as thermal, tactile, and proprioceptive senses. Nonnutritive sucking on a pacifier, with or without sucrose, is a common comfort measure used with newborns. Skin-to-skin contact with the mother during a painful procedure can help to

TABLE 17-4

CRIES Neonatal Postoperative Pain Scale*

	0	1	2
Crying	No	High pitched	Inconsolable
Requires oxygen for saturation >95%	No	<30%	>30%
Increased vital signs	Heart rate and blood pressure equal to or less than preoperative state	Heart rate and blood pressure <20% of preoperative state	Heart rate and blood pressure >20% of preoperative state
Expression	None	Grimace	Grimace and grunt
Sleepless	No	Wakes at frequent intervals	Constantly awake

CODING TIPS FOR USING CRIES

Crying	The characteristic cry of pain is high pitched. If no cry or cry that is not high pitched, score 0. If cry is high pitched but infant is easily consoled, score 1. If cry is high pitched and infant is inconsolable, score 2.
Requires oxygen for saturation >95%	Look for changes in oxygenation. Infants experiencing pain manifest decreases in oxygenation as measured by total carbon dioxide or oxygen saturation. (Consider other causes of changes in oxygenation, such as atelectasis, pneumothorax, oversedation.) If no oxygen is required, score 0. If <30% oxygen is required, score 1. If >30% oxygen is required, score 2.
Increased vital signs	NOTE: Measure blood pressure last because this may wake child, causing difficulty with other assessments. Use baseline preoperative parameters from a nonstressed period. Multiply baseline heart rate (HR) × 0.2, then add this to baseline HR to determine the HR that is 20% over baseline. Do likewise for blood pressure (BP). Use mean BP. If HR and BP are both unchanged or less than baseline, score 0. If HR or BP is increased but increase is <20% of baseline, score 1. If either one is increased >20% over baseline, score 2.
Expression	The facial expression most often associated with pain is a grimace. This may be characterized by brow lowering, eyes squeezed shut, deepening of the nasolabial furrow, open lips and mouth. If no grimace is present, score 0. If grimace alone is present, score 1. If grimace and noncry vocalization grunt is present, score 2.
Sleepless	This is scored based on the infant's state during the hour preceding this recorded score. If the child has been continuously asleep, score 0. If he or she has awakened at frequent intervals, score 1. If he or she has been awake constantly, score 2.

Source: Krechel, S. & Bildner, J. (1995). CRIES: A new neonatal postoperative pain measurement score: Initial testing of validity and reliability. *Paediatric Anaesthesia, 5*(1), 53-61.
*Neonatal pain assessment tool developed at the University of Missouri-Columbia.

reduce pain. Combining these nonpharmacologic methods results in more effective pain reduction. Distraction with visual, oral, auditory, or tactile stimulation may be helpful in term or older infants (Clifford, Stringer, Christensen, & Mountain, 2004; Walden & Franck, 2003).

Pharmacologic management

Pharmacologic agents are used to alleviate pain in neonates associated with procedures. Local anesthesia has become routine during procedures such as chest tube insertion and circumcision. Topical anesthesia has been used for circumcision, lumbar puncture, venipuncture, and heel sticks. Nonopioid analgesia (acetaminophen) is effective for mild to moderate pain from inflammatory conditions. Morphine and fentanyl are the most widely used opioid analgesics for pharmacologic management of neonatal pain. Continuous or bolus intravenous infusion of opioids provides effective and safe pain control. Ketorolac (Toradol) has been shown to be effective in the management of postoperative neonatal pain.

Postoperative neonatal pain should be managed with around-the-clock dosing or use of a continual drip. Dosing as needed (prn) is not considered to be an effective management of chronic or postoperative pain in infants. Traditional belief holds that the continued use of opioids for neonates in the postoperative period results in prolonged intubation. Consequently, traditional practice is to discontinue all opioids several hours before and after extubation, preventing pain relief. Furdon, Eastman, Benjamin, and

Horgan (1998) found that continuous opioid infusion in infants without an underlying pulmonary or neurologic pathologic condition actually shortened the time to extubation and caused no problems of respiratory depression that required reintubation.

Other methods for managing neonatal pain are epidural infusion, local and regional nerve blocks, and intradermal or topical anesthetics. A concentrated sucrose solution, especially when administered with a pacifier, can decrease pain associated with heel lance and venipuncture (Stevens, Yamada, & Ohlsson, 2004). Oral acetaminophen may be administered for painful procedures such as circumcision, venipuncture, and heel stick.

DISCHARGE PLANNING AND TEACHING

Infant care activities can cause much anxiety for new parents. Support from nursing staff members can be an important factor in determining whether new parents seek and accept help in the future. Whether this child is the woman's or the couple's first newborn or an adolescent whose mother will be the primary caregiver, and whether or not the parents attended parenthood preparation classes, parents appreciate anticipatory guidance in the care of their infant. The nurse should avoid trying to cover all the content at one time because the parents can be overwhelmed by too much information and become anxious. However, because early discharge of new mothers is currently common practice, teaching all the content that is necessary can be a challenge for the nurse because of time constraints. As a result, many institutions have developed home visitation programs that take the necessary teaching to the new parents, although the hospital nurse still provides most of the essential information for newborn care (see Community Activity box).

To set priorities for teaching the nurse follows parental cues. Deficient knowledge should be identified before beginning to teach. Normal growth and development and the changing needs of the infant (e.g., for personal interaction and stimulation, growth milestones, exercise, injury prevention, and social contacts), as well as the topics that follow, should be included during discharge planning with parents. Safety issues should be addressed (Box 17-6).

COMMUNITY ACTIVITY

Contact a community health nurse or a referral service in your community. Arrange a visit or interview with the health care team. Identify assessments that are made on follow-up visits for new mothers. Include information on teaching related to the following topics: car seat safety, sudden infant death syndrome, infant sleep patterns, immunizations, and cardiopulmonary resuscitation. Include key concepts related to each topic. Evaluate the effectiveness of the teaching that is provided.

BOX 17-6
Infant Safety

- Never leave your baby alone on a bed, couch, or table. Even newborns can move enough to eventually reach the edge and fall off.
- Never put your baby on a cushion, pillow, beanbag, or waterbed to sleep. Your baby may suffocate. Also, do not keep pillows, large floppy toys, or loose plastic sheeting in the crib.
- Do not place your infant on his or her stomach to sleep during the first few months of life. The American Academy of Pediatrics advises against this prone position because it has been associated with an increased incidence of sudden infant death syndrome (SIDS). The back-lying position is preferable.
- When using an infant carrier, stay within arm's reach when the carrier is on a high place, such as a table, sofa, or store counter. If at all possible, place the carrier on the floor near you.
- Infant carriers do not keep your baby safe in a car. Always place your baby in an approved car safety seat when traveling in a motor vehicle (car, truck, bus, or van). Car safety seats are recommended for travel on trains and airplanes as well. Use the car safety seat for *every* ride. Your baby should be in a rear-facing infant car safety seat from birth to 20 pounds, and the car safety seat should be in the back seat of the car (see Fig. 17-23). This precaution is especially important in vehicles with front passenger air bags because, when air bags inflate, they can be fatal for infants and toddlers.
- When bathing your baby, never leave him or her alone. Newborns and infants can drown in 1 to 2 inches of water.
- Be sure that your hot water heater is set at 120° F or less. Always check bathwater temperature with your elbow before putting your baby in the bath.
- Do not tie anything around your baby's neck. Pacifiers, for example, tied around the neck with a ribbon or string may strangle your baby.
- Check your baby's crib for safety. Slats should be no more than 2¼ inches apart. The space between the mattress and sides should be less than 2 fingerwidths. The bedposts should have no decorative knobs.
- Keep the crib or playpen away from window blind and drapery cords; your baby could strangle on them.
- Keep the crib and playpen well away from radiators, heat vents, and portable heaters. Linens in the crib or playpen could catch fire if they come in contact with these heat sources.
- Install smoke detectors on every floor of your home. Check them once a month to be sure they are working properly. Change batteries twice a year.
- Avoid exposing your baby to cigarette or cigar smoke in your home or other places. Passive exposure to tobacco smoke greatly increases the likelihood that your infant will have respiratory symptoms and illnesses.
- Be gentle with your baby. Do not pick your baby up or swing your baby by the arms or throw him or her up in the air.

e Spanish Guidelines: General Advice

Temperature

The following topics should be reviewed:

- The causes of elevation in body temperature (e.g., overwrapping, cold stress with resultant vasoconstriction, or minimal response to infection) and the body's response to extremes in environmental temperature
- Signs to be reported, such as high or low temperatures with accompanying fussiness, lethargy, irritability, poor feeding, and crying
- Ways to promote normal body temperature, such as dressing the infant appropriately for the environmental air temperature and protecting the infant from exposure to direct sunlight
- Use of warm wraps or extra blankets in cold weather
- Technique for taking the newborn's axillary temperature

Respirations

Review the following points:

- Normal variations in the rate and rhythm
- Reflexes such as sneezing to clear the airway
- The need to protect the infant from the following:
  - Exposure to people with upper respiratory tract infections and respiratory syncytial virus
  - Exposure to secondhand tobacco smoke
  - Suffocation from loose bedding, water beds, and beanbag chairs; drowning (in bath water); entrapment under excessive bedding or in soft bedding; anything tied around the infant's neck; poorly constructed playpens, bassinets, or cribs
- Sleep position–on back when put to sleep
- Avoid the use of baby powder which is a commonly aspirated substance. Parents are advised that, if they prefer to use a powder, a cornstarch preparation can be substituted. Whenever a powder is used, it should be placed in the caregiver's hand and then applied to the skin, never sprinkled directly onto the skin.
- Symptoms of the common cold, which include nasal congestion and excess drainage of mucus, coughing, sneezing, difficulty in swallowing or breathing, decreased vigor in feeding, and low-grade fever
  - Advise the parents on measures to help the infant, such as the following:
    - Feed smaller amounts more often to prevent overtiring the infant.
    - Hold the baby in an upright position to feed.
    - For sleeping, raise the infant's head and chest by raising the mattress 30 degrees. (Do *not* use a pillow.)
    - Avoid drafts; do not overdress the baby.
    - Use only medications prescribed by a physician. (Over-the-counter "cold" remedy medications are not appropriate for use in infants and should be avoided [Sharfstein, North, & Serwint, 2007].)
    - Use nasal saline drops in each nostril and suctioning well with bulb syringe to decrease and relieve secretions.

Feeding Schedules

Feeding practices and schedules for newborns are discussed in Chapter 18.

Elimination

A review includes the following reminders:

- Color of normal urine and number of voidings (2 to 6) to expect each day
- Changes to be expected in the color and consistency of the stool (i.e., meconium to transitional to soft yellow or golden yellow) and the number of bowel evacuations, plus the odor of stools for breastfed or bottle-fed infants (see Chapter 18)
- Formula-fed infants may have as few as one stool every other day after the first few weeks of life; stools are pasty to semi-formed
- Breastfed infants should have at least three stools every 24 hours for the first few weeks; the stools are looser and resemble mustard mixed with cottage cheese; the odor is less offensive than that of formula stools

Positioning and Holding

The AAP Task Force on Sudden Infant Death Syndrome (SIDS) (2011) recommends placing the infant in the supine position during the first year of life to prevent SIDS. Infants should lie on a firm surface, specifically on a firm crib mattress covered by a fitted sheet. Soft materials such as comforters, quilts, pillows, or sheepskins should not be placed in the crib.

Anatomically, the infant's shape–a barrel chest and flat, curveless spine–facilitates the infant to roll from the side to the prone position; therefore the side-lying position for sleep is not recommended. When the infant is awake, "tummy time" can be provided under parental supervision so the infant may begin to develop appropriate muscle tone for eventual crawling; this tummy time is also effective in the prevention of a misshaped head (positional plagiocephaly). Care must be taken to prevent the infant from rolling off flat, unguarded surfaces. When an infant is on such a surface the parent or nurse who must turn away from the infant even for a moment should always keep one hand placed securely on the infant. The infant is always held securely with the head supported because newborns are unable to maintain an erect head posture for more than a few moments. Fig. 17-21 illustrates various positions for holding an infant with adequate support.

Rashes

Diaper rash

The majority of infants will develop a diaper rash at some time. This dermatitis or skin inflammation appears as redness, scaling, blisters, or papules. Various factors contribute to diaper rash including: infrequent diaper changes, diarrhea, use of plastic pants to cover the diaper, a change in the infant's diet such as when solid

Critical Thinking/Clinical Decision Making

Sudden Infant Death Syndrome and Infant Sleep Position

Marlys gave birth to a full-term male infant named Daniel. They are being discharged today. The nurse has given her instructions about placing the baby on his back for sleep. Marlys said that she had noticed that the nurses placed Daniel on his side in the nursery and wondered why they did that when she was instructed to place Daniel on his back.

Michelle gave birth to Michael at 32 weeks. During the stay in the nursery the nurses placed Michael on his abdomen to sleep. At discharge, Michelle was instructed to place Michael on his back to sleep. Michelle asked why she had to place Michael on his back to sleep when he was used to sleeping on his abdomen. How should the nurses respond to these questions?

1. Evidence—Is evidence sufficient to draw conclusions about the safety and efficacy of the supine position for sleep in reducing the incidence of sudden infant death syndrome (SIDS)?
2. Assumptions—What assumptions can be made about the following factors related to infant positioning?
   a. Role modeling by nurses
   b. Sleep position in the nursery versus sleep position at home
   c. Sleep position for preterm versus term infants
   d. Nurses' knowledge and use of research evidence
3. What implications and priorities for nursing care can be drawn at this time?
4. Does the evidence objectively support your conclusion?
5. Do alternative perspectives to your conclusion exist?

foods are added, or when breast-feeding mothers eat certain foods.

Parents are instructed in measures to help prevent and treat diaper rash. Diapers should be checked often and changed as soon as the infant voids or stools. Plain water with mild soap is used to cleanse the diaper area; if baby wipes are used, they should be unscented and contain no alcohol. The infant's skin should be allowed to dry completely before applying another diaper. Exposing the buttocks to air can help dry up diaper rash. Because bacteria thrive in moist dark areas, exposing the skin to dry air decreases bacterial proliferation. Zinc oxide ointments can be used to protect the infant's skin from moisture and further excoriation.

While diaper rash can be alarming to parents and annoying to babies, most cases resolve within a few days with simple home treatments. There are instances when diaper rash is more serious and may require medical treatment.

The warm, moist atmosphere in the diaper area provides an optimal environment for *Candida albicans* growth; dermatitis appears in the perianal area, inguinal folds, and lower abdomen. The affected area is intensely erythematous with a sharply demarcated, scalloped edge, often with numerous satellite lesions that extend beyond the larger lesion. The usual source of infection is from handling by persons who do not practice adequate handwashing. It may also appear 2 to 3 days after an oral infection (thrush).

Therapy consists of applications of an anticandidal ointment, such as clotrimazole or miconazole, with each diaper change. Sometimes the infant is given an oral antifungal preparation such as nystatin or fluconazole to eliminate any gastrointestinal source of infection.

Other rashes

A rash on the cheeks may result from the infant's scratching with long unclipped fingernails or from rubbing the face against the crib sheets, particularly if regurgitated stomach contents are not washed off promptly. The newborn's skin begins a natural process of peeling and sloughing after birth. Dry skin may be treated with a neutral pH lotion, but this should be used sparingly. Newborn rash, erythema toxicum, is a common finding (see Fig. 16-6, *B*) and needs no treatment.

Clothing

Skill: Changing a Diaper

Parents commonly ask how warmly they should dress their infant. A simple suggestion is to dress the child as they dress themselves, adding or subtracting clothes and wraps for the child as necessary. A cotton shirt and diaper may be sufficient clothing for the young infant. A cap or bonnet is needed to protect the scalp and minimize heat loss if the weather is cool or to protect against sunburn. Wrapping the infant snugly in a blanket maintains body temperature and promotes a feeling of security. Overdressing in warm temperatures can cause discomfort, as can underdressing in cold weather. Parents are encouraged to dress the infant at all times in flame-retardant clothing. The eyes should be shaded if it is sunny and hot. Infant sunglasses are available to protect the infant's eyes when outdoors (Fig. 17-22).

Safety: Use of Car Seat

Infants should travel only in federally approved, rear-facing safety seats secured in the rear seat (Fig. 17-23). The safest area of the car is the back seat. A car safety seat that faces the rear gives the best protection for the disproportionately weak neck and heavy head of an infant. In this position the force of a frontal crash is spread over the head, neck, and back; the back of the car safety seat supports the spine.

NURSING ALERT Infants and toddlers should use a rear-facing seat until the age of 2 or for as long as possible up to the weight and height limit for their

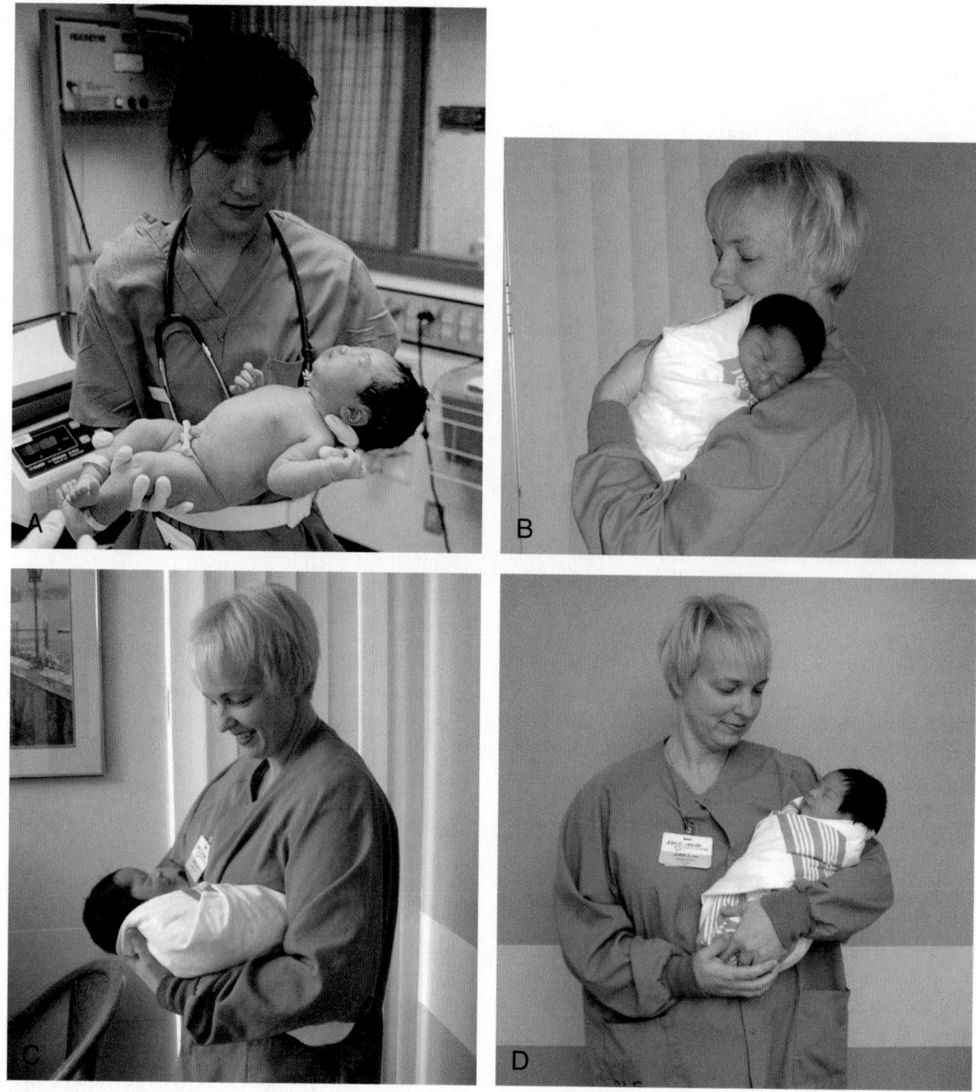

Fig. 17-21 Holding baby securely with support for head. **A,** Holding infant while moving infant from one place to another. Baby is undressed to show posture. **B,** Holding baby upright in "burping" position. **C,** "Football" hold. **D,** Cradling hold. (**A,** Courtesy Kim Molloy, Knoxville, IA. **B, C,** and **D,** Courtesy Julie Perry Nelson, Loveland, CO.)

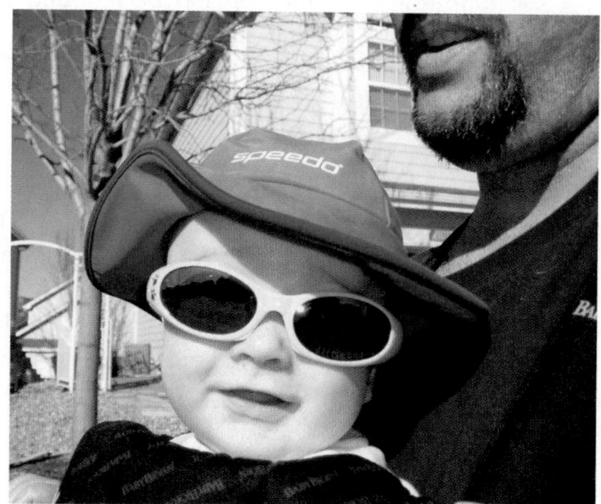

Fig. 17-22 Sunglasses protect the infant's eyes. (Courtesy Julie Perry Nelson, Loveland, CO.)

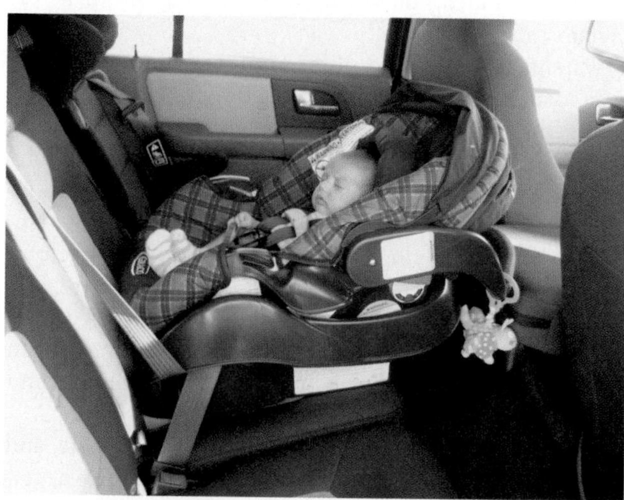

Fig. 17-23 Rear-facing car seat in rear seat of car. Infant is placed in seat when going home from the hospital. (Courtesy Brian and Mayannyn Sallee, Las Vegas, NV.)

particular car seat. The safest area of the car is the back seat. A car safety seat that faces the rear gives the best protection for the disproportionately weak neck and heavy head of an infant.

The car safety seat is secured using the vehicle seat belt; the infant is secured using the harness system in the car safety seat.

NURSING ALERT In cars equipped with air bags, rear-facing infant seats should not be placed in the front seat unless the air bag has been deactivated. Serious injury can occur if the air bag inflates because these types of infant seats fit closer to the dashboard.

Infants born at less than 37 weeks of gestation and with birth weight less than 2500 g should be observed in a car safety seat for a period (equal to the length of the car ride home) before discharge. The infant is monitored for apnea, bradycardia, and a decrease in oxygen saturation. Placing blanket rolls on either side of the infant may be necessary for support of the head and trunk. To prevent slumping the back-to-crotch strap distance should be 14 cm.

Nonnutritive Sucking

Sucking is the infant's chief pleasure. However, sucking needs may not be satisfied by breastfeeding or bottle-feeding alone. In fact, sucking is such a strong need that infants who are deprived of sucking, such as those with a cleft lip, will suck on their tongues. Some newborns are born with sucking pads on their fingers that developed during in utero sucking. Several benefits of nonnutritive sucking have been demonstrated, such as an increased weight gain in preterm infants, increased ability to maintain an organized state, and decreased crying.

There is compelling evidence that pacifiers prevent SIDS. The American Academy of Pediatrics (2005) suggests that parents consider offering a pacifier for naps and bedtime. The AAP recommends that the pacifier be used when the infant is placed down for sleep and that it should not be re-inserted once the infant falls asleep. No infant should be forced to take a pacifier. Pacifiers are to be cleaned often and replaced regularly and should not be coated with any type of sweet solution (AAP, 2005b). The AAP recommends that pacifier use be avoided in breastfeeding infants until breastfeeding is well established (AAP, 2005c).

Problems arise when parents are concerned about the sucking of fingers, thumb, or pacifier and try to restrain this natural tendency. Before giving advice, nurses should investigate the parents' feelings and base the guidance they give on the information solicited. For example, some parents may see no problem with the use of a finger but may find the use of a pacifier objectionable. In general, either practice need not be restrained unless thumb sucking persists past 4 years of age or past the time when the permanent teeth erupt. Parents are advised to consult with their pediatrician, pediatric dentist, or pediatric nurse practitioner about this topic.

A parent's excessive use of the pacifier to calm the infant should also be explored, however. Placing a pacifier in their infant's mouth as soon as the infant begins to cry is not unusual for parents, thus reinforcing a pattern of distress and relief.

If parents choose to let their infant use a pacifier, they need to be aware of certain safety considerations before purchasing one. A homemade or poorly designed pacifier can be dangerous because the entire object may be aspirated if it is small, or a portion may become lodged in the pharynx. Improvised pacifiers, such as those commonly made in hospitals from a padded nipple, also pose dangers because the nipple may separate from the plastic collar and be aspirated. Safe pacifiers are made of one piece that includes a shield or flange large enough to prevent entry into the mouth and a handle that can be grasped (Fig. 17-24).

Sponge Bathing, Cord Care, and Skin Care

Skill: Infant Bathing

Bathing serves several purposes. It provides opportunities for (1) completely cleansing the infant, (2) observing the infant's condition, (3) promoting comfort, and (4) parent-child-family socializing.

An important consideration in skin cleansing is the preservation of the skin's acid mantle, which is formed from the uppermost horny layer of the epidermis, sweat, superficial fat, metabolic products, and external substances such as amniotic fluid and microorganisms. At birth the skin has a pH of 6.4. Within 4 days the pH of the newborn's skin surface falls to within the bacteriostatic range (pH less than 5) (Krebs, 1998). Consequently, only plain, warm water should be used for the bath during this 4-day period. Alkaline soaps (such as Ivory) and oils, powder, and lotions should not be used during this time because they alter the acid mantle, thus providing a medium for bacterial growth.

Although the sponging technique is generally used, bathing the newborn by immersion has been found to allow less heat loss and provoke less crying. Immersion

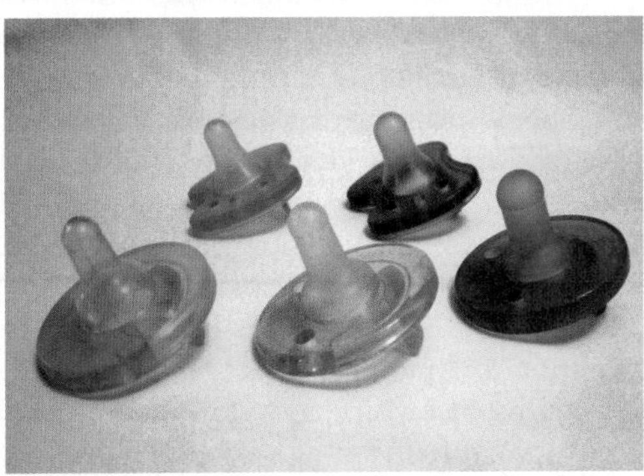

Fig. 17-24 Safe pacifiers for term and preterm infants. Note one-piece construction, easily grasped handle, and large shield with ventilation holes. (Courtesy Julie Perry Nelson, Loveland, CO.)

bathing is a safe alternative to sponge bathing, provided that the infant's condition is stable (no temperature instability, respiratory or cardiac illness) and that the infant is dried off immediately thereafter and kept warm (AWHONN, 2007). A daily bath is not necessary for achieving cleanliness and may do harm by disrupting the integrity of the newborn's skin; cleansing the perineum after a soiled diaper and daily cleansing of the face may suffice. Until the initial bath is completed, personnel must wear gloves to handle the newborn.

The infant bath time provides a wonderful opportunity for parent-infant social interaction. While bathing the baby, parents can talk to the infant, caress and cuddle the infant, and engage in arousal and imitation of facial expressions and smiling. Parents can pick a time for the bath that is easy for them and when the baby is awake, usually before a feeding.

Cord care

The umbilical cord begins to dry, shrivel, and blacken by the second or third day of life, depending in part on the cleansing method used. The umbilicus should be inspected often for signs of infection (e.g., foul odor, redness, purulent discharge), granuloma (i.e., small, red, raw-appearing polyp where the umbilical cord separates), bleeding, and discharge. The cord clamp is removed when the cord is dry in approximately 24 hours (see Fig. 17-4). The cord normally falls off in 10 to 14 days after birth but may remain attached for as long as 3 weeks in some cases. Parents are instructed in appropriate home cord care (per practitioner or institution protocol) and the expected time of cord separation.

The Teaching Guidelines box contains information regarding sponge bathing, skin care, cord care, cutting nails, and dressing the infant.

Infant Follow-Up Care

With shorter hospital stays the focus and site of infant care are changing. Home care may be provided either by a nurse as part of the routine follow-up care of patients or through a visiting nurse or community health nurse referral service. For infants discharged early, newborn home care is essential (Teaching Guidelines box).

Parents should plan for their infant's follow-up health care at the following ages: within 3 days if discharged early or breastfeeding to check for status of jaundice, feeding, and elimination (see also Physiologic Jaundice, pp. 491-493; 2 to 3 weeks of age for breastfeeding babies; 2 to 4 weeks of age for formula feeding babies; then every 2 months until 6 to 7 months of age; then every 3 months until 18 months; at 2 years; at 3 years; at preschool; and every 2 years thereafter.

Immunizations

The schedule for immunizations should be reviewed with parents (Table 17-5); HB vaccine is currently administered to newborns before hospital discharge (depending on maternal HB status) or within 1 month of birth. Nurses should become familiar with this schedule and should provide written instructions to the parents about when and where to obtain immunizations. (Immunization schedules change periodically and the nurse can update any information needed by checking with the website www.cdc.gov.) An infant's ability to protect him or herself against antigens by the formation of antibodies develops sequentially; therefore the infant must be developmentally capable of responding to these antibodies, which is the reason for planning sequential immunizations for infants.

TABLE 17-5

Immunization Schedule—2013*

IMMUNIZATION	AGE GIVEN
HBV (hepatitis B)	3 injections: before hospital discharge, 1 or 2 mo, final dose no earlier than age 24 weeks
HBIG (hepatitis B immunoglobulin—if mother is HBsAg positive)	Within 12 hours after birth
Rotavirus	2, 4, 6 mo
DTaP (diphtheria, tetanus, acellular pertussis)	2, 4, 6, 12-15 mo
Hib (*Haemophilus influenzae* b conjugate vaccine)	2, 4, 6, 12-15 mo
Pneumococcal	2, 4, 6, 12-15 mo
IPV (inactivated polio vaccine—injectable)	2, 4 mo
Influenza ("flu shot")	Yearly after 6 mo
MMR (measles, mumps, rubella)	12 to 15 mo
Varicella (chicken pox)	12 to 18 mo
Hepatitis A	12-23 mo (2 doses at least 6 mo apart)

Source: U.S. Department of Health and Human Services, Centers for Disease Control and Prevention. (2013). *Recommended immunization schedule for children from birth through 6 years.* Internet document available at http://www.cdc.gov/mmwr/preview/mmwrhtml/sub201a2.htm.

*This is the schedule for the first 18 months. For the full schedule, go to www.cdc.gov.

Cardiopulmonary resuscitation

All personnel working with infants must have current infant CPR certification. Parents should receive instruction in relieving airway obstruction (Emergency box) and CPR (Emergency box). Classes are often offered in hospitals and clinics during the prenatal period or to parents of newborns. Such instruction is especially important for parents whose infants were preterm or had cardiac or respiratory problems. Babysitters should also learn CPR.

TEACHING GUIDELINES

Sponge Bathing

FIT BATHS INTO THE FAMILY'S SCHEDULE

- Give a bath at any time convenient to you but not immediately after a feeding period because the increased handling may cause regurgitation.

PREVENT HEAT LOSS

- The temperature of the room should be 24° C (75° F), and the bathing area should be free of drafts.
- Control heat loss during the bath to conserve the infant's energy. Bathing the infant quickly, exposing only a portion of the body at a time, and drying thoroughly are all parts of the bathing technique.

GATHER SUPPLIES AND CLOTHING BEFORE STARTING

- Clothing suitable for wearing indoors: diaper, shirt; stretch suit or nightgown optional
- Unscented, mild soap
- Pins, if needed for diaper, closed and placed well out of the baby's reach
- Cotton balls
- Towels for drying the infant and a clean washcloth
- Receiving blanket
- Tub for water; fill only to 3 to 4 inches of water

BATHE THE BABY

- Bring the infant to the bathing area when all supplies are ready.
- Never leave the infant alone on bath table or in the bath water, not even for a second! If you have to leave, take the infant with you, or place the infant back into the crib.
- Test the temperature of the water. It should feel pleasantly warm to the inner wrist—36.6° to 37.2° C (98°-99° F).
- Do not hold the infant under running water—the water temperature may change, and the infant may be scalded or chilled rapidly. The baby may be tub bathed after the cord drops off and the umbilicus and circumcised penis are completely healed.
- If sponge bathing is to be performed, undress the baby and wrap in a towel with the head exposed. Uncover the parts of the body you are washing, taking care to keep the rest of the baby covered as much as possible to prevent heat loss.
- Begin by washing the baby's face with water; do not use soap on the face. Cleanse the eyes from the inner canthus outward using separate parts of a clean washcloth for each eye. For the first 2 to 3 days a discharge may result from the reaction of the conjunctiva to the substance (erythromycin) used as a prophylactic measure against infection. Any discharge should be considered abnormal and reported to the health care provider.
- Cleanse the ears and nose with twists of moistened cotton or a corner of the washcloth. Do not use cotton-tipped swabs because they may cause injury. The areas behind the ears need daily cleansing.
- Wash the body with mild soap; rinse and dry to decrease heat loss. Place your hand under the baby's shoulders and lift gently to expose the neck, lift the chin, and wash the neck, taking to care to cleanse between the skin folds. Wash between the fingers and toes, then rinse and dry thoroughly. Wash the genital area last.
- If the hair is to be washed, begin by wrapping the infant in a towel with the head exposed. Hold the infant in a football position (under the arm) with one hand, using the other hand to wash the hair. Wash the scalp with water, mild soap, and a soft brush; rinse well and dry thoroughly. Scalp desquamation, called *cradle cap,* can often be prevented by removing any scales with a fine-toothed comb or brush after washing. If the condition persists, the health care provider may prescribe a medicated shampoo to massage into the scalp. A blow dryer is never used on an infant because the temperature is too hot for a baby's skin.

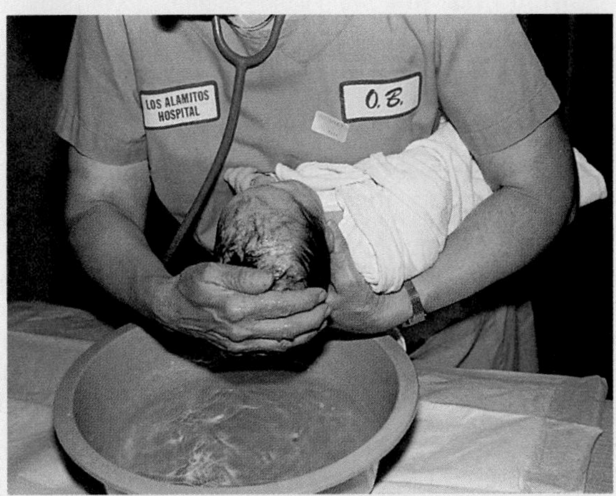

Wash hair with baby wrapped to limit heat loss. (Courtesy Marjorie Pyle, RNC, Lifecircle, Costa Mesa, CA.).

SKIN CARE

- The skin of a newborn is sensitive and should be cleaned only with water between baths. Soap has drying properties, and its use is limited to bathing. Creams, lotions, ointments, or powders are not recommended. If the skin seems excessively dry during the first 2 to 3 weeks after birth, an unscented, non–alcohol-based lotion may be used; checking with the health care provider for suggestions on skin care products is best. Experts advise that baby clothes be laundered separately using a mild laundry detergent (Dreft or Ivory Snow); clothes should be rinsed twice with plain water.
- The fragile skin can be injured by too vigorous cleansing. If stool or other debris has dried and caked on the skin, soak the area to remove it. Do not attempt to rub it off because abrasion may result. Gentleness, patting dry rather than rubbing, and using a mild soap without perfumes or coloring are recommended. Chemicals in

Continued

TEACHING GUIDELINES—cont'd

Sponge Bathing

the coloring and perfume can cause rashes on sensitive skin.

- Babies are very prone to sunburn and should be kept out of direct sunlight. Use of sunscreens should be discussed with the health care provider.
- Babies often develop rashes that are normal. Neonatal acne resembles pimples and may appear at 2 to 4 weeks of age, resolving without treatment by 6 to 8 months. Heat rash is common in warm weather, which appears as a fine red rash around creases or folds where the baby sweats.

CARE OF THE CORD

- Cleanse with soap and water around base of the cord where it joins the skin. Notify the health care provider of any odor, discharge, or skin inflammation around the cord. The clamp is removed when the cord is dry (approximately 24 hours). The diaper should not cover the cord because a wet or soiled diaper will slow or prevent drying of the cord and foster infection. When the cord drops off after 10 to 14 days, small drops of blood may be seen when the baby cries. This bleeding will heal by itself. It is not dangerous.

NAIL CARE

- Do not cut fingernails and toenails immediately after birth. The nails have to grow out far enough from the skin so that the skin is not cut by mistake. If the baby scratches him or herself, apply loosely fitted mitts over each of the baby's hands. Do so as a last resort, however, because it interferes with the baby's ability for self-consolation sucking on thumb or finger. When the nails have grown, the fingernails and toenails can be trimmed with manicure scissors or clippers; nails should be cut straight across. The ideal time to trim the nails is when the infant is sleeping. Soft emery boards may be used to file the nails. Nails should be kept short.

CLEANSE GENITALS

- Cleanse the genitals of infants daily and after voiding or defecating. For girls the genitals are cleansed by separating the labia and gently washing from the pubic area to the anus. For uncircumcised boys, gently pull back (retract) the foreskin. Stop when resistance is felt. In most newborns the inner layer of the foreskin adheres to the glans, and the foreskin cannot be retracted. Wash and rinse the tip (glans) with soap and warm water, and replace the foreskin. The foreskin must be returned to its original position to prevent constriction and swelling. By age 3 years in 90% of boys the foreskin can be retracted easily without causing pain or trauma. For others the foreskin is not retractable until adolescence. As soon as the foreskin is partly retractable and the child is old enough, he can be taught self-management. Once healed the circumcised penis does not require any special care other than cleansing with diaper changes.
- The infant's skin should be allowed to dry completely before applying another diaper. Exposing the buttocks to air can help dry up diaper rash. Because bacteria thrive in moist dark areas, exposing the skin to dry air decreases bacterial proliferation. Zinc oxide ointments can be used to protect the infant's skin from moisture and further excoriation.

TEACHING GUIDELINES

Newborn Progress after Early Discharge*

- Wet diapers: six to ten per day after day 3-4
- Breastfeeding: successful latch-on and feeding every 1.5 to 3 hours daily (8-12 times in 24 hours)
- Formula-feeding: successfully, voiding as noted above, taking approximately 3 to 4 ounces every 3 to 4 hours daily
- Circumcision: wash with warm water only; yellow exudate forming, nonbleeding, PlastiBell intact for 48 hours
- Stools: at least one every 48 hours for formula-fed infants and at least three per day for breastfeeding infants
- Color: pink to ruddy when crying; pink centrally when at rest or asleep
- Activity: has four or five wakeful periods per day and alerts to environmental sounds and voices
- Jaundice: physiologic jaundice (not appearing in first 24 hours), feeding, voiding, and stooling as noted above, or practitioner notification for suspicion of pathologic jaundice (appears within 24 hours of birth, ABO/Rh problem suspected; hemolysis); decreased activity; poor feeding; dark-orange skin color persisting beyond fifth day in light-skinned newborn
- Cord: kept above diaper line; drying; periumbilical area skin pink (erythematous circle at umbilical site may be sign of omphalitis)
- Vital signs: heart rate 120 to 140 beats/min at rest; respiratory rate 30 to 55 breaths/min at rest without evidence of retractions, grunting, or nasal flaring; temperature 36.5° to 37.5° C axillary
- Position of sleep: back

*Any deviation from the above or suspicion of poor newborn adaptation should be reported to the practitioner at once.

EMERGENCY

Relieving Airway Obstruction

- Back blow and chest thrusts are used to clear an airway obstructed by a foreign body.

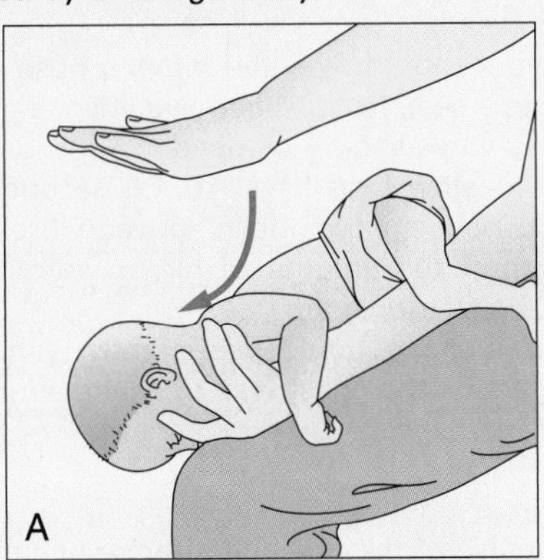

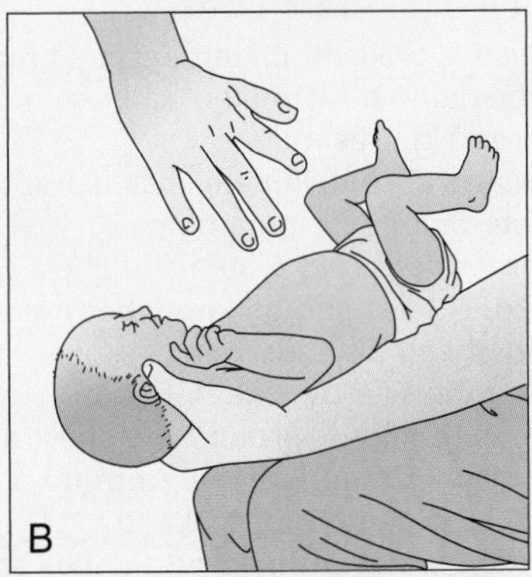

Back blows and chest thrust in infant to clear airway obstruction. **A**, Back blow. **B**, Chest thrust.

BACK BLOWS

- Position the infant prone over the forearm with the infant's head down and the jaw firmly supported.
- Rest the supporting arm on the thigh.
- Deliver four back blows forcefully between the infant's shoulder blades with the heel of the free hand.

TURN THE INFANT

- Place the free hand on the infant's back to sandwich the baby between both hands; one hand supports the neck, jaw, and chest, while the other supports the back.
- Turn the infant over, and place the infant's head lower than the chest, supporting the head and neck.
- Alternative position: Place the infant face down on your lap with the head lower than the trunk; firmly support the head. Apply back blows, and then turn the infant as a unit.

CHEST THRUSTS

- Provide four downward chest thrusts on the lower third of the sternum.
- Remove the foreign body, if it is visible.

OPEN THE AIRWAY

- Open the airway with the head tilt–chin lift maneuver, and attempt to ventilate.
- Repeat the sequence of back blows, turning, and chest thrusts.
- Continue these emergency procedures until signs of recovery occur:
  - Palpable peripheral pulses return.
  - The pupils become normal in size and are responsive to light.
  - Mottling and cyanosis disappear.
- Record the time and duration of the procedure and the effects of this intervention.

Practical Suggestions for the First Weeks at Home

Numerous changes occur during the first weeks of parenthood. Care management should be directed toward helping parents cope with infant care, role changes, altered lifestyle, and change in family structure resulting from the addition of a new baby. Developing skill and confidence in caring for an infant can be especially anxiety provoking. Anticipatory guidance can help prevent a shock of reality in the transition from hospital or birthing center to home that might negate the parents' joy or cause them undue stress. For example, the nurse can teach parents several strategies that help quiet a fussy baby, prevent crying, and induce quiet attention or sleep.

Instructions for the first days at home

Parents, especially first-time parents, must be helped to anticipate events during the transition from hospital to home. Even the simplest strategies can provide enormous support. Written information reinforcing education topics is helpful for parents, as is a list of available community resources, both local and national, and websites that provide reliable information about child care. Classes in the prenatal period or during the postpartum stay are helpful. Instructions for the first days at home should minimally include activities of daily living, dealing with visitors, and activity and rest.

Activities of daily living. Given the demands of a newborn, the mother's discomfort or fatigue associated with giving birth, and a busy homecoming day, even small details of daily life can become stressful. Measures such as using disposable diapers, preparing frozen or microwave dinners during pregnancy, or getting takeout meals can decrease stress by eliminating at least one or two parental responsibilities during the first few days at home.

Planning for discharge soon after an infant feeding increases the likelihood that the couple will have adequate

Cardiopulmonary Resuscitation (CPR) for Infants

- Wash hands before and after touching infant and equipment. Wear gloves, if possible.

ASSESS RESPONSIVENESS

- Observe color; tap or gently shake shoulders.
- Yell for help; if alone, perform CPR for 1 minute before calling for help again.

POSITION INFANT

- Turn the infant onto back, supporting the head and neck.
- Place the infant on firm, flat surface.

AIRWAY

- Open the airway with the head tilt-chin lift method.
- Place one hand on the infant's forehead, and tilt the head back.
- Place the fingers of the other hand under the bone of the lower jaw at the chin.

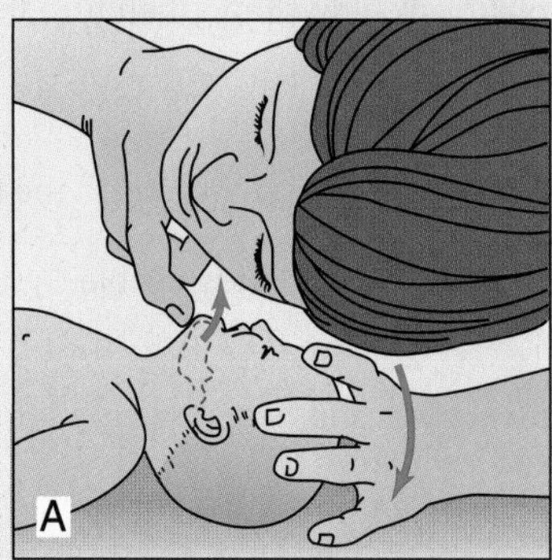

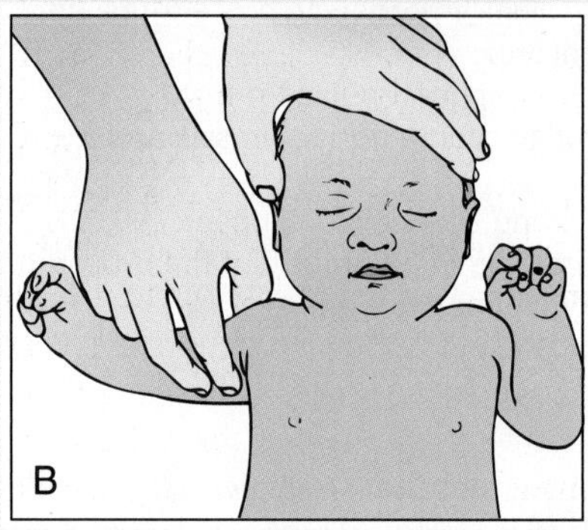

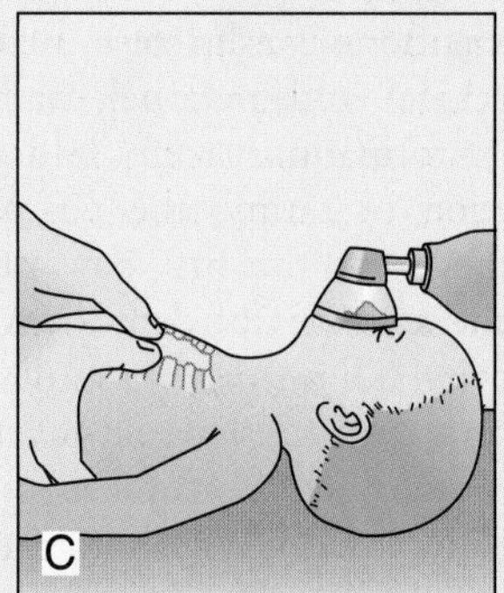

A, Opening airway with head tilt–chin lift method. **B**, Checking pulse of brachial artery. **C**, Side-by-side thumb placement for chest compression in newborn.

BREATHING

- Assess for evidence of breathing:
  - Observe for chest movement.
  - Listen for exhaled air.
  - Feel for exhaled air flow.
- To breathe for infant:
  - Take a breath.
  - Place your mouth over the infant's nose and mouth to create a seal. NOTE: When available, a mask with a one-way valve should be used.
  - Give two slow breaths (1 to 1.5 seconds for each breath), pausing to inhale between breaths. NOTE: Gently puff the volume of air in your cheeks into infant. Do not force air.
- The infant's chest should rise slightly with each puff; keep fingers on the chest wall to sense air entry.

CIRCULATION

- Assess circulation:
  - Check pulse of the brachial artery while maintaining the head tilt.
  - If the pulse is present, initiate rescue breathing. Continue procedure at 40 to 60 breaths/min until spontaneous breathing resumes.
  - If the pulse is absent, initiate chest compressions and coordinate them with breathing.
- Chest compression: Two systems of chest compression can be used. Nurses should know both methods.
- Maintain the head tilt and:
  1. Place thumbs side-by-side in the middle third of the sternum with fingers around the chest and supporting the back. Compress the sternum 1.25 to 2 cm (one third the depth of the chest).
  2. Place index finger of hand just under an imaginary line drawn between the nipples. Place the middle and ring fingers on the sternum adjacent to the index finger. Using the middle and ring fingers, compress the sternum approximately 1.25 to 2.5 cm (one third the depth of the chest).
- Avoid compressing the xiphoid process.
- Release the pressure without moving the thumbs and fingers from the chest.
- Use a 30:2 compression-ventilation ratio for one-rescuer CPR and 15:2 compression-ventilation ratio for two-rescuer CPR.
- Provide 100 compressions per minute
- Provide five cycles of three compressions and two ventilations of CPR (about 2 minutes) before leaving to call 911.
- After the cycles, check the brachial artery to determine whether a pulse can be felt.
- Discontinue compressions when the infant's spontaneous heart rate reaches or exceeds 80 beats/min.
- Record the time and duration of the procedure and the effects of intervention.

Source: Berg, M. D. et al. (2010). Part 13: Pediatric Basic Life Support: 2010 American Heart Association Guidelines for Cardiopulmonary Resuscitation and Emergency Cardiovascular Care. *Circulation, 122,* S862-S875.

time to get home and relatively settled before the next feeding. Offering a sample carton of premixed bottles for the formula-fed infant prevents the need for rushed preparation of formula.

Visitors. New parents are often inadequately prepared for the reality of bringing a new infant home because they romanticize the homecoming. One mother stated, "By the time we drove an hour through traffic, my stitches were hurting, and all I wanted was a warm sitz bath and some private time with Bill and the baby, in that order. Instead, a carload of visitors pulled into the driveway as we were unbuckling the baby from his car seat. I thought I would surely cry."

The nurse can help parents explore ways, in advance, to assert their need to limit visitors. When family and friends ask what they can do to help, new parents can suggest they prepare and bring them a meal, which might be used immediately or frozen for later, or pick up items at the store. Parents can work out a signal for alerting the partner that the mother is getting tired or uncomfortable and needs the partner to invite the visitors to another room or to leave. Some mothers find that wearing a robe and not appearing ready for company leads visitors to stay a shorter time. A sign on the front door saying "Mother and baby resting–please do not disturb" may be useful.

Activity and rest. Because mothers have reported fatigue to be a major problem during the first few weeks after giving birth, they need to be encouraged to limit their activities and be realistic about their level of fatigue. Activities should not be sustained for long periods. Family, friends, and neighbors can be solicited for support and help with meals, housecleaning, picking up other children, and so on. Rest periods throughout the day are important. Mothers can nap when the baby sleeps. Adequate nutrition is also important for postpartum recovery and in dealing with fatigue.

Anticipatory guidance regarding the newborn

Anticipatory guidance helps prepare new parents for what to expect as their newborn grows and develops. Parents with realistic expectations of infant needs and behavior are better prepared to adjust to the demands of a new baby and to parenthood itself.

New parents can be overwhelmed by a large volume of information and become anxious. Anticipatory guidance should include the following: newborn sleep-wake cycles, interpretation of crying and quieting techniques, infant developmental milestones, sensory enrichment and infant stimulation, recognizing signs of illness, and well-baby follow-up and immunizations. Printed materials and audiotapes or videotapes for parents to take home are helpful. With more and more use of the Internet, parents may also be given a list of websites that might be accessed for information.

Development of day-night routines. Nurses can help prepare new parents for the fact that most newborns cannot tell the difference between night and day and must learn the rhythm of day-night routines. Nurses should provide basic suggestions for settling a newborn and for helping him or her develop a predictable routine. Examples of such suggestions include the following:

- In the late afternoon, bring the baby out to the center of family activity. Keep the baby there for the rest of the evening. If the baby falls asleep, let the baby do so in the infant seat or in someone's arms. Save the crib or bassinet for nighttime sleep.
- Give the baby a bath right before bedtime. This activity soothes the baby and helps him or her expend energy.
- Feed the baby for the last evening time around 11:00 PM, and put him or her to bed in the crib or bassinet.
- For nighttime feedings and diaper changes, keep a small night-light on to avoid turning on bright lights. Talk in soft whispers (if at all), and handle the baby gently and only as absolutely necessary to feed and diaper. Nighttime feedings should be all business and no play! Babies usually go back to sleep if the room is quiet and dark.

A predictable, stable routine gradually develops for *most* babies; however, some babies *never* develop one. New parents will cope better if they are willing to be flexible and to give up some control during the early weeks.

Interpretation of crying and quieting techniques. Crying is an infant's first social communication. Some babies cry more than others, but all babies cry. They cry to communicate that they are hungry, uncomfortable, wet, ill, or bored and sometimes for no apparent reason at all. The longer parents are around their infants, the easier the task becomes of interpreting what a cry means. Many infants have a fussy period during the day, often in the late afternoon or early evening when everyone is naturally tired. Environmental tension adds to the length and intensity of crying spells. Babies also have periods of vigorous crying when no comforting can help. These periods of crying may last for long stretches until the infants seem to cry themselves to sleep. Possibly the infants are trying to discharge enough energy that they can settle themselves down. The nurse needs to reinforce for new parents that time and infant maturation will take care of these types of cries.

Crying because of colic is a common concern of new parents. Babies with colic cry inconsolably for several hours, pull their legs up to their stomach, and pass large amounts of gas. No one really knows what colic is or why babies get it. Parents can be encouraged to contact their nurse-practitioner or pediatrician if they are concerned that their baby has colic.

Certain types of sensory stimulation can calm and quiet infants and help them get to sleep. Important characteristics of this sensory stimulation–whether tactile, vestibular, auditory, or visual–appear to be that the stimulation is mild, slow, and rhythmic, and consistently and regularly

Spanish Guidelines: Infant Quieting Techniques
Assessment Video: Crying Female Neonate
Spanish Guidelines: Daily Care

Skill: Swaddling

presented. Tactile stimulation can include warmth, patting, back rubbing, and covering the skin with textured cloth. Swaddling (see Fig. 17-21, *D)* to keep arms and legs close to the body (as in utero) provides widespread and constant tactile stimulation and a sense of security. Vestibular stimulation is especially effective and can be accomplished by mild rhythmic movement such as rocking or by holding the infant upright, as on the parent's shoulder.

The nurse can teach parents several strategies that help quiet a fussy baby, prevent crying, and induce quiet attention or sleep (Box 17-7).

Developmental milestones. Knowledge of infant growth and development helps parents have realistic expectations of what an infant can do. When parents understand and appreciate the limitations and developing abilities of their infant, adjustment to parenthood can go more smoothly. Emphasizing the individuality of the infant enhances the capacity of the family to offer their infant an optimally nurturing environment.

Brazelton (1995) suggests the concept of "touch-points" for intervention, that is, points at which a change in the system (baby, parent, and family) is brought about by the baby's spurts in development (cognitive, motor, or emotional). Immediately before each spurt in development is a predictable short period of disorganization in the baby. Parents are likely to feel disorganized and stressed as well. Because these periods of disorganization are predictable, nurses can offer parents anticipatory guidance to help them understand what happens with infant development and to prepare them for the subsequent spurts in development.

The nurse should provide parents with information on month-by-month infant growth and development. Written information that parents can consult later is especially helpful. Table 17-6 provides a summary of infant growth and development during the first 2 to 3 months.

Infant stimulation. Interacting with their parents is an important way in which infants learn about themselves and their environment. Nurses can teach parents a variety of ways to stimulate their infant's development and to enrich the infant's learning environment. Home health nurses can evaluate the home environment and make suggestions to parents for promotion of their baby's physical, cognitive, and emotional development. Suggestions for teaching infants during the first few months are presented in Boxes 17-8 and 17-9. Table 17-7 presents suggestions for visual, auditory, tactile, and kinetic stimulation.

Recognizing signs of illness. In addition to explaining the need for well-baby follow-up visits, the nurse should discuss with parents the signs of illness in newborns (Box 17-10). Of particular importance is the parents' assessment of jaundice in newborns discharged early. Parents should be advised to call their nurse-practitioner or pediatrician immediately if they notice increasing jaundice or signs of illness and to ask about over-the-counter medications, such as acetaminophen for infants, to keep at home.

BOX 17-7

Infant Quieting Techniques

- Many newborns feel insecure in the center of a large crib. They prefer a small, warm, soft space that reminds them of intrauterine life. Try a smaller bed, such as a bassinet, portable crib, buggy, or cradle, or use a rolled-up blanket to turn a corner of the big crib into a smaller place.
- Carry your baby in a frontpack or backpack.
- Swaddle your newborn snugly in a receiving blanket. Swaddling keeps your newborn's arms and legs close to his or her body, similar to the intrauterine position; it also makes the newborn feel more secure.
- Prewarm the crib sheets with a hot water bottle or heating pad set on low that you remove before putting your baby to bed. Some babies startle when placed on a cold sheet.
- Some newborns need extra sucking to soothe themselves to sleep. Breastfeeding mothers may prefer to let their infant suckle at the breast as a soothing technique. Other mothers choose to use a pacifier. Stroke the pacifier against the roof of the baby's mouth to encourage him or her to suck it during the first 2 weeks. Around 3 months of age, infants become able to consistently find and suck their thumbs as a way of self-consoling.
- A rhythmic, monotonous noise simulating the intrauterine sounds of your heartbeat and blood flow may help your infant settle down. Some parents have found that putting the baby in a portable crib beside the dishwasher or washing machine helps settle a fussy baby.
- Movement often helps quiet a baby. Take your baby for a ride in the car, or take your baby for an outing in a stroller or carriage. Rock your baby in a rocking chair or cradle.
- Place your baby on his or her stomach across your lap; pat and rub his or her back while gently bouncing your legs or swaying them from left to right.
- Babies enjoy close skin-to-skin contact. A combination of this and warm water often helps soothe a fussy baby. Fill your tub with warm water. Get in and let the baby lie on your chest so that the baby is immersed in the water up to his or her neck. Cuddle the baby close.
- Let your baby see your face. Talk to your baby in a soothing voice.
- Your baby may simply be bored. Bring him or her into the room where you and the rest of the family are. Change your baby's position; many babies like to be upright, for example, by being held up on your shoulder.

TABLE 17-6

Growth and Development during Infancy

1 MONTH	2 MONTHS	3 MONTHS
PHYSICAL		
Weight gain of 5 to 7.5 oz (150-210 g) weekly for first 6 mo Height gain of 1 in (2.5 cm) monthly for first 6 mo Head circumference increases by 0.6 in (1.5 cm) monthly for first 6 mo Primitive reflexes present and strong Doll's eye reflex and dance reflex fading Preferential nose breathing (most infants)	Posterior fontanel closed Crawling reflex disappears	Primitive reflexes fading
GROSS MOTOR		
Assumes flexed position with pelvis high but knees not under abdomen when prone (at birth, knees flexed under abdomen)† Can turn head from side to side when prone, lifts head momentarily from bed† Has marked head lag, especially when pulled from lying to sitting position Holds head momentarily parallel and in midline when suspended in prone position Assumes asymmetric tonic neck reflex position when supine When held in standing position, body limp at knees and hips In sitting position, back is uniformly rounded; absence of head control	Assumes less flexed position when prone—hips flat, legs extended, arms flexed, head to side† Less head lag when pulled to sitting position Can maintain head in same plane as rest of body when held in ventral suspension When prone, can lift head almost 45 degrees off table When held in sitting position, head is held up but bobs forward Assumes asymmetric tonic neck reflex position intermittently	Able to hold head more erect when sitting, but still bobs forward Has only slight head lag when pulled to sitting position Assumes symmetric body positioning Able to raise head and shoulders from prone position to a 45- to 90-degree angle from table; bears weight on forearms When held in standing position, able to bear slight fraction of weight on legs Regards own hand
FINE MOTOR		
Hands predominantly closed Grasp reflex strong Hand clenches on contact with rattle	Hands often open Grasp reflex fading	Actively holds rattle but will not reach for it† Grasp reflex absent Hands kept loosely open Clutches own hand; pulls at blanket and clothes
SENSORY		
Able to fixate on moving object in range of 45 degrees when held at a distance of 8-10 in. Visual acuity approaches 20/100*† Follows light to midline Quiets when hears a voice	Binocular fixation and convergence to near objects beginning When supine, follows dangling toy from side to point beyond midline Visually searches to locate sounds Turns head to side when sound is made at level of ear	Follows object to periphery (180 degrees)† Locates sound by turning head to side and looking in same direction† Begins to have ability to coordinate stimuli from various sense organs
VOCALIZATION		
Cries to express displeasure Makes small throaty sounds Makes comfort sounds during feeding	Vocalizes, distinct from crying† Crying becomes differentiated Coos Vocalizes to familiar voice	Squeals aloud to show pleasure† Coos, babbles, chuckles Vocalizes when smiling "Talks" a great deal when spoken to Less crying during periods of wakefulness

*Degree of visual acuity varies according to vision measurement procedure used.
†Milestones that represent essential integrative aspects of development that lay the foundation for the achievement of more advanced skills.

Continued

TABLE 17-6

Growth and Development during Infancy—cont'd

1 MONTH	2 MONTHS	3 MONTHS
SOCIALIZATION AND COGNITION		
Is in sensorimotor phase—stage I, use of reflexes (birth-1 mo), and stage II, primary circular reactions (1-4 mo) Watches parent's face intently as she or he talks to infant	Demonstrates social smile in response to various stimuli†	Displays considerable interest in surroundings Ceases crying when parent enters room Can recognize familiar faces and objects, such as feeding bottle Shows awareness of strange situations

Source: Hockenberry, M. & Wilson, D. (2011). *Wong's nursing care of infants and children* (9th ed.). St. Louis: Mosby.

BOX 17-8

Teaching Your Newborn

- Newborns learn things every day. You can teach your newborn by playing with him or her and giving your newborn toys that help him or her to learn.
- Talk to your baby a lot. Tell your baby what is going on in the room ("Listen to the dog barking."). Label objects that you see or use ("Here's the washcloth."), and describe things you are doing ("Let's put the shirt over Kerry's head!").
- Look at your baby's face and make eye contact. Play face-making games: smile, stick out your tongue, open your eyes wide. As your baby gets older, he or she will try to imitate these facial expressions.
- Babies like music and rhythmic movement. Rock or swing your baby as you sing to him or her in a gentle voice.
- Acknowledge your baby's attempts to "answer" your talking and singing. He or she will respond to you by looking in your direction, making eye contact, moving his or her arms and legs, and making sounds.
- Babies like bright colors and vivid contrasts. Show your baby pictures and objects that are black and white, are bright primary colors (red, blue, yellow), and have large patterns. Keep colorful mobiles and toys where your baby can see them.
- Babies like to be held upright. Holding your newborn on your shoulder lets your baby look around his or her world and provides vestibular stimulation. Let your baby lift his or her head for a few seconds. Keep your hand ready to support your baby's head.

BOX 17-9

Teaching Your 1 Month Old

At 1 to 2 months of age, your infant is gaining more control of his or her movements; the infant has more head control and may even hold an object briefly in his or her hand. Your baby is also becoming more social. He or she demonstrates behaviors to engage you in interaction: smiling, cooing, making longer eye contact, and following you with his or her eyes.

During these months, you can help your baby learn if you:

- Put your baby on his or her stomach on a blanket on the floor. Lie on your stomach facing your baby. Talk to your baby to get him or her to raise his or her head to see you.
- Roll your baby onto his or her back and play with your baby's legs. Move the baby's legs in a bicycle-riding motion. Try to get your baby to kick his or her legs.
- Play hand games, such as pat-a-cake, with your baby; kiss your baby's fingers; place your baby's hands on your face. Bring your baby's hands in front of his or her eyes as you play; get your baby to look at his or her hands.
- Encourage your baby to watch and follow objects with his or her eyes. Use a noise-making toy, such as a rattle or a chime, or a brightly colored object approximately 12 inches from his or her eyes; move it slowly to one side and then the other. Objects hanging from a play frame are good for your baby to watch while he or she is on his or her back or sitting in an infant seat.
- Continue to talk and sing a lot to your baby. Continue to tell your baby what you are doing with him or her and what is going on in the immediate environment.
- Keep your baby near you during times when the family usually is together, such as at mealtimes. Infant seats, especially ones that bounce or rock, and infant swings are good to use at these times.

TABLE 17-7

Play during Infancy: Suggested Activities for Birth through 3 Months

AGE (MONTHS)	VISUAL STIMULATION	AUDITORY STIMULATION	TACTILE STIMULATION	KINETIC STIMULATION
Birth-1	Look at infant at close range Hang bright, shiny object within 9 to 10 inches of infant's face and in midline Hang mobiles with black-and-white contrast designs	Talk to infant, sing in soft voice Play music box, radio, television Have ticking clock or metronome nearby	Hold, caress, cuddle Keep infant warm Infant may like to be swaddled	Rock infant, place in cradle Use carriage for walks
2-3	Provide bright objects Make room bright with pictures or mirrors on walls Take infant to various rooms while doing chores Place infant in infant seat for vertical view of environment	Talk to infant Include in family gatherings Expose to various environmental noises other than those of home Use rattles, wind chimes	Caress infant while bathing, at diaper change Comb hair with a soft brush	Use infant swing Take in car for rides Exercise body by moving extremities in swimming motion Use cradle gym

Source: Hockenberry, M. & Wilson, D. (2011). *Wong's nursing care of infants and children* (9th ed.). St. Louis: Mosby.

BOX 17-10

Signs of Illness

- Fever: temperature above 38° C (100.4° F) axillary (under arm for 3 to 4 minutes); also a continual rise in temperature
- Hypothermia: temperature below 36.5° (97.7° F) axillary
- Poor feeding or little interest in food: refusal to eat for two feedings in a row
- Vomiting: more than one episode of forceful vomiting or frequent vomiting (over a 6-hour period)
- Diarrhea: two consecutive green, watery stools (NOTE: Stools of breastfed infants are normally looser than stools of formula-fed infants. Diarrhea will leave a water ring around the stool, whereas breastfed stools will not.)
- Decreased bowel movement: less than two soiled diapers per day after 48 hours or less than three soiled diapers per day by the fifth day of life
- Decreased urination: no wet diapers for 18 to 24 hours or less than six to eight wet diapers per day after 3-4 days.
- Breathing difficulties: labored breathing with flared nostrils or absence of breathing for more than 15 seconds (NOTE: A newborn's breathing is normally irregular and between 30 to 40 breaths/min. Count the breaths for a full minute.)
- Cyanosis whether accompanying a feeding or not
- Lethargy: sleepiness, difficulty waking, or periods of sleep longer than 6 hours (Most newborns sleep for short periods, usually from 1 to 4 hours, and wake to be fed.)
- Inconsolable crying (attempts to quiet not effective) or continuous high-pitched cry
- Bleeding or purulent drainage from umbilical cord or circumcision
- Drainage developing in the eyes

KEY POINTS

- Assessment of the newborn requires data from the prenatal, intrapartal, and postnatal periods.
- The immediate assessment of the newborn includes Apgar scoring and a general evaluation of physical status.
- Knowledge of biologic and behavioral characteristics is essential for guiding assessment and interpreting data.
- Nursing care immediately after birth includes maintaining an open airway, preventing heat loss, and promoting parent-infant interaction.
- Providing a protective environment is a key responsibility of the nurse and includes such measures as careful identification procedures, support of physiologic functions, ways to prevent infection, and restraining techniques.
- The newborn has social and physical needs.
- Circumcision is an elective surgical procedure.
- Pain in neonates must be assessed and managed.
- Anticipatory guidance helps prepare new parents for what to expect after hospital discharge.
- All parents should have instruction in infant CPR.

Audio Chapter Summaries: Access an audio summary of these Key Points on evolve

References

Albers, S. & Levy, H. (2005). Newborn screening. In H. Taeusch, R. Ballard, & C. Gleason (Eds.), *Avery's diseases of the newborn* (8th ed.). Philadelphia: Saunders.

Alexander, G., Himes, J., Kaufman, R., Mor, J., & Kogan, M. (1996). A United States national reference for fetal growth. *Obstetrics & Gynecology*, *87*(2),163-168.

American Academy of Pediatrics (AAP) Committee on Infectious Diseases. (2006). *Red book: 2006 report of the committee on infectious diseases* (27th ed.). Elk Grove Village, IL: AAP.

American Academy of Pediatrics (AAP) Subcommittee on Hyperbilirubinemia. (2004). Clinical practice guideline: Management of hyperbilirubinemia in the newborn infant 35 or more weeks of gestation. *Pediatrics*, *114*(1), 297-316.

American Academy of Pediatrics (AAP) Task Force on Circumcision. (2012). Circumcision policy statement. *Pediatrics*, *130*(3), 585-586.

American Academy of Pediatrics. (2005a). AAP publications retired and reaffirmed. *Pediatrics*, *116*(3), 796.

American Academy of Pediatrics (AAP) Section on Breastfeeding. (2005c). Breastfeeding and the use of human milk, Policy Statement. *Pediatrics*, *115*(23) 496-506.

American Academy of Pediatrics (AAP) & American College of Obstetricians and Gynecologists (ACOG). (2012). *Guidelines for perinatal care* (7th ed.). Elk Grove Village, IL: AAP.

American College of Obstetricians and Gynecologists (ACOG). (2001). Circumcision. ACOG Committee Opinion No. 260. *Obstetrics & Gynecology*, *98*(4), 707-708.

American Heart Association. (2005). 2005 American Heart Association guidelines for cardiopulmonary resuscitation and emergency cardiovascular care. *Circulation*, *112*(24) Supplement IV12-IV18.

American Medical Association Council on Scientific Affairs. (2005). *Report 10 of the Council on Scientific Affairs (1-99): Neonatal circumcision.* Internet document available at http://www.ama-assn.org/ama/no-index/about-ama/13585.shtml (accessed July 31, 2009).

Arbuckle, T., Wilkins, R., & Sherman, G. (1993). Birth weight percentiles by gestational age in Canada. *Obstetrics & Gynecology*, *81*(1), 39-48.

Association of Women's Health, Obstetric, and Neonatal Nurses (AWHONN). (2007). *Neonatal skin care: Evidence-based clinical practice guideline* (2nd ed.). Washington, DC: AWHONN.

Bakewell-Sachs, S. (2007). Near-term/late preterm infants. *Newborn & Infant Nursing Reviews*, *7*(2), 67-71.

Ballard, J., Khoury, J., Wedig, K., Wang, L., Eilers-Walsman, B., & Lipp, R. (1991). New Ballard score, expanded to include extremely premature infants. *Journal of Pediatrics*, *119*(3), 417-423.

Ballard, J., Novak, K., & Driver, M. (1979). A simplified score for assessment of fetal maturity of newly born infants. *Journal of Pediatrics*, *95*(5 Pt 1), 769-774.

Battaglia, F. & Lubchenco, L. (1967). A practical classification of newborn infants by weight and gestational age. *Journal of Pediatrics*, *71*(2), 159-163.

Berg, M. D., Schexnayder, S. M., Chameides, L., Terry, M., Donoghue, A., Hickey, R. W., Berg, R. A., Sutton, R. M., & Hazinski, M. F. (2010). Part 13: Pediatric Basic Life Support: 2010 American Heart Association Guidelines for Cardiopulmonary Resuscitation and Emergency Cardiovascular Care. *Circulation*, *122*, S862-S875.

Blackburn, S. (2007). *Maternal, fetal, and neonatal physiology: A clinical perspective* (3rd ed.). St. Louis: Saunders.

Brady-Fryer, B., Wiebe, N., & Lander, J. A. (2004). Pain relief for neonatal circumcision. *Cochrane Database of Systematic Reviews 2004*, Issue 3. CD004217.

Brazelton, T. B. (1995). Working with families: Opportunities for early intervention. *Pediatric Clinics of North America*, *42*(1), 1.

Clifford, P., Stringer, M., Christensen, H., & Mountain, D. (2004). Pain assessment and intervention for term newborns. *Journal of Midwifery & Women's Health*, *49*(6), 514-519.

Cornblath, M., Hawdon, J. M., Williams, A. F., Aynsely-Green, A., Ward-Platt, M. P., Schwartz, R., et al. (2000). Controversies regarding definition of neonatal hypoglycemia: Suggested operational thresholds. *Pediatrics*, *105*(5), 1141-1145.

D'Avanzo, C. E. (2008). *Mosby's pocket guide to cultural health assessment* (4th ed.). St. Louis: Mosby.

Engle, W. D., Jackson, G. L., Sendelbach, D., Manning, D., & Frawley, W. H. (2002). Assessment of a transcutaneous device in the evaluation of neonatal hyperbilirubinemia in a primarily Hispanic population. *Pediatrics*, *110*(1 Pt 1), 61-67.

Furdon, S., Eastman, M., Benjamin, K., & Horgan, M. (1998). Outcome measures after standardized pain management strategies in postoperative patients in the NICU. *Journal of Perinatal and Neonatal Nursing*, *12*(1), 58-69.

Gardner, S. L., Carter, B. S., Enzman-Hines, M. I., & Hernandez, J. A. (2011). *Merenstein & Gardner's handbook of neonatal intensive care* (7th ed.). St. Louis: Mosby.

Hagedorn, M. E. (2006). Respiratory distress. In G. B. Merenstein & S. L. Gardner (Eds.), *Handbook of neonatal intensive care* (6th ed.). St. Louis: Mosby.

Hoseth, E., Joergensen, A., Ebbesen, F., & Moeller, M. (2000). Blood glucose levels in a population of healthy, breast fed, term infants of appropriate size for gestational age. *Archives of Diseases in Childhood, Fetal and Neonatal Edition*, *83*(2), F117-F119.

Keren, R., Luan, X., Friedman, S., Saddlemire, S., Cnaan, A., & Bhutani, V. K. (2008). A comparison of alternative risk-assessment strategies for predicting significant neonatal hyperbilirubinemia in term and near-term infants. *Pediatrics*, *121*(1), e170-e179.

Kramer, M. S., Platt, R. W., Wen, S. W., Joseph, K. S., Allen, A., Abrahamowicz, M., et al. (2001). A new and improved population-based Canadian reference for birth weight for gestational age. *Pediatrics*, *108*(2), e35.

Krebs, T. (1998). Cord care: Is it necessary? *Mother Baby Journal*, *3*(2), 5-12, 18-20.

Krechel, S. & Bildner, J. (1995). CRIES: A new neonatal postoperative pain measurement score–initial testing of validity and reliability. *Paediatric Anaesthesia*, *5*(1), 53-61.

Lawrence, J., Alcock, D., McGrath, P., Kay, J., MacMurray, S., & Dulberg, C. (1993). The development of a tool to assess neonatal pain. *Neonatal Network*, *12*(6), 59-66.

Madan, A., Holland, S., Humbert, J. E., & Benitz, W. E. (2002). Racial differences in birth weight of term infants in a northern California population. *Journal of Perinatology*, *22*(3), 230-235.

Maisels, M. J. (2005). Jaundice. In M. G. MacDonald, M. D. Mullett, & M. M. Seshia (Eds), *Neonatology: Pathophysiology and management of the newborn* (6th ed.). Philadelphia: Lippincott Williams & Wilkins.

McConnell, T. P., Lee, C. W., Couillard, M., & Sherrill, W. W. (2004). Trends in umbilical cord care: Scientific evidence for practice. *Newborn & Infant Nursing Reviews*, *4*(4), 211-222.

Mincey, H. & Gonzaba, G. (2007). End tidal carbon monoxide: A new method to detect hyperbilirubinemia in newborns. *Newborn & Infant Nursing Reviews, 7*(2), 122-128.

Pasero, C. (2002). Pain assessment in infants and young children: Neonates. *American Journal of Nursing, 102*(8), 61, 63, 65.

Razmus, I., Dalton, M., & Wilson, D. (2004). Pain management for newborn circumcision. *Pediatric Nursing, 30*(5), 414-417, 427.

Sharfstein, J. M., North, M. N., & Serwint, J. R. (2007). Over the counter but no longer under the radar–pediatric cough and cold medications. *New England Journal of Medicine, 357*(23), 2321-2324.

Steffensrud, S. (2004). Hyperbilirubinemia in term and near-term infants: Kernicterus on the rise? *Newborn & Infant Nursing Reviews, 4*(4), 191-200.

Stevens, B., Johnston, C., Petryshen, P., & Taddio, A. (1996). Premature infant pain profile: Development and initial validation. *Clinical Journal of Pain, 12*(1), 13-22.

Stevens, B., Yamada, J., & Ohlsson, A. (2004). Sucrose for analgesia in newborn infants undergoing procedures. *Cochrane Database of Systematic Reviews* 2004, Issue 3. CD001069.

Stoll, B. J. (2007). The fetus and the neonatal infant. In R. M. Kliegman, R. E. Behrman, H. B. Jenson, & Stanton, B. F. (Eds.), *Nelson textbook of pediatrics* (18th ed.). Philadelphia: Saunders.

Thomas, P., Peabody, J., Turnier, V., & Clark, R. H. (2000). A new look at intrauterine growth and the impact of race, altitude, and gender, *Pediatrics, 106*(2). e21.

Visscher, M. O., Narendran, V., Pickens, W. L., LaRuffa, A. A., Meinzen-Derr, J., Allen, K., et al. (2005). Vernix caseosa in neonatal adaptation. *Journal of Perinatology, 25*(7), 440-446.

Walden, M. & Franck, L. (2003). Identification, management, and prevention of newborn/infant pain. In C. Kenner & J. Lott (Eds.), *Comprehensive neonatal nursing: A physiologic perspective* (3rd ed.). St. Louis: Saunders.

Walden, M. & Gibbins, S. (2008). *Pain assessment & management guideline for practice* (2nd ed.). Glenview, IL: National Association of Neonatal Nurses.

Zupan, J, Garner, P., & Omari, A. A. (2004). Topical umbilical cord care at birth, *Cochrane Database of Systematic Reviews* 2004, Issue 3. CD001057.

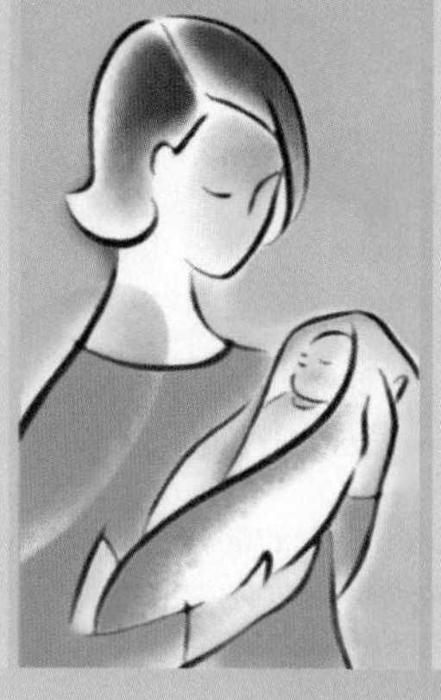

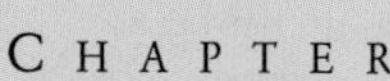
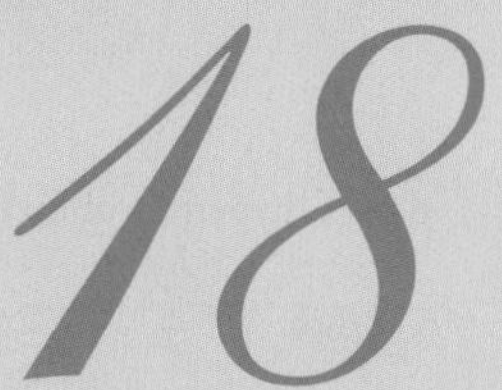

CHAPTER 18

Newborn Nutrition and Feeding

KATHRYN RHODES ALDEN

LEARNING OBJECTIVES

- Describe current recommendations for infant feeding.
- Explain the nurse's role in helping families choose an infant feeding method.
- Discuss benefits of breastfeeding for infants, mothers, families, and society.
- Describe nutritional needs of infants.
- Describe the anatomic and physiologic aspects of breastfeeding.
- Recognize newborn feeding-readiness cues.
- Explain maternal and infant indicators of effective breastfeeding.
- Examine nursing interventions to facilitate and promote successful breastfeeding.
- Analyze common problems associated with breastfeeding and nursing interventions to help resolve them.
- Compare powdered, concentrated, and ready-to-use forms of commercial infant formula.
- Develop a teaching plan for the formula-feeding family.

KEY TERMS AND DEFINITIONS

colostrum Early milk, produced from approximately 16 weeks of pregnancy into the first postpartum days; rich in antibodies, higher in protein, and lower in fat than mature milk, with laxative effect to clear meconium and promote excretion of bilirubin

demand feeding Feeding in response to feeding cues exhibited by the infant that indicate the presence of hunger

engorgement Painful swelling of breast tissue as a result of rapid increase in milk production and venous congestion causing interstitial tissue edema; impaired milk flow results in accumulation of milk in breasts; most often occurs between the third and fifth postpartum days

feeding-readiness cues Infant behaviors (mouthing motions, sucking fist, awakening, and crying) indicating that the infant is interested in feeding

growth spurts Times of increased neonatal growth that usually occur at approximately 6 to 10 days, 6 weeks, 3 months, and 6 months; increased caloric needs of the infant prompt more frequent feedings

inverted nipples Nipples invert rather than evert when stimulated; can interfere with effective latch

lactation consultant Health care professional who has specialized training and experience working with breastfeeding mothers and infants

lactogenesis Process of breast milk production

latch Placement of the infant's mouth over the nipple, areola, and breast, making a seal between the mouth and breast to create adequate suction for milk removal

mastitis Inflammation of the breast, often associated with infection, characterized by influenza-like symptoms and redness and tenderness in the affected breast

milk ejection reflex (MER) Release of milk caused by the contraction of the myoepithelial cells surrounding the milk glands in response to oxytocin; also called the let-down reflex

plugged milk duct Blockage of milk duct causing ineffective emptying of breast

rooting reflex Normal response of the newborn to move toward whatever touches the area around the mouth and to attempt to suck; usually disappears by 3 to 4 months of age

supply-meets-demand system Physiologic basis for milk production; milk volume is produced in response to amount removed from the breast

WEB RESOURCES

Additional related content can be found on the companion website at evolve
http://evolve.elsevier.com/Lowdermilk/Maternity/

- NCLEX Review Questions
- Case Study: Breastfeeding
- Critical Thinking Exercise: Breastfeeding
- Critical Thinking Exercise: Formula Preparation
- Nursing Care Plan: Breastfeeding and Infant Nutrition
- Nursing Care Plan: The Newborn with Insufficient Intake of Nutrients
- Skill: Infant Feeding
- Spanish Guidelines: Breastfeeding: Latching On
- Spanish Guidelines: Burping

Good nutrition in infancy fosters optimal growth and development. Infant feeding is more than the provision of nutrition; it is an opportunity for social, psychologic, and even educational interaction between parent and infant. It can also establish a basis for developing good eating habits that last a lifetime.

Through preconception and prenatal education and counseling, nurses play an instrumental role in assisting parents with the selection of an infant feeding method. Scientific evidence is clear that human milk provides the best nutrition for infants, and parents should be strongly encouraged to choose breastfeeding (American Academy of Pediatrics [AAP] Section on Breastfeeding, 2012). Although many health care providers and the general public may consider artificial baby milk (infant formula) to be equivalent to breast milk, this belief is erroneous. Human milk is species specific, uniquely designed to meet the needs of human infants. The composition of human milk changes to meet the nutritional needs of growing infants. It is highly complex, with antiinfective and nutritional components combined with growth factors, enzymes that aid in digestion and absorption of nutrients, and fatty acids that promote brain growth and development. Infant formulas are usually adequate in providing nutrition to maintain infant growth and development within normal limits, but they are not equivalent to human milk.

Whether the parents choose to breastfeed or to give their infant artificial baby milk (formula), nurses provide support and ongoing education. Parent education is necessarily based on current research findings and standards of practice.

This chapter focuses on meeting nutritional needs for normal growth and development from birth to age 6 months, with emphasis on the neonatal period, when feeding practices and patterns are established. Both breastfeeding and formula feeding are addressed.

RECOMMENDED INFANT NUTRITION

The AAP recommends exclusive breastfeeding or human milk feeding for the first 6 months of life and that breastfeeding or human milk feeding continue as the sole source of milk for the first year. During the second 6 months of life, appropriate complementary foods (solids) are added to the infant diet. If infants are weaned from breast milk before 12 months of age, they should receive iron-fortified infant formula, not cow's milk (AAP Section on Breastfeeding, 2012). According to the Global Strategy for Infant and Young Child Feeding, endorsed by the World Health Organization (WHO) and United Nations Children's Fund (UNICEF), infants should be exclusively breastfed for 6 months, and breastfeeding should continue for up to 2 years and beyond (WHO/UNICEF, 2003).

BREASTFEEDING RATES

Breastfeeding rates in the United States have risen steadily over the past decade. The Centers for Disease Control and Prevention (CDC, 2012) reported that the U.S. breastfeeding initiation rate in 2009 was 76.9%, which is the highest ever reported. Despite increases in breastfeeding rates, the U.S. continues to fall short of the *Healthy People 2020* goals (USDHHS, 2010). Trends remain unchanged in breastfeeding rates among minority groups in the United States. The lowest rates are among non-Hispanic black women, although the overall percentage has increased in recent years. The minority group most likely to breastfeed is Hispanic women (Scanlon, Grummer-Strawn, Li, et al, 2010).

BENEFITS OF BREASTFEEDING

Case Study: Breastfeeding

Numerous research studies have identified the beneficial effects of human milk for infants during the first year of life. Long-term epidemiologic studies have shown that these benefits do not cease when the infant is weaned; instead, these benefits extend into childhood and beyond. Breastfeeding has many advantages for mothers, for families, and for society in general (AAP Section on Breastfeeding, 2012; Lawrence & Lawrence, 2011; Ip et al., 2009). In discussing the benefits of breastfeeding with parents, nurses and other health care professionals must have a thorough understanding of these benefits from both a physiologic and a psychosocial perspective. Table 18-1 lists the benefits of breastfeeding.

CHOOSING AN INFANT FEEDING METHOD

Breastfeeding is a natural extension of pregnancy and childbirth; it is much more than simply a means of supplying nutrition for infants. Women most often breastfeed their babies because they are aware of the benefits to the infant (Nelson, 2012). Many women seek the unique bonding experience between mother and infant that is characteristic of breastfeeding. Women tend to select the same method of infant feeding for each of their children. If the first child was breastfed, subsequent children will likely also be breastfed (Taylor, Geller, Risica, Kirtania, & Cabral, 2008).

The support of the partner and family is a major factor in the mother's decision to breastfeed. Women who perceive their partners to prefer breastfeeding are more likely to choose this method of infant feeding. Women are more likely to breastfeed successfully when partners and family members are positive about breastfeeding and have the skills to support breastfeeding (Clifford & McIntyre, 2008).

Parents who choose to formula-feed often make this decision without complete information and understanding of the benefits of breastfeeding and the potential hazards of formula feeding. Even women who are educated about the advantages of breastfeeding may still decide to formula-feed. Cultural beliefs, as well as myths and misconceptions about breastfeeding, influence women's decision making. Many women see formula feeding as more convenient or less embarrassing than breastfeeding. Some view formula feeding as a way to ensure that the father, other family members, and day-care providers can feed the baby. Some women lack confidence in their ability to produce breast milk of adequate quantity or quality. Women who have had previous unsuccessful breastfeeding experiences may choose to formula feed subsequent infants. Some women see breastfeeding as incompatible with an active social life, or they think that it will prevent them from going back to work. Modesty issues and societal barriers exist against breastfeeding in public. A major barrier for many women is the influence of family and friends.

Breastfeeding is contraindicated in a few situations. Newborns who have galactosemia should not be breastfed. Mothers with active tuberculosis or human immunodeficiency virus infection and those who are positive for human T-cell lymphotropic virus type I or type II should not breastfeed. Breastfeeding is not recommended when mothers are receiving chemotherapy or radioactive isotopes (e.g., with diagnostic procedures). Maternal use of

TABLE 18-1

Benefits of Breastfeeding

BENEFITS FOR THE INFANT	BENEFITS FOR THE MOTHER	BENEFITS TO FAMILIES AND SOCIETY
• Decreased incidence and severity of infectious diseases: bacterial meningitis, bacteremia, diarrhea, respiratory infection, necrotizing enterocolitis, otitis media, urinary tract infection, late-onset sepsis in preterm infants • Reduced postneonatal infant mortality • Decreased rates of SIDS • Decreased incidence of type I and type 2 diabetes • Decreased incidence of lymphoma, leukemia, Hodgkin disease • Reduced risk of obesity and hypercholesterolemia • Decreased incidence and severity of asthma and other allergies • Slightly enhanced cognitive development • Enhanced jaw development and decreased problems with malocclusions and malalignment of teeth • Analgesic effect for infants undergoing painful procedures such as venipuncture	• Decreased postpartum bleeding and more rapid uterine involution • Reduced risk of breast cancer, uterine cancer, and ovarian cancer • Earlier return to prepregnancy weight • Decreased risk of postmenopausal osteoporosis • Unique bonding experience • Increased maternal role attainment	• Convenient; ready to feed • No bottles or other necessary equipment • Less expensive than infant formula • Reduced annual health care costs • Less parental absence from work because of ill infant • Reduced environmental burden related to disposal of formula cans

Sources: American Academy of Pediatrics Section on Breastfeeding. (2012). Breastfeeding and the use of human milk—policy statement. *Pediatrics, 129*(3), e827-e841; Ip, S., Chung, M., Raman, G., Trikalinos, T.A., & Lau, J. (2009). A summary of the Agency for Healthcare Research and Quality's evidence report on breastfeeding in developed countries. *Breastfeeding Medicine, 4*(Suppl 1), S17-S30.
SIDS, Sudden infant death syndrome.

EVIDENCE-BASED PRACTICE

The Usefulness of Prenatal Breastfeeding Education

Pat Gingrich

ASK THE QUESTIONS

Does prenatal education about breastfeeding promote initiation of breastfeeding and continuing exclusive breastfeeding for 3 and 6 months? If so, what prenatal education strategies are most effective?

SEARCH FOR EVIDENCE

Search Strategies: Professional organization guidelines, meta-analyses, systematic reviews, randomized controlled trials, nonrandomized prospective studies, and retrospective studies since 2006.

Search Databases: Cumulative Index to Nursing and Allied Health Literature, Cochrane, Medline, and the websites for the Association of Women's Health, Obstetric and Neonatal Nurses, the Centers for Disease Control and Prevention, the National Institute for Health and Clinical Excellence, and the Academy of Breastfeeding Medicine.

CRITICALLY ANALYZE THE EVIDENCE

After reviewing scientific literature indicating that health care provider attitude and ongoing support have a significant impact on the initiation and duration of exclusive breastfeeding, the Academy of Breastfeeding Medicine (2006) published a protocol calling for health care providers to discuss the benefits of breastfeeding, beginning with the first visit in the first trimester. The guidelines encourage an ongoing conversation with the patient and her family about feeding plans, attitudes, and previous experiences. Both parents are encouraged to attend prenatal breastfeeding classes before making a decision. Educational materials should include written, non–formula-advertising materials and may also include visual aids, books, and videos.

A *Cochrane Database of Systematic Review* of nine prenatal education trials totaling 2284 women found that the benefits and strategies of prenatal education are difficult to compare as a result of greatly differing interventions and outcome measures (Gagnon & Sandall, 2007). One particular challenge of studying this topic is the difficulty of randomizing women to the interventions or control, when randomization may contradict a woman's choice. The reviewers were not able to determine benefits or best strategies for prenatal education.

However, a subsequent randomized controlled trial (RCT) of 450 healthy women in Singapore who were over 34 weeks of gestation demonstrated that breastfeeding initiation and duration were significantly improved if the women were given either a prenatal education session (video, individual instruction and written materials) or two postnatal support sessions (individual instruction in hospital and at 2 weeks, with written materials), when compared with women receiving usual care (Su et al., 2007).

Group prenatal education sessions may also be effective, as well as efficient for the health care provider. In a more recent RCT of 1047 pregnant women, participants who were randomized to receive weekly group educational and facilitated support sessions with their gestational peers from 18 weeks until term had significantly increased breastfeeding initiation, more prenatal knowledge, more readiness for labor and birth, and increased satisfaction compared with women receiving usual treatment. No differences in costs were noted, and birthweights remained similar. Interestingly, the women in the support group also had significantly fewer preterm births (Ickovics et al., 2007).

IMPLICATIONS FOR PRACTICE

On balance, the literature and expert opinion does confirm the value of prenatal education for initiation and duration of exclusive breastfeeding. Especially for the primipara or the woman lacking social support for breastfeeding, starting the dialogue early in pregnancy, or possibly before pregnancy, and using each contact to further educate the expectant family on the many benefits of breastfeeding make sense for the health care provider. Information is sufficient to recommend combinations of individual instruction and noncommercial written and multimedia material. Group education sessions may provide cost-effective use of the educator's time, along with added emotional and social support for participating families at similar gestational ages.

References

Academy of Breastfeeding Medicine Protocol Committee. (2006). ABM clinical protocol no. 14: Breastfeeding-friendly physician's office, part 1: Optimizing care for infants and children. *Breastfeeding Medicine, 1*(2), 115-119.

Gagnon, A. J. & Sandall, J. (2007). Individual or group antenatal education for childbirth or parenthood, or both. In *The Cochrane Database of Systematic Reviews,* 2007, Issue 3, CD 002869.

Ickovics, J. R., Kershaw, T. S., Westdahl, C., Magriles, U., Massey, Z., Reynolds, H., et al. (2007). Group prenatal care and perinatal outcomes: A randomized, controlled trial, *Obstetrics and Gynecology, 110*(2 Pt 1), 330-339.

Su, L. L., Chong, Y. S., Chan, Y. H., Chan, Y. S., Fok, D., Tun, K. T., et al. (2007). Antenatal education and postnatal support strategies for improving rates of exclusive breastfeeding: Randomized controlled trial. *British Medical Journal, 335*(7620), 596.

drugs of abuse ("street drugs") is incompatible with breastfeeding (AAP Section on Breastfeeding, 2012; Lawrence & Lawrence, 2011).

The key to encouraging mothers to breastfeed is education and anticipatory guidance, beginning as early as possible during pregnancy and even before pregnancy. Each encounter with an expectant mother is an opportunity to educate, dispel myths, clarify misinformation, and address personal concerns. Prenatal education and preparation for breastfeeding influence feeding decisions, breastfeeding success, and the amount of time that women breastfeed (Rosen, Krueger, Carney, & Graham, 2008). Prenatal preparation ideally includes the father of the baby, partner, or another significant support person, providing information about benefits of breastfeeding and how he or she can participate in infant care and nurturing.

Connecting expectant mothers with women from similar backgrounds who are breastfeeding or have successfully breastfed is often helpful. Nursing mothers' support groups provide information about breastfeeding along with opportunities for breastfeeding mothers to interact with one another and share concerns (Fig. 18-1). Peer counseling programs, such as those instituted by Special Supplemental Nutrition Program for Women, Infants, and Children (WIC) programs, are beneficial.

For women with limited access to health care the postpartum period may provide the first opportunity for education about breastfeeding. Even women who have indicated the desire to bottle-feed may benefit from information about the benefits of breastfeeding and the potential hazards of infant formula. Offering these women the chance to try breastfeeding with the assistance of a nurse may influence a change in infant feeding practices.

Promoting feelings of competence and confidence in the breastfeeding mother and reinforcing the unequaled contribution she is making toward the health and well-being of her infant are the responsibility of the nurse and other health care professionals. Women who are optimistic, with a sense of breastfeeding self-efficacy, and faith in breast milk as the best nutrition for the infant are likely to breastfeed longer (O'Brien, Buikstra, & Hegney, 2008). The most common reasons for breastfeeding cessation are insufficient milk supply, painful nipples, and problems getting the infant to feed. Early and ongoing assistance and support from health care professionals to prevent and address problems with breastfeeding can help promote a successful and satisfying breastfeeding experience for mothers and infants (Renfrew & Hall, 2008). Many health care agencies have **lactation consultants** on staff. These health care professionals who are usually nurses have specialized training and experience in assisting breastfeeding mothers and infants. Evidence-based guidelines for supporting breastfeeding are available for use by health care professionals (Association of Women's Health, Obstetric and Neonatal Nurses [AWHONN], 2007; International Lactation Consultant Association [ILCA], 1999).

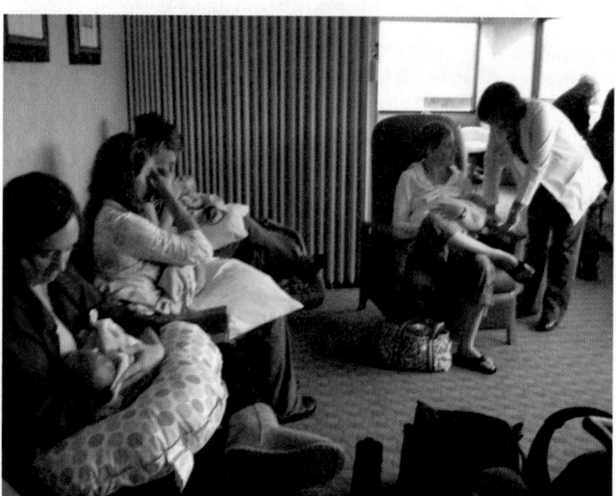

Fig. 18-1 Breastfeeding mothers support group with lactation consultant. (Courtesy Shannon Perry, Phoenix, AZ.)

Cultural Influences on Infant Feeding

Cultural beliefs and practices are significant influences on infant feeding methods. Although recognized cultural norms exist, one cannot assume that generalized observations about any cultural group hold true for all members of that group. Many regional and ethnic cultures can be found within the United States. Dealing effectively with these groups requires that nurses are knowledgeable and sensitive to the cultural factors influencing infant feeding practices.

In general, persons who have immigrated to the United States from poorer countries often choose to formula-feed their infants because they believe it is a better, more "modern" method or because they want to adapt to U.S. culture and perceive that bottle feeding is the custom. However, this notion is not always true. For example, Hispanic women born in the United States are less likely to breastfeed, whereas Hispanic women who have recently immigrated tend to choose the social norm of breastfeeding that is characteristic of their homeland (Ahluwalia, D'Angelo, Morrow, et al., 2012).

Breastfeeding beliefs and practices vary across cultures. For example, among the Muslim culture, breastfeeding for 24 months is customary. Before the first feeding, rubbing a small piece of softened date on the newborn's palate is a ritual practice. Because of the cultural emphasis on privacy and modesty, Muslim women may choose to bottle-feed formula or expressed breast milk while in the hospital (Shaikh & Ahmed, 2006).

Because of beliefs about the harmful nature or inadequacy of colostrum, some cultures apply restrictions on breastfeeding for a period of days after birth. Such is the case for many cultures in Southern Asia, the Pacific Islands, and parts of sub-Saharan Africa. Before the mother's milk is deemed to be "in," babies are fed prelacteal food such

COMMUNITY ACTIVITY

Explore the resources in your community for support of mothers who wish to breastfeed their infants. Find information related to cost, supplemental programs, and support groups. Are lactation consultants available in hospitals, pediatric offices, health departments, or private practice offices? Research the AWHONN web site and find what the position statement says in support of breastfeeding. Investigate support systems that are available for mothers who wish to bottle feed their infants. Are the support groups similar to the ones available for breastfeeding mothers?

as honey or clarified butter, in the belief that these substances will help to clear out the meconium (Laroia & Sharma, 2006; Shaikh & Ahmed, 2006). Other cultures begin breastfeeding immediately and offer the breast each time the infant cries.

A common practice among Latina women is to combine breastfeeding with formula feeding during the first week of life. This practice can potentially result in problems with milk supply and babies refusing to latch on to the breast, which can lead to early termination of breastfeeding (Bartick & Reyes, 2012).

Some cultures have specific beliefs and practices related to the mother's intake of foods that foster milk production. Korean mothers often eat seaweed soup and rice to enhance milk production. Hmong women believe that boiled chicken, rice, and hot water are the only appropriate nourishments during the first postpartum month. The balance between energy forces, hot and cold, or yin and yang is integral to the diet of the lactating mother. Hispanics, Vietnamese, Chinese, East Indians, and Arabs often use this belief in choosing foods. "Hot" foods are considered best for new mothers. This belief does not necessarily relate to the temperature or spiciness of foods. For example, chicken and broccoli are considered "hot," whereas many fresh fruits and vegetables are considered "cold." Families often bring desired foods into the health care setting.

NUTRIENT NEEDS

Fluids

During the first 2 days of life the fluid requirement for healthy infants (>1500 g) is 60 to 80 ml of water per kilogram of body weight per day. From day 3 to 7 the requirement is 100 to 150 ml/kg/day and from day 8 to day 30, 120 to 180 ml/kg/day (Dell & Davis, 2011). In general, neither breastfed nor formula-fed infants need to be given water, not even those living in very hot climates. Breast milk contains 87% water, which easily meets fluid requirements. Feeding water to infants may only decrease caloric consumption at a time when infants are growing rapidly.

Infants have room for little fluctuation in fluid balance and should be monitored closely for fluid intake and water loss. Infants lose water through excretion of urine and insensibly through respiration. Under normal circumstances, infants are born with some fluid reserve, and some of the weight loss during the first few days is related to fluid loss. In some cases, however, infants do not have this fluid reserve, possibly because of inadequate maternal hydration during labor or birth.

Energy

Infants require adequate caloric intake to provide energy for growth, digestion, physical activity, and maintenance of organ metabolic function. Energy needs vary according to age, maturity level, thermal environment, growth rate, health status, and activity level. For the first 3 months the infant needs 110 kcal/kg/day. From 3 months to 6 months the requirement is 100 kcal/kg/day. This level decreases slightly to 95 kcal/kg/day from 6 to 9 months and increases to 100 kcal/kg/day from 9 months to 1 year (AAP Committee on Nutrition, 2009).

Human milk provides 67 kcal/100 ml or 20 kcal/oz. The fat portion of the milk provides the greatest amount of energy. Infant formulas simulate the caloric content of human milk. Usually a standard formula contains 20 kcal/oz, though the composition differs among brands.

Carbohydrate

According to the Institute of Medicine (IOM) (2005), the adequate daily reference intake (DRI) for carbohydrate in the first 6 months of life is 60 g/day and 95 g/day for the second 6 months. Because newborns have only small hepatic glycogen stores, carbohydrates should provide at least 40% to 50% of the total calories in the diet. Moreover, newborns may have a limited ability to carry out gluconeogenesis (the formation of glucose from amino acids and other substrates) and ketogenesis (the formation of ketone bodies from fat), the mechanisms that provide alternative sources of energy.

As the primary carbohydrate in human milk and commercially prepared infant formula, lactose is the most abundant carbohydrate in the diet of infants up to age 6 months. Lactose provides calories in an easily available form. Its slow breakdown and absorption also increase calcium absorption. Corn syrup solids or glucose polymers are added to infant formulas to supplement the lactose in the cow's milk and thereby provide sufficient carbohydrates.

Oligosaccharides, another form of carbohydrates found in breast milk, are critical in the development of microflora in the intestinal tract of the newborn. These prebiotics promote an acidic environment in the intestines, preventing the growth of gram-negative and other pathogenic bacteria, thus increasing the infant's resistance to GI illness.

Fat

The average recommended DRI of fat for infants younger than 6 months is 31 g/day (IOM, 2005). For infants to acquire adequate calories from human milk or formula, at least 15% of the calories provided must come from fat (triglycerides).

The fat content of human milk is composed of lipids, triglycerides, and cholesterol; cholesterol is an essential element for brain growth. Human milk contains the essential fatty acids (EFAs), linoleic acid, and linolenic acid, as well as the long-chain polyunsaturated fatty acids, arachidonic acid (ARA), and docosahexaenoic acid (DHA). Fatty acids are important for growth, neurologic development, and visual function. Cow's milk contains fewer of the EFAs and no polyunsaturated fatty acids. Most formula companies are now adding DHA and ARA to their products. Studies of infants receiving supplements of DHA and ARA have shown mixed results in terms of visual acuity and cognitive function (Heird, 2007; Simmer, Patole, & Rao, 2008).

Modified cow's milk is used in most infant formulas, but the milk fat is removed, and another fat source such as corn oil, which the infant can digest and absorb, is added in its place. If whole milk or evaporated milk without added carbohydrate is fed to infants, the resulting fecal loss of fat (and therefore loss of energy) may be excessive because the milk moves through the infant's intestines too quickly for adequate absorption to take place. This circumstance can lead to poor weight gain.

Protein

High-quality protein from breast milk, infant formula, or other complementary foods is necessary for infant growth. The protein requirement per unit of body weight is greater in the newborn than at any other time of life. For infants younger than 6 months the average DRI for protein is 9.1 g/day (IOM, 2005).

Human milk contains the two proteins, whey (lactalbumin) and casein (curd), in a ratio of approximately 60 : 40, as compared with the ratio of 80 : 20 in most cow's milk–based formula. This whey/casein ratio in human milk makes it more easily digested and produces the soft stools seen in breastfed infants. The whey protein lactoferrin in human milk has iron-binding capabilities and bacteriostatic properties, particularly against gram-positive and gram-negative aerobes, anaerobes, and yeasts. The casein in human milk enhances the absorption of iron, thus preventing iron-dependent bacteria from proliferating in the gastrointestinal tract (Lawrence & Lawrence, 2011).

The amino acid components of human milk are uniquely suited to the newborn's metabolic capabilities. For example, cystine and taurine levels are high, whereas phenylalanine and methionine levels are low.

Vitamins

Human milk contains all of the vitamins required for infant nutrition, with individual variations based on maternal diet and genetic differences. Vitamins are added to cow's-milk formulas to resemble levels found in breast milk. Although cow's milk contains adequate amounts of vitamin A and vitamin B complex, vitamin C (ascorbic acid), vitamin E, and vitamin D must be added.

Vitamin D facilitates intestinal absorption of calcium and phosphorus, bone mineralization, and calcium reabsorption from bone. According to the AAP, all infants who are breastfed or partially breastfed should receive 400 international units of vitamin D daily, beginning the first few days of life. Nonbreastfeeding infants and older children who consume less than 1 quart per day of vitamin D–fortified milk should also receive 400 international units of vitamin D each day (Wagner, Grier, Section on Breastfeeding, & Committee on Nutrition, 2008).

Vitamin K, required for blood coagulation, is produced by intestinal bacteria. However, the gut is sterile at birth, and a few days are required for intestinal flora to become established and produce vitamin K. To prevent hemorrhagic problems in the newborn an injection of vitamin K is given at birth to all newborns, regardless of feeding method (AAP Section on Breastfeeding, 2012).

The breastfed infant's vitamin B_{12} intake is dependent on the mother's dietary intake and stores. Mothers who are on strict vegetarian (vegan) diets and those who consume few dairy products, eggs, or meat are at risk of vitamin B_{12} deficiency. Breastfed infants of vegan mothers should be supplemented with vitamin B_{12} from birth.

Minerals

The mineral content of commercial infant formula is designed to reflect that of breast milk. Unmodified cow's milk is much higher in mineral content than human milk, which also makes it unsuitable for infants during the first year of life. Minerals are typically highest in human milk during the first few days after birth and decrease slightly throughout lactation.

The ratio of calcium to phosphorus in human milk is 2 : 1, an optimal proportion for bone mineralization. Although cow's milk is high in calcium, the calcium-to-phosphorus ratio is low, resulting in decreased calcium absorption. Consequently, young infants fed unmodified cow's milk are at risk for hypocalcemia, seizures, and tetany. The calcium/phosphorus ratio in commercial infant formula is between that of human milk and cow's milk. The average DRI for calcium is 210 mg/day for infants younger than 6 months and 270 mg/day for infants between 7 months and 1 year (IOM, 2005).

Iron levels are low in all types of milk; however, iron from human milk is better absorbed than iron from cow's milk, iron-fortified formula, or infant cereals. Breastfed infants draw on iron reserves deposited in utero and benefit from the high lactose and vitamin C levels in human milk that facilitate iron absorption. Full-term infants have enough iron stores from the mother to last four months. After that time, exclusively breastfed infants are at risk for iron deficiency. They should receive an iron supplement until they are consuming complementary foods that contain iron (e.g., iron-fortified cereals). Formula-fed infants should receive an iron-fortified commercial infant formula until 12 months of age. Infants should not be fed low-iron formula (Baker, Greer, & AAP Committee on Nutrition, 2010).

Fluoride levels in human milk and commercial formulas are low. This mineral, which is important in the prevention of dental caries, may cause spotting of the permanent teeth (fluorosis) in excess amounts. Experts recommend that no fluoride supplements be given to infants younger than 6 months. From 6 months to 3 years, fluoride supplements are based on the concentration of fluoride in the water supply (AAP Section on Breastfeeding, 2012).

ANATOMY AND PHYSIOLOGY OF LACTATION

Anatomy of the Lactating Breast

Each female breast is composed of approximately 15 to 20 segments (lobes) embedded in fat and connective tissues and well supplied with blood vessels, lymphatic vessels, and nerves (Fig. 18-2). Within each lobe is glandular tissue consisting of alveoli, the milk-producing cells, surrounded by myoepithelial cells that contract to send the milk forward to the nipple during milk ejection. Each nipple has multiple pores that transfer milk to the suckling infant. The ratio of glandular tissue to adipose tissue in the lactating breast is approximately 2 : 1 compared with a 1 : 1 ratio in the nonlactating breast. Within each breast is a complex, intertwining network of milk ducts that transport milk from the alveoli to the nipple. The milk ducts dilate and expand at milk ejection. Previous thinking held that the milk ducts converged behind the nipple in lactiferous sinuses, which acted as reservoirs for milk. New research based on ultrasonography of lactating breasts has shown that these sinuses do not exist, and, in fact, glandular tissue can be found directly beneath the nipple (Geddes, 2007; Ramsay, Kent, Hartmann, & Hartmann, 2005) (Fig. 18-3).

The size and shape of the breast are not accurate indicators of its ability to produce milk. Although nearly every woman can lactate, a small number of women have insufficient mammary gland development to breastfeed their infants exclusively. Typically, these women experience few breast changes during puberty or early pregnancy. In some cases, women may still be able to breastfeed and offer supplemental nutrition to support optimal infant growth. Devices are available to allow mothers to offer supplements while the baby is nursing at the breast (Fig. 18-4).

Because of the effects of estrogen, progesterone, human placental lactogen, and other hormones of pregnancy, changes occur in the breasts in preparation for lactation. Breasts increase in size corresponding to growth of glandular and adipose tissue. Blood flow to the breasts nearly doubles during pregnancy. Sensitivity of the breasts increases, and veins become more prominent. The nipples become more erect, and the areola darken. Nipples and areola may enlarge. Around week 16 of gestation the

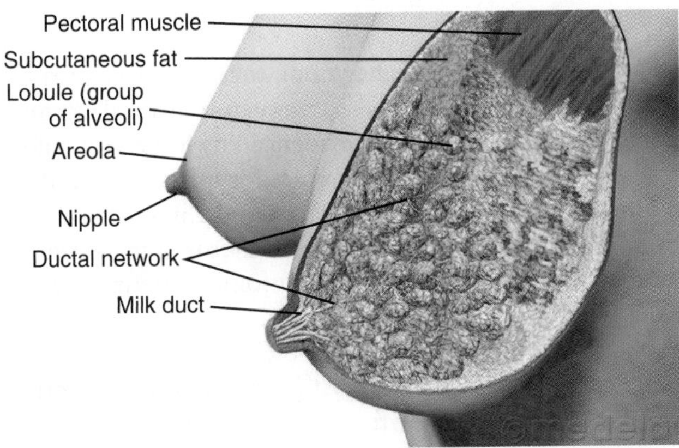

Fig. 18-2 Anatomy of the lactating breast. (Courtesy Medela, Inc.)

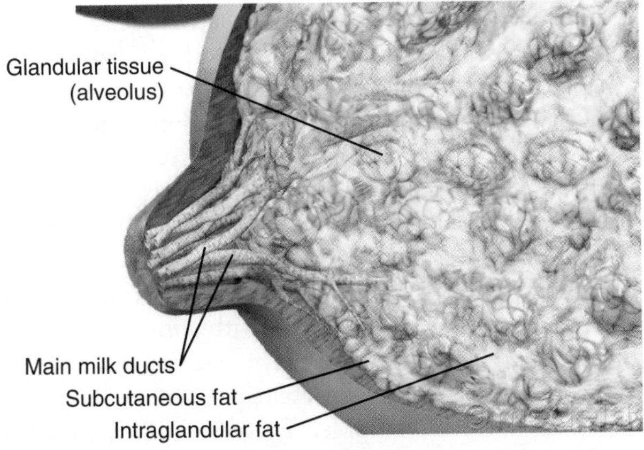

Fig. 18-3 Enhanced view of milk glands and milk ducts. (Courtesy Medela, Inc.)

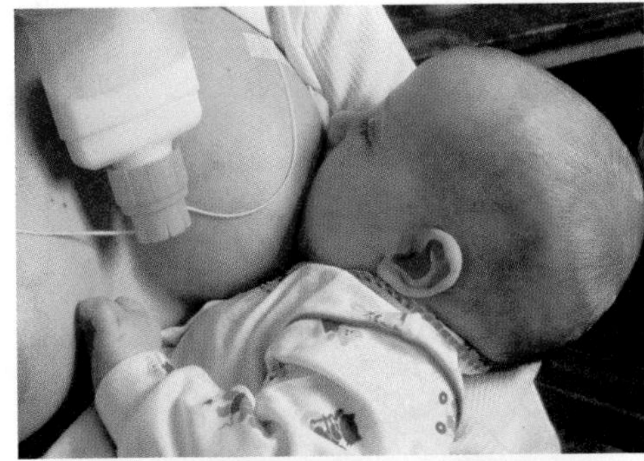

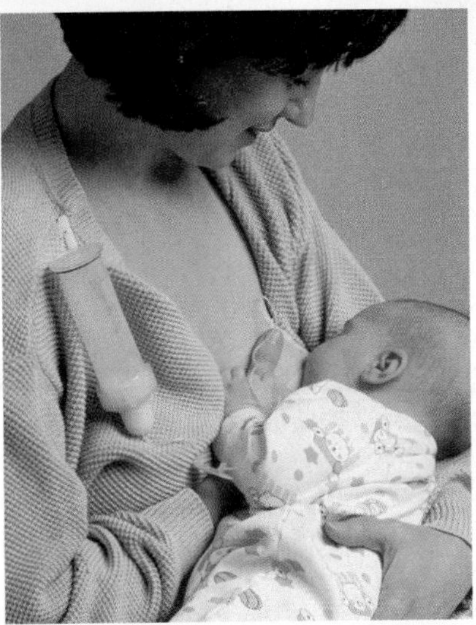

Fig. 18-4 Supplemental nursing system. (Courtesy Medela, Inc.)

alveoli begin producing colostrum (early milk). Montgomery glands on the areola increase in size and secretion. Secretions from these glands help provide protection against the mechanical stress of sucking and invasion by pathogens. The odor of the secretions may be a means of communication with the infant (Geddes, 2007).

Lactogenesis

After the mother gives birth a precipitous fall in estrogen and progesterone levels triggers the release of prolactin from the anterior pituitary gland. During pregnancy, prolactin prepares the breasts to secrete milk and, during lactation, to synthesize and secrete milk. Prolactin levels are highest during the first 10 days after birth, gradually declining over time but remaining above baseline levels for the duration of lactation. Prolactin is produced in response to infant suckling and emptying of the breasts (NOTE: Lactating breasts are never completely empty; the alveoli constantly produce milk as the infant feeds) (Fig. 18-5, *A*). Milk production is a **supply-meets-demand system;** that is, as milk is removed from the breast, more is produced. Incomplete emptying of the breasts can lead to decreased milk supply.

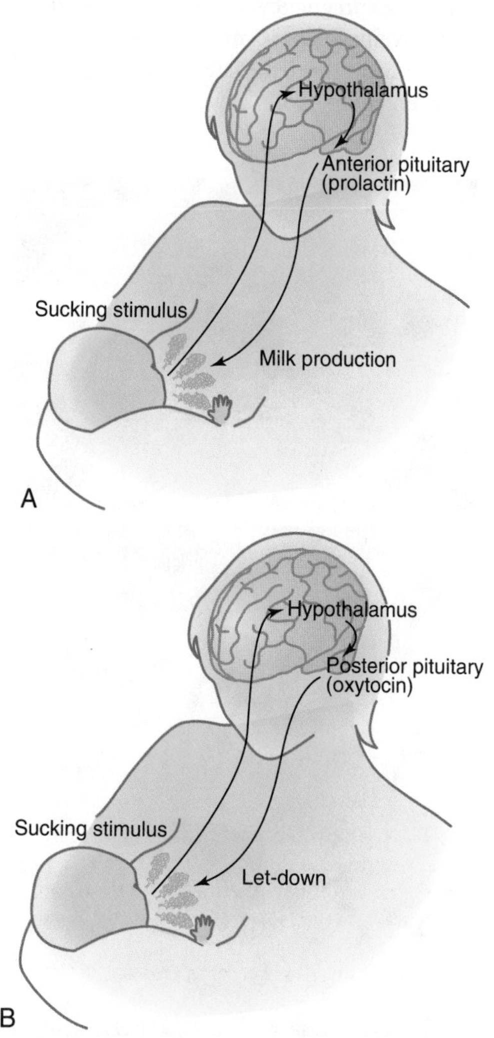

Fig. 18-5 Maternal breastfeeding reflexes. **A,** Milk production. **B,** Milk ejection (let-down).

Oxytocin is the other hormone essential to lactation. As the nipple is stimulated by the suckling infant the posterior pituitary is prompted by the hypothalamus to produce oxytocin. This hormone is responsible for the **milk ejection reflex (MER),** or let-down reflex (Fig. 18-5, *B*). The myoepithelial cells surrounding the alveoli respond to oxytocin by contracting and sending the milk forward through the ducts to the nipple. Many "let-downs" can occur with each feeding session. Thoughts, sights, sounds, or odors that the mother associates with her baby (or other babies), such as hearing the baby cry, can all trigger the MER. Many women report a tingling "pins and needles" sensation in the breasts as milk ejection occurs, although some mothers can detect milk ejection only by observing the sucking and swallowing of the infant. The milk ejection reflex also may occur during sexual activity because oxytocin is released during orgasm. The reflex can be inhibited by fear, stress, and alcohol consumption.

NURSING ALERT Be cautious in referring to the milk ejection reflex as "let-down." Some women may interpret let-down as being associated with feelings of depression.

Oxytocin is the same hormone that stimulates uterine contractions during labor. Consequently, the MER may be triggered during labor, as evidenced by leakage of colostrum. This reflex readies the breast for immediate feeding by the infant after birth. Oxytocin has the important function of contracting the mother's uterus after birth to control postpartum bleeding and promote uterine involution. Thus mothers who breastfeed are at decreased risk for postpartum hemorrhage. These uterine contractions, or "afterpains," that occur with breastfeeding are often painful during and after feeding for the first 3 to 5 days, particularly in multiparas, although they resolve within 1 week after birth.

Prolactin and oxytocin have been called the "mothering hormones" because they affect the postpartum woman's emotions, as well as her physical state. Many women report feeling thirsty or very relaxed during breastfeeding, probably as a result of these hormones.

The nipple-erection reflex is an important part of lactation. When the infant cries, suckles, or rubs against the breast, the nipple becomes erect, which assists in the propulsion of milk through the ducts to the nipple pores. Nipple sizes, shapes, and ability to become erect vary with individuals. Some women have flat or **inverted nipples** that do not become erect with stimulation; these women will likely need assistance with effective latch. However, babies are usually able to learn to breastfeed successfully with any nipple. These infants should not be offered bottles or pacifiers until breastfeeding is well established.

Uniqueness of Human Milk

Human milk is the ideal food for human infants. It is a dynamic substance with a composition that changes to meet the changing nutritional and immunologic needs of the infant as growth and development ensue. Breast milk is specific to the needs of each newborn; for example, the milk produced by mothers of preterm infants differs in composition from that of mothers who give birth at term.

Human milk contains immunologically active components that provide some protection against a broad spectrum of bacterial, viral, and protozoan infections. Secretory IgA is the major immunoglobulin in human milk; IgG, IgM, IgD, and IgE are also present. Human milk also contains T and B lymphocytes, epidermal growth factor, cytokines, interleukins, Bifidus factor, complement (C3 and C4), and lactoferrin, all of which have a specific role in preventing localized and systemic bacterial and viral infections (Lawrence & Lawrence, 2011) (Table 18-2).

Human milk composition and volumes vary according to the stage of lactation. In **lactogenesis** stage I, beginning at approximately 16 to 18 weeks of pregnancy, the breasts are preparing for milk production by producing colostrum. **Colostrum**, a clear yellowish fluid, is more concentrated than mature milk and is extremely rich in immunoglobulins. It has higher concentrations of protein and minerals but less fat than mature milk. The high protein level of colostrum facilitates binding of bilirubin, and the laxative action of colostrum promotes early passage of meconium. Colostrum gradually changes to mature milk; this transition is called "the milk coming in" or as lactogenesis stage II. By day 3 to 5 after birth, most women have had this onset of copious milk secretion. Breast milk continues to change in composition for approximately 10 days, when the mature milk is established in stage III of lactogenesis (Lawrence & Lawrence, 2011).

Composition of mature milk changes during each feeding. As the infant nurses, the fat content of breast milk increases. Initially, a bluish-white foremilk is released that is part skim milk (approximately 60% of the volume) and part whole milk (approximately 35% of the volume). It provides primarily lactose, protein, and water-soluble vitamins. The hindmilk, or cream (approximately 5%), is usually released 10 to 20 minutes into the feeding, although it may occur sooner. It contains the denser calories from fat necessary for ensuring optimal growth and contentment between feedings. Because of this changing composition of human milk during each feeding, breastfeeding the infant long enough to supply a balanced feeding is important.

TABLE 18-2

Summary of Immune Properties of Breast Milk

COMPONENT	ACTION
WHITE BLOOD CELLS	
B lymphocytes	Give rise to antibodies targeted against specific microbes
Macrophages	Kill microbes outright in baby's gut, produce lysozyme, and activate other components of the immune system
Neutrophils	May act as phagocytes, ingesting bacteria in baby's digestive system
T lymphocytes	Kill infected cells directly or send out chemical messages to mobilize other defenses Proliferate in the presence of organisms that cause serious illness in infants Manufacture compounds that can strengthen an infant's own immune response
MOLECULES	
Antibodies of secretory immunoglobulin A class	Bind to microbes in infant's digestive tract and thereby prevent them from passing through walls of the gut into body tissues
B_{12}-binding protein	Reduces amount of vitamin B_{12}, which bacteria need to grow
Bifidus factor	Promotes growth of *Lactobacillus bifidus,* a harmless bacterium, in infant's gut; growth of such nonpathogenic bacteria helps crowd out dangerous varieties
Fatty acids	Disrupts membranes surrounding certain viruses and destroys them
Fibronectin	Increases antimicrobial activity of macrophages; helps repair tissues that have been damaged by immune reactions in infant's gut
Gamma-interferon	Enhances antimicrobial activity of immune cells
Hormones and growth factors	Stimulates infant's digestive tract to mature more quickly; once the initially "leaky" membranes lining the gut mature, infants become less vulnerable to microorganisms
Lactoferrin	Binds to iron, a mineral many bacteria need to survive; by reducing the available amount of iron, lactoferrin thwarts growth of pathogenic bacteria
Lysozyme	Kills bacteria by disrupting their cell walls
Mucins	Adheres to bacteria and viruses, thus keeping such microorganisms from attaching to mucosal surfaces
Oligosaccharides	Binds to microorganisms and bars them from attaching to mucosal surfaces

From Newman, J. (1995). How breast milk protects newborns. *Scientific American, 273*(6), 76-79.

Milk production gradually increases as the baby grows so that by the time her infant is 2 weeks of age the mother produces 720 to 900 ml of milk every 24 hours. Babies have fairly predictable **growth spurts** (at approximately 10 days, 3 weeks, 6 weeks, 3 months, and 6 months), when more frequent feedings stimulate increased milk production. These growth spurts usually last 24 to 48 hours, and then the infants resume their usual feeding pattern.

CARE MANAGEMENT: THE BREASTFEEDING MOTHER AND INFANT

Critical Thinking Exercise: Breastfeeding

Skill: Infant Feeding

Effective management of the breastfeeding mother and infant requires that caregivers are knowledgeable about the benefits of breastfeeding, as well as about basic anatomic and physiologic aspects of breastfeeding. Caregivers also need to know how to assist the mother with feeding and interventions for common problems. Ongoing support of the mother enhances her self-confidence and promotes a satisfying and successful breastfeeding experience. During the time in the hospital the mother is encouraged to view each breastfeeding session as a "feeding lesson" or "practice session" that will foster her self-confidence and promote a satisfying breastfeeding experience for herself and her infant.

The mother needs to understand infant behaviors in relation to breastfeeding. When newborns feel hunger, they usually cry vigorously until their needs are met. Some infants, however, will withdraw into sleep because of discomfort associated with hunger. Babies exhibit **feeding-readiness cues** that a knowledgeable caregiver can recognize. Instead of waiting to feed until the infant is crying in a distraught manner or withdrawing into sleep, beginning a feeding when the baby exhibits some of these cues (even during light sleep) is preferable:

- Hand-to-mouth or hand-to-hand movements
- Sucking motions
- **Rooting reflex**–infant moves toward whatever touches the area around the mouth and attempts to suck
- Mouthing

Babies normally consume small amounts of milk during the first 3 days of life. As the baby adjusts to extrauterine life and the digestive tract is cleared of meconium, milk intake increases from 15 to 30 ml per feeding in the first 24 hours to 60 to 90 ml by the end of the first week.

At birth and for several months thereafter, all of the secretions of the infant's digestive tract contain enzymes especially suited to the digestion of human milk. The ability to digest foods other than milk depends on the physiologic development of the infant. The capacities for salivary, gastric, pancreatic, and intestinal digestion increase with age, indicating that the natural time for introduction of solid foods may be around 6 months of age.

Babies are born with a tongue extrusion reflex that causes them to push out of the mouth anything placed on the tongue. This reflex disappears by 6 months–another indication of physiologic readiness for solids.

Early introduction of solids may make the infant more prone to food allergies. Regular feeding of solids can lead to decreased intake of breast milk or formula and may be associated with early cessation of breastfeeding.

In the early days after birth, interventions focus on helping the mother and the newborn initiate breastfeeding and achieve some degree of success and satisfaction before discharge from the hospital or birthing center. Interventions to promote successful breastfeeding include basics such as latch and positioning, signs of adequate feeding, and self-care measures such as prevention of engorgement. An important intervention is to provide the parents with a list of resources that they may contact after discharge from the hospital.

The ideal time to begin breastfeeding is immediately after birth. Newborns without complications should be allowed to remain in direct skin-to-skin contact with the mother until the baby is able to breastfeed for the first time (AAP Section on Breastfeeding, 2012). Each mother should receive instruction, assistance, and support in positioning and latching on until she is able to do so independently (Nursing Process box).

Positioning

The four basic positions for breastfeeding are the football or clutch hold (under the arm), cradle, modified cradle or across-the-lap, and side-lying position (Fig. 18-6). Initially, it is advisable to use the position that most easily facilitates latch while allowing maximal comfort for the mother. The football or clutch hold is often recommended for early feedings because the mother can easily see the baby's mouth as she guides the infant onto the nipple.

NURSING ALERT To avoid confusion and misunderstanding, when working with Latina women, avoiding the term "football hold" to describe the under the arm or clutch position for breastfeeding is advisable. The word *football* refers to soccer in their culture.

Mothers who gave birth by cesarean often prefer the football or clutch hold. The modified cradle or across-the-lap hold also works well for early feedings, especially with smaller babies. The side-lying position allows the mother to rest while breastfeeding. Women with perineal pain and swelling often prefer this position. Cradling is the most common breastfeeding position for infants who have learned to latch on easily and feed effectively. Before discharge from the hospital a helpful measure may be to assist the mother to try all of the positions so that she will feel confident in her ability to vary positions at home.

During breastfeeding the mother should be as comfortable as possible. The nurse might suggest that the mother take time to empty her bladder and attend to other needs before starting a feeding session. The mother should place the infant at the level of the breast, supported by pillows

Nursing Care Plan: Breastfeeding and Infant Nutrition

NURSING CARE PLAN Breastfeeding and Infant Nutrition

NURSING DIAGNOSIS Ineffective breastfeeding related to knowledge deficit of the mother as evidenced by ongoing incorrect latch technique

Expected Outcomes *Mother will demonstrate the correct latch technique. Infant will latch on and suck with gliding jaw movements and audible swallowing. Mother will report "tugging" but no nipple pain with infant suckling. Mother will express increased satisfaction with breastfeeding, and neonate will exhibit satisfaction of hunger and sucking needs.*

Nursing Interventions/*Rationales*

- Assess the mother's knowledge and motivation for breastfeeding *to acknowledge the patient's desire for effective outcome and to provide a starting point for teaching.*
- Observe a breastfeeding session *to provide a baseline assessment for positive reinforcement and problem identification.*
- Describe and demonstrate ways to stimulate the sucking reflex, various positions for breastfeeding, and the use of pillows during a session *to promote maternal and neonatal comfort and effective latch.*
- Monitor the neonatal position of the mouth on the areola and position of the head and body *to give positive reinforcement for correct latch position or to correct poor latch position.*
- Teach the mother ways to stimulate neonate to maintain an awake state by diapering, unwrapping, massaging, or burping *to complete a breastfeeding session thoroughly and satisfactorily.*
- Give the mother information regarding lactation diet, expression of milk by hand or pump, and storage of expressed breast milk *to provide basic information.*
- Make sure the mother has written information on all aspects of breastfeeding *to reinforce oral instructions and demonstrations.*
- Refer to support groups, lactation consultant, or both, if needed, *to provide further information and group support.*

NURSING DIAGNOSIS Ineffective infant feeding pattern related to inability to coordinate sucking and swallowing

Expected Outcome *Neonate will coordinate sucking and swallowing to accomplish an effective feeding pattern.*

Nursing Interventions/*Rationales*

- Assess for factors that may contribute to ineffective sucking and swallowing *to provide a basis for a plan of care.*
- Teach the mother to observe feeding readiness cues *to enhance effective feeding.*
- Modify feeding methods as needed *to maintain hydration status and nutritional requirements.*
- Promote a calm, relaxed atmosphere *to provide a pleasant breastfeeding experience for the mother and neonate.*
- Refer to lactation consultant *to provide specialized support.*

NURSING DIAGNOSIS Anxiety related to ineffective infant feeding pattern

Expected Outcome *Mother will report a decrease in the anxiety level and express satisfaction with breastfeeding.*

Nursing Interventions/*Rationales*

- Monitor the maternal anxiety level during feeding sessions *to provide a basis for care planning.*
- Provide positive reinforcement for feeding pattern improvement *to decrease anxiety.*
- Monitor weight, intake, and output of the neonate *to provide information regarding effective feeding.*
- Enlist assistance of support persons *to provide positive feedback for increasing skill.*
- Provide information for lactation support *to decrease anxiety after discharge.*
- Initiate follow-up (telephone calls, follow-up with health care provider, outpatient lactation consultant) as needed *to assess progress, detect problems, and provide support.*

or folded blankets, turn the infant completely on his or her side, facing the mother so that the infant is "belly to belly," with the arms "hugging" the breast. The baby's mouth is directly in front of the nipple. The mother should support the baby's neck and shoulders with her hand and not push on the occiput. The baby's body is held in correct alignment (ears, shoulders, and hips are in a straight line) during latch-on and feeding.

Latch

Latch is defined as placement of the infant's mouth over the nipple, areola, and breast, making a seal between the mouth and breast to create adequate suction for milk removal. In preparation for latch during early feedings the mother should manually express a few drops of colostrum or milk and spread it over the nipple. This action lubricates the nipple and may entice the baby to open the mouth as the milk is tasted.

To facilitate latch the mother supports her breast in one hand with the thumb on top and four fingers underneath at the back edge of the areola. The breast is compressed slightly, as one might compress a large sandwich in preparing to take a bite, so that an adequate amount of breast tissue is taken into the mouth with latch (Weissinger, 1998). Most mothers need to support the breast during feeding for at least the first days until the infant is adept at feeding.

Spanish Guidelines: Breastfeeding: Latch On

With the baby held close to the breast with the mouth directly in front of the nipple the mother tickles the baby's lower lip with her nipple, stimulating the mouth to open. When the mouth is open wide and the tongue is down the mother quickly "hugs" the baby to the breast, bringing the baby onto the nipple. She brings the infant to the breast, not the breast to the infant (Fig. 18-7).

The amount of areola in the baby's mouth with correct latch depends on the size of the baby's mouth and the size

NURSING PROCESS *Breastfeeding Mother-Infant Pair*

ASSESSMENT

The assessment of the breastfeeding mother-newborn pair must include an assessment of infant feeding cues and the mother's physical and psychologic readiness to breastfeed.

NURSING DIAGNOSES

Nursing diagnoses for the breastfeeding woman and infant may include the following:

- *Effective breastfeeding* related to
  - Mother's knowledge of breastfeeding techniques
  - Mother's appropriate response to infant's feeding readiness cues
  - Mother's ability to facilitate efficient breastfeeding
- *Risk for ineffective breastfeeding* related to
  - Insufficient knowledge regarding newborn's reflexes and breastfeeding techniques
  - Lack of support by infant's father, family, friends
  - Lack of maternal self-confidence; presence of anxiety, fear of failure
  - Poor infant suckling reflex
  - Difficulty waking sleepy newborn
- *Risk for imbalanced nutrition: less than body requirements* related to
  - Increased caloric and nutrient needs for breastfeeding (mother)
  - Incorrect latch-on and inability to transfer milk (infant)
- *Risk for deficient fluid volume* related to
  - Ineffective suckling (infant)

EXPECTED OUTCOMES OF CARE

Infant

- Latch on and feed effectively at least eight times per day
- Gain weight appropriately
- Remain well hydrated (have one wet diaper per day until the fifth day of life and then six to eight wet diapers and at least three to four bowel movements every 24 hours)
- Sleep or seem contented between feedings

Mother

- Verbalize and demonstrate understanding of breastfeeding techniques, including positioning and latch-on, signs of adequate feeding, and self-care
- Report no nipple discomfort with breastfeeding
- Express satisfaction with the breastfeeding experience
- Consume a nutritionally balanced diet with appropriate caloric and fluid intake to support breastfeeding

Nursing interventions for the breastfeeding mother-infant pair are discussed on pp. 549-551.

EVALUATION

Evaluation is based on the expected outcomes, and the care plan is revised as needed based on the evaluation.

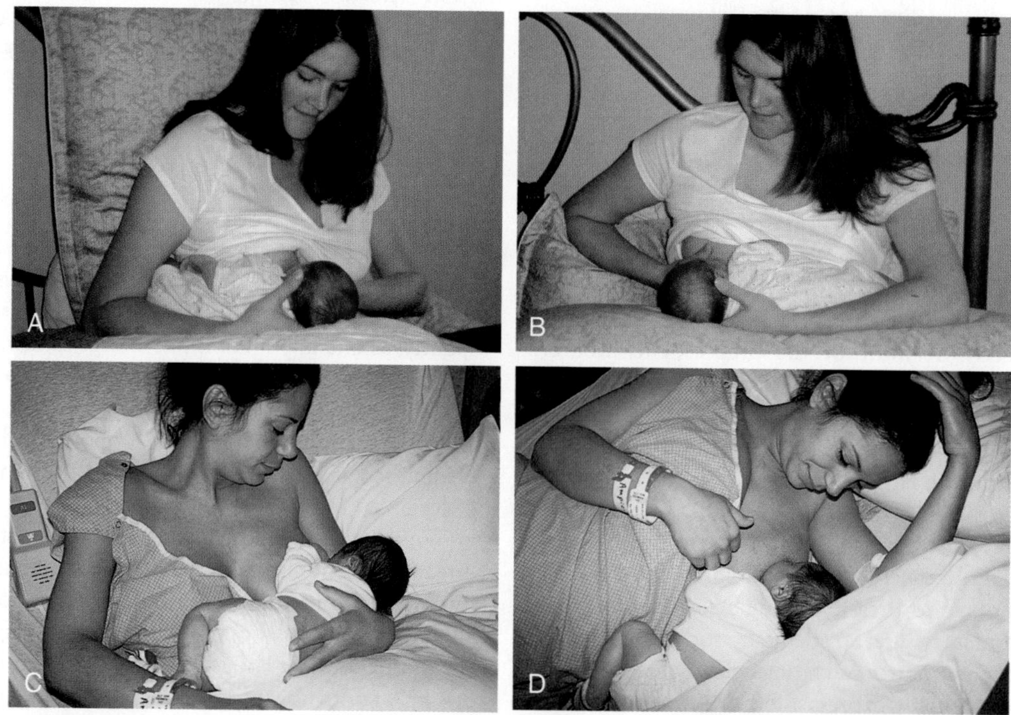

Fig. 18-6 Breastfeeding positions. **A,** Football or clutch (under the arm) hold. **B,** Across the lap (modified cradle). **C,** Cradling. **D,** Lying down. (**A** and **B** Courtesy Kathryn Alden, Chapel Hill, NC; **C** and **D** courtesy Marjorie Pyle, RNC, Lifecircle, Costa Mesa, CA.)

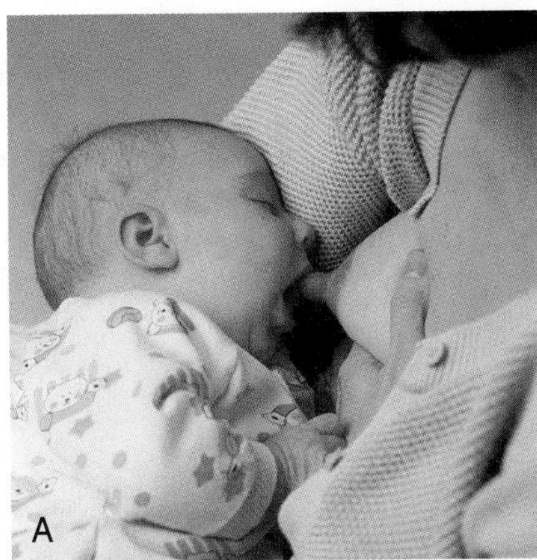

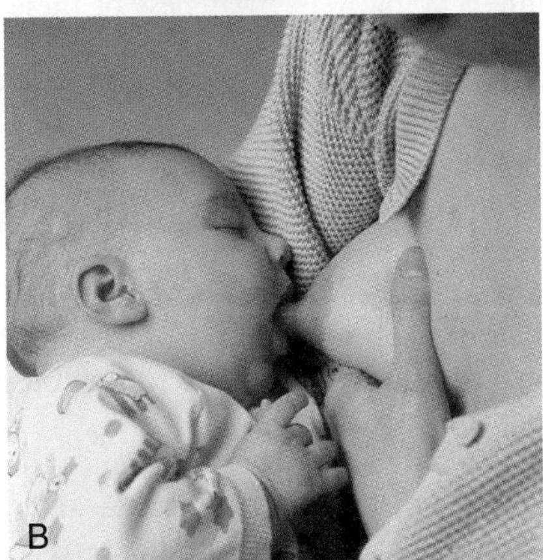

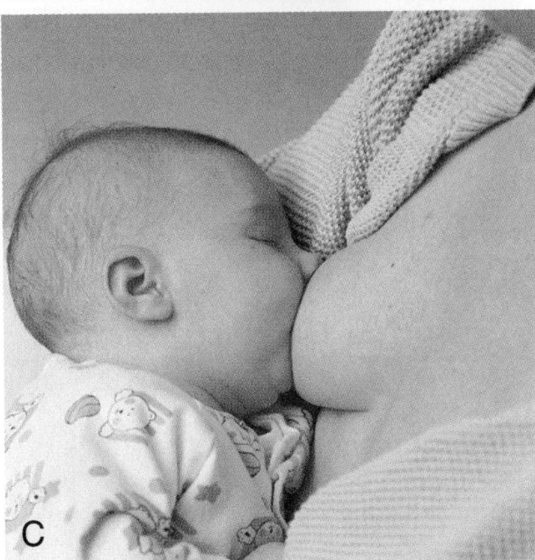

Fig. 18-7 Latch. **A,** Tickle baby's lower lip with your nipple until he or she opens wide. **B,** Once baby's mouth is opened wide, quickly pull baby onto breast. **C,** Baby should have as much areola (dark area around nipple) in his or her mouth as possible, not just the nipple. (Courtesy Medela, Inc.)

of the areola and the nipple. In general, the baby's mouth should cover the nipple and an areolar radius of approximately 2 to 3 cm all around the nipple. If breastfeeding is painful, the baby likely has not taken enough of the breast into the mouth, and the tongue is pinching the nipple.

When latched correctly, the baby's cheeks and chin are touching the breast. Depressing the breast tissue around the baby's nose to create breathing space is not necessary. If the mother is worried about the baby's breathing, she can raise the baby's hips slightly to change the angle of the baby's head at the breast. If the baby's nostrils happen to become occluded by the breast, reflexes will prompt the newborn to move the head and pull back to breathe.

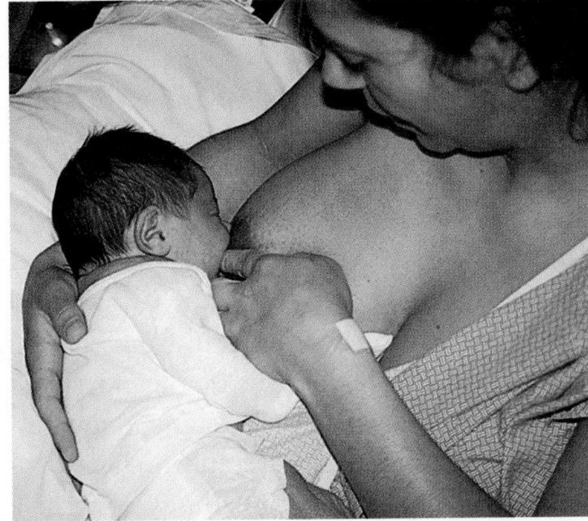

Fig. 18-8 Removing infant from the breast. (Courtesy Marjorie Pyle, RNC, Lifecircle, Costa Mesa, CA.)

If the baby is nursing appropriately, (1) the mother reports a firm tugging sensation on her nipples but feels no pinching or pain, (2) the baby sucks with cheeks rounded, not dimpled, (3) the baby's jaw glides smoothly with sucking, and (4) swallowing is usually audible. Sucking creates a vacuum in the intraoral cavity as the breast is compressed between the tongue and the palate. If the mother feels pinching or pain after the initial sucks or does not feel a strong tugging sensation on the nipple, the latch and positioning are evaluated. Any time the signs of adequate latch and sucking are not present the baby should be taken off the breast and latch attempted again. To prevent nipple trauma as the baby is taken off the breast the mother is instructed to break the suction by inserting a finger in the side of the baby's mouth between the gums and leaving it there until the nipple is completely out of the baby's mouth (Fig. 18-8).

Milk Ejection or Let-Down

As the baby begins sucking on the nipple the milk ejection, or let-down, reflex is stimulated (see Fig. 18-5, *B*). The following signs indicate that milk ejection has occurred:

- The mother may feel a tingling sensation in the nipples and in the breasts, although many women never feel their milk let down.
- The baby's suck changes from quick, shallow sucks to a slower, more drawing, sucking pattern.
- Audible swallowing is present as the baby sucks.
- In the early days the mother feels uterine cramping and may have increased lochia during and after feedings.
- The mother feels relaxed or drowsy during feedings.
- The opposite breast may leak.

Frequency of Feedings

Newborns need to breastfeed 8 to 12 times in a 24-hour period. Feeding patterns are variable because every baby is unique. Some infants will breastfeed every 2 to 3 hours throughout a 24-hour period. Others may cluster-feed, breastfeeding every hour or so for three to five feedings and then sleeping for 3 to 4 hours between clusters. During the first 24 to 48 hours after birth, most babies do not awaken this often to feed. Parents need to understand that they should awaken the baby to feed at least every 3 hours during the day and at least every 4 hours at night. (Feeding frequency is determined by counting from the beginning of one feeding to the beginning of the next.) Once the infant is feeding well and gaining weight adequately, going to **demand feeding** is appropriate, in which case the infant determines the frequency of feedings. (With demand feeding the infant should still receive at least eight feedings in 24 hours.) Caregivers should caution parents against attempting to place newborn infants on strict feeding schedules.

Infants should be fed whenever they exhibit feeding cues. Crying is a late sign of hunger, and babies may become frantic when they have to wait too long to feed. Some infants will go into a deep sleep when their hunger needs are not met. Keeping the baby close is the best way to observe and respond to infant feeding cues. Newborns should remain with mothers during the recovery period after birth and room-in during the hospital stay. At home, babies should be kept nearby so that parents can observe signs that the baby is ready to feed. One recommendation is that mother and breastfeeding infant sleep in close proximity to promote breastfeeding (AAP Section on Breastfeeding, 2012). The issue of bed-sharing (cobedding) has raised concerns because of the association between a higher incidence of sudden infant death syndrome (SIDS) and bed-sharing with an adult. Experts recommend that the breastfeeding infant be placed in a bassinet in close proximity to the mother, which would then allow for more convenient breastfeeding and at the same time prevent continuous bed-sharing (AAP Task Force on Sudden Infant Death Syndrome [SIDS], 2011).

Duration of Feedings

The duration of breastfeeding sessions is highly variable because the timing of milk transfer differs for each mother-baby pair. The average time for early feedings is 30 to 40 minutes or approximately 15 to 20 minutes per breast. As infants grow, they become more efficient at breastfeeding, and consequently the length of feedings decreases.

Some mothers prefer one-sided nursing, in which case the baby nurses only one breast at each feeding. The first breast offered should be alternated at each feeding to ensure that each breast receives equal stimulation and emptying. In reality, instructing mothers to feed for a set number of minutes is inappropriate. Mothers can determine when a baby has finished a feeding: The baby's sucking and swallowing pattern has slowed, the breast is softened, and the baby appears content and may fall asleep or release the nipple.

If a baby seems to be feeding effectively and the urine output is adequate but the weight gain is not satisfactory, the mother may be switching to the second breast too soon. The high-lactose, low-fat foremilk may cause the baby to have explosive stools, gas pains, and inconsolable crying. Feeding on the first breast until it softens ensures that the baby receives the higher fat hindmilk, which usually results in increased weight gain.

Indicators of Effective Breastfeeding

In the newborn period, when breastfeeding is becoming established, parents should be taught about the signs that breastfeeding is going well. Awareness of these signs will help them recognize when problems arise so that they may seek appropriate assistance (Box 18-1).

During the early days of breastfeeding, keeping a feeding diary may be helpful for parents, recording the time and length of feedings, as well as infant urine output and bowel movements. The data from the diary provide evidence of the effectiveness of breastfeeding and are useful to health care providers in assessing adequacy of feeding. Parents are instructed to take this feeding diary to the follow-up visit with the pediatric care provider.

While the number of wet diapers and bowel movements is highly indicative of feeding adequacy, it is also important that parents are aware of the expected changes in the characteristics of urine output and bowel movements during the early newborn period. As the volume of breast milk increases, urine becomes more dilute and should be light yellow in color; dark, concentrated urine

BOX 18-1

Signs of Effective Breastfeeding

MOTHER

- Onset of copious milk production (milk is "in") by day 3-4
- Firm tugging sensation on nipple as infant sucks, but no pain
- Uterine contractions and increased vaginal bleeding while feeding (first week or less)
- Feels relaxed and drowsy while feeding
- Increased thirst
- Breasts soften or lighten while feeding
- With milk ejection (let-down), may feel warm rush or tingling in breasts, leaking of milk from opposite breast

INFANT

- Latches on without difficulty
- Has bursts of 15-20 sucks/swallows at a time
- Audible swallowing is present
- Easily releases breast at end of feeding
- Infant appears contented after feeding
- Has at least three substantive bowel movements and six to eight wet diapers every 24 hours after day 4

can be associated with inadequate intake and possible dehydration (NOTE: Infants with jaundice may have darker urine as bilirubin is excreted). The first 1-2 days after birth, newborns pass meconium stools, which are greenish black, thick, and sticky. By day 2-3, the stools are becoming greener in color, thinner and less sticky. If the mother's milk has come in by day 3-4, the stools will start to appear greenish yellow and will be looser. By the end of the first week, breast milk stools are yellow, soft, and seedy (they resemble a mixture of mustard and cottage cheese). If an infant is still passing meconium stool by day 3-4, further assessment is needed to assess breastfeeding effectiveness and milk transfer.

For approximately the first month, breastfed infants typically have 5-10 bowel movements per day, often associated with feedings. The stooling pattern gradually changes; breastfed infants may continue to stool more than once per day or they may stool only every 2-3 days. As long as the baby continues to gain weight and appears healthy, this decrease in the number of bowel movements is normal.

Supplements, Bottles, and Pacifiers

The AAP recommends that, unless a medical indication exists, no supplements should be given to breastfeeding infants (AAP Section on Breastfeeding, 2012). With sound breastfeeding knowledge and practice, supplements are rarely needed. If a supplement is deemed necessary, giving the baby expressed breast milk is best.

Situations that may necessitate supplementary feeding include low birth weight, hypoglycemia, dehydration, weight loss, slow weight gain, or inborn errors of metabolism. Maternal indications for supplementation include delayed lactogenesis, intolerable pain during feedings, unavailability of mother because of severe illness or geographic separation, primary glandular insufficiency, or taking medications incompatible with breastfeeding (Table 18-3). Women who have had previous breast surgery such as augmentation or reduction may need to provide supplementary feedings for their infants.

Offering formula to a baby after breastfeeding just to "make sure the baby is getting enough" is normally unnecessary and should be avoided. This action can contribute to low milk supply because the baby becomes overly full and does not breastfeed often enough. Supplementation interferes with the supply-meets-demand system of milk production. The parents may interpret the baby's willingness to take a bottle to mean that the mother's milk supply is inadequate. They need to know that a baby will automatically suck from a bottle, as the easy flow of milk from the nipple triggers the suck-swallow reflex.

Newborns may become confused going from breast to bottle or bottle to breast when breastfeeding is first being established. Breastfeeding and bottle feeding require different oral motor skills. The way newborns use their tongues, cheeks, and lips, as well as the swallowing patterns, are very different. Even though some newborns can transition easily between breast and bottle, others may experience considerable difficulty. Because predicting which infants will adapt well and which ones will not is impossible, it is best to avoid bottles until breastfeeding is well established, usually after 3 to 4 weeks.

If supplementation is necessary, parents can use supplemental nursing devices, in which case the baby can be supplemented while breastfeeding (see Fig. 18-4). Infants can also be fed using a spoon, dropper, cup, or syringe. If parents choose to use bottles, a slow-flow nipple is recommended. Although some parents combine breastfeeding and bottle feeding, many babies never take a bottle and go directly from the breast to a cup as they grow.

TABLE 18-3

Selected Drugs Excreted in Milk

DRUG	AMERICAN ACADEMY OF PEDIATRICS RATING
Acetaminophen (Datril, Tylenol, Darvocet, Excedrin)	6
Alcohol (ethanol)	6
Aspirin (Bayer, Anacin, Bufferin, Excedrin, Fiorinal, Empirin)	5
Caffeine	6
Cocaine	2
Codeine	6
Heroin	2
Ibuprofen (Advil, Nuprin, Motrin)	6
Indomethacin (Indocin)	6
Ketorolac tromethamine (Toradol)	6
Marijuana	2
Medroxyprogesterone acetate (Depo-Provera)	6
Meperidine (Demerol, Mepergan)	6
Methadone	6
Morphine	6
Naproxen (Naproxyn, Anaprox, Naprosyn, Aleve)	6
Oxycodone	Not rated
Phenobarbital (Luminal, Donnatal, Tedral)	5
Phenytoin (Dilantin)	6
Propylthiouracil	6
Thyroid and thyroxine	6
Tolbutamide (Orinase)	6

American Academy of Pediatrics (AAP) Committee on Drugs rated drugs that transfer into human milk. The ratings are as follows:
1. Drugs that are contraindicated during breastfeeding
2. Drugs of abuse that are contraindicated during breastfeeding
3. Radioactive compounds that require temporary cessation of breastfeeding
4. Drugs with unknown effects on breastfeeding but may be of concern
5. Drugs that have been associated with significant effects on some breastfeeding infants and should be given to breastfeeding mothers with caution
6. Maternal medication usually compatible with breastfeeding
7. Food and environmental agents that have an effect of breastfeeding

Pacifier use with breastfeeding infants is discouraged until breastfeeding is well established. Studies have linked the early introduction of a pacifier with early termination of breastfeeding, decreased exclusive breastfeeding, and early weaning from the breast. Because a correlation has been identified between pacifier use at bedtime and a decreased risk of SIDS, experts recommend that the caregiver consider offering the infant a pacifier at nap time or regular bed time. In the breastfeeding infant the pacifier is not offered until after 1 month, at which time breastfeeding should be well established (AAP Task Force on SIDS, 2011; AWHONN, 2007).

Special Considerations

Sleepy baby

During the first few days of life, some babies need to be awakened for feedings. Parents are instructed to be alert for behavioral signs or feeding cues such as rapid eye movements under the eyelids, sucking movements, or hand-to-mouth motions. These signs, when present, indicate a good time to attempt breastfeeding. If the infant is awakened from a sound sleep, attempts at feeding are more likely to be unsuccessful. Unwrapping the baby, changing the diaper, sitting the baby upright, talking to the baby with variable pitch, gently massaging the baby's chest or back, and stroking the palms or soles may bring the baby to an alert state. Placing the sleepy baby skin-to-skin with the mother and moving to the breast when feeding readiness cues are apparent may be helpful (Box 18-2).

Fussy baby

Babies sometimes awaken from sleep crying frantically. Although they may be hungry, they cannot focus on feeding until they are calmed. Parents can swaddle the baby, hold the baby close, talk soothingly, and allow the baby to suck on a clean finger until calm enough to latch on to the breast. Placing the baby skin-to-skin with the mother can be very effective in calming the fussy infant (Box 18-3).

Infant fussiness during feeding may be the result of birth injury such as bruising of the head or fractured clavicle. Changing the feeding position may alleviate this problem.

Infants who were suctioned extensively or intubated at birth may demonstrate an aversion to oral stimulation. The baby may scream and stiffen if anything approaches the mouth. Parents may need to spend time holding and cuddling the baby before attempting to breastfeed.

An infant may become fussy and appear discontented when sucking if the nipple does not extend far enough into the mouth. The feeding may begin with well-organized sucks and swallows, but the infant soon begins to pull off the breast and cry. The mother should support her breast throughout the feeding so that the nipple stays in the same position as the feeding proceeds and the breast softens.

Fussiness may be related to GI distress (i.e., cramping, gas pains). It may occur in response to an occasional feeding of infant formula, or it may be related to something the mother has ingested, although most women are able to eat a normal diet without causing GI distress to the breastfeeding infant. No standard foods should be avoided by all mothers when breastfeeding because each mother-baby couple responds individually. However, an important point to note is that the flavor of breast milk changes according to the foods and spices ingested by the mother. If a food is suspected to cause GI problems in the infant, the mother should eliminate it from her diet for 2 weeks, reintroduce the food, and see if infant symptoms reappear. When a strong family history of milk protein intolerance exists, the baby may develop colic-like symptoms. Similarly, if the risk of allergy is high, breastfeeding mothers may be advised to avoid peanuts and other potent allergens (Becker & Scott, 2008).

Persistent crying or refusing to breastfeed can indicate illness, and parents are instructed to notify the health care provider if either circumstance occurs. Ear infections, sore throat, or oral thrush may cause the infant to be fussy and not breastfeed well.

Slow weight gain

Newborn infants typically lose 5% to 10% of body weight before they begin to demonstrate weight gain. Weight loss of 7% in a breastfeeding infant during the first 3 days of life needs to be investigated (Lawrence & Law-

BOX 18-2

Waking the Sleepy Newborn

- Lay the baby down and unwrap.
- Change the diaper.
- Hold the baby upright, turn from side to side.
- Talk to the baby.
- Gently, but firmly, massage the chest and back.
- Rub the baby's hands and feet.
- Gently rock the baby from a lying to sitting position and back again until the eyes open.
- Place the baby skin-to-skin on mother's chest.
- Adjust lighting up for stimulation or down to encourage the baby to open the eyes.

BOX 18-3

Calming the Fussy Baby

- Swaddle the baby.
- Hold closely.
- Place the baby skin-to-skin on mother's chest.
- Move or rock gently.
- Talk soothingly.
- Reduce environmental stimuli.
- Allow baby to suck on adult finger.

e Nursing Care Plan: The Newborn with Insufficient Intake of Nutrients

rence, 2011). After the early milk has transitioned to mature milk, infants should gain approximately 110 to 200 g/week or 20 to 28 g/day for the first 3 months. (Breastfed infants usually do not gain weight as quickly as formula-fed infants.) Health care providers should evaluate and monitor infants who continue to lose weight after 5 days, who do not regain birth weight by 14 days, or whose weight is below the 10th percentile by 1 month.

Parents are taught the warning signs of ineffective breastfeeding, including inadequate weight gain, minimal output, and feeding constantly (Box 18-4). If any of these warning signs are present, the parent should notify the health care provider.

At times, slow weight gain is related to inadequate breastfeeding. Feedings may be short or infrequent, or the infant may be latching incorrectly or sucking ineffectively or inefficiently. Other possibilities are illness or infection, malabsorption, or circumstances that increase the baby's energy needs, such as congenital heart disease, cystic fibrosis, or simply being small for gestational age. Slow weight gain must be differentiated from failure to thrive; this can be a serious problem that warrants medical intervention.

Maternal factors may be the cause of slow weight gain. The mother may have a problem with inadequate emptying of the breasts, pain with feeding, or inappropriate timing of feedings. Inadequate glandular breast tissue or previous breast surgery may affect milk supply. Severe intrapartum or postpartum hemorrhage, illness, or medications may decrease milk supply. Stress and fatigue also negatively affect milk production.

In most instances, the solution to slow weight gain is to improve the feeding technique. Positioning and latch are evaluated and adjustments are made. Adding a feeding or two in a 24-hour period may help. If the problem is a sleepy baby, parents are instructed in waking techniques.

BOX 18-4

Warning Signs of Ineffective Breastfeeding

- Baby has less than six wet diapers per day after the fourth day of life.
- Baby is having less than three stools per day after the fourth day of life.
- Stools are still meconium (black, tarry) by the fourth day of life.
- Mother's nipples are painful throughout feeding.
- Mother's nipples are damaged (bruised, cracked, bleeding).
- Milk supply has not increased (no breast fullness) by day 4.
- Baby seems to be feeding constantly.
- Baby is losing weight after the fourth day of life.
- Baby is gaining less than 0.5 ounce per day after the fourth day of life.
- Baby has not regained birth weight by the tenth day of life.

Using alternate breast massage during feedings may help increase the amount of milk going to the infant. With this technique the mother massages her breast from the chest wall to the nipple whenever the baby has sucking pauses. This technique also may increase the fat content of the milk, which aids in weight gain.

When babies are calorie deprived and need supplementation, they can receive expressed breast milk or formula with a nursing supplementer (see Fig. 18-4), spoon, cup, syringe, or bottle. In most cases, supplementation is necessary only for a short time until the baby gains weight and is feeding adequately.

Jaundice

Chapter 17 discusses jaundice (hyperbilirubinemia) in the newborn in detail. The type of jaundice most often seen in term newborns is physiologic jaundice. Hyperbilirubinemia is caused by bilirubin levels that rise steadily over the first 3 to 4 days, peak around day 5, and decrease thereafter. This condition has been called *early-onset jaundice* or *breastfeeding-associated jaundice*, which in the breastfed infant may be associated with insufficient feeding and infrequent stooling. Colostrum has a natural laxative effect and promotes early passage of meconium. Bilirubin is excreted from the body primarily through the intestines. Infrequent stooling allows bilirubin in the stool to be reabsorbed into the infant's system, thus promoting hyperbilirubinemia. Infants who receive water or glucose water supplements are more likely to have hyperbilirubinemia because only small amounts of bilirubin are excreted through the kidneys. Decreased caloric intake (less milk) is associated with decreased stooling and increased jaundice.

To prevent early-onset, breastfeeding-associated jaundice, newborns should be breastfed frequently during the first several days of life. Increased frequency of feedings is associated with decreased bilirubin levels.

To treat early-onset jaundice, breastfeeding is evaluated in terms of frequency and length of feedings, positioning, latch, and milk transfer. Factors such as a sleepy or lethargic infant or maternal breast engorgement may interfere with effective breastfeeding and should be corrected. If the infant's intake of milk needs to be increased, a supplemental feeding device can deliver additional breast milk or formula while the infant is nursing. Hyperbilirubinemia may reach levels that require treatment with phototherapy (see Chapter 17).

Late-onset jaundice or breast milk jaundice affects a few breastfed infants and develops in the second week of life, peaking between 6 and 14 days. Affected infants are typically thriving, gaining weight, and stooling normally; all pathologic causes of jaundice have been ruled out. In the presence of other risk factors, hyperbilirubinemia may be severe enough to require phototherapy. In most cases of breast milk jaundice, no intervention is necessary. Some health care providers may recommend temporary interruption of breastfeeding for 12 to 24 hours to allow bilirubin levels to decrease, although this approach is not preferred (Blackburn, 2013; Page-Goertz, 2008).

Any breastfeeding infant who develops jaundice should be carefully evaluated for weight loss greater than 7%, decreased milk intake, infrequent stooling (less than three to four stools/day by day 4), decreased urine output (fewer than four to six wet diapers/day), and serum bilirubin levels or transcutaneous monitoring (AAP Section on Breastfeeding, 2012).

Preterm infants

Human milk is the ideal food for preterm infants, with benefits that are unique and in addition to those received by term, healthy infants. Breast milk enhances retinal maturation in the preterm infant and improves neurocognitive outcomes; it also decreases the risk of necrotizing enterocolitis. Greater physiologic stability occurs with breastfeeding as compared with bottle feeding (Lawrence & Lawrence, 2011).

Initially, preterm milk contains higher concentrations of energy, fat, protein, sodium, chloride, potassium, iron, and magnesium than term milk. The milk is more similar to term milk by approximately 4 to 6 weeks. Human milk fortifier may be added to breast milk if growth of the preterm infant is inadequate (Lanese & Cross, 2008).

Depending on gestational age and physical condition, many preterm infants are capable of breastfeeding for at least some feedings each day. Mothers of preterm infants who are not able to breastfeed their infants should begin pumping their breasts as soon as possible after birth with a hospital-grade electric pump (Fig. 18-9). To establish optimal milk supply the mother should use a dual collection kit, pumping both breasts simultaneously 8 to 12 times daily for the first 10 to 14 days. These women are taught proper handling and storage of breast milk to minimize bacterial contamination and growth. Kangaroo care (skin-to-skin contact) is advised until the baby is able to breastfeed, and while breastfeeding is established, because it enhances milk production (Lanese & Cross, 2008).

The mothers of preterm infants often receive specific emotional benefits in breastfeeding or providing breast milk for their babies. They find rewards in knowing they can provide the healthiest nutrition for the infant and believe that breastfeeding enhances feelings of closeness to the infant.

Late preterm infants

Neonates born at $34\frac{0}{7}$ to $36\frac{6}{7}$ weeks of gestation are categorized as late preterm infants. These newborns are at risk of feeding difficulties because of their low energy stores and high energy demands. They tend to be sleepy, with minimal and short wakeful periods. Late preterm infants often tire easily while feeding, have a weak suck, and low tone; these factors can contribute to inadequate milk intake. Early and extended skin-to-skin contact promotes breastfeeding and helps to prevent hypothermia. Because these infants are more prone to positional apnea than term infants, mothers are advised to use the clutch (under the arm or football) hold for feeding, and to avoid flexing the head, which can impede breathing. Supplementation is often needed; expressed breast milk is the optimal supplement, preferably at the breast using a supplementer system (see Fig. 18-4) (Walker, 2008a).

Breastfeeding multiple infants

Breastfeeding is especially beneficial to twins, triplets, and other higher-order multiples because of the immunologic and nutritional advantages, as well as the opportunity for the mother to interact with each baby frequently. Most mothers are capable of producing an adequate milk supply for multiple infants. Parenting multiples may be overwhelming, and mothers, as well as fathers, need extra support and assistance learning how to manage feedings (Fig. 18-10).

Expressing and storing breast milk

Breast milk expression is a common practice, typically performed to obtain breast milk for someone else to feed

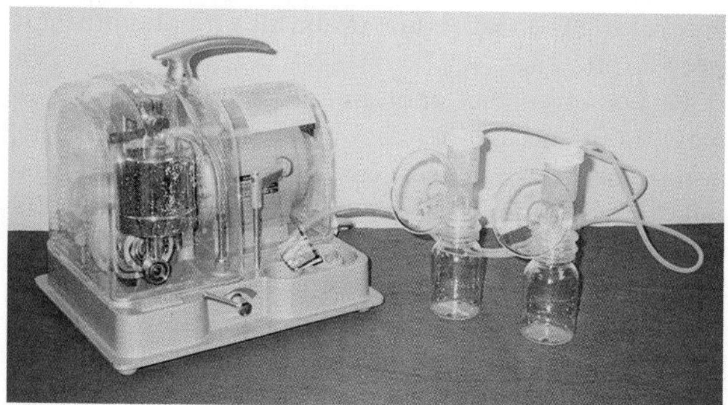

Fig. 18-9 Hospital-grade electric breast pump.

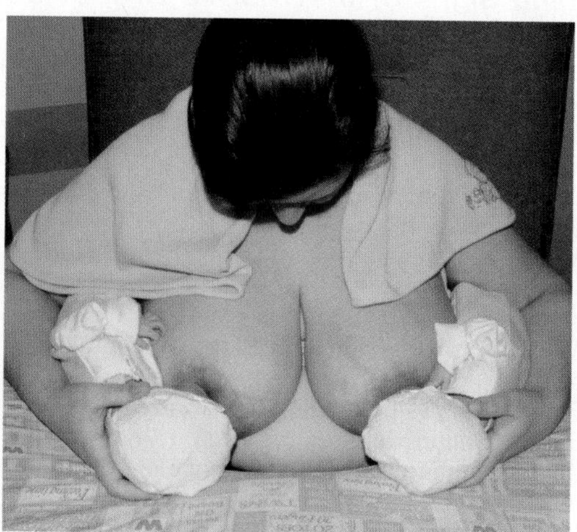

Fig. 18-10 Breastfeeding twins. (Courtesy Cheryl Briggs, RN, Annapolis, MD.)

to the baby. It is most often associated with maternal employment (Labiner-Wolfe, Fein, Shealy, & Wang, 2008). In some situations, expression of breast milk is necessary or desirable, such as when engorgement occurs, when the mother's nipples are sore or damaged, when the mother and baby are separated as in the case of a preterm infant who remains in the hospital after the mother is discharged, or when the mother leaves the infant with a caregiver and will not be present for feeding. Some women express milk to have an emergency supply (Labiner-Wolfe et al.). Some women choose to pump exclusively, providing breast milk for their infants, but never allowing the baby to suckle at the breast (Shealy, Scanlon, Labiner-Wolfe, Fein, & Grummer-Strawn, 2008).

Because pumping and hand expression are rarely as efficient as a baby in removing milk from the breast, the milk supply is never judged based solely on the volume expressed.

Hand expression. All mothers should be instructed in hand expression. After thoroughly washing her hands, the mother places one hand on her breast at the edge of the areola. With her thumb above and fingers below, she presses in toward her chest wall and gently compresses the breast while rolling her thumb and fingers forward toward the nipple. She repeats these motions rhythmically until the milk begins to flow. The mother simply maintains steady, light pressure while the milk is flowing easily. The thumb and fingers should not pinch the breast or slip down to the nipple, and the mother should rotate her hand to reach all sections of the breast.

Mechanical expression (pumping). For most women, recommendations are to initiate pumping only after the milk supply is well established and the infant is latching on and breastfeeding well. However, when breastfeeding is delayed after birth, such as when babies are ill or preterm, mothers should begin pumping with an electric breast pump as soon as possible and continue to pump regularly until the infant is able to breastfeed effectively.

Numerous approaches to pumping can be used. Some women pump on awakening in the morning or when the baby has fed but did not completely empty the breast. Others choose to pump after feedings or may pump one breast while the baby is feeding from the other. Double pumping (pumping both breasts at the same time) saves time and may stimulate the milk supply more effectively than single pumping (Fig. 18-11).

The amount of milk obtained when pumping depends on the type of pump being used, the time of day, the time since the baby breastfed, the mother's milk supply, how practiced she is at pumping, and her comfort level (pumping is uncomfortable for some women). Breast milk may vary in color and consistency, depending on the time of day, the age of the baby, and foods the mother has eaten.

Types of pumps. Many types of breast pumps are available, varying in price and effectiveness. Before purchasing or renting a breast pump the mother will benefit from counseling by a nurse or lactation consultant to determine which pump best suits her needs. The flange (funnel-shaped device that fits over the nipple or areola) should fit the nipple to prevent nipple pain, trauma, and possible reduction in milk supply. Mothers are advised to use the lowest suction setting on electric pumps, increasing gradually if needed. Breast massage before and during pumping can increase the amount of milk obtained (Mannel, 2008).

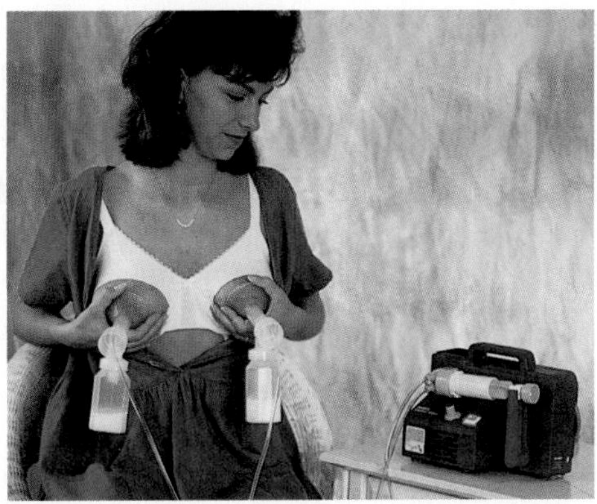

Fig. 18-11 Bilateral breast pumping. (Courtesy Medela, Inc.)

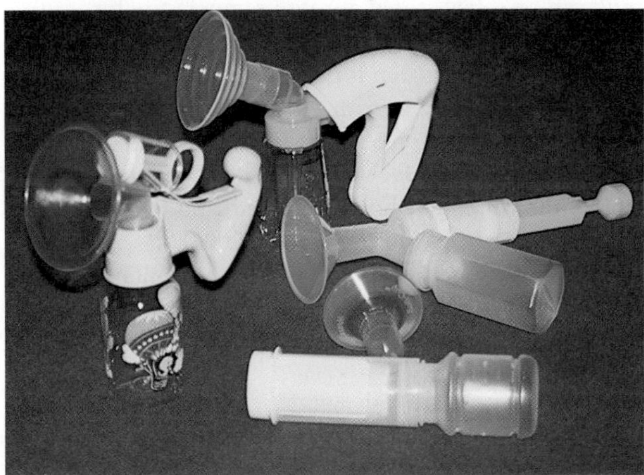

Fig. 18-12 Manual breast pumps. (Courtesy Marjorie Pyle, RNC, Lifecircle, Costa Mesa, CA.)

Manual or hand pumps are least expensive and may be the most appropriate where portability and quietness of operation are important. These pumps are most often used by mothers who are pumping for an occasional bottle (Fig. 18-12).

Full-service electric pumps, or hospital-grade pumps (see Fig. 18-9), most closely duplicate the sucking action and pressure of the breastfeeding infant. When breastfeeding is delayed after birth (e.g., preterm or ill newborn), or when mother and baby are separated for lengthy periods, these pumps are most appropriate. Because hospital-grade breast pumps are very heavy and expensive, portable versions of these pumps are available to rent for home use.

Electric, self-cycling double pumps are efficient and easy to use. These pumps are designed for working mothers. Some of these pumps come with carry bags containing coolers to store pumped milk.

Smaller electric or battery-operated pumps also are available. These pumps are typically used when pumping is performed occasionally, but some models are satisfactory for working mothers or others who pump on a regular basis.

Storage of breast milk. The preferred containers for long-term storage of breast milk are hard sided, such as hard plastic or glass, with an airtight seal. For short-term storage (<72 hours), plastic bags designed for human milk storage can be safely used.

For full-term, healthy infants, freshly expressed breast milk can be safely stored at room temperature for up to 8 hours, and it can be refrigerated safely for up to 5 to 8 days. Milk can be frozen for up to 6 months in the freezer section of a refrigerator with a separate door and for up to 12 months in a deep freezer. Storage guidelines for hospitalized infants are somewhat stricter. When breast milk is stored, the container should be dated, and the oldest milk should be used first (Jones & Tully, 2006).

Frozen milk is thawed by placing the container in the refrigerator for gradual thawing or in warm water for faster thawing. It cannot be refrozen and should be used within 24 hours. After thawing the container needs to be shaken so as to mix the layers that have separated (Academy of Breastfeeding Medicine [ABM], 2010; Jones & Tully, 2006) (see Patient Instructions for Self-Management Box).

NURSING ALERT Breast milk is never thawed or heated in a microwave oven. Microwaving does not heat evenly and can cause encapsulated boiling bubbles to form in the center of the liquid, which may not be detected when drops of milk are checked for temperature. Babies have sustained severe burns to the mouth, throat, and upper GI tract as a result of microwaved milk. In addition, microwaving (72°-98° C) significantly destroys the antiinfective factors and vitamin C content. The safety of low-temperature microwaving is questionable (Lawrence & Lawrence, 2011).

Being away from the infant (maternal employment)

Although returning to work is a common reason for early weaning, many women are able to combine breastfeeding successfully with employment, attending school, or other commitments. If feedings are missed, the milk supply can be affected. Some women's bodies adjust the milk supply to the times she is with the infant for feedings, whereas other women find they must pump otherwise the milk supply diminishes rapidly.

PATIENT INSTRUCTIONS FOR SELF-MANAGEMENT

Breast Milk Storage Guidelines for Home Use

- Before expressing or pumping breast milk, wash your hands.
- Containers for storing milk should be washed in hot, soapy water and rinsed thoroughly; they can also be washed in a dishwasher. If the water supply may not be clean, boil the containers after washing. Plastic bags designed specifically for breast milk storage can be used for short term storage (<72 hr).
- Write the date of expression on the container before storing the milk. A waterproof label is best.
- Store milk in serving sizes of 2 to 4 ounces to prevent waste.
- Storing breast milk in the refrigerator or freezer with other food items is acceptable.
- When storing milk in a refrigerator or freezer, place the containers in the middle or back of the freezer, not on the door.
- When filling a storage container that will be frozen, fill only ¾ full, allowing space at the top of the container for expansion.
- To thaw frozen breast milk, place the container in the refrigerator for gradual thawing, or place the container under warm, running water for quicker thawing. Never boil or microwave.
- Milk thawed in the refrigerator can be stored for 24 hours.
- Thawed breast milk should never be refrozen.
- Shake the milk container before feeding baby, and test the temperature of the milk on the inner aspect of your wrist.
- Any unused milk left in the bottle after feeding is discarded.

STORAGE GUIDELINES FOR HUMAN MILK

Method	Healthy Infant	Hospitalized Infant
Room temperature (77° F or 25° C)	<8 hours	<4 hours
Refrigerator (39° F or 4° C)	5-8 days	<8 days
Freezer compartment of a one door refrigerator	2 weeks	Not recommended
Freezer compartment of a two door refrigerator (23° F or −5° C) (not in door)	<6 months	<3 months
Deep freezer(−4° F or −20° C)	<12 months	<6 months

From: Jones, F. & Tully, M. R. (2006). *Best practice for expressing, storing and handling human milk in hospitals, homes, and child care settings.* Raleigh, NC: Human Milk Banking Association of America.

Women who are returning to work often face challenges in continuing to breastfeed. There may be issues in the workplace such as lack of flexibility in work schedules, inadequate breaks to allow time for pumping, lack of privacy, lack of space for pumping, and lack of support from supervisors or co-workers. Increasing numbers of women are working from home and may resume their jobs earlier than the traditional six week to three month maternity leave. Issues that may challenge continued breastfeeding while working include fatigue, child care concerns, competing demands, and household responsibilities.

Employed mothers can continue breastfeeding with appropriate guidance and support. Mothers are encouraged to set realistic goals for employment and breastfeeding, with accurate information regarding the costs, risks, and benefits of available feeding options.

Because women are a significant proportion of the workforce, many companies are making provisions for breastfeeding women returning to work after childbirth. Lactation rooms that provide space and privacy for pumping are available at many work sites and on college campuses. In some instances, breastfeeding women bring their babies to work. Since 1999, by law, women may breastfeed in federal buildings and on federal property. Some states have enacted legislation to ensure that mothers can breastfeed their babies in public places. These efforts may help mothers breastfeed longer and meet the recommendation of the AAP that breastfeeding continue for at least 1 year.

Weaning

Weaning is initiated when babies are introduced to foods other than breast milk and concludes with the last breastfeeding. Gradual weaning, over a period of weeks or months, is easier for mothers and infants than an abrupt weaning. Abrupt weaning is likely to be distressing for both mother and baby, as well as physically uncomfortable for the mother.

Weaning is initiated by either the infant or the mother. With infant-led weaning the infant moves at his or her own pace in omitting feedings, which usually facilitates a gradual decrease in the mother's milk supply. Mother-led weaning means that the mother decides which feedings to drop. This approach is most easily undertaken by omitting the feeding of least interest to the baby or the one through which the infant is most likely to sleep. Every few days thereafter the mother drops another feeding, and so on, until the infant is gradually weaned from the breast.

Infants can be weaned directly from the breast to a cup. Bottles are usually offered to infants younger than 6 months. If the infant is weaned before age 1 year, the infant should receive formula instead of cow's milk.

If abrupt weaning is necessary, breast engorgement often occurs. To relieve the discomfort the mother can take mild analgesics, wear a supportive bra, apply ice packs or cabbage leaves to the breasts, and pump small amounts if needed. Experts recommend avoiding pumping because the breasts should remain full enough to promote a decrease in the milk supply.

Weaning is often a very emotional time for mothers. Many women feel that weaning is the end to a special, satisfying relationship with the infant and benefit from time to adapt to the changes. Sudden weaning may evoke feelings of guilt and disappointment. Some women go through a grieving period after weaning. Nurses and others can assist the mother by discussing other ways to continue this nurturing relationship with the infant, such as skin-to-skin contact while bottle feeding or holding and cuddling the baby. Support from the father of the baby and other family members is essential at this time.

Milk banking

For infants who cannot be breastfed but who also cannot survive except on human milk, banked donor milk is critically important. Because of the antiinfective and growth-promoting properties of human milk, as well as its superior nutrition, donor milk is used in many neonatal intensive care units for preterm or sick infants when the mother's own milk is not available. Donor milk also is used therapeutically for a variety of medical conditions, such as in transplant recipients who are immunocompromised.

The Human Milk Banking Association of North America (HMBANA) (website: www.hmbana.org) has established annually reviewed guidelines for the operation of donor human milk banks. Donor milk banks collect, screen, process, and distribute the milk donated by breastfeeding mothers who are feeding their own infants and pumping a few ounces extra each day for the milk bank. All donors are screened both by interview and serologically for communicable diseases. Donor milk is stored frozen until it is heat processed to kill potential pathogens; it is then refrozen for storage until it is dispensed for use. The heat processing adds a level of protection for the recipient that is not possible with any other donor tissue or organ. Banked milk is dispensed only by prescription. A per-ounce fee is charged by the bank to pay for the processing costs, but the HMBANA guidelines prohibit payment to donors.

Care of the mother

Diet. In general, the breastfeeding mother should eat a healthy, well-balanced diet that includes an extra 200 to 500 calories per day over nonpregnant requirements. According to the IOM (2005) the estimated energy requirement (EER) for a lactating woman during the first 6 months is 2700 kcal/day; during the next 6 months the EER is 2768 kcal/day. Even with the increased caloric intake, women who are breastfeeding tend to lose weight more quickly than those who are formula feeding (Becker & Scott, 2008).

No specific foods have been identified that the breastfeeding mother must consume or avoid. In most cases the woman can consume a normal diet, according to her personal preferences and cultural practices. The ideal diet for the lactating mother is well balanced, consisting of nutrient-dense foods. The intake of calcium, minerals, and fat-soluble vitamins should be adequate. Women may be told to continue taking their prenatal vitamins as long as they are breastfeeding.

Mothers are encouraged to drink to quench thirst. Consumption of water by the mother does not increase milk supply, and overhydration can actually decrease milk production.

Weight loss. Medications or diets that promote weight loss are not recommended for breastfeeding mothers. Many women will experience a gradual weight loss while lactating as fat stores deposited during pregnancy are used. This factor can be an added incentive for breastfeeding. Rapid loss of large amounts of weight may be detrimental, given that fat-soluble contaminants to which the mother has been exposed are stored in body fat reserves, and these may be released into the breast milk. Another potential consequence of weight loss is reduced milk production. For most women, weight loss of 1 to 2 kilograms per month is safe; however, if weight loss exceeds this amount, careful evaluation of infant weight and feeding pattern is recommended (Lawrence & Lawrence, 2011).

Rest. The breastfeeding mother should rest as much as possible, especially in the first 1 or 2 weeks after birth. Fatigue, stress, and worry can negatively affect milk production and milk ejection (let-down). The nurse can encourage the mother to sleep when the baby sleeps. Breastfeeding in a side-lying position promotes rest for the mother. Assistance with household chores and caring for other children can be done by the father, grandparents or other relatives, and friends.

Breast care. The breastfeeding mother's normal routine bathing is all that is necessary to keep her breasts clean. Soap can have a drying effect on nipples; therefore the mother should avoid washing the nipples with soap.

Breast creams should not be used routinely because they may block the natural oil secreted by the Montgomery glands on the areola. Modified lanolin with reduced allergens is safe to use on dry or sore nipples. Lanolin can be beneficial in moist wound healing of sore nipples. Because lanolin is made from wool, women with wool allergies should be cautioned against its use. Lanolin is not recommended if nipple soreness is possibly related to monilial infection.

The mother with flat or inverted nipples will likely benefit from wearing breast shells in her bra. These hard plastic devices exert mild pressure around the base of the nipple to encourage nipple eversion. Women with flat or inverted nipples can begin wearing breast shells during the last month of pregnancy. Breast shells are also useful for sore nipples to keep the mother's bra or clothing from touching the nipples (Fig. 18-13).

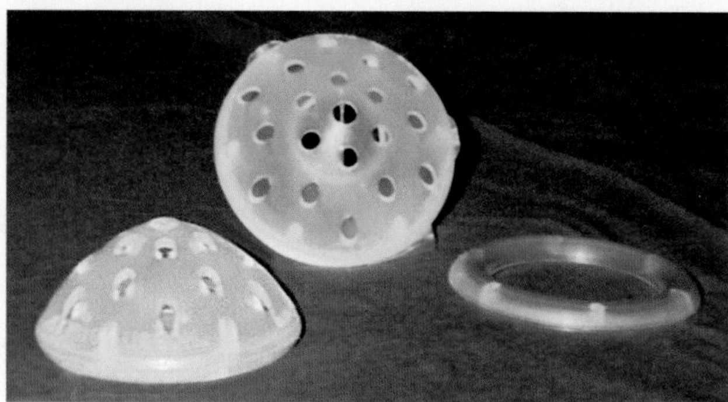

Fig. 18-13 Breast shells.

If a mother needs breast support, she will likely be uncomfortable unless she wears a bra because the ligament that supports the breast (Cooper's ligament) will otherwise stretch and be painful. Bras should fit well and provide nonbinding support. Underwire bras or improperly fitting bras can cause clogged milk ducts.

If leakage of milk between feedings is a problem, mothers can wear breast pads (disposable or washable) inside the bra. Plastic-lined breast pads are not recommended because they trap moisture and may contribute to sore nipples.

Sexual sensations. Some women experience rhythmic uterine contractions during breastfeeding. Such sensations are not unusual because uterine contractions and milk ejection are both triggered by oxytocin; however, they may be disturbing to some mothers who perceive them to resemble orgasm.

Breastfeeding and contraception. Although breastfeeding confers a period of infertility, it is not considered an effective method of contraception. Breastfeeding delays the return of ovulation and menstruation; however, ovulation may occur before the first menstrual period after birth. The contraceptive methods least likely to impact lactation are the lactational amenorrhea method, barrier methods (diaphragm/cap, spermicides, condoms), and intrauterine devices. Hormonal contraceptives, including pills, injectables, and implants, can cause a decrease in the milk supply. These contraceptives should be avoided during the first 6 postpartum weeks and in women with existing low milk supply, history of lactation failure, history of breast surgery, multiple birth, preterm birth, and in instances when the health of the mother or infant are compromised (ABM Protocol Committee, 2006). If hormonal contraceptives are used, progestin-only birth control pills or injections (Depo-Provera) are less likely to interfere with milk supply than other hormonal contraceptives. The etonogestrel implant Implanon is reported to be safe for use during lactation (Hohmann & Creinin, 2007).

Breastfeeding during pregnancy. Breastfeeding women can conceive and continue breastfeeding throughout the pregnancy if no medical contraindications exist (e.g., risk of preterm labor). For pregnant women who are breastfeeding, adequate nutrition is especially important to promote normal fetal growth.

Nipple tenderness associated with early pregnancy may cause discomfort when nursing the older child. The taste and composition of breast milk are altered during pregnancy, which may prompt some children to self-wean. Milk production may decrease about the fourth or fifth month of pregnancy (Lauwers & Swisher, 2011).

When the baby is born, colostrum is produced. The practice of breastfeeding a newborn and an older child is called *tandem nursing.* The nurse should remind the mother always to feed the infant first to ensure that the newborn is receiving adequate nutrition. The supply-meets-demand principle works in this situation, just as with breastfeeding multiples.

Medications and breastfeeding. Although much concern exists about the compatibility of drugs and breastfeeding, few drugs are absolutely contraindicated during lactation (see Table 18-3). Considerations in evaluating the safety of a specific medication during breastfeeding include the pharmacokinetics of the drug in the maternal system, as well as the absorption, metabolism, distribution, storage, and excretion in the infant. The gestational and chronologic age of the infant, body weight, and breastfeeding pattern are also considered. Breastfeeding mothers should be cautioned about taking any medications except those that are deemed essential. They are advised to check with their physician before taking any medication. If a breastfeeding mother is taking a medication that has a questionable effect on the infant, she is advised to take the medication just after nursing the baby or just before the infant is expected to sleep for a long time. References are available with specific information about medications and breastfeeding (Hale, 2012).

Alcoholic beverages are not recommended for breastfeeding mothers. However, if a mother chooses to consume alcohol, she can minimize its effects by having only one drink and by waiting 2 hours after drinking to breastfeed. The mother who is pumping for a sick or preterm infant should avoid alcohol entirely until her infant is healthy (Lawrence & Lawrence, 2011).

Smoking may impair milk production; it also exposes the infant to the risks of secondhand smoke. Nicotine is transferred to the infant in breast milk, whether the mother smokes or uses a nicotine patch, although the effect on the infant is uncertain. Lactating mothers who continue to smoke should be advised not to smoke within 2 hours before breastfeeding and never to smoke in the same room with the infant.

Caffeine intake may be associated with reduced iron concentration in milk and subsequent anemia in the infant. Maternal intake of caffeine may cause infant irritability and poor sleeping patterns. For most women, two servings of caffeine a day does not cause untoward effects; however, some infants are sensitive to even small amounts of caffeine. Mothers of such infants should limit caffeine intake. Caffeine is found in coffee, tea, chocolate, and many soft drinks.

Herbs and herbal teas are becoming more widely used during lactation. Although some herbs are considered safe, others contain pharmacologically active compounds that may have unfavorable effects. A thorough maternal history should include the use of any herbal remedies. Each remedy should then be evaluated for its compatibility with breastfeeding. The regional poison control center may provide information on the active properties of herbs.

Environmental contaminants. Human milk is often used to measure community exposure to environmental contaminants because there is a close correlation between milk levels and the levels in fat stores. Except under unusual circumstances, breastfeeding is not contraindicated because of exposure to environmental contaminants such as dichlorodiphenyltrichloroethane (DDT; an insecticide) and tetrachloroethylene (used in dry cleaning plants) (Lawrence & Lawrence, 2011).

Common concerns of the breastfeeding mother

The breastfeeding mother may experience some common problems. In the majority of cases, these complications are preventable if the mother receives appropriate education about breastfeeding. Early recognition and prompt resolution of these problems is important to prevent interruption of breastfeeding and to promote the mother's comfort and sense of well-being. Emotional support provided by the nurse or lactation consultant is essential to help allay the mother's frustration and anxiety and to prevent early cessation of breastfeeding.

Engorgement. Engorgement is a common response of the breasts to the sudden change in hormones and the onset of significantly increased milk volume. It usually occurs 3 to 5 days after birth when the milk "comes in" and lasts approximately 24 hours. Blood supply to the breasts increases and causes swelling of tissues surrounding the milk ducts. The milk ducts may be pinched shut so that milk cannot flow from the breasts. The breasts are firm, tender, and hot and may appear shiny and taut. The areolae are firm, and the nipples may flatten, creating difficulty for the infant in latching on to the breast. Because back pressure on full milk glands inhibits milk production, if milk is not removed from the breasts, the milk supply may diminish.

When engorgement occurs, it is a temporary condition that is usually resolved within 24 hours. The mother is instructed to feed every 2 hours, softening at least one breast, and pumping the other breast as needed to soften it. Pumping during engorgement will not cause a problematic increase in milk supply.

Because of the swelling of breast tissue surrounding the milk ducts, ice packs are recommended in a 15 to 20 minutes on, 45 minutes off rotation between feedings. The ice packs should cover both breasts. Large bags of frozen

Critical Thinking/Clinical Decision Making

Breastfeeding: Engorgement and Nipple Soreness

Mary was discharged from the birthing center at 48 hours postpartum with her newborn son, Matthew. He is now 4 days of age, and she has brought him to the clinic for a follow-up visit. Mary states that her milk came in yesterday, and her breasts have been hard and painful ever since. Latching the baby on has been difficult. She reports that breastfeeding is very painful and that her nipples are cracked and so sore that she "can hardly stand to feed the baby." Matthew has had only one wet diaper and no bowel movements in the last 24 hours. He is crying most of the time and never seems to settle down to sleep for very long. Mary states, "I am ready to give up on this breastfeeding thing and just switch to formula."

1. Evidence—Does the nurse have sufficient evidence at this time to draw conclusions about the feeding difficulties experienced by this mother and infant?
2. Assumptions—What assumptions can be made about the following issues?
   a. Mary's milk supply
   b. Mary's sore nipples
   c. Matthew's urinary output and bowel elimination pattern
   d. Mary's commitment to breastfeeding
3. What implications and priorities for nursing care can be identified at this time?
4. Does the evidence objectively support your conclusion?
5. Do alternative perspectives to your conclusion exist?

peas or niblet corn make easy packs and can be refrozen between uses.

Fresh, raw cabbage leaves placed over the breasts between feedings may help reduce the swelling. The cabbage leaves are washed, chilled in the refrigerator or freezer, and then placed over the breasts for 15 to 20 minutes (Fig. 18-14). This treatment can be repeated for two or three sessions. Frequent application of cabbage leaves can decrease milk supply. Cabbage leaves are often very effective for formula-feeding mothers who want their milk to "dry up"; they are advised to wear the cabbage leaves constantly while engorged, replacing the leaves with fresh ones as they become wilted. Cabbage leaves should not be used if the mother is allergic to cabbage or sulfa drugs or develops a skin rash.

Antiinflammatory medications, such as ibuprofen, may help reduce the pain and swelling associated with engorgement. Ibuprofen also helps reduce fever and aching in the breasts that are often associated with engorgement.

Because heat increases blood flow, application of heat to an already congested breast is usually counterproductive. Occasionally, however, standing in a warm shower will start the milk leaking, or the mother may be able to manually express enough milk to soften the areola sufficiently to allow the baby to latch on and feed.

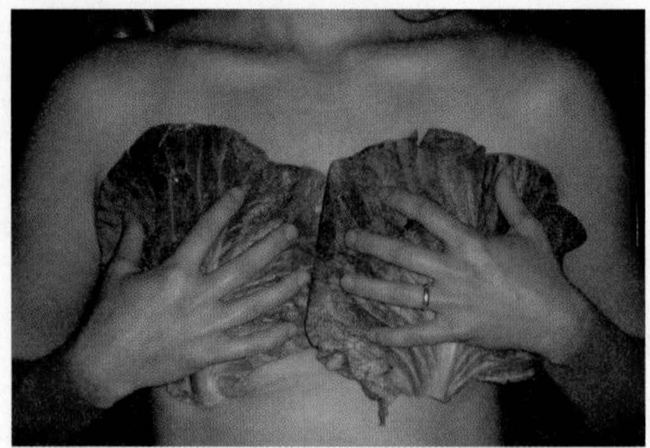

Fig. 18-14 Cabbage leaves to treat engorgement. (Courtesy Kathryn Alden, Chapel Hill, NC.)

Sore nipples. Mild nipple tenderness during the first few days of breastfeeding is common. Severe soreness or painful, abraded, cracked, or bleeding nipples are not normal and most often result from poor positioning, incorrect latch, improper suck, or monilial infection. Severe nipple pain may be related to vasospasm or Raynaud's phenomenon (Walker, 2008b). The key to preventing sore nipples is correct breastfeeding technique. Limiting the time at the breast will not prevent sore nipples.

For the first few days after birth the mother may experience some tenderness with the infant's initial sucks. This tenderness should quickly dissipate as the milk begins to flow and acts as a lubricant. To make the initial sucks less painful the mother can express a few drops of colostrum or milk to moisten the nipple and areola before latch. If the mother continues to experience nipple pain or discomfort after the first few sucks, helping the mother evaluate the latch and baby's position at the breast is necessary. If the nipple pain continues, the mother needs to remove the baby from the breast, breaking suction with her finger in the baby's mouth. Repositioning the mother or infant may be helpful in resolving the nipple discomfort. The mother then proceeds to attempt latch again, making sure the baby's mouth is open wide before the baby is pulled quickly to the breast (see Fig. 18-7). Sore nipples are often the result of the mother latching the baby onto the breast before the mouth is open wide.

The nurse or lactation consultant can assess the infant's suck by inserting a clean, gloved finger into the mouth and stimulating the infant to suck. If the tongue is not extruding over the lower gum and the mother reports pain or pinching with sucking, the baby may have ankyloglossia, which is a short or tight frenulum (commonly known as *tongue-tie*). In some instances, this condition is corrected surgically to free the tongue for less painful, more effective breastfeeding.

The treatment for sore nipples is first to correct the cause. Early assessment and intervention are essential to increase the likelihood that the mother will continue to breastfeed. Once the problem is identified and corrected, sore nipples should heal within a few days, even though the baby continues to breastfeed regularly. When sore nipples occur, the woman is advised to start the feeding on the least sore nipple. After feeding, have the mother wipe the nipples with water to remove the baby's saliva. A few drops of milk can be expressed, rubbed into the nipple, and allowed to air dry. Sore nipples should be open to air as much as possible. Breast shells worn inside the bra allow air to circulate while keeping clothing off sore nipples (see Fig. 18-13).

Rapid healing of sore nipples is critical to relieve the mother's discomfort, maintain breastfeeding, and prevent mastitis. Although numerous creams, ointments, gels, and gel pads have been used to treat sore nipples, there is a lack of conclusive evidence related to the effectiveness of any particular method. However, many health care professionals recommend their use because they have not been shown to cause harm. Some women report increased comfort for sore nipples with the application of purified lanolin or hydrogel pads. An antibiotic ointment may be recommended if nipples are cracked, abraded, or bleeding, but this must be washed off before the feeding (Smith & Riordan, 2010).

If nipples are extremely sore or damaged, and if the mother cannot tolerate breastfeeding, she may need to use an electric breast pump for 24 to 48 hours to allow the nipples to begin healing before resuming breastfeeding. The mother should use a pump that will effectively empty the breasts (see Fig. 18-9).

Monilial infections. Sore nipples that occur after the newborn period are often the result of a monilial (yeast) infection. The mother usually reports sudden onset of severe nipple pain and tenderness, burning, or stinging and may have sharp, shooting, burning pains into the breasts during and after feedings. The nipples appear somewhat pink and shiny or may be scaly or flaky; a visible rash, small blisters, or thrush may be seen. Most often the pain is out of proportion to the appearance of the nipple. Yeast infections of the nipples and breast are excruciatingly painful and can lead to early cessation of breastfeeding if not recognized and treated promptly.

Infants may or may not exhibit symptoms of monilial infection. Oral thrush and a red, raised diaper rash are common signs of a yeast infection. An affected infant is usually very fussy and gassy. When feeding, the infant is likely to pull off the breast soon after starting to feed, crying with apparent pain.

The most common predisposing factors for yeast infections of the breast include vaginal yeast infections, previous antibiotic use, and nipple damage. Oral thrush in the infant is a common cause of monilial infection in maternal nipples and breasts.

Mothers and infants must be treated simultaneously, even if the infant has no visible signs of infection. Treatment for mother is typically an antifungal cream such as miconazole applied to the nipples after feedings and, in some cases, a systemic antifungal medication such as fluconazole, taken for approximately 2 weeks. Most pediatricians prescribe an oral antifungal medication, such as nystatin, miconazole, or fluconazole, for infants. Treatment should continue for at least 7 days after symptoms begin to improve. Thorough handwashing is essential to prevent the spread of yeast (Walker, 2008b).

Plugged milk ducts. A milk duct may become plugged or clogged, causing an area of the breast to become swollen and tender. This area typically does not empty or soften with feeding or pumping. A small white pearl may also be visible on the tip of the nipple; this pearl is the curd of milk blocking the flow. The mother is afebrile and has no generalized symptoms.

Plugged milk ducts are most often the result of inadequate emptying of the breast, which may be caused by clothing that is too tight, a poorly fitting or underwire bra, or always using the same position for feeding. Application of warm compresses to the affected area and to the nipple before feeding helps promote emptying of the breast and release of the plug. (A disposable diaper filled with warm water makes an easy compress.)

Frequent feeding is recommended, with the baby beginning the feeding on the affected side to foster more complete emptying. The mother is advised to massage the affected area while the infant nurses or while she is pumping. Varying feeding positions and feeding without wearing a bra may be useful in resolving a plugged duct.

Plugged milk ducts may increase susceptibility to breast infection. For recurrent plugged ducts, taking lecithin, a fat emulsifier, may be useful for the mother (Walker, 2008b).

Mastitis. Although the term *mastitis* means inflammation of the breast, it is most often used to refer to infection of the breast. Mastitis is characterized by the sudden onset of influenza-like symptoms, including fever, chills, body aches, and headache. Localized breast pain and tenderness and a hot, reddened area on the breast, often resembling the shape of a pie wedge, are noted. Mastitis most commonly occurs in the upper outer quadrant of the breast; one or both breasts may be affected. The majority of cases occur during the first 6 weeks of breastfeeding, but mastitis can occur at any time (Academy of Breastfeeding Medicine (ABM) Protocol Committee, 2008).

Certain factors may predispose a woman to mastitis. Inadequate emptying of the breasts is common, which may be related to engorgement, plugged ducts, a sudden decrease in the number of feedings, abrupt weaning, or wearing underwire bras. Sore, cracked nipples may lead to mastitis by providing a portal of entry for causative organisms (*Staphylococcus, Streptococcus,* and *Escherichia coli* being most common). Stress and fatigue, maternal illness, ill family members, breast trauma, and poor maternal nutrition also are predisposing factors for mastitis. Women with insulin dependent diabetes may be at increased risk of mastitis (ABM Protocol Committee, 2008).

Breastfeeding mothers should be taught the signs of mastitis before they are discharged from the hospital after birth, and they need to know to call the health care provider promptly if the symptoms occur. Treatment includes antibiotics such as cephalexin or dicloxacillin for 10 to 14 days and analgesic and antipyretic medications such as ibuprofen. The mother is advised to rest as much as possible and to feed the baby or pump frequently, striving to empty the affected side adequately. Warm compresses to the breast before feeding or pumping may be useful. Adequate fluid intake and a balanced diet are important for the mother with mastitis (ABM Protocol Committee, 2008).

Complications of mastitis include breast abscess, chronic mastitis, or fungal infections of the breast. Most complications can be prevented by early recognition and treatment.

Follow-up after hospital discharge

Problems with sore nipples, engorgement, and jaundice are likely to occur after discharge. One of the nurse's roles is to educate and prepare the mother for problems she may encounter once she is home. The mother should be given a list of resources for help with breastfeeding concerns and instruction on when to call for assistance. Community resources for breastfeeding mothers include lactation consultants in hospitals, physician offices, or in private practice; nurses in pediatric or obstetric offices; support groups such as La Leche League; and peer counseling programs (e.g., those offered through WIC). Parents who utilize the Internet appreciate a list of websites containing current and correct information about breastfeeding.

Telephone follow-up by hospital, birth center, or office nurses within the first day or two after discharge can provide a means to identify any problems and offer needed advice and support. Breastfeeding infants should be seen by a health care provider at 3 to 5 days of age and again at 2 to 3 weeks to assess weight gain and offer encouragement and support to the mother (AAP Section on Breastfeeding, 2012).

FORMULA FEEDING

Parent Education

Inexperienced mothers and fathers who are formula feeding their infants usually need teaching, counseling, and support. They may need assistance with formula preparation, the feeding process, and with any problems they may experience. Some parents who are formula feeding may express concern that the baby will suffer as a result of their decision to bottle-feed. Emphasis on the beneficial use of feeding times for close contact and socializing with the infant can help relieve some of this concern.

Readiness for feeding

The first feeding of formula is ideally given after the initial transition to extrauterine life is made. Feeding-readiness cues include stability of vital signs, effective breathing pattern, presence of bowel sounds, an active sucking reflex, and those described earlier for breastfed infants.

Feeding patterns

In the first 24 to 48 hours of life a newborn will typically take 10 to 15 ml of formula at a feeding. Intake gradually increases during the first week of life. Most newborns are drinking 90 to 150 ml at a feeding by the end of the second week, or sooner. The newborn infant should be fed at least every 3 to 4 hours, even if waking the newborn is required for the feedings; rigid feeding schedules, however, are not recommended. The infant showing an adequate weight gain can be allowed to sleep at night and be fed only on awakening. Most newborns need six to eight feedings in 24 hours, and the number of feedings decreases as the infant matures. By 3 to 4 weeks after birth a fairly predictable feeding pattern has usually developed. Scheduling feedings arbitrarily at predetermined intervals may not meet a newborn's needs, but initiating feedings at convenient times often moves the newborn's feedings to times that work for the family.

Mothers will usually notice increases in the infant's appetite at 7 to 10 days, 3 weeks, 6 weeks, 3 months, and 6 months. These appetite spurts correspond to growth spurts. Mothers should increase the amount of formula per feeding by approximately 30 ml to meet the baby's needs at these times.

Feeding technique

Parents who choose formula feeding often need education regarding feeding techniques. Infants should be held for all feedings. During feedings, parents are encouraged to sit comfortably, holding the infant closely in a semi upright position with good head support. Feedings provide opportunities to bond with the baby through touching, talking, singing, or reading to the infant. Parents should consider feedings as a time of peaceful relaxation with the infant.

A bottle should never be propped with a pillow or other inanimate object and left with the infant. This practice may result in choking, and it deprives the infant of important interaction during feeding. Moreover, propping the bottle has been implicated in causing nursing-bottle caries, or decay of the first teeth resulting from continuous bathing of the teeth with carbohydrate-containing fluid as the infant sporadically sucks the nipple.

The bottle should be held so that fluid fills the nipple and none of the air in the bottle is allowed to enter the nipple (Fig. 18-15). The infant falls asleep, turns aside the head, or ceases to suck which usually indicates that enough formula has been taken to satisfy the baby. Teach parents to look for these cues and avoid overfeeding, which can contribute to obesity.

Most infants swallow air when fed from a bottle and need a chance to burp several times during a feeding. Parents are taught various positions that can be used for burping (Fig. 18-16).

Common concerns

Parents need to know what to do if the infant is spitting up. They may need to decrease the amount of feeding or feed smaller amounts more frequently. Burping the infant several times during a feeding, such as when the infant's sucking slows down or stops, may decrease spitting. Holding the baby upright for 30 minutes after feeding and avoiding bouncing or placing the infant on the abdomen soon after the feeding is finished may help. Spitting may be a result of overfeeding or may be symptomatic of gastroesophageal reflux. Parents should report vomiting one third or more of the feeding at most feeding sessions or projectile vomiting to the health care provider. Parents should be cautioned to refrain from changing the infant's formula without consulting the health care provider.

Bottles and nipples

Various brands and styles of bottles and nipples are available to parents. Most babies will feed well with any bottle and nipple. The bottles and nipples should be washed in warm soapy water, using a bottle and nipple brush to facilitate thorough cleansing. Boiling of bottles and nipples is not necessary unless some question exists about the safety of the water supply or if the infant has oral thrush. An angled bottle may be preferable to a straight bottle because the angled bottle encourages more physiologic positioning of the infant, improves the infant's comfort level, and decreases the need for burping (Fig. 18-15).

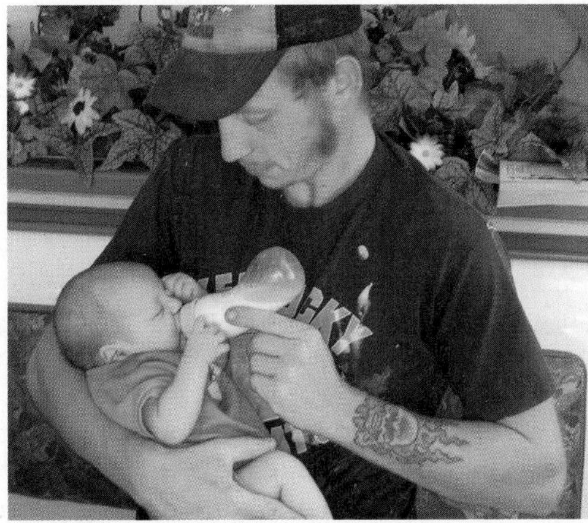

Fig. 18-15 Father bottle feeding infant son. Note angled bottle that ensures that milk covers nipple area. (Courtesy Eugene Doerr, Leitchfield, KY.)

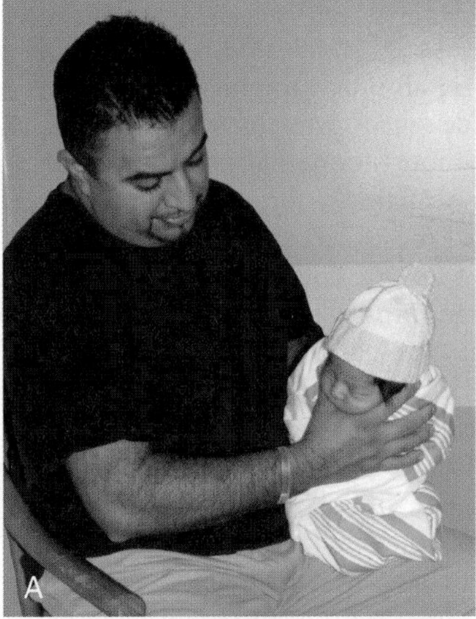

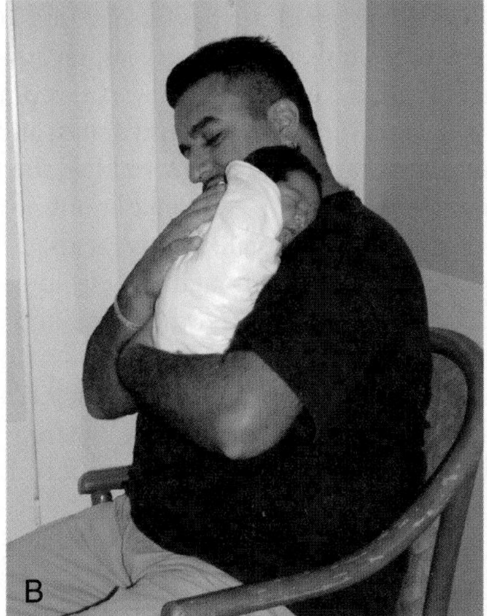

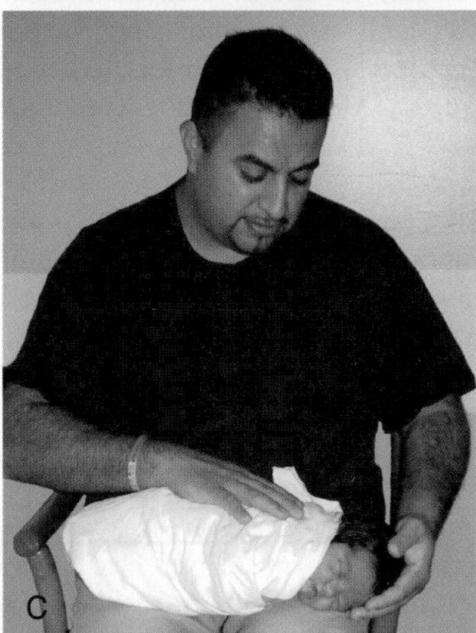

Fig. 18-16 Positions for burping an infant. **A,** Sitting. **B,** On the shoulder. **C,** Across the lap. (Courtesy Julie Perry Nelson, Loveland, CO.)

Spanish Guidelines: Burping

Critical Thinking Exercise: Formula Preparation

Infant formulas

Commercial formulas. Human milk is the "gold standard" for all infant formulas. Commercial infant formulas are designed to resemble human milk as closely as possible, although none has ever duplicated it. The exact composition of infant formula varies with the manufacturer, but all must meet specific standards.

Infants who are not breastfed should be given commercial iron-fortified formulas. Families with limited income may be eligible for services through the WIC program, which provides iron-fortified infant formula.

Commercially prepared formulas are cow's milk–based formulas that have been modified to closely resemble the nutritional content of human milk. These formulas are altered from cow's milk by removing butterfat, decreasing the protein content, and adding vegetable oil and carbohydrate. Some cow's milk–based formulas have demineralized whey added to yield a whey/casein ratio of 60:40. The standard cow's milk–based formulas, regardless of the commercial brand, have essentially the same compositions of vitamins, minerals, protein, carbohydrates, and essential amino acids, with minor variations such as the source of carbohydrate; nucleotides to enhance immune function; and long-chain polyunsaturated fatty acids, DHA, and arachidonic acid, which are thought to improve visual and cognitive function. Furthermore, the U.S. Food and Drug Administration regulates the manufacture of infant formula in the United States to ensure product safety. Standard cow's milk–based formulas are sold as low-iron and iron-fortified formulas; however, only the iron-fortified formulas meet the requirements of infants.

Four main categories of commercially prepared infant formulas are available: (1) *cow's milk–based formulas,* (2) *soy-based formulas,* commonly used for children who are lactose or cow's milk protein intolerant; (3) *casein-* or *whey-hydrolysate formulas,* used primarily for children who cannot tolerate or digest cow's milk or soy-based formulas; and (4) *amino acid formulas; used for infants with multiple food protein intolerances.*

The AAP Committee on Nutrition indicates that few solid indications exist for the use of soy protein–based formulas instead of cow's milk–based formulas (Bhatia, Greer, & AAP Committee on Nutrition, 2008). The soy-based milk formulas are recommended for infants with galactosemia and hereditary lactase deficiency; infants with secondary lactase deficiency may benefit as well. Infants with documented IgE allergies caused by cow's milk should be fed an extensively hydrolyzed protein formula because approximately 10% to 14% of infants with cow's milk–based intolerance will also have a soy protein allergy. Soy protein–based formulas have not been proved to be effective against colic or in the prevention of allergy in healthy or high risk infants.

Alternate milk sources such as goat's milk, skim or low fat milk, condensed milk, or raw, unpasteurized milk from any animal source should not be fed to infants because they are inadequate to support growth and may contain excess protein or an inadequate calcium/phosphorus ratio, which may cause seizures.

Formula preparation

Commercial formulas are available in three forms: powder, concentrate, and ready-to-feed. All forms are equivalent in terms of nutritional content, but they vary considerably in cost.

- Powdered formula is the least expensive type. It is easily mixed by using one scoop for every 60 ml of water.
- Concentrated formula is more expensive than powder. It is diluted with equal parts of water and can be stored in the refrigerator for 48 hours after opening.
- Ready-to-feed formula is the most expensive but the easiest to use. The desired amount is poured into the bottle. The opened can is safely refrigerated for 48 hours. This type of formula can be purchased in individual disposable bottles for the most convenient feeding.

The commercial infant formula must include label directions for preparation and use of the formula with pictures and symbols for the benefit of individuals who cannot read. Some manufacturers translate the directions into languages such as Spanish, French, Vietnamese, Chinese, and Arabic to prevent misunderstanding and errors in formula preparation. An important aspect to impress on families is that the proportions must not be altered–that is, neither diluted to extend the amount of formula nor concentrated to provide more calories. The newborn's kidneys are immature; giving the infant overly concentrated formula may provide protein and minerals in amounts that exceed the kidneys' excretory ability. In contrast, if the formula is diluted too much (sometimes done to save money), the infant does not consume sufficient calories and does not grow appropriately. The water used to mix either powdered or concentrated liquid formula need not contain any fluoride, especially in the first 6 months of life; excess fluoride can permanently stain the teeth once they do appear.

Sterilization of formula rarely is recommended when families have access to a safe public water supply. Instead, formula is prepared with attention to cleanliness. When water from a private well is used, parents should be advised to contact the health department to have a chemical and bacteriologic analysis of the water performed before using the water in formula preparation. The presence of nitrates, excess fluoride, or bacteria may be harmful to the infant.

If the sanitary conditions in the home appear unsafe, the nurse should recommend the use of ready-to-feed formula or to teach the mother to sterilize the formula. The two traditional methods for sterilization are terminal heating and the aseptic method. In the terminal heating method the prepared formula is placed in the bottles,

TEACHING GUIDELINES

Formula Preparation and Feeding

FORMULA PREPARATION

- Wash your hands and clean the bottle, nipple, and can opener thoroughly before preparing formula.
- If new nipples seem too firm or stiff, they can be softened by boiling them in water for 5 minutes before use.
- Note the expiration date on the formula container. It should be used before the expiration date. Any unopened expired formula should be returned to the place of purchase.
- Read the label on the container of formula and mix it exactly according to the directions.
- Use tap water to mix concentrated or powdered formula unless directed otherwise by your baby's physician or nurse.
- Test the size of the nipple hole by holding a prepared bottle upside down. The formula should drip from the nipple. If it runs in a stream, the hole is too big and should not be used. If it has to be shaken for the formula to come out, the hole is too small. You can either buy a new nipple or enlarge the hole by boiling the nipple for 5 minutes with a sewing needle inserted in the hole.
- If a nipple collapses when your baby sucks, loosen the nipple ring a little to let in air.
- Opened cans of ready-to-feed or concentrated formula should be covered and refrigerated. Any unused portions must be discarded after 48 hours.
- Bottles or cans of unopened formula can be stored at room temperature.
- If the formula is refrigerated, warm it by placing the bottle in a pan of hot water. Never use a microwave to warm any food to be given to a baby. Test the temperature of the formula by letting a few drops fall on the inside of your wrist. If the formula feels comfortably warm to you, the temperature is correct.

FEEDING TECHNIQUES AND TIPS

- Newborns should be fed at least every 3 to 4 hours and should never go longer than 4 hours without feeding until a satisfactory pattern of weight gain is established. This period may be as long as 2 weeks. If a baby cries or fusses between feedings, check to see if the diaper should be changed and if the baby needs to be picked up and cuddled. If the baby continues to cry and acts hungry, then feed the baby. Babies do not get hungry on a regular schedule.
- Infants gradually increase the amount of milk they drink with each feeding. The first day or so, most newborns consume 15 to 30 ml (0.5 to 1 ounce) with each feeding. This amount increases as the infant grows. If any formula remains in the bottle as the feeding ends, that milk must be thrown away because saliva from the baby's mouth can cause the formula to spoil.
- Keep a feeding diary, writing down the amount of formula the infant drinks with each feeding for the first week or so. Also, record the wet diapers and bowel movements the baby is having. Take this diary with you when you take the baby for the first pediatrician visit.
- For feeding, hold the infant close in a semi reclining position. Talk to the baby during the feeding. This time is ideal for social interaction and cuddling.
- Place the nipple in the infant's mouth on the tongue. It should touch the roof of the mouth to stimulate the baby's sucking reflex. Hold the bottle like a pencil. Keep the bottle tipped so that the nipple stays filled with milk and the baby does not suck in air.
- Taking a few sucks and then pausing briefly before continuing to suck again is normal for infants. Some infants take longer to feed than others. Be patient. Keeping the baby awake and encouraging sucking may be necessary. Moving the nipple gently in the infant's mouth may stimulate sucking.
- Newborns are apt to swallow air when sucking. Give the infant opportunities to burp several times during a feeding. As the infant gets older, you will know better when to stop for burping.
- After the first 2 or 3 days the stools of a formula-fed infant are yellow and soft but formed. The infant may have a stool with each feeding in the first 2 weeks, although this amount may decrease to one or two stools each day. It is not abnormal for formula fed infants to have only one stool every 48 hours.

SAFETY TIPS

- Infants should be held and never left alone while feeding. Never prop the bottle. The infant might inhale formula or choke on any that was spit up. Infants who fall asleep with a propped bottle of milk or juice may be prone to cavities when the first teeth come in.
- Know how to use the bulb syringe and how to help an infant who is choking.

which are topped with the nipples placed upside down and covered with the caps, and then sealed loosely with the rings. The bottles are then boiled together in a water bath for 25 minutes. In the aseptic method the bottles, rings, caps, nipples, and any other necessary equipment, such as a funnel, are boiled separately, after which the formula is poured into the bottles. Any formula left in the bottle after the feeding should be discarded because the infant's saliva has mixed with it. (Instructions for formula preparation and feeding are provided in the Teaching Guidelines box.)

Vitamin and mineral supplementation

Commercial iron-fortified formula has all of the nutrients that infants need for the first 6 months of life. After 6 months, fluoride supplementation of 0.25 mg per day is required if the local water supply is not fluoridated. Non-breastfeeding infants who consume less than 1 quart per day of vitamin D–fortified milk should receive 400 international units of vitamin D each day (Wagner, Grier, Section on Breastfeeding, & Committee on Nutrition, 2008).

Weaning

The bottle-fed infant will gradually learn to use a cup, and the parents will find that they are preparing fewer bottles. The bottle feeding before bedtime is often the last one to remain. Babies have a strong need to suck, and the baby who has the bottle taken away too early or abruptly will compensate with nonnutritive sucking on his or her fingers, thumb, a pacifier, or even his or her own tongue. Weaning from a bottle should therefore be attempted gradually because the baby has learned to rely on the comfort that sucking provides.

Introducing solid foods

The infant receives the right balance of nutrients from breast milk or formula during the first 4 to 6 months. The notion that the feeding of solids will help the infant sleep through the night is not true. Parents should not put cereal into the infant's bottle. Introduction of solid foods before the infant is 4 to 6 months of age may result in overfeeding and decreased intake of breast milk or formula. The infant cannot communicate feeling full as can an older child, who is able to turn the head away. The proper balance of carbohydrate, protein, and fat for an infant to grow properly is in the breast milk or formula.

The infant's individual growth pattern helps determine the right time to start solids. The primary health care provider will advise when to introduce solid foods. The schedule for introducing solid foods and the types of foods to serve will be discussed during well-baby supervision visits with the pediatrician or pediatric nurse practitioner.

KEY POINTS

- Human breast milk is species specific and is the recommended form of infant nutrition. It provides immunologic protection against many infections and diseases.
- Breast milk changes in composition with each stage of lactation, during each feeding, and as the infant grows.
- During the prenatal period, expectant parents should be informed of the benefits of breastfeeding for infants, mothers, families, and society.
- Infants should be breastfed as soon as possible after birth and at least 8 to 12 times per day thereafter.
- Specific, measurable indicators have been identified to show that the infant is breastfeeding effectively.
- Breast milk production is based on a supply-meets-demand principle: The more the infant nurses, the greater the milk supply.
- Commercial infant formulas provide satisfactory nutrition for most infants.
- Infants should be held for feedings.
- Parents should be instructed about the types of commercial infant formulas, proper preparation for feeding, and correct feeding technique.
- Solid foods should be started after age 4 to 6 months.
- Unmodified cow's milk is inappropriate during the first year of life.
- Nurses must be knowledgeable about feeding methods and provide education and support for families.

Audio Chapter Summaries Access an audio summary of these Key Points on evolve

References

Ahluwalia, I. B., D'Angelo, D., Morrow B., & McDonald, J. A. (2012). Association between acculturation and breastfeeding among Hispanic women: Data from the Pregnancy Risk Assessment and Monitoring System. *Journal of Human Lactation, 28*(2), 167-173.

American Academy of Pediatrics Section on Breastfeeding. (2012). Breastfeeding and the use of human milk. Policy Statement. *Pediatrics, 129*(3), e827-e841.

American Academy of Pediatrics Committee on Nutrition. (2009). *Pediatric nutrition handbook* (6th ed.). Elk Grove Village, IL: AAP.

American Academy of Pediatrics Task Force on Sudden Infant Death Syndrome. (2011). SIDS and other sleep-related infant deaths: Expansion of recommendations for a safe infant sleeping environment. *Pediatrics, 128*(5), e1341-e1367.

Academy of Breastfeeding Medicine (ABM). (2010). *Clinical protocol No. 8: Human milk storage information for home use for healthy full-term infants. Breastfeeding Medicine, 5*(3), 127-130.

Academy of Breastfeeding Medicine Protocol Committee. (2006). *ABM clinical protocol No. 13: Contraception during breastfeeding. Breastfeeding Medicine, 1*(1), 43-51.

Academy of Breastfeeding Medicine Protocol Committee. (2008). Clinical Protocol No. 4: Mastitis. *Breastfeeding Medicine, 3*(3), 177-180.

Association of Women's Health, Obstetric and Neonatal Nurses (AWHONN). (2007). *Breastfeeding and the role of the nurse in the promotion of breastfeeding.* Washington, DC: AWHONN.

Baker, R. D., Greer, F. R., & AAP Committee on Nutrition. (2010). Clinical report: Diagnosis and prevention of iron-deficiency and iron-deficiency anemia in infants and young children (0-3 years of age). *Pediatrics, 126*(5), 1-11.

Bartick, M., & Reyes, C. (2012). Las dos cosas: An analysis of attitudes of Latina women on non-exclusive breastfeeding. *Breastfeeding Medicine, 7*(1), 19-24.

Becker, G., & Scott, M. (2008). Nutrition for lactating women. In R. Mannel, P. J. Martens, & M. Walker (Eds.), *Core curriculum for lactation consultant practice* (2nd ed.). Sudbury, MA: Jones & Bartlett.

Bhatia, J., Greer, F., & American Academy of Pediatrics Committee on Nutrition. (2008). Use of soy protein-based formulas in infant feeding. *Pediatrics, 121*(5), 1062-1068.

Blackburn, S. (2013). *Maternal, fetal, and neonatal physiology: A clinical perspective* (4th ed.). St. Louis: Saunders.

Centers for Disease Control and Prevention (CDC) (2012). Breastfeeding report card–United States. Available at www.cdc.gov/breastfeeding/data/reportcard.htm (accessed June 21, 2013).

Clifford, J., & McIntyre, E. (2008). Who supports breastfeeding? *Breastfeeding Review, 16*(2), 9-19.

Dell, K. M., & Davis, I. D. (2011). Fluid, electrolyte, and acid-base homeostasis. In R. J. Martin, A. A. Fanaroff, & M. C. Walsh (Eds.), *Fanaroff and Martin's neonatal-perinatal medicine: Diseases of the fetus and infant* (9th ed.). Philadelphia: Mosby.

Geddes, D. T. (2007). Inside the lactating breast: The latest anatomy research. *Journal of Midwifery and Women's Health, 52*(6), 556-563.

Hale, T. W. (2012). *Medications and mothers' milk* (15th ed.). Amarillo, TX: Hale Publishing.

Heird, W. C. (2007). The feeding of infants and children. In R. M. Kliegman, R. E. Behrman, H. B. Jenson, & B. F. Stanton (Eds.), *Nelson textbook of pediatrics* (18th ed.). Philadelphia: Saunders.

Hohmann, H., & Creinin, M. D. (2007). The contraceptive implant. *Clinical Obstetrics and Gynecology, 50*(4), 907-917.

Institute of Medicine. (2005). *Dietary reference intakes for energy, carbohydrate, fiber, fatty acids, cholesterol, protein, and amino acids.* Washington, DC: Food and Nutrition Board, Institute of Medicine, National Academies Press.

International Lactation Consultant Association (ILCA). (1999). *Evidence-based guidelines for breastfeeding management during the first fourteen days.* Raleigh, NC: ILCA.

Ip, S., Chung, M., Raman, G., Trikalinos, T. A., & Lau, J. (2009). A summary of the Agency for Healthcare Research and Quality's evidence report on breastfeeding in developed countries. *Breastfeeding Medicine*, 4(Suppl 1), S17-S30.

Jones, F., & Tully, M. R. (2006). *Best practices for expressing, storing, and handling human milk in hospitals, homes, and child care settings* (2nd ed.). Raleigh, NC: Human Milk Banking Association of America.

Labiner-Wolfe, J., Fein, S. B., Shealy, K. R., & Wang, C. (2008). Prevalence of breast milk expression and associated factors. *Pediatrics, 122* (Suppl. 2), S63-S68.

Lanese, M. G., & Cross, M. (2008). Breastfeeding a preterm infant. In R. Mannel, P. J. Martens, & M. Walker (Eds.), *Core curriculum for lactation consultant practice.* (2nd ed.). Sudbury, MA: Jones and Bartlett.

Laroia, N., & Sharma, D. (2006). The religious and cultural bases for breastfeeding practices among the Hindus. *Breastfeeding Medicine, 1*(2), 94-98.

Lauwers, J., & Swisher, A. (2011). *Counseling the nursing mother* (5th ed.). Sudbury, MS: Jones and Bartlett.

Lawrence, R., & Lawrence, R. (2011). *Breastfeeding: A guide for the medical profession* (7th ed.). Philadelphia: Mosby.

Mannel, R. (2008). Milk expression, storage, and handling. In R. Mannel, P.J. Martens, & M. Walker (Eds.), *Core curriculum for lactation consultant practice* (2nd ed.). Sudbury, MA: Jones & Bartlett.

McDowell, M. M., Wang, C., & Kennedy-Stephenson, J. (2008). Breastfeeding in the United States: Findings from the national health and nutrition examination surveys, 1999-2006. *National Center for Health Statistics (NCHS) Data Brief, 5*, 1-7.

Nelson, A. M. (2012). A meta-synthesis related to infant feeding decision making. *MCN American Journal of Maternal Child Nursing, 37*(4), 249-252.

O'Brien, M., Buikstra, E., & Hegney, D. (2008). The influence of psychological factors on breastfeeding duration. *Journal of Advanced Nursing, 63*(4), 397-408.

Page-Goertz, S. (2008). Hyperbilirubinemia and hypoglycemia. In R. Mannel, P.J. Martens, & M. Walker (Eds.), *Core curriculum for lactation consultant practice* (2nd ed.). Sudbury, MA: Jones and Bartlett.

Ramsay, D. T., Kent, J. C., Hartmann, R. A., & Hartmann, P. E. (2005). Anatomy of the lactating human breast redefined with ultrasound imaging. *Journal of Anatomy, 206*, 525-534.

Renfrew, M., & Hall, D. (2008). Enabling women to breastfeed. *British Medical Journal, 337*, 1066-1067.

Rosen, I. M., Krueger, M. V., Carney, L. M., & Graham, J. A. (2008). Prenatal breastfeeding education and breastfeeding outcomes. *MCN: The American Journal of Maternal/Child Nursing, 33*(5), 315-319.

Scanlon, K. S., Grummer-Strawn, L., Li, R., et al. (2010). Racial and ethnic differences in breastfeeding initiation and duration, by state–National Immunization Survey, United States, 2004-2008. *MMWR Morbidity and Mortality Weekly Report, 59*(11), 327-334.

Shaikh, U., & Ahmed, O. (2006). Islam and infant feeding. *Breastfeeding Medicine, 1*(3), 164-167.

Shealy, K. R., Scanlon, K. S., Labiner-Wolfe, J., Fein, S. B., & Grummer-Strawn, L. M. (2008). Characteristics of breastfeeding practice among U.S. mothers. *Pediatrics, 122*(2), S50-S55.

Simmer, K., Patole, S., & Rao, S. C. (2007). Longchain polyunsaturated fatty acid supplementation in infants born at term. In *The Cochrane Database of Systematic Reviews*, 2007, CD 000376.

Smith, L. J., & Riordan J. (2010). Postpartum care. In J. Riodan & K. Wambach (Eds.). *Breastfeeding and human lactation* (4th ed.). Boston: Jones & Bartlett.

Taylor, J. S., Geller, L., Risica, P. M., Kirtania, U., & Cabral, H. J. (2008). Birth order and breastfeeding initiation: Results of a national survey. *Breastfeeding Medicine, 3*(1), 20-27.

U.S. Department of Health and Human Services (USDHHS). (2010). *Healthy People 2020.* Washington, DC: USDHHS. Available at www.healthypeople.gov/hp2020/ (accessed June 21, 2013).

Wagner, C. L., Grier, F. R., Section on Breastfeeding, & Committee on Nutrition. (2008). Prevention of rickets and vitamin D deficiency in infants, children and adolescents. *Pediatrics, 122*(5), 1142-1152.

Walker, M. (2008a). Breastfeeding the late preterm infant. *Journal of Obstetric, Gynecologic, and Neonatal Nursing, 37*(6), 692-701.

Walker, M. (2008b). Conquering common breastfeeding problems. *Journal of Perinatal Nursing, 22*(4), 267-274.

Weissinger, D. (1998). A breastfeeding teaching tool using a sandwich analogy for latch-on. *Journal of Human Lactation, 14*(1), 51-56.

World Health Organization (WHO); UNICEF. (2003). *Global strategy for infant and young child feeding.* Geneva: WHO. Internet document available at http://www.who.int/child_adolescent_health/documents/9241562218/en/ (accessed June 16, 2009).

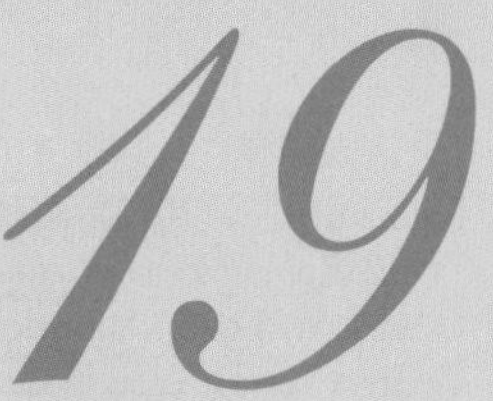

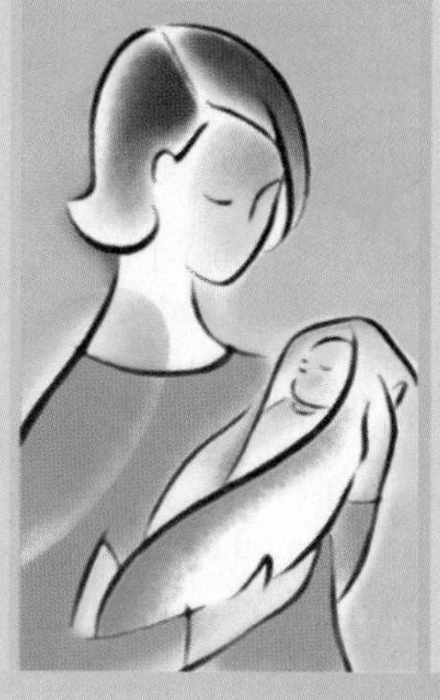

CHAPTER 19

Assessment of High Risk Pregnancy

KITTY CASHION

LEARNING OBJECTIVES

- Explore the biophysical, psychosocial, sociodemographic, and environmental aspects of high risk pregnancy.
- Examine risk factors identified through history, physical examination, and diagnostic techniques.
- Differentiate among diagnostic techniques, including when they are used in pregnancy and for what purposes.
- Develop a teaching plan to explain diagnostic techniques and implications of findings to patients and their families.

KEY TERMS AND DEFINITIONS

acoustic stimulation test Antepartum test to elicit fetal heart rate response to sound; performed by applying sound source (laryngeal stimulator) to the maternal abdomen over the fetal head

alpha-fetoprotein (AFP) Fetal antigen; elevated levels in amniotic fluid and maternal blood are associated with neural tube defects

amniocentesis Procedure in which a needle is inserted through the abdominal and uterine walls to obtain amniotic fluid; used for assessment of fetal health and maturity

amniotic fluid index (AFI) Estimation of amount of amniotic fluid by means of ultrasound to determine excess or decrease

biophysical profile (BPP) Noninvasive assessment of the fetus and its environment using ultrasonography and fetal monitoring; includes fetal breathing movements, gross body movements, fetal tone, reactive fetal heart rate, and qualitative amniotic fluid volume

chorionic villus sampling (CVS) Removal of fetal tissue from the placenta for genetic diagnostic studies

contraction stress test (CST) (also called oxytocin challenge test [OCT]) Test to stimulate uterine contractions for the purpose of assessing fetal response; a healthy fetus does not react to contractions, whereas a compromised fetus demonstrates late decelerations in the fetal heart rate that are indicative of uteroplacental insufficiency

daily fetal movement count (DFMC) Maternal assessment of fetal activity; the number of fetal movements within a specified time are counted; also called "kick count"

Doppler blood flow analysis Use of ultrasound for noninvasive measurement of blood flow in the fetus and placenta

magnetic resonance imaging (MRI) Noninvasive nuclear procedure for imaging tissues with high fat and water content; in obstetrics, uses include evaluation of fetal structures, placenta, and amniotic fluid volume

nonstress test (NST) Evaluation of fetal response (fetal heart rate) to natural contractile uterine activity or to an increase in fetal activity

percutaneous umbilical blood sampling (PUBS) (also called cordocentesis) Procedure during which a fetal umbilical vessel is accessed for blood sampling or for transfusions

uteroplacental insufficiency (UPI) Decline in placental function (exchange of gases, nutrients, and wastes) leading to fetal hypoxia and acidosis; evidenced by late decelerations of the fetal heart rate in response to uterine contractions

WEB RESOURCES

Additional related content can be found on the companion website at evolve

http://evolve.elsevier.com/Lowdermilk/Maternity/

- NCLEX Review Questions
- Spanish Guidelines: High Risk Factors

Approximately 500,000 of the 4 million births that occur in the United States each year are categorized as *high risk* because of maternal or fetal complications. A high risk pregnancy is one in which the life or health of the mother or fetus is jeopardized by a disorder coincidental with or unique to pregnancy. Care of these high risk patients requires the combined efforts of medical and nursing personnel. Factors associated with a diagnosis of a high risk pregnancy are identified in this chapter. Diagnostic techniques often used to monitor the maternal-fetal unit at risk are also described.

ASSESSMENT OF RISK FACTORS

Pregnancies can be designated as high risk for any of several undesirable outcomes. Those considered to be at risk for uteroplacental insufficiency (UPI), the gradual decline in delivery of needed substances by the placenta to the fetus, carry a serious threat for fetal growth restriction, intrauterine fetal death, intrapartum death, intrapartum fetal distress, and various types of neonatal morbidity.

In the past, risk factors were evaluated only from a medical standpoint; therefore only adverse medical, obstetric, or physiologic conditions were considered to place the woman at risk. Today, a more comprehensive approach to high risk pregnancy is used, and the factors associated with high risk childbearing are grouped into broad categories based on threats to health and pregnancy outcome. Categories of risk are biophysical, psychosocial, sociodemographic, and environmental (Gilbert, E.S., 2007) (Box 19-1). Risk factors are interrelated and cumulative in their effects.

Biophysical risks include factors that originate within the mother or fetus and affect the development or functioning of either one or both. Examples include genetic disorders, nutritional and general health status, and medical or obstetric-related illnesses. Box 19-2 lists common risk factors for several pregnancy-related problems.

Psychosocial risks consist of maternal behaviors and adverse lifestyles that have a negative effect on the health of the mother or fetus. These risks may include emotional distress and disturbed interpersonal relationships, as well as inadequate social support and unsafe cultural practices.

Sociodemographic risks arise from the mother and her family. These risks may place the mother and fetus at risk. Examples include lack of prenatal care, low income, marital status, and ethnicity (see Box 19-1). Environmental factors include hazards in the workplace and the woman's general environment and may include environmental chemicals (e.g., pesticides, lead, mercury), radiation, and pollutants (Silbergeld & Patrick, 2005).

Spanish Guidelines: High Risk Factors

Psychologic Considerations Related to High Risk Pregnancy

Once a pregnancy has been identified as high risk, the pregnant woman and her fetus will be monitored carefully throughout the remainder of the pregnancy. All women who undergo antepartal assessments are at risk for real and potential problems and may feel anxious. In most instances the tests are ordered because of suspected fetal compromise, deterioration of a maternal condition, or both. In the third trimester, pregnant women are most concerned about protecting themselves and their fetuses and consider themselves most vulnerable to outside influences. The label of *high risk* often increases this sense of vulnerability.

When a woman is diagnosed with a high risk pregnancy, she and her family will likely experience stress related to the diagnosis. The woman may exhibit various psychologic responses including anxiety, low self-esteem, guilt, frustration, and inability to function. A high risk pregnancy can also affect parental attachment, accomplishment of the tasks of pregnancy, and family adaptation to the pregnancy. If the woman is fearful for her own well-being, she

BOX 19-1

Categories of High Risk Factors

BIOPHYSICAL FACTORS

- *Genetic considerations.* Genetic factors may interfere with normal fetal or neonatal development, result in congenital anomalies, or create difficulties for the mother. These factors include defective genes, transmissible inherited disorders and chromosomal anomalies, multiple pregnancy, large fetal size, and ABO incompatibility.
- *Nutritional status.* Adequate nutrition, without which fetal growth and development cannot proceed normally, is one of the most important determinants of pregnancy outcome. Conditions that influence nutritional status include the following: young age; three pregnancies in the previous 2 years; tobacco, alcohol, or drug use; inadequate dietary intake because of chronic illness or food fads; inadequate or excessive weight gain; and hematocrit value less than 33%.
- *Medical and obstetric disorders.* Complications of current and past pregnancies, obstetric-related illnesses, and pregnancy losses put the patient at risk (see Box 19-2).

PSYCHOSOCIAL FACTORS

- *Smoking.* A strong, consistent, causal relation has been established between maternal smoking and reduced birth weight. Risks include low-birth-weight infants,

Continued

BOX 19-1

Categories of High Risk Factors—cont'd

higher neonatal mortality rates, increased miscarriages, and increased incidence of premature rupture of membranes. These risks are aggravated by low socioeconomic status, poor nutritional status, and concurrent use of alcohol.

- *Caffeine.* Birth defects in humans have not been related to caffeine consumption. However, pregnant women who consume more than 200 mg of caffeine daily (equivalent to about 12 ounces of coffee per day) may be at increased risk for miscarriage or for giving birth to infants with IUGR.
- *Alcohol.* Although the exact effects of alcohol in pregnancy have not been quantified and its mode of action is largely unexplained, it exerts adverse effects on the fetus, resulting in fetal alcohol syndrome, fetal alcohol effects, learning disabilities, and hyperactivity.
- *Drugs.* The developing fetus may be adversely affected by drugs through several mechanisms. They can be teratogenic, cause metabolic disturbances, produce chemical effects, or cause depression or alteration of CNS function. This category includes medications prescribed by a health care provider or bought over the counter, as well as commonly abused drugs such as heroin, cocaine, and marijuana. (See Chapter 20 for more information about drug and alcohol abuse.)
- *Psychologic status.* Childbearing triggers profound and complex physiologic, psychologic, and social changes, with evidence to suggest a relationship between emotional distress and birth complications. This risk factor includes conditions such as specific intrapsychic disturbances and addictive lifestyles; a history of child or spouse abuse; inadequate support systems; family disruption or dissolution; maternal role changes or conflicts; noncompliance with cultural norms; unsafe cultural, ethnic, or religious practices; and situational crises.

SOCIODEMOGRAPHIC FACTORS

- *Low income.* Poverty underlies many other risk factors and leads to inadequate financial resources for food and prenatal care, poor general health, increased risk of medical complications of pregnancy, and greater prevalence of adverse environmental influences.
- *Lack of prenatal care.* Failure to diagnose and treat complications early is a major risk factor arising from financial barriers or lack of access to care; depersonalization of the system resulting in long waits, routine visits, variability in health care personnel, and unpleasant physical surroundings; lack of understanding of the need for early and continued care or cultural beliefs that do not support the need; and fear of the health care system and its providers.
- *Age.* Women at both ends of the childbearing age spectrum have an increased incidence of poor outcomes; however, age may not be a risk factor in all cases. Both physiologic and psychologic risks should be evaluated.
  a. *Adolescents.* More complications are seen in young mothers (younger than 15 years), who have a 60% higher mortality rate than those older than 20 years and in pregnancies occurring less than 6 years after menarche. Complications include anemia, preeclampsia, prolonged labor, and contracted pelvis and cephalopelvic disproportion. Long-term social implications of early motherhood are lower educational status, lower income, increased dependence on government support programs, higher divorce rates, and higher parity.
  b. *Mature mothers.* The risks to older mothers are not from age alone but from other considerations such as number and spacing of previous pregnancies, genetic disposition of the parents, and medical history, lifestyle, nutrition, and prenatal care. The increased likelihood of chronic diseases and complications that arises from more invasive medical management of a pregnancy and labor combined with demographic characteristics put an older woman at risk. Medical conditions more likely to be experienced by mature women include hypertension and preeclampsia, diabetes, extended labor, cesarean birth, placenta previa, abruptio placentae, and death. Her fetus is at greater risk for low birth weight and macrosomia, chromosomal abnormalities, congenital malformations, and neonatal death.
- *Parity.* The number of previous pregnancies is a risk factor associated with age and includes all first pregnancies, especially a first pregnancy at either end of the childbearing age continuum. The incidence of preeclampsia and dystocia is increased with a first birth.
- *Marital status.* The increased mortality and morbidity rates for unmarried women, including an increased risk for preeclampsia, are often related to inadequate prenatal care and a young childbearing age.
- *Residence.* The availability and quality of prenatal care varies widely with geographic residence. Women in metropolitan areas have more prenatal visits than those in rural areas who have fewer opportunities for specialized care and consequently a higher incidence of maternal mortality. Health care in the inner city, where residents are usually poorer and begin childbearing earlier and continue for longer, may be of lower quality than in a more affluent neighborhood.
- *Ethnicity.* Although ethnicity by itself is not a major risk, race is an indicator of other sociodemographic risk factors. Non-Caucasian women are more than three times as likely as Caucasian women to die of pregnancy-related causes. African-American babies have the highest rates of prematurity and low birth weight, with the infant mortality rate among African-Americans being more than double that among Caucasians.

ENVIRONMENTAL FACTORS

- Various environmental substances can affect fertility and fetal development, the chance of a live birth, and the child's subsequent mental and physical development. Environmental influences include infections, radiation, chemicals such as pesticides, therapeutic drugs, illicit drugs, industrial pollutants, cigarette smoke, stress, and diet. Paternal exposure to mutagenic agents in the workplace has been associated with an increased risk of miscarriage.

BOX 19-2

Specific Pregnancy Problems and Related Risk Factors

POLYHYDRAMNIOS

- Diabetes mellitus
- Fetal congenital anomalies

INTRAUTERINE GROWTH RESTRICTION

- Maternal causes:
  Hypertensive disorders
  Diabetes
  Chronic renal disease
  Collagen vascular disease
  Thrombophilia
  Cyanotic heart disease
  Poor weight gain
  Smoking, alcohol use, illicit drug use
  Living at a high altitude
  Multiple gestation
- Fetoplacental causes:
  Chromosomal abnormalities
  Congenital malformations
  Intrauterine infection
  Genetic syndromes (e.g., trisomy 13 and trisomy 18)
  Abnormal placental development

OLIGOHYDRAMNIOS

- Renal agenesis (Potter syndrome)
- Premature rupture of membranes
- Prolonged pregnancy
- Uteroplacental insufficiency
- Maternal hypertensive disorders

CHROMOSOMAL ABNORMALITIES

- Maternal age 35 years or older
- Balanced translocation (maternal and paternal)

Sources: Baschat, A. A., Galan, H. L., Ross, M. G., & Gabbe, S. G. (2007). Intrauterine growth restriction. In S. Gabbe, J. Niebyl, & J. Simpson (Eds.), *Obstetrics: Normal and problem pregnancies* (5th ed.). Philadelphia: Churchill Livingstone; Gilbert, W. M. (2007). Amniotic fluid disorders. In S. Gabbe, J. Niebyl, & J. Simpson (Eds.), *Obstetrics: Normal and problem pregnancies* (5th ed.). Philadelphia: Churchill Livingstone; Resnik, R., & Creasy, R. K. (2009). Intrauterine growth restriction. In R. K. Creasy, R. Resnik, & J. D. Iams (Eds.), *Creasy and Resnik's maternal-fetal medicine: Principles and practice* (6th ed.). Philadelphia: Saunders; Simpson, J. L., & Otano, L. (2007). Prenatal genetic diagnosis. In S. Gabbe, J. Niebyl, & J. Simpson (Eds.), *Obstetrics: Normal and problem pregnancies* (5th ed.). Philadelphia: Churchill Livingstone.

may continue to feel ambivalence about the pregnancy or may not accept the reality of the pregnancy. She may not be able to complete preparations for the baby or go to childbirth classes if she is placed on restricted activity at home or hospitalized. The family may become frustrated because they cannot engage in activities that prepare them for parenthood. The nurse can help the woman and her family regain control and balance in their lives by providing support and encouragement, providing information about the pregnancy problem and its management, and providing opportunities to make as many choices as possible about the woman's care.

BOX 19-3

Common Maternal and Fetal Indications for Antepartum Testing

- Diabetes
- Chronic hypertension
- Preeclampsia
- Fetal growth restriction
- Multiple gestation
- Oligohydramnios
- Preterm premature rupture of membranes
- Postdate or postterm gestation
- Previous stillbirth
- Decreased fetal movement
- Systemic lupus erythematosus
- Renal disease
- Cholestasis of pregnancy

From Miller, L.A., Miller, D.A., & Tucker, S.M. (2013). *Mosby's pocket guide to fetal monitoring: A multidisciplinary approach* (7th ed.). St. Louis: Mosby.

Antepartum Testing

The major expected outcome of all antepartum testing is the detection of potential fetal compromise. Ideally, the technique used identifies fetal compromise before intrauterine asphyxia occurs so that the health care provider can take measures to prevent or minimize adverse perinatal outcomes. Antepartum testing is used primarily in patients at risk for disrupted fetal oxygenation. In most cases, monitoring begins by 32 to 34 weeks of gestation and continues regularly until birth. Assessment tests should be selected based on their effectiveness, and the results must be interpreted in light of the complete clinical picture. Box 19-3 lists common maternal and fetal indications for antepartum testing that are supported by currently available evidence (Miller, Miller, & Tucker, 2013).

The remainder of this chapter describes maternal and fetal assessment tests that are often used to monitor high risk pregnancies.

BIOPHYSICAL ASSESSMENT

Daily Fetal Movement Count

Assessment of fetal activity by the mother is a simple yet valuable method for monitoring the condition of the fetus. The **daily fetal movement count (DFMC)** (also called *kick count*) can be assessed at home and is noninvasive, inexpensive, simple to understand, and usually does not interfere with a daily routine. The DFMC is frequently used to monitor the fetus in pregnancies complicated by conditions that may affect fetal oxygenation (see Box 19-2). The presence of movements is generally a reassuring sign of fetal health.

Several different protocols are used for counting. One recommendation is to count once a day for 60 minutes. Another common recommendation is that mothers count fetal activity two or three times daily for 60 minutes each time. Except for establishing a very low number of daily fetal movements or a trend toward decreased motion, the clinical value of the absolute number of fetal movements has not been established, other than in the situation in which fetal movements cease entirely for 12 hours (the so-called *fetal alarm signal*). A count of fewer than three fetal movements within 1 hour warrants further evaluation by a nonstress test (NST) or contraction stress test (CST) (oxytocin challenge test [OCT]), biophysical profile (BPP), or a combination of these (see later discussion). Women should be taught the significance of the presence or absence of fetal movements (or both), the procedure for counting that is to be used, how to record findings on a daily fetal movement record, and when to notify the health care provider.

NURSING ALERT In assessing fetal movements, it is important to remember that they are usually not present during the fetal sleep cycle and that they may be temporarily reduced if the woman is taking depressant medications, drinking alcohol, or smoking a cigarette. They do not decrease as the woman nears term. Obesity decreases the ability of the mother to perceive fetal movement.

Ultrasonography

Sound is a form of wave energy that causes small particles in a medium to oscillate. The frequency of sound, which refers to the number of peaks or waves that move over a given point per unit of time, is expressed in hertz (Hz). Sound with a frequency of 1 cycle, or one peak per second, has a frequency of 1 Hz. When directional beams of sound strike an object, an echo is returned. The time delay between the emission of the sound and the return of the echo and the direction of the echo are noted. From these data the distance and location of an object can be calculated. Ultrasound is sound frequency higher than that detectable by humans (greater than 20,000 Hz). Ultrasound images are a reflection of the strength of the sending beam, the strength of the returning echo, and the density of the medium (e.g., muscle [uterus], bone, tissue [placenta], fluid, or blood) through which the beam is sent and returned.

Diagnostic ultrasonography is an important, safe technique in antepartum fetal surveillance. It provides critical information to health care providers regarding fetal activity and gestational age, normal versus abnormal fetal growth curves, visual assistance with which invasive tests may be performed more safely, fetal and placental anatomy, and fetal well-being (Richards, 2007). Ultrasound examination can be performed abdominally or transvaginally during pregnancy. Both methods produce a two- or three-dimensional view from which a pictorial image is obtained (Fig. 19-1, *A, B*). It is also possible to produce a four-dimensional image. Abdominal ultrasonography is more useful after the first trimester when the pregnant uterus becomes an abdominal organ. During the procedure, the woman usually should have a full bladder to displace the uterus upward to provide a better image of the fetus. Transmission gel or paste is applied to the woman's abdomen before a transducer is moved over the skin to enhance transmission and reception of the sound waves. She is positioned with small pillows under her head and knees. The display panel is positioned so that the woman or her partner (or both) can observe the images on the screen if they desire.

Transvaginal ultrasonography, in which the probe is inserted into the vagina, allows pelvic anatomic features to be evaluated in greater detail and intrauterine pregnancy to be diagnosed earlier. A transvaginal ultrasound examination is well tolerated by most pregnant women because it removes the need for a full bladder. It is especially useful in obese women whose thick abdominal layers cannot be penetrated adequately with an abdominal approach. A transvaginal ultrasound may be performed with the woman in a lithotomy position or with her pelvis elevated by towels, cushions or a folded pillow. This pelvic tilt is optimal to image the pelvic structures. A protective cover such as a condom, the finger of a clean rubber surgical glove, or a special probe cover provided by the manufacturer is used to cover the transducer probe. The probe is lubricated with a water-soluble gel and placed in the vagina either by the examiner or by the woman herself. During the examination the position of the probe or the tilt of the examining table may be changed so that the complete pelvis is in view. The procedure is not physically painful, although the woman will feel pressure as the probe is moved. Transvaginal ultrasonography is optimally used in the first trimester to detect ectopic pregnancies, monitor

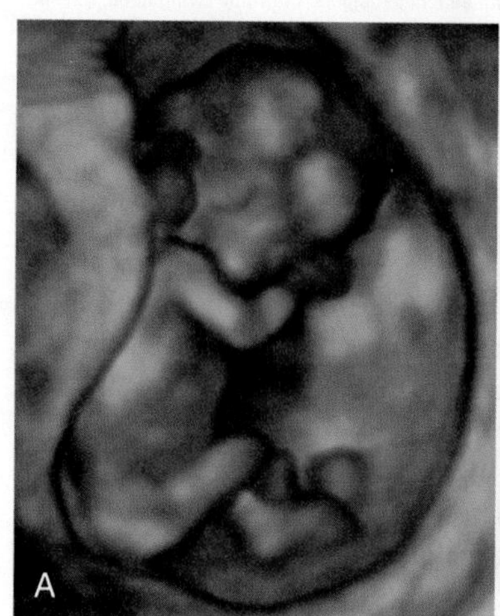

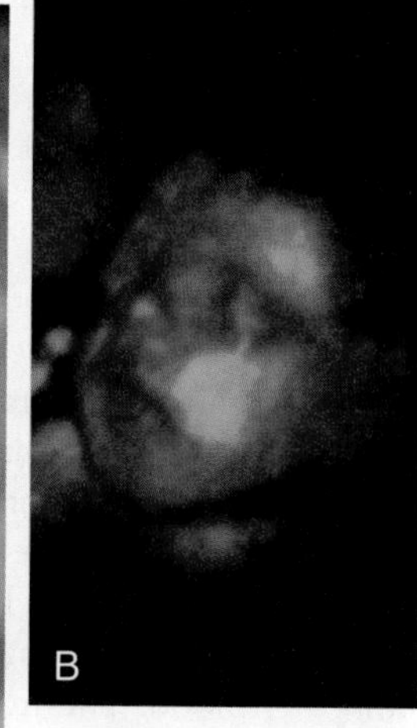

Fig. 19-1 Fetus seen on three-dimensional ultrasound. **A,** Full body view of fetus at 11 weeks and 6 days of gestation. **B,** Close-up view of fetal face later in pregnancy. (**A** Courtesy Shannon Perry, Phoenix, Az; **B** courtesy Margaret Spann, New Johnsonville, TN.)

the developing embryo, help identify abnormalities, and help establish gestational age. In some instances, it may be used as an adjunct to abdominal scanning to evaluate preterm labor in second- and third-trimester pregnancies.

Levels of ultrasonography

The American College of Obstetricians and Gynecologists (ACOG) (2004) describes three levels of ultrasonography. The *standard* examination is used most frequently and can be performed by ultrasonographers or other heath care professionals, including nurses, who have had special training. Indications for standard ultrasonography are described in detail in the next section. Its primary uses are to detect fetal viability, determine the presentation of the fetus, assess gestational age, locate the placenta, examine the fetal anatomic structures for malformations, and determine amniotic fluid volume (AFV). *Limited* examinations are performed for specific indications such as identifying fetal presentation during labor or evaluating fetal heart rate (FHR) activity when it is not detected by other methods (ACOG). *Specialized* or targeted examinations are performed if a woman is suspected of carrying an anatomically or a physiologically abnormal fetus. Indications for this comprehensive examination include abnormal findings on clinical examination, especially with polyhydramnios or oligohydramnios, elevated alpha-fetoprotein (AFP) levels, and a history of offspring with anomalies that can be detected by ultrasound examination. Specialized ultrasonography is performed by highly trained and experienced personnel (ACOG).

COMMUNITY ACTIVITY

Investigate the hospitals in your community to determine the level of treatment available for high risk obstetric patients. Identify criteria that would indicate that a patient would need to be transferred to a high risk facility. Describe ways to support family members through this process.

Indications for use

Major indications for obstetric sonography are listed by trimester in Table 19-1. During the first trimester, ultrasound examination is performed to obtain information regarding the number, size, and location of gestational sacs; the presence or absence of fetal cardiac and body movements; the presence or absence of uterine abnormalities (e.g., bicornuate uterus or fibroids) or adnexal masses (e.g., ovarian cysts or an ectopic pregnancy); and pregnancy dating (by measuring the crown-rump length).

During the second and third trimesters, information regarding the following conditions is sought: fetal viability, number, position, gestational age, growth pattern, and anomalies; AFV; placental location and maturity; presence of uterine fibroids or anomalies; presence of adnexal masses; and cervical length.

Ultrasonography provides earlier diagnoses, allowing therapy to be instituted sooner in the pregnancy, thereby decreasing the severity and duration of morbidity, both physical and emotional, for the family. For instance, early diagnosis of a fetal anomaly gives the family choices such as intrauterine surgery or other therapy for the fetus, termination of the pregnancy, or preparation for the care of an infant with a disorder.

Fetal heart activity. Fetal heart activity can be demonstrated as early as 6 to 7 weeks of gestation by real-time echo scanners and at 10 to 12 weeks by Doppler mode. Fetal death can be confirmed by lack of heart motion, the presence of fetal scalp edema, and maceration and overlap of the cranial bones.

TABLE 19-1

Major Uses of Ultrasonography during Pregnancy

FIRST TRIMESTER	SECOND TRIMESTER	THIRD TRIMESTER
Confirm pregnancy Confirm viability Determine gestational age Rule out ectopic pregnancy Detect multiple gestation Determine the cause of vaginal bleeding Use for visualization during chorionic villus sampling Detect maternal abnormalities such as bicornuate uterus, ovarian cysts, fibroids	Establish or confirm dates Confirm viability Detect polyhydramnios, oligohydramnios Detect congenital anomalies Detect intrauterine growth restriction (IUGR) Assess placental placement Use for visualization during amniocentesis	Confirm gestational age Confirm viability Detect macrosomia Detect congenital anomalies Detect IUGR Determine fetal position Detect placenta previa or abruptio placentae Use for visualization during amniocentesis, external version Biophysical profile Amniotic fluid volume assessment Doppler flow studies Detect placental maturity

Gestational age

Gestational dating by ultrasonography is indicated for conditions such as uncertain dates for the last normal menstrual period, recent discontinuation of oral contraceptives, bleeding episode during the first trimester, uterine size that does not agree with dates, and other high risk conditions. In fact, growing evidence suggests that pregnancies should be dated by an ultrasound performed before 22 weeks of gestation rather than by menstrual dates because the ultrasound dating is more accurate than even "sure" menstrual dates (Richards, 2007). The methods of fetal age estimation used include determination of gestational sac dimensions (at approximately 8 weeks), measurement of crown-rump length (between 7 and 12 weeks), measurement of the biparietal diameter (BPD) (after 12 weeks), and measurement of femur length (after 12 weeks) (Fig. 19-2). An ultrasound examination performed for pregnancy dating between 14 and 22 weeks of gestation is comparable to one performed during the first trimester in terms of accuracy. After that time, however, ultrasound dating is less reliable because of variability in fetal size (Richards).

Fetal growth. Fetal growth is determined by both intrinsic growth potential and environmental factors. Conditions that require ultrasound assessment of fetal growth include poor maternal weight gain or pattern of weight gain, previous pregnancy with intrauterine growth restriction (IUGR), chronic infections, ingestion of drugs (tobacco, alcohol, and over-the-counter and street drugs), maternal diabetes mellitus, hypertension, multifetal pregnancy, and other medical or surgical complications.

Serial evaluations of BPD, limb length, and abdominal circumference (AC) can allow differentiation among size discrepancy resulting from inaccurate dates, true IUGR, and macrosomia. IUGR may be symmetric (the fetus is small in all parameters) or asymmetric (head and body growth vary). Symmetric IUGR reflects a chronic or longstanding insult and may be caused by low genetic growth potential, intrauterine infection, undernutrition, heavy smoking, or chromosomal aberration. Asymmetric growth suggests an acute or late-occurring deprivation, such as placental insufficiency resulting from hypertension, renal disease, or cardiovascular disease. Reduced fetal growth is still one of the most frequent conditions associated with stillbirth. Macrosomic infants (those weighing 4000 g or more) are at increased risk for traumatic injury and asphyxia during birth. Macrosomia may also be characterized as symmetric or asymmetric.

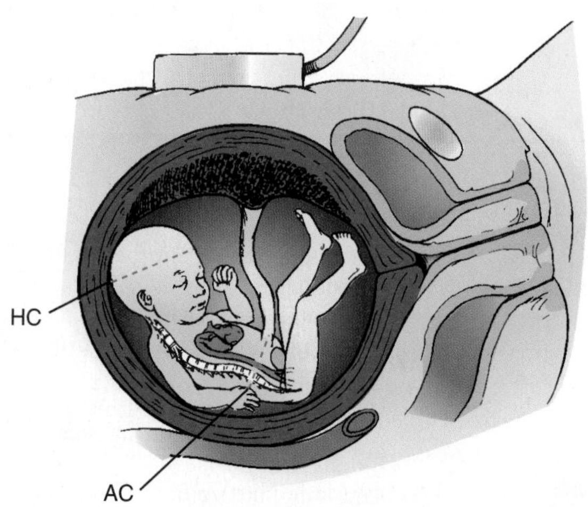

Fig. 19-2 Appropriate planes of sections *(dotted lines)* for head circumference (HC), and abdominal circumference (AC).

Fetal anatomy. Anatomic structures that can be identified by ultrasonography (depending on the gestational age) include the following: head (including ventricles and blood vessels), neck, spine, heart, stomach, small bowel, liver, kidneys, bladder, and limbs. Ultrasonography permits the confirmation of normal anatomy, as well as the detection of major fetal malformations. The presence of an anomaly may influence the location of birth (e.g., a subspecialty center versus a basic care center) and the method of birth (vaginal versus cesarean) to optimize neonatal outcomes. For example, plans are often made for a fetus with a condition that will require immediate surgery to be born in or nearby a hospital able to provide that care, rather than in a small community hospital that is totally unequipped to meet the newborn's needs.

The number of fetuses and their presentations also may be assessed by ultrasonography, allowing plans for therapy and mode of birth to be made in advance.

Fetal genetic disorders and physical anomalies. A prenatal screening technique called *nuchal translucency* (NT) screening uses ultrasound measurement of fluid in the nape of the fetal neck between 10 and 14 weeks of gestation to identify possible fetal abnormalities (Fig. 19-3). A fluid collection that is greater than 3 mm is considered abnormal. When combined with low maternal serum marker levels, an elevated NT indicates a possible increased risk of certain chromosomal abnormalities in the fetus, including trisomies 13, 18, and 21. An elevated NT alone indicates an increased risk of fetal cardiac disease. If the NT is abnormal, diagnostic genetic testing is recommended (ACOG, 2007; Gilbert, E.S., 2007).

Placental position and function. The pattern of uterine and placental growth and the fullness of the maternal bladder influence the apparent location of the placenta by ultrasonography. During the first trimester, differentiation between the endometrium and the small placenta is difficult. By 14 to 16 weeks the placenta is clearly defined; but if it is seen to be low lying, its relationship to the internal cervical os can sometimes be dramatically altered by varying the fullness of the maternal bladder. In approximately 4% to 6% of all pregnancies in which ultrasound scanning is performed during the second trimester the placenta seems to be overlying the os. However, more than 90% of cases of placenta previa diagnosed during the second trimester will have resolved by term, primarily because of the elongation of the lower uterine segment as

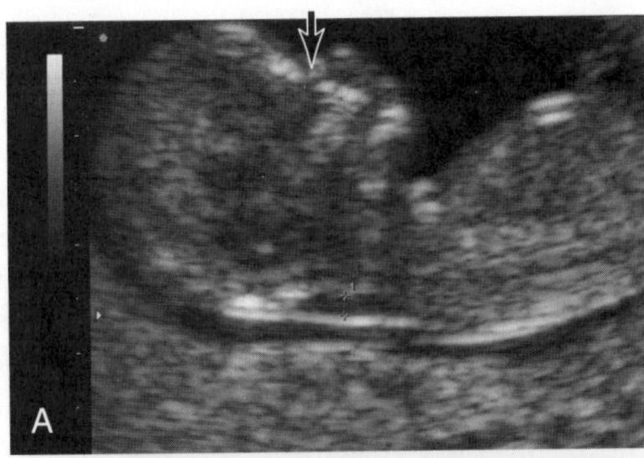

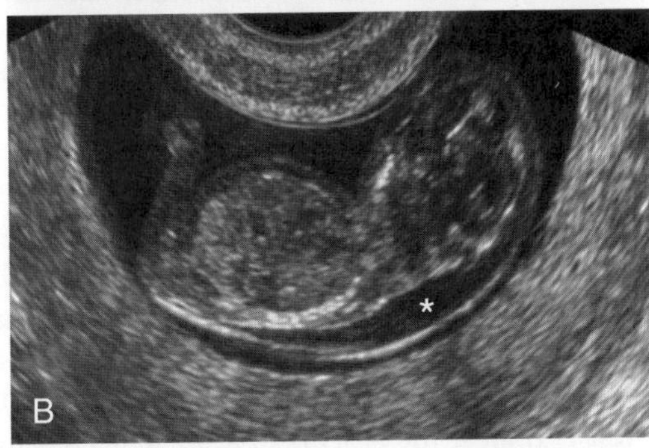

Fig. 19-3 Fetal nuchal translucency. **A**, Nuchal lucency (calipers) and nasal bone *(arrow)* in 12-week fetus. **B**, Increased nuchal translucency. Transvaginal ultrasound performed at 12 weeks demonstrates a sonolucent area *(asterisk)* over the posterior neck and upper thorax. (From Martin, R., Fanaroff, A., & Walsh, M. [2006]. *Fanaroff and Martin's neonatal-perinatal nursing: Diseases of the fetus and infant* [8th ed.]. Philadelphia: Mosby.)

pregnancy advances. Therefore, if placenta previa is diagnosed before 24 weeks of gestation, an ultrasound examination should be repeated between 28 and 32 weeks of gestation to confirm the diagnosis (Francois & Foley, 2007).

Another use for ultrasonography is grading of placental aging. Calcium deposits are of significance in postterm pregnancies because as they increase, the available surface area that can be adequately bathed by maternal blood decreases. Also, as blood vessels in the placenta age and thicken, oxygen transport is affected. Whether or not these placental changes adversely affect fetal outcomes in postterm pregnancies is unknown, however, given that most fetuses continue to grow (Gilbert, E.S., 2007).

Adjunct to other invasive tests. The safety of amniocentesis is increased when the positions of the fetus, placenta, and pockets of amniotic fluid can be identified accurately. Ultrasound scanning has reduced risks previously associated with amniocentesis, such as fetomaternal hemorrhage from a pierced placenta. Percutaneous umbilical blood sampling (PUBS) (also called cordocentesis) and chorionic villus sampling also are guided by ultrasonography to identify the cord and chorion frondosum accurately.

Fetal well-being

Physiologic parameters of the fetus that can be assessed with ultrasound scanning include AFV, vascular wave-

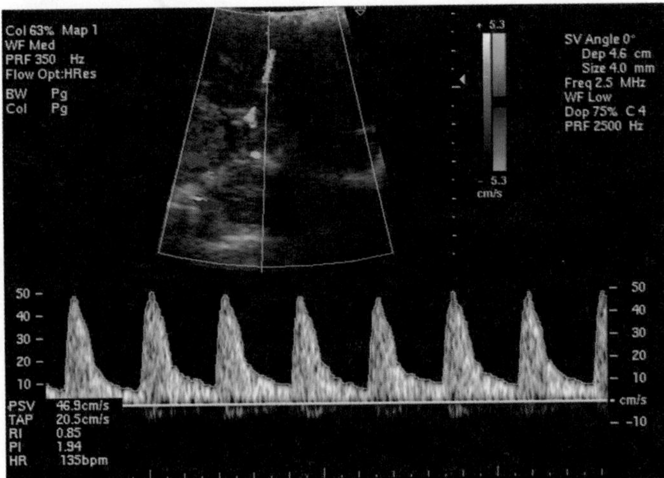

Fig. 19-4 Umbilical artery velocity waveform. (From Callen, P. [2000]. *Ultrasonography in obstetrics and gynecology* [4th ed.]. Philadelphia: Saunders.)

forms from the fetal circulation, heart motion, fetal breathing movements (FBMs), fetal urine production, and fetal limb and head movements. Assessment of these parameters, alone or in combination, yields a fairly reliable picture of fetal well-being. The significance of these findings is discussed in the following sections.

Doppler blood flow analysis. One of the major advances in perinatal medicine is the ability to study blood flow noninvasively in the fetus and placenta with ultrasound. Doppler blood flow analysis is a helpful adjunct in the management of pregnancies at risk because of hypertension, IUGR, diabetes mellitus, multiple fetuses, and preterm labor.

When a sound wave is reflected from a moving target, a change occurs in the frequency of the reflected wave relative to the transmitted wave, called the *Doppler effect.* An ultrasound beam scattered by a group of red blood cells (RBCs) is an example of this effect. The velocity of the RBCs can be determined by measuring the change in the frequency of the sound wave reflected off the cells (Fig. 19-4).

The shifted frequencies can be displayed as a plot of velocity versus time, and the shape of these waveforms can be analyzed to give information about blood flow and resistance in a given circulation. Velocity waveforms from umbilical and uterine arteries, reported as systolic/diastolic (S/D) ratios, can be first detected at 15 weeks of pregnancy. Because of the progressive decline in resistance in both the umbilical and uterine arteries, this ratio normally decreases as pregnancy advances. IUGR is seen more often in fetuses whose ratios remain elevated for their gestational age (Druzin, Smith, Gabbe, & Reed, 2007). Severely restricted uterine artery blood flow is indicated by absent or reversed flow during diastole (Tucker et al., 2009). In postterm pregnancies evaluated by Doppler umbilical flow studies an elevated S/D ratio indicates a poorly perfused placenta. Abnormal results also are seen with certain chromosome abnormalities (trisomy 13 and 18) and in the fetus of a mother who has systemic lupus erythematosus. Exposure to nicotine from maternal smoking also has been reported to increase the S/D ratio (see Fig. 19-4).

Amniotic fluid volume. Abnormalities in AFV are frequently associated with fetal disorders. Subjective determinants of oligohydramnios (decreased fluid) include the absence of fluid pockets in the uterine cavity and the impression of crowding of small fetal parts. An objective criterion of decreased AFV is met if the largest pocket of fluid measured in two perpendicular planes is less than 2 cm (Harman, 2009). Increased amniotic fluid is called *polyhydramnios* or sometimes just *hydramnios*. Subjective criteria for polyhydramnios include multiple large pockets of fluid, the impression of a floating fetus, and free movement of fetal limbs. Hydramnios is usually defined as pockets of amniotic fluid measuring more than 8 cm (Gilbert, W.M., 2007).

The total AFV can be evaluated by a method in which the vertical depth (in centimeters) of the largest pocket of amniotic fluid in all four quadrants surrounding the maternal umbilicus are totaled, providing an **amniotic fluid index (AFI).** A normal AFI is 10 cm or greater, with the upper range of normal around 25 cm. AFI values between 5 and 10 cm are considered to be low normal, whereas an AFI of less than 5 cm indicates oligohydramnios. With polyhydramnios the AFI would be above 25 cm (Tucker et al., 2009). Oligohydramnios is associated with congenital anomalies (e.g., renal agenesis), growth restriction, and fetal distress during labor. Polyhydramnios is associated with neural tube defects (NTDs), obstruction of the fetal gastrointestinal tract, multiple fetuses, and fetal hydrops.

Biophysical profile. Real-time ultrasound permits detailed assessment of the physical and physiologic characteristics of the developing fetus and cataloging of normal and abnormal biophysical responses to stimuli. The **biophysical profile (BPP)** is a noninvasive dynamic assessment of a fetus that is based on acute and chronic markers of fetal disease. The BPP includes AFV, FBMs, fetal movements, and fetal tone determined by ultrasound and FHR reactivity determined by means of NST. The BPP may therefore be considered a physical examination of the fetus, including determination of vital signs. FHR reactivity, FBMs, fetal movement, and fetal tone reflect current central nervous system (CNS) status, whereas the AFV demonstrates the adequacy of placental function over a longer period (Tucker et al., 2009). BPP scoring and management are detailed in Tables 19-2 and 19-3.

The BPP is used very frequently for antepartum fetal testing because it is a reliable predictor of fetal well-being. A BPP of 8 to 10 with a normal AFV is considered normal. Advantages of the test include excellent sensitivity and a low false-negative rate (Tucker et al., 2009). One limitation of the test is that, if the fetus is in a quiet sleep state, the BPP can require a long period of observation. Also, unless the ultrasound examination is videotaped, it cannot be reviewed (Druzin et al., 2007).

Nursing role

Although a growing number of nurses perform ultrasound scans and BPPs in certain centers, the main role of nurses is in counseling and educating women about the procedure. Ultrasound is widely used and, in fact, is considered a standard part of current prenatal care. Unlike

TABLE 19-2

Biophysical Profile Scoring

BIOPHYSICAL VARIABLE	NORMAL (SCORE = 2)	ABNORMAL (SCORE = 0)
Fetal breathing movements	At least one episode of >30 seconds' duration in 30 minutes' observation	Absent or no episode of ≥30 seconds' duration in 30 minutes
Gross body movement	At least 3 discrete body/limb movements in 30 minutes (episodes of active continuous movement considered a single movement)	Up to two episodes of body/limb movements in 30 minutes
Fetal tone	At least one episode of active extension with return to flexion of fetal limb(s) or trunk, opening and closing of hand considered normal tone	Either slow extension with return to partial flexion or movement of limb in full extension or absent fetal movement
Reactive fetal heart rate	At least two episodes of acceleration of ≥15 bpm and 15 seconds/duration associated with fetal movement in 30 minutes	Fewer than two accelerations or acceleration <15 bpm in 30 minutes
Qualitative amniotic fluid volume	At least one pocket of amniotic fluid measuring 2 cm in two perpendicular planes	Either no amniotic fluid pockets or a pocket <2 cm in two perpendicular planes

Source: Modified from Manning, F. A. (1992). Biophysical profile scoring. In J. Nijhuis (Ed.), *Fetal behavior.* New York: Oxford University Press. In Druzin, M., Smith, J., Gabbe, S., & Reed, K. (2007). Antepartum fetal evaluation. In S. Gabbe, J. Niebyl, & J. Simpson (Eds.), *Obstetrics: Normal and problem pregnancies* (5th ed.). Philadelphia: Churchill Livingstone.

TABLE 19-3

Biophysical Profile Management

SCORE	INTERPRETATION	MANAGEMENT
10	Normal infant; low risk of chronic asphyxia	Repeat testing at weekly intervals; repeat twice weekly in diabetic patients and patients at 41 weeks of gestation
8	Normal infant; low risk of chronic asphyxia	Repeat testing at weekly intervals; repeat testing twice weekly in diabetic patients and patients at 41 weeks of gestation; oligohydramnios is an indication for delivery
6	Suspect chronic asphyxia	If 36 weeks of gestation and conditions are favorable, deliver; if at >36 weeks and L/S <2.0, repeat test in 4-6 hours; deliver if oligohydramnios is present
4	Suspect chronic asphyxia	If 36 weeks of gestation, deliver; if <32 weeks of gestation, repeat score
0-2	Strongly suspect chronic asphyxia	Extend testing time to 120 minutes; if persistent score ≤4, deliver, regardless of gestational age

Source: Modified from Manning, F. A., Harman, C. R, Morrison, I., Menticoglou, S. M., Lange, I. R., & Johnson, J. M. (1990). Fetal assessment based on fetal biophysical profile scoring. *American Journal of Obstetrics and Gynecology, 162*, 703; Manning F. A. (1992). Biophysical profile scoring. In J. Nijhuis (Ed.), *Fetal behavior.* New York: Oxford University Press. In Druzin, M., Smith, J., Gabbe, S., & Reed, K. (2007). Antepartum fetal evaluation. In S. Gabbe, J. Niebyl, & J. Simpson (Eds.), *Obstetrics: Normal and problem pregnancies* (5th ed.). Philadelphia: Churchill Livingstone.
L/S, Lecithin/sphingomyelin.

many diagnostic tests, most women look forward to and enjoy their prenatal ultrasound. In the 30 years that diagnostic ultrasonography has been used, no evidence of any harmful effects on humans has emerged (Richards, 2007).

Magnetic Resonance Imaging

Magnetic resonance imaging (MRI) is a noninvasive radiologic technique used for obstetric and gynecologic diagnosis. Similar to computed tomography (CT), MRI provides excellent pictures of soft tissue. Unlike CT, ionizing radiation is not used; therefore vascular structures within the body can be visualized and evaluated without injecting an iodinated contrast medium, thus eliminating any known biologic risk. Similar to sonography, MRI is noninvasive and can provide images in multiple planes, but no interference occurs from skeletal, fatty, or gas-filled structures, and imaging of deep pelvic structures does not require a full bladder.

With MRI the examiner can evaluate fetal structure (CNS, thorax, abdomen, genitourinary tract, musculoskeletal system) and overall growth, the placenta (position, density, and presence of gestational trophoblastic disease), the quantity of amniotic fluid, maternal structures (uterus, cervix, adnexa, and pelvis), the biochemical status (pH, adenosine triphosphate content) of tissues and organs, and soft-tissue, metabolic, or functional anomalies.

The woman is placed on a table in the supine position and slid into the bore of the main magnet, which is similar in appearance to a CT scanner. Depending on the reason for the study the procedure may take from 20 to 60 minutes, during which time the woman must be perfectly still except for short respites. Because of the long time needed to produce MRIs, the fetus will probably move, which will obscure anatomic details. The only way to ensure that this problem does not occur is to administer a sedative to the mother, but this approach should be reserved for selected cases in which visualization of fetal detail is critical.

MRI has little effect on the fetus; concerns that the FHR or fetal movement would decrease have not been supported.

BOX 19-4

Fetal Rights

> Amniocentesis, percutaneous umbilical blood sampling (PUBS), and chorionic villus sampling (CVS) are prenatal tests used for diagnosing fetal defects in pregnancy. They are invasive and carry risks to the mother and fetus. A consideration of induced abortion is linked to the performance of these tests because no treatment for genetically affected fetuses has been developed; therefore the issue of fetal rights is a key ethical concern in prenatal testing for fetal defects.

BIOCHEMICAL ASSESSMENT

Biochemical assessment involves biologic examination (e.g., as chromosomes in exfoliated cells) and chemical determinations (e.g., lecithin/sphingomyelin [L/S] ratio and bilirubin level) (Table 19-4). Procedures used to obtain the needed specimens include amniocentesis, PUBS, chorionic villus sampling, and maternal sampling (Box 19-4).

Amniocentesis

Amniocentesis is performed to obtain amniotic fluid, which contains fetal cells. Under direct ultrasonographic visualization, a needle is inserted transabdominally into the uterus, amniotic fluid is withdrawn into a syringe, and the various assessments are performed (Fig. 19-5).

TABLE 19-4

Summary of Biochemical Monitoring Techniques

TEST	POSSIBLE FINDINGS	CLINICAL SIGNIFICANCE
MATERNAL BLOOD		
Coombs test	Titer of 1:8 and increasing	Significant Rh incompatibility
AFP	See AFP below	
AMNIOTIC FLUID ANALYSIS		
Color	Meconium	Possible hypoxia or asphyxia
Lung profile		Fetal lung maturity
L/S ratio	2:1	
Phosphatidylglycerol	Present	
S/A ratio (TDX FLM assay)	≥55 mg/g	
Creatinine	>2 mg/dl	Gestational age >36 weeks
Bilirubin (ΔOD, 450/nm)	<0.015	Gestational age >36 weeks, normal pregnancy
	High levels	Fetal hemolytic disease in Rh isoimmunized pregnancies
Lipid cells	>10%	Gestational age >35 weeks
AFP	High levels after 15 weeks of gestation	Open neural tube or other defect
Osmolality	Declines after 20 weeks of gestation	Advancing gestational age
Genetic disorders:	Dependent on cultured cells for karyotype and enzymatic activity	Counseling possibly required
Sex-linked		
Chromosomal		
Metabolic		

AFP, Alpha-fetoprotein; *L/S,* lecithin-sphingomyelin; *FLM,* fetal lung maturity; *S/A,* surfactant/albumin; *TDX FLM* assay, name of specific test used to determine S/A ratio.

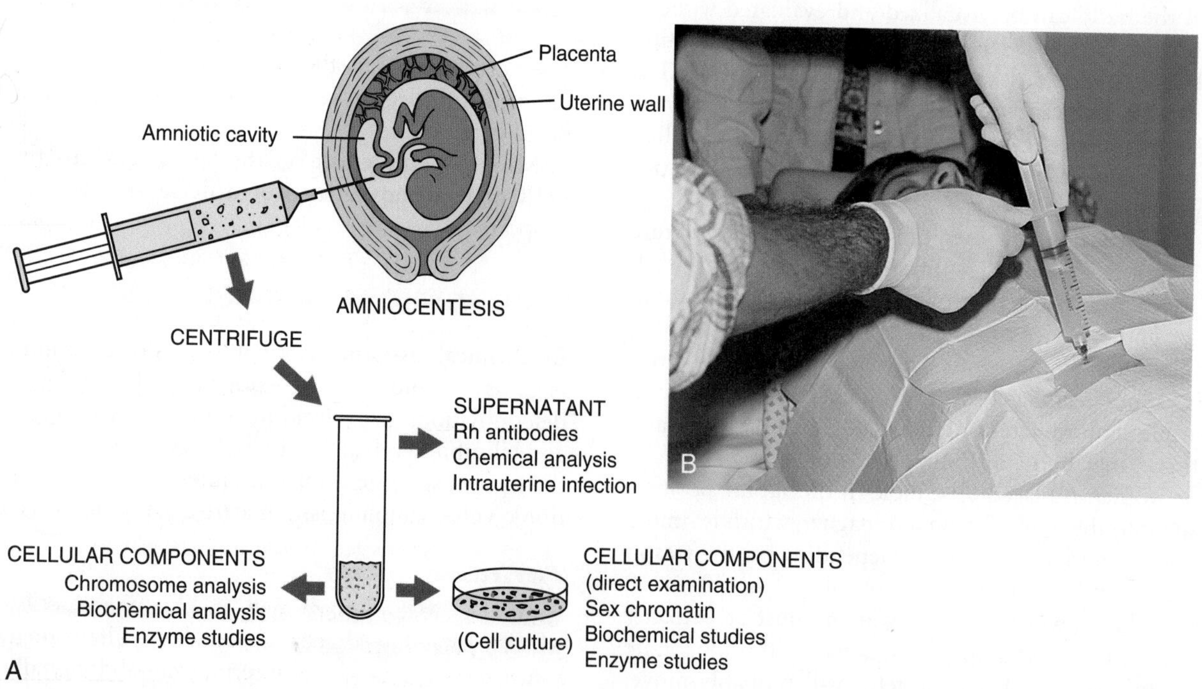

Fig. 19-5 **A,** Amniocentesis and laboratory use of amniotic fluid aspirant. **B,** Transabdominal amniocentesis. (**B,** Courtesy Marjorie Pyle, RNC, Lifecircle, Costa Mesa, CA.)

Amniocentesis is possible after week 14 of pregnancy, when the uterus becomes an abdominal organ, and sufficient amniotic fluid is available for testing. Indications for the procedure include prenatal diagnosis of genetic disorders or congenital anomalies (NTDs in particular), assessment of pulmonary maturity, and diagnosis of fetal hemolytic disease.

Complications in the mother and fetus occur in less than 1% of the cases and include the following:

- *Maternal:* hemorrhage, fetomaternal hemorrhage with possible maternal Rh isoimmunization, infection, labor, abruptio placentae, inadvertent damage to the intestines or bladder, and amniotic fluid embolism
- *Fetal:* death, hemorrhage, infection (amnionitis), direct injury from the needle, miscarriage or preterm labor, and leakage of amniotic fluid

NURSING ALERT Because of the possibility of fetomaternal hemorrhage, administering RhoD immune globulin to the woman who is Rh negative is standard practice after an amniocentesis.

Many of the complications have been minimized or eliminated by using ultrasonography to direct the procedure.

Indications for Use

Genetic concerns. Prenatal assessment of genetic disorders is indicated in women older than 35 years (Box 19-5), with a previous child with a chromosomal abnormality, or with a family history of chromosomal anomalies. Inherited errors of metabolism (such as Tay-Sachs disease, hemophilia, and thalassemia) and other disorders for which marker genes are known also may be detected. Fetal cells are cultured for karyotyping of chromosomes (see Chapter 5). Karyotyping also permits determination of fetal sex, which is important if an X-linked disorder (occurring almost always in a male fetus) is suspected.

Biochemical analysis of enzymes in amniotic fluid can detect inborn errors of metabolism. For example, AFP levels in amniotic fluid are assessed as a follow-up for elevated levels in maternal serum. High AFP levels in amniotic fluid help confirm the diagnosis of an NTD such as spina bifida or anencephaly or an abdominal wall defect such as omphalocele. The elevation results from the increased leakage of cerebrospinal fluid into the amniotic fluid through the closure defect. AFP levels may also be elevated in a normal multifetal pregnancy and with intestinal atresia, presumably caused by lack of fetal swallowing.

A concurrent test that finds the presence of acetylcholinesterase almost always indicates a fetal defect (Wapner, Jenkins, & Khalek, 2009). In such instances, follow-up ultrasound examination is recommended.

Fetal maturity. Accurate assessment of fetal maturity is possible through examination of amniotic fluid or its exfoliated cellular contents. The laboratory tests described are determinants of term pregnancy and fetal maturity (see Table 19-4). A quick means of determining an approximate L/S ratio is the *shake test* (foam test), or bubble stability test. Serial dilutions of fresh amniotic fluid are mixed with ethanol and shaken. After 15 minutes the amount of bubbles present at different dilutions indicates the presence of surfactant. Currently, the fetal lung maturity (FLM) assay is often used to determine fetal lung maturity because it is simple to perform. FLM test results are similar to those of the L/S ratio in terms of predicting pulmonary maturity (Mercer, 2009).

Fetal hemolytic disease. Another indication for amniocentesis is the identification and follow-up of fetal hemolytic disease in cases of isoimmunization. The procedure is usually not performed until the mother's antibody titer reaches 1:8 and is increasing. Although PUBS is still the procedure of choice to treat fetal hemolytic disease, it is now used less frequently for evaluating this condition. Doppler velocimetry of the fetal middle cerebral artery is currently used to predict anemia associated with fetal hemolytic disease accurately and noninvasively (Tucker et al., 2009).

BOX 19-5

Elimination of Maternal Age as an Indication for Invasive Prenatal Diagnosis

Maternal age of 35 years and older has been a standard indication for invasive prenatal testing since 1979. In January 2007, however, the American College of Obstetricians and Gynecologists (ACOG) published new guidelines stating that no specific age should be used as a threshold for invasive or noninvasive screening. Furthermore, all women, regardless of age, should have the option of invasive testing without first having screening (ACOG, 2007).

Chorionic Villus Sampling

The combined advantages of earlier diagnosis and rapid results have made chorionic villus sampling (CVS) a popular technique for genetic studies in the first trimester, although some risks to the fetus exist. Indications for CVS are similar to those for amniocentesis, although CVS cannot be used for maternal serum marker screening because no fluid is obtained. CVS performed in the second trimester carries no greater risk of pregnancy loss than amniocentesis, and it is considered equal to amniocentesis in terms of diagnostic accuracy (Simpson & Otano, 2007).

The procedure is performed between 10 and 12 weeks of gestation and involves the removal of a small tissue specimen from the fetal portion of the placenta (Figs. 19-6, 19-7). Because chorionic villi originate in the zygote, this tissue reflects the genetic makeup of the fetus.

CVS procedures can be accomplished either transcervically or transabdominally. In transcervical sampling a sterile catheter is introduced into the cervix under continuous ultrasonographic guidance, and a small portion of

EVIDENCE-BASED PRACTICE

Having a Baby Later In Life

Pat Gingrich

ASK THE QUESTION

What are the unique risks for advanced maternal age? Do differences exist in expectations and nursing care for older primiparas than for younger new mothers?

SEARCH FOR EVIDENCE

Search Strategies: Professional organization guidelines, meta-analyses, systematic reviews, randomized controlled trials, nonrandomized prospective studies, and retrospective studies since 2006.

Databases Searched: CINAHL, Cochrane, Medline, National Guideline Clearinghouse, TRIP Database Plus, and the websites for Association of Women's Health, Obstetric, and Neonatal Nurses (AWHONN) and Centers for Disease Control and Prevention.

CRITICALLY ANALYZE THE EVIDENCE

The childbearing years can span four decades of life. Many women are delaying childbirth well into their thirties or forties. Older mothers are more likely to be educated and have a higher socioeconomic status than younger mothers, but they may lack some of the robust physical resilience of youth.

Advanced maternal age is a risk factor for not only trisomy 21 (Down syndrome), but also increased stillbirths, preterm births, and small-for-gestational-age and low-birth-weight infants, particularly in primigravidas over 40 years of age (Delpisheh, Brabin, Attia, & Brabin, 2008). A systematic review of 37 studies confirms that the risk of stillbirth increases significantly over age 35 (Huang, Sauve, Birkett, Gergusson, & van Walraven, 2007).

Interestingly, even advanced age in the father may affect the offspring. A Danish study of 102,879 couples who gave birth from 1980 to 1996 demonstrated a significantly increased risk of mortality in offspring of fathers over age 45. The risk for mortality persisted into adulthood (Zhu, Vestergaard, Madsen, & Olsen, 2008).

IMPLICATIONS FOR PRACTICE

Most older mothers will have healthy and normal births. The nurse can ask open-ended questions about the baby and pregnancy so as to assess the psychosocial and emotional status of the patient. According to Suplee and associates (2007), older first-time mothers may have spent many years seeking pregnancy and therefore may bring a "last-chance" focus on this new role. The nurse needs to facilitate realistic expectations in the patient regarding life changes. Some older women expect a trouble-free, controlled, "no-risk" birth and a quick return to normal. They may need reminders of the need for flexibility about the birth process and the realities of postpartum adjustment. Others may be insecure about their physical and mental abilities and may see themselves as "high risk," requiring much care. The nurse can help her anxious patient focus on the normal and positive and encourage her to start envisioning holding her baby in her arms soon. Because these women may live far from extended family members, have aging parents, and their partners may work long hours, many older first-time mothers may not have an extensive social support system or even realize how isolated they will feel. Even after the birth, the nurse can provide the patient with resources about support groups and services, and encourage networking among new mothers and play groups (Suplee, Dawley, & Bloch, 2007).

References:

Delpisheh, A., Brabin, L., Attia, E., & Brabin, B. J. (2008). Pregnancy late in life: A hospital-based study of birth outcomes. *Journal of Women's Health*, 17(6), 965-970.

Huang, L., Sauve, R., Birkett, N., Gergusson, D., & van Walraven, C. (2007). Maternal age and risk of stillbirth: A systematic review. *Canadian Medical Association Journal*, 178(2), 165-172.

Suplee, P. D., Dawley, K., & Bloch, J. R. (2007). Tailoring peripartum nursing care for women of advanced maternal age. *Journal of Obstetric, Gynecologic, and Neonatal Nursing*, 36(6), 616-623.

Zhu, J. L., Vestergaard, M., Madsen, K. M., & Olsen, J. (2008). Paternal age and mortality in children. *European Journal of Epidemiology*, 23(7), 443-447.

the chorionic villi is aspirated with a syringe. The aspiration cannula and obturator must be placed at a suitable site, and rupture of the amniotic sac must be avoided (see Fig. 19-6).

If the abdominal approach is used, an 18-gauge spinal needle with stylet is inserted under sterile conditions through the abdominal wall into the chorion frondosum under ultrasound guidance. The stylet is then withdrawn, and the chorionic tissue is aspirated into a syringe (see Fig. 19-7).

Complications of the procedure include vaginal spotting or bleeding immediately afterward, miscarriage (in 0.3% of cases), rupture of membranes (in 0.1% of cases), and chorioamnionitis (in 0.5% of cases). Controversy exists concerning fetal limb reduction defects associated with CVS. Any increased risk appears to exist before 10 weeks of gestation. For this reason, CVS is usually not performed until after 9 menstrual weeks of gestation (Simpson & Otano, 2007).

NURSING ALERT Because of the possibility of fetomaternal hemorrhage, women who are Rh negative should receive immune globulin after CVS to prevent isoimmunization (Gilbert, E.S., 2007).

Use of amniocentesis and CVS is declining because of advances in noninvasive screening techniques. These techniques include measurement of NT, maternal serum screening tests in the first and second trimesters, and ultrasonography in the second trimester (Wapner et al., 2009).

Percutaneous Umbilical Blood Sampling

Direct access to the fetal circulation during the second and third trimesters is possible through percutaneous umbili-

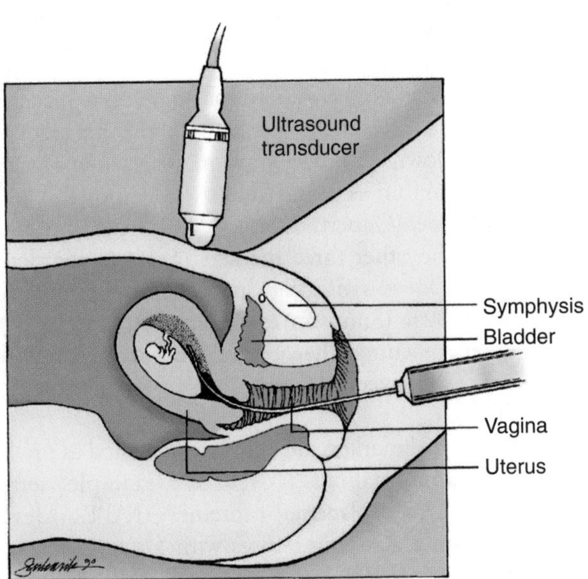

Fig. 19-6 Transcervical chorionic villus sampling. (From Gabbe, S., Niebyl, J., & Simpson, J. [2007]. *Obstetrics: Normal and problem pregnancies* [5th ed.]. Philadelphia: Churchill Livingstone.)

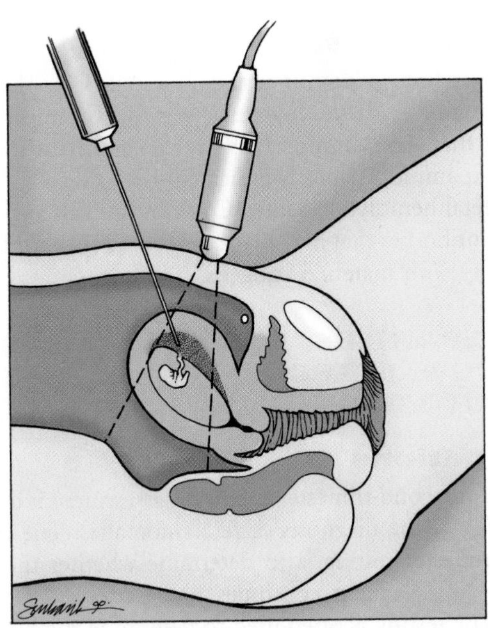

Fig. 19-7 Transabdominal chorionic villus sampling. (From Gabbe, S., Niebyl, J., & Simpson, J. [2007]. *Obstetrics: Normal and problem pregnancies* [5th ed.]. Philadelphia: Churchill Livingstone.)

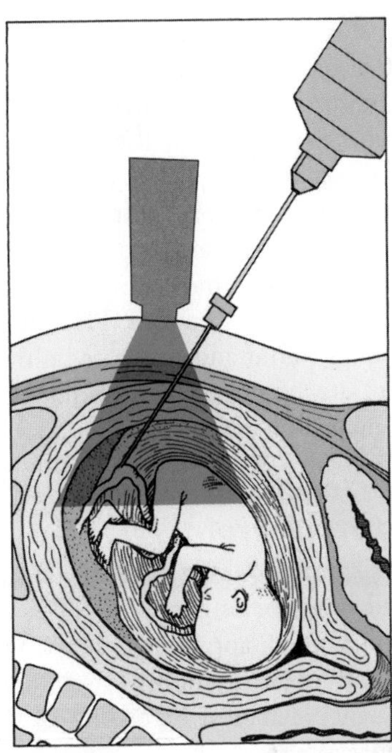

Fig. 19-8 Technique for percutaneous umbilical blood sampling guided by ultrasound.

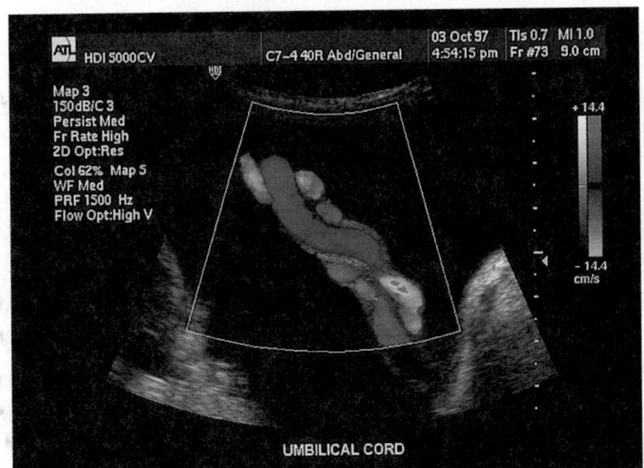

Fig. 19-9 Umbilical cord as seen on ultrasound at 26 weeks of gestation. (Courtesy Advanced Technology Laboratories, Bothell, WA.)

cal blood sampling (PUBS), or **cordocentesis**, which is the most widely used method for fetal blood sampling and transfusion. PUBS involves the insertion of a needle directly into a fetal umbilical vessel, preferably the vein, under ultrasound guidance. Ideally, the umbilical cord is punctured near its insertion into the placenta (Figs. 19-8, 19-9). At this point the cord is well anchored and will not move, and the risk of maternal blood contamination (from the placenta) is slight. Generally, a small amount of blood is removed and tested immediately by the Kleihauer-Betke procedure (Apt test) to ensure that it is fetal in origin (Simpson & Otano, 2007). Indications for use of PUBS include prenatal diagnosis of inherited blood disorders, karyotyping of malformed fetuses, detection of fetal infection, and assessment and treatment of isoimmunization and thrombocytopenia in the fetus (Wapner et al., 2009). Complications that can occur include loss of the pregnancy, hematomas, bleeding from the puncture site in the umbilical cord, transient fetal bradycardia, and fetomaternal hemorrhage. Maternal complications are rare, but include hemorrhage and transplacental hemorrhage (Simpson & Otano).

In fetuses at risk for isoimmune hemolytic anemia, PUBS permits precise identification of fetal blood type and RBC count and may prevent the need for further intervention. If the fetus is positive for the presence of maternal antibodies, a direct blood test can confirm the degree of anemia resulting from hemolysis. Intrauterine transfusion of severely anemic fetuses can be performed 4 to 5 weeks earlier than through the intraperitoneal route.

Follow-up includes continuous FHR monitoring for several minutes to 1 hour and a repeated ultrasound examination 1 hour later to ensure that no further bleeding or hematoma formation has occurred.

Maternal Assays

Alpha-fetoprotein

Maternal serum alpha-fetoprotein (MSAFP) levels have been used as a screening tool for NTDs in pregnancy. Through this technique, approximately 80% to 85% of all open NTDs and open abdominal wall defects can be detected early in pregnancy. Screening is recommended for all pregnant women.

The cause of NTDs is not well understood, but 95% of all affected infants are born to women with no family history of similar anomalies (Wapner et al., 2009). The defect occurs in approximately 2 of 1000 births in the United States. The rate of NTDs is decreasing as a result of the use of folate preconceptionally and during early pregnancy for prevention of this condition (Manning, 2009).

AFP is produced by the fetal liver, and increasing levels are detectable in the serum of pregnant women from 14 to 34 weeks. Although amniotic fluid AFP is diagnostic for NTD, MSAFP is a screening tool only and identifies candidates for the more definitive procedures of amniocentesis and ultrasound examination. MSAFP screening can be performed with reasonable reliability any time between 15 and 22 weeks of gestation (16 to 18 weeks being ideal) (Wapner et al., 2009).

Once the maternal level of AFP is determined, it is compared with normal values for each week of gestation. Values also should be correlated with maternal age, weight, race, and whether the woman has insulin-dependent diabetes. If findings are abnormal, follow-up procedures include genetic counseling for families with a history of NTD, repeated AFP, ultrasound examination, and possibly, amniocentesis.

Trisomy 21 (Down syndrome) and probably other autosomal trisomies are associated with lower-than-normal levels of MSAFP and amniotic fluid AFP. The *triple-marker test,* performed at 16 to 18 weeks of gestation, measures the levels of three maternal serum markers, MSAFP, unconjugated estriol, and human chorionic gonadotropin (hCG). In the presence of a fetus with Down syndrome the MSAFP and unconjugated estriol levels are low, whereas the hCG level is elevated. Low values in all three markers are associated with Trisomy 18 (Gilbert, E.S., 2007). Combining these three markers with the maternal age greatly increases detection of some trisomies.

The *quad-screen* adds an additional marker, a placental hormone called *inhibin A,* to increase the accuracy of screening for Down syndrome in women less than 35 years of age. Low inhibin A levels indicate the possibility of Down syndrome (Gilbert, E.S., 2007). The addition of inhibin A to the other three markers increases the detection rate for Down syndrome in the entire population from 70% to 80% (Simpson & Otano, 2007). Similar to triple marker screening, the optimal time to perform the quad-screen is between 16 and 18 weeks of gestation (Gilbert, E.S.).

Other maternal markers are being investigated as predictors of fetal abnormalities as well. For example, serum pregnancy-associated placental protein A (PAPP-A) levels are low in women carrying fetuses with Down syndrome (Simpson & Otano, 2007).

As with MSAFP, these tests are screening procedures only and are not diagnostic. A definitive examination of amniotic fluid for AFP and chromosomal analysis combined with ultrasound visualization of the fetus is necessary for diagnosis.

Coombs test

The indirect Coombs test is a screening tool for Rh incompatibility. If the maternal titer for Rh antibodies is greater than 1:8, amniocentesis for determination of bilirubin in amniotic fluid is indicated to establish the severity of fetal hemolytic anemia. Coombs test can also detect other antibodies that may place the fetus at risk for incompatibility with maternal antigens.

ANTEPARTAL ASSESSMENT USING ELECTRONIC FETAL MONITORING

Indications

First- and second-trimester antepartal assessment is directed primarily at the diagnosis of fetal anomalies. The goal of third-trimester testing is to determine whether the intrauterine environment continues to be supportive to the fetus. The testing is often used to determine the timing of childbirth for women at risk for UPI. Gradual loss of placental function results first in inadequate nutrient delivery to the fetus, leading to IUGR. Subsequently, respiratory function also is compromised, resulting in fetal hypoxia. Common indications for both the nonstress test (NST) and the contraction stress test (CST), sometimes called the oxytocin challenge test (OCT) are listed in Box 19-6.

No clinical contraindications exist for the NST, but results may not be conclusive if gestation is 26 weeks or less. In general the CST cannot be performed on women who should not deliver vaginally at the time the test is performed. Absolute contraindications for the CST are the following: preterm labor, placenta previa, vasa previa, cervical incompetence, multiple gestation, and previous classic incision for cesarean birth (Tucker et al., 2009).

Nonstress Test

The NST is the most widely applied technique for antepartum evaluation of the fetus. It is an ideal screening test and is the primary method of antepartum fetal assessment at most sites. The basis for the NST is that the normal fetus will produce characteristic heart rate patterns in response to fetal movement. In the term fetus, accelerations are associated with movement more than 85% of the time (Druzin et al., 2007). The most common reason for the absence of FHR accelerations is the quiet fetal sleep state. However, medications such as narcotics, barbiturates, and beta-blockers, maternal smoking, and the presence of fetal malformations can also adversely affect the test (Druzin; Gilbert, E.S., 2007). The NST can be performed easily and quickly in an outpatient setting because it is noninvasive, is relatively inexpensive, and has no known contraindications. Disadvantages include the requirement for twice-weekly testing and a high false-positive rate. The test also is slightly less sensitive in detecting fetal compromise than the CST or BPP (Tucker et al., 2009).

Procedure

The woman is seated in a reclining chair (or in semi-Fowler position) with a slight left tilt to optimize uterine perfusion and prevent supine hypotension. The FHR is recorded with a Doppler transducer, and a tocodynamometer is applied to detect uterine contractions or fetal movements. The tracing is observed for signs of fetal activity and a concurrent acceleration of FHR. If evidence of fetal movement is not apparent on the tracing, the woman may be asked to depress a button on a hand-held event marker connected to the monitor when she feels fetal movement. The movement is then noted on the tracing. Because almost all accelerations are accompanied by fetal movement, the movements need not be recorded for the test to be considered reactive. The test is usually completed within 20 to 30 minutes, but more time may be required if the fetus must be awakened from a sleep state.

Caregivers sometimes suggest that the woman drink orange juice or be given glucose to increase her blood sugar level and thereby stimulate fetal movements. This practice is common; however, research has not proven it to be effective (Druzin et al., 2007).

Vibroacoustic stimulation is often used to stimulate fetal activity if the initial NST result is nonreactive and thus hopefully shortens the time required to complete the test (Druzin et al.).

BOX 19-6

Indications for Electronic Fetal Monitoring Assessment Using the Nonstress Test and the Contraction Stress Test

- Maternal diabetes mellitus
- Chronic hypertension
- Hypertensive disorders in pregnancy
- Intrauterine growth restriction
- Sickle cell disease
- Maternal cyanotic heart disease
- Postmaturity
- History of previous stillbirth
- Decreased fetal movement
- Isoimmunization
- Hyperthyroidism
- Collagen disease
- Chronic renal disease

Interpretation

NST results are either reactive (Fig. 19-10) or nonreactive (Fig. 19-11). Box 19-7 lists criteria for both results.

A nonreactive test requires further evaluation. The testing period is often extended, usually for an additional 20 minutes, with the expectation that the fetal sleep state will change and the test will become reactive. During this time, vibroacoustic stimulation (see later discussion) may be used to stimulate fetal activity. If the test does not meet the criteria after 40 minutes, a CST or BPP will usually be performed. Once NST testing is initiated, it is usually repeated once or twice weekly for the remainder of the pregnancy (Druzin et al., 2007; Tucker et al., 2009).

Critical Thinking/Clinical Decision Making

Fetal Assessment Using the Nonstress Test

LaTonya is a 30-year-old G5 T3 P0 A1 L3 who is now at 41 weeks of gestation. Her physician has scheduled her for twice-weekly nonstress testing, and this appointment is her first. You are the nurse assigned to perform LaTonya's nonstress test (NST) today. As you help her get comfortable and attach the fetal heart rate and contraction monitors, LaTonya grumbles, "I don't see why I had to come get this test done. It was really hard to find a babysitter for my other kids, and I live on the other side of town!"

1. What is the purpose of performing fetal assessment tests, such as the NST, late in pregnancy?
2. What assumptions can be made about the following issues?
   a. The physiologic principle on which the NST is based
   b. Advantages of the NST
   c. Disadvantages of the NST
   d. The desired result of the NST
3. What implications and priorities for nursing care can be drawn at this time?
4. Does the evidence objectively support your conclusion?
5. Do alternative perspectives to your conclusion exist?

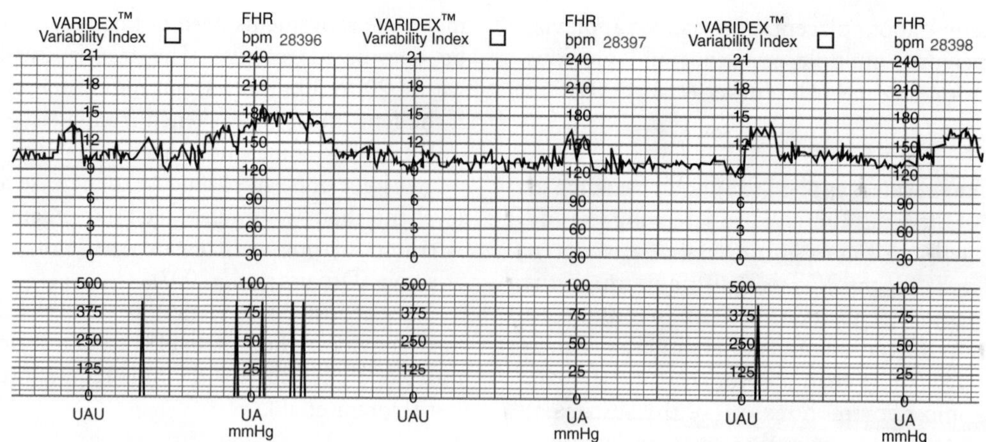

Fig. 19-10 Reactive nonstress test. (From Gabbe, S., Niebyl, J., & Simpson, J. [2007]. *Obstetrics: Normal and problem pregnancies* [5th ed.]. Philadelphia: Churchill Livingstone.)

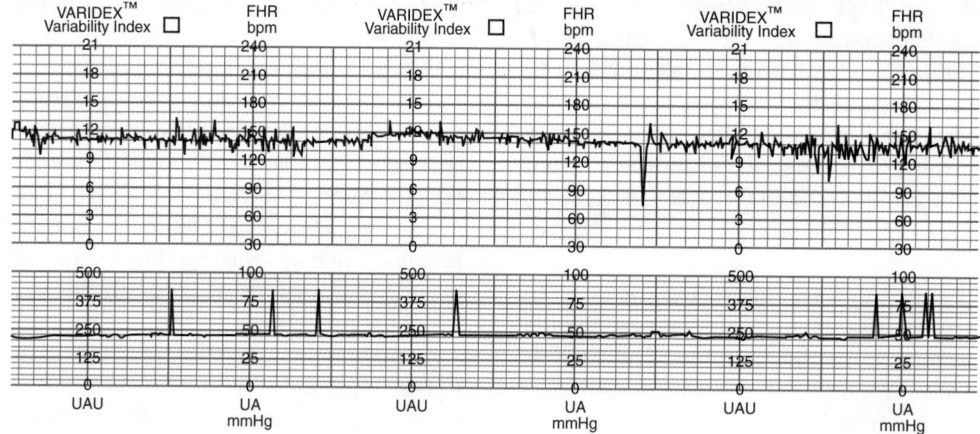

Fig. 19-11 Nonreactive nonstress test. (From Gabbe, S., Niebyl, J., & Simpson, J. [2007]. *Obstetrics: Normal and problem pregnancies* [5th ed.]. Philadelphia: Churchill Livingstone.)

BOX 19-7

Interpretation of the Nonstress Test

Reactive test: Two accelerations in a 20-minute period, each lasting at least 15 seconds and peaking at least 15 beats per minute above the baseline (Before 32 weeks of gestation, an acceleration is defined as an increase of at least 10 beats per minute and lasting at least 10 seconds.)

Nonreactive test: A test that does not produce two or more qualifying accelerations in a 20-minute period.

Source: Tucker, S. M., Miller, L. A, & Miller, D. A. (2009). *Mosby's pocket guide to fetal monitoring: A multidisciplinary approach* (6th ed.). St. Louis: Mosby.

Vibroacoustic Stimulation

Vibroacoustic stimulation (also called the *acoustic stimulation test*) is another method of testing antepartum FHR response. This test is generally performed in conjunction with the NST and uses a combination of sound and vibration to stimulate the fetus. Whether the acoustic or the vibratory component alters the fetal state is unclear. The test takes approximately 15 minutes to complete, with the fetus monitored for 5 to 10 minutes before stimulation to obtain a baseline FHR. If the fetal baseline pattern is nonreactive, the sound source (usually a laryngeal stimulator) is then activated for 3 seconds on the maternal abdomen over the fetal head. Monitoring continues for another 5 minutes, after which the monitor tracing is assessed. The desired result is a reactive NST. The accelerations produced may have a significant increase in duration (Fig. 19-12). The test may be repeated at 1-minute intervals up to three times when no response is noted. Further evaluation is needed with BPP or CST if the pattern is still nonreactive (Druzin et al., 2007).

Contraction Stress Test

The CST (or OCT) was the first widely used electronic fetal assessment test. It was devised as a graded stress test of the fetus, and its purpose was to identify the jeopardized

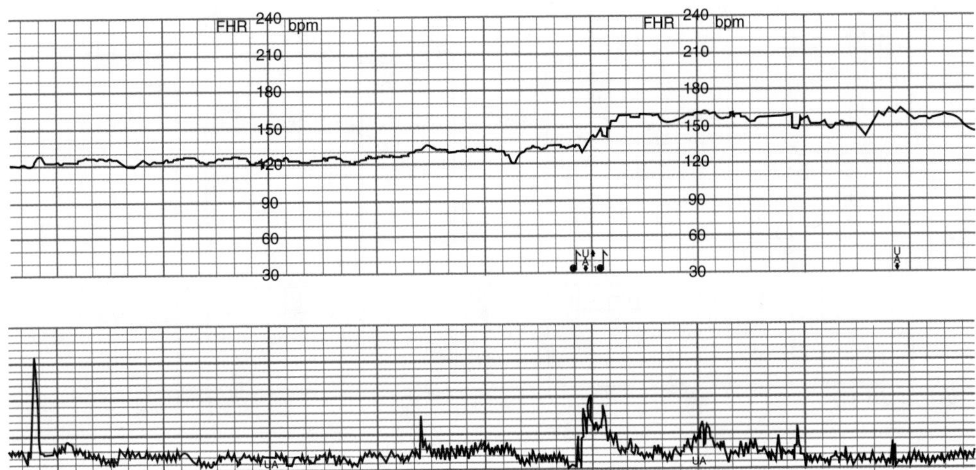

Fig. 19-12 Reactive NST after vibroacoustic stimulation. The stimulus was applied at the point marked by the musical notes. A sustained fetal heart rate acceleration was produced. (From Gabbe, S., Niebyl, J., & Simpson, J. [2007]. *Obstetrics: Normal and problem pregnancies* [5th ed.]. Philadelphia: Churchill Livingstone.)

fetus that was stable at rest but showed evidence of compromise after stress. Uterine contractions decrease uterine blood flow and placental perfusion. If this decrease is sufficient to produce hypoxia in the fetus, a deceleration in FHR will result.

NURSING ALERT In a healthy fetoplacental unit, uterine contractions do not usually produce late decelerations, whereas, if underlying UPI exists, contractions will produce late decelerations.

The CST provides an earlier warning of fetal compromise than the NST and with fewer false-positive results. However, in addition to the contraindications described earlier the CST is more time consuming and expensive than the NST. It is also an invasive procedure if oxytocin stimulation is required. Because of these disadvantages, the CST is infrequently used.

Procedure

The woman is placed in semi-Fowler position or sits in a reclining chair with a slight left tilt to optimize uterine perfusion and avoid supine hypotension. She is monitored electronically with the fetal ultrasound transducer and uterine tocodynamometer. The tracing is observed for 10 to 20 minutes for baseline rate and variability and the possible occurrence of spontaneous contractions. The two methods of CST are the nipple-stimulated contraction test and the oxytocin-stimulated contraction test.

Nipple-stimulated contraction test. Several methods of nipple stimulation have been described. In one approach the woman applies warm, moist washcloths to both breasts for several minutes. The woman is then asked to massage one nipple for 10 minutes. Massaging the nipple causes a release of oxytocin from the posterior pituitary. An alternative approach is for her to massage one nipple through her clothes for 2 minutes, rest for 5 minutes, and repeat the cycles of massage and rest as necessary to achieve adequate uterine activity. When adequate contractions or hyperstimulation (defined as uterine contractions lasting more than 90 seconds or five or more contractions in 10 minutes) occurs, stimulation should be stopped (Druzin et al., 2007).

Oxytocin-stimulated contraction test. Exogenous oxytocin also can be used to stimulate uterine contractions. An intravenous (IV) infusion is begun, and a dilute solution of oxytocin (e.g., 10 units in 1000 ml of fluid) is connected to the main line tubing through a piggyback port and delivered by an infusion pump to ensure an accurate dose. One method of oxytocin infusion is to begin at 0.5 milliunits/min and double the dose every 20 minutes until three uterine contractions of good quality, each lasting 40 to 60 seconds, are observed within a 10-minute period. A rate of 10 milliunits/min is usually adequate to elicit uterine contractions (Druzin et al., 2007).

Interpretation

CST results are either negative, positive, equivocal, suspicious, or unsatisfactory. If no late decelerations are observed with the contractions, the findings are considered negative (Fig. 19-13, *A*). Repetitive late decelerations render the test results positive (Fig. 19-13, *B*). Box 19-8 lists criteria for each possible test result.

The desired CST result is negative because it has consistently been associated with good fetal outcomes. With a negative result the test is repeated in 1 week. Positive CST results have been associated with intrauterine fetal death, late FHR decelerations in labor, IUGR, and meconium-stained amniotic fluid. A positive CST result usually leads to hospitalization for further close observation or

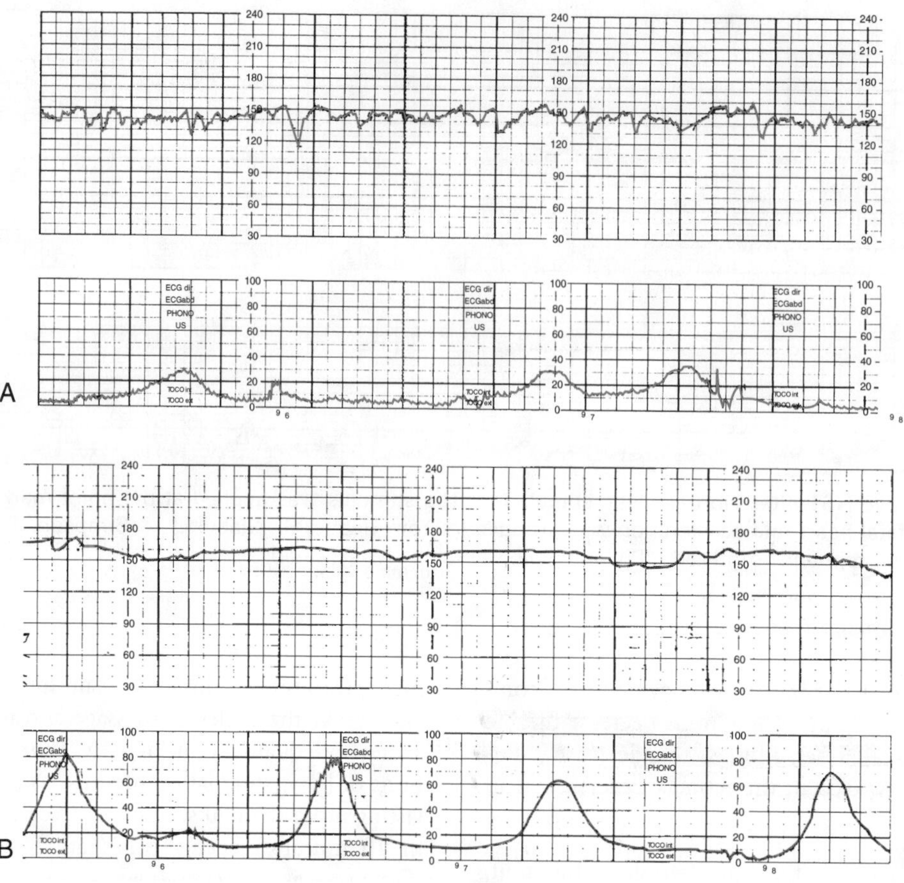

Fig. 19-13 Contraction stress test (CST). **A,** Negative CST. **B,** Positive CST. (From Tucker, S. [2004]. *Pocket guide to fetal monitoring and assessment* [5th ed.]. St. Louis: Mosby.)

BOX 19-8

Interpretation of the Contraction Stress Test

Negative test: At least three uterine contractions occur in a 10-minute period, with no late or significant variable decelerations.

Positive test: Late decelerations occur with 50% or more of contractions (even if fewer than three contractions occur in 10 minutes).

Equivocal-suspicious test: Prolonged decelerations, variable decelerations, or late decelerations occur with less than 50% of contractions.

Equivocal-hyperstimulatory test: Decelerations occur in the presence of contractions more frequent than every 2 minutes or lasting longer than 90 seconds.

Unsatisfactory test: Fewer than three uterine contractions in a 10-minute period or inability to obtain a continuous tracing of the fetal heart rate.

Source: Tucker, S. M., Miller, L. A., & Miller, D. A. (2009). *Mosby's pocket guide to fetal monitoring: A multidisciplinary approach* (6th ed.). St. Louis: Mosby.

delivery or both. Unsatisfactory, suspicious, and equivocal tests must be repeated within 24 hours (Druzin et al., 2007; Tucker et al., 2009).

NURSING ROLE IN ASSESSMENT OF THE HIGH RISK PREGNANCY

The nurse's role is primarily that of educator and support person when the woman is undergoing such examinations as ultrasonography, MRI, CVS, PUBS, and amniocentesis. In some instances the nurse may assist the physician with the procedure. In many settings, nurses perform NSTs, CSTs, and BPPs; conduct an initial assessment; and begin necessary interventions for nonreassuring results. These nursing procedures are accomplished after additional education and training, under guidance of established protocols, and in collaboration with obstetric providers. Patient teaching, which is an integral component of this role, involves preparing the woman for the procedure, interpreting the findings, and providing psychosocial support when needed.

KEY POINTS

- A high risk pregnancy is one in which the life or well-being of the mother or infant is jeopardized by a biophysical or psychosocial disorder coincidental with or unique to pregnancy.
- Biophysical, sociodemographic, psychosocial, and environmental factors place the pregnancy and fetus or neonate at risk.
- Biophysical assessment techniques include DFMCs, ultrasonography, and MRI.
- Biochemical monitoring techniques include amniocentesis, PUBS, CVS, and MSAFP.
- Reactive NSTs and negative CSTs suggest fetal well-being.
- Most assessment tests have some degree of risk for the mother and fetus and usually cause some anxiety for the woman and her family.

Audio Chapter Summaries Access an audio summary of these Key Points on evolve

References

American College of Obstetricians and Gynecologists (ACOG). (2007). *Screening for fetal chromosomal abnormalities. Practice Bulletin No. 77.* Washington, DC: ACOG.

American College of Obstetricians and Gynecologists (ACOG). (2004). *Ultrasonography in pregnancy. Practice Bulletin No. 58.* Washington, DC: ACOG.

Druzin, M., Smith, J., Gabbe, S., & Reed, K. (2007). Antepartum fetal evaluation. In S. Gabbe, J. Niebyl, & J. Simpson (Eds.), *Obstetrics: Normal and problem pregnancies* (5th ed.). Philadelphia: Churchill Livingstone.

Francois, K.E. & Foley, M.R. (2007). Antepartum and postpartum hemorrhage. In S. Gabbe, J. Niebyl, & J. Simpson (Eds.), *Obstetrics: Normal and problem pregnancies* (5th ed.). Philadelphia: Churchill Livingstone.

Gilbert, E. S. (2007). *Manual of high risk pregnancy & delivery* (4th ed.). St. Louis: Mosby.

Gilbert, W. M. (2007). Amniotic fluid disorders. In S. Gabbe, J. Niebyl, & J. Simpson (Eds.), *Obstetrics: Normal and problem pregnancies* (5th ed.). Philadelphia: Churchill Livingstone.

Harman, C. R. (2009). Assessment of fetal health. In R. K. Creasy, R. Resnik, & J. D. Iams (Eds.), *Creasy and Resnik's maternal-fetal medicine: Principles and practice* (6th ed.). Philadelphia: Saunders.

Manning, F. A. (2009). Imaging in the diagnosis of fetal anomalies. In R. K. Creasy, R. Resnik, & J. D. Iams (Eds.), *Creasy and Resnik's maternal-fetal medicine: Principles and practice* (6th ed.). Philadelphia: Saunders.

Mercer, B. M. (2009). Assessment and induction of fetal pulmonary maturity. In R. K. Creasy, R. Resnik, & J. D. Iams (Eds.), *Creasy and Resnik's maternal-fetal medicine: Principles and practice* (6th ed.). Philadelphia: Saunders.

Miller, L. A., Miller, D. A., & Tucker, S. M. (2013). *Mosby's pocket guide to fetal monitoring: A multidisciplinary approach* (7th ed.). St. Louis: Mosby.

Richards, D. S. (2007). Ultrasound for pregnancy dating, growth, and the diagnosis of fetal malformations. In S. Gabbe, J. Niebyl, & J. Simpson (Eds.), *Obstetrics: Normal and problem pregnancies* (5th ed.). Philadelphia: Churchill Livingstone.

Silbergeld, E., & Patrick, T. (2005). Environmental exposures, toxicologic mechanisms, and adverse pregnancy outcomes. *American Journal of Obstetrics and Gynecology, 192*(5), S11-121.

Simpson, J. L., & Otano, L. (2007). Prenatal genetic diagnosis. In S. Gabbe, J. Niebyl, & J. Simpson (Eds.), *Obstetrics: Normal and problem pregnancies* (5th ed.). Philadelphia: Churchill Livingstone.

Tucker, S. M., Miller, L. A, & Miller, D. A. (2009). *Mosby's pocket guide to fetal monitoring: A multidisciplinary approach* (6th ed.). St. Louis: Mosby.

Wapner, R. J., Jenkins, T. M., & Khalek, N. (2009). Prenatal diagnosis of congenital disorders. In R. K. Creasy, R. Resnik, & J. D. Iams (Eds.), *Creasy and Resnik's maternal-fetal medicine: Principles and practice* (6th ed.). Philadelphia: Saunders.

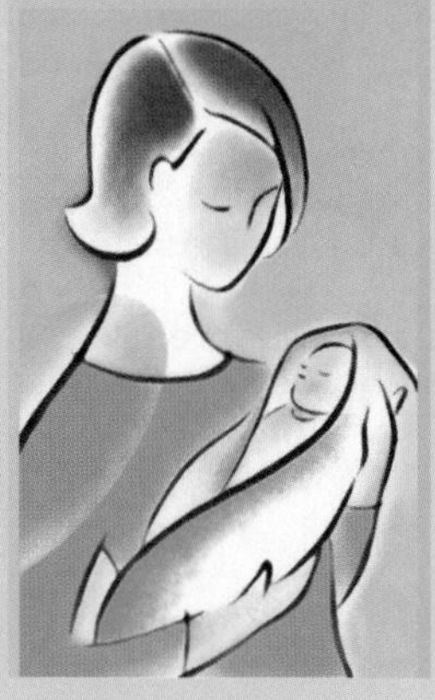

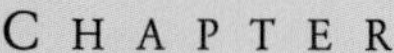

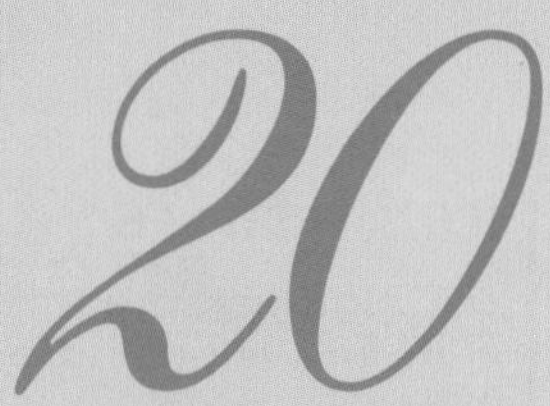

CHAPTER 20

Pregnancy at Risk: Preexisting Conditions

KITTY CASHION

LEARNING OBJECTIVES

- Differentiate the types of diabetes mellitus and their respective risk factors in pregnancy.
- Compare insulin requirements during pregnancy, postpartum, and with lactation.
- Identify maternal and fetal risks or complications associated with diabetes in pregnancy.
- Develop a plan of care for the pregnant woman with pregestational or gestational diabetes.
- Explain the effects of thyroid disorders on pregnancy.
- Differentiate the management for pregnant women with class I to class IV cardiac disease.
- Describe the different types of anemia and their effects during pregnancy.
- Explain the care of pregnant women with pulmonary disorders.
- Describe the effects of neurologic disorders on pregnancy.
- Outline the care of women whose pregnancies are complicated by autoimmune disorders.
- Discuss the care of pregnant women who use, abuse, or are dependent on alcohol or illicit or prescription drugs.

KEY TERMS AND DEFINITIONS

autoimmune disorders Group of diseases that disrupt the function of the immune system, causing the body to produce antibodies against itself, resulting in tissue damage

cardiac decompensation Condition of heart failure in which the heart is unable to maintain a sufficient cardiac output

euglycemia Pertaining to a normal blood glucose level; also called normoglycemia

gestational diabetes mellitus (GDM) Glucose intolerance first recognized during pregnancy

glycosylated hemoglobin A_{1c} Glycohemoglobin, a minor hemoglobin with glucose attached; the glycosylated hemoglobin concentration represents the average blood glucose level over the previous several weeks and is a measurement of glycemic control in diabetic therapy

hydramnios (polyhydramnios) Amniotic fluid in excess of 2000 ml

hyperglycemia Excess glucose in the blood, usually caused by inadequate secretion of insulin by the islet cells of the pancreas or inadequate control of diabetes mellitus

hyperthyroidism Excessive functional activity of the thyroid gland

hypoglycemia Less than a normal amount of glucose in the blood; usually caused by the administration of too much insulin, excessive secretion of insulin by the islet cells of the pancreas, or dietary deficiency

hypothyroidism Deficiency of thyroid gland activity with underproduction of thyroxine

ketoacidosis Accumulation of ketone bodies in the blood as a consequence of hyperglycemia; leads to metabolic acidosis

macrosomia Large body size as seen in neonates of mothers with pregestational or gestational diabetes

peripartum cardiomyopathy Inability of the heart to maintain an adequate cardiac output; congestive heart failure occurring during the peripartum

pregestational diabetes mellitus Diabetes mellitus type 1 or type 2 that exists before pregnancy

WEB RESOURCES

Additional related content can be found on the companion website at evolve

http://evolve.elsevier.com/Lowdermilk/Maternity/

- NCLEX Review Questions
- Case Study: Class III Cardiac Disorder
- Case Study: Pregestational Diabetes
- Critical Thinking Exercise: Gestational Diabetes
- Nursing Care Plan: Pregnancy Complicated by Pregestational Diabetes
- Nursing Care Plan: The Pregnant Woman with Heart Disease
- Nursing Care Plan: Substance Abuse during Pregnancy

For most women, pregnancy represents a normal part of life. This chapter discusses the care of women for whom pregnancy represents a significant risk because it is superimposed on a preexisting condition. However, with the active participation of well-motivated women in the treatment plan and careful management from a multidisciplinary health care team, positive pregnancy outcomes are often possible.

Providing safe and effective care for women experiencing high risk pregnancy and their fetuses is a challenge. Although unique needs related to the preexisting conditions are present, these high risk women also experience the feelings, needs, and concerns associated with a normal pregnancy. The primary objective of nursing care is to achieve optimal outcomes for both the pregnant woman and the fetus.

This chapter focuses on diabetes mellitus and other metabolic disorders and cardiovascular disorders. Select disorders of the respiratory system, gastrointestinal system, integumentary system, and central nervous system (CNS), as well as substance abuse are also discussed.

METABOLIC DISORDERS

Diabetes Mellitus

Around the world the incidence of diabetes mellitus is increasing at a rapid rate. In 2005 an estimated 20.8 million people (7% of the population) in the United States had been diagnosed with some form of diabetes. In the United States, experts predict a marked future increase in the number of women with preexisting diabetes who will become pregnant (Moore & Catalano, 2009). Diabetes mellitus is currently the most common endocrine disorder associated with pregnancy, occurring in approximately 4% to 14% of pregnant women (Gilbert, 2007). The perinatal mortality rate for well-managed diabetic pregnancies, excluding major congenital malformations, is approximately the same as for any other pregnancy (Landon, Catalano, & Gabbe, 2007). The key to an optimal pregnancy outcome is strict maternal glucose control before conception, as well as throughout the gestational period. Consequently, for women with diabetes, much emphasis is placed on preconception counseling.

Pregnancy complicated by diabetes is still considered high risk. It is most successfully managed by a multidisciplinary approach involving the obstetrician, perinatologist, internist or endocrinologist, ophthalmologist, nephrologist, neonatologist, nurse, nutritionist or dietitian, and social worker, as needed. A favorable outcome requires commitment and active participation by the pregnant woman and her family. Planning the pregnancy is preferable, working before conception with the woman and her family (Landon et al., 2007).

Pathogenesis

Diabetes mellitus refers to a group of metabolic diseases characterized by hyperglycemia resulting from defects in insulin secretion, insulin action, or both (American Diabetes Association [ADA], 2008). Insulin, produced by the beta cells in the islets of Langerhans in the pancreas, regulates blood glucose levels by enabling glucose to enter adipose and muscle cells, where it is used for energy. When insulin is insufficient or ineffective in promoting glucose uptake by the muscle and adipose cells, glucose accumulates in the bloodstream, and hyperglycemia results. Hyperglycemia causes hyperosmolarity of the blood, which attracts intracellular fluid into the vascular system, resulting in cellular dehydration and expanded blood volume. Consequently, the kidneys function to excrete large volumes of urine (polyuria) in an attempt to regulate excess vascular volume and to excrete the unusable glucose (glycosuria). Polyuria, along with cellular dehydration, causes excessive thirst (polydipsia).

The body compensates for its inability to convert carbohydrate (glucose) into energy by burning proteins (muscle) and fats. However, the end products of this metabolism are ketones and fatty acids, which, in excess quantities, produce ketoacidosis and acetonuria. Weight loss occurs as a result of the breakdown of fat and muscle tissue. This tissue breakdown causes a state of starvation that compels the individual to eat excessive amounts of food (polyphagia).

Over time, diabetes causes significant changes in both the microvascular and macrovascular circulations. These structural changes affect a variety of organ systems, particularly the heart, the eyes, the kidneys, and the nerves. Complications resulting from diabetes include premature atherosclerosis, retinopathy, nephropathy, and neuropathy.

Diabetes may be caused either by impaired insulin secretion, when the beta cells of the pancreas are destroyed by an autoimmune process, or by inadequate insulin action in target tissues at one or more points along the metabolic pathway. Both of these conditions are commonly present in the same person, and determining which, if either, abnormality is the primary cause of the disease is difficult (ADA, 2008). For additional information on diabetes, visit the American Diabetes Association's website at www.diabetes.org.

Classification

The current classification system includes four groups: type 1 diabetes, type 2 diabetes, other specific types (e.g., diabetes caused by genetic defects in B-cell function or insulin action, disease or injury of the pancreas, or drug-induced diabetes), and gestational diabetes mellitus (GDM) (ADA, 2008; Moore & Catalano, 2009). Approximately 90% of all pregnant women with diabetes have GDM (Gilbert, 2007). Of the women with pregestational diabetes, the majority (65%) of them have type 2 diabetes (Chan & Johnson, 2006).

Type 1 diabetes includes cases that are caused primarily by pancreatic islet beta cell destruction and that are prone to ketoacidosis. People with type 1 diabetes usually have an abrupt onset of illness at a young age and an absolute insulin deficiency. Type 1 diabetes includes cases currently thought to be caused by an autoimmune process, as well as those for which the cause is unknown (ADA, 2008; Landon et al., 2007).

Type 2 diabetes is the most prevalent form of the disease and includes individuals who have insulin resistance and usually relative (rather than absolute) insulin deficiency. Specific causes of type 2 diabetes are unknown at this time. Type 2 diabetes often goes undiagnosed for years because hyperglycemia develops gradually and is often not severe enough for the patient to recognize the classic signs of polyuria, polydipsia, and polyphagia. Most people who develop type 2 diabetes are obese or have an increased amount of body fat distributed primarily in the abdominal area. Other risk factors for the development of type 2 diabetes include aging, a sedentary lifestyle, family history and genetics, puberty, hypertension, and prior gestational diabetes. Type 2 diabetes often has a strong genetic predisposition (ADA, 2008; Moore & Catalano, 2009).

Pregestational diabetes mellitus is the label sometimes given to type 1 or type 2 diabetes that existed before pregnancy.

GDM is any degree of glucose intolerance with the onset or first recognition occurring during pregnancy. This definition is appropriate whether or not insulin is used for treatment or the diabetes persists after pregnancy. It does not exclude the possibility that the glucose intolerance preceded the pregnancy or that medication might be required for optimal glucose control. Women experiencing gestational diabetes should be reclassified 6 weeks or more after the pregnancy ends (ADA, 2008; Moore & Catalano, 2009).

White's classification of diabetes in pregnancy. Dr. Priscilla White, a physician who worked with pregnant women with diabetes during the 1940s, developed a classification system specifically for use with this group of women (Table 20-1). Dr. White's system was based on age at diagnosis, duration of illness, and presence of vascular disease (Landon et al., 2007; Moore & Catalano, 2009). Her classification system has been modified through the years but is still frequently used today to assess both maternal and fetal risk. Women in classes A through C generally have good pregnancy outcomes as long as their blood glucose levels are well controlled. Women in classes D through T, however, usually have poorer pregnancy outcomes because they have already developed the vascular damage that often accompanies long-standing diabetes.

Metabolic changes associated with pregnancy

Normal pregnancy is characterized by complex alterations in maternal glucose metabolism, insulin production,

TABLE 20-1

White's Classification of Diabetes in Pregnancy (Modified)

GESTATIONAL DIABETES	
Class A1	Patient has two or more abnormal values on the OGTT with a normal fasting blood sugar. Blood glucose levels are diet controlled.
Class A2	Patient was not known to have diabetes before pregnancy but requires medication for blood glucose control.
PREGESTATIONAL DIABETES	
Class B	Onset of disease occurs after age 20 and duration of illness <10 years.
Class C	Onset of disease occurs between 10 and 19 years of age or duration of illness for 10-19 years or both.
Class D	Onset of disease occurs <10 years of age or duration of illness >20 years or both.
Class F	Patient has developed diabetic nephropathy.
Class R	Patient has developed retinitis proliferans.
Class T	Patient has had a renal transplant.

Sources: Landon, M., Catalano, P., & Gabbe, S. (2007). Diabetes mellitus complicating pregnancy. In S. Gabbe, J. Niebyl, & J. Simpson (Eds.), *Obstetrics: Normal and problem pregnancies* (5th ed.). Philadelphia: Churchill Livingstone; Moore, T., & Catalano, P. (2009). Diabetes in pregnancy. In R. Creasy, R. Resnik, & J. Iams (Eds.), *Creasy and Resnik's maternal-fetal medicine: Principles and practice* (6th ed.). Philadelphia: Saunders.

OGTT, Oral glucose tolerance test.

and metabolic homeostasis. During normal pregnancy, adjustments in maternal metabolism allow for adequate nutrition for both the mother and the developing fetus. Glucose, the primary fuel used by the fetus, is transported across the placenta through the process of carrier-mediated facilitated diffusion, meaning that the glucose levels in the fetus are directly proportional to maternal levels. Although glucose crosses the placenta, insulin does not. Around the tenth week of gestation the fetus begins to secrete its own insulin at levels adequate to use the glucose obtained from the mother. Therefore, as maternal glucose levels rise, fetal glucose levels are increased, resulting in increased fetal insulin secretion.

During the first trimester of pregnancy the pregnant woman's metabolic status is significantly influenced by the rising levels of estrogen and progesterone. These hormones stimulate the beta cells in the pancreas to increase insulin production, which promotes increased peripheral use of glucose and decreased blood glucose, with fasting levels being reduced by approximately 10% (Fig. 20-1, *A*). At the same time, an increase in tissue glycogen stores and a decrease in hepatic glucose production occur, which further encourage lower fasting glucose levels. As a result of these normal metabolic changes of pregnancy, women with insulin-dependent diabetes are prone to hypoglycemia during the first trimester.

During the second and third trimesters, pregnancy exerts a "diabetogenic" effect on the maternal metabolic status. Because of the major hormonal changes, decreased tolerance to glucose, increased insulin resistance, decreased hepatic glycogen stores, and increased hepatic production of glucose occur. Rising levels of human chorionic somatomammotropin, estrogen, progesterone, prolactin, cortisol, and insulinase increase insulin resistance through their actions as insulin antagonists. Insulin resistance is a glucose-sparing mechanism that ensures an abundant supply of glucose for the fetus. Maternal insulin requirements gradually increase from approximately 18 to 24 weeks of gestation to approximately 36 weeks of gestation. Maternal insulin requirements may double or quadruple by the end of the pregnancy (Fig. 20-1, *B* and *C*).

At birth, expulsion of the placenta prompts an abrupt drop in levels of circulating placental hormones, cortisol, and insulinase (Fig. 20-1, *D*). Maternal tissues quickly regain their prepregnancy sensitivity to insulin. For the nonbreastfeeding mother the prepregnancy insulin-carbohydrate balance usually returns in approximately 7 to 10 days (Fig. 20-1, *E*). Lactation uses maternal glucose; therefore the breastfeeding mother's insulin requirements will remain low during lactation. On completion of weaning the mother's prepregnancy insulin requirement is reestablished (Fig. 20-1, *F*).

Pregestational Diabetes Mellitus

Case Study: Pregestational Diabetes

Approximately 2 per 1000 pregnancies are complicated by preexisting diabetes. Women who have **pregestational diabetes** may have either type 1 or type 2 diabetes, which may or may not be complicated by vascular disease, retinopathy, nephropathy, or other diabetic sequelae. Type 2 is the more common diagnosis compared with type 1. Almost all women with pregestational diabetes are insulin dependent during pregnancy. According to White's classification system, these women fall into classes B through T (see Table 20-1).

The diabetogenic state of pregnancy imposed on the compromised metabolic system of the woman with pregestational diabetes has significant implications. The normal hormonal adaptations of pregnancy affect

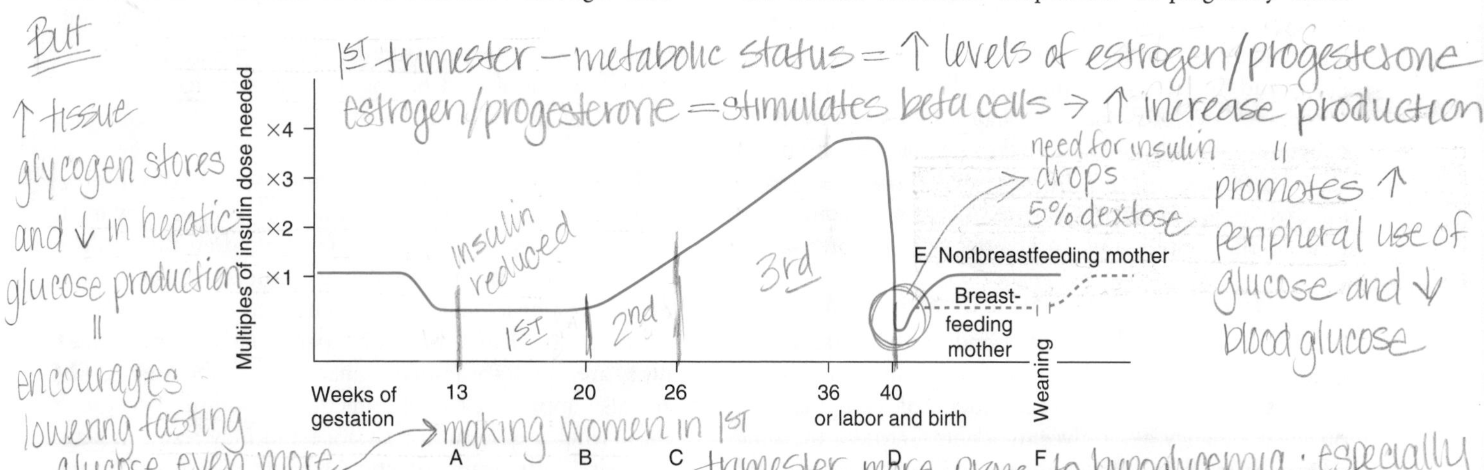

Fig. 20-1 Changing insulin needs during pregnancy. **A,** First trimester: Insulin need is reduced because of increased production by pancreas and increased peripheral sensitivity to insulin; nausea, vomiting, and decreased food intake by mother and glucose transfer to embryo or fetus contribute to hypoglycemia. **B,** Second trimester: Insulin needs begin to increase as placental hormones, cortisol, and insulinase act as insulin antagonists, decreasing insulin's effectiveness. **C,** Third trimester: Insulin needs may double or even quadruple but usually level off after 36 weeks of gestation. **D,** Day of birth: Maternal insulin requirements drop drastically to approach prepregnancy levels. **E,** Breastfeeding mother maintains lower insulin requirements, as much as 25% less than prepregnancy; insulin needs of nonbreastfeeding mother return to prepregnancy levels in 7 to 10 days. **F,** Weaning of breastfeeding infant causes mother's insulin needs to return to prepregnancy levels.

glycemic control, and pregnancy may accelerate the progress of vascular complications.

During the first trimester, when maternal blood glucose levels are normally reduced and the insulin response to glucose is enhanced, glycemic control is improved. The insulin dose for the woman with well-controlled diabetes may have to be reduced to prevent hypoglycemia. Nausea, vomiting, and cravings typical of early pregnancy result in dietary fluctuations that influence maternal glucose levels and may also necessitate a reduction in the insulin dose.

Because insulin requirements steadily increase after the first trimester, the insulin dose must be adjusted accordingly to prevent hyperglycemia. Insulin resistance begins as early as 14 to 16 weeks of gestation and continues to rise until it stabilizes during the last few weeks of pregnancy.

Preconception counseling

Preconception counseling is recommended for all women of reproductive age who have diabetes because it is associated with less perinatal mortality and fewer congenital anomalies (Moore & Catalano, 2009). Under ideal circumstances, women with pregestational diabetes are counseled before the time of conception to plan the optimal time for pregnancy, establish glycemic control before conception, and diagnose any vascular complications of diabetes. However, estimates indicate that fewer than 20% of women with diabetes in the United States participate in preconception counseling (Landon et al., 2007).

The woman's partner should be included in the counseling to assess the couple's level of understanding related to the effects of pregnancy on the diabetic condition and of the potential complications of pregnancy as a result of diabetes. The couple should also be informed of the anticipated alterations in management of diabetes during pregnancy and the need for a multidisciplinary team approach to health care. Financial implications of diabetic pregnancy and other demands related to frequent maternal and fetal surveillance should be discussed. Contraception is another important aspect of preconceptional counseling to assist the couple in planning effectively for pregnancy.

Maternal risks and complications

Although maternal morbidity and mortality rates have improved significantly, the pregnant woman with diabetes remains at risk for the development of complications during pregnancy. Poor glycemic control around the time of conception and in the early weeks of pregnancy is associated with an increased incidence of miscarriage. Women with good glycemic control before conception and in the first trimester are no more likely to miscarry than women who do not have diabetes (Moore & Catalano, 2009).

Poor glycemic control later in pregnancy, particularly in women without vascular disease, increases the rate of fetal macrosomia. **Macrosomia** has been defined in several different ways, including a birthweight more than 4000 to 4500 g, birthweight above the 90th percentile, and estimates of neonatal adipose tissue. Macrosomia occurs in approximately 40% of pregestational diabetic pregnancies and in up to 50% of pregnancies complicated by GDM (Landon et al., 2007; Moore & Catalano, 2009). Infants born to mothers with diabetes tend to have a disproportionate increase in shoulder, trunk, and chest size. Because of this tendency the risk of shoulder dystocia is greater in these babies than in other macrosomic infants. Women with diabetes therefore face an increased likelihood of cesarean birth because of failure of fetal descent or labor progress or of operative vaginal birth (birth involving the use of episiotomy, forceps, or vacuum extractor) (Landon et al.; Moore & Catalano).

Women with preexisting diabetes are at risk for several obstetric and medical complications. In general the risk of developing these complications increases with the duration and severity of the woman's diabetes. In one study the rates of preeclampsia, preterm birth, cesarean birth, and maternal mortality were much higher in women with preexisting diabetes than in women who did not have this disease. Approximately a third of women who have had diabetes for more than 20 years, for example, develop preeclampsia. Women with nephropathy and hypertension in addition to diabetes are also increasingly likely to develop preeclampsia. The rate of hypertensive disorders in all types of pregnancies complicated by diabetes is 15% to 30%. Chronic hypertension occurs in 10% to 20% of all diabetic pregnancies, and in up to 40% of those in women who have preexisting renal or retinal vascular disease (Moore & Catalano, 2009).

Hydramnios (polyhydramnios) occurs approximately 10 times more often in diabetic than in nondiabetic pregnancies. Hydramnios (amniotic fluid in excess of 2000 ml) is associated with premature rupture of membranes, onset of preterm labor, and postpartum hemorrhage (Cunningham, Leveno, Bloom, Hauth, Gilstrap, & Wenstrom, 2005).

Infections are more common and more serious in pregnant women with diabetes than in pregnant women without the disease. Disorders of carbohydrate metabolism alter the body's normal resistance to infection. The inflammatory response, leukocyte function, and vaginal pH are all affected. Vaginal infections, particularly monilial vaginitis, are more common. Urinary tract infections (UTIs) are also more prevalent. Infection is serious because it causes increased insulin resistance and may result in ketoacidosis. Postpartum infection is more common among women who are insulin dependent.

Ketoacidosis (accumulation of ketones in the blood resulting from hyperglycemia and leading to metabolic acidosis) occurs most often during the second and third trimesters, when the diabetogenic effect of pregnancy is the greatest. When the maternal metabolism is stressed by illness or infection, the woman is at increased risk for

EVIDENCE-BASED PRACTICE

Preconception Counseling for Women with Diabetes

Pat Gingrich

ASK THE QUESTION

What can we recommend for women with preexisting diabetes who desire pregnancy? What dietary advice can we offer to contribute to glycemic control?

SEARCH FOR EVIDENCE

Search Strategies: Professional organization guidelines, meta-analyses, systematic reviews, randomized controlled trials, nonrandomized prospective studies and retrospective studies since 2006.

Databases Searched: CINAHL, Cochrane, Medline, National Guideline Clearinghouse, TRIP Database and websites for Association of Women's Health, Obstetric, and Neonatal Nurses and Royal College of Obstetricians and Gynaecologists.

CRITICALLY ANALYZE THE DATA

The challenges of diabetes management become even greater during pregnancy, when hormonal changes, insulin resistance, and a growing fetus cause frequent shifts in glycemic control. Fetal risks associated with diabetes in pregnancy include anomalies, miscarriage, stillbirth, preterm birth, macrosomia leading to birth trauma or cesarean birth, and hypoglycemia. Maternal risks include increased retinopathy, nephropathy, preeclampsia, and injury from operative or cesarean birth.

The American Association of Clinical Endocrinologists (AACE, 2007) recommends that women be counseled before conception on the skills necessary to keep hemoglobin A_{1c} (Hgb A_{1c}) at less than 6%, blood glucose levels between 60 mg/dL fasting and 120 mg/dL at 1 hour after the first bite of a meal, and blood pressure under 130/80 mm Hg (AACE, 07). The guidelines further recommend evaluation of thyroid function, nephropathy, and retinopathy, as well as advice on healthy lifestyle and folic acid supplementation.

The professional guidelines on managing diabetes in pregnancy from the National Institute for Health and Clinical Excellence (Nice) (2008) recommend preconception counseling to optimize pregnancy outcomes. Good glycemic control should be established before conception and continue throughout pregnancy. The guidelines recommend counseling the diabetic woman seeking pregnancy about the role of diet, weight and exercise, the risks of hypoglycemia, the effects that nausea and vomiting can have on disease control, the risks of macrosomia, and assessment for retinopathy and nephropathy. Women should also know the risks to the neonate of hypoglycemia, as well as the possibility of obesity and diabetes later in life. They should understand the importance of glycemic control during labor and birth. The guidelines encourage women to attain a body mass index under 27 and a Hgb A_{1c} below 6.1% before conception (NICE).

All persons with diabetes should be counseled about the benefits of a low-glycemic diet. Low-glycemic foods slow down the digestion of food and moderate the postprandial glucose spike. The prevention of glucose extremes is especially importance in pregnancy. A Cochrane meta-analysis found that diabetic women and their babies can benefit from eating low-glycemic foods such as fruits, vegetables, whole grains, and legumes (Tieu, Crowther, & Middleton, 2008).

IMPLICATIONS FOR PRACTICE

Nurses are in an ideal position to counsel their patients with diabetes each year about the importance of glucose control and healthy habits before pregnancy. Women and their babies benefit from the skills that women learn about diet and exercise, as well as medical management of diabetes. Of particular benefit is the instruction in the low-glycemic diet. Women should be given the information they need to make informed decisions about their health and empowered by the knowledge to self-manage their care in partnership with the health team. Nurses should offer a positive message about their pregnancy and constant support, as well as frequent monitoring and follow-up. Women need emergency telephone numbers and other resources they can access anytime they have questions. Nurses can offer frequent encouragement and praise that pregnant women with diabetes are giving their babies the best possible start in life.

References:

American Association of Clinical Endocrinologists (AACE) Diabetes Mellitus Clinical Practice Guidelines Taskforce. (2007). AACE diabetes mellitus guidelines: diabetes and pregnancy. *Endocrine Practice, 13*(Supp. 1), 55-59.

National Institute for Health and Clinical Excellence (NICE). (2008). *Diabetes in pregnancy.* NICE Clinical Guideline No. 63. London: NICE.

Tieu, J., Crowther, C., & Middleton, P. (2008). Dietary advice in pregnancy for preventing gestational diabetes mellitus. In *The Cochrane Database of Systematic Reviews,* 2008, Issue 2, CD 006674.

COMMUNITY ACTIVITY

Research the March of Dimes website. Find out how the March of Dimes supports your community to prevent birth defects, prematurity, and infant mortality. Include efforts related to research, community service, education, and advocacy. Share findings and answer questions using a class discussion board. Inform classmates about volunteer opportunities that are available in the community related to these efforts.

diabetic ketoacidosis (DKA) DKA can also be caused by poor patient compliance with treatment or the onset of previously undiagnosed diabetes (Moore & Catalano, 2009). The use of beta-mimetic drugs such as terbutaline for tocolysis to arrest preterm labor may also contribute to the risk for hyperglycemia and subsequent DKA (Cunningham et al., 2005; Iams, Romero, & Creasy, 2009).

DKA may occur with blood glucose levels barely exceeding 200 mg/dl, as compared with 300 to 350 mg/dl in the nonpregnant state. In response to stress factors such as infection or illness, **hyperglycemia** occurs as a result of increased hepatic glucose production and decreased peripheral glucose use. Stress hormones, which act to impair insulin action and further contribute to insulin deficiency, are released. Fatty acids are mobilized from fat stores to enter into the circulation. As they are oxidized, ketone bodies are released into the peripheral circulation. The woman's buffering system is unable to compensate, and metabolic acidosis develops. The excessive blood glucose and ketone bodies result in osmotic diuresis with subsequent loss of fluid and electrolytes, volume depletion, and cellular dehydration. DKA is a medical emergency. Prompt treatment is necessary to prevent maternal coma or death. Ketoacidosis occurring at any time during pregnancy can lead to intrauterine fetal death. The incidence of DKA during pregnancy has decreased to approximately 2% from a rate of 20% or more in the past. The rate of intrauterine fetal demise (IUFD) with DKA, formerly approximately 35%, is currently 10% or less (Moore & Catalano, 2009) (Table 20-2).

The risk of **hypoglycemia** (a less-than-normal amount of glucose in the blood) is also increased. Early in pregnancy, when hepatic production of glucose is diminished and peripheral use of glucose is enhanced, hypoglycemia occurs frequently, often during sleep. Later in pregnancy, hypoglycemia may also result as insulin doses are adjusted to maintain **euglycemia** (a normal blood glucose level). Women with a prepregnancy history of severe hypoglycemia are at increased risk for severe hypoglycemia during gestation. Mild to moderate hypoglycemic episodes do not appear to have significant deleterious effects on fetal well-being (see Table 20-2).

Fetal and neonatal risks and complications

From the moment of conception the infant of a woman with diabetes faces an increased risk of complications that may occur during the antepartum, intrapartum, or neonatal periods. Infant morbidity and mortality rates associated with diabetic pregnancy are significantly reduced with strict control of maternal glucose levels before and during pregnancy.

Despite the improvements in care of pregnant women with diabetes, **intrauterine fetal demise (IUFD)** (sometimes known as *stillbirth*) is still a major concern. Approximately 2% to 5% of all fetal deaths occur in women whose pregnancies are complicated by preexisting diabetes. Hyperglycemia, ketoacidosis, congenital anomalies, infections, and maternal obesity are thought to be reasons for fetal death. In the third trimester, fetal acidosis is the most likely cause of fetal death (Paidas & Hossain, 2009).

The most important cause of perinatal loss in diabetic pregnancy is congenital malformations, which account for 30% to 50% of all perinatal loss (Lindsay, 2006). The incidence of congenital malformations is related to the severity and duration of the diabetes. Hyperglycemia during the first trimester of pregnancy, when organs and organ systems are forming, is the main cause of diabetes-associated birth defects. Anomalies commonly seen in infants affect primarily the cardiovascular system, the CNS, and the skeletal system (Cunningham et al., 2005; Moore & Catalano, 2009) (see Chapter 24).

The fetal pancreas begins to secrete insulin at 10 to 14 weeks of gestation. The fetus responds to maternal hyperglycemia by secreting large amounts of insulin (hyperinsulinism). Insulin acts as a growth hormone, causing the fetus to produce excess stores of glycogen, protein, and adipose tissue and leading to increased fetal size, or macrosomia. Birth injuries are more common in infants born to mothers with diabetes compared with mothers who do not have diabetes and macrosomic fetuses have the highest risk for this complication. Common birth injuries associated with diabetic pregnancies include brachial plexus palsy, facial nerve injury, humerus or clavicle fracture, and cephalhematoma. Most of these injuries are associated with difficult vaginal birth and shoulder dystocia (Moore & Catalano, 2009). Hypoglycemia at birth is also a risk for infants born to mothers with diabetes (for further discussion of neonatal complications related to maternal diabetes, see Chapter 24).

CARE MANAGEMENT

Antepartum

When a pregnant woman with diabetes initiates prenatal care, a thorough evaluation of her health status is completed. At the initial visit a complete physical examination is performed to assess the woman's current health status. In addition to the routine prenatal examination, specific efforts are made to assess the effects of the diabetes, specifically diabetic retinopathy, nephropathy, autonomic neuropathy, and coronary artery disease (Gilbert, 2007) (see Nursing Process box: Preexisting Diabetes).

In addition to routine prenatal laboratory tests, baseline renal function may be assessed with a 24-hour urine collection for total protein excretion and creatinine clearance. Urinalysis and culture are performed to assess for the presence of UTI, which is common in diabetic pregnancy. Because of the risk of coexisting thyroid disease, thyroid function tests may also be performed (see later discussion of thyroid disorders). The **glycosylated hemoglobin A_{1c}** level may be measured to assess recent glycemic control. With prolonged hyperglycemia, some of the hemoglobin remains saturated with glucose for the life of the red blood cell (RBC). Therefore a test for glycosylated hemoglobin provides a measure of glycemic control over time, specifically over the previous 4 to 6 weeks. Hemoglobin A_{1c} levels above 7 indicate elevated glucose during the previous 4 to 6 weeks (Gilbert, 2007). Fasting blood glucose or random (1 to 2 hours after eating) glucose levels may be assessed during antepartum visits (Fig. 20-2). Self-monitoring blood glucose records may also be reviewed.

TABLE 20-2

Differentiation of Hypoglycemia (Insulin Shock) and Hyperglycemia (Diabetic Ketoacidosis)

CAUSES	ONSET	SYMPTOMS	INTERVENTIONS
HYPOGLYCEMIA (INSULIN SHOCK)			
Excess insulin Insufficient food (delayed or missed meals) Excessive exercise or work Indigestion, diarrhea, vomiting	Rapid (regular insulin) Gradual (modified insulin or oral hypoglycemic agents)	Irritability Hunger Sweating Nervousness Personality change Weakness Fatigue Blurred or double vision Dizziness Headache Pallor; clammy skin Shallow respirations Rapid pulse Laboratory values Urine: negative for sugar and acetone Blood glucose: ≤60 mg/dl	Check blood glucose level when symptoms first appear. Eat or drink 15 g fast sugar (simple carbohydrate) immediately. Recheck blood glucose level in 15 min, and eat or drink another 15 g fast sugar (simple carbohydrate) if glucose remains low. Recheck blood glucose level in 15 min. Notify primary health care provider if no change in glucose level. If woman is unconscious, administer 50% dextrose IV push, 5% to 10% dextrose in water IV drip, or 1 mg glucagon subcutaneously. Obtain blood and urine specimens for laboratory testing.
HYPERGLYCEMIA (DKA)			
Insufficient insulin Excess or wrong kind of food Infection, injuries, illness Emotional stress Insufficient exercise	Slow (hours to days)	Thirst Nausea or vomiting Abdominal pain Constipation Drowsiness Dim vision Increased urination Headache Flushed, dry skin Rapid breathing Weak, rapid pulse Acetone (fruity) breath odor Laboratory value Urine: positive for sugar and acetone Blood glucose: ≥200 mg/dl	Notify primary health care provider. Administer insulin in accordance with blood glucose levels. Give IV fluids such as normal saline solution or one half normal saline solution; potassium when urinary output is adequate; bicarbonate for pH <7. Monitor laboratory testing of blood and urine.

DKA, Diabetic ketoacidosis; *IV,* intravenous.

Because of her high risk status, a woman with diabetes is monitored much more frequently and thoroughly than other pregnant women. During the first and second trimesters of pregnancy, her routine prenatal care visits will be scheduled every 1 to 2 weeks. In the last trimester, she will likely be seen one or two times each week. In the past, routine hospitalization for management of the diabetes, such as insulin dose changes, was common. With the availability of improved home glucose monitoring and the growing reluctance of third-party payers to reimburse for hospitalization, pregnant women with diabetes are now generally managed as outpatients. Some patient and family

NURSING PROCESS *Pregestational Diabetes*

ASSESSMENT

When a pregnant woman with diabetes initiates prenatal care, a thorough evaluation of her health status is completed. The assessment includes the following areas.

History

- Routine prenatal history
- Onset and course of diabetes
- Degree of glycemic control before pregnancy

Interview

- Learning needs:
  - Diabetes in pregnancy
  - Potential fetal complications
  - Plan of care
- Emotional status:
  - Coping with pregnancy superimposed on preexisting diabetes
  - Dealing with "high risk" status
  - Fear of maternal and fetal complications
  - Major changes in patterns of daily living so as to comply with plan of care
  - Support system
- Identifying significant persons and their roles:
  - Assess their reactions to the pregnancy and the management plan.
  - Assess their involvement in the treatment regimen.

Physical examination

- Assess current health status
- Perform routine prenatal examination
- Determine effects of diabetes on pregnancy:
  - Perform a baseline electrocardiogram to assess cardiovascular status.
  - Evaluate for retinopathy with follow-up as needed by an ophthalmologist each trimester and more often if retinopathy is diagnosed.
  - Monitor blood pressure.
  - Monitor weight gain.
  - Assess fundal height.

Laboratory tests

- Glycosylated hemoglobin (hemoglobin A_{1c})
- 24-hour urine collection for total protein excretion and creatinine clearance.
- Urinalysis and culture: initial prenatal visit and throughout the pregnancy
- Urine dipstick for ketones
- Thyroid function tests

NURSING DIAGNOSES

Nursing diagnoses for the woman with pregestational diabetes include the following:

- *Deficient knowledge* related to:
  - Diabetic pregnancy, management, and potential effects on the pregnant woman and fetus
- *Anxiety, fear, dysfunctional grieving, powerlessness, disturbed body image, situational low self-esteem, spiritual distress, ineffective role performance,* and *interrupted family processes* related to:
  - Stigma of being labeled *diabetic*
  - Effects of diabetes and its potential sequelae on the pregnant woman and the fetus
- *Risk for injury to fetus* related to:
  - Uteroplacental insufficiency
  - Birth trauma
- *Risk for injury to mother* related to:
  - Failure to follow a diabetic diet
  - Improper insulin administration
  - Hypoglycemia and hyperglycemia
  - Cesarean or operative vaginal birth
  - Postpartum infection

EXPECTED OUTCOMES OF CARE

Expected outcomes of care for the pregnant woman with pregestational diabetes include that she will do the following:

- Demonstrate or verbalize understanding of diabetic pregnancy, the plan of care, and the importance of glycemic control.
- Achieve and maintain glycemic control.
- Demonstrate effective coping.
- Experience no complications (maternal morbidity or mortality).
- Give birth to a healthy infant at term.

PLAN OF CARE AND INTERVENTIONS

Antepartum

- Routine prenatal visits every 1 to 2 weeks in first and second trimester and one to two times per week in the third trimester.
- Education:
  - Home glucose monitoring
  - Importance of a consistent daily schedule to maintain tight glucose control
  - Importance of good foot care and general skin care
- Diet:
  - Nutrition counseling by a registered dietitian
- Insulin therapy
- Exercise as prescribed by the primary health care provider
- Fetal surveillance:
  - Ultrasound examinations throughout pregnancy to determine gestational age, monitor fetal growth, and assess for hydramnios and anomalies
  - Maternal serum alpha-fetoprotein determination to screen for neural tube defects
  - Daily fetal movement counts (beginning at 28 weeks of gestation)
  - Nonstress tests, contraction stress tests, or biophysical profiles once or twice weekly (beginning at 34 weeks of gestation or sooner)

Intrapartum

- Determine blood glucose hourly.
- Administer regular insulin by intravenous drip as needed to maintain blood glucose levels in desired range.
- Monitor fetal heart rate (FHR) continuously.
- Observe for fetal dystocia.
- Ensure that a neonatal care provider is present at birth.

Postpartum

- Monitor blood glucose levels and adjust insulin dose as appropriate.
- Observe for complications (preeclampsia, hemorrhage, infection).
- Encourage breastfeeding.
- Provide family planning education.

EVALUATION

Evaluation of the effectiveness of care is based on the expected outcomes, which are closely associated with the degree of maternal metabolic control during pregnancy.

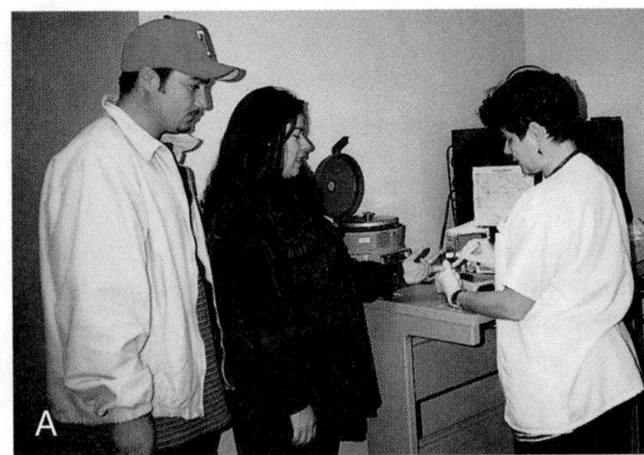
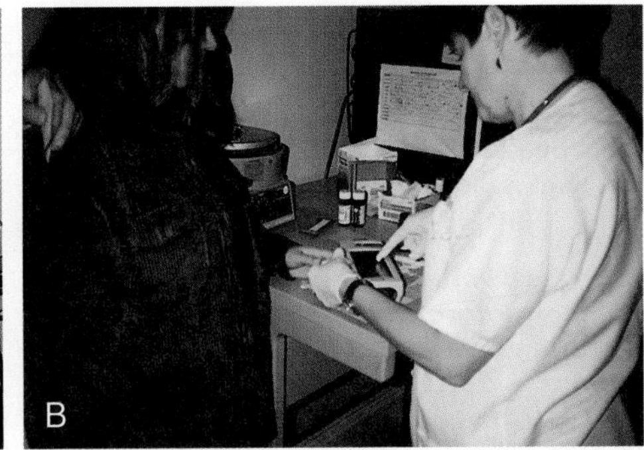

Fig. 20-2 **A,** Clinic nurse collects blood to determine glucose level. **B,** Nurse interprets glucose value displayed by monitor. (Courtesy Dee Lowdermilk, UNC Ambulatory Care Clinics, Chapel Hill, NC.)

TABLE 20-3

Target Blood Glucose Levels during Pregnancy

TIME OF DAY	TARGET PLASMA GLUCOSE LEVEL (mg/dL)
Premeal or fasting	>65 but <95
Postmeal (1 hr)	<130-140
Postmeal (2 hr)	<120

Sources: Landon, M., Catalano, P., & Gabbe, S. G. (2007). Diabetes mellitus complicating pregnancy. In S. Gabbe, J. Niebyl, & J. Simpson (Eds.), *Obstetrics: Normal and problem pregnancies* (5th ed.). Philadelphia: Churchill Livingstone; Moore, T., & Catalano, P. (2009). Diabetes in pregnancy. In R. Creasy, R. Resnik, & J. Iams (Eds.), *Creasy and Resnik's maternal-fetal medicine: Principles and practice* (6th ed.). Philadelphia: Saunders.

education and maternal and fetal assessment may be performed in the home, depending on the woman's insurance coverage and care provider preference.

Achieving and maintaining constant **euglycemia,** with plasma glucose levels in the range of 65 to 95 mg/dl preprandially and no higher than 130 to 140 mg/dl when measured 1 hour postprandially (Table 20-3), is the primary goal of medical therapy (Moore & Catalano, 2009). Euglycemia is achieved through a combination of diet, insulin, and exercise. Providing the woman with the knowledge, skill, and motivation she needs to achieve and maintain excellent blood glucose control is the primary nursing goal (see Nursing Care Plan: The Pregnant Woman with Pregestational Diabetes).

Achieving euglycemia requires commitment on the part of the woman and her family to make the necessary lifestyle changes, which can sometimes seem overwhelming. Maintaining tight blood glucose control necessitates that the woman follow a consistent daily schedule. She must get up and go to bed, eat, exercise, and take insulin at the same time each day. Blood glucose measurements are taken frequently to determine how well the major components of therapy (diet, insulin, and exercise) are working together to control blood glucose levels. The pregnant woman with diabetes should wear a medical identification bracelet at all times and carry insulin, syringes, and sources of fast sugar with her whenever she is away from home.

Because the woman with diabetes is at increased risk for infections, eye problems, and neurologic changes, foot care and general skin care are important. A daily bath that includes good perineal care and foot care is important. For dry skin, lotions, creams, or oils can be applied. Tight clothing should be avoided. Shoes or slippers that fit properly should be worn at all times and are best worn with socks or stockings. Feet should be inspected regularly; toenails should be cut straight across, and professional help should be sought for any foot problems. Extremes of temperature should be avoided.

Diet

The woman with pregestational diabetes has usually had nutritional counseling regarding management of her diabetes. However, because pregnancy produces special nutritional concerns and needs, the woman must be educated to incorporate these changes into dietary planning. For the woman who has "controlled" her diabetes for several years the changes in her insulin and dietary needs mandated by pregnancy may be difficult. Nutritional counseling is usually provided by a registered dietitian.

Dietary management during diabetic pregnancy must be based on blood (not urine) glucose levels. The diet is individualized to allow for increased fetal and metabolic requirements, with consideration of such factors as prepregnancy weight and dietary habits, overall health, ethnic background, lifestyle, stage of pregnancy, knowledge of nutrition, and insulin therapy. The dietary goals are to provide weight gain consistent with a normal pregnancy, to prevent ketoacidosis, and to minimize wide fluctuation of blood glucose levels.

For nonobese women, dietary counseling based on preconception body mass index (BMI) is 30 kcal/kg/day (Cunningham et al., 2005). In contrast, for obese women with a BMI greater than 30, experts recommend that the caloric intake total 25 kcal/kg/day (Moore & Catalano, 2009). The average diet includes 2200 calories (first trimester) to 2500 calories (second and third trimesters). Total calories may be distributed among three meals and one

Nursing Care Plan: Pregnancy Complicated by Pregestational Diabetes

NURSING CARE PLAN *The Pregnant Woman with Pregestational Diabetes*

NURSING DIAGNOSIS Deficient knowledge related to lack of recall of information as evidenced by the woman's questions and concerns

Expected Outcomes *Woman will be able to verbalize important information regarding diabetes, its management, and potential effects on the pregnancy and fetus.*

Nursing Interventions/*Rationales*

- Assess the woman's current knowledge base regarding the disease process, management, effects on pregnancy and fetus, and potential complications *to provide a database for further teaching.*
- Review the pathophysiologic aspects of diabetes, effects on pregnancy and fetus, and potential complications *to promote recall of information and compliance with the treatment plan.*
- Review the procedure for insulin administration, demonstrate the procedure for blood glucose monitoring and insulin measurement and administration, and obtain a return demonstration *to establish patient comfort and competence with procedures.*
- Discuss diet and exercise as prescribed *to promote self-management.*
- Review signs and symptoms of complications of hypoglycemia and hyperglycemia and appropriate interventions *to promote prompt recognition of complications and self-management.*
- Provide contact numbers for the health care team for prompt interventions and answers to questions on an ongoing basis *to promote comfort.*
- Review information on diagnostic tests, schedule of visits to the primary health care provider, and expected plan of care *to allay anxiety and enlist cooperation of the woman in her care.*

NURSING DIAGNOSIS Risk for fetal injury related to elevated maternal glucose levels

Expected Outcomes *Fetus will remain free of injury and be born at term in a healthy state.*

Nursing Interventions/*Rationales*

- Assess the woman's current diabetic control *to identify the risk for fetal mortality and congenital anomalies.*
- Monitor fundal height during each prenatal visit *to identify appropriate fetal growth.*
- Monitor for signs and symptoms of gestational hypertension *to identify early manifestations because pregnant women with diabetes are at increased risk.*
- Assess fetal movement and heart rate during each prenatal visit and perform fetal assessment tests as ordered during the third trimester *to assess fetal well-being.*
- Review the procedure for blood glucose testing and insulin administration and fetal movement counts *to promote self-management.*

NURSING DIAGNOSIS Anxiety related to threat to maternal and fetal well-being as evidenced by the woman's verbal expressions of concern

Expected Outcomes *Woman will identify sources of anxiety and report feeling less anxious.*

Nursing Interventions/*Rationales*

- Through therapeutic communication, promote an open relationship with woman *to promote trust.*
- Listen to the woman's feelings and concerns *to assess for any misconception or misinformation that may be contributing to anxiety.*
- Review potential dangers by providing factual information *to correct any misconceptions or misinformation.*
- Encourage the woman to share concerns with her health care team *to promote collaboration in her care.*

PATIENT INSTRUCTIONS FOR SELF-MANAGEMENT

Dietary Management of Diabetic Pregnancy

- Follow the prescribed diet plan.
- Eat a well-balanced diet, including daily food requirements for a normal pregnancy.
- Divide daily food intake among three meals and two to three snacks, depending on individual needs.
- Eat a substantial bedtime snack to prevent a severe drop in blood glucose level during the night.
- Take daily vitamins and iron as prescribed by the health care provider.
- Avoid foods high in refined sugar.
- Eat consistently each day; never skip meals or snacks.
- Eat foods high in dietary fiber.
- Avoid alcohol, nicotine, and caffeine.

evening snack or, more commonly, three meals and two or three snacks. Meals should be eaten on time and never skipped. Going more than 4 hours without food intake increases the risk for episodes of hypoglycemia. Snacks must be carefully planned in accordance with insulin therapy to prevent fluctuations in blood glucose levels. A large bedtime snack of at least 25 g of carbohydrate with some protein or fat is recommended to help prevent hypoglycemia and starvation ketosis during the night (Moore & Catalano).

The diet should consist of no more than 50% carbohydrates. The remaining 50% of calories should be equally divided between fats and protein (see Patient Instructions for Self-Management box: Dietary Management of Diabetic Pregnancy). Simple carbohydrates are limited. Complex carbohydrates that are high in fiber content are recommended because the starch and protein in such foods help regulate the blood glucose level by more sustained glucose release (Gilbert, 2007; Moore & Catalano, 2009).

Exercise

Although studies have shown that exercise enhances the use of glucose and decreases insulin need in women without diabetes, data regarding exercise in women with pregestational diabetes are limited. Any prescription of exercise during pregnancy for women with diabetes should be given by the primary health care provider and should be monitored closely to prevent complications, especially for women with vasculopathy. Women with vasculopathy usually depend completely on exogenous insulin and are at increased risk for wide fluctuations in blood glucose levels and ketoacidosis, which can be made worse by exercise.

When exercise is prescribed by the health care provider as part of the treatment plan, careful instructions are given to the woman. Exercise need not be vigorous to be beneficial; 15 to 30 minutes of walking four to six times a week is satisfactory for most pregnant women. Other exercises that may be recommended are non–weight-bearing activities such as arm exercises or use of a recumbent bicycle. The best time for exercise is after meals, when the blood glucose level is rising. To monitor the effect of insulin on blood glucose levels the woman can measure her blood glucose before, during, and after exercise.

NURSING ALERT Uterine contractions may occur during exercise; the woman should be advised to stop exercising immediately if they are detected, drink 2-3 glasses of water, and lie down on her side for an hour. If the contractions continue, she should contact her health care provider.

Insulin therapy

Adequate insulin is the primary factor in the maintenance of euglycemia during pregnancy, thus ensuring proper glucose metabolism of the woman and fetus. Insulin requirements during pregnancy change dramatically as the pregnancy progresses, necessitating frequent adjustments in the insulin dose. In the first trimester, from weeks 3 to 7 of gestation, insulin requirements are increased followed by a decrease between weeks 7 and 15 of gestation. However, the insulin dose may have to be decreased because of hypoglycemia. The commonly prescribed insulin dose is 0.7 units/kg in the first trimester for women with type 1 diabetes. During the second and third trimesters, because of insulin resistance, the dose must be increased significantly to maintain target glucose levels. Insulin requirements normally plateau after 35 weeks of gestation and often drop significantly after 38 weeks (Moore & Catalano, 2009).

For the woman with type 1 pregestational diabetes who has typically been accustomed to one injection per day of intermediate-acting insulin, multiple daily injections of mixed insulin are a new experience. The woman with type 2 diabetes previously treated with oral hypoglycemics is faced with the task of learning to self-administer injections of insulin. The nurse is instrumental in the education and support of pregestational diabetic women with regard to insulin administration and adjustment of the insulin dose to maintain euglycemia (see Patient Instructions for Self-Management box: Self-Administration of Insulin and Box 20-1).

Since 1982, most insulin preparations have been produced by inserting portions of DNA ("recombinant DNA") into special laboratory-cultivated bacteria or yeast cells. The cells then produce complete human insulin, which is less likely to cause antibody formation than animal-derived (beef or pork) insulin. More recently, insulin products called *insulin analogs,* in which the structure differs slightly from human insulin, have been produced. This small alteration in insulin structure results in changes in the onset and peak of action of the medication. Currently, the most commonly used insulin preparations include rapid-acting (lispro or aspart), short-acting (regular), intermediate-acting (N), and long-acting (glargine) (Landon et al., 2007) (Table 20-4). Mixtures of short- and intermediate-acting insulins in several proportions are also available.

Lispro (Humalog) and aspart (NovoLog) are commonly prescribed rapid-acting insulins with a shorter duration of action than regular insulin. Advantages of rapid-acting

BOX 20-1

Helpful Hints for Using Insulin

- The most common type of insulin used during pregnancy is a biosynthetic human insulin (Humulin) made by programming *Escherichia coli* bacteria to produce insulin.
- Insulin is classified either as rapid acting, short acting, intermediate acting, or long acting (see Table 20-4).
- Unused vials of insulin should be stored in the refrigerator until reaching their expiration date. Insulin should not be frozen. Vials currently in use can be stored at room temperature for up to a month. They should not be stored in direct sunlight.
- Regular insulin can be mixed with NPH insulin in the same syringe. Lispro insulin can also be mixed in a syringe with NPH or Ultralente insulin. Once mixed, the syringe can be used immediately or stored for future use. If it is used later, the syringe should be rotated 20 times before injection.
- Glargine insulin is administered at bedtime. It cannot be mixed with any other insulin in the same syringe. Prepared syringes are stable for 2 weeks in the refrigerator.
- Insulin may be administered by pen injector, jet injector, or insulin pump, in addition to syringe.
- The abdomen is the preferred injection site because insulin is best absorbed there. Other possible injection sites are the upper outer arm (not the deltoid area), the thighs, and the buttocks.
- Each injection should be given 1 inch from the previous injection. Each individual injection site should not be used more often than once in 30 days.

Source: Gilbert, E. (2007). *Manual of high risk pregnancy & delivery* (4th ed.). St. Louis: Mosby.

PATIENT INSTRUCTIONS FOR SELF-MANAGEMENT

Self-Administration of Insulin

PROCEDURE FOR MIXING NPH (INTERMEDIATE-ACTING) AND REGULAR (SHORT-ACTING) INSULIN

- Wash hands thoroughly and gather supplies. Be sure the insulin syringe corresponds to the concentration of insulin you are using.
- Check the insulin bottle to be certain it is the appropriate type, and check the expiration date.
- Gently rotate (do not shake) the insulin vial to mix the insulin.
- Wipe off rubber stopper of each vial with alcohol.
- Draw into syringe the amount of air equal to total dose.
- Inject air equal to NPH (intermediate-acting) dose into NPH vial. Remove syringe from vial.
- Inject air equal to regular insulin dose into regular insulin vial.
- Invert regular insulin bottle and withdraw regular insulin dose.
- Without adding more air to NPH vial, carefully withdraw NPH dose.

PROCEDURE FOR SELF-INJECTION OF INSULIN

- Select proper injection site.
- Injection site should be clean. No need to use alcohol. If alcohol is used, let it dry before injecting.
- Pinch the skin up to form a subcutaneous pocket and, holding the syringe as you would hold a pencil, puncture the skin at a 45- to 90-degree angle. If a great deal of fatty tissue is at the site, spread the skin taut and inject the syringe at a 90-degree angle.
- Slowly inject the insulin.
- As you withdraw the needle, cover the injection site with sterile gauze and apply gentle pressure to prevent bleeding.
- Record insulin dose and time of injection.

TABLE 20-4

Common Insulin Preparations

TYPE OF INSULIN	EXAMPLES GENERIC (TRADE) NAME	ONSET OF ACTION	PEAK OF ACTION	DURATION OF ACTION
Rapid-acting	Lispro (Humalog)	15 min	30-90 min	4-5 hr
	Aspart (NovoLog)	15 min	1-3 hr	3-5 hr
Short-acting	Humulin R	30 min	2-4 hr	5-7 hr
	Novolin R	30 min	2.5-5 hr	6-8 hr
Intermediate-acting	Humulin NPH	1-2 hr	6-12 hr	18-24 hr
	Novolin N	1.5 hr	4-20 hr	24 hr
	Humulin Lente	1-3 hr	6-12 hr	18-24 hr
	Novolin L	2.5 hr	7-15 hr	22 hr
Long-acting	Humulin Ultralente	4-6 hr	8-20 hr	>36 hr
	Glargine (Lantus)	1 hr	none	24 hr

Source: Landon, M., Catalano, P., & Gabbe, S. (2007). Diabetes mellitus complicating pregnancy. In S. Gabbe, J. Niebyl, & J. Simpson (Eds.), *Obstetrics: Normal and problem pregnancies* (5th ed.). Philadelphia: Churchill Livingstone.

insulins, such as lispro and aspart, include convenience, because they are injected immediately before mealtime, less hyperglycemia after meals, and fewer hypoglycemic episodes in some people. Because their effects last only 3 to 5 hours, most patients require a longer-acting insulin in addition to the rapid-acting insulin to maintain optimal blood glucose levels (Landon et al., 2007; Moore & Catalano, 2009) (see Table 20-4).

Glargine (Lantus) is a long-acting insulin lasting approximately 24 hours. Small amounts of glargine insulin are slowly released, with no pronounced peak. This insulin preparation is most often used with women who have insulin-resistant diabetes (type 2) requiring high doses of long-acting insulin. Glargine insulin is combined with a rapid-acting insulin to prevent hypoglycemia. Concerns associated with this medication include the need for monitoring for nocturnal hypoglycemia (Moore & Catalano, 2009) and a possible increase in the progression of retinopathy in some women (Landon et al., 2007). Glargine insulin provides a more stable basal blood glucose with less risk of nocturnal hypoglycemia than intermediate-acting insulin (Cianni et al., 2005). When glargine insulin is used, it is administered at bedtime. It cannot be mixed with any other insulin in the same syringe or at the same site (Gilbert, 2007) (see Table 20-4).

Most women with insulin-dependent diabetes are managed with two to three injections per day (Landon et al., 2007). Usually, two thirds of the daily insulin dose, with longer-acting (NPH) and shorter-acting (regular or lispro) insulin combined in a 2 : 1 ratio, is given before breakfast. The remaining one third, again a combination of longer- and shorter-acting insulin, is administered in the evening before dinner. To reduce the risk of hypoglycemia during the night, separate injections often are administered, with shorter-acting insulin given before dinner followed by longer-acting insulin at bedtime. An alternative insulin regimen that works well for some women is to administer shorter-acting insulin before each meal and longer-acting insulin at bedtime (Moore & Catalano, 2009).

Continuous subcutaneous insulin infusion (CSII) systems are increasingly used during pregnancy. The insulin pump is designed to mimic more closely the function of the pancreas in secreting insulin (Fig. 20-3). This portable, battery-powered device is worn, similar to a pager, during most daily activities. The pump infuses regular insulin at a set basal rate and has the capacity to deliver up to four different basal rates in 24 hours. It also delivers bolus doses of insulin before meals to control postprandial blood glucose levels. A fine-gauge plastic catheter is inserted into subcutaneous tissue, usually in the abdomen, and attached to the pump syringe by connecting tubing. The subcutaneous catheter and connecting tubing are changed every 2 to 3 days, although the infusion tubing can be left in place for several weeks without local complications. Although the insulin pump is convenient and generally provides good glycemic control, complications such as pump failure, precipitation of insulin inside the pump mechanism, abscess formation, and poor uptake from the infusion site can still occur. Therefore use of the insulin pump requires a knowledgeable, motivated patient, skilled health care providers, and prompt 24 hour availability of emergency assistance (Moore & Catalano, 2009).

Monitoring blood glucose levels

Blood glucose testing at home with a glucose reflectance meter is now considered the standard of care for monitoring blood glucose levels during pregnancy. It provides the most important tool available to the woman to assess her degree of glycemic control. Most of the newer reflectance meters are calibrated to provide plasma (rather than whole blood) glucose values. Plasma glucose values are 10% to 15% lower than those measured in whole blood from the same sample (Moore & Catalano, 2009).

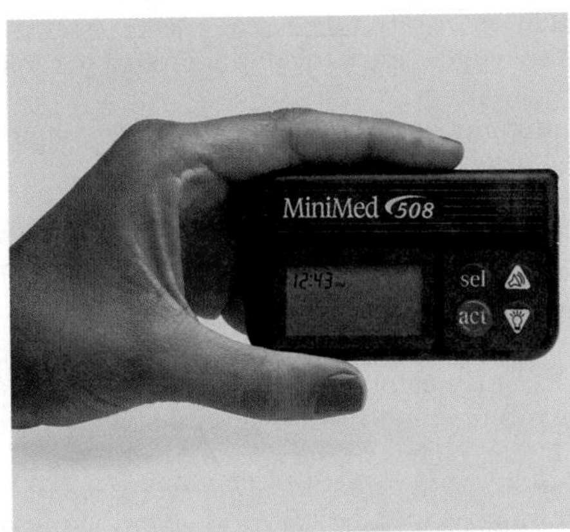

Fig. 20-3 Insulin pump shows basal rate for pregnant women with diabetes. (Courtesy MiniMed, Inc., Sylmar, CA.)

NURSING ALERT The nurse must be knowledgeable about the specific glucose reflectance meter that the patient uses because target glucose values depend on the type of meter used (Moore & Catalano, 2009).

To perform blood glucose monitoring an individual obtains a drop of blood by means of a finger stick and places it on a test strip. After a specified amount of time the glucose level can be read by the meter (see Patient Instructions for Self-Management box: Self-Testing of Blood Glucose Level). Blood glucose levels are routinely measured at various times throughout the day, such as before breakfast, lunch, and dinner; 2 hours after each meal; at bedtime; and in the middle of the night. When any readjustment in the insulin dose or diet is made, more frequent measurement of blood glucose is warranted. If nausea, vomiting, or diarrhea occurs, or if any infection is present, the woman will be asked to monitor her blood glucose levels more closely than usual.

NURSING ALERT Hyperglycemia will most likely be identified in 2-hour postprandial values because blood glucose levels peak approximately 2 hours after a meal.

Target levels of blood glucose during pregnancy are lower than nonpregnant values (see Table 20-3). Acceptable fasting levels are generally between 65 and 95 mg/dl, and 1-hour postprandial levels should be less than 130 to

PATIENT INSTRUCTIONS FOR SELF-MANAGEMENT

Self-Testing of Blood Glucose Level

- Gather supplies, check expiration date, and read instructions on testing materials. Prepare glucose reflectance meter for use according to manufacturer's directions.
- Wash hands in warm water (warmth increases circulation).
- Select site on side of any finger (all fingers should be used in rotation).
- Pierce site with lancet (may use automatic, spring-loaded, puncturing device). Cleaning the site with alcohol is not necessary.
- Drop hand down to side; with other hand gently squeeze finger from hand to fingertip.
- Allow blood to drop onto testing strip. Be sure to cover entire testing area.
- Determine blood glucose value using the glucose reflectance meter following manufacturer's instructions.
- Record results.
- Repeat as instructed by the health care provider and as needed for signs of hypoglycemia or hyperglycemia.

140 mg/dl (Moore & Catalano, 2009). Two-hour postprandial levels should be less than 120 mg/dl (Landon et al., 2007). The woman should be told to report episodes of hypoglycemia (less than 60 mg/dl) and hyperglycemia (more than 200 mg/dl) immediately to her health care provider so that adjustments in diet or insulin therapy can be made.

Pregnant women with diabetes are much more likely to develop hypoglycemia than hyperglycemia. Most episodes of mild or moderate hypoglycemia can be treated with oral intake of 15 g of simple carbohydrate (fast sugar) (see Patient Instructions for Self-Management box: Treatment for Hypoglycemia). If severe hypoglycemia occurs, in which case the woman experiences a decrease in or loss of consciousness or an inability to swallow, she will require a parenteral injection of glucagon or intravenous (IV) glucose. Because hypoglycemia can develop rapidly, and because impaired judgment can be associated with even moderate episodes, family members, friends, and work colleagues must be able to recognize signs and symptoms quickly and initiate proper treatment if necessary.

Hyperglycemia is less likely than hypoglycemia to occur, but it can rapidly progress to DKA, which is associated with an increased risk of fetal death (Cunningham et al., 2005; Moore & Catalano, 2009). Women and family members should be particularly alert for signs and symptoms of hyperglycemia, especially when infections or other illnesses occur (see Patient Instructions for Self-Management box: What to Do When Illness Occurs).

Urine testing

Even though urine testing for glucose is not beneficial during pregnancy, urine testing for ketones continues to have a place in diabetic management. Monitoring for urine ketones may detect inadequate caloric or carbohydrate intake (Gilbert, 2007). Women may be taught to perform ketone testing daily with the first morning urine. Testing may also be performed if a meal is missed or delayed, when illness occurs, or when the blood glucose level is greater than 200 mg/dl.

Complications requiring hospitalization. Occasionally, hospitalization is necessary to regulate insulin therapy and stabilize glucose levels. Infection, which can lead to hyperglycemia and DKA, is an indication for hospitalization, regardless of gestational age. Hospitalization during the third trimester for close maternal and fetal observation may be indicated for women whose diabetes is poorly controlled. In addition, women with diabetes are 10% to 20% more likely than women who do not have diabetes to also have preexisting hypertension or develop preeclampsia, which may necessitate hospitalization (Moore & Catalano, 2009).

Fetal surveillance. Diagnostic techniques for fetal surveillance are often performed to assess fetal growth and well-being. The goals of fetal surveillance are to detect fetal compromise as early as possible and to prevent intrauterine fetal death or unnecessary preterm birth.

Early in pregnancy the estimated date of birth is determined. A baseline sonogram is obtained during the first trimester to assess gestational age. Follow-up ultrasound

PATIENT INSTRUCTIONS FOR SELF-MANAGEMENT

Treatment for Hypoglycemia

- Be familiar with signs and symptoms of hypoglycemia (nervousness, headache, fatigue, shaking, irritability, tachycardia, hunger, blurred vision, sweaty skin, tingling of mouth or extremities).
- Check blood glucose level immediately when hypoglycemic symptoms occur.
- If blood glucose is below 60 mg/dl, immediately eat or drink something that contains 15 g of fast sugar (simple carbohydrate). Examples are:
  - ½ cup (4 ounces) unsweetened orange juice
  - ½ cup (4 ounces) regular (not diet) soda
  - 5 to 6 hard candies
  - 1 cup (8 ounces) skim milk
  - 2 to 3 glucose tablets
- Rest for 15 minutes, then recheck blood glucose.
- If glucose level is above 60 mg/dl, eat a meal to stabilize the sugar level.
- If glucose level is still below 60 mg/dl, eat or drink another serving of one of the fast sugars listed above.
- Wait 15 minutes, then recheck blood glucose. If the level is still under 60 mg/dl, notify your health care provider immediately.

Source: Gilbert, E. (2007). *Manual of high risk pregnancy & delivery* (4th ed.). St. Louis: Mosby.

PATIENT INSTRUCTIONS FOR SELF-MANAGEMENT

What to Do When Illness Occurs

- Be sure to take insulin even if unable to eat or appetite is less than normal. (Insulin needs are increased with illness or infection.)
- Call the health care provider and relay the following information:
  - Symptoms of illness (e.g., nausea, vomiting, diarrhea)
  - Elevated temperature
  - Most recent blood glucose level
  - Urine ketones
  - Time and amount of last insulin dose
- Increase oral intake of fluids to prevent dehydration.
- Rest as much as possible.
- If you are unable to reach your health care provider and blood glucose exceeds 200 mg/dl with urine ketones present, seek emergency treatment at the nearest health care facility. Do not attempt to self-treat for this condition.

examinations are usually performed during the pregnancy (as often as every 4 to 6 weeks) to monitor fetal growth, estimate fetal weight, and detect hydramnios, macrosomia, and congenital anomalies.

Because a fetus of a woman with diabetes is at increased risk for neural tube defects (e.g., spina bifida, anencephaly, microcephaly), measurement of maternal serum alpha-fetoprotein is performed between 15 and 20 weeks of gestation (ideally between 16 and 18 weeks of gestation) (Wapner, Jenkins, & Khalek, 2009). This assessment is often performed in conjunction with a detailed ultrasound study to examine the fetus for neural tube defects.

Fetal echocardiography may be performed between 20 and 22 weeks of gestation to detect cardiac anomalies, especially in women who had less-than-desirable glucose control early in pregnancy, as demonstrated by abnormal hemoglobin A_{1c} levels at the first prenatal visit (Moore & Catalano, 2009). Some practitioners repeat this fetal surveillance test at 34 weeks of gestation. Doppler studies of the umbilical artery may be performed in women with vascular disease to detect placental compromise.

The majority of fetal surveillance measures are concentrated in the third trimester, when the risk of fetal compromise is greatest. The goals of antepartum testing during the third trimester are to prevent IUFD and maximize the opportunity for the woman to safely give birth vaginally. Pregnant women should be taught how to make daily fetal movement counts, beginning at 28 weeks of gestation (see Chapter 19) (Moore & Catalano, 2009).

Biophysical testing (nonstress testing, contraction stress testing, or biophysical profile) once or twice weekly to evaluate fetal well-being, is typically begun around 34 weeks of gestation. This testing should begin around 28 weeks in women who have poor glucose control or significant hypertension (Moore & Catalano, 2009) (see Chapter 19).

Determination of birth date and mode of birth. The optimal time for birth is between 38.5 and 40 weeks of gestation, as long as good metabolic control is maintained and parameters of antepartum fetal surveillance remain within normal limits. Reasons to proceed with birth before term include poor metabolic control, worsening hypertensive disorders, fetal macrosomia, or fetal growth restriction (Cunningham et al., 2005; Moore & Catalano, 2009).

Many practitioners plan for elective labor induction between 38 and 40 weeks of gestation. To confirm fetal lung maturity an amniocentesis should be performed when birth will occur before 38.5 weeks of gestation. For the pregnancy complicated by diabetes, fetal lung maturation is best predicted by the amniotic fluid phosphatidylglycerol (>3%). If the fetal lungs are still immature, birth should be postponed until 40 weeks of gestation as long as fetal assessment test results remain reassuring. After that time, however, the benefits of conservative management are outweighed by the increasing risk of fetal compromise if the pregnancy is allowed to continue. Birth, despite poor fetal lung maturity, may be necessary when testing suggests fetal compromise or worsening maternal condition, such as deteriorating renal function or severe preeclampsia (Moore & Catalano, 2009).

Although vaginal birth is expected for most women with pregestational diabetes, the cesarean rate for these women ranges from 30% to 50%. Currently, the American College of Obstetricians and Gynecologists (ACOG) recommends that cesarean birth be considered when the estimated fetal weight is expected to be greater than 4500 g in an attempt to reduce the risk of shoulder dystocia. This recommendation appears to result in a small improvement in neonatal outcome (Moore & Catalano, 2009). Fetal distress and induction failures before term also contribute to the high rate of cesarean birth in these women (Gilbert, 2007).

Intrapartum

During the intrapartum period the woman with pregestational diabetes must be monitored closely to prevent complications related to dehydration, hypoglycemia, and hyperglycemia. Most women use large amounts of energy (calories) to accomplish the work and manage the stress of labor and birth. However, this calorie expenditure varies with the individual. Blood glucose levels and hydration must be carefully controlled during labor. An IV line is inserted for infusion of a maintenance fluid. Initially, this infusion may be normal saline or lactated Ringer's solution. The IV fluid will be changed to one containing 5% dextrose during active labor. Most commonly, insulin is administered by continuous infusion, piggybacked into the main intravenous line. Only regular insulin may be administered intravenously. Determinations of blood glucose levels are made every hour, and fluids and insulin are adjusted to maintain the blood glucose level at less than 140 mg/dl (Landon et al., 2007). Maintaining this target glucose level is essential because hyperglycemia during labor can cause metabolic problems in the neonate, particularly hypoglycemia.

During labor, continuous fetal heart monitoring is necessary. The woman should assume an upright or side-lying position during bed rest in labor to prevent supine hypotension because of a large fetus or polyhydramnios. Labor is allowed to progress provided normal rates of cervical dilation and fetal descent are maintained, and fetal well-being is evident. Failure to progress may indicate a macrosomic infant and cephalopelvic disproportion, necessitating a cesarean birth. The woman is observed and treated during labor for diabetic complications such as hyperglycemia, ketosis, and ketoacidosis. During second-stage labor, shoulder dystocia may occur with birth of a macrosomic infant (see Chapter 22). A neonatologist, pediatrician, or neonatal nurse practitioner will likely be present at the birth to initiate assessment and neonatal care.

If a cesarean birth is planned, it should be scheduled in the early morning to facilitate glycemic control. Women should take their full dose of NPH insulin the night before surgery. No morning insulin is given on the day of surgery, and the woman is given nothing by mouth. Epidural anesthesia is recommended because hypoglycemia can be detected earlier if the woman is awake. After surgery, glucose levels should be monitored carefully. Generally sliding scale insulin is used to control blood glucose levels until the woman resumes a regular diet (Moore & Catalano, 2009).

Postpartum

During the first 24 hours postpartum, insulin requirements decrease substantially because the major source of insulin resistance, the placenta, has been removed. Women with type 1 diabetes may require only one third to one half of their last pregnancy insulin dose on the first postpartum day, provided that they are eating a full diet (Landon et al., 2007). In women giving birth by cesarean an intravenous infusion of glucose and insulin may be required for type 1 diabetics until they resume a regular diet (Moore & Catalano, 2009). Several days after birth may be required to reestablish carbohydrate homeostasis (see Fig. 20-1, *D* and *E*). Blood glucose levels are carefully monitored in the postpartum period and the insulin dose is adjusted, often using a sliding scale. The woman who has insulin-dependent diabetes must realize the importance of eating on time even if the baby needs feeding or other pressing demands exist. Women with type 2 diabetes often require only 30% to 50% of their pregnancy insulin dose in the postpartum period (Moore & Catalano).

Possible postpartum complications include preeclampsia or eclampsia (or both), hemorrhage, and infection. Hemorrhage is a possibility if the mother's uterus was overdistended (hydramnios, macrosomic fetus) or overstimulated (oxytocin induction). Postpartum infections such as endometritis are more likely to occur in women with diabetes than in women who do not have diabetes.

Mothers are encouraged to breastfeed. In addition to the advantages of maternal satisfaction and pleasure, breastfeeding has an antidiabetogenic effect for the children of women with diabetes and for women with gestational diabetes (Lindsay, 2006; Moore & Catalano, 2009). This effect is important because a child born to a mother with type 2 diabetes has a 70% chance of also developing type 2 diabetes later in life. In addition, children who were exposed to hyperglycemia prenatally have an increased risk for obesity in childhood (Gilbert, 2007).

Insulin requirements in breastfeeding women may be one half of prepregnancy levels because of the carbohydrate used in human milk production. Because glucose levels are lower than normal, breastfeeding women are at increased risk for hypoglycemia, especially in the early postpartum period and after breastfeeding sessions, particularly after late night nursing (Moore & Catalano, 2009). Breastfeeding mothers with diabetes may be at increased risk for mastitis and yeast infections of the breast. The insulin dose, which is decreased during lactation, must be recalculated at weaning (see Fig. 20-1, *F*).

The mother may have early breastfeeding difficulties. Poor metabolic control may delay lactogenesis and contribute to decreased milk production (Moore & Catalano, 2009). Initial contact with and opportunity to breastfeed the infant may be delayed for mothers who gave birth by cesarean or if infants are placed in neonatal intensive care units or special care nurseries for observation during the first few hours after birth. Support and assistance from nursing staff and lactation specialists can facilitate the mother's early experience with breastfeeding and encourage her to continue.

The new mother needs information about family planning and contraception. Although family planning is important for all women, it is essential for the woman with diabetes so as to safeguard her own health and to promote optimal outcomes in future pregnancies. The risks and benefits of contraceptive methods should be discussed with the mother and her partner before discharge from the hospital. Barrier methods are often recommended as safe, inexpensive options that have no inherent risks for women with diabetes. The intrauterine device (IUD) may also be used by women who have diabetes without concerns about an increased risk of infection (Landon et al., 2007).

Use of oral contraceptives by women with diabetes is controversial because of the risk of thromboembolic and vascular complications and the effect on carbohydrate metabolism. In women without vascular disease or other risk factors, combination low-dose oral contraceptives may be prescribed. Progestin-only oral contraceptives also may be used because they minimally affect carbohydrate metabolism (Cunningham et al., 2005; Landon et al., 2007). Close monitoring of blood pressure and lipid levels is necessary to detect complications (Landon et al.).

Opinion is divided about the use of long-acting parenteral progestins, such as Depo-Provera. Some health care providers recommend their use, particularly in women who are noncompliant with daily dosing oral contraceptives. In contrast, other health care providers believe this method may adversely affect diabetic control. Transdermal (patch) and transvaginal (vaginal ring) administration are newer contraceptive methods, particularly effective in women who prefer weekly or every-third-week dosing, respectively. For women weighing more than 90 kg (198 pounds) the contraceptive failure rate with transdermal administration is higher than in normal-weight women (Cunningham et al., 2005). Therefore this method would be contraindicated in obese women. Limited data are available regarding their use in women with diabetes.

The risks associated with pregnancy increase with the duration and severity of diabetes. In addition, pregnancy may contribute to the vascular changes associated with diabetes. This information needs to be thoroughly discussed with the woman and her partner. Sterilization is often recommended for the woman who has completed her family, who has poor metabolic control, or who has significant vascular problems.

Gestational Diabetes Mellitus

Gestational diabetes mellitus (GDM), complicates approximately 3% to 9% of all pregnancies (Moore & Catalano, 2009) and accounts for more than 90% of all cases of diabetic pregnancy (Landon et al., 2007). According to White's classification system, these women fall into classes A_1 and A_2 (see Table 20-1). GDM is more likely to occur among Latina, Native American, Asian, and African-American women than in Caucasians (Moore & Catalano). GDM is likely to recur in future pregnancies, and the risk for development of overt diabetes in later life is also increased (Moore & Catalano). This tendency is especially true of women whose GDM is diagnosed early in pregnancy or who are obese (Landon et al.). Classic risk factors for GDM include maternal age over 25 years, previous macrosomic infant, previous unexplained IUFD, previous pregnancy with GDM, strong immediate family history of type 2 diabetes or GDM, obesity (weight >90 kg [198 pounds]), and fasting blood glucose above 140 mg/dl or random blood glucose above 200 mg/dl. Women at high risk for developing GDM should have glucola screening at the first prenatal visit and again at 24 to 28 weeks of gestation if the initial screen is negative (Landon et al.).

GDM is usually diagnosed during the second half of pregnancy. As fetal nutrient demands rise during the late second and the third trimesters, maternal nutrient ingestion induces greater and more sustained levels of blood glucose. At the same time, maternal insulin resistance is also increasing because of the insulin-antagonistic effects of the placental hormones, cortisol, and insulinase. Consequently, maternal insulin demands rise as much as threefold. Most pregnant women are capable of increasing insulin production to compensate for insulin resistance and to maintain euglycemia. When the pancreas is unable to produce sufficient insulin or the insulin is not used effectively, however, gestational diabetes can result.

Fetal risks

No increase in the incidence of birth defects has been found among infants of women who develop gestational diabetes after the first trimester because the critical period of organ formation has already passed by that time (Moore & Catalano, 2009). However, Anderson, Waller, Canfield, Shaw, Watkins, and Werler (2005) found that women who were obese before conception (BMI >30 kg/m^2) and developed gestational diabetes were at greater risk to give birth to infants with CNS defects.

Screening for gestational diabetes mellitus

All pregnant women should be screened for GDM by history, clinical risk factors, or laboratory screening of blood glucose levels. Based on history and clinical risk factors, some women are at low risk for the development of GDM. Therefore glucose testing for this low risk population is not cost effective (ADA, 2008). This group includes normal-weight women younger than 25 years of age who have no family history of diabetes, are not members of an ethnic or a racial group known to have a high prevalence of the disease, and have no previous history of abnormal glucose tolerance or adverse obstetric outcomes usually associated with GDM (ADA).

Critical Thinking Exercise: Gestational Diabetes

The screening test (glucola screening) most often used consists of a 50-g oral glucose load followed by a plasma glucose measurement 1 hour later. The woman need not be fasting. A glucose value of 130 to 140 mg/dl is considered a positive screen and should be followed by a 3-hour (100-g) oral glucose tolerance test (OGTT). The OGTT is administered after an overnight fast and at least 3 days of unrestricted diet (at least 150 g of carbohydrate) and physical activity. The woman is instructed to avoid caffeine because it will increase glucose levels and to abstain from smoking for 12 hours before the test. The 3-hour OGTT requires a fasting blood glucose level, which is drawn before giving a 100-gram glucose load. Blood glucose levels are then drawn 1, 2, and 3 hours later. The woman is diagnosed with gestational diabetes if two or more values are met or exceeded (Moore & Catalano, 2009) (Fig. 20-4).

Nursing diagnoses and expected outcomes of care for women with GDM are basically the same as those for women with pregestational diabetes except that the time frame for planning may be shortened with GDM because the diagnosis is usually made later in pregnancy (see Nursing Process box: Preexisting Diabetes).

CARE MANAGEMENT

Antepartum

When the diagnosis of gestational diabetes is made, treatment begins immediately, allowing little or no time for the woman and her family to adjust to the diagnosis before they are expected to participate in the treatment plan. With each step of the treatment plan the nurse and other health care providers should educate the woman and her family, providing detailed and comprehensive explanations to ensure understanding, participation, and adherence to the necessary interventions. Potential complications should be discussed, and the need for maintenance of euglycemia throughout the remainder of the pregnancy reinforced. Knowing that gestational diabetes typically disappears when the pregnancy is over may be reassuring for the woman and her family.

As with pregestational diabetes, the aim of therapy in women with GDM is strict blood glucose control. Fasting blood glucose levels should range from 65 to 95 mg/dl, and 1-hour postprandial blood glucose levels should be less than 130 to 140 mg/dl (Moore & Catalano, 2009).

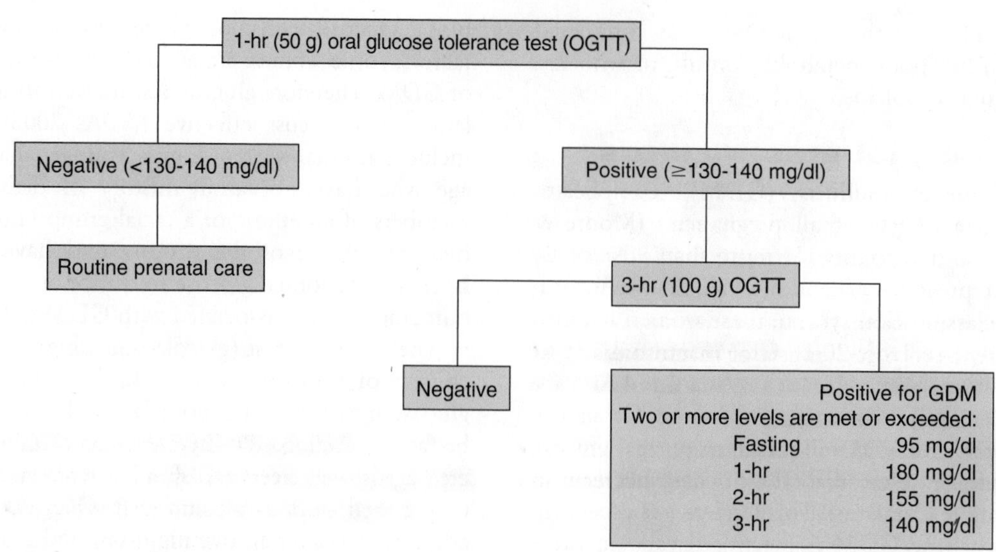

Fig. 20-4 Screening and diagnosis for gestational diabetes. (From American Diabetes Association. [2008]. Position statement: Diagnosis and classification of diabetes mellitus. *Diabetes Care, 31*[Suppl.], S55-S60; Moore, T. R., & Catalano, P. [2009]. Diabetes in pregnancy. In R. K. Creasy, R. Resnik, & J. D. Iams [Eds.], *Creasy and Resnik's maternal-fetal medicine: Principles and practice* [6th ed.]. Philadelphia: Saunders.)

Diet. Dietary modification is the mainstay of treatment for GDM. The woman with GDM is placed on a standard diabetic diet. The usual prescription is 30 kcal/kg/day based on a normal preconceptional weight. For obese women the usual prescription is up to 25 kcal/kg/day, which translates into 1500 to 2000 kcal/day for most women (Moore & Catalano, 2009). Carbohydrate intake is restricted to approximately 50% of caloric intake (Moore & Catalano). Dietary counseling by a nutritionist is recommended.

Exercise. Exercise in women with GDM helps lower blood glucose levels and may be instrumental in decreasing the need for insulin (Gilbert, 2007). Women with GDM who already have an active lifestyle should be encouraged to continue an exercise program.

Monitoring blood glucose levels. Blood glucose monitoring is necessary to determine whether euglycemia can be maintained by diet and exercise. Women are instructed to monitor their blood sugar daily. The frequency and timing of blood glucose monitoring should be individualized for each woman. However, a typical schedule for monitoring blood glucose is on rising in the morning, after breakfast, before and after lunch, after dinner, and at bedtime (Moore & Catalano, 2009). Women with GDM may perform self-monitoring at home, or monitoring may be performed at the clinic or office visit.

Medications for controlling blood glucose levels. Up to 20% of women with GDM will require insulin during the pregnancy to maintain adequate blood glucose levels, despite compliance with the prescribed diet. In contrast to women with insulin-dependent diabetes, women with gestational diabetes are initially managed with diet and exercise alone. If fasting plasma glucose levels are greater than 95 mg/dl or 2-hour postprandial levels are greater than 120 mg/dl, then insulin therapy is begun (Gilbert, 2007) (see Table 20-3). Glyburide, an oral hypoglycemic agent, is currently being used more frequently with women with GDM instead of insulin. The fact that only minimal amounts of glyburide cross the placenta to the fetus makes it a good drug for use during pregnancy. It has also been used in women with type 2 diabetes who required large amounts of insulin to achieve glucose control with smaller insulin doses. Recent studies have shown that glyburide should be taken at least 30 minutes (preferably 1 hour) before a meal so that its peak effect covers the 2-hour postprandial blood glucose level. Because episodes of hypoglycemia can occur between meals, women taking glyburide should always carry with them sources of fast sugar (Moore & Catalano, 2009). Women with diabetes who are unable or unwilling to take insulin by injection or are cognitively impaired may be candidates for glyburide use.

Fetal surveillance. No standard recommendation has been formulated for fetal surveillance in pregnancies complicated by GDM. Women whose blood glucose levels are well controlled by diet are at low risk for fetal complications. Limited antepartum fetal testing is performed in women with gestational diabetes as long as their fasting and 2-hour postprandial blood glucose levels remain within normal limits and they have no other risk factors. Women with hypertension, a history of a prior IUFD, or suspected macrosomia or those who require insulin for blood glucose control may have twice-weekly nonstress testing beginning at 32 weeks of gestation (Landon et al., 2007). In general, women with GDM can continue pregnancy until 40 weeks of gestation and the spontaneous onset of labor. However, fetal growth should be monitored carefully because the risk for macrosomia as the pregnancy approaches 40 weeks of gestation is apparently increased (Landon, et al.).

Intrapartum

During the labor and birth process, blood glucose levels are monitored hourly to maintain levels at 80 to 120 mg/dl (Moore & Catalano, 2009). Blood glucose levels within this range will decrease the incidence of neonatal hypoglycemia. Infusing regular insulin intravenously may be necessary during labor to maintain blood glucose levels within this range. IV fluids containing glucose are not commonly given during labor. Although gestational diabetes is not an indication for cesarean birth, this procedure may be necessary in the presence of preeclampsia or macrosomia.

Postpartum

Most women with GDM will return to normal glucose levels after childbirth. However, GDM is likely to recur in future pregnancies, and women with GDM are at significant risk for developing type 2 diabetes later in life. Assessment for carbohydrate intolerance with a 75 g oral glucose tolerance test should be performed at 6 to 12 weeks postpartum or after breastfeeding has stopped. Obesity is a major risk factor for the later development of diabetes. Women with a history of GDM, particularly those who are overweight, should be encouraged to make lifestyle changes that include weight loss and exercise to reduce this risk (Gilbert, 2007). Children born to women with GDM are also at risk for becoming obese in childhood or adolescence (Lindsay, 2006).

Thyroid Disorders

Hyperthyroidism

Hyperthyroidism in pregnancy is rare, occurring in approximately 1 or 2 of every 1000 pregnancies (Cunningham et al., 2005; Nader, 2009). In 90% to 95% of pregnant women, hyperthyroidism is caused by Graves disease (Nader). Clinical manifestations of hyperthyroidism include heat intolerance, diaphoresis, fatigue, anxiety, emotional lability, and tachycardia. Many of these symptoms also occur with pregnancy; thus the disorder can be difficult to diagnose. Signs that may help differentiate hyperthyroidism from normal pregnancy changes include weight loss, goiter, and a pulse rate greater than 100 beats/min (Nader). Laboratory findings include elevated free thyroxine (T_4) and triiodothyronine (T_3) levels and greatly suppressed thyroid-stimulating hormone (TSH) levels (Cunningham et al.; Nader). Moderate and severe hyperthyroidism must be treated during pregnancy; untreated or inadequately treated women have an increased risk of miscarriage, preterm birth, and giving birth to stillborn infants or infants with goiter, hyperthyroidism, or hypothyroidism. Most neonates born to women with hyperthyroidism, however, will have normal thyroid function. Women with hyperthyroidism are also at increased risk for developing severe preeclampsia and heart failure (Cunningham et al.; Nader).

The primary treatment of hyperthyroidism during pregnancy is drug therapy; the medication most often prescribed in the United States is propylthiouracil (PTU). The usual starting dose is 100 to 150 mg every 8 hours, with higher doses required for some women. Women generally show clinical improvement within 2 weeks of beginning therapy, but the medication requires 6 to 8 weeks to reach full effectiveness. During therapy the woman's free T_4 levels are measured monthly, and the results are used to taper the drug to the smallest effective dose to prevent development of unnecessary fetal or neonatal hypothyroidism. In many patients the medication can be discontinued by 32 to 36 weeks of gestation. PTU readily crosses the placenta and may cause fetal hypothyroidism, which is characterized by goiter, bradycardia, and intrauterine growth restriction (IUGR) (Mestman, 2007; Nader, 2009).

PTU is well tolerated by most women. Maternal side effects include pruritus, skin rash, drug-related fever, hepatitis, bronchospasm, and a lupus-like syndrome. The most severe side effect is agranulocytosis, which occurs very rarely and usually develops only in older women and in those taking high doses of PTU. Symptoms of agranulocytosis are fever and unexpected sore throat. These symptoms should be reported immediately to the health care provider, and the woman should stop taking the PTU. Leukopenia of a transient and benign nature may occur as a result of PTU therapy. Beta-adrenergic blockers such as propranolol (Inderal) or atenolol (Tenormin) may be used in severe hyperthyroidism to control maternal symptoms, especially heart rate. Long-term use of these medications is not recommended because of the potential for IUGR, bradycardia, and hypoglycemia (Nader, 2009).

After birth, women taking PTU who choose to breastfeed should be informed that the medication is not significantly concentrated in breast milk and does not appear to adversely affect the neonate's thyroid function. The woman should take her antithyroid medication just after breastfeeding, thus allowing a 3- to 4-hour period before nursing again (Nader, 2009).

Radioactive iodine must not be used in diagnosis or treatment of hyperthyroidism in pregnancy because therapeutic doses given to treat maternal thyroid disease may also destroy the fetal thyroid (Cunningham et al., 2005). In severe cases, surgical treatment of hyperthyroidism, subtotal thyroidectomy, may be performed during pregnancy. Surgery is best performed during the second trimester of pregnancy, although it can be performed during the first or third trimesters if necessary. Surgery is usually reserved for women with severe disease, those for whom drug therapy proves toxic, and those who are unable to follow the prescribed medical regimen. Risks associated with the surgery are hypoparathyroidism, recurrent laryngeal nerve paralysis, and anesthesia-related complications (Nader, 2009).

NURSING ALERT A serious but uncommon complication of undiagnosed or partially treated hyperthyroidism is thyroid storm, which may occur in response to stress such as labor and vaginal birth, infection, preeclampsia, or surgery. A woman with this emergency disorder may have fever, restlessness, tachycardia, vomiting, hypotension, or stupor. Prompt treatment is essential; IV fluids and oxygen are administered, along with high doses of PTU. After administration of PTU, iodide is given. Other medications include antipyretics, dexamethasone, and beta-blockers (Cunningham et al., 2005; Nader, 2009).

Hypothyroidism

Hypothyroidism during pregnancy is less common (1.3 per 1000) than hyperthyroidism. Hypothyroidism is often associated with menstrual and fertility problems, including an increased risk of miscarriage (Cunningham et al., 2005). Although iodine deficiency is rare in the United States, it is a common cause of maternal, fetal, and neonatal hypothyroidism in the world (Nader, 2009). Adult hypothyroidism is usually caused by glandular destruction by autoantibodies, most commonly because of Hashimoto thyroiditis. Characteristic symptoms of hypothyroidism include weight gain, lethargy, decrease in exercise capacity, and cold intolerance. Women who are moderately symptomatic can also develop constipation, hoarseness, hair loss, brittle nails, and dry skin. Laboratory values in pregnancy include elevated levels of TSH, with or without low T_4 levels (Nader).

Pregnant women with untreated hypothyroidism are at increased risk for miscarriage, preeclampsia, gestational hypertension, placental abruption, preterm birth, and stillbirth (Cunningham et al., 2005; Nader, 2009). Infants born to mothers with hypothyroidism may also be of low birth weight. These outcomes can be improved with early treatment (Nader).

Thyroid hormone supplements are used to treat hypothyroidism. Levothyroxine (e.g., l-thyroxine [Synthroid]) is most often prescribed during pregnancy. The usual beginning dosage is 0.1 to 0.15 mg per day, with adjustment by 25 to 50 mcg every 4 to 6 weeks as necessary based on the maternal TSH level (Cunningham et al., 2005; Nader, 2009). The aim of drug therapy is to maintain the woman's TSH level at the lower end of the normal range for pregnant women. Women with little or no functioning thyroid tissue will require higher doses of l-thyroxine. Also, as pregnancy progresses, increased doses of thyroid hormone are usually required. This increased demand during pregnancy may be related to increased estrogen levels (Cunningham et al.; Nader).

NURSING ALERT If taking iron supplementation, pregnant women should be told to take l-thyroxine at a different time of day than their iron tablets because ferrous sulfate decreases absorption of T_4 (Nader, 2009).

The fetus depends on maternal thyroid hormones until approximately 18 weeks of gestation, when fetal production begins. Normal maternal thyroxine levels early in pregnancy are important for proper fetal brain development. Studies have shown that even mild maternal hypothyroidism during the first trimester has been associated with long-term neuropsychologic damage in their children. More research needs to be conducted on this topic (Mestman, 2007).

Nursing care

Education of the pregnant woman with thyroid dysfunction is essential to promote compliance with the plan of treatment. Important points to discuss with the woman and her family include the disorder and its potential impact on her, her family, and her fetus; the medication regimen and possible side effects; the need for continuing medical supervision; and the importance of compliance.

The woman often needs assistance from the nurse in coping with the discomforts and frustrations associated with symptoms of the disorder. For example, the woman with hyperthyroidism who has nervousness and hyperactivity along with weakness and fatigue may benefit from suggestions to channel excess energies into quiet diversional activities such as reading or crafts. Discomfort associated with hypersensitivity to heat (hyperthyroidism) or cold intolerance (hypothyroidism) can be minimized by appropriate clothing and regulation of environmental temperatures, and by avoidance of temperature extremes.

Nutritional counseling with a registered dietitian may provide guidance in selecting a well-balanced diet. The woman with hyperthyroidism who has increased appetite and poor weight gain and the hypothyroid woman who has anorexia and lethargy need counseling to ensure adequate intake of nutritionally sound foods to meet both maternal and fetal needs.

Maternal Phenylketonuria

Phenylketonuria (PKU), a recognized cause of mental retardation, is an inborn error of metabolism caused by an autosomal recessive trait that creates a deficiency in the enzyme phenylalanine hydrolase. Absence of this enzyme impairs the body's ability to metabolize the amino acid phenylalanine, found in all protein foods. Consequently, toxic accumulation of phenylalanine in the blood occurs, which interferes with brain development and function. PKU affects 1 in every 15,000 live births in the United States (Cunningham et al., 2005).

PKU was the first inborn error of metabolism to be universally screened for in the United States. Since 1961, all newborns have been tested soon after birth for this disorder. Prompt diagnosis and therapy with a phenylalanine-restricted diet significantly decreases the incidence of mental retardation, but the optimal duration of treatment remains unclear (Aminoff, 2009).

The keys to the prevention of fetal anomalies caused by PKU are the identification of women in their reproductive years with the disorder and dietary compliance for women who are diagnosed. Screening for undiagnosed homozygous maternal PKU at the first prenatal visit may be warranted, especially in individuals with a family history of the disorder, with low intelligence of uncertain origin, or who have given birth to microcephalic infants. Ideally, women with PKU are placed on a dietary phenylalanine restriction before conception and throughout pregnancy. The dietary modification normally excludes all high-protein foods such as meat, milk, eggs, and nuts, as well as wheat products. Phenylalanine levels are monitored at least once and preferably twice a week throughout pregnancy (Gilbert, 2007). Experts recommend that maternal phenylalanine levels range between 2 and 6 mg/dl. These levels are associated with a decrease in fetal sequelae (Cunningham et al., 2005; Gilbert). High maternal phenylalanine levels are associated with microcephaly, mental retardation, and congenital heart defects in their children (Aminoff, 2009; Cunningham et al.). Ultrasound examinations are used for fetal surveillance beginning in the first trimester. A spontaneous vaginal birth is anticipated.

Women with PKU should be advised against breastfeeding because their milk will contain a high concentration of phenylalanine (Aminoff, 2009). If these women choose to breastfeed despite the risk, their phenylalanine blood levels must be monitored closely (Lawrence & Lawrence, 2005; Riordan, 2005). Breastfeeding mothers must still supplement the infant's diet with a special milk preparation: a phenylalanine-free formula that contains little or no phenylalanine (Riordan).

CARDIOVASCULAR DISORDERS

During a normal pregnancy the maternal cardiovascular system undergoes many changes that place a physiologic strain on the heart. The major cardiovascular changes that occur during a normal pregnancy and that affect the woman with cardiac disease are increased intravascular volume, decreased systemic vascular resistance, cardiac output changes occurring during labor and birth, and the intravascular volume changes that occur just after childbirth. The strain is present during pregnancy and continues for a few weeks after birth. The normal heart can compensate for the increased workload so that pregnancy, labor, and birth are generally well tolerated, but the diseased heart is hemodynamically challenged.

If the cardiovascular changes are not well tolerated, cardiac failure can develop during pregnancy, labor, or the postpartum period. In addition, if myocardial disease develops, valvular disease exists, or a congenital heart defect is present, **cardiac decompensation** (inability of the heart to maintain a sufficient cardiac output) may occur.

From 0.5% to 2% of pregnancies are complicated by heart disease. The rate of rheumatic fever, once responsible for the vast majority of cardiac disease in pregnancy, is now declining. Currently, congenital heart disease is an increasing cause of cardiac disease in pregnant women. Thanks to better management of congenital heart disease in childhood, pregnancy outcomes for women with these conditions are generally positive. However, cardiac disease accounts for 15% of maternal mortality during pregnancy (Gilbert, 2007). Box 20-2 lists maternal cardiac disease risk groups and their related mortality rates. Pregnancy is contraindicated in the presence of several cardiac conditions, including pulmonary hypertension, Marfan syndrome with aortic involvement, and Eisenmenger syndrome, because the maternal mortality rate is extremely high, approximately 50% (Gilbert).

The degree of disability experienced by the woman with cardiac disease is often more important in the treatment and prognosis during pregnancy than the diagnosis of the type of cardiovascular disease. The New York Heart Association (NYHA) functional classification of heart disease, is a widely accepted standard:

- Class I: asymptomatic without limitation of physical activity
- Class II: symptomatic with slight limitation of activity
- Class III: symptomatic with marked limitation of activity
- Class IV: symptomatic with inability to carry on any physical activity without discomfort

Case Study: Class III Cardiac Disorder

No classification of heart disease can be considered rigid or absolute, but the NYHA classification offers a basic practical guide for treatment, assuming that frequent prenatal visits, good patient cooperation, and appropriate

BOX 20-2

Maternal Cardiac Disease Risk Groups

GROUP I (MORTALITY RATE <1%)

- Atrial septal defect
- Patent ductus arteriosus
- Mitral valve prolapse with regurgitation
- Tetralogy of Fallot (corrected with good repair)
- Mitral stenosis or aortic regurgitation New York Heart Association (NYHA) class I and II

GROUP II (MORTALITY RATE 5%-20%)

- Mitral stenosis NYHA class III and IV or with atrial fibrillation
- Aortic stenosis
- Coarctation of aorta without valve involvement
- Uncorrected tetralogy of Fallot
- Previous myocardial infarction
- Marfan syndrome with normal aorta
- Artificial heart valve

GROUP III (MORTALITY RATE ~50%)

- Pulmonary hypertension
- Endocarditis
- Marfan syndrome with aortic involvement
- Eisenmenger syndrome

Source: Gilbert, E. (2007). *Manual of high risk pregnancy & delivery* (4th ed.). St. Louis: Mosby.

obstetric care occur. Medical therapy is conducted by a team approach and includes the cardiologist, the obstetrician, and nurses. The functional classification may change for the pregnant woman because of the hemodynamic changes that occur in the cardiovascular system. A 30% to 45% increase in cardiac output occurs, as compared with nonpregnancy resting values, with most of the increase in the first trimester and the peak at 20 to 26 weeks of gestation (Blanchard & Shabetai, 2009). The functional classification of the disease is determined at 3 months and again at 7 or 8 months of gestation. Pregnant women may progress from class I or II to III or IV during the pregnancy as cardiac output increases and more stress is placed on the heart.

Miscarriage and stillbirth both occur more often in the pregnant woman with cardiac problems than in healthy women. In addition, IUGR (a fetus smaller in size than would be expected for a particular gestational age) is common, probably because of low oxygen pressure in the mother (Blanchard & Shabetai, 2009).

A diagnosis of cardiac disease depends on the history, physical examination, radiographic and electrocardiographic findings, Holter monitoring, echocardiography, and, if indicated, ultrasonographic results. Most diagnostic studies are noninvasive and can be safely performed during pregnancy. The differential diagnosis of heart disease also involves ruling out respiratory problems and other potential causes of chest pain.

Selected Cardiovascular Disorders

Congenital cardiac diseases

Atrial septal defect. Atrial septal defect (ASD) is an abnormal opening between the atria. It is one of the causes of a left-to-right shunt and is the most common congenital defect seen during pregnancy. This defect may go undetected because the woman is usually asymptomatic. The pregnant woman with an ASD will most likely have an uncomplicated pregnancy. Some women may have right-sided heart failure or arrhythmias as the pregnancy progresses as a result of increased plasma volume.

Coarctation of the aorta. Coarctation of the aorta is a localized narrowing of the aorta near the insertion of the ductus. Patients with this lesion have hypertension in their upper extremities but hypotension in the lower extremities. Coarctation of the aorta is an example of an acyanotic congenital heart lesion. If at all possible, the lesion should be corrected surgically before pregnancy. However, pregnancy is usually relatively safe for the woman with uncomplicated, uncorrected coarctation. Maternal mortality rate is approximately 3% (Blanchard & Shabetai, 2009). Complications that can occur include hypertension, congestive heart failure, cerebrovascular accident (stroke), aortic dissection, aneurysm, and rupture (Blanchard & Shabetai; Easterling & Stout, 2007). The mainstays of treatment for uncorrected coarctation of the aorta during pregnancy are rest and antihypertensive medications, preferably beta-adrenergic blocking agents. Vaginal birth is possible with epidural anesthesia and shortening of the second stage with the assistance of vacuum or forceps use, if necessary. Beta-blockers should be continued throughout labor. Because of the risk of endocarditis, antibiotic prophylaxis is recommended at birth. The rate of fetal loss is approximately 10% (Cunningham et al., 2005; Setaro & Caulin-Glaser, 2004).

Tetralogy of Fallot. Tetralogy of Fallot is by far the most common cyanotic heart disease observed during pregnancy (Blanchard & Shabetai, 2009). Components of tetralogy of Fallot include a ventricular septal defect (VSD), pulmonary stenosis, overriding aorta, and right ventricular hypertrophy, leading to a right-to-left shunt. Women with tetralogy of Fallot are encouraged to have surgical repair preconceptionally because pregnancy does not cause a significant risk once the VSD and pulmonary stenosis have been repaired. Women with uncorrected tetralogy of Fallot, on the other hand, experience more right-to-left shunting during pregnancy, resulting in reduced blood flow through the pulmonary circulation and increasing hypoxemia, which can cause syncope or death. Maintenance of venous return in women with uncorrected tetralogy of Fallot is critical. Therefore the most dangerous time for these women is the late third trimester of pregnancy and the early postpartum period, when venous return is reduced by the large pregnant uterus and by peripheral venous pooling after birth. Use of pressure-graded support hose is recommended. Blood loss during birth may also adversely affect venous return, thus blood volume must be adequately maintained. Prophylactic antibiotics should be given during the intrapartum period (Blanchard & Shabetai).

Acquired cardiac diseases

Mitral valve prolapse. Mitral valve prolapse (MVP) is a fairly common, usually benign, condition. Recently, more specific echocardiographic diagnostic criteria have resulted in significantly reduced prevalence estimates for MVP (perhaps 1% of the female population) than previously thought (Blanchard & Shabetai, 2009). In MVP the mitral valve leaflets prolapse into the left atrium during ventricular systole, allowing some backflow of blood. Midsystolic click and late systolic murmur are hallmarks of this syndrome. Most cases are asymptomatic. A few women have atypical chest pain (sharp and located in the left side of the chest) that occurs at rest and does not respond to nitrates. They may also have anxiety, palpitations, dyspnea on exertion, and syncope. Specific treatment is generally not necessary except for symptomatic tachyarrhythmias and, rarely, heart failure (Cunningham et al., 2005). Chest pain and arrhythmias are usually treated with beta-blockers such as atenolol or metoprolol (Lopressor). If symptoms are unusually severe, thyroid function should also be checked (Blanchard & Shabetai). Pregnancy and its associated hemodynamic changes may change or alleviate the murmur and click of MVP, as well as symptoms. Pregnancy is generally well tolerated unless bacterial endocarditis occurs. Antibiotic prophylaxis is usually given before birth to prevent bacterial endocarditis (Cunningham et al.; Easterling & Stout, 2007).

Mitral stenosis. Mitral stenosis is almost always caused by rheumatic heart disease (RHD), a consequence of rheumatic fever (Easterling & Stout, 2007). Rheumatic fever develops suddenly, often several symptom-free weeks after an inadequately treated group A β-hemolytic streptococcal throat infection. Episodes of rheumatic fever create an autoimmune reaction in the heart tissue, leading to permanent damage of heart valves (usually the mitral valve) and the chordae tendineae cordis. This damage is classified as RHD. RHD may be evident during acute rheumatic fever or discovered years later. Recurrences of rheumatic fever are common, each with the potential to increase the severity of heart damage.

Mitral stenosis is a narrowing of the opening of the mitral valve caused by stiffening of valve leaflets, which obstructs blood flow from the atrium to the ventricle. As the mitral valve narrows, dyspnea worsens, occurring first on exertion and eventually at rest. A tight stenosis plus the increase in blood volume and cardiac output of normal pregnancy may cause pulmonary edema, atrial fibrillation, right-sided heart failure, infective endocarditis, pulmonary embolism, and massive hemoptysis (Blanchard & Shabetai, 2009; Cunningham et al., 2005). Approximately 25% of women with mitral valve stenosis may become symptomatic for the first time during pregnancy. Maternal mortality is related to functional capacity. Almost all maternal deaths related to mitral stenosis occur in women who are classified as NYHA class III or class IV (Cunningham et al.).

Pharmacologic treatment for women with a history of RHD includes prophylaxis with daily oral penicillin G or monthly benzathine penicillin (Bicillin) injections, diuretics to prevent pulmonary edema, and beta-blockers or calcium channel blockers to prevent tachycardia (Easterling & Stout, 2007). A combination of drugs will most likely be needed. Cardioversion may be needed for new-onset atrial fibrillation. Women who have chronic atrial fibrillation may need digoxin or beta-blockers to control the heart rate. In addition, anticoagulant therapy may be needed to prevent embolism (Blanchard & Shabetai, 2009).

The care of the woman with mitral stenosis is typically managed by reducing her activity, restricting dietary sodium, and increasing bed rest, in addition to the pharmacologic management discussed previously. The pregnant woman with mitral stenosis should be monitored clinically for symptoms and with echocardiograms to monitor the atrial and ventricular size, as well as heart valve function. Prophylaxis for intrapartum endocarditis and pulmonary infections may be given to women at high risk (Blanchard & Shabetai, 2009; Easterling & Stout, 2007).

During labor, adequate pain control is required to prevent tachycardia. Epidural analgesia for labor is preferred (Easterling & Stout, 2007). Encourage the woman to labor and give birth in the lateral decubitus position and avoid the supine and lithotomy positions. Shortening the second stage of labor by vacuum- or forceps-assisted birth is also important to decrease the cardiac workload. Cesarean birth should be performed only for obstetric indications. Aggressive diuresis is initiated immediately after birth because fluid shifts can place the woman at risk for pulmonary edema (Blanchard & Shabetai, 2009; Easterling & Stout).

For women with NYHA class III or IV cardiac disease, surgical intervention may be necessary. Valve replacement and open commissurotomy have been performed during pregnancy successfully. Currently, balloon valvotomy is likely to be the procedure of choice. Surgical intervention should be considered only when symptoms cannot be controlled by medical therapy.

Aortic stenosis. Aortic stenosis is a narrowing of the opening of the aortic valve leading to an obstruction to left ventricular ejection. It is rarely encountered as a complication of pregnancy because most women who develop this condition do so after their childbearing years are over. In the past the maternal mortality rate was reported to be as high as 17%, but it has decreased over the last several decades (Easterling & Stout, 2007). Medical management is similar to that for mitral stenosis.

Myocardial infarction. Myocardial infarction (MI), an acute ischemic event, rarely occurs in women of childbearing age. It is estimated to occur in only 1 of 10,000 pregnancies (Blanchard & Shabetai, 2009). Authorities anticipate that the incidence will rise, however, considering the increase in the age of childbearing women and of other risk factors such as stress, smoking, and cocaine use. Frequently, women with coronary artery disease have classic risk factors such as cigarette smoking, hyperlipidemia, obesity, and hypertension (Cunningham et al., 2005). Finally, the cardiac changes that normally occur in a pregnant woman may provoke symptoms for the first time.

MI occurs most frequently in the last trimester and in women older than 33 years. The maternal mortality rate from an MI during pregnancy is approximately 20%. Women are most likely to die at the time of the infarction or during labor and birth (Blanchard & Shabetai, 2009). The risk of maternal death increases if women give birth within 2 weeks of an MI (Easterling & Stout, 2007). Women who have MIs during pregnancy or the postpartum period should be assessed for thrombophilias (deficiency of proteins involved in coagulation inhibition), such as antiphospholipid antibody.

Medical management for pregnant women with MI is the same as that for nonpregnant women and includes the administration of oxygen, aspirin, beta-blockers, nitrates, and heparin. Women who have had symptomatic cardiac disease during the pregnancy should continue cardiac medications and receive oxygen during labor. Because pain can lead to tachycardia and increased cardiac demands, pain control during labor is crucial. The side-lying position is preferred to prevent pressure on the vena cava. Vaginal birth is preferable, with avoidance of maternal pushing and a vacuum- or forceps-assisted birth (Easterling & Stout, 2007).

Other cardiac diseases and conditions

Peripartum cardiomyopathy. Peripartum cardiomyopathy (PCM) is congestive heart failure with cardiomyopathy. The classic criteria for the diagnosis of PCM include development of congestive heart failure during the last month of pregnancy or within the first 5 postpartum months, absence of heart disease before the last month of pregnancy, a left ventricular ejection fraction of less than 45%, and, most importantly, lack of another cause for heart failure. The cause of the disease is unknown (Blanchard & Shabetai, 2009). Theories suggest a genetic predisposition or autoimmunity as a cause. A nutritional mechanism may be involved as well. At one time, viral infections were considered to be a possible cause, but the prevalence of antibodies to echovirus and Coxsackie virus has not been found to be greater in women with cardiomyopathy than in women who do not have the disease (Easterling & Stout, 2007). The incidence of PCM is 1 per 3000 to 4000 live births in the United States (Blanchard & Shabetai).

Associated risk factors include maternal age older than 35 years, multifetal gestation, preeclampsia, gestational hypertension, multiparity, African descent, and prolonged tocolytic therapy (Klein & Galan, 2004). Clinical findings are those of congestive heart failure (left ventricular failure). Clinical manifestations include dyspnea, fatigue, and edema, as well as radiologic findings of cardiomegaly.

Medical management of PCM includes a regimen used for congestive heart failure: diuretics, sodium and fluid restriction, afterload-reducing agents, and digoxin. Anticoagulation may be necessary if the cardiac chambers are significantly dilated and contract poorly because of the increased risk for clot formation. Angiotensin-converting enzyme inhibitors, often prescribed to achieve afterload reduction, can be used only in the postpartum period because they are associated with fetal renal dysfunction. During labor, epidural anesthesia is often used for pain control to decrease the cardiac workload and reduce tachycardia. Cesarean birth should be performed only for obstetric indications (Easterling & Stout, 2007).

In one half of all women with PCM, left ventricular dysfunction resolves within 6 months. These women generally do well. If left ventricular dysfunction does not resolve within 6 months, however, approximately 85% of women with PCM will die in the next 4 to 5 years. Death is usually the result of progressive congestive heart failure, arrhythmia, or thromboembolism (Easterling & Stout, 2007). The recurrence rate for cardiomyopathy in a subsequent pregnancy is high, anywhere from 20% to 50%. The risk of recurrence is increased in women who did not have complete recovery of left ventricular function after the initial episode of PCM (Blanchard & Shabetai, 2009).

Infective endocarditis. Infective endocarditis, or inflammation of the innermost lining (endocardium) of the heart caused by invasion of microorganisms, is an uncommon disorder during pregnancy (Cunningham et al., 2005). It may be seen in women taking street drugs intravenously. Bacterial endocarditis, leading to incompetence of heart valves and thus congestive heart failure and cerebral emboli, can result in death. Treatment is with antibiotics.

Eisenmenger syndrome. Eisenmenger syndrome is a right-to-left or bidirectional shunting that can be at either the atrial or the ventricular level of the heart and is combined with elevated pulmonary vascular resistance. It is associated with an underlying structural cardiac defect, either a ventricular septal defect (most common) or a patent ductus arteriosus (Blanchard & Shabetai, 2009). Eisenmenger syndrome is associated with high mortality (50% in mothers and 50% in fetuses). Because of the poor pregnancy outcomes, pregnancy should be avoided by women with Eisenmenger syndrome. Although sudden death can occur at any time, the intrapartum and early postpartum periods seem to be the most dangerous (Blanchard & Shabetai). Maternal morbidity is associated with right ventricular failure and associated cardiogenic shock (Cunningham et al., 2005). If pregnancy occurs, termination may be recommended if the woman has significant pulmonary hypertension.

In women who continue pregnancy despite the risks, management includes measures to maintain pulmonary blood flow. Physical activity is strictly limited. Other interventions include the use of pressure-graded elastic support hose and oxygen therapy. Hospitalization may be necessary to provide optimal care (Blanchard & Shabetai, 2009). During labor and birth, narcotic-based regional anesthesia provides pain relief without causing excessive hemodynamic instability. Hypotension must be prevented at all costs because it results in more right-to-left shunting, thereby increasing hypoxemia, increasing pulmonary vascular resistance, and worsening the shunt. Volume overload or excessive systemic resistance must also be prevented because it further stresses the failing right side of the heart. Cesarean birth should be performed only for obstetric indications and avoided whenever possible (Easterling & Stout, 2007).

Marfan syndrome. Marfan syndrome is an autosomal dominant disorder characterized by generalized weakness of the connective tissue, resulting in the characteristic feature of the disease, aortic root dilation. Other signs and symptoms associated with Marfan syndrome include dislocation of the optic lens, deformity of the anterior thorax, scoliosis, long limbs, joint laxity, and arachnodactyly. Diagnosis is usually based on family history and physical examination, including ocular, cardiovascular, and skeletal features (Easterling & Stout, 2007).

The majority of deaths from Marfan syndrome are caused by aortic dissection and rupture. Excruciating chest pain is the most common symptom of aortic dissection. Aortic dissection most often occurs in the third trimester of pregnancy or postpartum. Overall, the maternal mortality rate associated with Marfan's syndrome is greater than 50%. However, the mortality rate is significantly increased if the aortic root diameter measures more than 4.0 cm than if it is smaller in size (Easterling & Stout, 2007).

Preconception counseling for women with Marfan syndrome is essential to make women aware of the risks of pregnancy with this disease. Because the condition is inherited, 50% of the children born to women with Marfan syndrome will also have the disorder. An accurate assessment of the aortic root using noninvasive imaging with transesophageal echocardiography, computed tomography, or magnetic resonance imaging must be obtained to assess the woman's specific risk and make management recommendations. Elective repair of the aorta is recommended when the aortic root diameter measures 5.5 to 6.0 cm. Therefore women with an aortic root diameter greater than 5.5 cm should be counseled to have it repaired before becoming pregnant. Women with an aortic root diameter less than 4.0 cm, on the other hand, can attempt pregnancy with only modest risk (Easterling & Stout, 2007).

Management during pregnancy includes restricted activity and use of beta-blockers to maintain a resting heart rate of approximately 70 beats/min. Tachycardia should also be prevented during labor. Women with aortic root diameters less than 4.0 cm can give birth vaginally, reserving cesarean birth for obstetric indications. Some authorities, however, recommend that women with larger aortic root diameters give birth by elective cesarean because of concerns about increased pressure in the aorta during labor (Blanchard & Shabetai, 2009; Easterling & Stout, 2007).

Heart Transplantation

Increasing numbers of heart recipients are successfully completing pregnancies. Before conception the woman should be assessed for quality of ventricular function and potential rejection of the transplant. The woman should also be considered to be stabilized on her immunosuppressant regimen. Women who have no evidence of rejection and have normal cardiac function at the beginning of the pregnancy appear to do well during pregnancy, labor, and birth. Complications that are common in women who have had a heart transplant include hypertension, an episode of rejection, and preterm birth (Cunningham et al., 2005). Conception should be postponed for at least 1 year after transplantation to prevent acute rejection episodes (Blanchard & Shabetai, 2009). During labor, beta-blocking agents may be needed to prevent tachycardia resulting from vagal denervation from the transplant surgery. Vaginal birth is desired, but transplant recipients have an increased rate of cesarean births. Management of the intrapartal period requires the coordination of care among all health care providers involved in the care of the woman and her fetus. After birth the neonate may exhibit immunosuppressive effects during the first week of life. Though information is limited, breastfeeding infants of mothers who are taking cyclosporine absorb undetectable amounts (Weiner & Buhimschi, 2004).

CARE MANAGEMENT

The presence of cardiac disease makes the decision to become pregnant more difficult. Planned pregnancy requires that the woman understand the peripartum risks. If the pregnancy is unplanned, the nurse needs to explore the woman's desire to continue the pregnancy after examining the risks in relation to the status of her cardiac condition. The woman's partner and family should be included in the discussion. Women with significant cardiac compromise may choose to terminate the pregnancy. If she chooses to continue the pregnancy, the high risk pregnant woman's condition may be assessed as often as weekly (see Nursing Process box: Cardiac Disease). For additional information on cardiac disease, visit the American Heart Association's website at www.americanheart.org.

Antepartum

Therapy for the pregnant woman with heart disease is focused on minimizing stress on the heart. This stress is greatest between 28 and 32 weeks of gestation as the hemodynamic changes of pregnancy reach their maximum. Factors that increase the risk of cardiac decompensation are avoided. The workload of the cardiovascular system is reduced by appropriate treatment of any coexisting emotional stress, hypertension, anemia, hyperthyroidism, or obesity.

Signs and symptoms of cardiac decompensation are taught at the first prenatal visit and reviewed at each subsequent visit (see Signs of Potential Complications box; see also the Nursing Process box: Cardiac Disease for other information to include in patient teaching).

Infections are treated promptly because respiratory, urinary, or gastrointestinal (GI) tract infections can complicate the condition by accelerating the heart rate and by direct spread of organisms (e.g., streptococci) to the heart structure. The woman should notify her physician at the first sign of infection or exposure to an infection. Vaccination against influenza and pneumococcus may be given. Prophylactic antibiotics against bacterial endocarditis during pregnancy are not recommended by the American Heart Association, but their use is optional in high risk patients who give birth vaginally. Because bacteremia is common during both vaginal and cesarean birth, many

NURSING PROCESS *Cardiac Disease*

ASSESSMENT

The assessment of a pregnant woman with cardiac disease may include the following:

Interview

- Personal and family medical history: diseases of cardiovascular significance, including congenital heart disease, streptococcal infections, rheumatic fever, valvular disease, endocarditis, congestive heart failure, angina, or myocardial infarction
- Factors that would increase stress on the heart:
  - Anemia
  - Infection
  - Edema
- Symptoms of cardiac decompensation (see Signs of Potential Complications box: Cardiac Decompensation)
- Current medications
- Current stressors

Physical examination

- Monitor:
  - Amount and pattern of edema
  - Vital signs
  - Amount and pattern of weight gain.
- Observe for signs of cardiac decompensation (see Signs of Potential Complications Box: Cardiac Decompensation)
- Review results of laboratory and diagnostic tests:
  - Routine urinalysis and blood work (complete blood count and blood chemistry)
  - Perform baseline 12-lead electrocardiogram at the beginning of the pregnancy, if not before pregnancy
  - Perform echocardiograms and pulse oximetry studies as indicated

NURSING DIAGNOSES

Possible nursing diagnoses include the following:

Prenatal period

- *Fear* related to:
  - Increased peripartum risk
- *Deficient knowledge* related to:
  - Cardiac condition
  - Pregnancy and how it affects cardiac condition
  - Requirements to alter self-management activities
- *Activity intolerance* related to:
  - Cardiac condition
- *Risk for self-care deficit (bathing, grooming, and dressing)* related to:
  - Fatigue or activity intolerance
  - Need for bed rest
- *Impaired home maintenance* related to:
  - Woman's confinement to bed or limited activity level

Intrapartum period

- *Anxiety* related to:
  - Fear for infant's safety during birth
- *Fear of dying* related to:
  - Perceived physiologic inability to cope with stress of labor
- *Risk for impaired gas exchange* related to:
  - Cardiac condition

Postpartum period

- *Risk for impaired gas exchange* related to:
  - Cardiac condition
- *Risk for excess fluid volume* related to:
  - Extravascular fluid shifts
- *Ineffective breastfeeding* related to:
  - Fatigue from cardiac condition

EXPECTED OUTCOMES OF CARE

Expected outcomes are that the woman (and family, if appropriate) will do the following:

- Verbalize understanding of the disorder, management, and probable outcome.
- Describe her role in management, including when and how to take medication, adjust diet, and prepare for and participate in treatment.
- Cope with emotional reactions to pregnancy and an infant at risk.
- Adapt to the physiologic stressors of pregnancy, labor, and birth.
- Identify and use support systems.
- Carry her fetus to viability or to term.

PLAN OF CARE AND INTERVENTIONS

- Review signs and symptoms of cardiac decompensation with the pregnant woman and her family.
- Provide patient teaching as follows, based on the woman's NYHA classification:

The woman with Class I or II heart disease

- Needs 8 to 10 hours of sleep every night and should take 30-minute naps after meals.
- Should restrict activities (limit housework, shopping, and exercise) to the amount recommended for the functional classification of her heart disease.

The woman with Class II cardiac disease

- Should avoid heavy exertion; stop any activity that causes even minor signs and symptoms of cardiac decompensation.
- Will likely be admitted to the hospital near term (or earlier if signs of cardiac overload or dysrhythmia develop) for evaluation and treatment.

The woman with Class III cardiac disease

- Needs bed rest for much of the day

Other considerations

- Treat infections promptly; administer prophylactic antibiotics against bacterial endocarditis as ordered.
- Provide nutrition counseling. Refer to a registered dietitian as necessary.
- Teach the woman how to avoid constipation and resulting straining with bowel movements (Valsalva maneuver).
- Administer cardiac medications as prescribed.
- Monitor drug levels.
- Monitor the woman's blood work.
- Review results of tests for fetal maturity and well-being and placental sufficiency.
- Reinforce the need for close medical supervision.

EVALUATION

The nurse uses the previously stated expected outcomes as criteria to evaluate the care of the woman with cardiac disease.

signs of POTENTIAL COMPLICATIONS

Cardiac Decompensation

PREGNANT WOMAN: SUBJECTIVE SYMPTOMS

- Increasing fatigue or difficulty breathing, or both, with her usual activities
- Feeling of smothering
- Frequent cough
- Palpitations; feeling that her heart is "racing"
- Generalized edema: swelling of face, feet, legs, fingers (e.g., rings do not fit anymore)

NURSE: OBJECTIVE SIGNS

- Irregular, weak, rapid pulse (≥100 beats/min)
- Progressive, generalized edema
- Crackles at base of lungs after two inspirations and exhalations that do not clear after coughing
- Orthopnea; increasing dyspnea
- Rapid respirations (≥25 breaths/min)
- Moist, frequent cough
- Cyanosis of lips and nail beds

practitioners routinely give antibiotic prophylaxis to all high risk patients (Easterling & Stout, 2007).

Nutrition counseling is necessary, optimally with the woman's family present. The pregnant woman needs a well-balanced diet with iron and folic acid supplementation, high protein, and adequate calories to gain weight. Iron supplements tend to cause constipation. The pregnant woman should increase her intake of fluids and fiber. A stool softener may also be prescribed. The woman with a cardiac disorder should avoid straining during defecation, thus causing the Valsalva maneuver (forced expiration against a closed airway, which when released, causes blood to rush to the heart and overload the cardiac system). The woman's intake of potassium is monitored to prevent hypokalemia, especially if she is taking diuretics. A referral to a registered dietitian is recommended.

Cardiac medications are prescribed as needed for the pregnant woman, with attention to fetal well-being. The hemodynamic changes that occur during pregnancy, such as increased plasma volume and increased renal clearance of drugs, can alter the amount of medication needed to establish and maintain a therapeutic drug level.

If anticoagulant therapy is required during pregnancy for conditions such as recurrent venous thrombosis, pulmonary embolus, RHD, or prosthetic valves, heparin should be used because this large-molecule drug does not cross the placenta. The nurse should be aware of the goals of therapy and closely monitor the prothrombin time (e.g., International Normalized Ratio [INR]) accordingly. The woman may need to learn to self-administer injectable agents such as heparin or low–molecular-weight heparin (Lovenox). A woman taking warfarin (Coumadin) requires specific nutritional teaching to avoid foods high in vitamin K, such as raw, dark green leafy vegetables, which counteract the effects of warfarin.

Tests for fetal maturity and well-being and placental sufficiency may be necessary. Other therapy is directly related to the functional classification of heart disease. The nurse must reinforce the need for close medical supervision (see Nursing Care Plan: The Pregnant Woman with Heart Disease).

Intrapartum

For all pregnant women the intrapartum period is the time that evokes the most apprehension in patients and caregivers. The woman with impaired cardiac function has additional reasons to be anxious because labor and giving birth place an extra burden on her already compromised cardiovascular system.

Assessments include the routine assessments for all laboring women, as well as assessment for cardiac decompensation (see Signs of Potential Complications box). In addition, arterial blood gases (ABGs) may be needed to assess for adequate oxygenation. A Swan-Ganz catheter may be inserted to accurately monitor hemodynamic status during labor and birth. Electrocardiographic monitoring and continuous monitoring of blood pressure and oxygen saturation (pulse oximetry) are usually instituted for the woman, and the fetal heart rate is continuously monitored electronically.

NURSING ALERT A pulse rate of 100 beats/min or greater or a respiratory rate greater than 24 breaths/min is a concern. Check the respiratory status frequently for developing dyspnea, coughing, or crackles at the base of the lungs. Note the color and temperature of the skin as well. Pale, cool, clammy skin may indicate cardiac shock.

Nursing care during labor and birth focuses on the promotion of cardiac function. Minimize anxiety by maintaining a calm atmosphere in the labor and birth rooms. Provide anticipatory guidance by keeping the woman and her family informed of labor progress and events that will probably occur, as well as answering any questions they have. Support the woman's childbirth preparation method to the degree it is feasible for her cardiac condition. Nursing techniques that promote comfort, such as back massage, are also used.

Cardiac function is supported by keeping the woman's head and shoulders elevated and body parts resting on pillows. The side-lying position usually facilitates positive hemodynamics during labor. Discomfort is relieved with medication and supportive care. Epidural regional anesthesia provides better pain relief than narcotics and causes fewer alterations in hemodynamics (Cunningham et al., 2005).

LEGAL TIP **Cardiac and Metabolic Emergencies**
The management of emergencies such as maternal cardiopulmonary distress or arrest or maternal metabolic crisis should be documented in policies,

NURSING CARE PLAN *The Pregnant Woman with Heart Disease*

NURSING DIAGNOSIS Activity intolerance related to effects of pregnancy on the woman with rheumatic heart disease with mitral valve stenosis

Expected Outcome *Woman will verbalize a plan to change lifestyle throughout pregnancy so as to reduce the risk of cardiac decompensation.*

Nursing Interventions/*Rationales*

- Assist the woman in identifying factors that decrease activity tolerance and explore extent of limitations *to establish a baseline for evaluation.*
- Help the woman develop an individualized program of activity and rest, taking into account the living and working environment, as well as support of family and friends, *to maintain sufficient cardiac output.*
- Teach the woman to monitor physiologic responses to activity (e.g., pulse rate, respiratory rate) and reduce activity that causes fatigue or pain *to maintain sufficient cardiac output and prevent potential injury to fetus.*
- Enlist the woman's family and friends to assist her in pacing activities and to provide support in performing role functions and self-management activities that are too strenuous *to increase the chances of compliance with activity restrictions.*
- Suggest that the woman maintain an activity log that records activities, time, duration, intensity, and physiologic response *to evaluate effectiveness of and adherence to the activity program.*
- Discuss various quiet diversional activities that the woman can or may perform *to decrease the potential for boredom during rest periods.*

NURSING DIAGNOSIS Risk for ineffective therapeutic regimen management related to the woman's first pregnancy and perceived sense of wellness

Expected Outcome *Woman will participate in an effective therapeutic regimen for pregnancy complicated by heart disease.*

Nursing Interventions/*Rationales*

- Identify factors, such as insufficient knowledge about the effect of cardiac disease on pregnancy, that might inhibit the woman from participating in a therapeutic regimen *to promote early interventions, such as teaching about the importance of rest.*
- Teach the woman and her family about factors such as lack of rest or not taking prescribed medications that might adversely affect the pregnancy *to provide information and promote empowerment over the situation.*
- Encourage expression of feelings about the disease and its potential effect on the pregnancy *to promote a sense of trust.*
- Identify resources in the community *to provide a shared sense of common experiences.*
- Encourage the woman to verbalize her plan for carrying out the regimen of care *to evaluate the effects of teaching.*

NURSING DIAGNOSIS Decreased cardiac output related to increased circulatory volume secondary to pregnancy and cardiac disease

Expected Outcome *Woman will exhibit signs of adequate cardiac output (i.e., normal pulse and blood pressure; normal heart and breath sounds; normal skin color, tone, and turgor; normal capillary refill; normal urine output; no evidence of edema).*

Nursing Interventions/*Rationales*

- Reinforce the importance of activity and rest cycles *to prevent cardiac complications.*
- Reinforce the importance of the frequent visit schedule to the caregiver *to provide adequate surveillance of the high risk pregnancy.*
- Teach the woman and her family members the signs of cardiac decompensation *to provide information about when to contact the health care provider.*
- Teach the woman to lie on her side *to increase uteroplacental blood flow* and to elevate legs while sitting *to promote venous return.*
- Monitor intake and output and check for *edema to assess for renal complications or venous return problems.*
- Monitor fetal heart rate and fetal activity and perform a nonstress test as indicated *to assess fetal status and detect uteroplacental insufficiency.*

procedures, and protocols. Any independent nursing actions appropriate to the emergency should be clearly identified.

Beta-adrenergic agents such as terbutaline (Brethine) are associated with various side effects, including tachycardia, irregular pulse, myocardial ischemia, and pulmonary edema. A synthetic oxytocin, Syntocinon, can be used for induction of labor. This drug does not appear to cause significant coronary artery constriction in doses prescribed for labor induction or control of postpartum uterine atony. Cervical ripening agents containing prostaglandin are usually tolerated well, but they should be used cautiously.

If no obstetric problems exist, vaginal birth is recommended and may be accomplished with the woman in the side-lying position to facilitate uterine perfusion. If the supine position is used, position a pad under one hip to displace the uterus laterally and minimize the danger of supine hypotension. Have the woman flex her knees and place her feet flat on the bed. To prevent compression of popliteal veins and an increase in blood volume in the chest and trunk as a result of the effects of gravity, do not use stirrups. Open-glottis pushing is recommended. Avoid the Valsalva maneuver when pushing in the second stage of labor because it reduces diastolic ventricular filling and obstructs left ventricular outflow. Mask oxygen is important. Episiotomy and vacuum extraction or outlet forceps may be used to decrease the length of the second stage of labor and decrease the workload of the heart in second stage labor. Cesarean birth is not routinely recommended for women who have cardiovascular disease because of the risks of dramatic fluid shifts, sustained hemodynamic changes, and increased blood loss.

Penicillin prophylaxis may be ordered for nonallergic pregnant women with class II or higher cardiac disease to protect against bacterial endocarditis in labor and during the early puerperium. Women who are allergic to penicillin may receive vancomycin instead. Dilute IV oxytocin immediately after birth may be given to prevent hemorrhage caused by uterine atony. Ergot products should not be used because they increase blood pressure. Fluid balance should be maintained and blood loss replaced. If tubal sterilization is desired, surgery is delayed at least several days to ensure homeostasis.

Postpartum

Monitoring for cardiac decompensation in the postpartum period is essential. The first 24 to 48 hours postpartum are the most hemodynamically difficult for the woman. Hemorrhage or infection, or both, may worsen the cardiac condition. The woman with a cardiac disorder may continue to require a Swan-Ganz catheter and ABG monitoring.

NURSING ALERT The immediate postbirth period is hazardous for a woman whose heart function is compromised. Cardiac output increases rapidly as extravascular fluid is remobilized into the vascular compartment. At the moment of birth, intraabdominal pressure is reduced drastically; pressure on veins is removed, the splanchnic vessels engorge, and blood flow to the heart is increased.

Care in the postpartum period is tailored to the woman's functional capacity. Postpartum assessment of the woman with cardiac disease includes vital signs, oxygen saturation levels, lung and heart auscultation, edema, amount and character of bleeding, uterine tone and fundal height, urinary output, pain (especially chest pain), the activity-rest pattern, dietary intake, mother-infant interactions, and emotional state. The head of the bed is elevated, and the woman is encouraged to lie on her side. Bed rest may be ordered, with or without bathroom privileges. Progressive ambulation may be permitted as tolerated. The nurse may need to help the woman meet her grooming and hygiene needs and other activities. Bowel movements without stress or strain for the woman are promoted with stool softeners, diet, and fluids.

The woman may need a family member to help in the care of the infant. Breastfeeding is not contraindicated, but not all women with heart disease (particularly those with life-threatening disease) will be able to do so (Lawrence & Lawrence, 2005; Riordan, 2005). The woman who chooses to breastfeed will need the support of her family and the nursing staff to be successful. For example, she may need assistance in positioning herself or the infant for feeding. To conserve the woman's energy further the infant may need to be brought to the mother and taken from her after the feeding. Women who breastfeed may need less medication than usual for their cardiac condition, especially diuretics. Because diuretics can cause neonatal diuresis that can lead to dehydration, lactating women must be monitored closely to determine if medication doses can be reduced and still be effective.

If the woman is unable to breastfeed and her energy is not sufficient to allow her to bottle-feed the infant, the baby can be kept at the bedside so she can look at and touch her baby to establish an emotional bond with her baby with a low expenditure of energy. The infant should be held at the mother's eye level and near her lips and brought to her fingers. At the same time, involving the mother passively in her infant's care helps the mother feel vitally important–as she is–to the infant's well-being (e.g., "You can offer something no one else can: provide your baby with your sounds, touch, and rhythms that are so comforting."). Perhaps the woman can be encouraged to make a tape recording of her talking, singing, or whispering, which can be played for the baby in the nursery to help the infant feel her presence and be in contact with her voice. This measure also enhances maternal-infant bonding.

Preparation for discharge is carefully planned with the woman and family. Provision of help for the woman in the home by relatives, friends, and others must be addressed. If necessary, the nurse refers the family to community resources (e.g., for homemaking services). Rest and sleep periods, activity, and diet must be planned. The couple may also need information about reestablishing sexual relations and contraception or sterilization.

Women with congenital heart disease should be offered contraceptive counseling. In general, for women with congenital heart disease, the complications associated with pregnancy are usually greater than the risks associated with any form of contraception (Easterling & Stout, 2007). Surgery to achieve permanent sterilization, however, is often not a safe procedure for women with class III or class IV cardiac disease (Gilbert, 2007). Women at particular risk for thromboembolism should avoid combined estrogen-progestin oral contraceptives, but progestin-only pills can be used. Parenteral progestins (e.g., Depo-Provera) are safe and effective for women with cardiac disease. The IUD may be used by some women with congenital heart lesions. Although a theoretical risk exists of developing endocarditis, the actual risk for women using the IUD is probably very minimal (Easterling & Stout).

Monitoring for cardiac decompensation continues through the first few weeks after birth because of hormonal shifts that affect hemodynamics. Maternal cardiac output is usually stabilized by 2 weeks postpartum (Easterling & Stout, 2007).

Both men and women with congenital heart disease are at increased risk for having children who also have congenital heart disease. The risk for affected mothers is greater, approximately two to more than three times that of affected fathers. Children born with congenital heart disease to parents with congenital heart defects appear to inherit the risk for cardiac maldevelopment in general because they often do not have the same defect as the parent (Easterling & Stout, 2007). Therefore preconception counseling and genetic counseling before a subsequent pregnancy are essential.

ANEMIA

Anemia is a common medical disorder of pregnancy, affecting from 20% to 60% of pregnant women (Kilpatrick, 2009). Anemia results in a reduction of the oxygen-carrying capacity of the blood. Because the oxygen-carrying capacity of the blood is decreased, the heart tries to compensate by increasing the cardiac output. This effort increases the workload of the heart and stresses ventricular function. Therefore anemia that occurs with any other complication (e.g., preeclampsia) may result in congestive heart failure.

An indirect index of the oxygen-carrying capacity is the packed RBC volume, or hematocrit level. The normal hematocrit range in nonpregnant women is 37% to 47%. However, normal values for pregnant women with adequate iron stores may be as low as 33%. According to the Centers for Disease Control and Prevention (CDC), anemia in pregnancy is defined as hemoglobin below 11 g/dl in the first and third trimesters and less than 10.5 g/dl in the second trimester (Kilpatrick, 2009). A hemoglobin level less than 6 to 8 mg/dl is considered severe anemia (Blackburn, 2007).

When a woman has anemia during pregnancy, the loss of blood at birth, even if minimal, is not well tolerated. She is at an increased risk for requiring blood transfusions. Women with anemia have a higher incidence of puerperal complications, such as infection, than pregnant women with normal hematologic values.

Care of the anemic pregnant woman requires that the health care provider distinguish between the normal physiologic anemia of pregnancy and the disease states. The majority of cases of anemia in pregnancy are caused by iron deficiency. The other types include a considerable variety of acquired and hereditary anemias, such as folic acid deficiency, sickle cell anemia, and thalassemia.

Iron Deficiency Anemia

Iron deficiency anemia is the most common anemia of pregnancy. It is diagnosed by checking the woman's serum ferritin level in addition to her hemoglobin and hematocrit levels. The serum ferritin level reflects iron reserves. A serum ferritin value less than 12 mcg/dl in the presence of a low hemoglobin value indicates iron deficiency anemia. An association appears to exist between maternal iron deficiency anemia, especially severe anemia, and preterm birth and low-birthweight infants, although whether these poor pregnancy outcomes are caused by iron deficiency anemia is uncertain (Samuels, 2007). Usually, even the fetus of an anemic woman will receive adequate iron stores from the mother, at the cost of further depleting the mother's iron level (Blackburn, 2007).

Generally, iron deficiency anemia is preventable or easily treated with iron supplements. Because of the increased amounts of iron needed for fetal development and maternal stores, pregnant women are often encouraged to take prophylactic iron supplementation (Blackburn, 2007; Gilbert, 2007). One 325-mg tablet of ferrous sulfate taken daily provides adequate iron prophylaxis. Each tablet contains 60 mg of elemental iron, 10% of which is absorbed. Most women with iron deficiency anemia can absorb as much iron as they need by taking one 325-mg tablet of ferrous sulfate twice each day (Samuels, 2007). An important aspect to teach the pregnant woman is the significance of the iron therapy. Some pregnant women cannot tolerate the prescribed oral iron because of nausea and vomiting associated with the pregnancy and as a side effect of iron therapy. In such cases the woman may be given parenteral iron therapy by intramuscular or intravascular injection. Women who are severely anemic may require blood transfusions (Samuels).

Teach the importance of iron supplements for preventing or treating iron deficiency anemia (see Patient Instructions for Self-Management box: Iron Supplementation).

PATIENT INSTRUCTIONS FOR SELF-MANAGEMENT

Iron Supplementation

- Vitamin C (in citrus fruits, tomatoes, melons, and strawberries) and heme iron (in meats) increase the absorption of the iron supplement; therefore include these foods in the diet often.
- Bran, tea, coffee, other caffeinated beverages, milk, oxalates (in spinach and Swiss chard), and egg yolk decrease iron absorption. Avoid consuming them at the same time as the supplement.
- Iron is absorbed best if it is taken when the stomach is empty; that is, take it between meals with a drink other than tea, coffee, other caffeinated beverage, or milk.
- Iron can be taken at bedtime if abdominal discomfort occurs when it is taken between meals.
- If an iron dose is missed, take it as soon as it is remembered if within 13 hours of the scheduled dose. Do not double the dose.
- Keep the supplement in a childproof container and out of the reach of any children in the household.
- The iron may cause stools to be black or dark green.
- Constipation is common with iron supplementation. A diet high in fiber with adequate fluid intake is recommended.

In addition, teach dietary ways to decrease the GI side effects of iron therapy.

Folate Deficiency

Folate is a water-soluble vitamin found naturally in dark-green leafy vegetables, citrus fruits, eggs, legumes, and whole grains. Even in well-nourished women, folate deficiency is common. Poor diet, cooking with large volumes of water, and increased alcohol use may contribute to folate deficiency. During pregnancy the need for folate increases, both because of fetal demands and because folate is less well absorbed from the GI tract during gestation. Folic acid is the form of the vitamin used in vitamin supplements. The recommended daily intake of folic acid for pregnant women is 600 mcg per day. Both prescription and nonprescription prenatal vitamins contain more than this amount of folic acid and should be sufficient to prevent and treat folate deficiency. Women at particular risk for folate deficiency include those who have significant hemoglobinopathies, take anticonvulsant medication, or are pregnant with a multifetal gestation. These women will require larger-than-normal doses of folic acid (Samuels, 2007).

Folate deficiency is the most common cause of megaloblastic anemia during pregnancy, but a vitamin B_{12} deficiency must also be considered. Megaloblastic anemia rarely occurs before the third trimester of pregnancy (Kilpatrick, 2009; Samuels, 2007). Women with megaloblastic anemia caused by folic acid deficiency have the usual presenting symptoms and signs of anemia: pallor, fatigue, and lethargy, as well as glossitis and skin roughness, which are associated specifically with megaloblastic anemia (Kilpatrick). Folate deficiency usually improves rapidly with folic acid therapy. It rarely occurs in the fetus and is not a significant cause of perinatal morbidity. Iron deficiency is often associated with folate deficiency (Samuels).

Sickle Cell Hemoglobinopathy

Sickle cell hemoglobinopathy is a disease caused by the presence of abnormal hemoglobin in the blood. Sickle cell trait (SA hemoglobin pattern) is sickling of the RBCs but with a normal RBC life span. Most people with sickle cell trait are asymptomatic. Approximately 1 in 12 African-American adults in the United States have sickle cell trait (Samuels, 2007). Women with sickle cell trait require genetic counseling and partner testing to determine their risk of producing children with sickle cell trait or disease.

Women with sickle cell trait usually do well in pregnancy. However, they are at increased risk for preeclampsia, IUFD, preterm birth and low-birthweight infants, and postpartum endometritis. They are also at increased risk for UTIs and may be deficient in iron (Kilpatrick, 2009; Samuels, 2007).

Sickle cell anemia (sickle cell disease) is a recessive, hereditary, familial hemolytic anemia that affects persons of African or Mediterranean ancestry. These individuals usually have abnormal hemoglobin types (SS or SC). The average life span of RBCs in a person with sickle cell anemia is only 5 to 10 days, in comparison to the 120 day life span of a normal RBC. Sickle cell anemia (SS disease) occurs in 1 in 708 African-Americans in the United States (Samuels, 2007). Persons with sickle cell anemia have recurrent attacks (crises) of fever and pain, most often in the abdomen, joints, or extremities, although virtually all organ systems can be affected. These attacks are attributed to vascular occlusion when RBCs assume a characteristic sickled shape. Crises are usually triggered by dehydration, hypoxia, or acidosis (Samuels).

Women with sickle cell anemia require genetic counseling before pregnancy. All children born to a woman with sickle cell anemia will be affected in some way by the disease. The woman's partner must be tested to determine the couple's risk of producing children with sickle cell disease rather than sickle cell trait. Women with sickle cell anemia are at risk for poor pregnancy outcomes, including miscarriage, IUGR, and stillbirth. Although maternal mortality is rare, maternal morbidity is significant and includes an increased risk for preeclampsia and infection, particularly in the urinary tract and in the lungs. The frequency of painful crises also appears to be increased during pregnancy (Samuels, 2007).

The woman will be monitored carefully during pregnancy for the development of urinary tract infection or preeclampsia. In addition, she will have serial ultrasound examinations to monitor fetal growth and will likely have antepartum fetal testing performed regularly during the third trimester. Infections are treated aggressively with antibiotics. If crises occur, they are managed with analgesia,

Critical Thinking/Clinical Decision Making

Sickle Cell Hemoglobinopathy

Latasha is a 23-year-old G1 P0 with sickle cell anemia who is hospitalized with a crisis at 16 weeks of gestation. Latasha says, "I've been in and out of the hospital all my life because of my sickle cell disease. I sure hope my baby won't have this disease!"

1. What additional information is necessary to counsel Latasha regarding her baby's chance of having sickle cell disease?
2. What assumptions can be made about the following issues?
   a. The chance that Latasha's baby will inherit either sickle cell trait or sickle cell disease
   b. Pregnancy risks related to sickle cell disease
3. What implications and priorities for nursing care can be drawn at this time?
4. Does the evidence objectively support your conclusion?
5. Do alternative perspectives to your conclusion exist?

oxygen, and hydration. Some authorities recommend prophylactic transfusions as a way to improve oxygen-carrying capacity and suppress the synthesis of sickle hemoglobin. Others, however, believe that prophylactic transfusions do not improve fetal or neonatal outcome (Samuels, 2007).

NURSING ALERT Women with sickle cell anemia are not iron deficient. Therefore routine iron supplementation, even that found in prenatal vitamins, should be avoided because these women can develop iron overload (Samuels, 2007).

If no complications occur, pregnancy can continue until term. Intrapartum, women with sickle cell disease should be encouraged to labor in a side-lying position. They may require supplemental oxygen. Adequate hydration should be maintained while preventing fluid overload. Conduction anesthesia (e.g., epidural or combined spinal epidural anesthesia) is recommended because it provides excellent pain relief. Vaginal birth is preferred. Cesarean birth should be performed only for obstetric indications (Samuels, 2007).

Thalassemia

Thalassemia is a relatively common anemia in which an insufficient amount of hemoglobin is produced to fill the RBCs. Thalassemia is a hereditary disorder that involves the abnormal synthesis of the alpha or beta chains of hemoglobin. Beta thalassemia is the more common variety in the United States and usually occurs in persons of Mediterranean, North African, Middle Eastern, and Asian descent (Kilpatrick, 2009).

Beta thalassemia minor is the heterozygous form of this disorder. Persons with heterozygous beta thalassemia are carriers of the disorder and are usually asymptomatic (Samuels, 2007). They can expect to have a normal lifespan despite a moderately reduced hemoglobin level. Pregnancy will not worsen beta thalassemia minor. Neither does the disorder adversely affect pregnancy. Women with beta thalassemia minor do not require antepartum fetal testing (Samuels). Iron therapy should only be prescribed for patients who are iron deficient, although folic acid supplementation is recommended for all women with beta thalassemia minor.

The homozygous form of beta thalassemia is known as thalassemia major, or Cooley anemia. Persons with this form of the disease usually have hepatosplenomegaly and bone deformities caused by massive marrow tissue expansion. These individuals usually die of infection or cardiovascular complications fairly early in life. If they live to reach childbearing age, infertility is common. If women with this disorder do become pregnant, they usually experience severe anemia and congestive heart failure, although successful full-term pregnancies have been reported. Women with beta thalassemia major are managed much like those with sickle cell anemia during pregnancy (Samuels, 2007).

PULMONARY DISORDERS

As pregnancy advances and the enlarged uterus presses on the thoracic cavity, any pregnant woman may experience increased respiratory difficulty. This difficulty will be compounded by pulmonary disease.

Asthma

Asthma is a chronic inflammatory disorder involving the tracheobronchial airways, with increased airway responsiveness to a variety of stimuli. It is characterized by periods of exacerbations and remissions. Exacerbations are triggered by allergens, marked change in ambient temperature, or emotional tension. In many cases the actual cause may be unknown, although a family history of allergy is common. In response to stimuli, narrowing of the hyperreactive airways is widespread, causing difficulty with breathing; the condition is, however, reversible. The clinical manifestations are expiratory wheezing, productive cough, thick sputum, dyspnea, or any combination.

Asthma may be the most common potentially serious medical condition to complicate pregnancy. It affects 4% to 8% of all pregnancies. The prevalence and morbidity rates are increasing, although the asthma-related mortality has dropped in recent years (Whitty & Dombrowski, 2009). African-Americans aged 15 to 44 are twice as likely to be hospitalized with asthma and five times more likely to die from asthma compared with Caucasians (Whitty & Dombrowski, 2007).

The effect of pregnancy on asthma is unpredictable. The severity of the disease is unchanged in one third, improved in one third, and worsened in one third of pregnant women. If the disease worsens, the more severe symptoms usually occur during gestational weeks 24 to 36 (Gilbert, 2007). Asthma appears to be associated with intrauterine growth restriction and preterm birth (Whitty & Dombrowski, 2009).

The ultimate goal of asthma therapy in pregnancy is maintaining adequate oxygenation of the fetus by preventing hypoxic episodes in the mother. Achieving this goal requires monitoring lung function objectively (e.g., peak expiratory flow rate and forced expiratory volume in one second), avoiding or controlling asthma triggers (e.g., dust mites, animal dander, pollen, wood smoke), educating patients about the importance of controlling asthma during pregnancy, and drug therapy. Current drug therapy for asthma emphasizes treatment of airway inflammation to decrease airway hyperresponsiveness and prevent asthma symptoms. Decreasing airway inflammation with inhaled corticosteroids is currently the preferred treatment for managing persistent asthma during pregnancy (Whitty & Dombrowski, 2009).

During pregnancy, women with moderate or severe asthma will need ultrasound examinations to determine fetal growth and to date the pregnancy. Repeat ultrasound examinations should be performed after an asthma exacerbation to evaluate fetal activity, growth, and amniotic fluid volume. Women with moderate or severe asthma will probably begin antepartum fetal testing by 32 weeks of gestation (Whitty & Dombrowski, 2009). Respiratory infections should be treated, and mist or steam inhalation used to aid expectoration of mucus. Acute exacerbations may require albuterol, steroids, aminophylline, beta-adrenergic agents, and oxygen. Women with severe exacerbations unresponsive to treatment may require intubation and mechanical ventilation (Whitty & Dombrowski, 2007).

Asthma attacks can occur in labor; therefore medications for asthma are continued during labor and the postpartum period. Pulse oximetry should be instituted during labor. Epidural anesthesia reduces oxygen consumption and is recommended for pain relief. Fentanyl, a non–histamine-releasing narcotic may be used also for pain control and is not associated with bronchospasm (Cunningham et al., 2005; Whitty & Dombrowski, 2009).

During the postpartum period, women who have asthma are at increased risk for hemorrhage. If excessive bleeding occurs, oxytocin is the recommended drug. If prostaglandin E_2 or E_1 is used instead, the woman's respiratory status should be monitored (Whitty & Dombrowski, 2009). In general, only small amounts of asthma medications enter breast milk; therefore their use is not considered a contraindication to breastfeeding. In sensitive individuals, however, theophylline in breast milk can cause vomiting, feeding difficulties, jitteriness, and cardiac arrhythmias in neonates (Whitty & Dombrowski). The woman usually returns to her prepregnancy asthma status within 3 months after giving birth.

Cystic Fibrosis

Cystic fibrosis is a common autosomal recessive genetic disorder in which the exocrine glands produce excessive viscous secretions, which causes problems with both respiratory and digestive functions. Most persons with cystic fibrosis have chronic obstructive pulmonary disease, pancreatic exocrine insufficiency, and elevated sweat electrolytes. Morbidity and mortality is usually caused by progressive chronic bronchial pulmonary disease (Whitty & Dombrowski, 2009).

Since the gene for cystic fibrosis was identified in 1989, data can be collected for the purposes of genetic counseling for couples regarding carrier status. In the United States, approximately 4% of the Caucasian population are carriers of the cystic fibrosis gene. Cystic fibrosis occurs in 1 in 3200 live Caucasian births (Whitty & Dombrowski, 2009). Persons with cystic fibrosis now live longer than they did in the past because of earlier diagnosis of the disease and advances in antibiotic therapy and nutritional support. Men tend to live a little longer (median age of survival is 29.6 years) as compared with women, whose median age of survival is 27.3 years. Although most men with cystic fibrosis are infertile, women with the disease are often fertile and thus able to become pregnant (Whitty & Dombrowski, 2007).

In women with good nutrition, mild obstructive lung disease, and minimal lung impairment, pregnancy is tolerated well (Cunningham et al., 2005; Whitty & Dombrowski, 2009). In women with severe disease the pregnancy is often complicated by chronic hypoxemia and frequent pulmonary infections. Risk factors that may predict a poor pregnancy outcome are poor prepregnancy nutritional status, significant pulmonary disease with hypoxemia, pulmonary hypertension, liver disease, and diabetes mellitus (Whitty & Dombrowski). Increased maternal and perinatal mortality is related to severe pulmonary infection. The incidence of preterm birth, IUGR, and uteroplacental insufficiency is increased (Whitty & Dombrowski).

Care of the pregnant woman with cystic fibrosis requires a team effort. Ideally, the woman should reach 90% of her ideal body weight before becoming pregnant. A weight gain of 11 to 12 kg (24-26 lb) is recommended during pregnancy. Women who are unable to achieve the recommended weight gain through oral supplements may require nasogastric tube feedings at night. If malnutrition is severe, parenteral hyperalimentation may be necessary. Throughout pregnancy, frequent monitoring of the woman's weight, blood glucose, hemoglobin, total protein, serum albumin, prothrombin time, and fat-soluble vitamins A and E is suggested. Pancreatic enzymes should be adjusted as necessary (Whitty & Dombrowski, 2009).

Baseline pulmonary function tests should ideally be completed before pregnancy and continued as needed during pregnancy. Early detection and treatment of infection is critical. Management of infection includes intravenous antibiotics along with chest physical therapy and bronchial drainage (Whitty & Dombrowski, 2009).

Fetal assessment is essential, given that the fetus is at risk for uteroplacental insufficiency, which can result in IUGR. Maternal nutritional status and weight gain during pregnancy significantly affect fetal growth. Fundal height should be measured routinely and ultrasound examinations performed to evaluate fetal growth and amniotic fluid volume. Fetal movement counts are often recommended, starting at 28 weeks of gestation. Nonstress tests should be initiated at 32 weeks of gestation or sooner if evidence of fetal compromise exists (Whitty & Dombrowski, 2009).

During labor, monitoring for fluid and electrolyte balance is required. Increased cardiac output can lead to cardiopulmonary failure in the woman with pulmonary hypertension or cor pulmonale. The amount of sodium lost through sweat can be significant, and hypovolemia can occur. On the other hand, if any degree of cor pulmonale is present, fluid overload is a concern. Oxygen is given by facemask during labor, and oxygen saturation monitoring is recommended. Epidural or local analgesia is the preferred analgesic for birth, with vaginal birth recommended. Cesarean birth should be reserved for obstetric indications.

Breastfeeding appears to be safe as long as the sodium content of the milk is not abnormal (Lawrence & Lawrence, 2005). Pumping and discarding the milk is continued until the sodium content has been determined. Milk samples should be tested periodically for sodium, chloride, and total fat, and the infant's growth pattern should be monitored.

INTEGUMENTARY DISORDERS

The skin surface may exhibit many physiologic conditions during pregnancy. Dermatologic disorders induced by pregnancy include melasma (chloasma), herpes gestationis, noninflammatory pruritus of pregnancy, vascular "spiders," palmar erythema, and striae gravidarum. Skin problems generally aggravated by pregnancy are acne vulgaris (acne) (in the first trimester), erythema multiforme, herpetiform dermatitis (fever blisters and genital herpes), granuloma inguinale (Donovan bodies), condylomata acuminata (genital warts), neurofibromatosis (von Recklinghausen disease), and pemphigus. Dermatologic disorders usually improved by pregnancy include acne vulgaris (in the third trimester), seborrheic dermatitis (dandruff), and psoriasis (Cunningham et al., 2005). An unpredictable course during pregnancy may be expected in atopic dermatitis, lupus erythematosus, and herpes simplex. Explanation, reassurance, and commonsense measures should suffice for normal skin changes. In contrast, disease processes during and soon after pregnancy may be extremely difficult to diagnose and treat.

NURSING ALERT Isotretinoin (Accutane), commonly prescribed for cystic acne, is highly teratogenic. A risk exists for craniofacial, cardiac, and CNS malformations in exposed fetuses. This drug should not be taken during pregnancy.

Pruritus is a major symptom in several pregnancy-related skin diseases. Pruritus gravidarum, generalized itching without the presence of a rash, develops in up to 14% of pregnant women. It is often limited to the abdomen and is usually caused by skin distention and development of striae. Pruritus gravidarum is not associated with poor perinatal outcomes. It is treated symptomatically with skin lubrication, topical antipruritics, and oral antihistamines. Ultraviolet light and careful exposure to sunlight decrease itching. Pruritus gravidarum usually disappears shortly after birth but can recur in approximately one half of all subsequent pregnancies (Rapini, 2009).

Another common pregnancy-specific cause of pruritus is pruritic urticarial papules and plaques of pregnancy (PUPPP) (Fig. 20-5), also known as polymorphic eruption of pregnancy. PUPPP classically appears in primigravidas during the third trimester. The abdomen is usually affected, but lesions can spread to the arms, the thighs, the back,

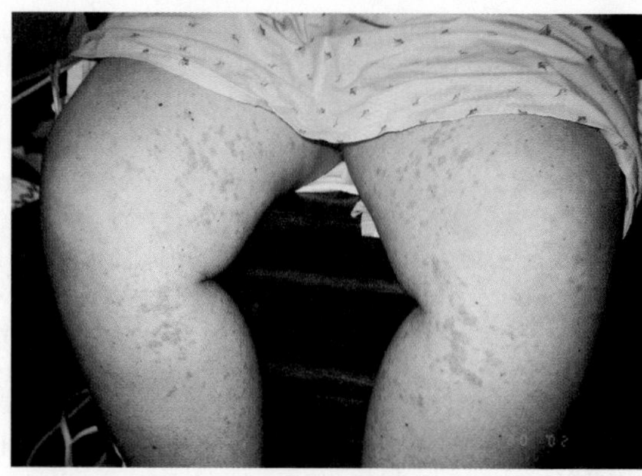

Fig. 20-5 Woman with pruritic urticarial papules and plaques of pregnancy (PUPPP). Lesions also are present on her arms, back, abdomen, and buttocks. (Courtesy Shannon Perry, Phoenix, AZ.)

and the buttocks. PUPPP almost always causes pruritus, and the itching is severe in 80% of cases. It is not, however, associated with poor maternal or fetal outcomes. Therefore the goal of therapy is simply to relieve maternal discomfort. Antipruritic topical medications, topical steroids, and oral antihistamines usually provide relief. Women with severe symptoms may require oral prednisone. PUPPP usually resolves before birth or within several weeks after birth. Rarely, however, it may persist or even begin after birth. PUPPP does not usually recur in subsequent pregnancies (Papoutsis & Kroumpouzos, 2007; Rapini, 2009).

Intrahepatic cholestasis of pregnancy (ICP) is a liver disorder unique to pregnancy that is characterized by generalized pruritus. The itching commonly affects the palms and soles but can occur on any part of the body. No skin lesions are present. Women with ICP have elevated serum bile acids and elevated liver function tests. Jaundice may or may not be present. Up to one half of patients with ICP develop dark urine and light colored stools. The cause of ICP is unknown, but approximately half of patients have a family history of the disorder. ICP occurs more frequently during the winter months than at other times of the year. A geographic variance in the prevalence of the disease also occurs. ICP occurs most often in South Asia, Chile, Bolivia, and Scandinavia, although it is seen less frequently now in Chile and in Scandinavia than in the past (Cappell, 2007; Williamson & Mackillop, 2009).

The major risks associated with ICP are meconium staining, stillbirth, and preterm birth. The cause of these complications is likely related to increased levels of fetal serum bile levels. Treatment consists of giving ursodeoxycholic acid, which effectively controls the pruritus and laboratory abnormalities associated with ICP, and continued monitoring of liver function tests and bile acids (Cappell, 2007; Williamson & Mackillop, 2009). Antepartum fetal testing is mandatory. If liver function tests do not improve, induction of labor is considered at 36 to 37 weeks of gestation if fetal lung maturity is present.

Symptoms usually disappear and laboratory abnormalities resolve within 2 to 4 weeks postpartum. ICP can recur in subsequent pregnancies, however, or with oral contraceptive use (Cappell).

NEUROLOGIC DISORDERS

The pregnant woman with a neurologic disorder needs to deal with potential teratogenic effects of prescribed medications, changes of mobility during pregnancy, and impaired ability to care for the baby. The nurse should be aware of all drugs the woman is taking and the associated potential for producing congenital anomalies. As the pregnancy progresses, the woman's center of gravity shifts and causes balance and gait changes. The nurse should advise the woman of these expected changes and suggest safety measures as appropriate. Family and community resources may be needed to assist in providing infant care for the neurologically impaired woman.

Epilepsy

Epilepsy (often called seizure disorder) is a disorder of the brain that causes recurrent seizures and is the most common major neurologic disorder accompanying pregnancy. Less than 1% of all pregnant women have a seizure disorder (Aminoff, 2009). Seizure disorders are either acquired (less than 15% of all cases) or idiopathic (more than 85% of all cases), which means that a specific cause for the seizures cannot be identified. The majority of women with a seizure disorder who become pregnant have an uneventful pregnancy with an excellent outcome (Samuels & Niebyl, 2007).

Women with epilepsy should receive preconception counseling if at all possible. A detailed history of medication use and seizure frequency should be obtained. If the woman has frequent seizures before conception, she is likely to continue this pattern during pregnancy. Therefore achieving effective seizure control is extremely important before conception, even if changing medications is required. Many studies have reported an increased incidence of congenital anomalies, including cleft lip and palate, congenital heart disease, and neural tube defects (NTDs), in infants born to women taking anticonvulsant medications. In particular, carbamazepine (Tegretol) and valproate (Depakote) should be avoided if possible because their use is associated with neural tube defects in the fetus. Several new anticonvulsant medications have been developed for use within the last decade. More information is needed regarding the fetal effects of these medications. Any anticonvulsant medication required to achieve good seizure control in a woman with epilepsy should be used, however, regardless of the increased risk of fetal anomalies, because the most important goal during pregnancy is the prevention of seizures (Samuels & Niebyl, 2007).

Women with epilepsy are advised to take a folic acid supplement of 4 mg daily, which may decrease the incidence of NTDs. They are also encouraged to take a prenatal vitamin containing vitamin D daily, because anticonvulsant medications can interfere with production of the active form of this vitamin (Samuels & Niebyl, 2007).

During pregnancy, only one anticonvulsant medication–at the lowest dose level that is effective at keeping the woman seizure free–should be prescribed. The increase in plasma volume that is a normal pregnancy change can affect drug metabolism and distribution. Therefore blood levels of anticonvulsant medications should be checked and drug dosages adjusted as necessary. With patient cooperation and close monitoring, most women with epilepsy should experience no change or even have fewer seizures during pregnancy. An increase in seizure frequency is usually related either to noncompliance with taking prescribed anticonvulsant medications or with sleep deprivation (Samuels & Niebyl, 2007). If an increase in seizure activity does occur during pregnancy, it is usually in women who had frequent seizures (more than one per month) before pregnancy (Aminoff, 2009).

In addition to congenital anomalies, the fetus of a woman with epilepsy is also at risk for IUGR. Determining an accurate gestational age as early as possible is important. This information will decrease any confusion later in pregnancy in regard to fetal growth issues. Maternal serum screening around 16 weeks of gestation and ultrasound examination at 18 to 22 weeks of gestation should be performed to assess for the presence of an NTD or other fetal anomalies. Nonstress testing later in pregnancy is not necessary, unless the woman has other medical or obstetric factors that increase the risk for stillbirth (Samuels & Niebyl, 2007).

Management of anticonvulsant therapy during prolonged labor is challenging. During labor, absorption of medications given orally is unpredictable, especially if vomiting occurs. Women who are maintained on phenytoin (Dilantin) or phenobarbital may be given these medications parenterally during labor. No parenteral form of carbamazepine has been developed; therefore women maintained on this medication may be given phenytoin intravenously instead to carry them through labor. Vaginal birth is preferred (Samuels & Niebyl, 2007).

After birth the levels of anticonvulsant medications must be monitored frequently for the first few weeks because they can rise rapidly. If medication dose levels were increased during pregnancy, they will need to be decreased quickly to prepregnancy levels. All of the major anticonvulsant medications are found in breast milk, but the use of these medications is not a contraindication to breastfeeding. Neonatal sedation may be a side effect of carbamazepine, primidone (Mysoline), and phenobarbital (Samuels & Niebyl, 2007).

During the neonatal period, infants can have a hemorrhagic disorder associated with exposure to anticonvulsant medications in utero, which causes vitamin K deficiency.

Some authorities recommend giving vitamin K daily during the last few weeks of pregnancy to women taking anticonvulsant medications, but this practice is not considered the standard of care (Samuels & Niebyl, 2007).

All methods of contraception can be used by women with an idiopathic seizure disorder. Commonly prescribed anticonvulsant medications such as carbamazepine, phenobarbital, and phenytoin, however, reduce the effectiveness of oral contraceptives. Women taking low-dose oral contraceptives especially may have more breakthrough bleeding and be at risk for an unplanned pregnancy (Samuels & Niebyl, 2007). Valproic acid and the newer anticonvulsant medications have not been reported to cause oral contraceptive failure (Aminoff, 2009). In terms of planning for future childbearing, couples should be informed that children born to women with a seizure disorder of unknown cause have a four times greater chance of developing an idiopathic seizure disorder compared with the general population. Interestingly, epilepsy in the father does not appear to increase a child's risk for developing a seizure disorder (Samuels & Niebyl).

Multiple Sclerosis

Multiple sclerosis (MS), a patchy demyelinization of the spinal cord and CNS, may be a viral disorder. MS occurs equally in men and women. Onset of symptoms, which include weakness of one or both lower extremities, visual complaints, and loss of coordination, is subtle and usually occurs between the ages of 20 and 40 years. The disease is characterized by exacerbations and remissions. Pregnancy does not seem to worsen the disease (Samuels & Niebyl, 2007).

Remissions during pregnancy are common. If an exacerbation occurs, it is more likely to do so during the third trimester of pregnancy or postpartum. Treatment may include corticosteroids and immunosuppressive agents. Several new drugs and biopharmaceuticals are available for treating MS. Because of the lack of experience, however, these agents should be used during pregnancy only if the benefits clearly appear to outweigh the potential risks (Samuels & Niebyl, 2007).

Women who have become paraplegic or have lumbosacral lesions as a result of MS may have little pain during labor. Determining when labor begins may be difficult for them. Uterine contractions occur normally, but these women may have difficulty pushing effectively during second stage labor. Therefore vacuum- or forceps-assisted birth may be necessary (Samuels & Niebyl, 2007).

Bell Palsy

Bell palsy is an acute idiopathic facial paralysis. The cause is unknown, but it occurs fairly often, especially in women of reproductive age. Women are affected two to four times more often than men. An association between Bell palsy and pregnancy was first cited by Bell in 1830. Pregnant women are affected three to four times more often than nonpregnant women. The incidence usually peaks during the third trimester and the puerperium. Women who develop Bell palsy during pregnancy have an increased risk for preeclampsia as well (Cunningham et al., 2005).

The clinical manifestations of Bell palsy include the sudden development of a unilateral facial weakness, with maximal weakness within 48 hours after onset (Ahmed, 2005; Cunningham et al., 2005), pain surrounding the ear, difficulty closing the eye on the affected side, hyperacusis (abnormal acuteness of the sense of hearing), and occasionally a loss of taste (Aminoff, 2009).

No effects of maternal Bell palsy have been observed in infants. Maternal outcome is generally good unless a complete block in nerve conduction occurs. Steroid therapy may improve outcome, although its benefits have not always been proven in past research studies. To be effective, steroids should be administered within the first 5 to 6 days after the paralysis develops (Aminoff, 2009). Supportive care includes prevention of injury to the constantly exposed cornea, facial muscle massage, and reassurance. Although 80% of affected men and nonpregnant women recover to a satisfactory level within a year, only approximately one half of women who develop the disorder during pregnancy do so (Cunningham et al., 2005).

AUTOIMMUNE DISORDERS

Autoimmune disorders make up a large group of diseases that disrupt the function of the immune system of the body. In these types of disorders the body's immune system is unable to distinguish "self" from "nonself." As a result, antibodies develop that attack its normally present antigens, causing tissue damage. Autoimmune disorders can occur during pregnancy because 70% of patients with an autoimmune disease are women of childbearing age (Gilbert, 2007). Common autoimmune diseases include systemic lupus erythematosus (SLE), antiphospholipid syndrome, rheumatoid arthritis, and systemic sclerosis (Holmgren & Branch, 2007).

Systemic Lupus Erythematosus

SLE is a chronic, multisystem inflammatory disease that affects the skin, joints, kidneys, lungs, nervous system, liver, and other body organs. The exact cause is unknown but probably involves the interaction of several factors, including immunologic, environmental, hormonal, and genetic factors. SLE is the most common serious autoimmune disease affecting women of reproductive age. It occurs two to four times more often in African-American and Latina women than in Caucasian women and is at least 5 to 10 times more common in women than in men. Most cases of SLE occur in adolescence or young adulthood (Gilbert, 2007; Holmgren & Branch, 2007).

The most common presenting symptoms of SLE include fatigue, weight loss, arthralgias, arthritis, and myalgias. Although a diagnosis of SLE is suspected based on clinical signs and symptoms, it is confirmed by laboratory testing that demonstrates the presence of circulating autoantibodies. As is the case with other autoimmune diseases, SLE is characterized by a series of exacerbations (flares) and remissions (Holmgren & Branch, 2007).

If the diagnosis has been established and the woman desires a child, she is advised to wait until she has been in remission for at least 6 months before attempting to become pregnant (Gilbert, 2007). A lupus flare occurs during pregnancy or postpartum in 15% to 60% of women with SLE. In addition to an exacerbation, other maternal risks include an increased rate of miscarriage, nephritis, preeclampsia, possible need to give birth at a preterm gestation, and an increased risk of cesarean birth. Fetal risks include stillbirth, IUGR, and preterm birth (Holmgren & Branch, 2007).

Medical therapy during pregnancy is kept to a minimum in women who are in remission or who have a mild form of SLE. Immunosuppressive medications should be discontinued before conception. Nonsteroidal antiinflammatory drugs and aspirin are ordinarily the most commonly used antiinflammatory drugs, but they are not recommended for use during pregnancy. Aspirin should not be used after 24 weeks of gestation because of an increased risk of premature closure of the fetal ductus arteriosus (Cunningham et al., 2005). Maintenance therapy with hydroxychloroquine or low doses of glucocorticoids can continue. Hydroxychloroquine, an antimalarial drug, may be the best medication for maintenance SLE therapy during pregnancy because it significantly reduces SLE disease activity but appears to cause no adverse effects on the fetus (Holmgren & Branch, 2007).

Prenatal care otherwise focuses on close monitoring to detect common pregnancy complications, such as hypertension, proteinuria, and IUGR. Ultrasound examinations are performed frequently to monitor fetal growth. Fetal assessment tests, including daily fetal movement counts, nonstress tests, and amniotic fluid volume assessment, will likely begin at 30 to 32 weeks of gestation. More frequent ultrasound examinations and fetal testing are necessary if the woman develops a SLE flare, hypertension, proteinuria, or evidence of IUGR (Holmgren & Branch, 2007).

Women with SLE can develop an exacerbation during labor. Even if a flare does not occur, all women who have received chronic steroid therapy within the year will need larger (stress) doses of steroids during labor (Holmgren & Branch, 2007). Vaginal birth is preferred, but cesarean birth is common because of maternal and fetal complications.

Because determining which, if any, patients are at risk for a SLE flare after birth is difficult, close follow-up with all of these women during the postpartum period is necessary. Any maintenance medications that were discontinued during the intrapartum period should be restarted immediately at doses similar to those used during pregnancy (Holmgren & Branch, 2007).

Women with SLE should limit their number of pregnancies because of increased adverse perinatal outcomes, as well as the guarded maternal prognosis (Cunningham et al., 2005). If desired, the safest time for tubal sterilization is during the postpartum period or when the disease is in remission. Oral contraceptives should be used cautiously because of the vascular disease that often accompanies SLE. An IUD increases the risk for infection and probably should not be prescribed for women receiving immunosuppressive therapy. Progestin-only implants and injections provide effective contraception with no known effects on lupus flares (Cunningham et al.; Gilbert, 2007).

SUBSTANCE ABUSE

The term *substance abuse* refers to the continued use of substances despite related problems in physical, social, or interpersonal areas (American Psychiatric Association, 2000). Recurrent abuse results in failure to fulfill major role obligations, and substance-related legal problems and ethical issues may exist (ACOG, 2004). Any use of alcohol or illicit drugs during pregnancy is considered abuse (APA). Chapter 2 discusses the commonly abused illicit and prescription drugs, and Chapter 24 discusses neonatal effects of maternal substance abuse. This discussion focuses on care of the pregnant woman who is a substance abuser.

Because many pregnant women are reluctant to reveal their use of substances or the extent of their use, data on prevalence are highly variable. Approximately 15% of all pregnant women have a substance abuse problem (Gilbert, 2007). Blinded urine drug screens conducted at hospitals across the United States revealed that similar rates of substance use during pregnancy occurred in women of different ages, races, and social classes, although the specific substances used differed by race and social class. African-American and poor women were more likely to use illicit substances, particularly cocaine, whereas Caucasian women were more likely to use alcohol (Wisner et al., 2007). Among pregnant women responding to a national survey, 10% reported alcohol use, 4% reported binge alcohol use, and almost 1% reported heavy alcohol use in the month before the survey (Brady & Ashley, 2005).

The damaging effects of alcohol and illicit drugs on pregnant women and their unborn babies are well documented (Gilbert, 2007; Wisner et al., 2007). Alcohol and other drugs easily pass from a mother to her baby through the placenta. Smoking during pregnancy has serious health risks, including bleeding complications, miscarriage, stillbirth, prematurity, low birth weight, and sudden infant death syndrome (Gilbert; Wisner et al.). Congenital abnormalities have occurred in infants of mothers who have taken drugs. With one exception, the safest pregnancy is one in which the woman is drug and alcohol free. For women addicted to opioids, methadone maintenance treatment is the current standard of care during pregnancy (Wisner et al.).

Less than 10% of pregnant women who are substance abusers receive treatment for their addictions. Social stigma, labeling, and guilt are significant barriers (Brady & Ashley, 2005). Women often do not seek help because of the fear of losing custody of their child or children or criminal prosecution. Pregnant women who abuse substances commonly have little understanding of the ways in which these substances affect them, their pregnancies, and their babies. In many instances, pregnant mothers who use psychoactive substances receive negative feedback from society, as well as from health care providers, who not only may condemn them for endangering the life of the fetus, but may also even withhold support as a result. Barriers within the drug treatment system may also deter these women from receiving the help they need. Traditionally, substance abuse treatment programs have not addressed issues that affect pregnant women, such as concurrent need for obstetric care and child care for other children. Long waiting lists and lack of health insurance present further barriers to treatment. Pregnant women with co-occurring substance abuse and psychiatric disorders face unique barriers because of the social stigma attached to both conditions and insufficient knowledge and training to manage coexisting disorders (Brady & Ashley).

Because of the risks to the unborn children, pregnant women who abuse substances may face criminal charges under expanded interpretations of child abuse and drug-trafficking statutes. Some states prosecute pregnant women on charges of child abuse because they became pregnant while addicted to drugs. Some policy makers have proposed that pregnant women who abuse substances be jailed, placed under house arrest, or committed to psychiatric hospitals for the remainder of their pregnancies (Stuart & Laraia, 2005). Nurses should become involved in efforts to block punitive legislation dealing with childbearing women who are substance abusers. If these women are punished legally, they will most likely avoid involvement with the health care system and thus will not receive the help they need (Gilbert, 2007).

LEGAL TIP Drug Testing during Pregnancy

Federal law provides no requirement for a health care provider to test either the pregnant woman or the newborn for the presence of drugs. However, nurses need to know the practices of the states in which they are working. In some states a woman whose urine drug screen test is positive at the time of labor and birth must be referred to child protective services. If the mother is not in a drug treatment program or is judged unable to provide care, the infant may be placed in foster care. In 2001, the U.S. Supreme Court ruled that, in all states, testing for drug use without the pregnant woman's permission is unlawful.

CARE MANAGEMENT

Screening

Screening questions for alcohol and drug abuse should be included in the overall assessment of the first prenatal visit of all women. The *4 Ps Plus* is a screening tool designed specifically to identify pregnant women who need in-depth assessment (Box 20-3). It consists of five questions and takes less than a minute to complete. Because women frequently deny or greatly underreport usage when asked about drug or alcohol consumption during pregnancy, asking about substance use before pregnancy is often an effective screening method (Wisner et al., 2007).

Urine toxicologic testing is often performed to screen for illicit drug use. Drugs may be found in urine days to weeks after ingestion, depending on how quickly they are metabolized and excreted from the body. Meconium (from the neonate) and hair can also be analyzed to determine past drug use over a longer period (Gilbert, 2007).

Assessment

After screening results indicate that substance abuse is a problem for an individual woman, the nursing process is used to deal with that problem (see Nursing Process box: Substance Abuse). Because of the lifestyle often associated with drug use, substance-abusing women are at risk for sexually transmitted infections (STIs), including human immunodeficiency virus (HIV). Laboratory assessments will likely include screening for syphilis, hepatitis B and C, and HIV. A skin test to screen for tuberculosis may also be ordered. Initial and serial ultrasound studies are usually performed to determine gestational age because the woman may have had amenorrhea as a result of her drug use or may have no idea when her last menstrual period occurred.

Initial Care

Intervention with the pregnant substance abuser begins with education about specific effects on pregnancy, the

BOX 20-3

Screening with the 4Ps Plus

Parents: Did either of your parents ever have a problem with alcohol or drugs?
Partner: Does your partner have a problem with alcohol or drugs?
Past: Have you ever had any beer or wine or liquor?
Pregnancy: In the month before you knew you were pregnant, how many cigarettes did you smoke? In the month before you knew you were pregnant, how much beer, wine, or liquor did you drink?

Sources: Chasnoff, I., McGourty, R. F., Bailey, G. W., Hutchins, E., Lightfoot, S. O., Pawson, L. L., et al. (2005). The 4 Ps Plus screen for substance use in pregnancy: Clinical application and outcomes. *Journal of Perinatology, 25*(6), 368-374. In Wisner, K., Sit, D., Reynolds, S., Altemus, M., Bogen, D., Sunder, K., et al. (2007). Psychiatric disorders. In S. Gabbe, J. Niebyl, & J. Simpson (Eds.), *Obstetrics: Normal and problem pregnancies* (5th ed.). Philadelphia: Churchill Livingstone.

NURSING PROCESS Substance Abuse

ASSESSMENT

The assessment of a pregnant woman who is a substance abuser may include the following:

- Interview:
  - Screen for current alcohol and drug abuse during the first prenatal visit. Document approximate frequency and amount for each drug used. Ask in this order:
    Over-the-counter and prescribed medications
    Legal drugs (e.g., caffeine, nicotine, alcohol)
    Illicit drugs (e.g., marijuana, cocaine, methamphetamines, heroin, etc.)
  - Assess for past or current physical abuse.
  - Assess for past or current sexual abuse.
  - Assess for history of psychiatric illness.
  - Assess for barriers to care, such as peer pressure, socioeconomic status, psychologic stress, or other environmental factors.
- Comprehensive physical examination
- Laboratory tests:
  - Complete blood cell count
  - Syphilis
  - Hepatitis B and C serology
  - Human immunodeficiency virus
  - Tuberculosis
  - Urine toxicologic testing for suspected drugs used or drugs commonly abused in the community
  - Liver function tests if alcohol abuse is suspected
- Pregnancy and fetal assessment:
  - Ultrasound to determine gestational age and fetal weight
  - Nonstress testing

NURSING DIAGNOSES

Nursing diagnoses for the woman who is a substance abuser may include the following:

- *Risk for infection* related to:
  - Lifestyle
  - Malnutrition
  - Method of drug administration
- *Self-care deficit, bathing or hygiene,* related to:
  - Effects of substance used
- *Ineffective coping* related to:
  - Lack of support system
  - Low self-esteem
  - Denial
- *Risk for impaired parent-infant attachment* related to:
  - Guilt
  - Continued substance abuse
- *Powerlessness* related to:
  - Lack of resources
  - Relationship with one or more abusive partners
- *Risk for suicide* related to:
  - Depression
  - Impulsivity while using substances

EXPECTED OUTCOMES OF CARE

The ideal long-term outcome is total abstinence, but this outcome may not be possible. The woman should participate in setting short-term outcomes such as the following:

- The woman will keep appointments for prenatal and postpartum care for herself and well-baby care for the infant.
- Fetal effects related to maternal substance abuse will be minimized.
- The infant will be cared for in a safe environment.
- The woman's physiologic symptoms will stabilize, and she will be able to care for herself and her infant.
- The woman will develop an attachment to her infant.
- The woman will become involved in a substance abuse treatment program.

PLAN OF CARE AND INTERVENTIONS

- Develop a trusting relationship.
- Maintain a nonjudgmental, nonpunitive attitude.
- Determine the woman's readiness for change.
- Motivate the woman to make lifestyle changes by providing her with information about health risks and the effects of substance abuse on her fetus.
- Refer to community and social services as needed.
- Refer to local clinics dealing with pregnant substance abusers when the woman is ready for treatment.
- Provide ongoing encouragement and support.
- Reinforce importance of keeping prenatal appointments.
- Promote maternal-infant bonding after the birth.

EVALUATION

Evaluation is difficult in pregnant women with substance abuse problems because the long-range effects cannot be projected. Short-term positive achievements are indicative of some success.

fetus, and the newborn for each drug used. Consequences of perinatal drug use should be clearly communicated and abstinence recommended as the safest course of action, unless the woman is abusing opioids. Women are frequently more receptive to making lifestyle changes during pregnancy than at any other time in their lives. The casual, experimental, or recreational drug user is frequently able to achieve and maintain sobriety when she receives education, support, and continued monitoring throughout the remainder of the pregnancy. Periodic screening throughout pregnancy of women who have admitted to drug use may help them to continue abstinence.

Treatment for substance abuse will be individualized for each woman, depending on the type of drug used and the frequency and amount of use. Women are more likely to attempt to stop smoking during pregnancy than at any other time in their lives. Quitting before conception is ideal, but even quitting before 16 weeks of gestation significantly decreases the adverse risks. Smoking cessation programs during pregnancy are effective and should be offered to all pregnant smokers. Many smoking cessation resources are available, both in print and online (Gilbert, 2007; Wisner et al., 2007). For more information on smoking cessation, visit the American Lung Association's website at www.lungusa.org. Detoxification, short-term inpatient or outpatient treatment, long-term residential treatment, aftercare services, and self-help support groups are all possible options for alcohol and drug abuse. Women for Sobriety may be a more helpful organization for women than Alcoholics Anonymous or Narcotics Anonymous, which were developed for male substance abusers. In general, long-term treatment of any sort is becoming increasingly difficult to obtain, particularly for women who lack insurance coverage. Although some programs allow a woman to keep her children with her at the treatment facility, far too few of them are available to meet the demand.

The pregnant woman with alcoholism requires referral to an appropriate detoxification program. Alcohol withdrawal treatment during pregnancy consists of the administration of benzodiazepines (diazepam [Valium], lorazepam [Ativan]). Disulfiram (Antabuse) is teratogenic; therefore its use in aversion therapy is contraindicated during pregnancy (Wisner et al., 2007). Attention should also be paid to the woman's nutritional status (Gilbert, 2007; Wisner et al.).

Methadone maintenance treatment (MMT) is currently considered the standard of care for pregnant women who are dependent on heroin or other narcotics. It should be offered as part of a comprehensive care program that includes behavior therapy and support services. MMT has been shown to decrease opioid and other drug abuse, reduce criminal activity, improve individual functioning, and decrease HIV infection rates. In addition, birthweight and head circumference are increased in infants born to women receiving MMT. However, 30% to 80% of infants exposed to opioids, including methadone, in utero require treatment for neonatal abstinence syndrome (NAS) (Wisner et al., 2007). Pregnant women who use cocaine should be advised to stop using immediately. Such women will need a great deal of assistance, such as an alcohol and drug treatment program, individual or group counseling, and participation in self-help support groups, to accomplish this major lifestyle change successfully.

Methamphetamines are stimulants with vasoconstrictive characteristics similar to cocaine and are used similarly. As is the case with cocaine users, methamphetamine users are urged to immediately stop all use during pregnancy. Unfortunately, because methamphetamine users are extremely psychologically addicted, the rate of relapse is very high.

Although substance abusers may be difficult to care for at any time, they are often particularly challenging during the intrapartum and postpartum periods because of manipulative and demanding behavior. Typically, these women display poor control over their behavior and a low threshold for pain. Increased dependency needs and poor parenting skills may also be apparent.

Nurses must understand that substance abuse is an illness and that these women deserve to be treated with patience, kindness, consistency, and firmness when necessary. Even women who are actively abusing drugs will experience pain during labor and after giving birth and may need pain medication, as well as nonpharmacologic interventions. Developing a standardized plan of care so that patients have limited opportunities to play staff members against one another is helpful. Mother-infant attachment should be promoted by identifying the woman's strengths and reinforcing positive maternal feelings and behaviors. Staffing should be sufficient to ensure strict surveillance of visitors and prevent unsupervised drug use.

Advice regarding breastfeeding must be individualized. Although all abused substances appear in breast milk, some in greater amounts than others (Lawrence & Lawrence, 2005), breastfeeding is definitely contraindicated in women who use amphetamines, alcohol, cocaine, heroin, or marijuana. Methadone use, however, is not a contraindication to breastfeeding. The baby's nutrition and safety needs are of primary importance in this consideration. For some women a desire to breastfeed may provide strong motivation to achieve and maintain sobriety.

Smoking can interfere with the let-down reflex. Women who smoke in the postpartum period and breastfeed should avoid smoking for 2 hours before a feeding to minimize the nicotine in the milk and improve the let-down reflex. All smokers should be discouraged from smoking in the same room with the infant because exposure to secondhand smoke can increase the likelihood that the infant will experience behavioral and respiratory health problems (Lawrence & Lawrence, 2005).

Follow-Up Care

Before a known substance abuser is discharged with her baby, the home situation must be assessed to determine that the environment is safe and that someone will be available to meet the infant's needs if the mother proves unable to do so. The hospital's social services department will usually be involved in interviewing the mother before discharge to ensure that the infant's needs will be met. Family members or friends will sometimes be asked to become actively involved with the mother and infant after discharge. A home care or public health nurse may be asked to make home visits to assess the mother's ability to care for the baby and provide guidance and support. If serious questions about the infant's well-being exist, the case will probably be referred to the state's child protective services agency for further action.

KEY POINTS

- Lack of maternal glycemic control before conception and in the first trimester of pregnancy may be responsible for fetal congenital malformations.
- Maternal insulin requirements increase as the pregnancy progresses and may quadruple by term as a result of insulin resistance created by placental hormones, insulinase, and cortisol.
- Poor glycemic control before and during pregnancy can lead to maternal complications such as miscarriage, infection, and dystocia (difficult labor) caused by fetal macrosomia.
- Close glucose monitoring, insulin administration when necessary, and dietary counseling are used to create a normal intrauterine environment for fetal growth and development in the pregnancy complicated by diabetes mellitus.
- Because GDM is asymptomatic in most cases, all women undergo routine screening by history or glucola administration (or both) during pregnancy.
- Thyroid dysfunction during pregnancy requires close monitoring of thyroid hormone levels to regulate therapy and prevent fetal insult.
- The stress of the normal maternal adaptations to pregnancy on a heart whose function is already taxed may cause cardiac decompensation.
- Maternal morbidity or mortality is a significant risk in a pregnancy complicated by mitral stenosis.
- Anemia, a common medical disorder of pregnancy, affects at least 20% of pregnant women.
- Asthma may be the most common potentially serious medical condition to complicate pregnancy. The prevalence and morbidity rates are increasing.
- Pruritus is a common symptom in pregnancy-specific inflammatory skin diseases.
- A pregnant woman with epilepsy should take only one anticonvulsant medication at the lowest dose level that is effective at keeping her seizure free, if at all possible.
- SLE is the most common serious autoimmune disease affecting women of reproductive age.
- Much support from a variety of sources, including family and friends, health care providers, and the recovery community, is needed to help perinatal substance abusers achieve and maintain sobriety.
- Health care providers must provide compassionate, nonjudgmental care to substance abusers.

Audio Chapter Summaries Access an audio summary of these Key Points on evolve

References

Ahmed, A. (2005). When is facial paralysis Bell palsy? Current diagnosis and treatment. *Cleveland Clinic Journal of Medicine*, *72*(5), 398-405.

American College of Obstetricians and Gynecologists (ACOG). (2004). *At risk drinking and illicit drug use: Ethical issues in obstetric practice.* ACOG Committee Opinion No. 294. Washington, DC: ACOG.

American Diabetes Association. (2008). Position statement: Diagnosis and classification of diabetes mellitus. *Diabetes Care*, *31*(Suppl.), S55-S60.

American Psychiatric Association. (2000). *Diagnostic and statistical manual of mental disorders (DSM-IV-TR)* (4th ed., text revision). Washington, DC: American Psychiatric Association Press.

Aminoff, M. (2009). Neurologic disorders. In R. Creasy, R. Resnik, & J. Iams (Eds.), *Creasy and Resnik's maternal-fetal medicine: Principles and practice* (6th ed.). Philadelphia: Saunders.

Anderson, J., Waller, D., Canfield, M., Shaw G., Watkins, M., & Werler, M. (2005). Maternal obesity, gestational diabetes, and central nervous system birth defects. *Epidemiology*, *16*(1), 87-92.

Blackburn, S. (2007). *Maternal, fetal, and neonatal physiology: A clinical perspective* (3rd ed.). St. Louis: Saunders.

Blanchard, D., & Shabetai, R. (2009). Cardiac diseases. In R. Creasy, R. Resnik, & J. Iams (Eds.), *Creasy and Resnik's maternal-fetal medicine: Principles and practice* (6th ed.). Philadelphia: Saunders.

Brady, T., & Ashley, O. (2005). *Women in substance abuse treatment: Results from alcohol and drug services study (ADSS).* DHHS Publication No. SMA 04-3968 Analytic Series A-26. Rockville MD: Substance and Mental Health Services Administration, Office of Applied Studies.

Cappell, M. (2007). Hepatic and gastrointestinal diseases. In S. Gabbe, J. Niebyl, & J. Simpson (Eds.), *Obstetrics: Normal and problem pregnancies* (5th ed.). Philadelphia: Churchill Livingstone.

Chan, P., & Johnson, S. (2006). *Gynecology and obstetrics: Current clinical strategies.* Laguna Hills, CA: CCS Publishing.

Cianni, G., Volpe, L., Lencioni, C., Chatzianagnostou, K., Cuccuru, J., Ghio, A., et al. (2005). Use of insulin glargine during the first weeks of pregnancy in five type 1 diabetic women. *Diabetes Care*, *28*(4), 982-983.

Cunningham, F., Leveno, K., Bloom, S., Hauth, J., Gilstrap, L., & Wenstrom, K. (Eds.). (2005). *Williams obstetrics* (22nd ed.). New York: McGraw-Hill.

Easterling, T., & Stout, K. (2007). Heart disease. In S. Gabbe, J. Niebyl, & J. Simpson (Eds.), *Obstetrics: Normal and problem pregnancies* (5th ed.). Philadelphia: Churchill Livingstone.

Gilbert, E. (2007). *Manual of high risk pregnancy & delivery* (4th ed.). St. Louis: Mosby.

Holmgren, C., & Branch, D. (2007). Collagen vascular diseases. In S. Gabbe, J. Niebyl, & J. Simpson (Eds.), *Obstetrics: Normal and problem pregnancies* (5th ed.). Philadelphia: Churchill Livingstone.

Iams, J., Romero, R., & Creasy, R. (2009). Preterm labor and birth. In R. Creasy, R. Resnik, & J. Iams (Eds.), *Creasy and Resnik's maternal-fetal medicine: Principles and practice* (6th ed.). Philadelphia: Saunders.

Kilpatrick, S. (2009). Anemia and pregnancy. In R. Creasy, R. Resnik, & J. Iams (Eds.), *Creasy and Resnik's maternal-fetal medicine: Principles and practice* (6th ed.). Philadelphia: Saunders.

Klein, L., & Galan, H. (2004). Cardiac disease in pregnancy. *Obstetrics and*

Gynecology Clinics of North America, 31(2), 429-459.

Landon, M., Catalano, P., & Gabbe, S. (2007). Diabetes mellitus complicating pregnancy. In S. Gabbe, J. Niebyl, & J. Simpson (Eds.), *Obstetrics: Normal and problem pregnancies* (5th ed.). Philadelphia: Churchill Livingstone.

Lawrence, R., & Lawrence, R. (2005). *Breastfeeding: A guide for the medical profession* (6th ed.). St. Louis: Mosby.

Lindsay, C. (2006). Pregnancy complicated by diabetes mellitus. In R. Martin, A. Fanaroff, & M. Walsh (Eds.), *Fanaroff and Martin's neonatal-perinatal medicine: Diseases of the fetus and infant* (8th ed.). Philadelphia: Mosby.

Mestman, J. (2007). Thyroid and parathyroid diseases in pregnancy. In S. Gabbe, J. Niebyl, & J. Simpson (Eds.), *Obstetrics: Normal and problem pregnancies* (5th ed.). Philadelphia: Churchill Livingstone.

Moore, T., & Catalano, P. (2009). Diabetes in pregnancy. In R. Creasy, R. Resnik, & J. Iams (Eds.), *Creasy and Resnik's maternal-fetal medicine: Principles and practice* (6th ed.). Philadelphia: Saunders.

Nader, S. (2009). Thyroid disease and pregnancy. In R. Creasy, R. Resnik, & J. Iams (Eds.), *Creasy and Resnik's maternal-fetal medicine: Principles and practice* (6th ed.). Philadelphia: Saunders.

Paidas, M., & Hossain, N. (2009). Embryonic and fetal demise. In R. Creasy, R. Resnik, & J. Iams (Eds.), *Creasy and Resnik's maternal-fetal medicine: Principles and practice* (6th ed.). Philadelphia: Saunders.

Papoutsis, J., & Kroumpouzos, G. (2007). Dermatologic disorders of pregnancy. In S. Gabbe, J. Niebyl, & J. Simpson (Eds.), *Obstetrics: Normal and problem pregnancies* (5th ed.). Philadelphia: Churchill Livingstone.

Rapini, R. (2009). The skin and pregnancy. In R. Creasy, R. Resnik, & J. Iams (Eds.), *Creasy and Resnik's maternal-fetal medicine: Principles and practice* (6th ed.). Philadelphia: Saunders.

Riordan, J. (2005). *Breastfeeding and human lactation* (3rd ed.). Boston: Jones & Bartlett.

Samuels, P. (2007). Hematologic complications of pregnancy. In S. Gabbe, J. Niebyl, & J. Simpson (Eds.), *Obstetrics: Normal and problem pregnancies* (5th ed.). Philadelphia: Churchill Livingstone.

Samuels, P., & Niebyl, J. (2007). Neurological disorders. In S. Gabbe, J. Niebyl, & J. Simpson (Eds.), *Obstetrics: Normal and problem pregnancies* (5th ed.). Philadelphia: Churchill Livingstone.

Setaro, J., & Caulin-Glaser, T. (2004). Pregnancy and cardiovascular disease. In G. Burrow, T. Duffy, & J. Copel (Eds.), *Medical complications during pregnancy* (6th ed.). Philadelphia: Saunders.

Stuart, G., & Laraia, M. (2005). *Principles and practice of psychiatric nursing* (8th ed.). St. Louis: Mosby.

Wapner, R., Jenkins, T., & Khalek, N. (2009). Prenatal diagnosis of congenital disorders. In R. Creasy, R. Resnik, & J. Iams (Eds.), *Creasy and Resnik's maternal-fetal medicine: Principles and practice* (6th ed.). Philadelphia: Saunders.

Weiner, C., & Buhimschi, C. (2004). *Drugs for pregnant and lactating women.* New York: Churchill Livingstone.

Whitty, J., & Dombrowski, M. (2007). Respiratory diseases in pregnancy. In S. Gabbe, J. Niebyl, & J. Simpson (Eds.), *Obstetrics: Normal and problem pregnancies* (5th ed.). Philadelphia: Churchill Livingstone.

Whitty, J., & Dombrowski, M. (2009). Respiratory diseases in pregnancy. In R. Creasy, R. Resnik, & J. Iams (Eds.), *Creasy and Resnik's maternal-fetal medicine: Principles and practice* (6th ed.). Philadelphia: Saunders.

Williamson, C., & Mackillop, L. (2009). Diseases of the liver, biliary system, and pancreas. In R. K. Creasy, R. Resnik, & J. D. Iams (Eds.), *Creasy and Resnik's maternal-fetal medicine: Principles and practice* (6th ed.). Philadelphia: Saunders.

Wisner, K., Sit, D., Reynolds, S., Altemus, M., Bogen, D., Sunder, K., et al. (2007). Psychiatric disorders. In S. Gabbe, J. Niebyl, & J. Simpson (Eds.), *Obstetrics: Normal and problem pregnancies* (5th ed.). Philadelphia: Churchill Livingstone.

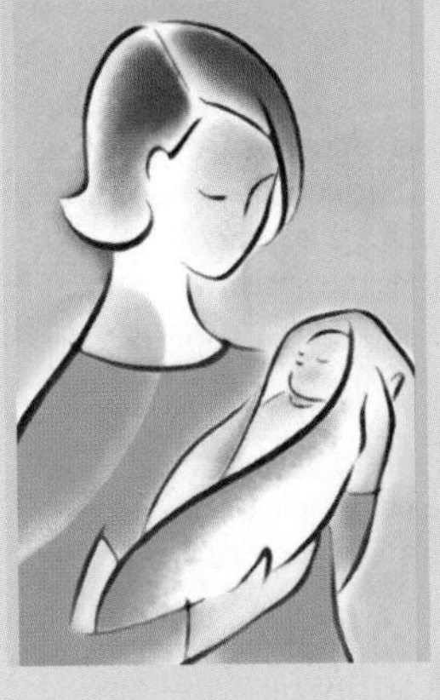

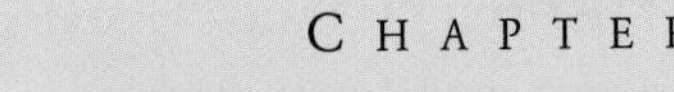

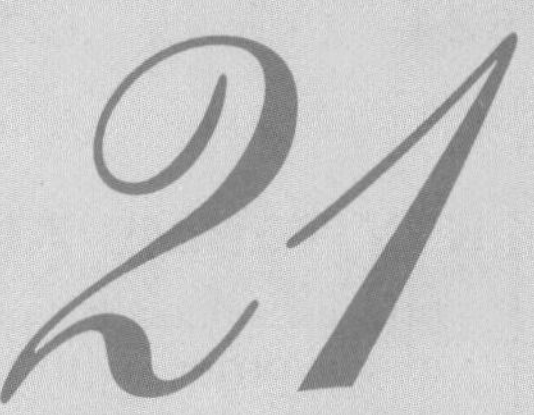

CHAPTER 21

Pregnancy at Risk: Gestational Conditions

KITTY CASHION

LEARNING OBJECTIVES

- *Differentiate the defining characteristics of gestational hypertension, preeclampsia and eclampsia, and chronic hypertension.*
- *Describe the pathophysiologic mechanisms of preeclampsia and eclampsia.*
- *Discuss the antepartum, intrapartum, and postpartum management of the woman with mild or severe gestational hypertension.*
- *Discuss the antepartum, intrapartum, and postpartum management of the woman with mild or severe preeclampsia.*
- *Discuss the preconception, antepartum, intrapartum, and postpartum management of the woman with chronic hypertension.*
- *Identify the priorities for the management of eclamptic seizures.*
- *Explain the effects of hyperemesis gravidarum on maternal and fetal well-being.*
- *Discuss the management of the woman with hyperemesis gravidarum in the hospital and at home.*
- *Differentiate among the causes, signs and symptoms, possible complications, and management of miscarriage, ectopic pregnancy, premature dilation of the cervix, and hydatidiform mole.*
- *Compare and contrast placenta previa and abruptio placentae in relation to signs and symptoms, complications, and management.*
- *Discuss the diagnosis and management of disseminated intravascular coagulation.*
- *Differentiate signs and symptoms, effects on pregnancy and the fetus, and management during pregnancy of common sexually transmitted infections and other infections.*
- *Explain the basic principles of care for a pregnant woman undergoing abdominal surgery.*
- *Discuss implications of trauma on the mother and fetus during pregnancy.*
- *Identify the priorities in assessment and stabilization measures for the pregnant trauma victim.*
- *Explain how performing cardiopulmonary resuscitation on a pregnant woman differs from performing this procedure on other adults.*

KEY TERMS AND DEFINITIONS

abruptio placentae Partial or complete premature separation of a normally implanted placenta

cerclage Use of a nonabsorbable suture to keep a premature dilating cervix closed; usually removed when pregnancy is at term

cervical funneling Effacement of the internal cervical os

chronic hypertension Systolic pressure of 140 mm Hg or higher or diastolic pressure of 90 mm Hg or higher that is present preconceptionally or occurs before 20 weeks of gestation

clonus Spasmodic alternation of muscular contraction and relaxation; counted in beats

Couvelaire uterus Interstitial myometrial hemorrhage after premature separation (abruption) of placenta; purplish-blue discoloration of the uterus is noted

disseminated intravascular coagulation (DIC) Pathologic form of coagulation in which clotting factors are consumed to such an extent that generalized bleeding can occur; associated with abruptio placentae, eclampsia, intrauterine fetal demise, amniotic fluid embolism, and hemorrhage

eclampsia Severe complication of pregnancy of unknown cause and occurring more often in the primigravida than in multiparous women;

KEY TERMS AND DEFINITIONS—cont'd

characterized by new-onset grand mal seizures in a woman with preeclampsia occurring during pregnancy or shortly after birth

ectopic pregnancy Implantation of the fertilized ovum outside of the uterine cavity; locations include the uterine tubes, ovaries, and abdomen

gestational hypertension The new onset of hypertension without proteinuria after week 20 of pregnancy

HELLP syndrome A laboratory diagnosis for a variant of severe preeclampsia that involves hepatic dysfunction, characterized by hemolysis, elevated liver enzymes, and low platelet count

hydatidiform mole (molar pregnancy) Gestational trophoblastic neoplasm usually resulting from fertilization of an egg that has no nucleus or an inactivated nucleus

hyperemesis gravidarum Abnormal condition of pregnancy characterized by protracted vomiting, weight loss, and fluid and electrolyte imbalance

miscarriage Loss of pregnancy that occurs naturally without interference or known cause; also called spontaneous abortion

placenta previa Placenta that is abnormally implanted in the thin, lower uterine segment. The condition is further classified as complete placenta previa, marginal placenta previa, or low-lying placenta according to gestational age and placental location in relation to the internal cervical os.

preeclampsia Disease encountered after 20 weeks of gestation or early in the puerperium; a vasospastic disease process characterized by hypertension and proteinuria

premature dilation of the cervix Cervix that is unable to remain closed until a pregnancy reaches term because of a mechanical defect in the cervix; also called incompetent cervix

superimposed preeclampsia New-onset proteinuria in a woman with hypertension before 20 weeks of gestation, sudden increase in proteinuria if already present in early gestation, sudden increase in hypertension, or the development of HELLP syndrome

TORCH infections Infections caused by organisms that damage the embryo or fetus; acronym for toxoplasmosis, other (e.g., syphilis), rubella, cytomegalovirus, and herpes simplex virus

WEB RESOURCES

Additional related content can be found on the companion website at evolve
http://evolve.elsevier.com/Lowdermilk/Maternity/

- NCLEX Review Questions
- Case Study: Preeclampsia
- Critical Thinking Exercise: Preeclampsia
- Nursing Care Plan: Hyperemesis Gravidarum
- Nursing Care Plan: Mild Preeclampsia: Home Care
- Nursing Care Plan: Placenta Previa
- Nursing Care Plan: Severe Preeclampsia: Hospital Care
- Spanish Guidelines: Assessment of Bleeding in Early Pregnancy

Some women experience significant problems during the months of gestation that can greatly affect pregnancy outcome. Some of these conditions develop as a result of the pregnant state; others are problems that can happen to anyone at any time of life but occur in this case during pregnancy. This chapter discusses a variety of disorders that did not exist before pregnancy, all of which have at least one thing in common: their occurrence in pregnancy puts the woman and fetus at risk. Hypertension in pregnancy, hyperemesis gravidarum, hemorrhagic complications of early and late pregnancy, surgery during pregnancy, trauma, and infections are discussed.

HYPERTENSION IN PREGNANCY

Significance and Incidence

Hypertensive disorders are the most common medical complication of pregnancy, occurring in 5% to 10% of all pregnancies. The incidence varies among hospitals, regions, and countries. Hypertensive disorders are a major cause of maternal and perinatal morbidity and mortality worldwide (Sibai, 2007). The four most common types of hypertensive disorders occurring in pregnancy are (1) gestational hypertension, (2) preeclampsia, (3) chronic hypertension, and (4) preeclampsia superimposed on chronic hypertension (Gilbert, 2007).

Classification

The classification of hypertensive disorders in pregnancy is confusing because standard definitions are not consistently used by all health care providers. The classification system most commonly used in the United States today is based on reports from the American College of Obstetricians and Gynecologists (ACOG) (2002) and the National High Blood Pressure Education Program Working Group on High Blood Pressure in Pregnancy (Working Group) (2000). This classification system is summarized in Table 21-1.

TABLE 21-1

Classification of Hypertensive States of Pregnancy

TYPE	DESCRIPTION
GESTATIONAL HYPERTENSIVE DISORDERS	
Gestational hypertension	Development of mild hypertension after week 20 of pregnancy in previously normotensive woman without proteinuria
Preeclampsia	Development of hypertension and proteinuria in previously normotensive woman after 20 weeks of gestation or in early postpartum period; in presence of trophoblastic disease, preeclampsia can develop before 20 weeks of gestation
Eclampsia	Development of convulsions or coma not attributable to other causes in preeclamptic woman
CHRONIC HYPERTENSIVE DISORDERS	
Chronic hypertension	Hypertension or proteinuria (or both) in pregnant woman present before pregnancy or diagnosed before 20 weeks of gestation and persistent after 6 weeks postpartum
Superimposed preeclampsia or eclampsia	• In women with hypertension before 20 weeks of gestation: new-onset proteinuria (≥0.5 g protein in a 24-hr collection) • In women with both hypertension and proteinuria before 20 weeks of gestation: significant increase in hypertension, plus one of the following: new onset of symptoms, thrombocytopenia, or elevated liver enzymes

Sources: American College of Obstetricians and Gynecologists (ACOG). (2002). *Diagnosis and management of preeclampsia and eclampsia.* ACOG Practice Bulletin No. 33. Washington DC: ACOG; Sibai, B. M. (2007). Hypertension. In S. Gabbe, J. Niebyl, & J. Simpson (Eds.), *Obstetrics: Normal and problem pregnancies* (5th ed.) Philadelphia: Churchill Livingstone.

Gestational hypertension

Gestational hypertension is the onset of hypertension without proteinuria after week 20 of pregnancy (ACOG, 2002; Working Group, 2000). Hypertension is defined as a systolic blood pressure (BP) greater than 140 mm Hg or a diastolic BP greater than 90 mm Hg. The hypertension should be recorded on at least two separate occasions at least 4 to 6 hours apart but within a maximum of a 1-week period (ACOG, 2002; Sibai, 2007; Working Group, 2000). Both the Working Group and the American Heart Association (AHA) have published extensive recommendations

BOX 21-1

Blood Pressure Measurement

- Measure blood pressure with the woman seated (ambulatory) or in the left lateral recumbent position with the arm at heart level.
- After positioning, allow the woman at least 10 minutes of quiet rest before blood pressure measurement to encourage relaxation.
- Instruct the woman to refrain from tobacco or caffeine use 30 minutes before blood pressure measurement.
- Use the right arm each time for blood pressure measurement.
- Hold the arm in a horizontal position at heart level.
- Use the proper-sized cuff (cuff should cover approximately 80% of the upper arm or be 1½ times the length of the upper arm).
- Maintain a slow, steady deflation rate.
- Take the average of two readings at least 6 hours apart to minimize recorded blood pressure variations across time.
- Use Korotkoff phase V (disappearance of sound) for recording the diastolic value.
- Use accurate equipment. The mercury sphygmomanometer is the most accurate device.
- If interchanging manual and electronic devices, use caution in interpreting different blood pressure values.

for accurately measuring BP (Pickering et al., 2005; Working Group, 2000). Box 21-1 provides detailed instructions for measuring BP.

Gestational hypertension is the most frequent cause of hypertension during pregnancy, with an incidence of 6% to 17% in primigravidas and 2% to 4% in multiparous women. It occurs much more frequently in women with multifetal pregnancies than in other women (Sibai, 2007). Gestational hypertension usually develops at or after 37 weeks of gestation. Women with gestational hypertension have no evidence of preexisting hypertension, and their BPs return to normal levels within 6 weeks after giving birth. Women with mild gestational hypertension usually have good pregnancy outcomes. Some women who are initially thought to have gestational hypertension will eventually be diagnosed with chronic hypertension instead. Others will go on to develop proteinuria, thereby changing their diagnosis to preeclampsia. Women who are diagnosed with gestational hypertension before 35 weeks of gestation are more likely to progress to preeclampsia than women whose onset of hypertension occurs closer to term (Sibai).

Critical Thinking Exercise: Preeclampsia

Preeclampsia

Preeclampsia is a pregnancy-specific condition in which hypertension and proteinuria develop after 20 weeks of gestation in a previously normotensive woman. A significant contributor to maternal and perinatal morbidity

Case Study: Preeclampsia

and mortality, preeclampsia complicates approximately 3% to 7% of all pregnancies (American Academy of Pediatrics [AAP] & ACOG, 2007). Preeclampsia is a vasospastic, systemic disorder and is usually categorized as mild or severe for purposes of management (ACOG, 2002; Working Group, 2000). Table 21-2 lists criteria for mild and severe preeclampsia, and Table 21-3 gives common laboratory changes that occur in mild and severe preeclampsia.

Proteinuria is defined as a concentration at or above 30 mg/dl (≥1+ on dipstick measurement) or more in at least two random urine specimens collected at least 6 hours apart with no evidence of urinary tract infection. In a 24-hour specimen, proteinuria is defined as a concentration at or above 300 mg/24 hours. Because of the discrepancy between random protein determinations the diagnosis of proteinuria should be based on a 24-hour urine collection if possible or a timed collection corrected for creatinine excretion if a 24-hour specimen is not feasible (ACOG, 2002; Longo, Dola, & Pridjian, 2003). To ensure accurate results, proteinuria should be determined using only a urine specimen that has been collected either by catheterization or by a thorough clean-catch technique.

Eclampsia

Eclampsia is the onset of seizure activity or coma in a woman with preeclampsia but with no history of a preexisting abnormality that can result in seizure activity (ACOG, 2002). The initial presentation of eclampsia varies, with one third of the women developing eclampsia during the pregnancy, one third during labor, and one third within 72 hours postpartum (Emery, 2005).

Chronic hypertension

Chronic hypertension is defined as hypertension that occurs before the pregnancy or is diagnosed before the twentieth week of gestation. Hypertension initially diagnosed during pregnancy that persists longer than 6 weeks postpartum is also classified as chronic hypertension (Sibai, 2007). Other authorities believe that a diagnosis of chronic hypertension can be made only if the BP has not returned to normal levels by 12 weeks after birth (Roberts & Funai, 2009).

Chronic hypertension with superimposed preeclampsia

Women with chronic hypertension may develop **superimposed preeclampsia,** which increases the morbidity for

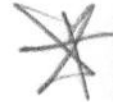

TABLE 21-2

Differentiation between Mild and Severe Preeclampsia

	MILD PREECLAMPSIA	SEVERE PREECLAMPSIA
MATERNAL EFFECTS		
Blood pressure (BP)	BP reading ≥140/90 mm Hg × two, at least 4-6 hr apart but within a maximum of a 1-week period	Rise to ≥160/110 mm Hg on two separate occasions 6 hr apart with pregnant woman on bed rest
Proteinuria		
Qualitative dipstick	≥1+ on dipstick	≥3+ on dipstick
Quantitative 24-hr analysis	Proteinuria of ≥300 mg in a 24-hr specimen	Proteinuria of ≥5 g in 24-hr specimen
Urine output	Output matching intake, ≥25-30 ml/hr	<400-500 ml/24 hr
Headache	Absent or transient	Persistent or severe
Visual problems	Absent	Blurred, photophobia
Irritability or changes in affect	Transient	May be severe
Epigastric or right upper quadrant pain, nausea, and vomiting	Absent	May be present
Thrombocytopenia	Absent	May be present
Impaired liver function	Normal	May be present
Pulmonary edema	Absent	May be present
FETAL EFFECTS		
Placental perfusion	Reduced	Decreased perfusion expressing as IUGR in fetus; nonreassuring fetal status on antepartum testing

Sources: American College of Obstetricians and Gynecologists (ACOG). (2002). *Diagnosis and management of preeclampsia and eclampsia.* ACOG Practice Bulletin No. 33. Washington, DC: ACOG; Sibai, B. M. (2007). Hypertension. In S. Gabbe, J. Niebyl, & J. Simpson (Eds.), *Obstetrics: Normal and problem pregnancies* (5th ed.) Philadelphia: Churchill Livingstone.

FHR, Fetal heart rate; *IUGR,* intrauterine growth restriction.

TABLE 21-3

Common Laboratory Changes in Preeclampsia

	NORMAL NONPREGNANT	PREECLAMPSIA	HELLP
Hemoglobin, hematocrit	12-16 g/dl, 37%-47%	May ↑	↓
Platelets (cells/mm³)	150,000-400,000/mm³	Unchanged or <100,000/mm³	<100,000/mm³
Prothrombin time (PT), partial thromboplastin time (PTT)	12-14 sec, 60-70 sec	Unchanged	Unchanged
Fibrinogen	200-400 mg/dl	300-600 mg/dl	↓
Fibrin split products (FSP)	Absent	Absent or present	Present
Blood urea nitrogen (BUN)	10-20 mg/dl	↑	↑
Creatinine	0.5-1.1 mg/dl	>1.2 mg/dl	↑
Lactate dehydrogenase (LDH)*	45-90 units/L	↑	↑ (>600 units/L)
Aspartate aminotransferase (AST), serum glutamic oxaloacetic transaminase (SGOT)	4-20 units/L	Unchanged to minimal ↑	↑ (>70 units/L)
Alanine aminotransferase (ALT)	3-21 units/L	Unchanged to minimal ↑	↑
Creatinine clearance	80-125 ml/min	130-180 ml/min	↓
Burr cells or schistocytes	Absent	Absent	Present
Uric acid	2-6.6 mg/dl	>5.9 mg/dl	>10 mg/dl
Bilirubin (total)	0.1-1 mg/dl	unchanged or ↑	↑ (>.1.2 mg/dl)

Sources: American College of Obstetricians and Gynecologists (ACOG). (2002). *Diagnosis and management of preeclampsia and eclampsia.* ACOG Practice Bulletin No. 33. Washington, DC: ACOG; Cunningham, F., Leveno, K., Bloom, S., Hauth, J., Gilstrap, L., & Wenstrom, K. (Eds.). (2005). *Williams obstetrics* (22nd ed.). New York: McGraw-Hill; Dildy, G. (2004). Complications of preeclampsia. In G. Dildy, M. Belfort, G. Saade, J. Phelan, G. Hankins, & S. Clark (Eds.), *Critical care obstetrics* (4th ed.). Malden, MA: Blackwell Science; Sibai, B. M. (2007). Hypertension. In S. Gabbe, J. Niebyl, & J. Simpson (Eds.), *Obstetrics: Normal and problem pregnancies* (5th ed.). Philadelphia: Churchill Livingstone.
*LDH values differ according to the test or assays being performed.

both the mother and the fetus. A diagnosis of superimposed preeclampsia is made with the following findings (Sibai, 2007):

- In women with hypertension before 20 weeks of gestation
  - New-onset proteinuria (≥0.5 g protein in a 24-hour collection)
- In women with both hypertension and proteinuria before 20 weeks of gestation
  - Significant increase in hypertension, plus one of the following:
    - New onset of symptoms
    - Thrombocytopenia
    - Elevated liver enzymes

Preeclampsia

Etiology

Preeclampsia is a condition unique to human pregnancy; signs and symptoms develop only during pregnancy and disappear quickly after birth of the fetus and placenta. The cause of preeclampsia is not known. Although preeclampsia is generally a disease of primigravidas, its cause may not be the same for all women. For example, the pathogenesis for a healthy nulliparous woman who develops mild preeclampsia near term or in labor may be very different than that of the woman who has preexisting vascular disease or diabetes, a multifetal pregnancy, or who develops severe preeclampsia earlier in the pregnancy (Sibai, 2007). Box 21-2 lists risk factors for the development of preeclampsia.

Many theories have been suggested to explain the cause of preeclampsia. Current theories that are still being considered include abnormal trophoblast invasion, coagulation abnormalities, vascular endothelial damage, cardiovascular maladaptation, and dietary deficiencies or excesses. Immunologic factors and genetic predisposition may also play an important role (Sibai, 2007).

Pathophysiology

Preeclampsia can progress along a continuum from mild to severe preeclampsia to eclampsia. Current thought is that the pathologic changes that occur in the woman with preeclampsia are caused by disruptions in placental perfusion and endothelial cell dysfunction (Gilbert, 2007; Peters, 2008). These pathologic changes are present long before the clinical diagnosis of preeclampsia is made (Roberts & Funai, 2009). Normally in pregnancy the spiral arteries in the uterus widen from thick-walled muscular vessels to thinner, saclike vessels with much larger diameters. This change increases the capacity of the vessels, allowing them to handle the increased blood volume of pregnancy. Because this vascular remodeling does not occur or only partially develops in women with preeclampsia, decreased placental perfusion and hypoxia result (Peters). Placental ischemia is thought to cause endothelial cell dysfunction by stimulating the release of a substance

Edema is assessed for distribution, degree, and pitting. Dependent edema is edema of the lowest or most dependent parts of the body, where hydrostatic pressure is greatest. If a pregnant woman is ambulatory, the edema may first be evident in the feet and ankles. If she is confined to bed, the edema is more likely to occur in the sacral region. Pitting edema is edema that leaves a small depression or pit after finger pressure is applied to the swollen area. The pit, which is caused by movement of fluid to adjacent tissue away from the point of pressure, normally disappears within 10 to 30 seconds. Although the amount of edema is difficult to quantify, the method shown in Fig. 21-3 may be used to record relative degrees of edema formation.

Deep tendon reflexes (DTRs) are evaluated as a baseline and to detect any changes. The biceps and patellar reflexes and ankle clonus are assessed and the findings recorded (Fig. 21-4; Table 21-4). To elicit the biceps reflex the examiner strikes a downward blow with a percussion hammer over the thumb, which is situated over the biceps tendon (Fig. 21-4, *A*). Normal response is flexion of the arm at the elbow, described as a 2+ response. The patellar reflex is elicited with the woman's legs hanging freely over the end of the examining table or with the woman lying on her side with the knee slightly flexed (Fig. 21-4, *B*). A blow with a percussion hammer is dealt directly to the patellar tendon, inferior to the patella. Normal response is the extension or kicking out of the leg. To assess for hyperac-

EVIDENCE-BASED PRACTICE

Preeclampsia Risk Factors and Prevention

Pat Gingrich

ASK THE QUESTION

What risk factors predict preeclampsia? Once risk is identified, can anything prevent its onset?

SEARCH FOR EVIDENCE

Search Strategies: Professional organization guidelines, meta-analyses, systematic reviews, randomized controlled trials since 2007.

Databases Searched: CINAHL, Cochrane, Medline, National Guideline Clearinghouse, TRIP database, AHRQ database, and the websites for Association of Women's Health, Obstetric, and Neonatal Nurses; National Institute for Health and Clinical Excellence; and the Society of Obstetricians and Gynaecologists of Canada.

CRITICALLY ANALYZE THE DATA

Preeclampsia can endanger the fetus by impeding uteroplacental perfusion while risking maternal harm from hypertension and seizures. In addition to established risk factors based on medical history, a systematic review of the association between maternal infections and the occurrence of preeclampsia revealed that periodontal disease and urinary tract infection were risk factors (Conde-Agudelo, Villar, & Lindheimer, 2008). Another systematic analysis of 16 studies found that maternal bacterial or viral infections was associated with twice the risk of preeclampsia when compared with similar women who had no infection (Rustveld, Kelsey, & Sharma, 2008). The authors suggest that this association is related to the inflammation of preeclampsia.

Prevention of preeclampsia in women at increased risk has had variable success. Professional guidelines of the SOGC (2008) recommend low-dose aspirin started before 16 weeks of gestation plus calcium supplementation for women with low calcium intake. A Cochrane meta-analysis of 10 randomized controlled trials involving 65,000 women found that antioxidants vitamins A and E are not effective at decreasing the risk of preeclampsia (Rumbold, Duley, Crowther, & Haslam, 2008). The SOGC guidelines specifically do not recommend calorie or sodium restrictions during pregnancy or treatment with prostaglandins or thiazide diuretics. Evidence reinforces the importance for pregnant women at risk for preeclampsia to avoid alcohol and smoking, engage in regular exercise, and take multivitamins with folate. Avoiding interpregnancy weight gain may be beneficial, as may increasing rest and decreasing stress during the third trimester (SOGC, 2008).

IMPLICATIONS FOR PRACTICE

The woman at risk for preeclampsia, especially severe or early preeclampsia, may suffer harm to her own health and compromise of the growing fetus, resulting in preterm or small-for-gestational-age birth. Screening for risk factors enables more diligent observation for the onset of preeclampsia and perhaps even prevention. Women at risk need education about any prescription or over-the-counter supplements and the signs and symptoms of the disease. Women who have experienced infections, especially periodontal disease and urinary tract infection, should be thoroughly assessed at their prenatal visits for any sign of preeclampsia. Women benefit from decreasing free-radical production by avoiding alcohol, smoking, and stress. Some treatments, such as low-dose aspirin, work best if started before 16 weeks or even before conception.

Health care workers will need to keep informed about the evidence, which can sometimes be contradictory. Finally, women at risk for preeclampsia and especially those who have been diagnosed should have the opportunity to ask questions and voice their fears about this poorly understood disease.

References:

Conde-Agudelo, A., Villar, J., & Lindheimer, M. (2008). Maternal infections and risk of preeclampsia: systematic review and metaanalysis. *American Journal of Obstetrics and Gynecology*, 198(1), 7–22.

Rumbold, A., Duley, L., Crowther, C. A., & Haslam, R. R. (2008). Antioxidants for preventing pre-eclampsia. In *The Cochrane Database of Systematic Reviews* 2008, Issue1, CD 004227.

Rustveld, L. O., Kelsey, S. F., & Sharma, R. (2008). Association between maternal infections and preeclampsia: a systematic review of epidemiological studies. *Maternal Child Health Journal*, 12(2), 223–242.

Society of Obstetricians and Gynaecologists of Canada. (2008). Diagnosis, evaluation, and management of the hypertensive disorders of pregnancy. *Journal of Obstetric, Gynaecology Canada*, 30(3), s1–s6.

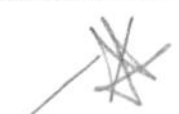

tive reflexes (clonus) at the ankle joint the examiner supports the leg with the knee flexed (Fig. 21-4, *C*). With one hand the examiner sharply dorsiflexes the foot, maintains the position for a moment, and then releases the foot. Normal (negative clonus) response is elicited when no rhythmic oscillations (jerks) are felt while the foot is held in dorsiflexion. When the foot is released, no oscillations are seen as the foot drops to the plantar-flexed position. Abnormal (positive clonus) response is recognized by rhythmic oscillations of one or more "beats" felt when the foot is in dorsiflexion and seen as the foot drops to the plantar-flexed position.

Mild Gestational Hypertension and Mild Preeclampsia

The goals of therapy for women with mild gestational hypertension or mild preeclampsia are to ensure maternal safety and to deliver a healthy newborn as close to term as possible. At or near term the plan of care for a woman with gestational hypertension or mild preeclampsia is most likely to be the induction of labor preceded, if necessary, by cervical ripening. When mild gestational or mild preeclampsia is diagnosed earlier in gestation, however, immediate birth may not be in the best interest of the fetus. Management of women with these disorders before 37 weeks of gestation is controversial (Sibai, 2007).

Home care

Women with mild gestational hypertension and mild preeclampsia may be safely managed at home, provided they have frequent maternal and fetal evaluation. Successful home care requires the woman to be well educated about preeclampsia and highly motivated to follow the plan of care. All teaching should include the woman and

Nursing Care Plan: Mild Preeclampsia: Home Care

TABLE 21-4

Assessing Deep Tendon Reflexes

GRADE	DEEP TENDON REFLEX RESPONSE
0	No response
1+	Sluggish or diminished
2+	Active or expected response
3+	More brisk than expected, slightly hyperactive
4+	Brisk, hyperactive, with intermittent or transient clonus

Source: Seidel, H., Ball, J., Dains, J., & Benedict, G. (2006). *Mosby's guide to physical examination* (6th ed.). St. Louis: Mosby.

COMMUNITY ACTIVITY

Contact the nearest health department, perinatal clinic, or private office. Assess the educational and recommended screening tools available for women with hypertensive disorders of pregnancy. Are tools available in languages other than English? Suggest ways to make tools more available to pregnant women in the community. Gather data related to the number of women who have hypertensive disorders in your local area and compare with national statistics.

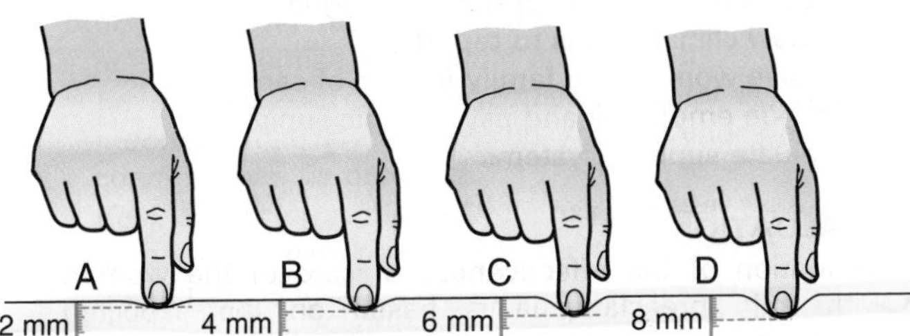

Fig. 21-3 Assessment of pitting edema of lower extremities. **A,** +1; **B,** +2; **C,** +3; **D,** +4.

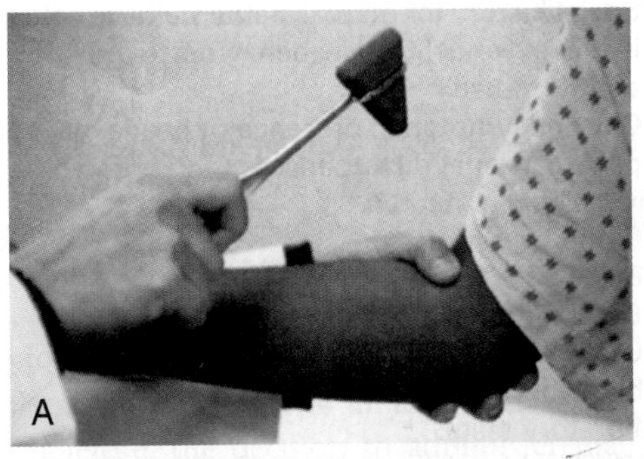

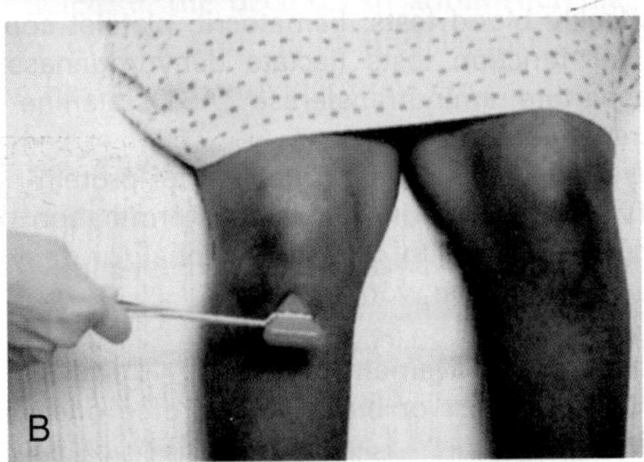

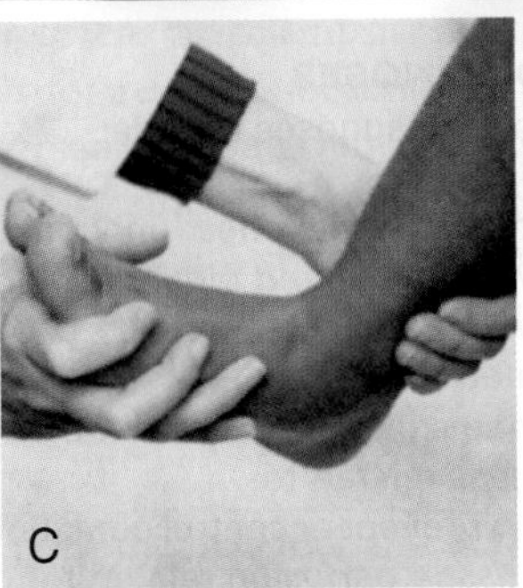

Fig. 21-4 **A,** Biceps reflex. **B,** Patellar reflex with patient's legs hanging freely over end of examining table. **C,** Test for ankle clonus. (From Seidel, H., Ball, J., Dains, J., Benedict, G. [2006]. *Mosby's guide to physical examination* [6th ed.]. St. Louis: Mosby.)

BOX 21-3

Hospital Precautionary Measures

- Environment:
  Quiet
  Nonstimulating
  Lighting subdued
- Seizure precautions:
  Suction equipment tested and ready to use
  Oxygen administration equipment tested and ready to use
- Call button within easy reach
- Emergency medications available on the unit
  Hydralazine
  Labetalol
  Nifedipine
  Magnesium sulfate
  Calcium gluconate
- Emergency birth pack accessible

for the development of vaginal bleeding. Continuous FHR monitoring is also important because the fetuses of these women are at risk for hypoxia and intolerance of labor (Sibai, 2007).

Magnesium sulfate. One of the important goals of care for the woman with severe preeclampsia is prevention or control of convulsions. Magnesium sulfate is the drug of choice in the prevention and treatment of convulsions caused by preeclampsia or eclampsia (Cunningham, Leveno, Bloom, Hauth, Gilstrap, & Wenstrom, 2005; Sibai, 2007). The routine use of magnesium sulfate is indicated for severe preeclampsia, HELLP syndrome, or eclampsia. Magnesium sulfate is administered as a secondary infusion (piggyback) to the main intravenous (IV) line by volumetric infusion pump. An initial loading dose of 4 to 6 g of magnesium sulfate per protocol or physician's order is infused over 15 to 30 minutes. This dose is followed by a maintenance dose of magnesium sulfate that is diluted in an IV solution per physician's order (e.g., 40 g of magnesium sulfate in 1000 ml of lactated Ringer's solution) and administered by infusion pump at 2 g/hour (Cunningham et al.). This dose should maintain a therapeutic serum magnesium level of 4 to 7 mEq/L (Cunningham et al.; Gilbert, 2007). After the loading dose, a transient lowering of the arterial BP may occur secondary to relaxation of smooth muscle by the magnesium sulfate (Cunningham et al.; Gilbert) (Box 21-4).

Magnesium sulfate is rarely given intramuscularly because the absorption rate cannot be controlled, injections are painful, and tissue necrosis may occur. However, the intramuscular (IM) route may be used with some women who are being transported to a tertiary-care center. The IM dose is 4 to 5 g given in each buttock, a total of 10 g (with 1% procaine possibly being added to the solution to reduce injection pain) and can be repeated at 4-hour intervals. The Z-track technique should be used for the deep IM injection followed by gentle massage at the site.

Magnesium sulfate interferes with the release of acetylcholine at the synapses, decreasing neuromuscular irritability, depressing cardiac conduction, and decreasing CNS irritability. Because magnesium circulates in a free state and unbound to protein and is excreted in the urine, accurate recordings of maternal urine output must be obtained. If renal function declines, all of the magnesium sulfate will not be excreted and can cause magnesium toxicity. Given that magnesium sulfate is a CNS depressant, the nurse assesses for signs and symptoms of magnesium toxicity. Expected side effects of magnesium sulfate are a feeling of warmth, flushing, and burning at the IV site. Symptoms of mild toxicity include lethargy, muscle weakness, decreased or absent DTRs, and slurred speech. Increasing toxicity may be indicated by maternal hypotension, bradycardia, bradypnea, and cardiac arrest (Gilbert, 2007). Blood may be drawn to precisely determine the serum magnesium level if mild or severe toxicity is suspected (see Box 21-4).

NURSING ALERT Loss of patellar reflexes, respiratory depression, oliguria, and decreased level of consciousness are signs of magnesium toxicity. Actions are needed to prevent respiratory or cardiac arrest. If magnesium toxicity is suspected, the infusion should be discontinued immediately. Calcium gluconate, the antidote for magnesium sulfate, may also be ordered (10 ml of a 10% solution, or 1 g) and given by slow IV push (usually by the physician) over at least 3 minutes to prevent undesirable reactions such as arrhythmias, bradycardia, and ventricular fibrillation (Cunningham et al., 2005; Gilbert, 2007).

Magnesium sulfate does not seem to affect the FHR in a healthy term fetus. Neonatal serum magnesium levels approximate the levels of the mother. Doses of magnesium sulfate that prevent maternal seizures have been determined to be safe for the fetus (Roberts & Funai, 2009). Toxic levels in the newborn can cause depressed respirations and hyporeflexia at birth (Cunningham et al., 2005). The neonatal team should attend the birth to provide resuscitation measures as needed.

NURSING ALERT Because magnesium sulfate is also a tocolytic agent, its use may increase the duration of labor. A preeclamptic woman receiving magnesium sulfate may need augmentation with oxytocin during labor. The amount of oxytocin needed to stimulate labor may be more than that needed for a woman who is not receiving magnesium sulfate.

Control of blood pressure. For the severely hypertensive preeclamptic woman, antihypertensive medications may be ordered to lower the diastolic BP. Initiation of antihypertensive therapy reduces maternal morbidity and mortality rates associated with left ventricular failure and cerebral hemorrhage. Because a degree of maternal

BOX 21-4

Care of the Patient with Preeclampsia Receiving Magnesium Sulfate

PATIENT AND FAMILY TEACHING

- Explain technique, rationale, and reactions to expect:
  Route and rate
  Purpose of "piggyback" infusion
- Reasons for use:
  Tailor information to woman's readiness to learn.
  Explain that magnesium sulfate is used to prevent disease progression.
  Explain that magnesium sulfate is used to prevent seizures, *not* to decrease blood pressure.
- Reactions to expect from medication:
  Initially, the woman will appear flushed and will feel hot, sedated, nauseated. She may experience burning at the IV site, especially during the bolus.
  Sedation will continue.
- Monitoring to anticipate:
  Maternal: blood pressure, pulse, respiratory rate, DTRs, level of consciousness, urine output (indwelling catheter), presence of headache, visual disturbances, epigastric pain
  Fetal: FHR and activity

ADMINISTRATION

- Verify physician order.
- Position woman in side-lying position.
- Prepare solution and administer with an infusion control device (pump).
- Piggyback a solution of 40 g of magnesium sulfate in 1000 ml lactated Ringer's solution with an infusion control device at the ordered rate: loading dose—initial bolus of 4-6 g over 15-30 min; maintenance dose—2 g/hr, according to unit protocol or specific physician's order.

MATERNAL AND FETAL ASSESSMENTS

- Monitor blood pressure, pulse, respiratory rate, FHR, and contractions every 15-30 min, depending on woman's condition.
- Monitor intake and output, proteinuria, DTRs, presence of headache, visual disturbances, level of consciousness, and epigastric pain at least hourly.
- Restrict hourly fluid intake to a total of 100-125 ml/hr; urinary output should be at least 25-30 ml/hr.

REPORTABLE CONDITIONS

- Blood pressure: systolic ≥160 mm Hg, diastolic ≥110 mm Hg, or both
- Respiratory rate: <12 breaths/min
- Urinary output <25-30 ml/hr
- Presence of headache, visual disturbances, decrease in level of consciousness, or epigastric pain
- Increasing severity or loss of DTRs, increasing edema, proteinuria
- Any abnormal laboratory values (magnesium levels, platelet count, creatinine clearance, levels of uric acid, AST, ALT, prothrombin time, partial thromboplastin time, fibrinogen, fibrin split products)
- Any other significant change in maternal or fetal status

EMERGENCY MEASURES

- Keep emergency drugs and intubation equipment immediately available.
- Keep side rails up.
- Keep lights dimmed, and maintain a quiet environment.

DOCUMENTATION

- All of the above

ALT, Alanine aminotransferase; *AST*, aspartate aminotransferase; *DTRs*, deep tendon reflexes; *FHR*, fetal heart rate; *IV*, intravenous.

hypertension is necessary to maintain uteroplacental perfusion, antihypertensive therapy must not decrease the arterial pressure too much or too rapidly. Many health care providers use a target range of less than 110 mm Hg for the diastolic pressure and less than 160 mm Hg for the systolic pressure (Cunningham et al., 2005; Sibai et al., 2005). No universal agreement has been reached on the level of hypertension that requires treatment to prevent complications. In general, however, sustained systolic pressures of 160 to 180 mm Hg or more, sustained diastolic pressures of 105 to 110 mm Hg or a mean BP of 130 mm Hg or greater are treated (Sibai, 2007).

IV hydralazine remains the antihypertensive agent of choice for the intrapartum treatment of hypertension in severe preeclampsia (Cunningham et al., 2005; Sibai, 2007). Recent research has shown that intravenous labetalol hydrochloride or oral nifedipine are as effective as hydralazine at controlling BP but have fewer side effects (Sibai). Nifedipine, labetalol, or methyldopa may be used during pregnancy or the postpartum period for BP control. (ACOG, 2002; Cunningham et al.; Sibai). The choice of agent used depends on patient response and physician preference. Table 21-5 compares antihypertensive agents used to treat hypertension in pregnancy.

Postpartum care

Throughout the postpartum period the woman will need careful assessment of her vital signs, intake and output, DTRs, level of consciousness, uterine tone, and lochial flow. The magnesium sulfate infusion is continued for 12 to 24 hours after birth for seizure prophylaxis. Assessments for effects and side effects continue until the medication is discontinued. Given that magnesium sulfate potentiates the action of narcotics, CNS depressants, and calcium channel blockers, these drugs must be administered with caution. Even if no convulsions occurred before the birth, they may occur during the postpartum period. The nurse should also assess the woman for any symptoms of preeclampsia such as headaches, visual disturbances, or epigastric pain.

The preeclamptic woman is unable to tolerate excessive postpartum blood loss because of hemoconcentration.

TABLE 21-5

Pharmacologic Control of Hypertension in Pregnancy

ACTION	TARGET TISSUE	EFFECTS: MATERNAL EFFECTS	EFFECTS: FETAL EFFECTS	NURSING ACTIONS
HYDRALAZINE (APRESOLINE, NEOPRESOL)				
Arteriolar vasodilator	Peripheral arterioles: to decrease muscle tone, decrease peripheral resistance; hypothalamus and medullary vasomotor center for minor decrease in sympathetic tone	Headache, flushing, palpitations, tachycardia, some decrease in uteroplacental blood flow, increase in heart rate and cardiac output, increase in oxygen consumption, nausea and vomiting	Tachycardia; late decelerations and bradycardia if maternal diastolic pressure <90 mm Hg	Assess for effects of medication; alert mother (family) to expected effects of medication; assess blood pressure frequently because precipitous drop can lead to shock and perhaps abruptio placentae; if giving multiple doses, wait at least 20 minutes after the first dose is given to administer an additional dose to allow time to assess the effects of the initial dose; assess urinary output; maintain bed rest in a lateral position with side rails up; use with caution in presence of maternal tachycardia.
LABETALOL HYDROCHLORIDE (NORMODYNE, TRANDATE)				
Beta-blocking agent causing vasodilation without significant change in cardiac output	Peripheral arterioles (see hydralazine)	Minimal: flushing, tremulousness; minimal change in pulse rate	Minimal, if any	See hydralazine; less likely to cause excessive hypotension and tachycardia; less rebound hypertension than hydralazine. Do not use in women with asthma or heart failure.
METHYLDOPA (ALDOMET)				
Maintenance therapy if needed: 250-500 mg orally every 8 hr (α_2-receptor agonist)	Postganglionic nerve endings: interferes with chemical neurotransmission to reduce peripheral vascular resistance; causes CNS sedation	Sleepiness, postural hypotension, constipation; rare: drug-induced fever in 1% of women and positive Coombs test result in 20% of women	After 4 mo maternal therapy, positive Coombs test result in infant	See hydralazine.
NIFEDIPINE (ADALAT, PROCARDIA)				
Calcium channel blocker	Arterioles: to reduce systemic vascular resistance by relaxation of arterial smooth muscle	Headache, flushing; may interfere with labor	Minimal	See hydralazine; avoid concurrent use with magnesium sulfate because skeletal muscle blockade can result.

CNS, Central nervous system.

Oxytocin or prostaglandin products are used to control bleeding. Ergot products (e.g., Ergotrate, Methergine) are contraindicated because they increase BP.

NURSING ALERT The woman is at risk for a boggy uterus and a large lochia flow as a result of the magnesium sulfate therapy. Uterine tone and lochia flow should be assessed frequently.

Hypertension may persist for days or weeks after birth. Women with severe gestational hypertension or severe preeclampsia are frequently discharged from the hospital on an antihypertensive medication such as labetalol or nifedipine. If such is the case, their BP needs to be checked frequently either at home or at the health care provider's office. In many instances, BP returns to normal within a few weeks after birth, and antihypertensive medications can be discontinued.

The nurse provides important emotional support to the woman and her family during this stressful period. Coping mechanisms should be assessed and appropriate referrals initiated. If the preeclampsia was severe, the infant may be premature and in a special care nursery. The woman and her family may be worried about their infant's survival, and the day-to-day fluctuations in the infant's status can be emotionally draining (Simpson & James, 2005). Emotional stress can also decrease the woman's ability to process information. Thus the nurse should include the family during all discharge teaching and provide them with written information.

The woman should be informed that the chance of developing preeclampsia or eclampsia in a future pregnancy is increased sevenfold and that comprehensive prenatal care is essential for assessment and early intervention (Duckitt & Harrington, 2005). Women with preeclampsia are also at increased risk for chronic hypertension later in life, especially if preeclampsia was diagnosed at a preterm gestation. Women who developed preeclampsia before 30 weeks of gestation are increasingly likely to have underlying renal disease. In addition, recent evidence suggests that women who develop preeclampsia may be at increased risk for future coronary artery disease. Therefore the postpartum period may provide an excellent opportunity to educate women about lifestyle changes that could decrease the risk for developing these future problems (Sibai, 2007).

Eclampsia

Eclampsia is usually preceded by various premonitory symptoms and signs, including persistent headache, blurred vision, severe epigastric or right upper quadrant abdominal pain, and altered mental status. However, convulsions can appear suddenly and without warning in a seemingly stable woman with only minimal BP elevations (Sibai, 2007). The convulsions that occur in eclampsia are frightening to observe. Tonic contraction of all body muscles (seen as arms flexed, hands clenched, legs inverted) precedes the tonic-clonic convulsions. During this stage, muscles alternately relax and contract. Respirations are halted and then begin again with long, deep, stertorous inhalations. Hypotension follows, and coma ensues. Nystagmus and muscular twitching persist for a time. Disorientation and amnesia cloud the immediate recovery. Seizures may recur within minutes of the first convulsion, or the woman may never have another. During the convulsion the pregnant woman and fetus are not receiving oxygen; thus eclamptic seizures produce a marked metabolic insult to both the woman and the fetus (Cunningham et al., 2005).

Immediate care

The immediate goal of care during a convulsion is to ensure a patent airway (see Emergency box: Eclampsia). Patient safety is a major concern. When convulsions occur, turn the woman onto her side to prevent aspiration of vomitus and supine hypotension syndrome. Make certain that the side rails on the bed are raised; pad them with a folded blanket or pillow if possible. Women with eclampsia have been known to sustain fractures due to falling out of bed during the seizure.

After the convulsion ceases, suction food and fluids from the glottis, and administer 10 L of oxygen by a nonrebreather facemask. If an IV infusion is not in place, insert one with an 18-gauge needle. If an IV line was in place before the seizure, it may have infiltrated and will need to be restarted immediately. A loading dose of 6 g magnesium sulfate is infused intravenously over 15 to 30 minutes followed by a maintenance dose of 2 g per hour given by continuous infusion (Sibai, 2007). If eclampsia develops after the initiation of magnesium sulfate therapy, additional magnesium sulfate or another anticonvulsant (e.g., diazepam [Valium]) may be administered (Sibai et al., 2005; Sibai). Fetal and neonatal effects of diazepam include decreased FHR variability, neonatal hypotonia, decreased respirations, and depressed sucking reflex. With adequate blood magnesium levels, the eclamptic woman will rarely continue to have seizures (Chan & Winkle, 2006; Cunningham et al., 2005).

A rapid assessment of uterine activity, cervical status, and fetal status is performed after a convulsion. During the convulsion, membranes may have ruptured, the cervix may have dilated because the uterus becomes hypercontractile and hypertonic, and birth may be imminent. The FHR tracing may demonstrate bradycardia, late decelerations, absent or minimal baseline variability, or any combination. These findings usually resolve within a few minutes after the convulsion ends and the woman's hypoxia is corrected (Sibai, 2007).

NURSING ALERT Immediately after a seizure the woman may be very confused and can be combative, necessitating the temporary use of restraints. Maintain a quiet, darkened environment. Several hours may be needed for the woman to regain her usual level of

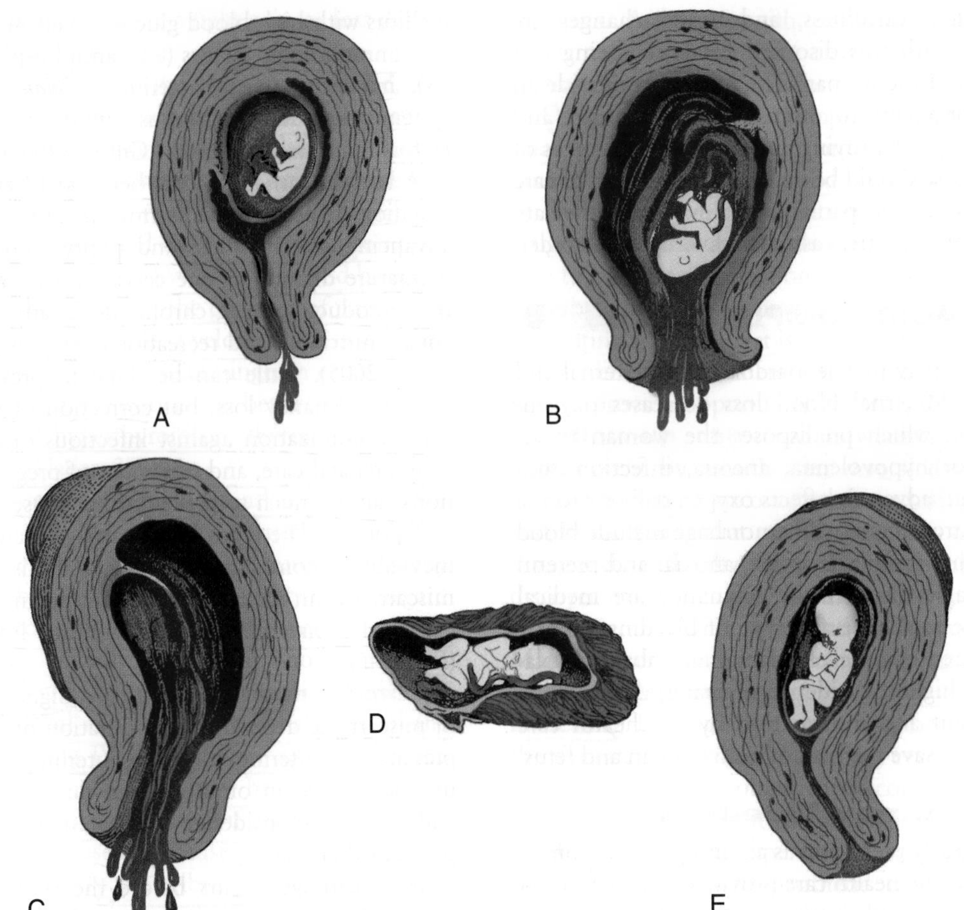

Fig. 21-5 Miscarriage. **A,** Threatened. **B,** Inevitable. **C,** Incomplete. **D,** Complete. **E,** Missed.

There may be no bleeding or cramping, and the cervical os remains closed.

Recurrent early (habitual) miscarriage is three or more spontaneous pregnancy losses before 20 weeks of gestation. The cause is often unclear but is thought to be multifactorial in nature (Pandey, Rani, & Agrawal, 2005). Anticardiolipin antibodies are also being investigated for their impact on pregnancy and as an indicator for recurrent spontaneous abortion (Velayuthaprabhu & Archunan, 2005). Women with a history of recurrent miscarriage are at increased risk for preterm birth, placenta previa, and fetal anomalies in subsequent pregnancies (Cunningham et al., 2005).

Miscarriages can become septic, although this occurrence is uncommon. Symptoms of a septic miscarriage include fever and abdominal tenderness. Vaginal bleeding, which may be slight to heavy, is usually malodorous.

Management

Initial care. Management (see Table 21-6) depends on the classification of the miscarriage and on signs and symptoms. Traditionally, threatened miscarriages have been managed expectantly with supportive care. Repetitive measurement of hCG levels may be performed to evaluate the viability of the pregnancy. In early pregnancy the concentration of this hormone should double every 1.4 to 2.0 days until approximately 60 or 70 days of gestation (Cunningham et al., 2005). If miscarriage is suspected, measurement of two serum quantitative β-hCG levels is performed 48 hours apart. If a normal pregnancy is present, the β-hCG level doubles in this time. A falling or inappropriately rising β-hCG level indicates pregnancy loss.

Follow-up treatment depends on whether the threatened miscarriage progresses to actual miscarriage or symptoms subside and the pregnancy remains intact (see Nursing Process box: Miscarriage). Dilation and curettage (D&C) is a surgical procedure in which the cervix is dilated and a curette is inserted to scrape the uterine walls and remove uterine contents. A D&C is commonly performed to treat inevitable and incomplete miscarriage. The nurse reinforces explanations, answers any questions or concerns, and prepares the woman for surgery.

Dilation and evacuation, performed after 16 weeks of gestation, consists of wide cervical dilation followed by instrumental removal of the uterine contents.

Before either surgical procedure is performed, a full history should be obtained and general and pelvic examinations should be performed. General preoperative and

TABLE 21-6

Assessing Miscarriage and the Usual Management

TYPE OF MISCARRIAGE	AMOUNT OF BLEEDING	UTERINE CRAMPING	PASSAGE OF TISSUE	CERVICAL DILATION	MANAGEMENT
Threatened	Slight, spotting	Mild	No	No	Bed rest (controversial), sedation, and avoidance of stress, sexual stimulation, and orgasm usually recommended. Acetaminophen-based analgesics may be given. Further treatment depends on woman's response to treatment.
Inevitable	Moderate	Mild to severe	No	Yes	Bed rest if no pain, fever or bleeding. If rupture of membranes (ROM), bleeding, pain, or fever is present, then prompt termination of pregnancy is accomplished usually by dilation and curettage.
Incomplete	Heavy, profuse	Severe	Yes	Yes, with tissue in cervix	May or may not require additional cervical dilation before curettage. Suction curettage may be performed.
Complete	Slight	Mild	Yes	No (Cervix has already closed after tissue passed)	No further intervention may be needed if uterine contractions are adequate to prevent hemorrhage and no infection is present. Suction curettage may be performed to ensure no retained fetal or maternal tissue.
Missed	None, spotting	None	No	No	If spontaneous evacuation of the uterus does not occur within 1 month, uterus is emptied by method appropriate to duration of pregnancy. Blood clotting factors are monitored until uterus is empty. Disseminated intravascular coagulation (DIC) and incoagulability of blood with uncontrolled hemorrhage may develop in cases of fetal death after the twelfth week, if products of conception are retained for longer than 5 weeks. May be treated with dilation and curettage or misoprostol (Cytotec) given orally or vaginally.
Septic	Varies, usually malodorous	Varies	Varies	Yes, usually	The uterus is emptied immediately by a method appropriate for the gestational age. Cervical culture and sensitivity studies are performed, and broad-spectrum antibiotic therapy (e.g., ampicillin) is started. Treatment for septic shock is initiated if necessary.
Recurrent (generally defined as three or more consecutive miscarriages)	Varies	Varies	Yes	Yes, usually	Varies; depends on type. Prophylactic cerclage may be performed if premature cervical dilation is the cause. Tests of value include: parental cytogenetic analysis and lupus anticoagulant and anticardiolipin antibodies assays on the woman.

Sources: Cunningham, F., Leveno, K., Bloom, S., Hauth, J., Gilstrap, L., & Wenstrom, K. (2005). *Williams obstetrics* (22nd ed.). New York: McGraw-Hill; Gilbert, E. (2007). *Manual of high risk pregnancy & delivery* (4th ed.). St. Louis: Mosby.

NURSING PROCESS *Miscarriage*

ASSESSMENT
- History:
  - Pregnancy history: last menstrual period, previous pregnancies, pregnancy losses
- Interview:
  - Pain (type, location)
  - Bleeding (quantity, appearance)
  - Allergies
  - Emotional status
- Physical examination:
  - Vital signs
  - Speculum vaginal examination
  - Ultrasonography
- Laboratory tests:
  - β-hCG (pregnancy)
  - Hemoglobin (anemia)
  - White blood cell (infection)

NURSING DIAGNOSES
Possible nursing diagnoses include:
- *Anxiety* or *fear* related to:
  - Unknown outcome and unfamiliarity with medical procedures
- *Deficient fluid volume* related to:
  - Excessive bleeding secondary to miscarriage
- *Acute pain* related to:
  - Uterine contractions
- *Anticipatory grieving* related to:
  - Unexpected pregnancy outcome
- *Situational low self-esteem* related to:
  - Inability to successfully carry a pregnancy to term gestation
- *Risk for infection* related to:
  - Surgical treatment
  - Dilated cervix

EXPECTED OUTCOMES OF CARE
Expected outcomes are that the woman will do the following:
- Discuss the impact of the loss on her and her family.
- Identify and use available support systems.
- Develop no signs and symptoms of physiologic or psychologic complications (e.g., hemorrhage, infection, depression).
- Verbalize relief from pain.

PLAN OF CARE AND INTERVENTIONS
- Physiologic stabilization:
  - Initiate an intravenous line.
  - Initial laboratory tests: blood type and Rh, hemoglobin, hematocrit, indirect Coombs test.
- Administer medications as ordered (antiemetics, uterotonics, antibiotics, analgesics).
- Prepare woman for manual or surgical evacuation of uterus if products of conception have not passed.
- Explain procedures.
- Offer the option of seeing the products of conception.
- Provide education on recognition of grief responses and how to manage these responses.
- Provide discharge teaching (medications, need for rest, normal physical findings, resumption of sexual activity, family planning). (See Teaching Guidelines: Discharge Teaching for the Woman after Early Miscarriage.)
- Refer to support group or counseling as necessary. (See text.)
- Follow up with telephone calls. (See text.)

EVALUATION
Evaluation is based on the predetermined patient-centered outcomes.

postoperative care is appropriate for the woman requiring surgical intervention for miscarriage. Analgesics or anesthesia that are appropriate to the procedure are used.

Outpatient management of first-trimester pregnancy loss may be accomplished with the use of misoprostol intravaginally for up to 2 days (Moodliar, Bagratee, & Moodley, 2005; Zhang et al., 2005). No difference in short-term psychologic outcomes has been noted between expectant and surgical management. If evidence of infection, unstable vital signs, or uncontrollable bleeding exists, a surgical evacuation is performed (Butler, Kelsberg, St. Anna, & Crawford, 2005).

For late incomplete, inevitable, or missed miscarriages (16 to 20 weeks of gestation), prostaglandins may be administered into the amniotic sac or by vaginal suppository to induce or augment labor and cause the products of conception to be expelled. IV oxytocin may also be used.

Nursing care is similar to the care for any woman whose labor is being induced (see Chapter 22). Special care may be needed for management of side effects of prostaglandin, such as nausea, vomiting, and diarrhea. If the products of conception are not passed in entirety, the woman may be prepared for manual or surgical evacuation of the uterus.

After evacuation of the uterus, 10 to 20 units of oxytocin in 1000 ml of IV fluids may be given to prevent hemorrhage. For excessive bleeding after the miscarriage, ergot products such as ergonovine (Methergine) or a prostaglandin derivative such as carboprost tromethamine (Hemabate) may be given to contract the uterus. (See Medication Guide: Drugs Used to Manage Postpartum Hemorrhage, on p. 727 in Chapter 23. Antibiotics are given as necessary. Analgesics, such as antiprostaglandin agents, may decrease discomfort from cramping. Transfusion therapy may be required for shock or anemia. The woman who is Rh negative and is not isoimmunized is given an IM injection of $Rh_o(D)$ immune globulin within 72 hours of the miscarriage (Cunningham et al., 2005).

Psychosocial aspects of care focus on what the pregnancy loss means to the woman and her family. Grief from perinatal loss is complex and unique to each individual (Hutti, 2005). Explanations are provided regarding the nature of the miscarriage, expected procedures, and possible future implications for childbearing.

As with other fetal or neonatal losses, the woman should be offered the option of seeing the products of conception. She may also want to know what the hospital does with the products of conception or whether she needs to make a decision about final disposition of fetal remains.

NURSING ALERT Procedures for disposition of the fetal remains vary from hospital to hospital and state to state. The nurse should know what the usual procedures are in his or her setting.

Follow-up care at home. The woman will likely be discharged home within a few hours after a D&C or as soon as her vital signs are stable, vaginal bleeding remains minimal, and she has recovered from anesthesia. Discharge teaching emphasizes the need for rest. If significant blood loss has occurred, iron supplementation may be ordered. Teaching includes information about normal physical findings, such as cramping, type and amount of bleeding, resumption of sexual activity, and family planning (see Nursing Process box: Miscarriage, p. 646). Frequently the woman and her partner want to know when she may become pregnant again. Discuss with them the importance of completely resolving the loss before attempting another pregnancy (Gilbert, 2007). Follow-up care should assess the woman's physical and emotional recovery. Referrals to local support groups should be provided as needed (see Teaching Guidelines box). Share Pregnancy and Infant Loss Support, Inc. (www.nationalshare.org) is an excellent on-line resource for families that have experienced an early pregnancy loss.

Follow-up telephone calls after a loss are important. The woman may appreciate a telephone call on what would have been her due date. These calls provide opportunities for the woman to ask questions, seek advice, and receive information to help process her grief.

> **TEACHING GUIDELINES**
>
> **Discharge Teaching for the Woman after Early Miscarriage**
>
> - Clean the perineum after each voiding or bowel movement and change perineal pads often.
> - Shower (avoid tub baths) for 2 weeks.
> - Avoid tampon use, douching, and vaginal intercourse for 2 weeks.
> - Notify physician if an elevated temperature or a foul-smelling vaginal discharge develops.
> - Eat foods high in iron and protein to promote tissue repair and red blood cell replacement.
> - Seek assistance from support groups, clergy, or professional counseling as needed.
> - Allow yourself (and your partner) to grieve the loss before becoming pregnant again.
>
> Source: Gilbert, E. (2007). *Manual of high risk pregnancy & delivery* (4th ed.). St. Louis: Mosby.

Recurrent Premature Dilation of the Cervix (Incompetent Cervix)

Another cause of late miscarriage is recurrent **premature dilation of the cervix (incompetent cervix)**, which has traditionally been defined as passive and painless dilation of the cervix during the second trimester. This definition assumes an "all-or-nothing" role for the cervix; it is either "competent" or "incompetent." Current research contends that cervical competence is variable and exists as a continuum that is determined in part by cervical length. Other related causative factors include composition of the cervical tissue and the individual circumstances associated with the pregnancy in terms of maternal stress and lifestyle. Iams (2009) refers to this condition as *cervical insufficiency.*

Etiology

Etiologic factors include a history of previous cervical trauma such as lacerations during childbirth, excessive cervical dilation for curettage or biopsy, or ingestion of diethylstilbestrol (DES) by the woman's mother while pregnant with the woman. Because DES has not been used since the early 1970s, however, this risk factor should soon be only of historic interest (Ludmir & Owen, 2007). Multiple gestation alone does not produce cervical incompetency or justify prophylactic cervical cerclage (Ludmir & Owen). Other causes are a congenitally short cervix and cervical or uterine anomalies.

A short cervix = cervical competence

Diagnosis

Reduced cervical competence is a clinical diagnosis, based on history. Short labors, recurring loss of the pregnancy at progressively earlier gestational ages, advanced cervical dilation at the time of first presentation, and a history of prior cervical surgery or trauma are characteristics that suggest reduced cervical competence (Iams, 2009). Ultrasound examination during pregnancy is used to diagnose this condition objectively. A short cervix (less than 25 mm in length) is indicative of reduced cervical competence. Often, but not always, the short cervix is accompanied by **cervical funneling** (beaking) or effacement of the internal cervical os (Iams; Ludmir & Owen, 2007; Rust, Atlas, Kimmel, Roberts, & Hess, 2005).

Management

Medical management consists of bed rest, pessaries, antibiotics, antiinflammatory drugs, and progesterone supplementation (Iams, 2009). Surgical management, with placement of a cervical **cerclage,** may be chosen instead. During pregnancy the McDonald technique is often the procedure of choice. In this procedure a band of homologous fascia or nonabsorbable ribbon (Mersilene polyester fiber mesh) may be placed around the cervix beneath the mucosa to constrict the internal os of the cervix (Fig. 21-6)

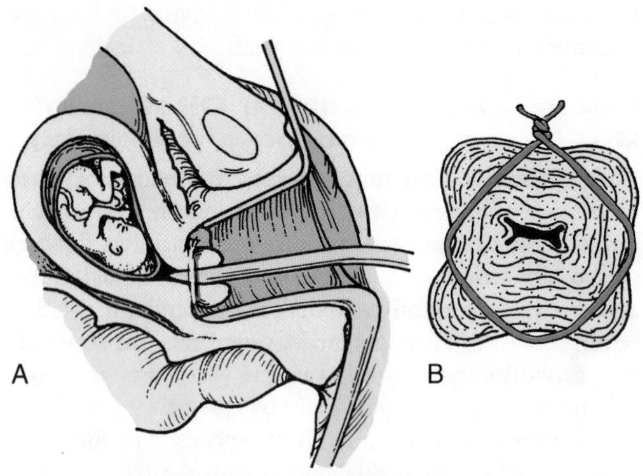

Fig. 21-6 **A,** Cerclage correction of premature dilation of the cervical os. **B,** Cross-sectional view of closed internal os.

(Cunningham et al., 2005). A cerclage procedure can be classified according to time or whether it is elective (prophylactic), urgent, or emergent (Rust & Roberts, 2005).

A prophylactic cerclage is usually placed at 11 to 15 weeks of gestation. The cerclage is electively removed (usually an office or a clinic procedure) when the woman reaches 37 weeks of gestation, or it may be left in place until spontaneous labor begins. Occasionally the cerclage is left in place and a cesarean birth performed. The best treatment for reduced cervical competence is uncertain at this time. Current research results indicate that selective cerclage placement during pregnancy based on repeated ultrasound examination of the cervix may produce pregnancy outcomes that are just as good as those obtained after prophylactic cerclage placement. Ultrasound surveillance begins at 15 to 16 weeks of gestation. Cerclage placement is offered if the cervical length falls to less than 20 to 25 mm before 23 to 24 weeks (Iams, 2009). Risks of the procedure include premature rupture of membranes (PROM), preterm labor, and chorioamnionitis. Although no consensus has been reached, 24 weeks is often used as the upper gestational age limit for cerclage placement (Iams).

The nurse assesses the woman's feelings about her pregnancy and her understanding of reduced cervical competence. Evaluating the woman's support systems is also important. Because the diagnosis of reduced cervical competence is usually not made until the woman has lost one or more pregnancies, she may feel guilty or to blame for this impending loss. Assessing for previous reactions to stresses and appropriateness of coping responses is therefore important. The woman needs the support of her health care providers, as well as that of her family.

If a cerclage is performed, the nurse monitors the woman postoperatively for contractions, PROM, and signs of infection. Discharge teaching focuses on continued monitoring of these aspects at home.

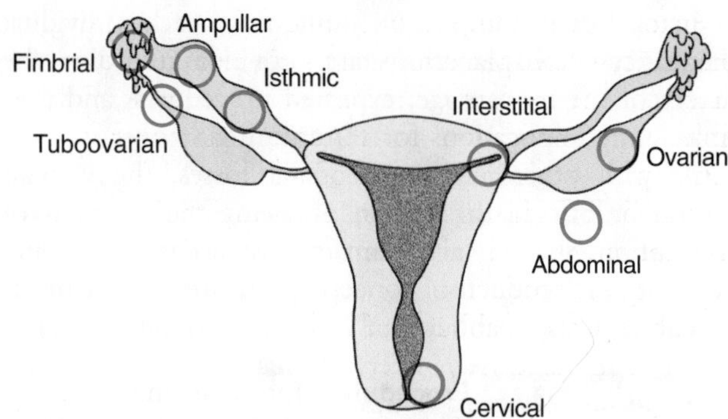

Fig. 21-7 Sites of implantation of ectopic pregnancies. Order of frequency of occurrence is ampulla, isthmus, interstitium, fimbria, tuboovarian ligament, ovary, abdominal cavity, and cervix (external os).

Follow-up care at home

The woman will likely be on bedrest for a least a few days immediately following cerclage placement. She will also probably be advised to avoid sexual intercourse until after a postoperative check. Thereafter, decisions about physical activity and intercourse are individualized, based on the status of the woman's cervix, as determined by digital and ultrasound examination (Ludmir & Owen, 2007). The woman must understand the importance of initial activity restriction at home and the need for close observation and supervision. Tocolytic medications may be prescribed to prevent uterine contractions and further dilation of the cervix. If so, the woman must be instructed on the expected response and possible side effects. Additional instruction includes the need to watch for and report signs of preterm labor, ROM, and infection. Finally, the woman should know the signs that would warrant an immediate return to the hospital, including strong contractions less than 5 minutes apart, ROM, severe perineal pressure, and an urge to push. If management is unsuccessful and the fetus is born before viability, appropriate grief support should be provided. If the fetus is born prematurely, appropriate anticipatory guidance and support will be necessary.

Ectopic Pregnancy

Incidence and etiology

An **ectopic pregnancy** is one in which the fertilized ovum is implanted outside the uterine cavity (Fig. 21-7). The incidence of ectopic pregnancy in the general population is 2% (Gilbert, 2007). Ectopic pregnancies are often called *tubal pregnancies* because approximately 95% are located in the fallopian tube. Although they are much less common, however, ectopic pregnancies can also occur in the abdominal cavity, on an ovary, or on the cervix. Of all tubal ectopic pregnancies, more than half (approximately 55%) are located in the ampulla, or largest portion of the tube (Gilbert, 2007).

Ectopic pregnancy is responsible for 10% to 15% of all pregnancy-related maternal deaths (Gilbert, 2007). It is the most common cause of maternal mortality in the first trimester (Cunningham et al., 2005). Moreover, ectopic pregnancy is a leading cause of infertility. Women have increased difficulty conceiving after an ectopic pregnancy and are at an increased risk of developing a subsequent ectopic pregnancy.

The reported incidence of ectopic pregnancy is rising. Some of the increase is likely because of improved diagnostic techniques, such as more sensitive β-hCG measurement and transvaginal ultrasound, resulting in the identification of more cases. Other causes for the rise include an increased incidence of sexually transmitted tubal infection and damage, popularity of contraceptive methods that predispose failures to be ectopic (e.g., the intrauterine device [IUD]), use of tubal sterilization methods that increase the chance of ectopic pregnancy, increasing use of assisted reproductive techniques, and increased use of tubal surgery (Cunningham et al., 2005; Gilbert, 2007).

Ectopic pregnancy is classified according to site of implantation (e.g., tubal, ovarian, or abdominal). The uterus is the only organ capable of containing and sustaining a term pregnancy. Only approximately 5% of abdominal pregnancies reach viability. Surgery to remove the embryo or fetus is usually performed as soon as an abdominal pregnancy is identified, however, because of the high risk for hemorrhage at any time during the pregnancy (Gilbert, 2007). The risk for fetal deformity in an abdominal pregnancy is also high as a result of pressure deformities caused by oligohydramnios. The most common problems include facial or cranial asymmetry, various joint deformities, limb deficiency, and central nervous system anomalies (Fig. 21-8) (Cunningham et al., 2005; Gilbert).

Clinical manifestations

Most cases of ectopic (tubal) pregnancy are diagnosed before rupture based on the three most classic symptoms: (1) abdominal pain, (2) delayed menses, and (3) abnormal vaginal bleeding (spotting) that occurs approximately 6 to 8 weeks after the last normal menstrual period (Gilbert, 2007). Abdominal pain occurs in almost every case. It usually begins as a dull, lower quadrant pain on one side. The discomfort can progress from a dull pain to a colicky pain when the tube stretches, to sharp, stabbing pain (Cunningham et al., 2005; Gilbert). It progresses to a diffuse, constant, severe pain that is generalized throughout the lower abdomen (Gilbert). Up to 90% of women with an ectopic pregnancy report a period that is delayed 1 to 2 weeks or is lighter than usual, or an irregular period. Mild to moderate dark red or brown intermittent vaginal bleeding occurs in up to 80% of women.

If the ectopic pregnancy is not diagnosed until after rupture has occurred, referred shoulder pain may be present in addition to generalized, one-sided, or deep lower quadrant acute abdominal pain. Referred shoulder pain results from diaphragmatic irritation caused by blood in the peritoneal cavity. The woman may exhibit signs of shock, such as faintness and dizziness, related to the amount of bleeding in the abdominal cavity and not necessarily related to obvious vaginal bleeding. An ecchymotic blueness around the umbilicus (Cullen sign), indicating hematoperitoneum, may also develop in an undiagnosed, ruptured intraabdominal ectopic pregnancy.

Tubal Pregnancy Management

The differential diagnosis of ectopic pregnancy involves consideration of numerous disorders that share many signs and symptoms. Many of these women come into the emergency department experiencing first-trimester bleeding or pain. Miscarriage, ruptured corpus luteum cyst, appendicitis, salpingitis, ovarian cysts, torsion of the ovary, and urinary tract infection are all possible diagnoses. The key to early detection of ectopic pregnancy is having a high index of suspicion for this condition. *Every* woman with abdominal pain, vaginal spotting or bleeding, and a positive pregnancy test should undergo screening for ectopic pregnancy.

The most important screening tools for ectopic pregnancy are serial quantitative β-hCG levels and transvaginal ultrasound. Laboratory screening includes determination of serum progesterone and β-hCG levels. If either of these values is lower than would be expected for a normal pregnancy, the woman is asked to return within 48 hours

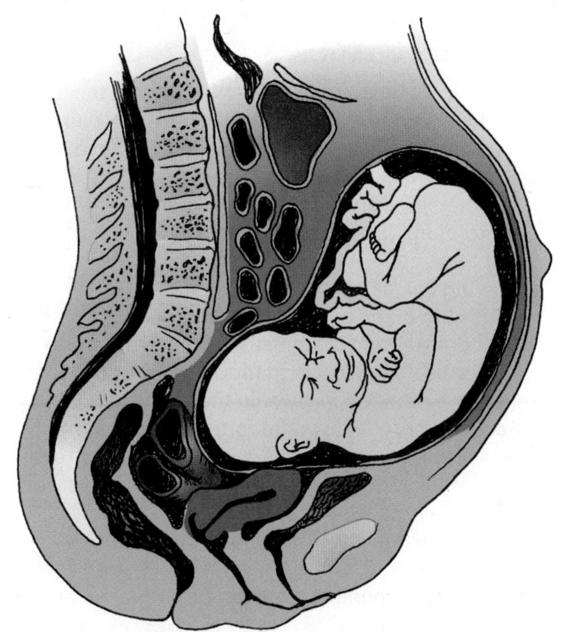

Fig. 21-8 Ectopic pregnancy, abdominal.

for serial measurements. Transvaginal ultrasonography is performed to confirm intrauterine or tubal pregnancy (Farquhar, 2005). An intrauterine sac should be visible by abdominal ultrasound at 5 to 6 menstrual weeks or 28 days after ovulation. A transvaginal ultrasound can identify an intrauterine gestation as early as 1 week after a missed period. When the β-hCG level is greater than 1000 milli-international units/ml a gestational sac is seen one half of the time (Cunningham et al., 2005).

The woman should also be assessed for the presence of active bleeding, which is associated with tubal rupture. If internal bleeding is present, assessment may reveal vertigo, shoulder pain, hypotension, and tachycardia. A vaginal examination should be performed only once, and then with great caution. Approximately 20% of women with a tubal pregnancy have a palpable mass on examination. Rupturing the mass is possible during a bimanual examination; thus a gentle touch is critical.

Immediate care

Surgical management. Surgical management depends on the location and cause of the ectopic pregnancy, the extent of tissue involvement, and the woman's desires regarding future fertility. One option is removal of the entire tube (salpingectomy). If the tube has not ruptured and the woman desires future fertility, salpingostomy may be performed instead. In this procedure an incision is made over the pregnancy site in the tube and the products of conception are gently and very carefully removed. The incision is not sutured but left to close by secondary intention instead, given that this method results in less scarring.

Critical Thinking/Clinical Decision Making

Ectopic Pregnancy

Kendra is a 19-year-old G1 P0 who enters the emergency department with lower abdominal pain and vaginal spotting. She reports that her last menstrual period was 6 weeks ago. A pregnancy test is positive.

1. Does the nurse have sufficient evidence at this time to diagnose ectopic pregnancy?
2. What assumptions can be made about the following issues?
   a. Possible diagnoses for Kendra
   b. Laboratory and diagnostic tests necessary to diagnose ectopic pregnancy
   c. If her examination reveals that Kendra has an ectopic pregnancy, criteria that must be met to treat this condition medically with methotrexate
3. What implications and priorities for nursing care can be drawn at this time?
4. Does the evidence objectively support your conclusion?
5. Do alternative perspectives to your conclusion exist?

If surgery is planned, general preoperative and postoperative care is appropriate for the woman with an ectopic pregnancy. Before surgery, vital signs (pulse, respirations, and BP) are assessed every 15 minutes or as needed, according to the severity of the bleeding and the woman's condition. Preoperative laboratory tests include determination of blood type and Rh factor, complete blood cell count, and serum quantitative β-hCG level. Ultrasonography is used to confirm an extrauterine pregnancy. Blood replacement may be necessary. The nurse verifies the woman's Rh and antibody status and administers $Rh_o(D)$ immune globulin if appropriate.

Medical management. Medical management involves giving methotrexate to dissolve the tubal pregnancy. Methotrexate is an antimetabolite and folic acid antagonist that destroys rapidly dividing cells. Hemodynamically stable women with ectopic pregnancies are eligible for methotrexate therapy if the mass is unruptured and measures less than 3.5 cm in diameter by ultrasound, if no fetal cardiac activity is noted on ultrasound, if the serum β-hCG level is less than 5000 international units/L, and if the woman is willing to comply with posttreatment monitoring (Cunningham et al., 2005; Murray, Baakdah, Bardell, & Tulandi, 2005). Methotrexate therapy avoids surgery and is a safe, effective, and cost-effective way of managing many cases of tubal pregnancy. The woman is informed of how the medication works, possible side effects, whom to call if she has concerns or if problems develop, and the importance of follow-up care (Box 21-5).

NURSING ALERT The woman on methotrexate therapy who drinks alcohol and takes vitamins containing folic acid (such as prenatal vitamins) increases her risk of having side effects of the drug or exacerbating the ectopic rupture.

Follow-up care. The woman and her family should be encouraged to share their feelings and concerns related to the loss. Future fertility should be discussed. A contraceptive method should be used for at least three menstrual cycles to allow time for the woman's body to heal (Gilbert, 2007). Every woman who has been diagnosed with an ectopic pregnancy should be told to contact her health care provider as soon as she suspects that she might be pregnant because of the increased risk for recurrent ectopic pregnancy. These women may need referral to grief or infertility support groups. In addition to the loss of the current pregnancy, they are faced with the possibility of future pregnancy losses or infertility.

Hydatidiform Mole (Molar Pregnancy)

Hydatidiform mole (molar pregnancy), is a benign proliferative growth of the placental trophoblast in which the chorionic villi develop into edematous, cystic, avascular transparent vesicles that hang in a grapelike cluster.

BOX 21-5

Nursing Considerations for Women Undergoing Methotrexate Treatment for Ectopic Pregnancy

ADMINISTRATION

- Obtain woman's current height and weight.
- Check to make sure laboratory and diagnostic tests have been completed, including:
  - Complete blood cell count and blood type and Rh-antibody status
  - Liver and renal function tests
  - Serum β-hCG levels (should be <5000 mIU/L)
  - Transvaginal ultrasound confirming size of mass and absence of fetal cardiac activity
- Administer methotrexate 50 mg/m^2 intramuscularly (IM).
- Administer $Rh_o(D)$ immune globulin (150 mcg to 300 mcg IM as ordered if woman has Rh-negative blood).

PATIENT AND FAMILY TEACHING

- Review how methotrexate works.
- Inform the woman of possible side effects—gas pain, stomatitis and conjunctivitis are common; rare effects include pleuritis, gastritis, dermatitis, alopecia, enteritis, increased liver enzymes, and bone marrow suppression.
- Advise the woman to discontinue folic acid supplements.
- Advise the woman to avoid "gas forming" foods.
- Advise the woman to avoid sun exposure because the drug will make her more photosensitive.
- Advise the woman to refrain from strenuous activities.
- Advise the woman to avoid putting anything in her vagina—no tampons, douches, or vaginal intercourse.
- Advise the woman to report to her health care provider immediately if she has severe abdominal pain that may be a sign of impending or actual rupture.

FOLLOW-UP

- Inform the woman to return to the clinic or office as instructed by her health care provider for measurement of β-hCG level.
- If β-hCG level does not drop appropriately, a second dose of methotrexate may be necessary.
- Advise the woman that she will need to return to the clinic or office for weekly measurements of β-hCG until the level is <15 mIU/L. Weekly followup visits may be required for several months until the desired β-hCG level is reached.

Sources: Gilbert, E. (2007). *Manual of high risk pregnancy & delivery* (4th ed.). St. Louis: Mosby; Murray, H., Baakdah, H., Bardell, T., & Tulandi, T. (2005). Diagnosis and treatment of ectopic pregnancy. *Canadian Medical Association Journal, 173*(8), 905–912.

Hydatidiform mole is a gestational trophoblastic disease. Gestational trophoblastic disease (GTD) is a spectrum of pregnancy-related trophoblastic proliferative disorders without a viable fetus. In addition to hydatidiform mole, GTD includes gestational trophoblastic neoplasia (GTN). GTN refers to persistent trophoblastic tissue that is presumed to be malignant (Gilbert, 2007). Once almost invariably fatal, because of early diagnosis and treatment, GTN is now the most successfully treated gynecologic cancer (Cohn, Ramaswamy, & Blum, 2009).

Incidence and etiology

Hydatidiform mole occurs in 1 in 1000 pregnancies in the United States (Cohn et al., 2009). The cause is unknown, although it may be related to an ovular defect or a nutritional deficiency. Women at increased risk for hydatidiform mole formation are those who have had ovulation stimulation with clomiphene (Clomid) and those who are in their early teens or over 40 years of age. Other risk factors include history of miscarriage and nutritional factors (e.g., deficient intake of carotene and animal fats) (Bess & Wood, 2006; Cohn et al., 2009).

Types

A hydatidiform mole may be further categorized as a complete or partial mole. The complete mole results from fertilization of an egg in which the nucleus has been lost or inactivated (Fig. 21-9, *A*). The nucleus of a sperm (23,X) duplicates itself (resulting in the diploid number 46,XX) because the ovum has no genetic material or the material is inactive. The mole resembles a bunch of white grapes (Fig. 21-9, *B*). The hydropic (fluid-filled) vesicles grow rapidly, causing the uterus to be larger than expected for the duration of the pregnancy. Usually the complete mole contains no fetus, placenta, amniotic membranes, or fluid. Maternal blood has no placenta to receive it; therefore hemorrhage into the uterine cavity and vaginal bleeding occur. In approximately 20% of women with a complete mole, choriocarcinoma or GTN occurs (Cunningham et al., 2005).

For a partial mole, chromosomal studies often show a karyotype of 69,XXY; 69,XXX; or 69,XYY. This arrangement occurs as a result of two sperm fertilizing an apparently normal ovum (Fig. 21-10). Partial moles often have embryonic or fetal parts and an amniotic sac. Congenital anomalies are usually present (Cunningham et al., 2005). The potential for malignant transformation is 5% to 10% (Cunningham et al.).

Clinical manifestations

In the early stages the clinical manifestations of a complete hydatidiform mole cannot be distinguished from those of normal pregnancy. Later, vaginal bleeding occurs in almost 95% of cases. The vaginal discharge may be dark brown (resembling prune juice) or bright red and either scant or profuse. It may continue for only a few days or intermittently for weeks. Early in pregnancy the uterus in approximately one half of affected women is significantly larger than expected from menstrual dates. The percentage of women with an excessively enlarged uterus increases as length of time since the last menstrual period

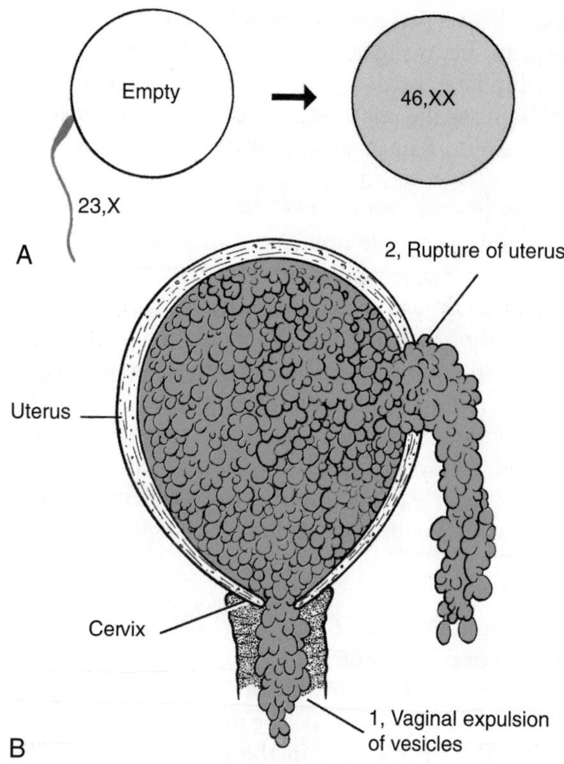

Fig. 21-9 **A,** Chromosomal origin of complete mole. Single sperm (color) fertilizes an "empty" ovum. Reduplication of sperm's 23,X set gives completely homozygous diploid 46,XX. Similar process follows fertilization of empty ovum by two sperm with two independently drawn sets of 23,X or 23,Y; both karyotypes of 46,XX and 46,XY can therefore result. **B,** Uterine rupture with hydatidiform mole. *1,* Evacuation of mole through cervix. *2,* Rupture of uterus and spillage of mole into peritoneal cavity (rare).

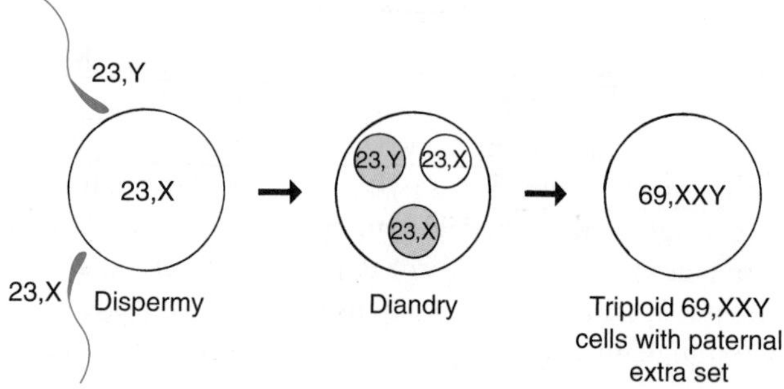

Fig. 21-10 Chromosomal origin of triploid partial mole. Normal ovum with 23,X haploid set is fertilized by two sperms to give a total of 69 chromosomes. Sex configuration of XXY, XXX, or XYY is possible.

increases. Approximately 25% of affected women have a uterus smaller than would be expected from menstrual dates.

Anemia from blood loss, excessive nausea and vomiting (hyperemesis gravidarum), and abdominal cramps caused by uterine distention are relatively common findings. Women may also pass vesicles from the uterus, which are frequently avascular edematous villi. Preeclampsia occurs in approximately 70% of women with large, rapidly growing hydatidiform moles and occurs earlier than usual in the pregnancy. If preeclampsia is diagnosed before 24 weeks of gestation, hydatidiform mole should be suspected and ruled out. Hyperthyroidism is another serious complication of hydatidiform mole. Usually treatment of the hydatidiform mole restores thyroid function to normal. Partial moles cause few of these symptoms and may be mistaken for an incomplete or missed miscarriage (Cohn et al., 2009; Nader, 2009; Roberts & Funai, 2009).

Diagnosis

Transvaginal ultrasound and serum hCG levels are used for diagnosis. Transvaginal ultrasound is the most accurate tool for diagnosing a hydatidiform mole. A characteristic pattern of multiple diffuse intrauterine masses, often called a *snowstorm pattern,* is seen in place of, or along with, an embryo or a fetus. The trophoblastic tissue secretes the hCG hormone. In a molar pregnancy, hCG levels are persistently high or rising beyond 10 to 12 weeks of gestation, the time they would begin to decline in a normal pregnancy (Gilbert, 2007).

Management

Although most moles abort spontaneously, suction curettage offers a safe, rapid, and effective method of evacuating a hydatidiform mole if necessary (Cunningham et al., 2005; Gilbert, 2007). Induction of labor with oxytocic agents or prostaglandins is not recommended because of the increased risk of embolization of trophoblastic tissue (Gilbert). Administration of Rh_o(D) immune globulin to women who are Rh negative is necessary to prevent isoimmunization.

The nurse provides the woman and her family with information about the disease process, the necessity for a long course of follow-up, and the possible consequences of the disease. The nurse helps the woman and her family cope with the pregnancy loss and recognize that the pregnancy was not normal. In addition, the woman and her family are encouraged to express their feelings, and information is provided about support groups or counseling resources as needed. Explanations about the importance of postponing a subsequent pregnancy and contraceptive counseling are provided to emphasize the need for consistent and reliable use of the method chosen.

NURSING ALERT To avoid confusion with signs of pregnancy, pregnancy should be avoided for 6 months to 1 year. Any contraceptive method except an IUD is acceptable. Oral contraceptives are preferred because they are highly effective.

Follow-up care

Follow-up management includes frequent physical and pelvic examinations along with biweekly measurements of β-hCG level until the level decreases to normal and remains normal for 3 weeks. Monthly measurements are taken for 6 months and then every 2 months for a total of 1 year. A rising titer and an enlarging uterus may indicate choriocarcinoma (malignant GTD). Women with a complete hydatidiform molar pregnancy are at a 15% to 28% risk of requiring further management with chemotherapy for persistent trophoblastic disease (Wolfberg, Berkowitz, Goldstein, Feltmate, & Lieberman, 2005). Referral to community support resources may be needed. Internet resources such as Share: Pregnancy and Infant Loss Support, Inc., at www.nationalshare.org and the International Society for the Study of Trophoblastic Disease at www.isstd.org may also be useful.

Late Pregnancy Bleeding

The major causes of bleeding in late pregnancy are placenta previa and premature separation of the placenta (abruptio placentae or placental abruption). Expedient assessment for and diagnosis of the cause of bleeding is essential to reduce risk of maternal and perinatal morbidity and mortality (Table 21-7).

Placenta previa = painless

Because of advances in ultrasonography, especially transvaginal ultrasound, and an increased understanding of the changing relationship between the placenta and the internal cervical os as pregnancy progresses, definitions

Nursing Care Plan: Placenta Previa

TABLE 21-7

Summary of Findings: Abruptio Placentae and Placenta Previa

	ABRUPTIO PLACENTAE			
	GRADE 1 MILD SEPARATION (10%-20%)	GRADE 2 MODERATE SEPARATION (20%-50%)	GRADE 3 SEVERE SEPARATION (>50%)	PLACENTA PREVIA
Bleeding, external, vaginal	Minimal	Absent to moderate	Absent to moderate	Minimal to severe and life-threatening
Total amount of blood loss	<500 ml	1000-1500 ml	>1500 ml	Varies
Color of blood	Dark red	Dark red	Dark red	Bright red
Shock	Rare; none	Mild shock	Common, often sudden, profound	Uncommon
Coagulopathy	Rare, none	Occasional DIC	Frequent DIC	None
Uterine tonicity	Normal	Increased, may be localized to one region or diffuse over uterus, uterus fails to relax between contractions	Tetanic, persistent uterine contractions, boardlike uterus	Normal
Tenderness (pain)	Usually absent	Present	Agonizing, unremitting uterine pain	Absent
ULTRASONOGRAPHIC FINDINGS				
Location of placenta	Normal, upper uterine segment	Normal, upper uterine segment	Normal, upper uterine segment	Abnormal, lower uterine segment
Station of presenting part	Variable to engaged	Variable to engaged	Variable to engaged	High, not engaged
Fetal position	Usual distribution*	Usual distribution*	Usual distribution*	Commonly transverse, breech, or oblique
Gestational or chronic hypertension	Usual distribution*	Commonly present	Commonly present	Usual distribution*
Fetal effects	Normal fetal heart rate pattern	Abnormal fetal heart rate pattern	Abnormal fetal heart rate pattern; fetal death can occur	Normal fetal heart rate pattern

*Usual distribution refers to the usual variations of incidence seen when there is no concurrent problem.
DIC, Disseminated intravascular coagulation.

and classifications of placental previa have recently changed. In **placenta previa,** the placenta is implanted in the lower uterine segment such that it completely or partially covers the cervix or is close enough to the cervix to cause bleeding when the cervix dilates or the lower uterine segment effaces (Fig. 21-11) (Hull & Resnik, 2009). When transvaginal ultrasound is used, the placenta is classified as a *complete placenta previa* if it totally covers the internal cervical os. In a *marginal placenta previa* the edge of the placenta is seen on transvaginal ultrasound to be 2.5 cm or closer to the internal cervical os. When the exact relationship of the placenta to the internal cervical os has not been determined or in the case of apparent placenta previa in the second trimester, the term *low-lying placenta* is used (Hull & Resnik).

Incidence and etiology. Placenta previa affects approximately 1 in 200 pregnancies at term. Some evidence suggests that the incidence of placenta previa is increasing, perhaps as a result of the increasing cesarean birth rate. In addition to a history of previous cesarean birth, other risk factors for placenta previa include advanced maternal age (>35-40 years of age), multiparity, history of prior suction curettage, and smoking (Hull & Resnik, 2009). Cigarette smoking leads to a decrease in uteroplacental oxygenation and thus a need for increased placental surface area. Placenta previa is more likely to occur in women with multiple gestations because of the larger placental area associated with these pregnancies. Women who had placenta previa in a previous pregnancy are more likely than others to develop the problem in a subsequent pregnancy, perhaps as a result of a genetic predisposition. Previous cesarean birth and curettage in the past for miscarriage or induced abortion are risk factors for placenta previa because both result in endometrial damage and uterine scarring (Francois & Foley, 2007; Hull & Resnik).

Clinical manifestations. Placenta previa is typically characterized by painless, bright-red vaginal bleeding during the second or third trimester. In the past, placenta previa was usually diagnosed after an episode of bleeding. Currently, however, most cases are diagnosed by ultrasound before significant vaginal bleeding occurs (Francois & Foley, 2007). This bleeding is associated with the disruption of placental blood vessels that occurs with stretching and thinning of the lower uterine segment (Francois & Foley). The initial bleeding is usually a small amount and stops as clots form; however, it can recur at any time (Gilbert, 2007).

Vital signs may be normal, even with heavy blood loss, because a pregnant woman can lose up to 40% of her blood volume without showing signs of shock. Clinical presentation and decreasing urinary output may be better indicators of acute blood loss than vital signs alone. The FHR is reassuring unless a major detachment of the placenta occurs.

Abdominal examination usually reveals a soft, relaxed, nontender uterus with normal tone. The presenting part of the fetus usually remains high because the placenta occupies the lower uterine segment. Thus the fundal height is often greater than expected for gestational age. Because of the abnormally located placenta, fetal malpresentation (breech and transverse or oblique lie) is common.

Maternal and fetal outcomes. Complications associated with placenta previa include PROM, preterm labor and birth, surgery-related trauma to structures adjacent to the uterus, anesthesia complications, blood transfusion reactions, overinfusion of fluids, abnormal placental attachments, postpartum hemorrhage, anemia, thrombophlebitis, and infection (Cunningham et al., 2005).

The greatest risk of fetal death is caused by preterm birth. Other fetal risks include malpresentation and fetal anemia (Gilbert, 2007). Infants who are small for gestational age or have IUGR have been associated with placenta previa. This association may be related to poor placental exchange or hypovolemia resulting from maternal blood loss and maternal anemia (Gilbert).

Diagnosis. All women with painless vaginal bleeding after 20 weeks of gestation should be assumed to have a placenta previa until proven otherwise. A transabdominal ultrasound examination should be performed initially followed by a transvaginal scan, unless the transabdominal ultrasound clearly shows that the placenta is not located

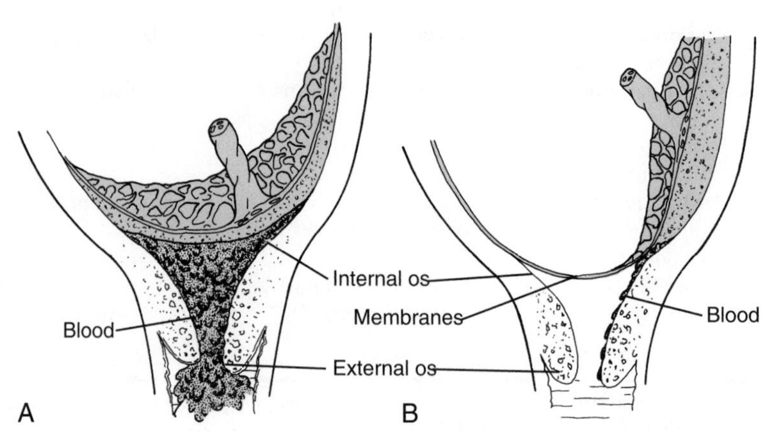

Fig. 21-11 Types of placenta previa. **A,** Complete. **B,** Marginal.

in the lower uterine segment. A transvaginal ultrasound is better than a transabdominal scan for accurately determining placental location (Hull & Resnik, 2009). If ultrasonographic scanning reveals a normally implanted placenta, a speculum examination may be performed to rule out local causes of bleeding (e.g., cervicitis, polyps, carcinoma of the cervix), and a coagulation profile is obtained to rule out other causes of bleeding.

Management

Once placenta previa has been diagnosed, a management plan is developed. The woman will be managed either expectantly or actively, depending on the gestational age, amount of bleeding, and fetal condition (see Nursing Process box: Placenta Previa.)

Expectant management. Expectant management (observation and bed rest) is implemented if the fetus is at less than 36 weeks of gestation and has a reassuring FHR tracing, the bleeding is mild (<250 ml) and stops, and the patient is not in labor. The purpose of expectant management is to allow the fetus time to mature (Gilbert, 2007). The woman will initially be hospitalized in a labor and birth unit for continuous FHR and contraction monitoring. Large-bore intravenous access should be initiated immediately. Initial laboratory tests include hemoglobin, hematocrit, platelet count, and coagulation studies. A "type and screen" blood sample should be maintained at all times in the blood bank to allow for immediate crossmatch of blood component therapy if necessary. If the woman is at less than 34 weeks of gestation, antenatal corticosteroids should be administered (Francois & Foley, 2007; Gilbert).

If the bleeding stops, the woman will most likely be placed on bedrest with bathroom privileges and limited

NURSING PROCESS *Placenta Previa*

ASSESSMENT

- History:
  - Pregnancy (gravidity, parity, estimated date of birth)
- Interview:
  - General status
  - Bleeding (quantity, precipitating event, associated pain)
- Physical examination:
  - Vital signs
  - Fetal status
  - Abdominal exam (soft, relaxed, nontender, with normal tone)
- Laboratory tests:
  - Complete blood cell count
  - Blood type and Rh factor
  - Coagulation profile
  - Possible type and cross match
- Abdominal or transvaginal ultrasound or both

NURSING DIAGNOSES

Possible nursing diagnoses include:

- *Decreased cardiac output* related to:
  - Excessive blood loss secondary to placenta previa
- *Deficient fluid volume* related to:
  - Excessive blood loss secondary to placenta previa
- *Ineffective peripheral tissue perfusion* related to:
  - Hypovolemia and shunting of blood to central circulation
- *Anxiety* or *fear* related to:
  - Maternal condition and pregnancy outcome
- *Anticipatory grieving* related to:
  - Actual or perceived threat to self, pregnancy, or infant

EXPECTED OUTCOMES OF CARE

Expected outcomes are that the woman will do the following:

- Verbalize understanding of her condition and its management.
- Identify and use available support systems.
- Demonstrate compliance with prescribed activity limitations.
- Develop no complications related to bleeding.
- Give birth to a healthy term infant.

PLAN OF CARE AND INTERVENTIONS: EXPECTANT MANAGEMENT

- Place on bedrest with bathroom privileges and limited activity.
- Monitor maternal vital signs.
- Monitor blood loss:
  - Estimate and record amount of blood on disposable pads, perineal pads, and bed linens.
  - Obtain serial hematocrit or hemoglobin levels.
- Maintain a "type and screen" sample in the hospital blood bank at all times.
- Monitor fetal condition: Perform a nonstress test or biophysical profile once or twice per week.
- Place on "pelvic rest."
  - No vaginal examinations!
  - No douching.
  - No vaginal intercourse.
- Provide emotional support to the woman and her family.
- Administer medications as ordered.
- Provide diversionary activities.
- Notify hospital chaplain or other support services as desired by the woman.
- Be prepared for an emergency cesarean birth at any time.

EVALUATION

The expected outcomes of care are used to evaluate the care for the woman with placenta previa.

activity (able to use the bathroom, shower, and move around her hospital room for 15 to 30 minutes at a time, four times a day). No vaginal or rectal examinations are performed, and the woman is placed on "pelvic rest" (nothing in the vagina). Ultrasonographic examinations may be performed every 2 to 3 weeks. Fetal surveillance may include an NST or BPP once or twice weekly. Bleeding is assessed by checking the amount of blood on perineal pads, bed pads, and linens. Serial laboratory values are evaluated for decreasing hemoglobin and hematocrit levels and changes in coagulation values. The woman should also be monitored for signs of preterm labor. Magnesium sulfate can be given for tocolysis if uterine contractions are identified (Francois & Foley, 2007; Gilbert, 2007).

The woman with placenta previa should always be considered a potential emergency because massive blood loss with resulting hypovolemic shock can occur quickly if bleeding resumes. The possibility always exists that she will require an emergency cesarean for birth. Placenta previa in a preterm gestation may be an indication for transfer to a tertiary-care perinatal center, given that a neonatal intensive care unit may be necessary for care of the preterm neonate. Also, because many community hospitals are not prepared to perform emergency surgery 24 hours per day, 7 days per week, transfer to a tertiary-care center may be necessary to ensure constant access to cesarean birth.

Home care. Occasionally, women with placenta previa are discharged from the hospital before giving birth to be managed at home. The woman's condition should be stable, and she should have experienced no vaginal bleeding for at least 48 hours before discharge (Hull & Resnik, 2009). A candidate for home care must meet other strict criteria as well. She should be able and willing to comply with activity restrictions (bedrest with bathroom privileges and pelvic rest), have access to a telephone, close supervision by family or friends in the home, and constant access to transportation. If bleeding resumes, she will need to return to the hospital immediately. She must also be able to keep all appointments for fetal testing, laboratory assessments, and prenatal care. Visits by a perinatal home care nurse may be arranged.

If hospitalization or home care with activity restriction is prolonged, the woman may have concerns about her work- or family-related responsibilities or may become bored with inactivity. She should be encouraged to participate in her own care and decisions about care as much as possible. Provision of diversionary activities or encouragement to participate in activities she enjoys and can perform during bed rest is needed. Participation in a support group made up of other women on bed rest while hospitalized or online if at home may be a helpful coping mechanism. (See Patient Instructions for Self-Management box: Coping with Activity Restrictions, p. 634).

Active management. If the woman is at or beyond 36 weeks of gestation or bleeding is excessive or persistent, immediate cesarean birth is indicated (Hull & Resnik, 2009). Expectant management will be terminated as soon as the fetus is mature, if excessive bleeding develops, active labor begins, or any other obstetric reason to terminate the pregnancy (e.g., chorioamnionitis) develops (Gilbert, 2007). Cesarean birth is indicated in all women with ultrasound evidence of placenta previa (Francois & Foley, 2007; Hull & Resnik). In women with placental "migration" or movement of the placenta in relationship to the internal os, a vaginal birth may be attempted (Cunningham et al., 2005).

If cesarean birth is planned, the nurse continuously assesses maternal and fetal status while preparing the woman for surgery. Maternal vital signs are assessed frequently for decreasing BP, increasing pulse rate, changes in level of consciousness, and oliguria. Fetal assessment is maintained by continuous EFM to assess for signs of hypoxia.

Blood loss may not cease with the birth of the infant. The large vascular channels in the lower uterine segment may continue to bleed because of that segment's diminished muscle content. The natural mechanism to control bleeding so characteristic of the upper part of the uterus–the interlacing muscle bundles, the "living ligature" contracting around open vessels–is absent in the lower part of the uterus. Postpartum hemorrhage may therefore occur even if the fundus is contracted firmly.

Emotional support for the woman and her family is extremely important. The actively bleeding woman is concerned not only for her own well-being, but also for the well-being of her fetus. All procedures should be explained, and a support person should be present. The woman should be encouraged to express her concerns and feelings. If the woman and her support person or family desire pastoral support, the nurse can notify the hospital chaplain service or provide information about other supportive resources.

Premature separation of placenta (abruptio placentae)

Premature separation of the placenta, or **abruptio placentae**, is the detachment of part or all of a normally implanted placenta from the uterus (Fig. 21-12). Separation occurs in the area of the decidua basalis after 20 weeks of gestation and before the birth of the infant.

Incidence and etiology. Premature separation of the placenta is a serious complication that accounts for significant maternal and fetal morbidity and mortality. Approximately 1 in 75 to 1 in 226 of pregnancies is complicated by abruptio placentae. The range in incidence likely reflects both variable criteria for diagnosis and an increased recognition of milder forms of abruption. Approximately one third of all antepartum bleeding is caused by placental abruption (Francois & Foley, 2007).

Maternal hypertension, whether chronic or pregnancy related, is the most consistently identified risk factor for abruption. Cocaine use is also a risk factor because it

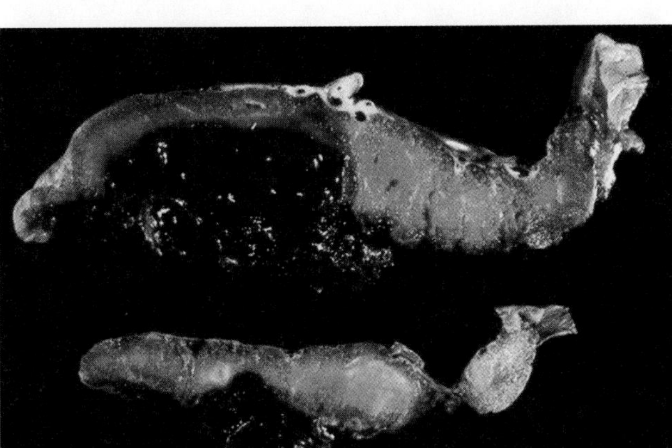

Fig. 21-12 Abruptio placentae. Premature separation of normally implanted placenta. A large retroplacental clot is present. (From Creasy, R, Resnik, R., and Iams, J. [2009]. *Creasy & Resnik's maternal-fetal medicine: Principles and practice* [6th ed.]. Philadelphia: Saunders.)

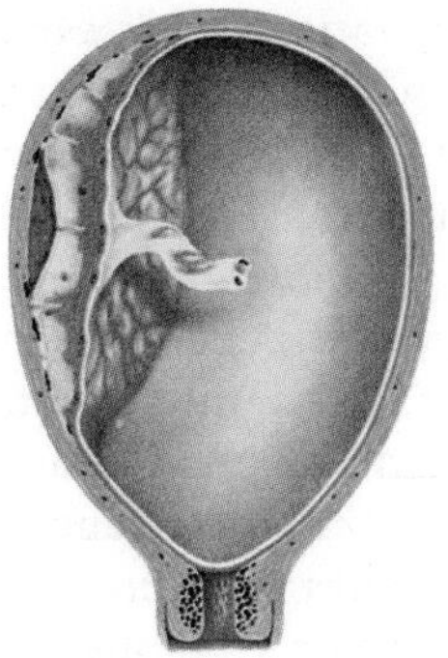

Partial separation (concealed hemorrhage)

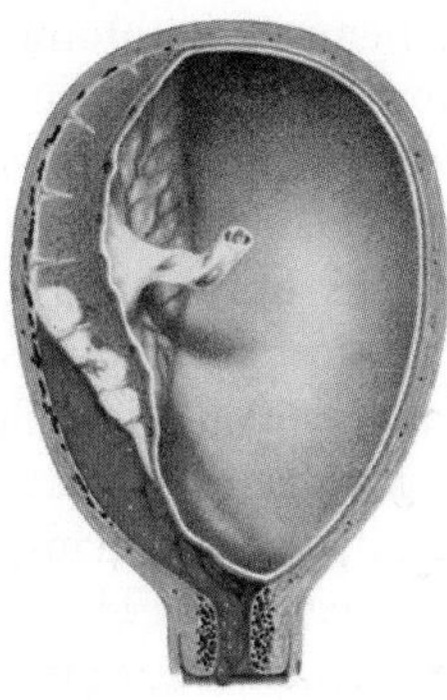

Partial separation (apparent hemorrhage)

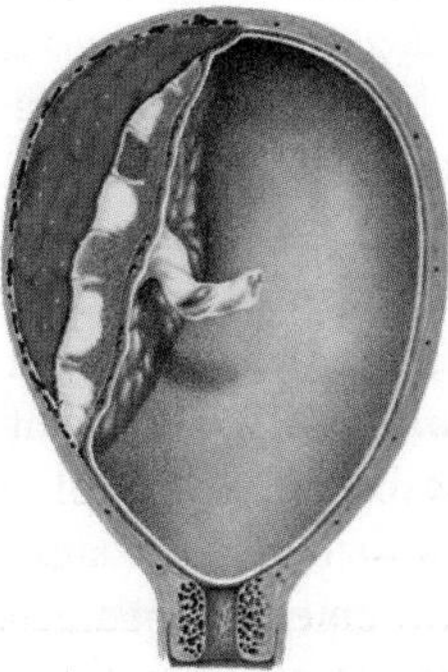

Complete separation (concealed hemorrhage)

Fig. 21-13 Abruptio placentae, showing partial and complete placental separation.

causes vascular disruption in the placental bed. Blunt external abdominal trauma, most often the result of motor-vehicle accidents (MVAs) or maternal battering, is another frequent cause of placental abruption (Francois & Foley, 2007). Other risk factors include cigarette smoking, a history of abruption in a previous pregnancy and PROM (Cunningham et al., 2005; Hull & Resnik, 2009). Abruption is more likely to occur in twin gestations than in singletons (Francois & Foley). Women who have had two previous abruptions have a recurrence risk of 25% in the next pregnancy (Hull & Resnik).

Classification. The most common classification of placental abruption is according to type and severity. This classification system is summarized in Table 21-7.

Clinical manifestations. The separation may be partial or complete, or only the margin of the placenta may be involved. Bleeding from the placental site may dissect (separate) the membranes from the decidua basalis and flow out through the vagina (70%-80%), it may remain concealed (retroplacental hemorrhage) (10%-20%), or both (Fig. 21-13) (Francois & Foley, 2007; Gilbert, 2007). Clinical symptoms vary with degree of separation (see Table 21-7). If cesarean birth is performed, blood clots may be noted on entry into the uterus. Blood clot will often be attached to the posterior surface of the placenta (referred to as a retroplacental clot) (see Fig. 21-12).

Classic symptoms of abruptio placentae include vaginal bleeding, abdominal pain, and uterine tenderness and contractions (Cunningham et al., 2005; Hull & Resnik, 2009). Bleeding may result in maternal hypovolemia (i.e., shock, oliguria, anuria) and coagulopathy. Mild to severe uterine hypertonicity is present. Pain is mild to severe and localized over one region of the uterus or diffuse over the uterus with a boardlike abdomen.

Extensive myometrial bleeding damages the uterine muscle. If blood accumulates between the separated placenta and the uterine wall, it may produce a **Couvelaire uterus.** The uterus appears purple or blue, rather than its usual "bubble gum pink" color and contractility is lost. Shock may occur and is out of proportion to blood loss. Laboratory findings include a positive Apt test result (blood in the amniotic fluid), a decrease in hemoglobin and hematocrit levels, which may appear later, and a decrease in coagulation factor levels. Clotting defects (e.g., DIC) are present in approximately 40% of women who develop a large abruption (Francois & Foley, 2007). A Kleihauer-Betke (KB) test may be ordered to determine the presence of fetal-to-maternal bleeding (transplacental hemorrhage), although this test appears to have no value in the general workup of patients with abruption. The KB test may be useful to guide Rh_o(D) immune globulin therapy in Rh-negative women who have had an abruption (Hull & Resnik, 2009).

Maternal and fetal outcomes. The mother's prognosis depends on the extent of placental detachment, overall blood loss, degree of coagulopathy present and time between placental detachment and birth. Maternal complications are associated with the abruption or its treatment. Hemorrhage, hypovolemic shock, hypofibrinogenemia, and thrombocytopenia are associated with severe abruption. Renal failure and pituitary necrosis may result from ischemia. In rare cases, women who are Rh negative can become sensitized if fetal-to-maternal hemorrhage occurs and the fetal blood type is Rh positive.

Placental abruption is associated with a perinatal mortality rate of 20% to 30%. If more than 50% of the placenta is involved, fetal death is likely to occur. Other fetal and neonatal risks include IUGR and preterm birth (Francois & Foley, 2007; Hull & Resnik, 2009). Risks for neurologic defects and death from sudden infant death syndrome are also increased in newborns following placental abruption (Cunningham et al., 2005; Francois & Foley).

Diagnosis. Placental abruption is primarily a clinical diagnosis. Although ultrasound can be used to rule out placenta previa, it cannot detect all cases of abruption. A retroplacental mass may be detected with ultrasonographic examination, but negative findings do not rule out a life-threatening abruption. In fact, at least 50% of abruptions cannot be identified on ultrasound (Hull & Resnik, 2009). Hypofibrinogenemia and evidence of DIC support the diagnosis, but many women with placental abruption do not develop coagulopathy. The diagnosis of abruption is confirmed after birth by visual inspection of the placenta. Adherent clot on the maternal surface of the placenta and depression of the underlying placental surface are usually present (see Fig. 21-12) (Francois & Foley, 2007; Gilbert, 2007).

Abruptio placentae should be highly suspected in the woman with a sudden onset of intense, usually localized, uterine pain, with or without vaginal bleeding. Initial assessment is much the same as for placenta previa. Physical examination usually reveals abdominal pain, uterine tenderness, and contractions. The fundal height may be measured over time because an increasing fundal height indicates concealed bleeding. Approximately 60% of live fetuses exhibit nonreassuring FHR patterns, and elevated uterine resting tone may also be noted on the monitor tracing (Francois & Foley, 2007). Coagulopathy, as evidenced by abnormal clotting studies (fibrinogen, platelet count, PTT, fibrin split products), may be present if a large or complete abruption has occurred.

Management

Expectant management. Management depends on the severity of blood loss and fetal maturity and status. If the abruption is mild and the fetus is less than 36 weeks of gestation and not in distress, expectant management may be implemented. The woman is hospitalized and observed closely for signs of bleeding and labor. The fetal status is also monitored with intermittent FHR monitoring and NSTs or BPPs until fetal maturity is determined or until the woman's condition deteriorates and immediate birth is indicated. Corticosteroids should be given to accelerate fetal lung maturity (Cunningham et al., 2005). Women who are Rh negative may be given $Rh_o(D)$ immune globulin if fetal-to-maternal hemorrhage occurs.

Active management. Immediate birth is the management of choice if the fetus is at term gestation or if the bleeding is moderate to severe and the mother or fetus is in jeopardy. At least one large-bore (16- to 18-gauge) IV line should be started. Maternal vital signs are monitored frequently to observe for signs of declining hemodynamic status, such as increasing pulse rate and decreasing BP. Serial laboratory studies include hematocrit or hemoglobin determinations and clotting studies. Continuous EFM is mandatory. An indwelling Foley catheter is inserted for continuous assessment of urine output, an excellent indirect measure of maternal organ perfusion. Blood and fluid volume replacement may be necessary, along with administering blood products to correct any coagulation defects.

Vaginal birth is usually feasible and is desirable, especially in cases of fetal death. Labor induction or augmentation may initiated so long as the mother and fetus are closely monitored for any evidence of compromise. Cesarean birth should be reserved for cases of fetal distress or other obstetric complications. Cesarean birth should not be attempted when the women has severe and uncorrected coagulopathy because it may result in uncontrollable bleeding (Francois & Foley, 2007).

Nursing care of patients experiencing moderate to severe abruption is demanding because it requires constant close monitoring of the maternal and fetal condition. Information about abruptio placentae, including the cause, treatment, and expected outcome, is given to the woman and her family. Emotional support is also extremely important because the woman and her family may be experiencing fetal loss in addition to the woman's critical illness.

Cord insertion and placental variations

Velamentous insertion of the cord *(vasa previa)* is a rare placental anomaly associated with placenta previa and multiple gestation. The cord vessels begin to branch at the membranes and then course onto the placenta (Fig. 21-14). ROM or traction on the cord may tear one or more of the fetal vessels. As a result the fetus may rapidly bleed to death. *Battledore* (marginal) insertion of the cord (Fig. 21-15, *A*) increases the risk of fetal hemorrhage, especially after marginal separation of the placenta.

In rare instances the placenta may be divided into two or more separate lobes, resulting in *succenturiate* placenta (Fig. 21-15, *B*). Each lobe has a distinct circulation. The vessels collect at the periphery, and the main trunks eventually unite to form the vessels of the cord. Blood vessels joining the lobes may be supported only by the fetal membranes and are therefore in danger of tearing during labor, birth, or expulsion of the placenta. During expulsion of the placenta, one or more of the separate lobes may remain attached to the decidua basalis, preventing uterine contraction and increasing the risk of postpartum hemorrhage.

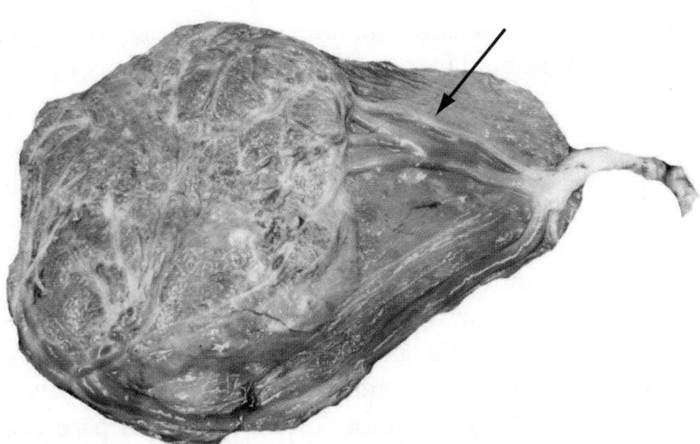

Fig 21-14 Vasa previa (velamentous insertion of cord). Arrow shows velamentous cord insertion in the placenta. (From Creasy, R, Resnik, R., & Iams, J. [2009]. *Creasy & Resnik's maternal-fetal medicine: Principles and practice* [6th ed.]. Philadelphia: Saunders.)

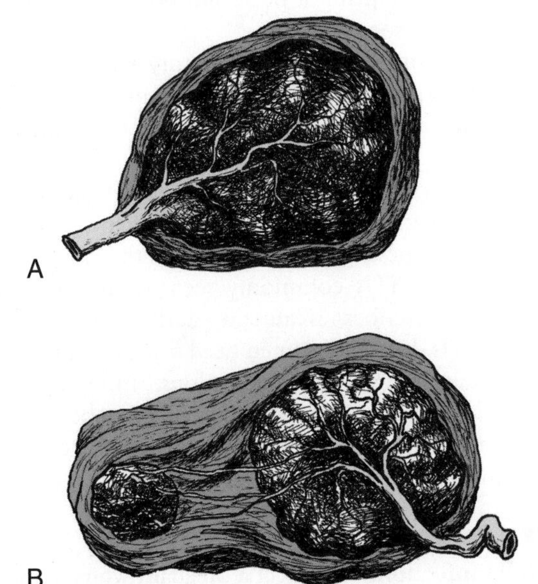

Fig. 21-15 Cord insertion and placental variations **A,** Battledore placenta. **B,** Placenta succenturiate.

CLOTTING DISORDERS IN PREGNANCY

Normal Clotting

Normally a delicate balance (homeostasis) exists between the opposing hemostatic and fibrinolytic systems. The hemostatic system stops the flow of blood from injured vessels, first by a platelet plug, which is followed by the formation of a fibrin clot. The coagulation process involves an interaction of the coagulation factors that constantly circulate in the bloodstream in which each factor sequentially activates the factor next in line, the "cascade effect" sequence. The fibrinolytic system is the process through which the fibrin clot is split into fibrinolytic degradation products and circulation is restored.

Clotting Problems

Disseminated intravascular coagulation

Disseminated intravascular coagulation (DIC), or consumptive coagulopathy, is a pathologic form of clotting that is diffuse and consumes large amounts of clotting factors, causing widespread external bleeding, internal bleeding, or both, and clotting (Cunningham et al., 2005). DIC is never a primary diagnosis. Instead, it results from some problem that triggered the clotting cascade, either extrinsically, by the release of large amounts of tissue thromboplastin, or intrinsically, by widespread damage to vascular integrity.

In the obstetric population, DIC is most often triggered by the release of large amounts of tissue thromboplastin, which occurs in abruptio placentae and in retained dead fetus and anaphylactoid syndrome of pregnancy (amniotic fluid embolus) syndromes. Severe preeclampsia, HELLP syndrome, and gram-negative sepsis are examples of conditions that can trigger DIC because of widespread damage to vascular integrity (Cunningham et al., 2005; Gilbert, 2007). DIC is an overactivation of the clotting cascade and the fibrinolytic system, resulting in depletion of platelets and clotting factors, which results in the formation of multiple fibrin clots throughout the body's vasculature, even in the microcirculation. Blood cells are destroyed as they pass through these fibrin choked vessels. Thus DIC results in a clinical picture of clotting, bleeding, and ischemia (Cunningham et al.; Labelle & Kitchens, 2005). Clinical manifestations and laboratory test results are summarized in Box 21-6.

Management. Medical management in all cases of DIC involves correction of the underlying cause (e.g., removal of the dead fetus, treatment of existing infection or of preeclampsia or eclampsia, or removal of a placental abruption). Volume replacement, blood component therapy, optimization of oxygenation and perfusion status, and continued reassessment of laboratory parameters are the usual forms of treatment (Francois & Foley, 2007). Vitamin K administration and recombinant activated factor VIIa also may be considered as adjuvant therapies (Francois & Foley).

Nursing interventions include assessment for signs of bleeding (see Box 21-6) and signs of complications from the administration of blood and blood products, administering fluid or blood replacement as ordered, cardiac and hemodynamic monitoring, and protecting the woman from injury. Because renal failure is one consequence of DIC, urinary output is closely monitored by using an indwelling Foley catheter. Urinary output must be maintained at more than 30 ml/hr (Gilbert, 2007). Vital signs are assessed frequently. If DIC develops before birth, the woman should be maintained in a side-lying tilt to maximize blood flow to the uterus. Oxygen may be administered through a nonrebreather facemask at 8 to 10 L/min or per hospital protocol or physician order. Fetal

BOX 21-6

Clinical Manifestations and Laboratory Screening Results for Women with Disseminated Intravascular Coagulation

POSSIBLE PHYSICAL EXAMINATION FINDINGS

- Spontaneous bleeding from gums, nose
- Oozing, excessive bleeding from venipuncture site, intravenous access site, or site of insertion of urinary catheter
- Petechiae, for example, on the arm where blood pressure cuff was placed
- Other signs of bruising
- Hematuria
- Gastrointestinal bleeding
- Tachycardia
- Diaphoresis

LABORATORY COAGULATION SCREENING TEST RESULTS

- Platelets—decreased
- Fibrinogen—decreased
- Factor V (proaccelerin)—decreased
- Factor VIII (antihemolytic factor)—decreased
- Prothrombin time—prolonged
- Partial prothrombin time—prolonged
- Fibrin degradation products—increased
- D-dimer test (specific fibrin degradation fragment) —increased
- Red blood smear—fragmented red blood cells

Sources: Cunningham, F., Leveno, K., Bloom, S., Hauth, J., Gilstrap, L., & Wenstrom, K. (2005). *Williams obstetrics* (22nd ed.). New York: McGraw-Hill; Labelle, C., & Kitchens, C. (2005). Disseminated intravascular coagulation: Treat the cause, not the lab values. *Cleveland Clinic Journal of Medicine, 72*(5), 377–397; Roberts, J., & Funai, E. (2009). Pregnancy-related hypertension. In R. Creasy, R. Resnik, & J. Iams (Eds.), *Creasy and Resnik's maternal-fetal medicine: Principles and practice* (6th ed.). Philadelphia: Saunders.

assessments are performed to monitor fetal well-being (Labelle & Kitchens, 2005). DIC usually is "cured" with the birth and as coagulation abnormalities resolve.

The woman and her family will be anxious and concerned about her condition and prognosis. The nurse offers explanations about care and provides emotional support to the woman and her family through this critical time.

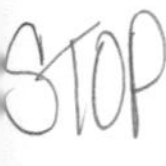

INFECTIONS ACQUIRED DURING PREGNANCY

Sexually Transmitted Infections

Sexually transmitted infections (STIs) in pregnancy are responsible for significant morbidity rates. Some consequences of maternal infection, such as infertility and sterility, last a lifetime. Psychosocial sequelae may include altered interpersonal relationships and lowered self-esteem. Congenitally acquired infection may affect the length and quality of a child's life.

Chapter 3 discusses the diagnosis and management of STIs, and Chapter 24 discusses neonatal effects and management. This discussion focuses only on the effects of several common STIs on pregnancy and the fetus (Table 21-8). Effects on pregnancy and the fetus also vary according to whether the infection has been treated at the time of labor and birth.

Management

Currently, more than 20 STIs are known to affect the outcome of pregnancy (Gilbert, 2007). Factors that influence the development and management of STIs during pregnancy include a previous history of STI or pelvic inflammatory disease, number of current sexual partners, frequency of intercourse, and anticipated sexual activity during pregnancy. Lifestyle choices also may affect STIs in the perinatal period. Risk factors include use of IV drugs or having a partner who uses IV drugs. Other lifestyle factors that increase susceptibility to STIs (through suppressive effects on the immune system) include smoking, alcohol use, inadequate or poor nutrition, and high levels of fatigue or personal stress.

Physical examination and laboratory studies to determine the presence of STIs in the pregnant woman are the same as those performed in nonpregnant women (see Chapter 3).

Treatment of specific STIs may be different for the pregnant woman and may even be different at different stages of pregnancy. Table 21-8 describes the maternal and fetal effects for STIs commonly seen during pregnancy. Table 21-9 describes treatment during pregnancy of common STIs. Infected women need instruction regarding how to take prescribed medications, information on whether their partner or partners also need to be evaluated and treated, and a review of preventive measures to prevent reinfection.

TORCH Infections

TORCH infections can affect a pregnant woman and her fetus. Toxoplasmosis, other infections (e.g., hepatitis), rubella virus, cytomegalovirus, and herpes simplex virus, known collectively as *TORCH infections,* are a group of organisms capable of crossing the placenta and adversely affecting the development of the fetus. Generally, all TORCH infections produce influenza-like symptoms in the woman, but fetal and neonatal effects are more serious. TORCH infections and their maternal and fetal effects are described in Table 21-10. Neonatal effects are discussed in Chapter 24.

Urinary Tract Infections

Urinary tract infections (UTIs) are a common medical complication of pregnancy, occurring in approximately 20% of all pregnancies. They are also responsible for 10% of all hospitalizations during pregnancy (Duff, Sweet, & Edwards, 2009). UTIs include asymptomatic bacteriuria, cystitis, and pyelonephritis. UTIs are usually caused by coliform organisms that are a normal part of the perineal

TABLE 21-8

Maternal and Fetal Effects of Common Sexually Transmitted Infections

INFECTION	MATERNAL EFFECTS	FETAL EFFECTS
Chlamydia	Premature rupture of membranes Preterm labor Postpartum endometritis	Low birth weight
Gonorrhea	Miscarriage Preterm labor Premature rupture of membranes Amniotic infection syndrome Chorioamnionitis Postpartum endometritis Postpartum sepsis	Preterm birth IUGR
Group B *Streptococcus*	Urinary tract infection Chorioamnionitis Postpartum endometritis Sepsis Meningitis (rare)	Preterm birth
Herpes simplex virus	Intrauterine infection (rare)	Congenital infection (rare)
Human papilloma virus (HPV)	Dystocia from large lesions Excessive bleeding from lesions after birth trauma	
Syphilis	Miscarriage Preterm labor	IUGR Preterm birth Stillbirth Congenital infection

Sources: Gilbert, E.. (2007). Manual of high risk pregnancy and delivery (4th ed.). St. Louis: Mosby; Duff, P., Sweet, R., & Edwards, R. (2009). Maternal and fetal infections. In R. Creasy, R. Resnik, & J. Iams (Eds.). *Creasy and Resnik's maternal-fetal medicine: Principles and practice* (6th ed.). Philadelphia: Saunders.
IUGR, Intrauterine growth restriction.

TABLE 21-9

Treatment of Common Sexually Transmitted Infections in Pregnancy

SEXUALLY TRANSMITTED INFECTION	RECOMMENDED TREATMENT	NURSING CONSIDERATIONS
Chlamydia	Azithromycin 1 g PO in a single dose; or amoxicillin 500 mg PO three times a day × 7 days	Screening is performed at first prenatal visit. Instruct woman to take after meals and with 8 oz water; instruct partner to be tested and treated if needed.
Herpes simplex virus	Acyclovir 400 mg three times a day beginning at 36 weeks of gestation and continuing until birth for women with recurrent herpes, as suppressive therapy to prevent an outbreak during labor Oral analgesics and topical anesthetics may be ordered for severe discomfort.	Instruct woman in comfort measures: keep lesions clean and dry; bathe frequently and then thoroughly dry affected area with a hair dryer on a low setting; use compresses on lesions (cold milk, colloidal oatmeal) every 2 to 4 hr, sitz baths; woman should abstain from intercourse while lesions are present; if woman has active lesions at time of labor, a cesarean birth will usually be performed to prevent perinatal transmission.
Gonorrhea	Ceftriaxone 125 mg IM × one dose or Cefixime 400 mg PO × one dose plus treatment for chlamydia as listed above	Screening is performed at first prenatal visit; repeated in third trimester if high risk. Instruct partner to be tested and treated if needed.

Continued

TABLE 21-9

Treatment of Common Sexually Transmitted Infections in Pregnancy—cont'd

SEXUALLY TRANSMITTED INFECTION	RECOMMENDED TREATMENT	NURSING CONSIDERATIONS
Group B *Streptococcus*	Penicillin G 5 million units IV initial dose followed by 2.5 million units IV every 4 hr until birth. For women with penicillin allergy but not at high risk for anaphylaxis, the drug of choice is cephazolin 2 g IV initially followed by 1 g every 8 hr until birth.	Pregnant women should be screened at 35-37 weeks of gestation; if positive or status unknown at time of labor, the woman is treated. Accurate rapid polymerase chain reaction testing is now available for use if no antepartum screening results are available when the woman is admitted to give birth.
Hepatitis B	None for infected pregnant women	Screening should be at first prenatal visit, with rescreening in third trimester for high risk patients; treatment is supportive—bed rest, high-protein, low-fat diet, increased fluid intake; the woman should avoid medications that are metabolized in the liver.
Human papilloma virus	Trichloracetic acid (TCA) or bichloracetic acid (BCA) 80%-90% applied topically to warts once a week; lesions may also be removed with scissors, scalpel, curettage, electrosurgery, or cryosurgery Treat only patients who have multiple confluent lesions.	Podophyllin resin, podofilox, and imiquimod have not been shown to be safe for use during pregnancy; xylocaine jelly can be applied for burning sensations; inform partners to be tested and treated if needed; couples should use condoms for intercourse; inform women that smoking can decrease effects of therapy.
Syphilis	Benzathine penicillin G 2.4 million units IM once; if syphilis of more than one year duration or duration is unknown, then 2.4 million units IM (one dose per week × 3 weeks) for a total of 7.2 million units benzathine penicillin G. No proven alternatives to penicillin in pregnancy exist; women who have a history of allergy to penicillin should be desensitized and treated with penicillin	Treatment cures maternal infection and prevents congenital syphilis 98% of the time; women treated during the second trimester are at risk for preterm labor if the Jarisch-Herxheimer reaction occurs; routine screening during pregnancy should be at the first prenatal visit and in the third trimester in women at high risk; partners should be tested and treated if needed.
Trichomonas	Metronidazole 2 grams PO × one dose	Symptomatic pregnant women should be treated but routine screening and treatment of all pregnant women is not recommended. Inform partners to be treated; women should avoid alcohol and vinegar products to avoid nausea and vomiting, intestinal cramping, and headaches; not recommended during lactation; stop breastfeeding, treat; resume in 48 hours after last dose. Women may use breast pump and discard milk to prevent interruption of milk supply.
Candidiasis	Over-the-counter topical agents; butoconazole, clotrimazole, miconazole, or terconazole × 7 days	Treatment of partners is not recommended because candidiasis is not usually acquired through intercourse. Medications may be used during lactation.
Bacterial vaginosis	Metronidazole PO for at least 7 days in women at high risk for preterm labor (e.g., those with a history of previous preterm birth)	Routine screening and treatment in women at low risk for preterm labor is not recommended. Screening of women at high risk for preterm labor (e.g., those with a history of previous preterm birth) should be done at the first prenatal visit.

Source: Duff, P., Sweet, R., & Edwards, R. K. (2009). Maternal and fetal infections. In R. Creasy, R. Resnik, & J. Iams (Eds.), *Creasy and Resnik's maternal-fetal medicine: Principles and practice* (6th ed.). Philadelphia: Saunders.
IM, Intramuscularly; *IV,* intravenously; *PO,* by mouth.

TABLE 21-10

Maternal Infection: TORCH

INFECTION	MATERNAL EFFECTS	FETAL EFFECTS	COUNSELING: PREVENTION, IDENTIFICATION, AND MANAGEMENT
Toxoplasmosis (protozoa)	Most infections asymptomatic Acute infection similar to mononucleosis Woman immune after first episode (except in immunocompromised patients)	Congenital infection is most likely to occur when maternal infection develops during the third trimester. The risk of fetal injury, however, is greatest when maternal infection occurs during the first trimester.	Good handwashing technique should be used. Eating raw or rare meat and exposure to litter used by infected cats should be avoided; toxoplasma titer should be checked if there are cats in the house. If titer is rising during early pregnancy, abortion may be considered an option.
OTHER INFECTIONS			
Hepatitis A (infectious hepatitis) (virus)	Liver failure (extremely rare) Low-grade fever, malaise, poor appetite, right upper quadrant pain and tenderness, jaundice, and light-colored stools	Perinatal transmission virtually never occurs.	Spread by fecal-oral contact especially by culinary workers; gamma-globulin can be given as prophylaxis for hepatitis A. Hepatitis A vaccine is now available.
Hepatitis B (serum hepatitis) (virus)	May be transmitted sexually. Approximately 10% of patients become chronic carriers. Some people with chronic hepatitis B eventually develop severe chronic liver disease, such as cirrhosis or hepatocellular carcinoma.	Infection occurs during birth. Maternal vaccination during pregnancy should present no risk for fetus (however, data are not available).	Generally passed by contaminated needles, syringes, or blood transfusions; also can be transmitted orally or by coitus (but incubation period is longer); hepatitis B immune globulin can be given prophylactically after exposure. Hepatitis B vaccine recommended for populations at risk. Populations at risk are women from Asia, Pacific islands, Indochina, Haiti, South Africa, Alaska (women of Eskimo descent); other women at risk include health care providers, users of intravenous drugs, those sexually active with multiple partners or single partner with multiple risks.
Rubella (3-day or German measles) (virus)	Rash, fever, mild symptoms such as headache, malaise, myalgias, and arthralgias; postauricular lymph nodes may be swollen; mild conjunctivitis	Approximately 50%-80% of fetuses exposed to the virus within 12 weeks after conception will show signs of congenital infection. Very few fetuses are affected if infection occurs after 18 weeks of gestation. The most common fetal anomalies associated with congenital rubella syndrome are deafness, eye defects (e.g., cataracts or retinopathy), central nervous system defects, and cardiac defects.	Vaccination of pregnant women contraindicated; pregnancy should be prevented for 1 month after vaccination. Women may breastfeed after vaccination and the vaccine can be administered along with immunoglobulin preparations such as Rh immune globulin.

Continued

TABLE 21-10

Maternal Infection: TORCH—cont'd

INFECTION	MATERNAL EFFECTS	FETAL EFFECTS	COUNSELING: PREVENTION, IDENTIFICATION, AND MANAGEMENT
Cytomegalovirus (CMV) (a herpes virus)	Most adults are asymptomatic or have only mild influenza-like symptoms. The presence of CMV antibodies does not totally prevent reinfection.	The fetus can be infected transplacentally. Infection is much more likely with a primary maternal infection. The most common indications of congenital infection include hepatosplenomegaly, intracranial calcifications, jaundice, growth restriction, microcephaly, chorioretinitis, hearing loss, thrombocytopenia, hyperbilirubinemia, and hepatitis.	The virus is transmitted by transplantation of an infected organ, transfusion of infected blood, sexual contact, or contact with contaminated saliva or urine. Virus may be reactivated and cause disease in utero or during birth in subsequent pregnancies; fetal infection may occur during passage through infected birth canal. Prevention includes use of CMV-negative blood products if transfusion of pregnant women is necessary and teaching all women to wash hands carefully after handling infant diapers and toys.
Herpes genitalis (herpes simplex virus, type 1 or type 2 [HSV-1 or HSV-2])	Primary infection with painful blisters, tender inguinal lymph nodes, fever, viral meningitis (rare) Recurrent infections are much milder and shorter.	Transplacental infection resulting in congenital infection is rare and usually occurs with primary maternal infection. The risk mainly exists with infection late in pregnancy.	As many as two-thirds of women with HSV-2 antibodies acquired the infection asymptomatically; however, asymptomatic women can give birth to seriously infected neonates. Risk of transmission is greatest during vaginal birth if woman has active lesions; thus cesarean birth is recommended. Acyclovir can be used to treat recurrent outbreaks during pregnancy or as suppressive therapy late in pregnancy to prevent an outbreak during labor and birth.

Source: Duff, P., Sweet, R., & Edwards, R. (2009). Maternal and fetal infections. In R. Creasy, R. Resnik, & J. Iams (Eds.), *Creasy and Resnik's maternal-fetal medicine: Principles and practice* (6th ed.). Philadelphia: Saunders.

flora. By far the most common cause of UTIs is *Escherichia coli,* a gram-negative bacteria responsible for 85% of cases. Another gram-negative bacteria that causes UTIs is *Klebsiella pneumoniae.* The gram-positive organisms group B streptococci, enterococci, and staphylococci account for less than 10% of all infections (Gilbert, 2007).

Asymptomatic bacteriuria

Asymptomatic bacteriuria refers to the persistent presence of bacteria within the urinary tract of women who have no symptoms. A clean-voided urine specimen containing more than 100,000 organisms per ml is diagnostic. If asymptomatic bacteriuria is not treated, up to 40% of infected women will subsequently develop symptomatic infection during the pregnancy (Colombo & Samuels, 2007). Therefore ACOG recommends that all women be screened for asymptomatic bacteriuria at their first prenatal visit (Colombo & Samuels). Asymptomatic bacteriuria has been associated with preterm birth and low-birth-weight infants (AAP & ACOG, 2007; Cunningham et al., 2005).

Asymptomatic bacteriuria should be treated with an antibiotic. Antibiotics that are often prescribed include amoxicillin, ampicillin, cephalexin (Keflex), ciprofloxacin (Cipro), levofloxacin (Levaquin), nitrofurantoin (Macrodantin), and trimethoprim-sulfamethoxazole (Bactrim DS). Several different regimens, including single dose, 3-day, and 10-day treatment may be used (Cunningham et al., 2005). A repeat urine culture is usually ordered 1 to 2 weeks after completing therapy because approximately 15% of women will not respond to therapy or will have a reinfection (Colombo & Samuels, 2007). Women who have persistent or frequent recurrences of bacteriuria may be placed on suppressive therapy, often nitrofurantoin each night at bedtime, for the remainder of the pregnancy (Cunningham et al.).

Cystitis

Cystitis (bladder infection) is characterized by dysuria, urgency, and frequency, along with lower abdominal or suprapubic pain. Usually, white blood cells, as well as bacteria, will be found in the urine. Microscopic or gross hematuria may also be present. Typically, symptoms are confined to the bladder rather than becoming systemic. Cystitis is usually uncomplicated, but it may lead to ascending UTI if untreated. Approximately 40% of pregnant women with pyelonephritis experienced symptoms of bladder infection before developing pyelonephritis (Cunningham et al., 2005).

Cystitis is often treated with a 3-day course of antibiotic therapy, which is usually 90% effective in curing the infection. Antibiotics often prescribed include amoxicillin, ampicillin, cephalexin (Keflex), ciprofloxacin (Cipro), levofloxacin (Levaquin), nitrofurantoin (Macrodantin), and trimethoprim-sulfamethoxazole (Bactrim DS) (Cunningham et al., 2005). Phenazopyridine (Pyridium), a urinary analgesic, is often prescribed along with an antibiotic for relief of symptoms caused by irritation of the urinary tract. Although phenazopyridine is effective at relieving dysuria, urgency, and frequency, women should be taught that the medication colors urine and tears orange. Women should be instructed to avoid wearing contact lenses while taking this medication and warned that it will stain underwear.

Pyelonephritis

Renal infection (pyelonephritis) is the most common serious medical complication of pregnancy and the most common nonobstetric cause of hospitalization during pregnancy (Colombo & Samuels, 2007; Cunningham et al., 2005). The most common maternal complications associated with pyelonephritis include anemia, septicemia, transient renal dysfunction, and pulmonary insufficiency. Women with pyelonephritis can develop urosepsis, sepsis syndrome, and renal dysfunction. In addition, pulmonary injury resembling adult respiratory distress syndrome (ARDS) can occur in pregnant women with acute pyelonephritis, most likely the result of damage to alveolar tissue caused by the release of endotoxins from gram-negative bacteria (Colombo & Samuels; Cunningham et al.). Recurrent pyelonephritis is thought to cause fetal death and IUGR. Acute pyelonephritis is associated with preterm labor (Colombo & Samuels).

Pyelonephritis develops most often during the second trimester of pregnancy and is most often caused by the *E. coli* organism. Infection develops only in the right kidney in more than one half of all cases. The onset of pyelonephritis is often abrupt, with fever, shaking chills, and aching in the lumbar area of the back. Anorexia and nausea and vomiting may also be present. Usually, one or both costovertebral angles will be tender to palpation.

Women diagnosed with pyelonephritis are admitted to the hospital immediately. Treatment with intravenous antibiotics will be started as soon as urine and blood samples for culture and sensitivity have been collected. Ampicillin, gentamycin, cefazolin (Ancef), or ceftriaxone (Rocephin) are often ordered initially because they are broad-spectrum antibiotics that are usually effective. The woman must be monitored closely for the possible development of sepsis (Cunningham et al., 2005).

Clinical symptoms generally resolve within a couple of days after antibiotic therapy is begun. The antibiotic may need to be changed based on the results of the initial culture and sensitivity testing, or if the woman has not responded to therapy within 48 hours (Gilbert, 2007). Most women become afebrile within 72 hours. If no clinical improvement is seen within 48 to 72 hours, an ultrasound should be performed to assess for a urinary tract obstruction. Once the woman is afebrile, she will be changed from intravenous to oral antibiotics (Cunningham, et al., 2005).

Usually, antibiotic therapy will be continued for 7 to 10 days after the woman is discharged from the hospital. A urine culture will likely be repeated 1 to 2 weeks after antibiotic therapy has been completed. Recurrent infection develops in 30% to 40% of women after completion of treatment for pyelonephritis. Therefore urine cultures should be obtained each trimester for the remainder of the pregnancy. Many women will be maintained on a prophylactic antibiotic (often nitrofurantoin once or twice daily) for the remainder of the pregnancy (Colombo & Samuels, 2007; Cunningham et al., 2005).

Patient education

Nurses are often responsible for teaching patients about taking medications safely and effectively. This education is especially important in regard to antibiotics because this type of medication is so often misused by the general public. The woman should be instructed to finish the entire course of prescribed antibiotic therapy rather than stopping the medication as soon as she feels better. Failure to do so can ultimately lead to the creation of additional drug-resistant organisms. Antibiotics should be taken on time and around the clock so that medication levels in the body remain constant. Finally, many women will develop a yeast infection while taking antibiotics because the medication kills normal flora in the genitourinary tract, as well as pathologic organisms. Therefore they should be encouraged to include yogurt, cheese, or milk containing active acidophilus cultures in their diet while on antibiotics.

Woman should also be taught simple ways to prevent future urinary tract infections. See Patient Instructions for Self-Management box: Prevention of Urinary Tract Infections for several suggestions.

SURGICAL EMERGENCIES DURING PREGNANCY

Pregnant patients may certainly develop any medical or surgical disease that can occur in nonpregnant women of childbearing age. The need for abdominal surgery occurs as frequently among pregnant women as among nonpregnant women of comparable age. However, pregnancy may make diagnosis difficult. An enlarged uterus and displaced internal organs may make abdominal palpation difficult, alter the position of an affected organ, or change the usual signs and symptoms associated with a particular disorder. The most common nongynecologic abdominal conditions requiring surgery during pregnancy are appendicitis and symptomatic cholelithiasis (Lu & Curet, 2007).

Appendicitis

Appendicitis is the most common nongynecologic cause of an acute surgical abdomen during pregnancy, occurring in as many as 1 in 1500 pregnancies (Lu & Curet, 2007). The diagnosis of appendicitis is often delayed because the usual signs and symptoms mimic some normal changes of pregnancy such as nausea and vomiting and increased white blood cell (WBC) count (Cunningham et al., 2005). As pregnancy progresses the appendix is pushed upward and to the right of its usual anatomic location. Because of these changes, rupture of the appendix and the subsequent development of peritonitis occur two to three times more often in pregnant women than in nonpregnant women.

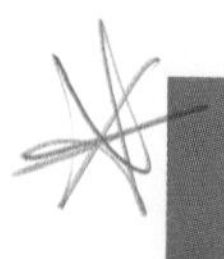

PATIENT INSTRUCTIONS FOR SELF-MANAGEMENT

Prevention of Urinary Tract Infections

- Wipe from front to back after voiding or having a bowel movement.
- Choose underwear or hosiery with a cotton crotch.
- Avoid tight-fitting clothing, especially jeans.
- Limit time spent in damp exercise clothes (especially swimsuits and leotards or tights).
- Avoid bath salts or bubble bath.
- Avoid colored or scented toilet tissue.
- If sensitive, discontinue use of feminine hygiene deodorant sprays.
- Don't ignore the urge to void.
- Void before and after intercourse and before going to bed at night.
- Drink at least 8 glasses of fluid (especially water) every day.

The most common symptom of appendicitis in pregnant women is right lower quadrant abdominal pain, regardless of gestational age. Nausea and vomiting is often present, but loss of appetite is not a reliable indicator of appendicitis. Fever, tachycardia, a dry tongue, and localized abdominal tenderness are commonly found in nonpregnant persons with appendicitis, but they are less likely indicators for the disorder in pregnant women. Because of the physiologic increase in WBCs that occurs in pregnancy, this test is not helpful in making the diagnosis. A urinalysis and a chest x-ray examination should be performed to rule out UTI and right lower lobe pneumonia, given that both of these conditions can cause lower abdominal pain (Kelly & Savides, 2009).

Ultrasound is useful during the first and second trimesters of pregnancy for diagnosing appendicitis. It is less accurate during the third trimester than earlier in pregnancy because the examination is technically more difficult to perform. In the third trimester of pregnancy, helical computerized tomography (CT) scanning may be more useful than other imaging modalities (Lu & Curet, 2007). Magnetic resonance imaging (MRI) may be used if appendicitis has not been confirmed by other imaging techniques (Kelly & Savides, 2009).

Prompt surgical intervention to remove the appendix is still the standard treatment (Kelly & Savides, 2009). Appendectomy before rupture usually does not require either antibiotic or tocolytic therapy. If surgery is delayed until after rupture, multiple antibiotics are ordered. Rupture is likely to result in preterm labor and perhaps fetal loss.

Cholelithiasis and Cholecystitis

Cholelithiasis (the presence of gallstones in the gallbladder) and cholecystitis (inflammation of the gallbladder) are both more common during pregnancy, probably because of increased hormone levels, along with pressure from the enlarged uterus that interferes with the normal circulation and drainage of the gallbladder. In fact, the second most common nongynecologic condition requiring surgery during pregnancy is symptomatic cholelithiasis, occurring in 1 of 1600 pregnancies (Blackburn, 2007; Lu & Curet, 2007).

Women with acute cholecystitis usually have fatty food intolerance along with colicky abdominal pain radiating to the back or shoulder, nausea, and vomiting. Fever may also be present. Ultrasound is often used to detect the presence of stones or dilation of the common bile duct (Lu & Curet, 2007).

Generally, gallbladder surgery should be postponed until the puerperium. The woman can usually be managed conservatively for the remainder of the pregnancy. Therapy generally includes intravenous hydration, bowel rest with nasogastric suction and no oral intake, and narcotics. Morphine should not be used as an analgesic because it may cause ductal spasm. Antibiotics are given if evidence of cholecystitis or infection exists (Lu & Curet, 2007).

Patients with obstructive jaundice, gallstone pancreatitis, suspected peritonitis or those for whom conservative (medical) management has not been successful should be treated surgically with cholecystectomy or cholecystotomy. The safest time to operate on a pregnant patient is during the second trimester, when the risks of teratogenesis, miscarriage, and preterm birth are lowest. Laparoscopic cholecystectomy at that time appears to be safe (Lu & Curet, 2007).

Gynecologic Problems

Pregnancy predisposes a woman to ovarian problems, especially during the first trimester. Ovarian cysts and twisting (torsion) of ovarian cysts or twisting of adnexal tissues may occur. Other problems include retained or enlarged cystic corpus luteum of pregnancy, and bacterial invasion of reproductive or other intraperitoneal organs. Serial ultrasounds, MRIs, and transvaginal color Doppler are used to diagnose most ovarian abnormalities (Cunningham et al., 2005). Ovarian masses generally regress by 16 to 20 weeks of gestation, but, if not, then elective surgery may be performed to remove masses. Laparotomy or laparoscopy may be required to discriminate between ovarian problems and early ectopic pregnancy, appendicitis, or an infectious process.

Management

Initial assessment of the pregnant woman requiring surgery focuses on her presenting signs and symptoms. A thorough history is obtained, and a physical examination is performed. Laboratory testing includes, at a minimum, a complete blood count with differential and a urinalysis. Additional laboratory and other diagnostic tests may be necessary to reach a diagnosis. In addition, FHR and activity, along with uterine activity, should be monitored. Constant vigilance for symptoms of impending obstetric complications should be maintained. The extent of preoperative assessment is determined by the immediacy of surgical intervention and the specific disorder that requires surgery.

When surgery becomes necessary during pregnancy, the woman and her family are concerned about the effects of the procedure and medication on fetal well-being and the course of the pregnancy. An important part of preoperative nursing care is encouraging the woman to express her fears, concerns, and questions.

Preoperative care for a pregnant woman differs from that for a nonpregnant woman in one significant aspect: the presence of at least one other person, the fetus. Continuous FHR and uterine contraction monitoring should be performed if the fetus is considered viable. Procedures such as preparation of the operative site and time of insertion of IV lines and urinary retention catheters vary with the physician and the facility. However, in every instance a total restriction of solid foods and liquids or a clear specification of the type, amount, and time at which clear liquids may be taken before surgery is ordered. Some bowel preparation, such as clear liquids and laxatives, may be required before surgery. Food by mouth is restricted for several hours before a scheduled procedure. Even if she has had nothing by mouth–but more importantly, if surgery is unexpected–the woman is in danger of vomiting and aspirating, and special precautions are taken before anesthetic is administered (e.g., administering an antacid).

Intraoperatively, perinatal nurses may collaborate with the surgical staff to increase their knowledge about the special needs of pregnant women undergoing surgery. One intervention to improve fetal oxygenation is positioning the woman on the operating table with a lateral tilt to prevent maternal compression of the vena cava. Continuous fetal and uterine monitoring during the surgical procedure is recommended because of the risk for preterm labor. Monitoring may be accomplished using sterile aquasonic gel and a sterile sleeve for the transducer. During abdominal surgery, uterine contractions may be palpated manually.

In the immediate recovery period, general observations and care pertinent to postoperative recovery are initiated. Frequent assessments are carried out for several hours after surgery. Whether the woman is cared for in the surgical postanesthesia recovery area or in the labor and birth unit, continuous fetal and uterine monitoring will likely be initiated or resumed because of the increased risk of preterm labor. Tocolysis may be necessary if preterm labor occurs (see Chapter 22).

Plans for the woman's return home and for convalescent care should be completed as early as possible before discharge. Depending on her insurance coverage, nursing care may be provided through a home health agency. If not, the woman and other support persons must be taught necessary skills and procedures, such as wound care. Ideally the woman and other caregivers should have opportunities for supervised practice before discharge so that they can feel comfortable with their knowledge and ability before being totally responsible for providing care. Box 21-7 lists information that should be included in discharge teaching for the postoperative patient. The woman may also need referrals to various community agencies for evaluation of the home situation, child care, home health care, and financial or other assistance.

TRAUMA DURING PREGNANCY

Trauma is a common complication during pregnancy because the majority of pregnant women in the United States continue their usual activities. Therefore pregnant women are at the same risk as other women for vehicular crashes, falls, industrial mishaps, violence, and other injuries in the home and community. Treatment of pregnant trauma victims is complicated because trauma health care providers seldom have the same level of expertise in the care of pregnant women as they do in care of nonpregnant trauma victims (Lutz, 2005).

BOX 21-7

Discharge Teaching for Home Care after Surgery

- Care of incision site
- Diet and elimination related to gastrointestinal function
- Signs and symptoms of developing complications: wound infection, thrombophlebitis, pneumonia
- Equipment needed and technique for assessing temperature
- Recommended schedule for resumption of activities of daily living
- Treatments and medications ordered
- List of resource persons and their telephone numbers
- Schedule of follow-up visits
- If birth has not occurred:
  - Assessment of fetal activity (kick counts)
  - Signs of preterm labor

Significance

Approximately 8% of pregnancies are complicated by major trauma, and trauma is the leading cause of nonobsteteric maternal death. As pregnancy progresses the risk of trauma increases because more cases of trauma are reported in the third trimester than earlier in gestation. Motor vehicle accidents (MVAs) falls, and violence are the leading causes of blunt trauma during pregnancy. Gunshot and stab wounds are the most common causes of penetrating trauma in pregnant women (Gilbert, 2007; Lu & Curet, 2007).

The effect of trauma on pregnancy is influenced by the length of gestation, type and severity of the trauma, and degree of disruption of uterine and fetal physiologic features. Trauma increases the incidence of miscarriage, preterm labor, abruptio placentae, and stillbirth (Cunningham et al., 2005; Mattox & Goetzl, 2005). Other common fetal effects of trauma include PROM, fetomaternal transfusion, skull injuries, and hypoxic compromise. Trauma results in fetal death more often than in maternal death (Gilbert, 2007).

Special considerations for mother and fetus are necessary when trauma occurs during pregnancy because of the physiologic alterations that accompany pregnancy and because of the presence of the fetus. Fetal survival depends on maternal survival; therefore the pregnant woman must receive immediate stabilization and appropriate care for optimal fetal outcome.

Maternal Physiologic Characteristics

Providing optimal care for the pregnant woman after trauma depends on understanding the physiologic state of pregnancy and its effects on trauma. The pregnant woman's body will exhibit responses different from those of a nonpregnant person to the same traumatic insults. Because of the different responses to injury during pregnancy, management strategies must be adapted for appropriate resuscitation, fluid therapy, positioning, assessments, and most other interventions. Significant maternal adaptations and the relation to trauma are summarized in Table 21-11.

The uterus and bladder are confined to the bony pelvis during the first trimester of pregnancy and are at reduced risk for injury in cases of abdominal trauma. After pregnancy progresses beyond the fourteenth week, however, the uterus becomes an abdominal organ, and the risk for injury in cases of abdominal trauma increases. During the second and third trimesters the distended bladder becomes an abdominal organ and is at increased risk for injury and rupture. Bowel injuries occur less often during pregnancy than other times because of the protection provided by the enlarged uterus.

The elevated levels of progesterone that accompany pregnancy relax smooth muscle and profoundly affect the gastrointestinal tract. Gastrointestinal motility decreases, with a resultant increased time required for gastric emptying. Airway management of the unconscious pregnant woman therefore is of critical importance because of this increased risk for pulmonary aspiration of gastric contents (Lu & Curet, 2007).

A pregnant woman has decreased tolerance for hypoxia and apnea because of her decreased functional residual capacity and increased renal loss of bicarbonate. Acidosis develops more quickly in the pregnant than in the nonpregnant state.

Cardiac output increases 44% to 50% over prepregnancy values and is position dependent in the third trimester. Because of compression of the inferior vena cava and descending aorta by the pregnant uterus, cardiac output will decrease dramatically if the woman is placed in the supine position. Therefore the supine position must be avoided, even in women with cervical spine injuries.

Circulating blood volume increases 50% during gestation, and pregnant women can tolerate a large blood loss readily without demonstrating clinical signs. Hemodynamic instability that indicates the need for transfusion may not be apparent until blood loss nears 1000 to 2000 ml. Clinical signs of hemorrhage do not appear until after a 30% loss of circulating volume occurs (Lu & Curet, 2007).

Fetal Physiologic Characteristics

Perfusion of the uterine arteries, which provide the primary blood supply to the uteroplacental unit, depends on adequate maternal arterial pressure because these vessels lack autoregulation. Therefore maternal hypotension decreases uterine and fetal perfusion. Maternal shock results in splanchnic and uterine artery vasoconstriction, which decreases blood flow and oxygen transport to the fetus. EFM can assist in the evaluation of maternal status after trauma because it reflects fetal cardiac responses to hypoxia and hypoperfusion. Hypoperfusion may be present in the pregnant woman before she exhibits clinical signs of shock

TABLE 21-11

Maternal Adaptations during Pregnancy and Relation to Trauma

SYSTEM	ALTERATION	CLINICAL RESPONSES
Respiratory	↑ Oxygen consumption	↑ Risk of acidosis
	↑ Tidal volume	↑ Risk of respiratory mismanagement
	↓ Functional residual capacity	
	Chronic compensated alkalosis	↓ Blood-buffering capacity
	↓ $Paco_2$	
	↓ Serum bicarbonate	
Cardiovascular	↑ Circulating volume, 1600 ml	Can lose 1000 ml blood
	↑ CO	No signs of shock until blood loss >30% total blood volume
	↑ Heart rate	
	↓ SVR	
	↓ Arterial blood pressure	↓ Placental perfusion in supine position
	Heart displaced upward to left	Point of maximal impulse, fourth intercostal space
Renal	↑ Renal plasma flow	
	Dilation of ureters and urethra	↑ Risk of stasis, infection
	Bladder displaced forward	↑ Risk of bladder trauma
Gastrointestinal	↓ Gastric motility	↑ Risk of aspiration
	↑ Hydrochloric acid production	
	↓ Competency of gastroesophageal sphincter	Passive regurgitation of stomach acids if head lower than stomach
Reproductive	↑ Blood flow to organs	Source of ↑ blood loss
	Uterine enlargement	Vena caval compression in supine position
Musculoskeletal	Displacement of abdominal viscera	↑ Risk of injury, altered rebound response
	Pelvic venous congestion	Altered pain referral
	Cartilage softened	↑ Risk of pelvic fracture
		Center of gravity changed
	Fetal head in pelvis	↑ Risk of fetal injury
Hematologic	↑ Clotting factors	↑ Risk of thrombus formation
	↓ Fibrinolytic activity	

such as increased heart rate and decreased BP. The FHR tracing may reveal the earliest evidence of maternal compromise when it shows signs of fetal hypoxia, including tachycardia or late or prolonged decelerations, especially when associated with absent or minimal baseline variability.

Mechanisms of Trauma

Blunt-force abdominal trauma

MVAs account for the great majority of blunt-force abdominal trauma during pregnancy. Maternal and fetal mortality and morbidity rates after an MVA are directly correlated with whether the mother remains inside the vehicle or is ejected. Maternal death is usually the result of a head injury or exsanguination from a major vessel rupture. Serious retroperitoneal hemorrhage after lower abdominal and pelvic trauma is reported more frequently than normal during pregnancy. Serious maternal abdominal injuries are usually the result of splenic rupture or liver or renal injury. When the mother survives, abruptio placentae is the most common cause of fetal death (Gilbert, 2007). Placental separation is thought to be a result of deformation of the elastic myometrium around the relatively inelastic placenta. Shearing of the placental edge from the underlying decidua basalis results and is worsened by the increased intrauterine pressure resulting from the impact. All pregnant victims must be thoroughly evaluated for signs and symptoms of abruptio placentae after even minor blunt abdominal trauma.

Pelvic fracture may result from severe injury and may produce bladder trauma or retroperitoneal bleeding with the two-point displacement of pelvic bones that usually occurs. One point of displacement is commonly at the symphysis pubis, and the second point is posterior because of the structure of the pelvis. A thorough evaluation for clinical signs of internal hemorrhage is indicated.

Direct fetal injury as a complication of trauma during pregnancy most often involves the fetal skull and brain (Lu & Curet, 2007). Most commonly this injury accompanies maternal pelvic fracture in late gestation after the fetal head becomes engaged. When the force of the impact is great enough to fracture the maternal pelvis, the fetus will often sustain a skull fracture. Evaluation for fetal skull fracture or intracranial hemorrhage is indicated.

Uterine rupture as a result of trauma is rare, occurring in less than 1% of all reported cases of trauma during pregnancy. The likelihood of uterine rupture depends on numerous factors, including gestational age, the intensity of the impact, and the presence of a predisposing factor such as a distended uterus caused by polyhydramnios or multiple gestation or the presence of a uterine scar resulting from previous uterine surgery (Cunningham et al., 2005). When uterine rupture occurs, the force responsible is usually a direct, high-energy blow. Fetal death is common with traumatic uterine rupture. However, maternal death occurs less than 10% of the time, and, when it does, it is usually the result of massive injuries sustained from an impact severe enough to rupture the uterus.

Penetrating abdominal trauma

Bullet wounds are the most frequent cause of penetrating abdominal injury, followed by stab wounds. Penetrating abdominal wounds have disparate prognoses for mother and fetus in almost 66% of cases; that is, the woman survives, but the fetus does not. The enlarged uterus may protect other maternal organs, but the fetus is more vulnerable than the mother (Cunningham et al., 2005).

Numerous factors determine the extent and severity of maternal and fetal injury from a bullet wound, including size and velocity of the bullet, anatomic region penetrated, angle of entry, path of the bullet, organs damaged, gestational age, and exit wound. Once the bullet enters the body, it may ricochet several times as it encounters organs or bone, or it may sever a large blood vessel. During the second half of pregnancy the fetus usually sustains a direct injury from the bullet. Gunshot wounds require surgical exploration to determine the extent of injury and repair the damage as needed.

Stab wounds are limited by the length and width of the penetrating object and are usually confined to the pathway of the weapon. Maternal and fetal injury are less if the stab wound is located in the upper abdomen and from movement of the penetrating object from above the head downward toward the abdomen than from movement of the penetrating object from the ground upward toward the lower abdomen. Stab wounds usually require surgical exploration to clean out debris, determine extent of injury, and repair the damage.

Thoracic trauma

Thoracic trauma is reported to produce 25% of all trauma deaths. Pulmonary contusion results from nearly 75% of blunt thoracic trauma and is a potentially life-threatening condition. Pulmonary contusion can be difficult to recognize, especially if flail chest is also present or if no evidence of thoracic injury is noted. Pulmonary contusion should be suspected in cases of thoracic injury, especially after blunt-force acceleration or deceleration trauma, such as that occurring when a rapidly moving vehicle crashes into an immovable object.

Penetrating wounds into the chest can result in pneumothorax or hemothorax. This type of injury is usually caused by a vehicular crash that results in impalement by the steering column or a loose article in the vehicle that became a projectile with the force of impact. Stab wounds into the chest also may occur as a result of violence.

Management

Immediate stabilization

Immediate priorities for stabilization of the pregnant woman after trauma should be identical to those of the nonpregnant trauma patient. Pregnancy should not result in any restriction of the diagnostic, pharmacologic, or resuscitative procedures or maneuvers usually provided to trauma victims (AAP & ACOG, 2007). The initial response of many trauma team members when caring for the pregnant woman is to assess fetal status first because of the concern for a healthy neonate. Instead the trauma team should follow a methodical evaluation of maternal status to ensure complete assessment and stabilization of the mother. Fetal survival depends on maternal survival, and stabilization of the mother improves the chance of fetal survival.

NURSING ALERT Priorities of care for the pregnant woman after trauma must be to resuscitate the woman and stabilize her condition first and then consider fetal needs.

Primary survey

The systematic evaluation begins with a *primary survey* and the initial CABDs of resuscitation: *compressions, airway, breathing,* and *defibrillation.* If defibrillation is needed, the paddles need to be placed one rib interspace higher than usual because the heart is displaced slightly by the enlarged uterus.

NURSING ALERT Avoid hyperextension of the neck in the trauma victim; instead, use jaw thrust to establish an airway.

Once an airway is established, assessment should focus on adequacy of oxygenation. The chest wall is observed for movement. If breathing is absent, ventilations and endotracheal intubation are initiated. Guidelines for intubation and mechanical ventilation in pregnant women are similar to those for nonpregnant persons. Pregnant women, however, should be managed as high risk for aspiration because they are more likely to aspirate gastric contents than nonpregnant women (Lu & Curet, 2007). Supplemental oxygen should be administered with a tight-fitting, nonrebreathing facemask at 10 to 12 L/min to maintain adequate oxygen availability to the fetus. The chest wall is assessed for penetrating chest wound or flail chest. Breathing with a flail chest will be rapid and labored, chest wall movements will be uncoordinated and asymmetric, and crepitus from bony fragments may be palpated.

Rapid placement of two large-bore (14- to 16-gauge) IV lines is necessary in the majority of seriously injured patients. Placing the lines while veins are still distended is important. Cardiac arrest during the immediate stabilization period is usually the result of profound hypovolemia, necessitating massive fluid resuscitation. Because of the 50% increase in blood volume during pregnancy, published formulas for nonpregnant adults used for estimating crystalloid and blood replacement to counter blood loss must be adjusted upward.

Replacement of red blood cells and other blood components is anticipated, and blood is drawn for type, crossmatch, complete blood cell count, and platelet count. Infusion of type-specific whole blood or packed red blood cells is usually necessary to improve fetal oxygenation status and to replace blood loss. During an extreme emergency, type O Rh-negative blood may be administered without matching.

Vasopressor drugs to restore maternal arterial BP should be avoided, if possible, until volume replacement is administered. Although vasopressor agents result in decreased perfusion to the uterus, they should be given if needed for successful resuscitation of the mother (Lu & Curet, 2007).

After 24 weeks of gestation, venous return to the heart is best accomplished by positioning the uterus to one side to eliminate the weight of the uterus compressing the inferior vena cava or the descending aorta. This facilitates efforts to establish the forward flow of blood through resuscitation and stabilization (Lu & Curet, 2007). If a lateral position is not possible because of resuscitative efforts or cervical spine immobilization, manually deflect the uterus to the left, or place a wedge or rolled blanket or towel underneath the right side of the backboard or stretcher.

Cardiopulmonary resuscitation (CPR) for the pregnant woman

Fortunately, cardiac arrest is rare during pregnancy. Besides trauma, another common reason for performing CPR on a pregnant woman is airway obstruction caused by choking (Emergency box: Cardiopulmonary Resuscitation for the Pregnant Woman; Fig. 21-16). In nonpregnant persons, chest compressions are not particularly effective in establishing adequate cardiac output. Such is even more the case in pregnant women because of aortocaval compression caused by the gravid uterus. Therefore some authorities recommend open cardiac massage early in the resuscitation process to increase organ perfusion. If CPR is not effective within 4 to 5 minutes, perimortem cesarean birth is often recommended to facilitate resuscitative efforts (Cunningham et al., 2005; Lu & Curet, 2007). Removal of the stressor of pregnancy early in the process of resuscitation may increase the chances for both mater-

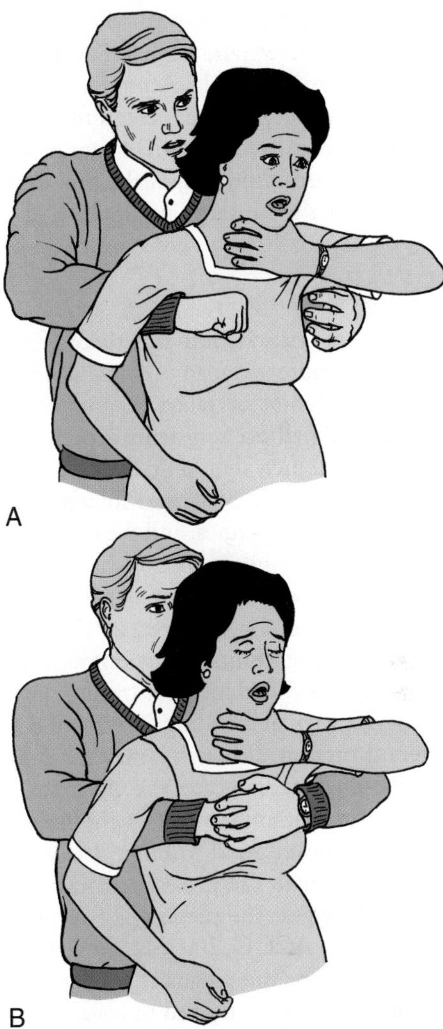

Fig. 21-16 Clearing airway obstruction in woman in late stage of pregnancy. **A,** Standing behind victim, place your arms under woman's armpits and across chest. Place thumb side of your clenched fist against middle of sternum, and place other hand over fist. **B,** Perform backward chest thrusts until foreign body is expelled or woman becomes unconscious (see Emergency box below).

EMERGENCY

Relief of Foreign Body Airway Obstruction

If the pregnant woman is unable to speak or cough, perform chest thrusts. Stand behind the woman and place your arms under her armpits to encircle her chest. Press backward with quick thrusts until the foreign body is expelled (see Fig. 21-16). If the woman becomes unconscious, carefully support her to the ground, immediately activate EMS, and begin CPR.

Data from Aufderheide T.P., Cave, D.M., Hazinski, M. F., et al: Part 5: Adult Basic Life Support: 2010 American Heart Association Guidelines for Cardiopulmonary Resuscitation and Emergency Cardiovascular Care Science. *Circulation 122*(Suppl 3), S685-S705.
CPR, cardiopulmonary resuscitation; *EMS,* emergency medical services.

nal and fetal survival. Cesarean birth should also be performed if the fetus is viable and maternal cardiopulmonary arrest appears to be untreatable. According to one study, 98% of infants born within 5 minutes of maternal cardiac arrest were neurologically normal. The rate of intact neonatal survival decreases, however, as the time from maternal arrest to delivery increases (Cunningham et al.; Lu & Curet).

Secondary survey

After immediate resuscitation and successful stabilization measures, a more detailed *secondary survey* of the mother and fetus should be taken. A complete physical assessment including all body systems is performed.

The maternal abdomen should be evaluated thoroughly because a large percentage of serious injuries involve the uterus, intraperitoneal structures, and the retroperitoneum. The greatest clinical concern after vehicular crashes is abruptio placentae, given that up to 40% of these women will have an abruption (Lu & Curet, 2007). Assessments should focus on recognition of this complication, with thorough evaluation of fetal monitor tracings, uterine tenderness, labor, or vaginal bleeding. Ultrasound does not reliably detect abruption, although it may be useful to help establish gestational age, locate the placenta, evaluate cardiac activity (to determine whether the fetus is alive), and determine amniotic fluid volume. Ultrasound may also be used to evaluate the presence of intraabdominal fluid that would suggest the presence of intraabdominal hemorrhage (AAP & ACOG, 2007; Lu & Curet).

Peritoneal lavage for the pregnant woman after blunt-force abdominal trauma has proved to be a safe procedure and can be helpful in the early diagnosis of intraperitoneal injury or hemorrhage. Under direct visualization the peritoneum is incised, and a peritoneal dialysis catheter is positioned. If aspiration yields free-flowing blood, the test is considered positive, and a laparotomy should be performed. This procedure is not necessary before laparotomy if intraperitoneal bleeding is clinically apparent. Indications for peritoneal lavage include abdominal symptoms or signs suggestive of intraperitoneal bleeding, alteration in mental status, unexplained shock, and multiple severe injuries (Cunningham et al., 2005).

If trauma is the result of a penetrating wound, the woman should be completely undressed and thoroughly examined for all entrance and exit wounds. A bullet may be located on x-ray films. Exploratory laparotomy is necessary after a gunshot wound to explore the abdominal cavity for organ damage and to repair any damage present, with full examination of all organs, the entire bowel, and posterior vessels. If uterine injury is determined, a thorough evaluation of the risks and benefits of cesarean birth is quickly accomplished. A cesarean birth is desirable if the fetus is alive and near term and may be necessary for the preterm fetus because of the high incidence of fetal injury in these cases. The fetus usually tolerates surgery and anesthesia if adequate uterine perfusion and oxygenation are maintained.

EMERGENCY

Cardiopulmonary Resuscitation for the Pregnant Woman

ASSESSMENT

- Determine unresponsiveness and no breathing or no normal breathing.
- Activate emergency medical system and get AED if available.
- Return to victim and check for pulse.
- Begin chest compressions if no pulse is felt.

COMPRESSIONS

- Position the woman on a flat, firm surface with her uterus displaced laterally with a wedge (e.g., a rolled towel placed under her hip) or manually or place her in a lateral position.
- Begin chest compressions at a rate of 100/min. Push hard and push fast1 AT the end of each compression allow chest to recoil (reexpand) completely.
  - Chest compressions may be performed slightly higher on the sternum if the uterus is enlarged enough to displace the diaphragm into a higher position.
- After five cycles of 30 compressions and two breaths (or approximately 2 min), check for a pulse. If no pulse is present, continue CPR.

AIRWAY

- Open airway using head tilt-chin lift maneuver.

BREATHING

- Deliver breaths using a face mask or bag-mask device if possible
- Deliver each breath over 1 second, watching for shec rise.
- Deliver breaths using a ratio of 30 chest compressions to 2 breaths.

DEFIBRILLATION

- Use an AED according to standard protocol to analyze heart rhythm and deliver shock if indicated.

Data from Aufderheide T.P., Cave, D.M., Hazinski, M. F., et al: Part 5: Adult Basic Life Support: 2010 American Heart Association Guidelines for Cardiopulmonary Resuscitation and Emergency Cardiovascular Care Science. *Circulation 122*(Suppl 3), S685-S705. *AED*, Automated external defibrillator; *CPR*, cardiopulmonary resuscitation.

Uterine contraction and FHR monitoring should be initiated soon after the woman is stable because abruptio placentae usually becomes apparent shortly after the injury. Even if frequent contractions are not present, the FHR tracing is reassuring, and no clinical evidence of placental abruption is seen, monitoring should still be continued for a minimum of 4 to 6 hours. Even with a reassuring FHR tracing, a small risk of abruption persists for up to several days following the trauma (Lu & Curet, 2007).

Ten to thirty percent of all pregnant trauma patients have some level of fetomaternal hemorrhage. Hemorrhage can lead to fetal anemia, distress, or even death. If the pregnant trauma victim is Rh negative, fetomaternal hemorrhage can result in sensitization and hemolytic disease of the neonate. All Rh-negative, unsensitized women should receive $Rh_o(D)$ immune globulin. KB testing is recommended for all Rh-negative women to determine the amount of hemorrhage and calculate the correct dose of $Rh_o(D)$ immune globulin. (AAP & ACOG, 2007; Lu & Curet, 2007).

In addition to assisting with stabilization of the woman, the nurse will likely be providing emotional support for the injured woman and her family. Other family members may also have been critically injured or killed. The nurse collaborates with staff members in other units of the same hospital, as well as at other hospitals, to make sure that questions are answered and consistent information is given. Grief support may also be necessary.

Follow-up care

With minor trauma the woman may be discharged home after an adequate period of EFM that demonstrates fetal reassurance and absence of uterine contractions (Cunningham et al., 2005). Her vital signs should be stable, with no evidence of bleeding at the time of discharge. No uterine contractions should be noted, and the FHR tracing should be reassuring before monitoring is discontinued and the woman discharged (Cunningham et al., 2005). The woman should be instructed to contact her health care provider immediately if changes in fetal movement or signs and symptoms indicative of preterm labor, PROM, or placental abruption develop.

If the trauma occurred as a result of an MVA, the woman should be reminded about the importance of using the seat belt harness for every trip, no matter how short, and given directions for positioning it properly. During pregnancy the shoulder strap should cross between the breasts and over the upper abdomen above the uterus. The lap belt should cross over the pelvis below the uterus (Gilbert, 2007) (see Fig. 7-17). If the trauma occurred as a result of domestic violence, the woman may need information about intimate partner violence (see Chapter 2); referral to a crisis center, law enforcement agency, or counseling center; and help in forming a safety plan.

KEY POINTS

- Hypertensive disorders during pregnancy are a leading cause of infant and maternal morbidity and mortality worldwide.
- The cause of preeclampsia is unknown, and no known reliable tests have been developed for predicting which women are at risk for this condition.
- Preeclampsia is a multisystem disease rather than only an increase in BP.
- HELLP syndrome, which usually becomes apparent during the third trimester, is a variant of severe preeclampsia, not a separate illness.
- Magnesium sulfate, the anticonvulsive agent of choice for preventing eclampsia, requires close monitoring of reflexes, respirations, and urinary output; its antidote, calcium gluconate, should be available on the unit.
- The intent of emergency interventions for eclampsia is to prevent self-injury, ensure adequate oxygenation, reduce aspiration risk, establish seizure control with magnesium sulfate, and correct maternal acidemia.
- The woman with hyperemesis gravidarum may have significant weight loss and dehydration; management focuses on restoring fluid and electrolyte balance and preventing recurrence of nausea and vomiting.
- Some miscarriages occur for unknown reasons, but fetal or placental maldevelopment and maternal factors account for many others.
- The type of miscarriage and signs and symptoms direct care management.
- Recurrent premature dilation of the cervix (incompetent cervix) may be treated with a cervical cerclage; the woman is instructed on activity restriction and recognizing the warning signs of preterm labor, PROM, and infection.
- Ectopic pregnancy is a significant cause of maternal morbidity and mortality.
- The two categories of gestational trophoblastic disease are (1) hydatidiform mole and (2) GTN. β-hCG titers are measured to confirm the diagnosis and to follow up after treatment.
- Premature separation of the placenta (abruptio placentae) and placenta previa are differentiated by the type of bleeding, uterine tonicity, and the presence or absence of pain.
- UTIs are the most common medical complication of pregnancy.
- Pyelonephritis is a serious medical complication of pregnancy and the most common nonobstetric cause of hospitalization during pregnancy.
- An enlarged uterus, displaced internal organs, and altered laboratory values may confound the differential diagnosis in the pregnant woman when the need for immediate abdominal surgery occurs.
- Preoperative care for a pregnant woman differs from that for a nonpregnant woman in one significant aspect: the presence of at least one other person, the fetus.
- MVAs, falls, and violence are the leading causes of blunt-force trauma during pregnancy.
- Fetal survival depends on maternal survival; after trauma the first priority is resuscitation and stabilization of the pregnant woman before consideration of fetal concerns.
- Even minor trauma can be associated with major complications for the pregnancy, including abruptio placentae, fetomaternal hemorrhage, preterm labor and birth, and fetal death.
- In the case of a cardiac arrest in a pregnant woman, the standard advanced cardiac life support guidelines should be implemented with a few slight modifications. The uterus must be displaced laterally and the defibrillation paddles should be placed one rib interspace higher.

Audio Chapter Summaries Access an audio summary of these Key Points on evolve

References

American College of Obstetricians and Gynecologists (ACOG). (2002). *Diagnosis and management of preeclampsia and eclampsia. ACOG Practice Bulletin No. 33.* Washington, DC: ACOG.

American College of Obstetricians and Gynecologists (ACOG) & American Academy of Pediatrics (AAP). (2007). Guidelines for perinatal care (6th ed.). Washington, DC: ACOG.

Bess, K. & Wood, T. (2006). Understanding gestational trophoblastic disease: How nurses can help those dealing with a diagnosis. *AWHONN Lifelines, 10*(4), 320-326.

Blackburn, S. (2007). *Maternal, fetal, & neonatal physiology: A clinical perspective* (3rd ed.). St. Louis: Saunders.

Butler, C., Kelsberg, G., St. Anna, L., & Crawford, P. (2005). How long is expectant management safe in first-trimester miscarriage? *Journal of Family Practice, 54*(10), 889-890.

Chan, P., & Winkle, C. (2006). *Gynecology and obstetrics: Current clinical strategies.* Laguna Hills, CA: CCS Publishing.

Cockey, C. (2005). Predicting preclampsia. *AWHONN Lifelines, 9*(1), 25-26.

Cohn, D., Ramaswamy, B., & Blum, K. (2009). Malignancy and pregnancy. In R. K. Creasy, R. Resnik, & J. D. Iams (Eds.), *Creasy and Resnik's maternal-fetal medicine: Principles and practice* (6th ed.). Philadelphia: Saunders.

Colombo, D., & Samuels, P. (2007). Renal disease. In S. Gabbe, J. Niebyl, & J. Simpson (Eds.), *Obstetrics: Normal and problem pregnancies* (5th ed.). Philadelphia: Churchill Livingstone.

Cunningham, F., Leveno, K., Bloom, S., Hauth, J., Gilstrap, L., & Wenstrom, K. (2005). *Williams obstetrics* (22nd ed.). New York: McGraw-Hill.

Davis, M. (2004). Nausea and vomiting of pregnancy: An evidence-based review. *Journal of Perinatal and Neonatal Nursing 18*(4), 312-328.

Duckitt, K., & Harrington, D. (2005). Risk factors for pre-eclampsia at antenatal booking: Systematic review of controlled studies. *British Medical Journal, 330*(7491), 565.

Duff, P., Sweet, R., & Edwards, R. (2009). Maternal and fetal infections.. In R. Creasy, R. Resnik, & J. Iams (Eds.), *Creasy and Resnik's maternal-fetal medicine: Principles and practice* (6th ed.). Philadelphia: Saunders.

Emery, S. (2005). Hypertensive disorders of pregnancy: Overdiagnosis is appropriate. *Cleveland Clinic Journal of Medicine, 72*(4), 345-352.

Farquhar, C. (2005). Ectopic pregnancy. *Lancet, 366*(9485), 583-591.

Francois, K., & Foley, M. (2007). Antepartum and postpartum hemorrhage. In S. Gabbe, J. Niebyl, & J. Simpson (Eds.), *Obstetrics: Normal and problem pregnancies* (5th ed.). Philadelphia: Churchill Livingstone.

Gilbert, E. (2007). *Manual of high risk pregnancy & delivery* (4th ed.). St. Louis: Mosby.

Gordon, M. (2007). Maternal physiology. In S. Gabbe, J. Niebyl, & J. Simpson (Eds.), *Obstetrics: Normal and problem pregnancies* (5th ed.). Philadelphia: Churchill Livingstone.

Hull, A., & Resnik, R. (2009). Placenta previa, placenta accrete, abruptio placentae, and vasa previa. In R. K. Creasy, R. Resnik, & J. D. Iams (Eds.), *Creasy and Resnik's maternal-fetal medicine: Principles and practice* (6th ed.). Philadelphia: Saunders.

Hutti, M. (2005). Social and professional support needs of families after perinatal loss. *Journal of Obstetric, Gynecologic, and Neonatal Nursing, 34*(5), 630-638.

Iams, J. (2009). Cervical insufficiency. In R. Creasy, R. Resnik, & J. Iams (Eds.), *Creasy and Resnik's maternal-fetal medicine: Principles and practice* (6th ed.). Philadelphia: Saunders.

Kelly, T., & Savides, T. (2009). Gastrointestinal disease in pregnancy. In R. Creasy, R. Resnik, & J. Iams (Eds.), *Creasy and Resnik's maternal-fetal medicine: Principles and practice* (6th ed.). Philadelphia: Saunders.

Labelle, C., & Kitchens, C. (2005). Disseminated intravascular coagulation: Treat the cause, not the lab values. *Cleveland Clinic Journal of Medicine, 72*(5), 377-397.

Longo, S., Dola, C., & Pridjian, G. (2003). Preeclampsia and eclampsia revisited. *Southern Medical Journal, 96*(9), 891-898.

Lu, E., & Curet, M. (2007). Surgical procedures in pregnancy. In S. Gabbe, J. Niebyl, & J. Simpson (Eds.). *Obstetrics: Normal and problem pregnancies* (5th ed.). Philadelphia: Churchill Livingstone.

Ludmir, J., & Owen, J. (2007). Cervical incompetence. In S. Gabbe, J. Niebyl, & J. Simpson (Eds.). *Obstetrics: Normal and problem pregnancies* (5th ed.). Philadelphia: Churchill Livingstone.

Lutz, K. (2005). Abused pregnant women's interactions with health care providers during the childbearing year. *Journal of Obstetric, Gynecologic, and Neonatal Nursing, 34*(2), 151-162.

Mattox, K., & Goetzl, L. (2005). Trauma in pregnancy. *Critical Care Medicine, 33*(10S), S385-S389.

Moodliar, S., Bagratee, J., & Moodley, J. (2005). Medical versus surgical evacuation of first-trimester spontaneous abortion. *International Journal of Gynecology and Obstetrics, 91*(1), 21-26.

Murray, H., Baakdah, H., Bardell, T., & Tulandi, T. (2005). Diagnosis and treatment of ectopic pregnancy. *Canadian Medical Association Journal, 173*(8), 905-912.

Nader, S. (2009). Thyroid disease and pregnancy. In R. Creasy, R. Resnik, & J. Iams (Eds.), *Creasy and Resnik's maternal-fetal medicine: Principles and practice* (6th ed.). Philadelphia: Saunders.

National High Blood Pressure Education Program Working Group on High Blood Pressure in Pregnancy. (2000). Report of the national high blood pressure education program working group on high blood pressure in pregnancy. *American Journal of Obstetrics and Gynecology, 183*(1), S1-S22.

Pandey, M., Rani, R., & Agrawal, S. (2005). An update in recurrent spontaneous abortion. *Archives of Gynecology and Obstetrics, 272*(2), 95-108.

Peters, R. (2008). High blood pressure in pregnancy. *Nursing for Women's Health, 12*(5), 410-421.

Pickering, T., Hall, J., Appel, L., Falkner, B., Graves, J., Hill, M., et al. (2005). Recommendations for blood pressure measurement in humans and experimental animals. Part I: Blood pressure measurement in humans: A statement for professionals from the subcommittee of professional and public education of the American Heart Association Council on High Blood Pressure Research. *Hypertension, 45*, 142-161.

Roberts, J., & Funai, E. (2009). Pregnancy-related hypertension. In R. Creasy, R. Resnik, & J. Iams (Eds.), *Creasy and Resnik's maternal-fetal medicine: Principles and practice* (6th ed.). Philadelphia: Saunders.

Rust, O., Atlas, R., Kimmel, S., Roberts, W., & Hess, L. (2005). Does the presence of a funnel increase the risk of adverse perinatal outcome in a patient with a short cervix? *American Journal of Obstetrics and Gynecology, 192*(4), 1060-1066.

Rust, O., & Roberts, W. (2005). Does cerclage prevent preterm birth? *Obstetric and Gynecology Clinics of North America, 32*(3), 441-456.

Sibai, B. (2007). Hypertension. In S. Gabbe, J. Niebyl, & J. Simpson (Eds.), *Obstetrics:*

Normal and problem pregnancies (5th ed.). Philadelphia: Churchill Livingstone.

Sibai, B., Dekker, G., & Kupferminc, M. (2005). Pre-eclampsia. *Lancet, 365*(9461), 785-799.

Simpson, J., & Jauniaux, E. (2007). Pregnancy loss. In S. Gabbe, J. Niebyl, & J. Simpson (Eds.), *Obstetrics: Normal and problem pregnancies* (5th ed.). Philadelphia: Churchill Livingstone.

Simpson, K., & James, D. (2005). *Postpartum care.* White Plains, NY: March of Dimes.

Velayuthaprabhu, S., & Archunan, G. (2005). Evaluation of anticardiolipin antibodies and antiphosphatidylserine antibodies in women with recurrent abortion. *Indian Journal of Medical Science, 59*(8), 347-352.

Wolfberg, A., Berkowitz, R., Goldstein, D., Feltmate, C., & Lieberman, E. (2005). Postevacuation hCG levels and risk of gestational trophoblastic neoplasia in women with complete molar pregnancy. *Obstetrics and Gynecology, 106*(3), 548-552.

Zhang, J., Gilles, J., Barnhart, K., Creinin, M., Westhoff, C., Frederick, M., et al. (2005). A comparison of medical management with misoprostol and surgical management for early pregnancy failure. *New England Journal of Medicine, 353*(8), 761-769.

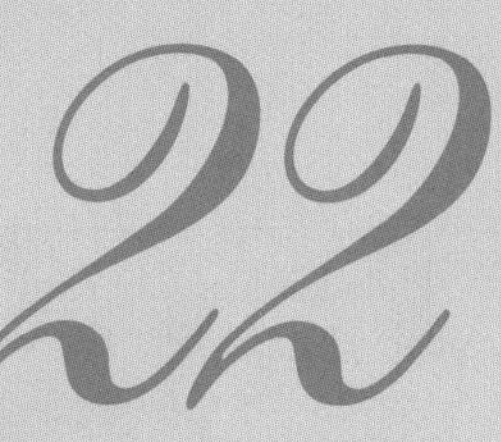

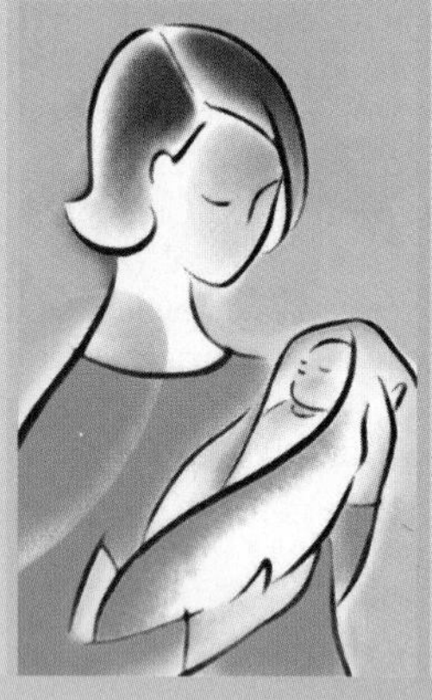

CHAPTER 22

Labor and Birth at Risk

KITTY CASHION

LEARNING OBJECTIVES

- *Differentiate between preterm birth and low birth weight.*
- *Identify the major risk factors associated with spontaneous preterm birth.*
- *Analyze current interventions to prevent spontaneous preterm birth.*
- *Discuss the use of tocolytics and antenatal glucocorticoids in preterm labor.*
- *Evaluate the effects of prescribed bed rest on pregnant women and their families.*
- *Design a nursing care plan for women with preterm premature rupture of membranes (preterm PROM).*
- *Summarize the nursing care for women having induction or augmentation of labor, forceps- and vacuum-assisted birth, cesarean birth, and vaginal birth after a cesarean birth.*
- *Explain the care of a woman with postterm pregnancy.*
- *Discuss obstetric emergencies and their appropriate management.*

KEY TERMS AND DEFINITIONS

anaphylactoid syndrome of pregnancy (ASP) Rare complication of pregnancy characterized by the sudden, acute onset of hypoxia, hypotension, or cardiac arrest and coagulopathy that can occur either during labor or during birth or immediately after birth; also known as amniotic fluid embolism

antenatal glucocorticoids Medications administered to the mother for the purpose of accelerating fetal lung maturity when an increased risk exists for preterm birth between 24 and 34 weeks of gestation

augmentation of labor Stimulation of ineffective uterine contractions after labor has started spontaneously but is not progressing satisfactorily

Bishop score Rating system to evaluate inducibility (ripeness) of the cervix; a higher score increases the likelihood of a successful induction of labor

cephalopelvic disproportion (CPD) Condition in which the infant's head is of such a shape, size, or position that it cannot pass through the mother's pelvis, or the maternal pelvis is too small, abnormally shaped, or deformed to allow the passage of a fetus of average size

cesarean birth Birth of a fetus by an incision through the abdominal wall and uterus

chorioamnionitis Inflammatory reaction in fetal membranes to bacteria or viruses in the amniotic fluid, which then become infiltrated with polymorphonuclear leukocytes

dysfunctional labor Abnormal uterine contractions that prevent normal progress of cervical dilation, effacement, or descent

dystocia Prolonged, painful, or otherwise difficult labor caused by various conditions associated with the five factors affecting labor (powers, passage, passenger, maternal position, and maternal emotions)

external cephalic version (ECV) Turning of the fetus to a vertex presentation by external exertion of pressure on the fetus through the maternal abdomen

forceps-assisted birth Vaginal birth in which forceps (i.e., curved-bladed instruments) are used to assist in the birth of the fetal head

hypertonic uterine dysfunction Uncoordinated, painful, frequent uterine contractions that do not cause cervical dilation and effacement; primary dysfunctional labor

hypotonic uterine dysfunction Weak, ineffective uterine contractions usually occurring in the active phase of labor; often related to cephalopelvic disproportion or malposition of the fetus; secondary uterine inertia

KEY TERMS AND DEFINITIONS—cont'd

late preterm birth Birth that occurs between 34 and 36 weeks of gestation

oxytocin Hormone produced by the posterior pituitary gland that stimulates uterine contractions and the release of milk in the mammary glands (let-down reflex); synthetic oxytocin is a medication that mimics the uterine stimulating action of oxytocin

postterm pregnancy Pregnancy that extends past 42 weeks of gestation

precipitous labor Rapid or sudden labor lasting less than 3 hours from the onset of uterine contractions to complete birth of the fetus

premature rupture of membranes (PROM) Rupture of the amniotic sac and leakage of amniotic fluid before the onset of labor at any gestational age

preterm birth Birth occurring before the completion of 37 weeks of gestation

preterm labor Uterine contractions causing cervical change that occur between 20 weeks and 37 weeks of pregnancy

preterm premature rupture of membranes (preterm PROM) Premature rupture of membranes that occurs before 37 weeks of gestation

prolapse of the umbilical cord Protrusion of the umbilical cord in advance of the presenting part

shoulder dystocia Condition in which the head is born but the anterior shoulder cannot pass under the pubic arch

therapeutic rest Administration of analgesics and implementation of comfort or relaxation measures to decrease pain and induce rest for management of hypertonic uterine dysfunction

tocolytics Medications used to suppress uterine activity and relax the uterus in cases of hyperstimulation or preterm labor

trial of labor (TOL) Period of observation to determine whether a laboring woman is likely to be successful in progressing to a vaginal birth

vacuum-assisted birth Birth involving attachment of a vacuum cap to the fetal head (occiput) and application of negative pressure to assist in birth of the fetus

vaginal birth after cesarean (VBAC) Giving birth vaginally after having had a previous cesarean birth

WEB RESOURCES

Additional related content can be found on the companion website at evolve

http://evolve.elsevier.com/Lowdermilk/Maternity/

- NCLEX Review Questions
- Animation: Breech Birth
- Animation: Breech Examination
- Animation: Cord Prolapse
- Animation: Shoulder Dystocia
- Case Study: Postdate Pregnancy
- Case Study: Preterm Labor
- Nursing Care Plan: Dysfunctional Labor: Hypotonic Uterine Dysfunction with Protracted Active Phase
- Nursing Care Plan: Preterm Labor
- Spanish Guidelines: Cesarean Birth
- Spanish Guidelines: Induction of Labor
- Video: Childbirth (Cesarean)

When complications arise during labor and birth, the risk of perinatal morbidity and mortality increases. Some complications are anticipated, especially if the woman is identified as high risk during the antepartum period; others are unexpected or unforeseen. A crucial responsibility for nurses is to understand the normal birth process to prevent and detect deviations from normal labor and birth and to implement nursing measures when complications arise. Optimal care of the laboring woman, fetus, and family experiencing complications is possible only when the nurse and other members of the obstetric team use their knowledge and skills in a concerted effort to provide competent and compassionate care. This chapter focuses on the problems of preterm labor and birth, dystocia, postterm pregnancy, and obstetric emergencies.

PRETERM LABOR AND BIRTH

Preterm labor is defined as cervical changes and uterine contractions occurring between 20 and 37 weeks of pregnancy. **Preterm birth** is any birth that occurs before the completion of 37 weeks of gestation (Iams & Romero, 2007). It occurs in approximately 12.8% of all live births, and the rate has been increasing for the last several years. Preterm birth is the major unsolved problem in perinatal medicine today (Iams, Romero, & Creasy, 2009).

Case Study: Preterm Labor

Approximately 75% of all preterm births are termed **late preterm births** because they occur between 34 and 36 weeks of gestation. Although these babies experience significant complications, the great majority of infant deaths and the most serious morbidity occur among the 16% of all preterm infants who are born before 32 weeks of gestation (Iams et al., 2009). See Chapters 18 and 24 for more discussion of problems related to late preterm birth.

Preterm Birth versus Low Birth Weight

Although they have distinctly different meanings, the terms *preterm birth* or *prematurity* and *low birth weight* were often used interchangeably in the past. Preterm birth describes the length of gestation (i.e., less than 37 weeks regardless of the weight of the infant), whereas low birth weight describes only weight at the time of birth (i.e., ≤2500 g). Because birth weight was far easier to determine than gestational age, in many settings and publications, low birth weight was used as a substitute term for preterm birth. Preterm birth, however, is a more dangerous health condition for an infant than low birth weight because a decreased length of time in the uterus correlates with immaturity of body systems. Low birth weight babies can be, but are not necessarily, preterm; low birth weight can be caused by conditions other than preterm birth, such as intrauterine growth restriction (IUGR), a condition of inadequate fetal growth not necessarily correlated with initiation of labor. On the other hand, infants born at a preterm gestation can weigh more than 2500 g at birth. Today, thanks to advances in pregnancy dating, outcomes related to gestational age can be increasingly distinguished from outcomes related to birth weight (Iams et al., 2009).

The incidence of preterm birth in developed countries has increased mainly as a result of more late preterm births and multifetal gestations. An increased use of assisted reproductive technologies has led to the rise in multifetal gestations (Iams et al., 2009). An increasing willingness on the part of health care providers to end the pregnancy when maternal or obstetric conditions threaten the health of mother or fetus after 32 to 34 weeks of gestation also contributes to the rise in preterm births (Iams & Romero, 2007).

Increasingly, preterm births are being divided into two categories, spontaneous and indicated. Spontaneous preterm births occur after an early initiation of the labor process. Conditions such as preterm labor with intact membranes, preterm premature rupture of membranes (preterm PROM), cervical insufficiency, or amnionitis often result in preterm birth. Approximately 75% of all preterm births in the United States are spontaneous (Iams et al., 2009). Box 22-1 lists risk factors for the development of spontaneous preterm birth.

Indicated preterm births, on the other hand, occur as a means to resolve maternal or fetal risk related to continuing the pregnancy. Approximately 25% of all preterm births in the United States are indicated because of medical or obstetric conditions that affect the mother, the fetus, or both. An increase in the number of indicated preterm births accounts for much of the recent rise in late preterm births (Iams et al., 2009). Box 22-2 lists common causes of indicated preterm births.

BOX 22-1

Risk Factors for Spontaneous Preterm Birth

- Genital tract infection
- African-American race
- Multifetal gestation
- Second-trimester bleeding
- Low prepregnancy weight
- History of previous spontaneous preterm birth

Source: Iams, J., Romero, R., & Creasy, R. (2009). Preterm labor and birth. In R. Creasy, R. Resnik, & J. Iams (Eds.), *Creasy and Resnik's maternal-fetal medicine: Principles and practice* (6th ed.). Philadelphia: Saunders.

BOX 22-2

Common Causes of Indicated Preterm Birth

- Preeclampsia
- Fetal distress
- Intrauterine growth restriction IUGR
- Abruptio placentae
- Intrauterine fetal demise
- Pregestational and gestational diabetes
- Renal disease
- Rh sensitization
- Congenital malformations

Source: Iams, J., Romero, R., & Creasy, R. (2009). Preterm labor and birth. In R. Creasy, R. Resnik, & J. Iams (Eds.), *Creasy and Resnik's maternal-fetal medicine: Principles and practice* (6th ed.). Philadelphia: Saunders.

The remainder of this section deals with spontaneous preterm labor and birth.

Predicting Spontaneous Preterm Labor and Birth

A history of previous preterm birth, multiple gestation, bleeding after the first trimester of pregnancy, and a low maternal body mass index have been shown to be major risk factors for spontaneous preterm birth (Iams & Romero, 2007). Other risk factors include non-Caucasian race (especially African-American), low socioeconomic and educational status, living with chronic stress, smoking, substance abuse, physically demanding working conditions, and periodontal disease (Iams et al., 2009). A recent study found that perceived levels of stress measured at 28 weeks of gestation in African-American women experiencing preterm labor were higher in those who gave birth prematurely than in those whose pregnancies reached term (Gennaro, Shults, & Garry, 2008). In addition, the risk for preterm birth appears to be genetically related. Relatives of women who were born prematurely or gave birth prematurely also have an increased risk for spontaneous preterm birth (Iams et al., 2009).

Many risk scoring systems have been developed in an attempt to determine which women might go into labor prematurely. None of these systems has been very successful, however, because at least 50% of all women who ultimately give birth prematurely have no identifiable risk factors (Iams & Romero, 2007; Iams et al., 2009). Therefore all women should be educated about prematurity not only in early pregnancy, but also in the preconceptional period.

Biochemical markers

Fetal fibronectin has been studied extensively and is currently marketed in the United States as a diagnostic test for preterm labor. Fetal fibronectin is a glycoprotein found in plasma produced during fetal life. The test is performed by collecting fluid from the woman's cervix and vagina using a swab during a vaginal examination. Fetal fibronectin is normally present in cervical and vaginal fluid early in pregnancy and then again in late pregnancy.

The presence of fetal fibronectin during the late second and early third trimesters of pregnancy may be related to placental inflammation, which is thought to be one cause of spontaneous preterm labor. The presence of fetal fibronectin is not very sensitive as a predictor of preterm birth, however. Before 35 weeks of gestation a positive fetal fibronectin test predicts preterm birth only approximately 25% of the time. The test's sensitivity may be better earlier in pregnancy. In one study the fetal fibronectin test predicted 65% of preterm births occurring before 28 weeks of gestation when it was performed between 22 and 24 weeks. The test is often used to predict who will *not* go into preterm labor because preterm birth is very unlikely to occur in women with a negative result. Use of the fetal fibronectin test in women who are at low risk for preterm birth as a screening tool is not recommended (Iams et al., 2009).

Cervical length

Another possible predictor of preterm birth is endocervical length. Changes in cervical length occur before uterine activity; therefore cervical measurement can identify women in whom the labor process has begun. However, because preterm cervical shortening occurs over a period of weeks, neither digital nor ultrasound cervical examination is very sensitive at predicting imminent preterm birth (Iams et al., 2009). Women whose cervical length is more that 30 mm are unlikely to give birth prematurely even if they have symptoms of preterm labor (Iams & Romero, 2007; Iams et al., 2009).

Causes of spontaneous preterm labor and birth

Infection is currently the only factor that has been definitely shown to cause preterm labor. Another proposed cause of preterm labor and birth is bleeding at the site of placental implantation in the uterus in the first or second trimester of pregnancy. The resulting uteroplacental ischemia or hemorrhage at the decidual layer of the placenta may somehow activate the preterm labor process. Intrauterine inflammation is associated with infection, uterine vascular compromise, and decidual hemorrhage, and may contribute to preterm labor. Maternal and fetal stress, uterine overdistention, allergic reaction, and a decrease in progesterone are other factors that may play a part in initiating preterm labor. That preterm labor is caused by multiple pathologic processes that eventually result in uterine contractions, cervical changes, or membrane rupture is becoming increasingly clear (Iams et al., 2009; Romero & Lockwood, 2009).

Two recent research studies suggest that recurrent preterm birth can be prevented in some women by administering prophylactic progesterone supplementation. In one study, women were given vaginal suppositories daily. In the other, women received weekly intramuscular injections of 17-alpha hydroxyprogesterone caproate. In both studies the risk of recurrent preterm birth was reduced by approximately one third. Exactly how progesterone works to prevent recurrent preterm birth is unclear; thus more study is necessary. Another important point to note is that prophylactic supplemental progesterone administration is recommended only for women who have previously given birth prematurely (Meis & Society for Maternal-Fetal Medicine, 2005; Romero & Lockwood, 2009).

CARE MANAGEMENT

Because all pregnant women must be considered at risk for preterm labor, assessment regarding knowledge of this condition begins early in pregnancy and continues throughout the prenatal period. Nursing diagnoses, interventions, and expected outcomes of care will be established for each woman based on her assessment findings (see the Nursing Process box: Preterm Labor and the Nursing Care Plan box: Preterm Labor).

Prevention

Primary prevention strategies that address risk factors associated with preterm labor and birth are less costly in human and financial terms than the high-tech and often lifelong care required by preterm infants and their families. Programs aimed at health promotion and disease prevention that encourage healthy lifestyles for the population in general and women of childbearing age in particular should be developed. Preconceptional counseling for women with a history of preterm birth may identify correctable risk factors. Smoking cessation, for example, has been shown to prevent preterm labor and birth (Freda, 2006; Iams et al., 2009). Many interventions intended to prevent spontaneous preterm birth have been recommended in the past and are still often prescribed. However, some of these interventions have not been shown to reduce the rate of preterm birth. Ongoing research is needed, especially given that our understanding of the pathophysiologic mechanisms of preterm birth is increasing (Iams et al., 2009).

NURSING PROCESS *Preterm Labor*

ASSESSMENT

Each pregnant woman should be assessed in regard to her knowledge of:

- Dangers of preterm birth
- Symptoms of preterm labor
- What to do if symptoms of preterm labor occur

- Also assess women experiencing preterm labor in regard to their:
  - Psychosocial status
  - Emotional status
  - Impact of diagnosis and treatment on family dynamics

NURSING DIAGNOSES

Nursing diagnoses that are relevant for women at risk for preterm birth include the following:

- *Risk for imbalanced fluid volume (maternal)* related to:
  - the administration of tocolytics to suppress preterm labor
- *Interrupted family processes* related to:
  - the required limitation on maternal activity associated with preterm labor
- *Anticipatory grieving* related to:
  - the potential for birth of the preterm infant
- *Risk for impaired parent-infant attachment* related to:
  - care requirements of the preterm infant

EXPECTED OUTCOMES OF CARE

Expected outcomes include that the woman will do the following:

- Learn the signs and symptoms of preterm labor and be able to assess herself and her need for intervention.
- Follow teaching suggestions and call her primary health care provider if symptoms occur.
- Not experience symptoms of preterm labor, or if she does, will take appropriate action.
- Maintain her pregnancy for at least 37 completed weeks.
- Give birth to a healthy, full-term infant.

PLAN OF CARE AND INTERVENTIONS

- Teach the symptoms of preterm labor (see Box 22-3).
- Teach appropriate responses if symptoms of preterm labor occur (see Teaching for Self-Management: What to Do if Symptoms of Preterm Labor Occur).
- Administer medications (e.g., corticosteroids and tocolytics) as ordered (see Medication Guides).
- Assist the woman and her family in making lifestyle modifications, if necessary, to decrease the risk of preterm birth.
- Assist in making plans to transport the pregnant woman-fetus to a hospital that is capable of providing care for the infant if preterm birth appears likely.
- Prepare to assist with stabilization and initial care of a preterm infant if birth appears imminent.

EVALUATION

The nurse can be reasonably assured that care was effective to the extent that the expected outcomes for care have been achieved.

Early Recognition and Diagnosis

Although preterm birth is often not preventable, early recognition of preterm labor is still essential in the effort to implement interventions that have been demonstrated to reduce neonatal morbidity and mortality These interventions include transfer of the mother before birth to a hospital equipped to care for her preterm infant, giving antibiotics in labor to prevent neonatal group B *Streptococcus* infection, and giving antenatal corticosteroids to the woman in preterm labor to prevent or reduce neonatal morbidity or mortality from conditions including respiratory distress syndrome, intraventricular hemorrhage, and necrotizing enterocolitis (Iams & Romero, 2007).

Because more than half of preterm births occur in women without obvious risk factors, all pregnant women should be taught the symptoms of preterm labor (Box 22-3). Pregnant women must also be taught what to do if the symptoms of preterm labor occur. Interventions must be initiated promptly to allow time for corticosteroid administration and transfer to a hospital capable of providing care for the infant. See Patient Instructions for Self-Management box: What to Do If Symptoms of Preterm Labor Occur for recommended actions. In particular,

BOX 22-3

Signs and Symptoms of Preterm Labor

UTERINE ACTIVITY

- Uterine contractions that occur more frequently than every 10 minutes persisting for 1 hour or more
- Uterine contractions that may be painful or painless

DISCOMFORT

- Lower abdominal cramping similar to gas pains; may be accompanied by diarrhea
- Dull, intermittent low back pain (below the waist)
- Painful, menstrual-like cramps
- Suprapubic pain or pressure
- Pelvic pressure or heaviness
- Urinary frequency

VAGINAL DISCHARGE

- Change in character and amount of usual discharge: thicker (mucoid) or thinner (watery); bloody, brown, or colorless; increased amount; odor
- Rupture of amniotic membranes

NURSING CARE PLAN *Preterm Labor*

NURSING DIAGNOSIS Deficient knowledge related to the recognition of preterm labor

Expected Outcome *Woman and significant other will verbalize the signs and symptoms of preterm labor.*

Nursing Interventions/*Rationales*

- Assess what the partners know about abnormal signs and symptoms during pregnancy *to identify areas of deficit.*
- Discuss signs and symptoms that serve as warning signs of preterm labor *so that the woman or her partner has adequate information to identify problems early.*
- Provide written supplemental materials that include a list of warning signs and instructions regarding what to do if any of the listed signs occur *so that the couple can reinforce and review learning and act swiftly and appropriately should a sign occur.*
- Discuss and demonstrate how to assess and time the contractions *to provide needed skills to assess the signs of labor.*

NURSING DIAGNOSIS Risk for maternal or fetal injury related to the recurrence of preterm labor

Expected Outcome *Woman demonstrates the ability to assess self for signs of recurring labor; maternal-fetal well-being is maintained.*

Nursing Interventions/*Rationales*

- Teach the woman and partner how to monitor uterine contraction activity daily *to provide immediate evidence of a worsening condition.*
- Teach the woman or partner to report rupture of membranes, vaginal bleeding, cramping, pelvic pressure, or low backache to the appropriate health care resource immediately *because such symptoms are signs of labor.*
- Teach the woman to monitor her weight, diet, fluid intake, and vital signs on a daily basis *to evaluate for potential problems.*
- Reinforce limitations of modified bed rest (resting most of the day on a couch, in a recliner, or in bed; bathroom privileges; up to the table for meals; allowed to shower daily) *to decrease the likelihood of the onset of labor.*
- Encourage the woman to use a side-lying position *to enhance placental perfusion.*
- Remind the couple to abstain from sexual intercourse and nipple stimulation if these activities cause uterine contractions *to decrease the likelihood of the onset of labor.*
- Teach relaxation techniques *to decrease uterine tone and decrease anxiety and stress.*
- Teach the woman to take tocolytic or other medications per physician's orders *to inhibit uterine contractions.*
- Teach the woman and partner about, and have them report, any medication side effects immediately *to prevent medication-induced complications.*
- Have the family arrange for alternative strategies for carrying out the woman's usual roles and functions *to decrease stress and limit temptations to increase activity.*
- If small children are part of the household, encourage the family to make alternative arrangements for child care *to enhance the woman's compliance with modified bed rest.*

NURSING DIAGNOSIS Anxiety related to preterm labor and potentially premature neonate

Expected Outcome *Feelings and symptoms of fear or anxiety are decreased.*

Nursing Interventions/*Rationales*

- Provide a calm, soothing atmosphere, and teach the family *to provide emotional support to facilitate coping.*
- Encourage the verbalization of fears *to decrease the intensity of emotional responses.*
- Involve the woman and family in the home management of her condition *to promote an increased sense of control.*
- Help the woman identify and use appropriate coping strategies and support systems *to reduce fear and anxiety.*
- Explore the use of desensitization strategies such as progressive muscle relaxation, visual imagery, or thought-stopping *to reduce fear-related emotions and related physical symptoms.*
- Provide information about online support groups *to reduce fear and anxiety.*

NURSING DIAGNOSIS Deficient diversional activity related to modified bed rest

Expected Outcome *The woman will verbalize diminished feelings of boredom.*

Nursing Interventions/*Rationales*

- Assist the woman in creatively exploring personally meaningful activities that can be pursued on modified bed rest *to ensure activities that have meaning, purpose, and value to the individual.*
- Maintain the emphasis on personal choices of the woman *because doing so promotes control and minimizes imposition of routines by others.*
- Evaluate the support and system resources that are available in the environment *to assist in providing diversional activities.*
- Explore ways for the woman to remain an active participant in home management and decision making *to promote control.*
- Engage support of the family and friends in carrying out chosen activities and making necessary environmental alterations *to ensure success.*
- Teach the woman about stress management and relaxation techniques *to help manage the tension of confinement.*

patient education regarding any symptoms of uterine contractions or cramping between 20 and 37 weeks of gestation should be directed toward telling the woman that these symptoms are not just normal discomforts of pregnancy, but rather indications of possible preterm labor (Fig. 22-1).

The diagnosis of preterm labor is based on three major diagnostic criteria:

1. Gestational age between 20 and 37 weeks
2. Uterine activity (e.g., contractions)
3. Progressive cervical change (e.g., effacement of 80%, or cervical dilation of 2 cm or greater)

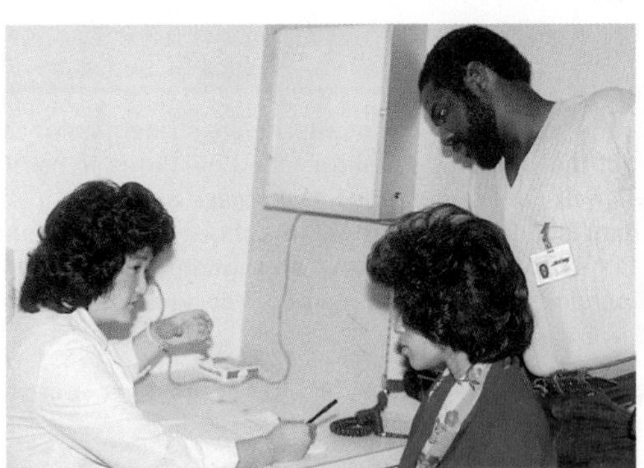

Fig. 22-1 Nurse teaching woman signs and symptoms of preterm labor. (Courtesy Marjorie Pyle, RNC, Lifecircle, Costa Mesa, CA.)

PATIENT INSTRUCTIONS FOR SELF-MANAGEMENT

What to Do if Symptoms of Preterm Labor Occur

- Empty your bladder.
- Drink two to three glasses of water or juice.
- Lie down on your side for 1 hour.
- Palpate for contractions.
- If symptoms continue, call your health care provider, or go to the hospital.
- If symptoms go away, resume light activity but not what you were doing when the symptoms began.
- If symptoms return, call your health care provider, or go to the hospital.
- If any of the following symptoms occur, call your health care provider immediately:
  - Uterine contractions every 10 minutes or less for 1 hour or more
  - Vaginal bleeding
  - Odorous vaginal discharge
  - Fluid leaking from the vagina

BOX 22-4

Adverse Effects of Bed Rest

MATERNAL EFFECTS (PHYSICAL)

- Weight loss
- Muscle wasting, weakness
- Bone demineralization and calcium loss
- Decreased plasma volume and cardiac output
- Increased clotting tendency; risk for thrombophlebitis
- Cardiac deconditioning
- Alteration in bowel function
- Sleep disturbance, fatigue
- Prolonged postpartum recovery

MATERNAL EFFECTS (PSYCHOSOCIAL)

- Loss of control associated with role reversals
- Dysphoria-anxiety, depression, hostility, anger
- Guilt associated with difficulty in complying with activity restriction and the inability to meet role responsibilities
- Boredom, loneliness
- Emotional lability (mood swings)

EFFECTS ON SUPPORT SYSTEM

- Stress associated with role reversals, increased responsibilities, disruption of family routines
- Financial strain associated with loss of maternal income and cost of treatment
- Fear and anxiety regarding the well-being of the mother and fetus

If the presence of fetal fibronectin is used as another diagnostic criterion, a sample of cervical mucus for testing should be obtained before an examination for cervical changes because the lubricant used to examine the cervix can reduce the accuracy of the test for fetal fibronectin.

Lifestyle Modifications

Activity restriction

Activity restriction, including bed rest and limited work, is a commonly prescribed intervention for the prevention of preterm birth. Bed rest, however, is not a benign intervention, and no evidence has been published in the literature to support the effectiveness of this intervention in reducing preterm birth rates (Iams et al., 2009). In fact, the American College of Obstetricians and Gynecologists (ACOG) (2003) states in its practice bulletin on management of preterm labor that bed rest should not be routinely recommended. Research indicates that bed rest causes adverse physical effects, including risk of thrombus formation, muscle atrophy, osteoporosis, and cardiovascular deconditioning (Iams & Romero, 2007). In many instances, these symptoms are not resolved by 6 weeks postpartum (Maloni & Park, 2005). Additionally, bed rest also affects women and their families psychologically, emotionally, socially, and financially. Box 22-4 lists adverse effects of bed rest.

Restriction of sexual activity

Restriction of sexual activity is also frequently recommended for women at risk for preterm birth. This intervention has not been shown to be effective at preventing preterm birth. However, sexual abstinence has not been studied in women with specific risk factors for preterm birth, such as a short cervix. Therefore more research is indicated (Iams et al., 2009). If, however, symptoms of preterm labor occur after sexual activity, then that activity may need to be curtailed until 37 weeks of gestation.

Home care

Women who are at high risk for preterm birth are commonly told that "taking it easy" at home for weeks or months would be best for them. Many health care providers now recommend only modified bed rest. The home care of the woman at risk for preterm birth is a challenge, however, for the nurse, who must assist the woman and her family in dealing with the many difficulties faced by families in which one member is incapacitated.

The woman's environment can be modified for convenience by using tables and storage units around her bed or couch to keep essential items within reach (e.g., telephone, television, radio, tape or compact disc player, computer with Internet access, snacks, books, magazines, newspapers, items for hobbies) (Fig. 22-2). Ensuring that the bed or couch is near a window and the bathroom is also helpful. Covering the bed with an egg crate mattress can relieve discomfort. Women often find that following a daily schedule of meals, activities, and hygiene and grooming (e.g., shower, dressing in street clothes, applying make-up) reduces boredom and helps them maintain control and normalcy. See the Patient Instructions for Self-Management box: Coping with Activity Restriction (in Chapter 21) for more information. With modified bed rest, women are usually allowed bathroom privileges for toileting and showering and can be up to the table for meals.

Suppression of Uterine Activity

Tocolytics are medications given to arrest labor after uterine contractions and cervical change have occurred. Usually, tocolytic therapy will not prolong the pregnancy long enough for further fetal growth or maturation to occur. Rather, the goal of tocolytic therapy is to delay birth long enough to institute interventions that have been demonstrated to reduce neonatal morbidity and mortality (Iams et al., 2009). Maternal and fetal contraindications to tocolytic therapy are listed in Box 22-5. Box 22-6 describes nursing care for women receiving tocolytic therapy.

Selecting the appropriate tocolytic medication requires consideration of each drug's effectiveness, risks, and side effects. No medication currently used for tocolysis in the United States has been approved by the U.S. Food and Drug Administration (FDA) for the purpose of arresting preterm labor. Instead, drugs marketed for other purposes, such as treatment of asthma or hypertension or as antiinflammatory or analgesic agents, are used on an "off-label" basis (i.e., drugs known to be effective for a specific purpose, although not specifically developed and tested for this purpose) (Iams et al., 2009). Important contraindications exist to the use of all tocolytics (see Box 22-5).

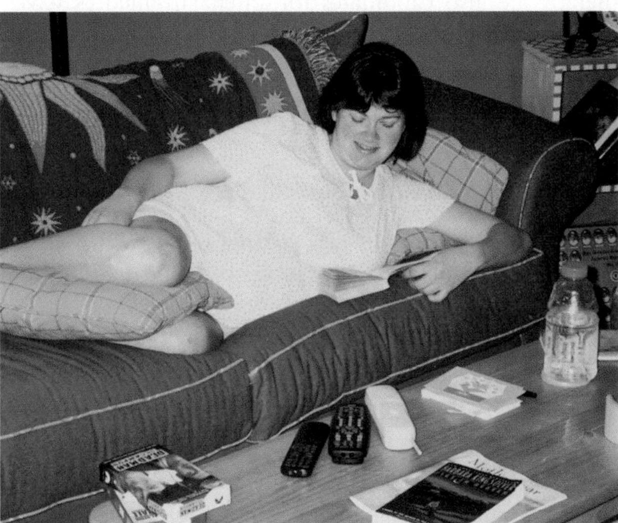

Fig. 22-2 Woman at home on restricted activity for preterm labor prevention. Note how she has arranged her daytime resting area so that needed items are close at hand. (Courtesy Amy Turner, Cary, NC.)

BOX 22-5

Contraindications to Tocolysis

MATERNAL
- Hypertension
- Significant vaginal bleeding
- Cardiac disease

FETAL
- Gestational age of 36 weeks or more
- Fetal demise
- Lethal fetal anomaly
- Chorioamnionitis
- Evidence of acute or chronic fetal compromise

Source: Iams, J., Romero, R., & Creasy, R. (2009). Preterm labor and birth. In R. Creasy, R. Resnik, & J. Iams (Eds.), *Creasy and Resnik's Maternal-fetal medicine: Principles and practice* (6th ed.). Philadelphia: Saunders.

BOX 22-6

Nursing Care for Women Receiving Tocolytic Therapy

- Explain the purpose and side effects of the tocolytic medication or medications ordered for the woman.
- Position the woman on her side to enhance placental perfusion and reduce pressure on the cervix.
- Monitor maternal vital signs, fetal heart rate, and labor status according to hospital protocol and professional standards.
- Assess the mother and fetus for signs of adverse reactions related to the tocolytic medication or medications being administered (see Medication Guide: Tocolytic Therapy for Preterm Labor).
- Determine maternal fluid balance by measuring daily weight and intake and output.
- Limit fluid intake to 2500-3000 ml/day, especially if a beta-adrenergic agonist is being administered.
- Provide psychosocial support and opportunities for the woman and family to express feelings and concerns.
- Offer comfort measures as necessary.
- Encourage diversional activities and relaxation techniques.

Magnesium sulfate is the most commonly used tocolytic agent because clinicians are familiar with its use as treatment of preeclampsia and its presumed safety as compared with beta-adrenergic agonists. Evidence for its effectiveness as a tocolytic is weak, however. Magnesium sulfate apparently promotes smooth-muscle relaxation by competing with calcium in cells (Iams & Romero, 2007; Rideout, 2005). Magnesium sulfate is administered intravenously. It may be a good choice for use in patients in whom other tocolytic agents are contraindicated (see Medication Guide: Tocolytic Therapy for Preterm Labor) (Iams & Romero, 2007; Iams et al., 2009).

Beta$_2$-adrenergic agonists have been widely used in the past as tocolytics. However, they have many maternal and fetal cardiopulmonary and metabolic adverse reactions in part related to beta$_1$-stimulation. Therefore they are increasingly being replaced by medications that are safer and have fewer side effects. Beta$_2$-adrenergic agonists should not be used in women with known or suspected heart disease, severe preeclampsia or eclampsia, pregestational or gestational diabetes, or hyperthyroidism (Iams & Romero, 2007; Iams et al., 2009) (see Medication Guide: Tocolytic Therapy for Preterm Labor).

Terbutaline (Brethine), the best-known beta-adrenergic agonist medication used for tocolysis, works by relaxing uterine smooth muscle as a result of stimulation of beta$_2$-receptors on uterine smooth muscle. A single dose of terbutaline given subcutaneously may help diagnose preterm labor. In one study, women whose contractions persisted or recurred after a single injection of terbutaline were more likely to actually be in preterm labor than those whose contractions ceased. Terbutaline is often given subcutaneously to facilitate maternal transfer to a tertiary-care center or to initiate tocolytic therapy while another agent with a slower onset of action is being administered concurrently. Long-term oral or subcutaneous administration of terbutaline has not been proven to be effective at reducing prematurity or neonatal morbidity (Iams & Romero, 2007; Iams et al., 2009).

Nifedipine (Adalat, Procardia), a calcium channel blocker, is another tocolytic agent that can suppress contractions. It works by inhibiting calcium from entering smooth-muscle cells, thus reducing uterine contractions. Because of its ease of administration and low incidence of significant maternal and fetal side effects, nifedipine's use is increasing. The drug is rapidly absorbed after oral administration. Maternal side effects, which include headache, flushing, dizziness, and nausea, are generally mild and relate primarily to hypotension that occurs with administration. However, at least one myocardial infarction has been reported in a young healthy woman who received a second dose of nifedipine. Nifedipine should not be combined with magnesium sulfate, given that concurrent administration can cause skeletal muscle blockade. It should also not be given along with or immediately after giving beta-mimetics (Iams & Romero, 2007; Iams et al., 2009). (see Medication Guide: Tocolytic Therapy for Preterm Labor).

Indomethacin (Indocin), a nonsteroidal antiinflammatory drug (NSAID), has been shown in some trials to suppress preterm labor by blocking the production of prostaglandins. Serious maternal side effects are uncommon, and indomethacin is usually well tolerated. However, three serious fetal or neonatal side effects have caused major concerns about its use as a tocolytic. These side effects include constriction of the ductus arteriosus, oligohydramnios, and neonatal pulmonary hypertension. Therefore limiting the use of indomethacin to a short duration of treatment in women with preterm labor at less than 32 weeks of gestation is recommended (Iams & Romero, 2007; Iams et al., 2009) (see Medication Guide: Tocolytic Therapy for Preterm Labor).

Promotion of Fetal Lung Maturity

Antenatal glucocorticoids

Antenatal glucocorticoids given as intramuscular injections to the mother to accelerate fetal lung maturity are now considered one of the most effective and cost-efficient interventions for preventing morbidity and mortality associated with preterm labor. Antenatal glucocorticoids have been shown to reduce significantly the incidence of respiratory distress syndrome, intraventricular hemorrhage, necrotizing enterocolitis, and death in neonates without increasing the risk of infection in either mothers or newborns (Mercer, 2009a). The National Institutes of Health consensus panel recommended that all women at 24 to 34 weeks of gestation be given a single course of antenatal glucocorticoids when preterm birth is threatened, unless evidence indicates that corticosteroids will have an adverse effect on the mother or birth is imminent. In general, women who are candidates for tocolytic therapy are also candidates for antenatal glucocorticoids (Mercer, 2009a). The regimen for the administration of antenatal glucocorticoids is given in the Medication Guide: Antenatal Glucocorticoid Therapy with Betamethasone, Dexamethasone.

NURSING ALERT All women between 24 and 34 weeks of pregnancy who are at risk for preterm birth within 7 days should receive treatment with a single course of antenatal glucocorticoids. Because optimal benefit begins 24 hours after the first injection, timely administration is essential (Mercer, 2009a).

Management of Inevitable Preterm Birth

Labor that has progressed to a cervical dilation of 4 cm or more is likely to lead to inevitable preterm birth. If birth appears imminent, preparations to care for a small, immature neonate should be made. Remember that women in preterm labor may rapidly progress to birth and that a very small fetus may be born through a cervix that is not completely dilated. Also, malpresentation (e.g., breech presen-

beta-adrenergic agonist = terbutaline

Medication Guide

Tocolytic Therapy for Preterm Labor

Medication and Action	Dosage and Route	Adverse Effects	Nursing Considerations
MAGNESIUM SULFATE			
• CNS depressant; relaxes smooth muscles including uterus	• Intravenous fluid should contain 40 g in 1000 ml, piggyback to primary infusion, and administer using controller pump • Loading dose: 4-6 g over 20-30 min • Maintenance dose: 1-4 g/hr • Use for stabilization only • Discontinue within 24-48 hours at the maintenance dose or if intolerable adverse reactions occur	Maternal adverse reactions: • Hot flushes, sweating, burning at the IV insertion site, nausea and vomiting, dry mouth, drowsiness, blurred vision, diplopia, headache, ileus, generalized muscle weakness, lethargy, dizziness • Hypocalcemia • SOB • Transient hypotension • Some reactions may subside when loading dose is completed Intolerable adverse reactions: • Respiratory rate fewer than 12 breaths/min • Pulmonary edema • Absent DTRs • Chest pain • Severe hypotension • Altered level of consciousness • Extreme muscle weakness • Urine output less than 25-30 ml/hr or less than 100 ml/4 hours • Serum magnesium level of 10 mEq/L (9 mg/dl) or greater Fetal (uncommon): • Decreased breathing movement, reduced FHR variability, nonreactive NST	• Assess woman and fetus to obtain baseline before beginning therapy and then before and after each incremental change; follow frequency of agency protocol • Monitor serum magnesium levels with higher doses; therapeutic range is between 4 and 7.5 mEq/L or 5-8 mg/dl • Discontinue infusion and notify physician if intolerable adverse reactions occur • Ensure that calcium gluconate 1 g (10 ml of 10% solution) or calcium chloride (normal dose is 500 mg IV infused over 30 min) is available for emergency administration to reverse magnesium sulfate toxicity • Should not be given to women with myasthenia gravis • Total IV intake should be limited to 125 ml/hr
BETA-ADRENERGIC AGONIST (BETA-MIMETIC)			
Terbutaline (Brethine) • Relaxes smooth muscles, inhibiting uterine activity, and causing bronchodilation	• Subcutaneous injection of 0.25 mg every 4 hrs • Treatment should last no longer than 24 hrs • Discontinue use if intolerable side effects occur	Maternal: (most are mild and of limited duration) • Tachycardia, chest discomfort, palpitations, arrhythmias • Tremors, dizziness, nervousness • Headache • Nasal congestion, • Nausea and vomiting • Hypokalemia • Hyperglycemia • Hypotension Intolerable adverse reactions: • Tachycardia greater than 130 beats/min • BP less than 90/60 mm Hg • Chest pain • Cardiac dysrhythmias • Myocardial infarction • Pulmonary edema	• Should not be used in women with a history of cardiac disease, pregestational or gestational diabetes, severe gestational hypertension, preeclampsia, eclampsia, migraine headaches or hyperthyroidism, or with significant hemorrhage • Myocardial infarction leading to death has been reported after use • Validate that woman is in PTL and is over 20 weeks and less than 35 weeks of gestation

Continued

Medication Guide

Tocolytic Therapy for Preterm Labor—cont'd

Medication and Action	Dosage and Route	Adverse Effects	Nursing Considerations

		Fetal:
		• Tachycardia
		• Hyperinsulinemia
		• Hyperglycemia
			• Assess woman and fetus according to agency protocol, being alert for adverse reactions
			• Assess maternal glucose and potassium levels before treatment is initiated and on occasion during treatment. Significant hyperglycemia (greater than 180 mg/dl) and hypokalemia (less than 2.5 mEq/L) may occur
			• Notify physician if the woman exhibits the following:
			  • Maternal heart rate greater than 130 beats/min; dysrhythmias, chest pain
			  • BP less than 90/60 mm Hg
			  • Signs of pulmonary edema (e.g., dyspnea, crackles, decreased Sao_2)
			  • Fetal heart rate greater than 180 beats/min
			• Hyperglycemia occurs more frequently in women who are being treated simultaneously with corticosteroids
			• Ensure that propranolol (Inderal) is available to reverse adverse effects related to cardiovascular function

CALCIUM CHANNEL BLOCKERS			
Nifedipine (Adalat, Procardia) • Relax smooth muscles including the uterus by blocking calcium entry	• Initial dose: 10-20 mg, orally, every 3 to 6 hours until contractions are rare, followed by long-acting formulations of 30 or 60 mg every 8–12 hrs for 48 hrs while corticosteroids are being given (however, the ideal dose has not been established)	Maternal (most effects are mild) • Hypotension • Headache • Flushing • Dizziness, • Nausea Fetal: • Hypotension (questionable)	• Avoid concurrent use with magnesium sulfate because skeletal muscle blockade can result • Should not be given simultaneously with or immediately after terbutaline because of effects on heart rate and blood pressure • Assess woman and fetus according to agency protocol, being alert for adverse reactions • Do not use sublingual route of administration

Medication Guide

Tocolytic Therapy for Preterm Labor—cont'd

Medication and Action	Dosage and Route	Adverse Effects	Nursing Considerations
PROSTAGLANDIN SYNTHETASE INHIBITORS (NSAIDs)			
Indomethacin (Indocin) • Relaxes uterine smooth muscle by inhibiting prostaglandins	• Loading dose: 50 mg orally, then 25-50 mg orally every 6 hours for 48 hours	Maternal (common) • Nausea and vomiting • Heartburn Less common, but more serious: • Gastrointestinal bleeding • Prolonged bleeding time • Thrombocytopenia • Asthma in aspirin-sensitive patients Fetal: • Constriction of ductus arteriosus • Oligohydramnios, caused by reduced fetal urine production • Neonatal pulmonary hypertension	• The long acting formulations decrease the incidence of adverse effects • Used only if gestational age is less than 32 weeks • Administer for 48 hours or less • Do not use in women with renal or hepatic disease, active peptic ulcer disease, poorly controlled hypertension, asthma, or coagulation disorders • Can mask maternal fever • Assess woman and fetus according to agency policy, being alert for adverse reactions • Determine amniotic fluid volume and function of fetal ductus arteriosus before initiating therapy and within 48 hours of discontinuing therapy; assessment is critical if therapy continues for more than 48 hours • Administer with food to decrease GI distress • Monitor for signs of postpartum hemorrhage

Sources: Gilbert, E., (2007). *Manual of high risk pregnancy and delivery* (4th ed.). St. Louis: Mosby; Iams, J., & Romero, R. (2007). Preterm birth. In S. Gabbe, J. Niebyl, & J. Simpson (Eds.), *Obstetrics: Normal and problem pregnancies* (5th ed.). Philadelphia: Churchill Livingstone; Iams, J., Romero, R., & Creasy, R. (2009). Preterm labor and birth. In R. Creasy, R. Resnik, & J. Iams (Eds.), *Creasy and Resnik's maternal-fetal medicine: Principles and practice* (6th ed.). Philadelphia: Saunders.

CNS, Central nervous system; *DTRs,* deep tendon reflexes; *FHR,* fetal heart rate; *GI,* gastrointestinal; *NSAIDs,* nonsteroidal antiinflammatory drugs; *NST,* nonstress test; *PTL,* preterm labor; *Sao_2,* arterial oxygen saturation; *SOB,* shortness of breath.

Medication Guide

Antenatal Glucocorticoid Therapy with Betamethasone, Dexamethasone

ACTION

- Stimulates fetal lung maturation by promoting release of enzymes that induce production or release of lung surfactant. NOTE: The U.S. Food and Drug Administration has not approved these medications for this use (i.e., this is an unlabeled use for obstetrics).

INDICATION

- To accelerate lung maturity in fetuses between 24 and 34 weeks of gestation

DOSAGE AND ROUTE

- Betamethasone: 12 mg intramuscularly (IM) for two doses 24 hr apart
- Dexamethasone: 6 mg IM for four doses 12 hr apart

ADVERSE REACTIONS

- Pulmonary edema (if given with beta-adrenergic medications)
- May worsen maternal condition (diabetes, hypertension).

NURSING CONSIDERATIONS

- Give deep IM injection in gluteal or vastus lateralis muscle.
- Medication *must* be given by IM injection; oral administration is *not* an acceptable alternative.
- Injection is painful.
- Assess blood glucose levels. Women with diabetes whose blood sugars previously have been well controlled may require increased insulin doses for several days.

EVIDENCE-BASED PRACTICE

Corticosteroids for Lung Maturity in Preterm Labor: One Course or Two?

Pat Gingrich

ASK THE QUESTION

What can we tell our patients about the use of antenatal corticosteroids (betamethasone) to accelerate fetal lung maturity in women at risk for preterm birth?

SEARCH FOR EVIDENCE

Search Strategies: Professional organization guidelines, meta-analyses, systematic reviews, randomized controlled trials, nonrandomized prospective studies, and retrospective studies since 2006.

Databases Searched: CINAHL, Cochrane, Medline, National Guideline Clearinghouse, and TRIP Database Plus.

CRITICALLY ANALYZE THE EVIDENCE

Preterm infants are at increased risk for respiratory distress syndrome if they are born before their lungs are producing adequate surfactant. To mature the fetal lungs before birth, women at risk for preterm birth are given an antenatal course of corticosteroids. A Cochrane systematic review of 21 trials involving 3885 women and 4269 infants examined outcomes when women were given a course of corticosteroids before the birth. The reviewers found a decrease in the following unwanted outcomes: neonatal death, cerebral hemorrhage, necrotizing enterocolitis, need for respiratory support, neonatal intensive care unit admission, and infection in the first 48 hours (Roberts & Dalziel, 2006). In addition, corticosteroids improved outcomes in the presence of premature rupture of membranes and gestational hypertension. The benefits were so great that the reviewers supported this single course of corticosteroids as a routine for nearly all women at risk for preterm birth.

One dramatic retrospective cohort study of 23-week gestation newborns (an age usually considered only marginally viable) found an 82% reduction in deaths if the woman completed a course of corticosteroids before the birth (Hayes et al., 2008).

When treated women manage to remain pregnant for another week or more, do therapy benefits remain? A retrospective cohort study of 357 women, treated initially at 26 to 34 weeks of gestation, looked at infant outcomes. The authors found that when the interval between treatment and birth exceeded 14 days, the need for ventilatory support and surfactant use was significantly higher than when the treatment-to-birth interval was 2 to 14 days (Ring, Garland, Stafeil, Carr, Peckman, & Percon, 2007).

If therapy benefits diminish across time while remaining pregnant, should therapy be repeated, and when? Another Cochrane systematic review examined five randomized, controlled trials involving 2000 women who were 23 to 33 weeks pregnant at the time of their first course of corticosteroids and who remained pregnant at least another 7 days. The authors found that repeat courses of corticosteroids after 7 days decreased the occurrence and severity of neonatal lung disease during the first few weeks of life (Crowther & Harding, 2007). However, retreatment was also associated with reduced size at birth and an increased risk for cesarean birth. These reviewers still recommended the second course because of the short-term benefit but called for more long-term studies.

IMPLICATIONS FOR PRACTICE

The prospect of preterm birth can be terribly unsettling to prospective parents who worry about their baby being born at risk for complications. Here is a treatment that offers dramatically improved odds of survival, with fewer complications. Although the decisions to treat women at risk for preterm birth with corticosteroids once or twice remain in the medical domain, labor and birth nurses who give the medications need to understand the current evidence and be able to communicate the risks and benefits to their patients.

References:

Crowther, C. A., & Harding, J. E. (2007). Repeat doses of prenatal corticosteroids for women at risk for preterm birth for preventing neonatal respiratory disease. In *The Cochrane Database of Systematic Reviews,* 2007, Issue 3, Art. No.: CD 003935.

Hayes, E. J., Paul, D. A., Stahl, G. E., Seibel-Seamon, J., Dysart, K., Leiby, B. E., et al. (2008). Effect of antenatal corticosteroids on survival for neonates at 23 weeks gestation. *Obstetrics and Gynecology, 111*(4), 921-926.

Ring, A. M., Garland, J. S., Stafeil, B. R., Carr, M. N., Peckman, G. S., & Percon, R. A. (2007). The effect of a prolonged time interval between antenatal corticosteroid administration and delivery on outcomes in preterm neonates: A cohort study. *American Journal of Obstetrics and Gynecology, 196*(5), 457, e1-e6.

Roberts, D., & Dalziel, S. (2006). Antenatal corticosteroids for accelerating fetal lung maturation for women at risk for preterm birth. In *The Cochrane Database of Systematic Reviews,* 2006, Issue 3, Art. No.: CD 004454.

tation) occurs much more frequently in preterm than in term fetuses. Therefore nurses must be prepared to handle the emergency birth of a preterm infant, from either cephalic or breech presentation, without the woman's health care provider being present. Personnel skilled at neonatal resuscitation should be present at the time of birth. Equipment, supplies, and medications used for neonatal resuscitation should be gathered in advance and prepared for immediate use. If birth occurs in a hospital that is not prepared to provide continuing care for a preterm neonate, plans for transfer of the baby to a higher level of care should be made immediately.

Fetal and Early Neonatal Loss

Preterm birth or the presence of congenital anomalies or genetic disorders incompatible with life are major reasons for intrauterine fetal demise (stillbirth) or early neonatal death. In many of these situations, the parents will have already been told that the fetus has died or that the baby has a condition that is incompatible with life and will most likely die very soon after birth. Sometimes, however, the fetal death will be unexpected, diagnosed only after the woman has been admitted to the labor and birth unit. Whatever the case, labor and birth nurses must be prepared to provide sensitive care to these patients and their families.

If fetal or early neonatal death is expected, the parents and members of the health care team need to discuss the situation before the birth and decide on a management plan that is acceptable to everyone. One major decision that must be made is whether the parents desire cesarean birth if an abnormal fetal heart rate (FHR) tracing is detected. If cesarean birth is not desired, usually the FHR will not be monitored during labor.

Another major decision is whether to attempt neonatal resuscitation, and to what lengths resuscitation should go. Sometimes the feasibility of neonatal resuscitation cannot be determined until the baby's size and physical appearance have been assessed after birth. If the baby is too small, too immature, or too malformed for effective resuscitation, comfort care can be provided instead. The baby is kept warm and comfortable, either at the mother's bedside or in the nursery, depending on the parents' desires, until death occurs. Parents can choose to view and hold the baby as they wish.

After the birth, the woman should be given the opportunity to decide if she wants to stay on the maternity unit or be moved to another hospital unit instead. She may prefer to be away from the sound of crying babies and exposure to other families who have had healthy infants. On the other hand, postpartum care and grief support may not be as good on another hospital unit where the staff is not experienced in postpartum and bereavement care.

Whether death occurs in utero or after birth, parents are faced with the same needs. See Chapter 24 for additional information on dealing with families experiencing a perinatal loss.

PREMATURE RUPTURE OF MEMBRANES

Premature rupture of membranes (PROM) is the spontaneous rupture of the amniotic sac and leakage of amniotic fluid beginning before the onset of labor at any gestational age (Mercer, 2007). **Preterm premature rupture of membranes (preterm PROM)** (i.e., membranes rupture before 37 weeks of gestation) is responsible for approximately one third of all preterm births (Mercer, 2007). Preterm PROM most likely results from pathologic weakening of the fetal membranes caused by inflammation, stress from uterine contractions, or other factors that cause increased uterine pressure. Infection of the urogenital tract is associated with preterm PROM (Mercer, 2007; Mercer, 2009b). Preterm PROM is diagnosed after the woman reports either a sudden gush of fluid or a slow leak of fluid from the vagina.

Chorioamnionitis (i.e., infection of the amniotic cavity) is the most common maternal complication of preterm PROM. Other less-common but serious maternal complications include placental abruption, sepsis, and death (Mercer, 2007; Mercer, 2009b). Fetal complications from preterm PROM are related primarily to intrauterine infection, umbilical cord compression, and placental abruption. Another possible fetal complication when preterm PROM occurs before 20 weeks of gestation is pulmonary hypoplasia (Mercer, 2009b).

Management

Management of PROM is determined individually for each woman based on an assessment of the estimated risk of maternal, fetal, and neonatal complications if pregnancy is allowed to continue or immediate labor and birth are attempted. At term, because infection is the greatest maternal, fetal, and neonatal risk, birth is the best option. Labor will most likely be induced if it does not begin spontaneously soon after PROM occurs (Mercer, 2009b).

Preterm PROM is often managed expectantly or conservatively if the risks to the fetus and newborn associated with preterm birth are considered to be greater than the risks of infection. Women with preterm PROM are usually hospitalized in an attempt to prolong the pregnancy and allow additional time for fetal maturation unless intrauterine infection, significant vaginal bleeding, placental abruption, preterm labor, or fetal compromise occurs (Mercer, 2009b).

Conservative management of preterm PROM includes daily fetal assessment, usually by a nonstress test (NST) and a biophysical profile (BPP). (See Chapter 19 for further discussion of these tests.) In addition the woman will be monitored for labor, placental abruption, and the development of intrauterine infection. Antenatal corticosteroids will be administered to women who are at less than 32 weeks of gestation, because they have been proven to decrease the risk of several neonatal complications including respiratory distress syndrome, intraventricular hemorrhage, and necrotizing enterocolitis. In addition, a 7-day course of broad-spectrum antibiotics (e.g., ampicillin, erythromycin) will be administered to treat or prevent intrauterine infection (Mercer, 2007; Mercer, 2009b).

Vigilance for signs of infection is a major part of the nursing care and patient education after preterm PROM. The woman must be taught how to keep her genital area clean and that nothing should be introduced into her vagina. Signs of infection (e.g., fever, foul-smelling vaginal discharge, rapid pulse) should be reported to the primary health care provider immediately (see Patient Instructions for Self-Management box: The Woman with Preterm Premature Rupture of Membranes). If chorioamnionitis develops, labor will be induced. Should preterm labor occur, tocolytic medications may be administered in an attempt to gain time for transporting the woman to a hospital capable of providing care to a preterm infant or for antenatal corticosteroids or antibiotics to reach effective levels (Gilbert, 2007; Mercer, 2007).

PATIENT INSTRUCTIONS FOR SELF-MANAGEMENT

The Woman with Preterm Premature Rupture of Membranes

- Take your temperature every 4 hours when awake.
- Report temperature of more than 38° C (100.4° F).
- Remain on modified bed rest.
- Insert nothing in the vagina.
- Do not engage in sexual activity.
- Assess for uterine contractions.
- Do fetal movement counts daily.
- Do not take tub baths.
- Watch for foul-smelling vaginal discharge or if uterus becomes tender or sore when touched.
- Wipe front to back after urinating or having a bowel movement.
- Take antibiotics if prescribed.
- See primary health care provider as scheduled.

DYSTOCIA

A long, difficult, or abnormal labor is known as *dysfunctional labor,* or *dystocia;* it is caused by various conditions associated with the five factors affecting labor. Estimates suggest that dysfunctional labor occurs in approximately 8% to 11% of all births (Gilbert, 2007). Dystocia is the second most common indication for cesarean birth after previous cesarean birth (Nielsen, Galan, Kilpatrick, & Garrison, 2007). Dystocia can be caused by any one of the following:

- Ineffective uterine contractions or maternal bearing-down efforts (the powers), the most common cause of dystocia (Cunningham, Leveno, Bloom, Hauth, Gilstrap, & Wenstrom, 2005)
- Alterations in the pelvic structure (the passage)
- Fetal causes that include abnormal presentation or position, anomalies, excessive size, and number of fetuses (the passenger)
- Maternal position during labor and birth
- Psychologic responses of the mother to labor related to past experiences, preparation, culture and heritage, and support system

These five factors are interdependent. In assessing the woman for an abnormal labor pattern, the nurse must consider the way in which these factors interact and influence labor progress. Dystocia is suspected when the characteristics of uterine contractions are altered or when progress in the rate of cervical dilation or progress in fetal descent and expulsion is lacking.

e Nursing Care Plan: Dysfunctional Labor

Dysfunctional Labor

Dysfunctional labor is described as abnormal uterine contractions that prevent the normal progress of cervical dilation, effacement (primary powers), or descent (secondary powers). Gilbert (2007) cited several factors that seem to increase a woman's risk for uterine dystocia, including the following:

- Overweight
- Short stature
- Advanced maternal age
- Infertility difficulties
- Uterine abnormalities (e.g., congenital malformations; overdistention, as with multiple gestation; or polyhydramnios)
- Malpresentations and positions of the fetus
- Cephalopelvic disproportion (or fetopelvic disproportion)
- Uterine overstimulation with oxytocin
- Maternal fatigue, dehydration and electrolyte imbalance, and fear
- Inappropriate timing of analgesic or anesthetic administration

Abnormal uterine activity can be further described as being *hypertonic or hypotonic.* Contractions may be frequent and painfully strong with hypertonic uterine activity but are ineffective at promoting cervical effacement and dilation. With hypotonic uterine activity, on the other hand, the rise in uterine pressure generated during contractions is insufficient to promote cervical effacement and dilation (Gilbert, 2007).

Hypertonic uterine dysfunction

The woman experiencing **hypertonic uterine dysfunction,** or primary dysfunctional labor, is often an anxious first-time mother who is having painful and frequent contractions that are ineffective in causing cervical dilation or effacement to progress. These contractions usually occur in the latent phase of first stage labor (cervical dilation of less than 4 cm) and are usually uncoordinated. The force of the contractions may be in the midsection of the uterus rather than in the fundus. Therefore the uterus is unable to apply downward pressure to push the presenting part against the cervix. The uterus may not relax completely between contractions.

Women with hypertonic uterine dysfunction may be exhausted and express concern about loss of control because of the intense pain they are experiencing and the lack of progress. **Therapeutic rest,** which is achieved with a warm bath or shower and the administration of analgesics such as morphine, meperidine (Demerol), or nalbuphine (Nubain) or sedatives such as zolpidem (Ambien) to inhibit uterine contractions, reduce pain, and encourage sleep, is usually prescribed for the management of hypertonic uterine dysfunction (Battista & Wing, 2007; Gilbert, 2007). (See Nursing Care Plan: Dysfunctional Labor: Hypotonic Uterine Dysfunction with Protracted Active Phase on this book's Evolve website).

Hypotonic uterine dysfunction

The second and more common type of uterine dysfunction is **hypotonic uterine dysfunction,** or secondary uterine inertia. The woman initially makes normal progress into the active phase of labor; then the contractions become weak and inefficient or stop altogether. The uterus is easily indented, even at the peak of contractions. Intrauterine pressure during the contraction is insufficient for progress of cervical effacement and dilation. Cephalopelvic disproportion and malposition are common causes of this type of uterine dysfunction.

A woman with hypotonic uterine dysfunction may become exhausted and be at increased risk for infection. Management usually consists of inserting an intrauterine pressure catheter (IUPC) to evaluate uterine activity accurately. If the contractions are not strong enough to cause cervical change, then labor is augmented with oxytocin (Pitocin) (Battista & Wing, 2007).

Secondary powers

Secondary powers, or bearing-down efforts, are compromised when large amounts of analgesic medications are given. Anesthesia may also block the bearing-down reflex and, as a result, alter the effectiveness of voluntary efforts. Exhaustion resulting from lack of sleep or long labor and fatigue resulting from inadequate hydration and food intake reduce the effectiveness of the woman's voluntary efforts. Maternal position can work against the forces of gravity and decrease the strength and efficiency of the contractions.

Nursing interventions to improve maternal bearing-down efforts include helping the woman to find comfortable positions for pushing and coaching her to push effectively. See Chapter 12 for further discussion of second stage labor management. If the woman is unable to give birth spontaneously, assisted vaginal birth using a vacuum or forceps or cesarean birth will be necessary. See discussion of forceps- and vacuum-assisted vaginal birth and cesarean birth later in this chapter.

Abnormal labor patterns

Six abnormal labor patterns were identified and classified by Friedman (1989) according to the nature of the cervical dilation and fetal descent. These patterns include (1) prolonged latent phase, (2) protracted active phase dilation, (3) secondary arrest: no change, (4) protracted descent, (5) arrest of descent, and (6) failure of descent. Table 22-1 further describes these abnormal labor patterns. These abnormal labor patterns may result from a variety of causes, including ineffective uterine contractions, pelvic contractures, cephalopelvic disproportion, abnormal fetal presentation or position, early use of analgesics, nerve block analgesia or anesthesia, and anxiety and stress. Progress in either the first or the second stage of labor can be protracted (prolonged) or arrested (stopped). Abnormal progress can be identified by plotting cervical dilation and fetal descent on a labor graph (partogram) at various intervals after the onset of labor and comparing the resulting curve with the expected labor curve for a nulliparous or multiparous labor. If a woman exhibits an abnormal labor pattern, the primary health care provider should be notified.

TABLE 22-1

Abnormal Labor Patterns

PATTERN	NULLIPARAS	MULTIPARAS
Prolonged latent phase	>20 hr	>14 hr
Protracted active phase dilation	<1.2 cm/hr	<1.5 cm/hr
Secondary arrest: no change	≥2 hr	≥2 hr
Protracted descent	<1 cm/hr	<2 cm/hr
Arrest of descent	≥1 hr	≥½ hr
Failure of descent	No change during deceleration phase and second stage	
Precipitous labor	>5 cm/hr	10 cm/hr

Precipitous labor. Precipitous labor is defined as labor that lasts less than 3 hours from the onset of contractions to the time of birth. This abnormal labor pattern occurs in approximately 2% of all births in the United States. Precipitous birth alone is not usually associated with significant maternal or infant morbidity or mortality (Battista & Wing, 2007).

Precipitous labor may result from hypertonic uterine contractions that are tetanic in intensity. Conditions often associated with this type of uterine contractions include placental abruption, an excessive number of uterine contractions, and recent cocaine use (Battista & Wing, 2007). Maternal complications can include uterine rupture, lacerations of the birth canal, anaphylactoid syndrome of pregnancy (amniotic fluid embolism) and postpartum hemorrhage. Fetal complications include hypoxia, caused by decreased periods of uterine relaxation between contractions, and in rare instances, intracranial trauma related to rapid birth (Cunningham et al., 2005).

Women who have experienced precipitous labor often describe feelings of disbelief that their labor began so quickly, alarm that their labor progressed so rapidly, panic about the possibility they would not make it to the hospital in time to give birth, and finally relief when they arrived at the hospital. In addition, women have expressed frustration when nurses did not believe them when they reported their readiness to push.

Alterations in Pelvic Structure

Pelvic dystocia

Pelvic dystocia can occur whenever contractures of the pelvic diameters occur that reduce the capacity of the bony pelvis, including the inlet, midpelvis, outlet, or any combination of these planes.

Disproportion of the pelvis is the least common cause of dystocia (Cunningham et al., 2005). Pelvic contractures may be caused by congenital abnormalities, maternal malnutrition, neoplasms, or lower spinal disorders. An immature pelvic size predisposes some adolescent mothers to pelvic dystocia. Pelvic deformities also may be the result of motor vehicle accidents or other trauma.

Soft-tissue dystocia

Soft-tissue dystocia results from obstruction of the birth passage by an anatomic abnormality other than that involving the bony pelvis. The obstruction may result from placenta previa (low-lying placenta) that partially or completely obstructs the internal os of the cervix. Other causes, such as leiomyomas (uterine fibroids) in the lower uterine segment, ovarian tumors, and a full bladder or rectum, may prevent the fetus from entering the pelvis. Occasionally, cervical edema occurs during labor when the cervix is caught between the presenting part and the symphysis pubis or when the woman begins bearing-down efforts prematurely, thereby inhibiting complete dilation. Sexually transmitted infections (e.g., human papillomavirus) can alter cervical tissue integrity and thus interfere with adequate effacement and dilation.

Fetal Causes

Dystocia of fetal origin may be caused by anomalies, excessive fetal size, malpresentation, malposition, or multifetal pregnancy. Complications associated with dystocia of fetal origin include neonatal asphyxia, fetal injuries or fractures, and maternal vaginal lacerations. Although spontaneous vaginal birth is possible in these instances, a forceps-assisted, vacuum-assisted, or cesarean birth is often necessary.

Anomalies

Gross ascites, large tumors, open neural tube defects (e.g., myelomeningocele), and hydrocephalus are examples of fetal anomalies that can cause dystocia. The anomalies affect the relationship of the fetal anatomy to the maternal pelvic capacity, with the result that the fetus is unable to descend through the birth canal.

Cephalopelvic disproportion

Cephalopelvic disproportion (CPD), also called *fetopelvic disproportion* (FPD), is disproportion between the size of the fetus and the size of the mother's pelvis. When CPD is present, the fetus cannot fit through the maternal pelvis to be born vaginally. Although CPD is often related to excessive fetal size, or *macrosomia* (i.e., 4000 g or more), the problem in many cases is malposition of the fetal presenting part rather than true CPD (Battista & Wing, 2007). Fetal macrosomia is associated with maternal diabetes mellitus, obesity, multiparity, or the large size of one or both parents. If the maternal pelvis is too small, abnormally shaped, or deformed, CPD may be of maternal origin. In this case the fetus may be of average size or even smaller. Unfortunately, CPD cannot be accurately predicted (Battista & Wing).

Malposition

The most common fetal malposition is persistent occipitoposterior position (i.e., right occipitoposterior or left occipitoposterior; see Chapter 9), occurring in approximately 15% of all labors during the latent phase of first stage labor. Approximately 5% of all fetuses are in this position at birth (Gilbert, 2007). Labor, especially the second stage, is prolonged. The woman typically complains of severe back pain from the pressure of the fetal head (occiput) pressing against her sacrum. Box 22-7 iden-

BOX 22-7

Back Labor—Occiput Posterior Position Measures to Relieve Back Pain and Facilitate Rotation of Fetal Head

Measures to Reduce Back Pain during a Contraction

- *Counterpressure:* Apply fist or heel of the hand to sacral area.
- *Heat or cold applications:* Apply to sacral area.
- *Double hip squeeze:*
  - Woman assumes a position with hip joints flexed, such as the knee-chest position.
  - Partner, nurse, or doula places hands over gluteal muscles and presses with palms of hands up and inward toward the center of the pelvis.
- *Knee press:*
  - Woman assumes a sitting position with knees a few inches apart and feet flat on the floor or on a stool.
  - Partner, nurse, or doula cups a knee in each hand with heels of hands on top of tibia then presses the knees straight back toward the woman's hips while leaning forward toward the woman.

Measures to Facilitate the Rotation of the Fetal Head (May Also Relieve Back Pain)

- *Lateral abdominal stroking:* Stroke the abdomen in the direction that the fetal head should rotate.
- *Hands-and-knees position* (all-fours): Can also be accomplished by kneeling while leaning forward over a birth ball, padded chair seat, bed, or over-the-bed table.
- Squatting
- Pelvic rocking
- Stair climbing
- *Lateral position:* Lie on side toward which the fetus should turn.
- *Lunges:* Widens pelvis on side toward which woman lunges:
  - Woman stands, facing forward, next to or alongside a chair, so that she can lunge toward the side the fetal back is on or in the direction of the fetal occiput.
  - Woman places foot on seat of chair with toes pointed toward the back of the chair, then lunges.
  - Alternative position for lunge: kneeling.

tifies suggested measures to relieve back pain and encourage rotation of the fetal occiput to an anterior position, which will facilitate birth (Gilbert, 2007; Stremler, Hodnett, Petryshen, Stevens, Weston, & Willan, 2005).

Malpresentation

Malpresentation (the fetal presentation is something other than cephalic, or head first) is another commonly reported complication of labor and birth. Breech presentation is the most common form of malpresentation, occurring in 3% to 4% of all labors (Lanni & Seeds, 2007). The three types of breech presentation are (1) frank breech (hips flexed, knees extended), (2) complete breech (hips and knees flexed), and (3) footling breech (when one foot [single footling] or both feet [double footling] present before the buttocks) (Gilbert, 2007) (Fig. 22-3). Breech presentations are associated with multifetal gestation, preterm birth, fetal and maternal anomalies, hydramnios, and oligohydramnios. High rates of breech presentation are also noted in fetuses with certain genetic disorders (e.g., trisomies 13, 18, and 21; Potter syndrome [renal agenesis]; myotonic dystrophy). Fetuses with neuromuscular disorders have a high rate of breech presentation perhaps because they are less capable of movement within the uterus. Diagnosis is made by abdominal palpation and vaginal examination and usually confirmed by ultrasound scan (Lanni & Seeds, 2007; Thorp, 2009).

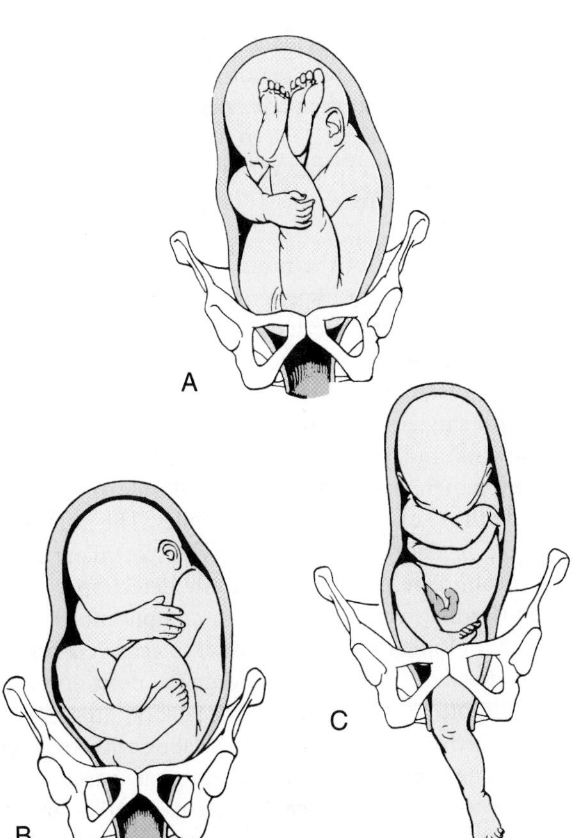

Fig. 22-3 Breech presentation. **A**, Frank breech. **B**, Complete breech. **C**, Single footling breech. (From Gilbert, E. [2007]. *Manual of high risk pregnancy & delivery* [4th ed.]. St. Louis: Mosby.)

During labor the descent of the fetus in a breech presentation may be slow because the breech is not as good a dilating wedge as is the fetal head. A risk of prolapse of the cord exists if the membranes rupture in early labor. The presence of meconium in amniotic fluid is not necessarily a sign of fetal distress because it results from pressure on the fetal abdominal wall as it traverses the birth canal. The heart tones of fetuses in a breech presentation are best heard at or above the umbilicus.

Animation: Breech Birth

Vaginal birth is accomplished by mechanisms of labor that manipulate the buttocks and lower extremities as they emerge from the birth canal (Fig. 22-4). Risks associated with vaginal birth from a breech presentation include prolapse of the umbilical cord (especially in single or double footling breech presentations) and trapping of the aftercoming fetal head (especially with preterm infants). Safe vaginal birth from a breech presentation is largely dependent on the experience, judgment, and skill of the health care provider who performs the delivery. Criteria for attempting a vaginal birth from a breech presentation are (Thorp, 2009):

Animation: Breech Examination

- Frank or complete breech presentation
- Estimated fetal weight between 2000 and 3800 g
- Normal (gynecoid) maternal pelvis
- Flexed fetal head

External cephalic version (ECV) (see later discussion) may be tried to turn the fetus to a vertex presentation (see Fig. 22-5). If the attempt at ECV is unsuccessful, the woman usually gives birth by cesarean (Gilbert, 2007).

Face and brow presentations are uncommon and are associated with fetal anomalies, pelvic contractures, and CPD. Vaginal birth is possible if the fetus flexes to a vertex presentation, although forceps are often used. Cesarean birth is indicated if the presentation persists, if fetal distress occurs, or if labor stops progressing.

Cesarean birth is usually necessary for a fetus in a transverse lie (i.e., shoulder) presentation, although ECV may be attempted after 36 to 37 weeks of gestation (Thorp, 2009).

Multifetal pregnancy

Multifetal pregnancy is the gestation of twins, triplets, quadruplets, or more infants. Multiple gestations now account for more than 3% of all live births in the United States. Over the last several decades the rate of twin births in the United States has increased every year. Currently, 32.3 twin births occur in every 1000 births in the United States (Malone & D'Alton, 2009). This increase has been attributed to the use of fertility-enhancing medications and procedures and the older age of childbearing women. When compared with younger women, those 35 years of age and older are naturally more likely to have a multifetal pregnancy. Although the twin birth rate continues to rise,

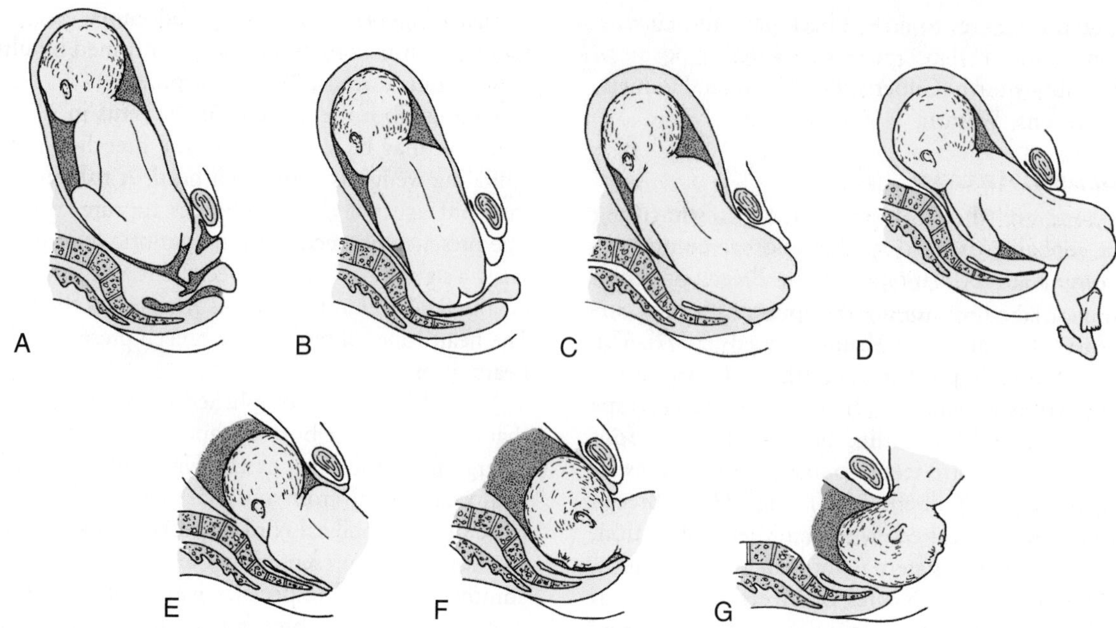

Fig. 22-4 Mechanism of labor in breech presentation. **A,** Breech before onset of labor. **B,** Engagement and internal rotation. **C,** Lateral flexion. **D,** External rotation or restitution. **E,** Internal rotation of shoulders and head. **F,** Face rotates to sacrum when occiput is anterior. **G,** Head is born by gradual flexion during elevation of fetal body.

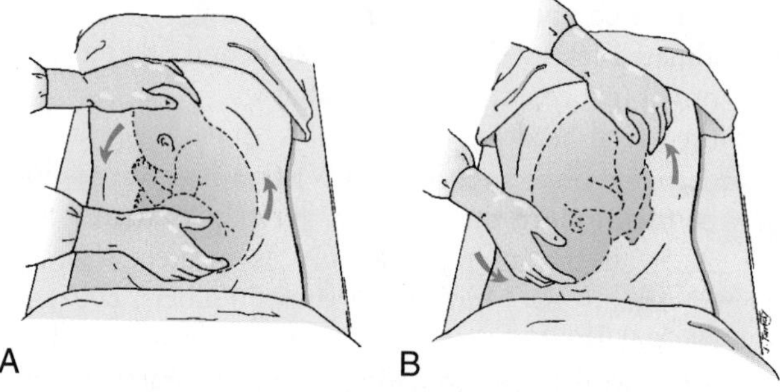

Fig. 22-5 External version of fetus from breech to vertex presentation. This must be achieved without force. **A,** Breech is pushed up out of pelvic inlet while head is pulled toward inlet. **B,** Head is pushed toward inlet while breech is pulled upward.

refinements in the treatments used for infertility are probably reducing the incidence of higher-order multiple births, which seem to have stabilized (Cleary-Goldman, Chitkara, & Berkowitz, 2007; Malone & D'Alton, 2009).

Multiple births are associated with more complications (e.g., dysfunctional labor) than are single births. The higher incidence of fetal and newborn complications and higher risk of perinatal mortality primarily stem from the birth of low birth weight infants resulting from preterm birth or IUGR (or both) in part related to placental dysfunction and twin-to-twin transfusion. Fetuses may experience distress and asphyxia during the birth process as a result of cord prolapse and the onset of placental separation with the birth of the first fetus. As a result, the risk for long-term problems such as cerebral palsy is higher among infants who were part of a multiple birth.

In addition, fetal complications such as congenital anomalies and abnormal presentations can result in dystocia and an increased incidence of cesarean birth. For example, in only 40% to 45% of all twin pregnancies do both fetuses present in the vertex position, the most favorable for vaginal birth. In 35% to 40% of the pregnancies, one twin may present in the vertex position and the other in a breech or transverse lie presentation (Malone & D'Alton, 2009).

The health status of the mother may be compromised by an increased risk for hypertension, anemia, and hemorrhage associated with uterine atony, abruptio placentae, and multiple or adherent placentas. Duration of the phases and stages of labor may vary from the duration experienced with singleton births.

Teamwork and planning are essential components of the management of childbirth in multiple pregnancies, especially those of higher-order multiples. The nurse plays a key role in coordinating the activities of many highly skilled health care professionals. Early detection and care of the maternal, fetal, and newborn complications associated with multiple births are essential to achieve a positive outcome for mother and babies. Maternal positioning and active support are used to enhance labor progress and placental perfusion. Stimulation of labor with oxytocin, epidural anesthesia, internal or external version, and forceps or vacuum assistance may be used to accomplish the vaginal birth of twins. Cesarean birth is almost always planned for higher-order multiple births. Each infant will have its own team of health care providers present at the birth. Emotional support that includes expression of feelings and full explanations of events as they occur and of the status of the mother and the fetuses and newborns is important to reduce the anxiety and stress that the mother and her family experience.

Position of the Woman

The functional relationship among the uterine contractions, the fetus, and the mother's pelvis are altered by the maternal position. In addition, the position can provide either a mechanical advantage or disadvantage to the mechanisms of labor by altering the effects of gravity and the body-part relationships that are important to the progress of labor. For example, the use of upright positions in second stage labor is associated with a shorter interval to birth, less pain and perineal damage, and less operative vaginal births compared with other positions (Roberts & Hanson, 2007).

Discouraging maternal movement or restricting labor to the recumbent or lithotomy position may compromise progress. The incidence of dystocia in women confined to these positions is increased, resulting in an increased need for augmentation of labor or forceps-assisted, vacuum-assisted, or cesarean birth.

Psychologic Responses

Hormones and neurotransmitters released in response to stress (e.g., catecholamines) can cause dystocia. Sources of stress vary for each woman, but pain and the absence of a support person are two factors often related to dystocia. Confinement to bed and restriction of maternal movement can be a source of psychologic stress that compounds the physiologic stress caused by immobility in the unmedicated laboring woman. When anxiety is excessive, it can inhibit cervical dilation and result in prolonged labor and increased pain perception. Anxiety also causes increased levels of stress-related hormones (e.g., beta-endorphin, adrenocorticotropic hormone, cortisol, epinephrine). These hormones act on the smooth muscles of the uterus. Increased levels can cause dystocia by reducing uterine contractility.

CARE MANAGEMENT

Risk assessment is a continuous process in the laboring woman. By reviewing the woman's labor history and observing her physical and psychologic responses to the current labor, any factors that might contribute to dystocia should be identified. Nursing diagnoses, interventions, and expected outcomes of care are then established for each woman based on her assessment findings. Many interventions for dystocia (e.g., ECV, cervical ripening, induction or augmentation of labor, and operative procedures [forceps- or vacuum-assisted birth, cesarean birth]) are implemented collaboratively with other members of the health care team. Commonly performed interventions are discussed in detail in the Obstetric Procedures section (see Nursing Process box: Dystocia).

When providing care for a woman who is experiencing labor or birth complications, all members of the health care team are responsible for complying with professional standards of care.

LEGAL TIP **Standard of Care—Labor and Birth Complications**

- Document all assessment findings, interventions, and patient responses in the patient record according to unit protocols, procedures, and policies and professional standards.
- Assess whether the woman (and her family, if appropriate) is fully informed about the procedures to which she is consenting.
- Provide full explanations regarding events that are taking place and interventions that are needed to help her and her baby.
- Maintain safety by administering medications and treatments correctly.
- Have telephone orders signed as soon as possible.
- Provide care at the acceptable standard (e.g., according to hospital protocols and professional standards).
- If short staffing occurs in the unit and the nurse is assigned additional patients, the nurse should document that rejecting this additional assignment would have placed these patients in danger as a result of abandonment.
- Maternal and fetal monitoring continues until birth according to the policies, procedures, and protocols of the birthing facility, even when a decision to carry out cesarean birth is made.

Obstetric Procedures

Version

Version is the turning of the fetus from one presentation to another. It may be accomplished either externally or internally by the physician.

External cephalic version. External cephalic version (EVC) is used in an attempt to turn the fetus from a breech or shoulder presentation to a vertex presentation for birth. It may be attempted in a labor and birth setting after 37 weeks of gestation. ECV is accomplished by the exertion of gentle, constant pressure on the abdomen (Fig. 22-5). Before ECV is attempted, ultrasound scanning is performed to determine the fetal position, locate the umbilical cord, rule out placenta previa, evaluate the adequacy of the maternal pelvis, and assess the amount of amniotic fluid, the gestational age, and the presence of any anomalies. An NST is performed to confirm fetal well-being, or the fetal heart rate (FHR) is monitored for a period (e.g., 10-20 minutes). Informed consent is obtained. A tocolytic agent such as terbutaline is often given to relax the uterus and to facilitate the maneuver (Thorp, 2009). Contraindications to ECV include (Thorp):

- Uterine anomalies
- Third-trimester bleeding
- Multiple gestation

NURSING PROCESS *Dystocia*

ASSESSMENT

Women in labor are continuously assessed for signs that labor is progressing normally:

Past history

- Dystocia in a previous pregnancy

Physical

- Characteristics of uterine contractions (frequency, intensity, duration)
- Progress of cervical effacement and dilation
- Characteristics of fetal heart rate tracing (baseline rate, variability, presence of decelerations)
- Presentation, position, and station of fetus
- Status of amniotic membranes (intact or ruptured)
- Characteristics of maternal pelvis

Psychologic

- Anxiety

NURSING DIAGNOSES

Possible nursing diagnoses for women experiencing dystocia include:

- *Risk for maternal or fetal injury* related to:
  - Interventions implemented for dystocia
- *Powerlessness* related to:
  - Loss of control
- *Risk for infection* related to:
  - Premature rupture of membranes
  - Operative procedures
- *Ineffective individual coping* related to:
  - Inadequate support system
  - Exhaustion
  - Pain

EXPECTED OUTCOMES OF CARE

Expected outcomes include that the woman will do the following:

- Understand the causes and treatment of dysfunctional labor.
- Implement or assist with interventions recommended by the health care team to enhance the progress of labor and birth.
- Express relief of pain.
- Experience labor and birth with minimal or no complications, such as infection, injury, or hemorrhage.
- Give birth to a healthy infant who has experienced no fetal distress or birth injury.

PLAN OF CARE AND INTERVENTIONS

- Communicate pertinent assessment findings to the woman's primary health care provider immediately.
- Implement or assist with interventions as ordered or per unit protocol.
- Ensure that the woman and one or more of her significant others receive an explanation regarding the reason or reasons for performing a particular intervention. (See the Obstetric Procedures section beginning on p. 695 for information regarding specific interventions.)
- Ensure that all questions are answered to the woman's (or support person or persons) satisfaction.
- Provide support and encouragement to the woman and her support persons during the labor and birth.

EVALUATION

The nurse can be reasonably assured that care was effective to the extent that the expected outcomes for care have been achieved.

- Oligohydramnios
- Evidence of uteroplacental insufficiency
- A nuchal cord (identified by ultrasound)
- Previous cesarean birth or other significant uterine surgery
- Obvious CPD

ECV is most successful in a multiparous woman who has a normal amount of amniotic fluid and whose fetus is not yet engaged in the pelvis (Cunningham et al., 2005). If ECV is not successful, ACOG recommends that the woman undergo planned cesarean birth (Thorp, 2009).

During an attempted ECV the nurse continuously monitors the FHR (especially for bradycardia and variable decelerations), checks the maternal vital signs, and assesses the woman's level of comfort because the procedure may cause discomfort. After the procedure is completed the nurse continues to monitor maternal vital signs and uterine activity and to assess for vaginal bleeding. FHR monitoring should also continue for 1 hour. Women who are Rh negative should receive Rh_o(D) immune globulin because the manipulation can cause fetomaternal bleeding (Lanni & Seeds, 2007; Thorp, 2009).

Spanish Guidelines: Induction of Labor

Internal version. With internal version the fetus is turned by the physician, who inserts a hand into the uterus and changes the presentation to cephalic (head) or podalic (foot). Internal version is only rarely used, most often in twin pregnancies to deliver the second fetus. The safety of this procedure has not been documented; maternal and fetal injury is possible. Cesarean birth is the usual method for managing malpresentation in multifetal pregnancies. The nurse's role in this situation is to monitor the status of the fetus and provide support to the woman.

Induction of labor

Induction of labor is the chemical or mechanical initiation of uterine contractions before their spontaneous onset for the purpose of bringing about the birth. Labor may be induced either electively or for indicated reasons. The number of labor inductions in the United States has more than doubled in recent years to a rate of 22.3% in 2005 (Mahlmeister, 2008). The rate of elective inductions is likely increasing more rapidly than the rate of indicated inductions (Thorp, 2009).

Induction of labor is indicated if continuing the pregnancy could be dangerous for either the woman or the fetus and if no contraindications exist to artificial rupture of membranes or augmenting uterine contractions (Thorp, 2009). Box 22-8 lists indications and contraindications for labor induction.

An elective induction is one in which labor is initiated without a medical indication. Many of these elective inductions are purely for the convenience of the woman or her health care practitioner. At times, however, labor may be electively induced in unusual situations, such as to allay maternal fears or anxieties caused by prior perinatal losses or to ensure that experienced multispecialty personnel are available to handle anticipated maternal or neonatal complications immediately following birth (Battista & Wing, 2007). The two major risks associated with elective labor induction at term are increased rates of cesarean birth and iatrogenic prematurity (Battista & Wing). To prevent iatrogenic prematurity, elective induction of labor should not be initiated until the woman reaches 39 completed weeks of gestation (ACOG, 1999; Cherouny, Federico, Haradan, Leavitt Gullo, & Resar, 2005).

Both chemical and mechanical methods are used to induce labor. Intravenous oxytocin and amniotomy are the most common methods used in the United States. Prostaglandins are also increasingly used for inducing labor (see Medication Guides: Prostaglandin E_1 and Prostaglandin E_2). Prostaglandin E_1 (misoprostol [Cytotec]), inserted intravaginally, has proven to be more effective for cervical ripening and labor induction than either intravaginal or intracervical prostaglandin E_2. Misoprostol was originally approved for use in preventing gastric ulcers induced by NSAIDs. Although the drug's manufacturer has acknowledged for several years that misoprostol is effective for cervical ripening and labor induction, it has not yet been approved by the FDA for these uses (Thorp, 2009). Ingesting herbal preparations (e.g., blue or black cohosh, evening primrose oil, raspberry leaves) is a complementary measure that has been shown to enhance cervical ripening or induce labor (Gilbert, 2007; Moleti, 2009).

Success rates for the induction of labor are increased when the condition of the cervix is favorable, or inducible. A rating system such as the **Bishop score** (Table 22-2) can be used to evaluate inducibility. For example, a score of 8 or more on this 13-point scale indicates that the cervix is soft, anterior, 50% or more effaced, and dilated 2 cm or more and that the presenting part is engaged. When the Bishop score totals 8 or more, induction is usually successful (Gilbert, 2007).

BOX 22-8

Indications and Contraindications for Labor Induction

INDICATIONS
- Hypertensive complications of pregnancy
- Fetal death
- Chorioamnionitis
- Diabetes mellitus
- Postterm pregnancy, especially when oligohydramnios is present
- Intrauterine growth restriction
- Premature rupture of membranes with established fetal maturity

CONTRAINDICATIONS
- Acute, severe fetal distress
- Shoulder presentation (transverse lie)
- Floating fetal presenting part
- Uncontrolled hemorrhage
- Placenta previa
- Previous uterine incision that prohibits a trial of labor

RELATIVE CONTRAINDICATIONS
- Grand multiparity (five or more pregnancies that ended after 20 weeks of gestation)
- Multiple gestation
- Suspected cephalopelvic disproportion
- Breech presentations
- Inability to adequately monitor fetal heart rate or contractions (or both) throughout labor

Source: Thorp, J. (2009). Clinical aspects of normal and abnormal labor. In R. Creasy, R. Resnik, & J. Iams (Eds.), *Creasy and Resnik's maternal-fetal medicine: Principles and practice* (6th ed.). Philadelphia: Saunders.

TABLE 22-2

Bishop Score

	SCORE			
	0	1	2	3
Dilation (cm)	0	1-2	3-4	≥5
Effacement (%)	0-30	40-50	60-70	≥80
Station (cm)	−3	−2	−1, 0	+1, +2
Cervical consistency	Firm	Medium	Soft	Soft
Cervix position	Posterior	Mid-position	Anterior	Anterior

meconium = earliest stool for infant.

Medication Guide

Prostaglandin E_1 (PGE_1): Misoprostol (Cytotec)

ACTION

- PGE_1 ripens the cervix, making it softer and causing it to begin to dilate and efface; it stimulates uterine contractions.

INDICATIONS

- PGE_1 is used for preinduction cervical ripening (ripen the cervix before oxytocin induction of labor when the Bishop score is 4 or less) and for inducement of labor or abortion (abortifacient agent); it has not yet been approved by the FDA for cervical ripening or labor induction (i.e., this is an unlabeled use for obstetrics).
- It should not be used if the woman has a history of previous cesarean birth or other major uterine surgery.

DOSAGE AND ADMINISTRATION

- Misoprostol is available either as a 100-mcg or a 200-mcg tablet. Therefore tablets must be broken to prepare the correct dose. This preparation should take place in the pharmacy to ensure accurate doses.
- Recommended initial dose is 25 mcg. Insert intravaginally into the posterior vaginal fornix using the tips of index and middle fingers without the use of a lubricant. Repeat every 3 to 6 hours up to 6 doses in a 24-hour period or until an effective contraction pattern is established (three or more uterine contractions in 10 minutes), the cervix ripens (Bishop score of 8 or greater), or significant adverse effects occur.

ADVERSE EFFECTS

- Higher doses (e.g., 50 mcg every 6 hours) are more likely to result in adverse reactions such as nausea and vomiting, diarrhea, fever, uterine tachysystole with or without an abnormal FHR and pattern, or fetal passage of meconium. The risk for adverse reactions is reduced with lower dosages and longer intervals between doses.

NURSING CONSIDERATIONS

- Explain the procedure to the woman and her family; ensure that an informed consent has been obtained as per agency policy.
- Assess the woman and fetus before each insertion and during treatment following agency protocol for frequency. Assess maternal vital signs and health status, FHR and pattern, and status of pregnancy, including indications for cervical ripening or induction of labor, signs of labor or impending labor, and the Bishop score. Recognize that an abnormal FHR and pattern; maternal fever, infection, vaginal bleeding, or hypersensitivity; and regular, progressive uterine contractions contraindicate the use of misoprostol.
- Avoid giving aluminum hydroxide and magnesium-containing antacids along with misoprostol.
- Use with caution in women with renal failure because the medication is eliminated through the kidneys.
- Have the woman void before insertion.
- Assist the woman to maintain a supine position with a lateral tilt or a side-lying position for 30 to 40 minutes after insertion.
- Prepare to (1) swab the vagina to remove unabsorbed medication using a saline-soaked gauze wrapped around fingers or (2) administer terbutaline 0.25 mg subcutaneously if significant adverse effects occur.
- Initiate oxytocin for induction of labor no sooner than 4 hours after the last dose of misoprostol was administered, following agency protocol, if ripening has occurred and labor has not begun.
- Document all assessment findings and administration procedures.

Data from Hill, W., Harvey, C. (2013). Induction of labor. In N. Troiano, C. Harvey, B. Chez, (Eds.). *AWHONN's high risk & critical care obstetrics* (3rd ed.). Philadelphia: Wolters Kluwer/Lippincott Williams & Wilkins; Moleti, C. (2009). Trends and controversies in labor induction. *MCN American Journal of Maternal Child Nursing, 34*(1), 40-47; Thorp, J.M.: (2009). Clinical aspects of normal and abnormal labor. In R. Creasy, R. Resnik. J. Iams (Eds.). *Creasy and Resnik's maternal-fetal medicine: Principles and practice* (6th ed.). Philadelphia: Saunders.

FDA, Food and Drug Administration; *FHR,* fetal heart rate.

Cervical ripening methods

Chemical agents. Preparations of prostaglandin E_1 and prostaglandin E_2 have been shown to be effective when used before induction to "ripen" (soften and thin) the cervix (see Medication Guides: Prostaglandin E_1 and Prostaglandin E_2). Advantages of prostaglandin use for cervical ripening include a decreased need for oxytocin induction, decreased oxytocin induction time, and a decrease in the amount of oxytocin required for successful induction (Gilbert, 2007). Prostaglandin E_1, although much less expensive and more effective than prostaglandin E_2 for inducing labor and birth, is associated with an increased risk for hyperstimulation of the uterus with FHR changes and meconium-stained amniotic fluid (Battista & Wing, 2007).

Mechanical methods. Mechanical dilators ripen the cervix by stimulating the release of endogenous prostaglandins. Balloon catheters (e.g., Foley catheter) can be inserted into the intracervical canal to ripen and dilate the cervix. Hydroscopic dilators (substances that absorb fluid from surrounding tissues and then enlarge) also can be used for cervical ripening. Laminaria tents (natural cervical dilators made from desiccated seaweed) and synthetic dilators containing magnesium sulfate (Lamicel) are inserted into the endocervix without rupturing the membranes. As these dilators absorb fluid, they expand and cause cervical dilation. When compared with prostaglandins, these mechanical methods achieved a lower rate of birth within 24 hours but caused no increase in the cesarean birth rate. Additionally, they were less likely to cause uterine hyperstimulation (Thorp, 2009).

Several other methods that have been recommended over the years for cervical ripening include breast stimulation, sexual intercourse, ingestion of castor oil, and stripping membranes. All of these methods, however, have either not been proven to be effective and safe or their use

Medication Guide

Prostaglandin E_2 (PGE_2): Dinoprostone (Cervidil Insert; Prepidil Gel)

ACTION

- PGE_2 ripens the cervix, making it softer and causing it to begin to dilate and efface; it stimulates uterine contractions. Dinoprostone is the only FDA-approved medication for cervical ripening or labor induction.

INDICATIONS

- PGE_2 is used for preinduction cervical ripening (ripen the cervix before oxytocin induction of labor when the Bishop score is 4 or less) and for inducement of labor or abortion (abortifacient agent).
- It is not recommended for use if the woman has a history of previous cesarean birth or other major uterine surgery.

DOSAGE AND ROUTE

Cervidil Insert:

- Dosage is 10 mg of dinoprostone designed to be gradually released (approximately 0.3 mg/hr) over 12 hours. Insert is placed transvaginally into the posterior fornix of the vagina. The insert is removed after 12 hours or at the onset of active labor or earlier if tachysystole or abnormal FHR and patterns occur.

Prepidil Gel:

- Dosage is 0.5 mg of dinoprostone in a 2.5-mL syringe. Gel is administered through a catheter attached to the syringe into the cervical canal just below the internal cervical os. Dose may be repeated every 6 hours as needed for cervical ripening up to a maximum cumulative dose of 1.5 mg (3 doses) in a 24-hour period.

ADVERSE EFFECTS

- Potential adverse effects include headache, nausea and vomiting, diarrhea, fever, hypotension, uterine tachysystole with or without an abnormal FHR and pattern, or fetal passage of meconium.

NURSING CONSIDERATIONS

- Explain the procedure to the woman and her family. Ensure that an informed consent has been obtained as per agency policy.
- Assess the woman and fetus before each insertion and during treatment following agency protocol for frequency. Assess maternal vital signs and health status, FHR and pattern, and status of pregnancy, including indications for cervical ripening or induction of labor, signs of labor or impending labor, and the Bishop score. Recognize that an abnormal FHR and pattern; maternal fever, infection, vaginal bleeding, or hypersensitivity; and regular, progressive uterine contractions contraindicate the use of dinoprostone.
- Avoid use in women with asthma, glaucoma, and hypotension or hypertension.
- Use with caution if the woman has cardiac, renal, or hepatic disease, anemia, jaundice, diabetes, epilepsy, or genitourinary (GU) infections.
- Bring the gel to room temperature just before administration. Do not force the warming process by using a warm-water bath or other source of external heat such as microwave because heat may cause inactivation.
- Keep the insert frozen until just before insertion. No warming is needed.
- Have the woman void before insertion.
- Assist the woman to maintain a supine position with a lateral tilt or a side-lying position for at least 30 minutes after insertion of the gel or for 2 hours after placement of the insert.
- Allow the woman to ambulate after the recommended period of bedrest and observation.
- Prepare to pull the string to remove the insert and to administer terbutaline 0.25 mg subcutaneously if significant adverse effects occur. There is no effective way to remove the gel from the vagina if uterine tachysystole or abnormal FHR and patterns occur.
- Delay the initiation of oxytocin for induction of labor for 6 to 12 hours after the last instillation of the gel or for 30 to 60 minutes after removal of the insert, or follow agency protocol for induction if ripening has occurred but labor has not begun.
- Document all assessment findings and administration procedures.

Data from Hill, W., Harvey, C. (2013). Induction of labor. In N. Troiano, C. Harvey, B. Chez (Eds.). *AWHONN's high risk & critical care obstetrics* (3rd ed.). Philadelphia: Wolters Kluwer/Lippincott Williams & Wilkins; Moleti, C. (2009). Trends and controversies in labor induction. *MCN American Journal of Maternal Child Nursing, 34*(1), 40-47.
FDA, Food and Drug Administration; *FHR,* fetal heart rate.

is associated with undesirable side effects (Moleti, 2009; Thorp, 2009).

Amniotomy. Amniotomy (i.e., artificial rupture of membranes) can be used to induce labor when the condition of the cervix is favorable (ripe) or to augment labor if progress begins to slow. Amniotomy decreases the length of some labors, even without the use of oxytocin. However, risks of amniotomy include intraamniotic infection and variable fetal heart rate decelerations (Gilbert, 2007). Other potential risks include umbilical cord prolapse and fetal injury. Once an amniotomy is performed the woman is committed to labor with an unknown outcome for how and when she will give birth.

Before the procedure the woman should be told what to expect. She also should be assured that the actual rupture of the membranes is painless for her and the fetus, although she may experience some discomfort when the Amnihook or other sharp instrument is inserted through the vagina and cervix (see Procedure box: Assisting with Amniotomy). The presenting part of the fetus should be engaged and well applied to the cervix before the procedure to prevent cord prolapse (Battista & Wing, 2007). The woman should also be free of active infection of the genital tract (e.g., herpes) and should be human immunodeficiency virus (HIV) negative.

NURSING ALERT The FHR is assessed before and immediately after the amniotomy to detect any changes (e.g., transient tachycardia is common, but bradycardia and variable decelerations are not) that may indicate cord compression or prolapse.

Procedure

Assisting with Amniotomy

PROCEDURE

- Explain the procedure to the woman.
- Assess fetal heart rate (FHR) before the procedure begins to obtain a baseline reading.
- Place several underpads under the woman's buttocks to absorb the fluid.
- Position the woman on a padded bed pan, fracture pan, or rolled up towel to elevate her hips.
- Assist the health care provider who is performing the procedure by providing sterile gloves and lubricant for the vaginal examination.
- Unwrap sterile package containing Amnihook or Allis clamp and pass instrument to the primary health care provider, who inserts it alongside the fingers and then hooks and tears the membranes.
- Reassess the FHR.
- Assess the color, consistency, and odor of the fluid.
- Assess the woman's temperature every 2 hours or per protocol.
- Evaluate the woman for signs and symptoms of infection.

DOCUMENTATION

- Record the following:
  - Time of rupture
  - Color, odor, and consistency of the fluid
  - FHR before and after the procedure
  - Maternal status (how well procedure was tolerated)

LEGAL TIP **Performing Amniotomy**

Nurses should not perform amniotomy. This procedure should be performed by the primary health care provider.

The woman's temperature should be checked at least every 2 hours after membranes rupture, more frequently if signs or symptoms of infection are noted. If her temperature is 38° C or higher, notify the primary health care provider. The nurse assesses for other signs and symptoms of infection, such as maternal chills, uterine tenderness on palpation, foul-smelling vaginal drainage, and fetal tachycardia (Gilbert, 2007). Comfort measures, such as frequently changing the woman's underpads and perineal cleansing, are implemented.

Oxytocin. Oxytocin is a hormone normally produced by the posterior pituitary gland that stimulates uterine contractions and aids in milk let-down. Synthetic oxytocin (Pitocin) may be used either to induce labor or to augment a labor that is progressing slowly because of inadequate uterine contractions. Oxytocin is currently used in the majority of all births in the United States; it is also the drug most commonly associated with adverse events during childbirth. In fact, oxytocin was recently added to the list of high-alert medications designated by the Institute for Safe Medication Practices because it has the potential to cause significant harm when used inappropriately. The most common errors involving oxytocin administration during labor are dose related (Clark, Simpson, Knox, & Garite, 2009; Mahlmeister, 2008; Simpson & Knox, 2009).

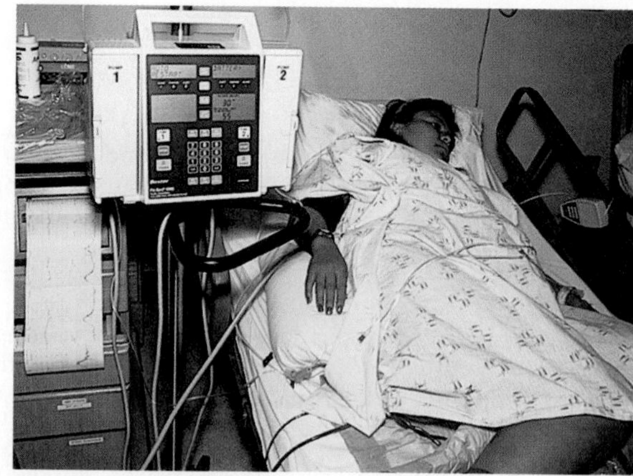

Fig. 22-6 Woman in side-lying position receiving oxytocin. (Courtesy Michael S. Clement, MD, Mesa, AZ.)

Oxytocin use can present hazards to both the mother and fetus. Maternal hazards include pain, abruptio placentae, uterine rupture, unnecessary cesarean birth caused by nonreassuring FHR patterns, postpartum hemorrhage, and infection. If the contractions are too frequent or prolonged, the fetus can experience hypoxemia and acidemia, which eventually results in late decelerations and minimal or absent baseline variability. The goal of oxytocin use is to produce contractions of normal intensity, duration, and intensity while using the lowest dose of medication possible (Simpson & Knox, 2009).

Currently the recommended protocol for administering oxytocin is to begin with a starting dose of 1 milliunit/min and increase by 1 to 2 milliunits no more frequently than every 30 to 60 minutes (Simpson & Knox, 2009). This recommendation is based on research findings related to the pharmacokinetics of oxytocin. The uterus responds to oxytocin within 3 to 5 minutes of intravenous administration. The half-life of oxytocin (the time required to metabolize and eliminate one half the dose) is approximately 10 to 12 minutes. Finally, approximately 40 minutes is required to reach a steady state of oxytocin, the point in time when the rate of oxytocin administered intravenously equals the rate of oxytocin elimination (Mahlmeister, 2008). (See Medication Guide: Oxytocin) (Fig. 22-6). Low-dose (physiologic) protocols such as the one described previously result in less uterine hyperstimulation, decreased fetal compromise, and significantly reduced use of oxytocin without affecting the duration of labor or cesarean birth rate (Battista & Wing, 2007; Gilbert, 2007).

High-dose protocols, in which the initial dose of oxytocin is larger and the dose level is increased more rapidly than in low-dose protocols, have been found to result in reduced lengths of labor and fewer forceps-assisted and cesarean births caused by dystocia. However, high-dose

Medication Guide

Oxytocin (Pitocin)

ACTION

- Oxytocin is a hormone produced in the posterior pituitary gland that stimulates uterine contractions and aids in milk let-down. Pitocin is a synthetic form of this hormone.

INDICATIONS

- Oxytocin is used primarily for labor induction and augmentation. It is also used to control postpartum bleeding.

DOSAGE

- The intravenous solution containing oxytocin should be mixed in a standard concentration. Concentrations often used are 10 units in 1000 mL of fluid, 20 units in 1000 mL of fluid, or 30 units in 500 mL of fluid.
- Use isotonic intravenous solutions (e.g., 0.9% sodium chloride, lactated Ringer's [LR]) to avoid electrolyte imbalance.
- Oxytocin is administered intravenously through a secondary line connected to the main line at the proximal port (connection closest to the intravenous insertion site). Oxytocin is always administered by pump.
- Begin oxytocin administration at 1 milliunit/min. Increase the rate by 1 to 2 milliunits/min, no more frequently than every 30 to 60 minutes based on the response of the woman and fetus and the progress of labor.
- The goal of oxytocin administration is to produce acceptable uterine contractions as evidenced by:
  - Consistent achievement of 200 to 220 MVUs *or*
  - A consistent pattern of one contraction every 2 to 3 minutes, lasting 80 to 90 seconds, and strong to palpation

ADVERSE EFFECTS

- Possible maternal adverse effects include uterine tachysystole, placental abruption, uterine rupture, unnecessary cesarean birth caused by abnormal FHR and patterns, postpartum hemorrhage, infection, and death from water intoxication (e.g., severe hyponatremia).
- Possible fetal adverse effects include hypoxemia and acidosis, eventually resulting in abnormal FHR and patterns.

NURSING CONSIDERATIONS

- Patient and partner teaching and support:
  - Reasons for use of oxytocin (e.g., start or improve labor)
  - Reactions to expect concerning the nature of contractions: the intensity of the contraction increases more rapidly, holds the peak longer, and ends more quickly; contractions will come regularly and more often
  - Monitoring to anticipate
- Continue to keep woman and her partner informed regarding progress.
- Remember that women vary greatly in their response to oxytocin; some require only very small amounts of medication to produce adequate contractions, whereas others need larger doses.
- Assessment
  - Fetal status using electronic fetal monitoring; evaluate tracing every 15 minutes and with every change in dose during the first stage of labor and every 5 minutes during the active pushing phase of the second stage of labor.
  - Monitor the contraction pattern and uterine resting tone every 15 minutes and with every change in dose during the first stage of labor and every 5 minutes during the second stage of labor.
  - Monitor blood pressure, pulse, and respirations every 30 to 60 minutes and with every change in dose.
  - Assess intake and output; limit IV intake to 1000 mL in 8 hours; urine output should be 120 mL or more every 4 hours.
  - Perform vaginal examination as indicated.
  - Monitor for side effects, including nausea, vomiting, headache, hypotension.
  - Observe emotional responses of woman and her partner.
- Use a standard definition for uterine tachysystole that does not include an abnormal FHR and pattern or the woman's perception of pain (see the Emergency Box on p. 702).
- The rate of oxytocin infusion should be continually titrated to the lowest dose that achieves acceptable labor progress. Usually the oxytocin dose can be decreased or discontinued after rupture of membranes and in the active phase of first-stage labor.
- Documentation
  - The time the oxytocin infusion is begun, and each time the infusion is increased, decreased, or discontinued
  - Assessment data as described above
  - Interventions for uterine tachysystole and abnormal FHR and patterns and the response to the interventions
  - Notification of the primary health care provider and that person's response

Data from American College of Obstetricians and Gynecologists (ACOG). (2009). *Induction of labor* (ACOG Practice Bulletin No. 107). Washington: DC; Clark, S., Simpson, K, Knox, G., et al. (2009). Oxytocin: New perspectives on an old drug. *American Journal of Obstetrics and Gynecology, 200*(1), 35, e1-e6; Hill, W., Harvey, C. (2013). Induction of labor. In N. Troiano, C. Harvey, B. Chez (Eds.). *AWHONN's high risk & critical care obstetrics* (3rd ed.). Philadelphia: Wolters Kluwer/Lippincott Williams & Wilkins; Mahlmeister, L. (2008). Best practices in perinatal care: Evidence-based management of oxytocin induction and augmentation of labor. *Journal of Perinatal and Neonatal Nursing, 22*(4), 259-263; Simpson, K. (2008). Labor and birth. In K. Simpson, P. Creehan (Eds.). *AWHONN's perinatal nursing* (3rd ed.). Philadelphia: Lippincott Williams & Wilkins; Simpson, K., Knox, G. (2009). Oxytocin as a high-alert medication: Implications for perinatal patient safety. *MCN American Journal of Maternal Child Nursing, 34*(1), 8-15.
FHR, Fetal heart rate; *IV*, intravenous; *MVUs*, Montevideo units.

protocols have been associated with increased uterine hyperstimulation and increased cesarean births related to fetal stress (Battista & Wing, 2007; Gilbert, 2007; Simpson & Knox, 2009). Some practitioners administer oxytocin in 10-minute pulsed infusions rather than as a continuous infusion. This method, which more closely resembles the endogenous release of oxytocin than the others, is reported to be effective for labor induction but requires significantly less oxytocin use than continuous infusion (Battista & Wing; Gilbert).

Nursing considerations. An evidence-based written protocol for the preparation and administration of oxytocin should be established by the obstetric department (physicians, nurse midwives, and nurses) in each institution. Other safety measures recommended for use of this high-alert drug include using a standard concentra-

EMERGENCY

Uterine Tachysystole with Oxytocin

SIGNS

- More than five contractions in 10 minutes
- A series of single contractions lasting more than 2 minutes
- Contractions of normal duration occurring within 1 minute of each other

INTERVENTIONS (WITH REASSURING FHR)

- Reposition or maintain woman in side-lying position (either side).
- Administer IV fluid bolus with 500 ml of lactated Ringer's solution.
- If uterine activity has not returned to normal after 10 minutes, decrease the oxytocin dose by at least one half. If uterine activity has not returned to normal after another 10 minutes, discontinue the oxytocin infusion until fewer than five contractions occur in 10 minutes.

INTERVENTIONS (WITH NONREASSURING FHR)

- Discontinue oxytocin infusion immediately.
- Reposition or maintain woman in side-lying position (either side).
- Administer IV fluid bolus with 500 ml of lactated Ringer's solution.
- Consider giving oxygen at 10 L/min by nonrebreather face mask if the above interventions do not resolve the nonreassuring FHR pattern.
- If no response, consider giving 0.25 mg terbutaline subcutaneously.
- Notify primary health care provider of actions taken and maternal and fetal response.

RESUMPTION OF OXYTOCIN AFTER RESOLUTION OF TACHYSYSTOLE

- If the oxytocin infusion has been discontinued for less than 20-30 minutes, resume at no more than one half the rate that caused the tachysystole.
- If the oxytocin infusion has been discontinued for more than 30-40 minutes, resume at the initial starting dose.

Sources: Mahlmeister, L. (2008). Best practices in perinatal care: Evidence-based management of oxytocin induction and augmentation of labor. *Journal of Perinatal and Neonatal Nursing, 22*(4), 259-263; Simpson, K., & Knox, G. (2009). Oxytocin as a high-alert medication: Implications for perinatal patient safety. *MCN: The American Journal of Maternal Child Nursing, 34*(1), 8-15.
FHR, Fetal heart rate; *IV,* intravenous.

tion of oxytocin and a standard definition of uterine tachysystole that does not include a nonreassuring FHR pattern or the woman's perception of pain. Additionally, standardized treatment of oxytocin-induced uterine tachysystole is recommended (Simpson & Knox, 2009) (see Emergency box: Uterine Tachysystole with Oxytocin).

Much confusion has existed regarding the definition of *excessive uterine contractions.* The Eunice Kennedy Shriver National Institute of Child Health and Human Development, along with ACOG and the Society for Maternal-Fetal Medicine, sponsored a workshop in April 2008 to review definitions, interpretation, and research recommendations for intrapartum fetal monitoring. The workshop participants also recommended standardizing definitions regarding uterine contractions for use in clinical practice. This group defined uterine tachysystole as more than five contractions in 10 minutes averaged over a 30-minute window. The term *tachysystole* applies to both spontaneous and stimulated labor. Workshop participants also recommended that use of the terms hyperstimulation and hypercontractility be abandoned because they are not defined (Macones, Hankins, Spong, Hauth, & Moore, 2008). ACOG (2009) has recently published a practice bulletin that supports use of the 2008 NICHD workshop recommendations.

NURSING ALERT If uterine tachysystole occurs, interventions are implemented immediately (see Emergency box: Uterine Tachysystole with Oxytocin). The primary health care provider is informed of the interventions initiated and the maternal and fetal response.

Augmentation of labor

Augmentation of labor is the stimulation of uterine contractions after labor has started spontaneously but progress is unsatisfactory. Augmentation is usually implemented for the management of hypotonic uterine dysfunction, resulting in a slowing of the labor process (protracted active phase). Common augmentation methods include oxytocin infusion and amniotomy. Noninvasive methods such as emptying the bladder, ambulation and position changes, relaxation measures, and nourishment and hydration should be attempted before invasive interventions are initiated. The administration procedure and nursing assessment and care measures for augmentation of labor with oxytocin are similar to those used for induction of labor with oxytocin (see Medication Guide: Oxytocin).

Some physicians advocate *active management of labor,* that is, the augmentation of labor to establish efficient labor with the aggressive use of oxytocin so that the woman gives birth within 12 hours of admission to the labor unit. Advocates of active management believe that intervening early (as soon as a nulliparous labor is not progressing at least 1 cm/hr) with use of higher-than-normal (pharmacologic) oxytocin doses administered at frequent increment intervals (e.g., a starting dose of 6 milliunits/min with increases of 6 milliunits/min every 15 minutes) shortens labor (Gilbert, 2007).

Additional components of the active management of labor include strict criteria to diagnose that the woman is indeed in active labor with 100% effacement, amniotomy within 1 hour of admission of a woman in labor if spontaneous rupture of the membranes has not occurred, and continuous presence of a personal nurse who provides one-on-one care for the woman while she is in labor. Many obstetricians in the United States emphasize the use of high-dose oxytocin protocols but do not implement all the other components of active management. At least one large review of published studies on the effectiveness of active management of labor protocols concluded that the presence of a personal nurse who provides constant emotional and physical support is the only component associated with shorter labors and lower rates of cesarean birth (Clark et al., 2009; Gilbert, 2007).

The original active management of labor protocols were written for nulliparous women who began laboring spontaneously. However, active management of labor protocols have been implemented by some providers in the United States on women who were not appropriate candidates (Mahlmeister, 2008).

Operative vaginal birth

Operative vaginal births are accomplished with the assistance of forceps or vacuum extractor. Indications and prerequisites for the use of both instruments are similar. The decision to use forceps or vacuum is made based on the experience and personal preference of the operator (physician) performing the procedure. Several types of operative vaginal births exist, defined primarily by the station and position of the fetal head in relationship to the maternal pelvis (Table 22-3) (American Academy of Pediatrics [AAP] & ACOG, 2007).

Forceps-assisted birth

A **forceps-assisted birth** is one in which an instrument with two curved blades is used to assist in the birth of the fetal head. The cephalic-like curve of the forceps commonly used is similar to the shape of the fetal head, with a pelvic curve to the blades conforming to the curve of the pelvic axis. The blades are joined by a pin, screw, or groove arrangement. These locks prevent the forceps from compressing the fetal skull (Fig. 22-7). (See Table 22-3.)

Maternal indications for forceps-assisted birth include a prolonged second stage of labor and the need to shorten the second stage of labor for maternal reasons (e.g., maternal exhaustion or maternal cardiopulmonary or cerebrovascular disease) (Nielsen et al., 2007). Fetal indications for this procedure include birth of a fetus in distress or in certain abnormal presentations, arrest of rotation, or delivery of the head in a breech presentation. The use of forceps during childbirth has been decreasing, replaced by vacuum extraction or cesarean birth (Nielsen et al.; Thorp, 2009).

TABLE 22-3

Definitions for Forceps- and Vacuum-Assisted Births

TYPE	DESCRIPTION
Outlet	Fetal scalp is visible on the perineum without manually separating the labia
Low	Fetal head is at least at the +2 station
Midpelvis	Fetal head is engaged (no higher than 0 station) but above the +2 station

Source: American Academy of Pediatrics (AAP) & American College of Obstetricians and Gynecologists (ACOG). (2007). *Guidelines for perinatal care* (6th ed.). Washington, DC: ACOG.

Certain conditions are required for a forceps-assisted birth to be successful. The woman's cervix must be fully dilated to prevent lacerations and hemorrhage. The bladder should be empty. The presenting part must be engaged. Membranes must be ruptured so that the position and station of the fetal head can be precisely determined and the forceps can firmly grasp the head during birth (Fig. 22-8). In addition, the size of the maternal pelvis must be assessed as adequate for the estimated fetal weight.

Management. Both blades are positioned by the physician, and the handles are locked. Traction is usually applied during contractions. The mother may or may not be instructed to push during contractions, depending on physician preference. If a decrease in FHR occurs, the forceps are removed and reapplied.

Nursing considerations. When a forceps-assisted birth is deemed necessary, the nurse obtains the type of forceps requested by the physician. The nurse may explain to the mother that the forceps blades fit the same way two tablespoons fit around an egg, with the blades placed in front of the baby's ears.

NURSING ALERT Because compression of the cord between the fetal head and the forceps will cause a decrease in FHR, the FHR is assessed, reported, and recorded before and after application of the forceps.

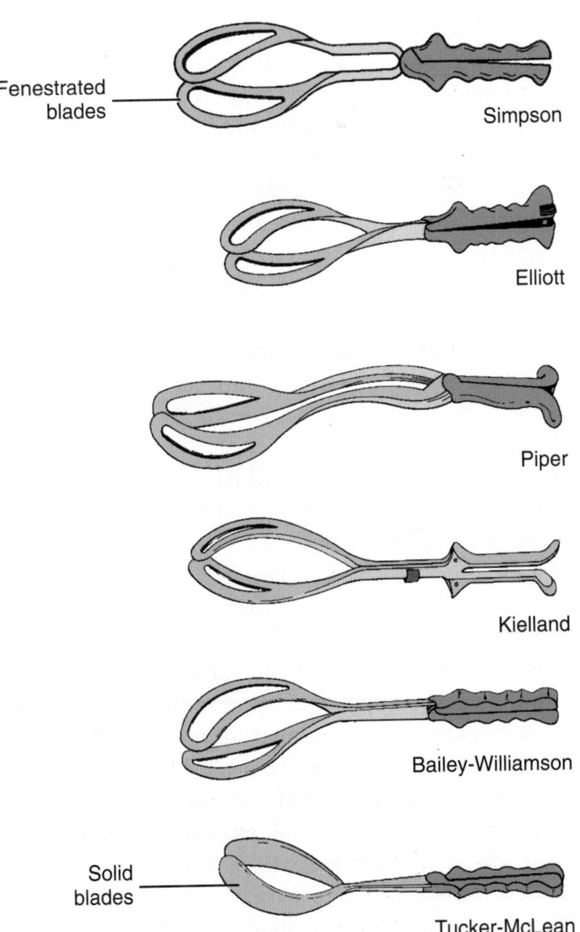

Fig. 22-7 Types of forceps. Piper forceps are used to assist delivery of the head in a breech birth.

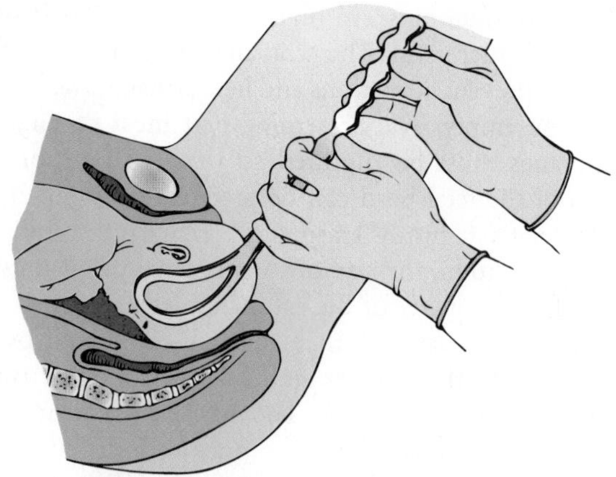

Fig. 22-8 Outlet forceps-assisted extraction of the head.

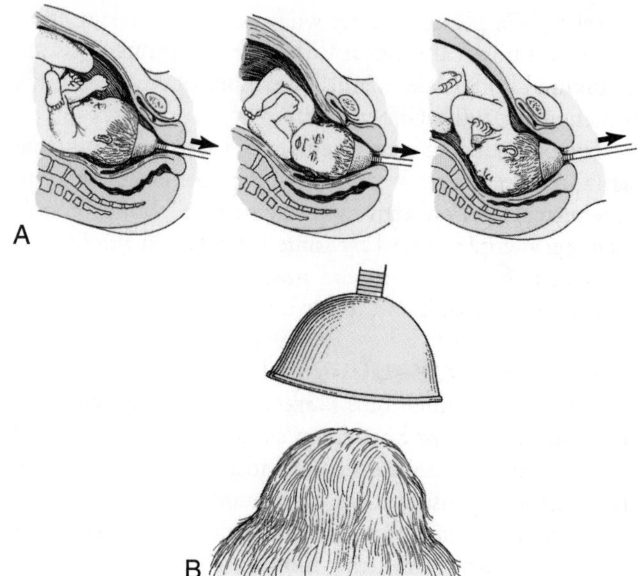

Fig. 22-9 Use of vacuum extraction to rotate fetal head and assist with descent. **A,** Arrow indicates direction of traction on the vacuum cup. **B,** Caput succedaneum formed by the vacuum cup.

After birth the woman should be assessed for any vaginal or cervical lacerations, urinary retention, and hematoma formation in the pelvic soft tissues. The infant should be checked for bruising or abrasions at the site of the blade applications, facial palsy resulting from pressure of the blades on the facial nerve, and subdural hematoma. Newborn and postpartum caregivers should be told that a forceps-assisted birth was performed.

Vacuum-assisted birth

Vacuum-assisted birth, or vacuum extraction, is a birth method involving the attachment of a vacuum cup to the fetal head, using negative pressure to assist in the birth of the head (Fig. 22-9). It is generally not used to assist birth before 34 weeks of gestation (Cunningham et al., 2005; Nielsen et al., 2007) (see Table 22-3). Advantages of vacuum-assisted birth as compared with forceps-assisted birth are the ease with which the vacuum can be placed and the need for less anesthesia; it is also far easier to learn the skills necessary to safely use the vacuum than to gain a similar level of skill with forceps (Thorp, 2009).

Management. The vacuum cup is applied to the fetal head by the physician. From a nursing perspective, basically, two types of vacuum devices are currently in use. One is a self-contained unit, which allows the physician to both position the cup on the baby's head and generate the desired amount of negative pressure to create a vacuum. When the other type of vacuum device is used, the physician applies the cup to the baby's head, after which the nurse connects the suction tubing attached to the cup to wall suction or a separate hand pump and generates the amount of pressure requested by the physician. With both types of vacuum devices, a caput develops inside the cup as the pressure is initiated (see Fig. 22-9). The woman is encouraged to push as traction is applied by the physician. The vacuum cup is released and removed after birth of the head. If vacuum extraction is not successful, a forceps-assisted or cesarean birth is usually performed.

Risks to the newborn include cephalhematoma, scalp lacerations, and subdural hematoma. Neonatal complications can be reduced by strict adherence to the manufacturer's recommendations for method of application, amount of pressure to be generated, and duration of application. Maternal risks include perineal, vaginal, or cervical lacerations and soft-tissue hematomas.

Nursing considerations. The nurse's role for the woman who has a vacuum-assisted birth is primarily one of a support person and educator. Documentation of the procedure in the patient's medical record is important and is often the nurse's responsibility (Box 22-9). Neonatal caregivers should be told that the birth was vacuum assisted. After birth the newborn must be observed for signs of trauma and infection at the application site and for cerebral irritation (e.g., poor sucking or listlessness). The newborn may also be at risk for neonatal jaundice as bruising resolves. The parents may need to be reassured that the caput succedaneum usually disappears in 3 to 5 days (Fig. 22-9, *B*) (Gilbert, 2007).

BOX 22-9

Assisting with Birth by Vacuum Extraction

- Assess fetal heart rate frequently during the procedure.
- Encourage the woman to push during contractions.
- If responsible for generating pressure for the vacuum, do not exceed the "green zone" indicated on the pump. Verify with the physician the amount of pressure to be generated.
- Document the number of pulls attempted, maximal pressure used, and any pop-offs that occur.

Cesarean birth

Cesarean birth is the birth of a fetus through a transabdominal incision in the uterus. Whether cesarean birth is planned (scheduled) or unplanned (emergency), the loss of the experience of giving birth to a child in the traditional manner may have a negative effect on a woman's self-concept. An effort is therefore made to maintain the focus on the birth of a child rather than on the operative procedure.

The purpose of cesarean birth is to preserve the life or health of the mother and her fetus; it may be the best choice for birth when evidence exists of maternal or fetal complications. Since the advent of modern surgical methods and care and the use of antibiotics, maternal and fetal morbidity and mortality have decreased. In addition, incisions are usually made in the lower uterine segment rather than in the muscular body of the uterus, thus promoting effective healing. However, despite these advances, cesarean birth still poses threats to the health of the mother and infant.

The incidence of cesarean births escalated to 31.1% of live births in 2006, the highest rate ever reported in the United States (Martin et al., 2009). Part of the reason for this rise is that several common risk factors for cesarean birth are increasing in frequency, especially in developed countries. These factors include fetal macrosomia, advanced maternal age, obesity, gestational diabetes, and multifetal pregnancy (Thorp, 2009). Malpractice concerns are another factor related to the elevated incidence, along with an increase in the number of cesareans performed on maternal request, currently estimated to be 2.5% of all births in the United States (ACOG, 2007; Landon, 2007). An international estimate of the elective cesarean birth rate is much higher compared with the United States, between 4% and 18% (Collard, Diallo, Habinsky, Hentschell, & Vezeau, 2008/2009).

Approaches for the management of labor and birth to reduce the rate of cesarean births while increasing the rate of vaginal birth after cesarean (VBAC) are presented in Box 22-10. However, the rate of VBAC is decreasing. Currently, only approximately 9% of women in the United States with a prior cesarean birth undergo a trial of labor (TOL) with the goal of a VBAC (Landon, 2007). This decline may be related to concerns regarding an increased risk of uterine rupture and other complications of VBAC with resulting poor outcomes for women and infants (Landon; Thorp, 2009).

The type of nursing care given also may influence the rate of cesarean births. A labor-management approach that uses one-to-one support and emphasizes ambulation, maternal position changes, and nonpharmacologic pain relief supports the physiologic progression of labor and a spontaneous vaginal birth (Albers, 2007). Several studies have found that the labor-management approach that most consistently reduces cesarean birth rates is one-to-one support of the laboring woman by another woman, such

BOX 22-10

Selected Measures to Reduce Cesarean Birth Rate and Increase Rate of Vaginal Birth after Cesarean

EDUCATE THE WOMAN REGARDING
- Advantages and safety of the home environment for early or latent labor
- Indicators for hospital admission
- Management techniques to use during labor to enhance progress
- Nonpharmacologic measures to reduce pain and discomfort and enhance relaxation
- Safety and effectiveness of TOL and VBAC

ESTABLISH ADMISSION CRITERIA FOR WOMEN IN LABOR
- Distinguish clinical manifestations for false labor, latent or early labor, and active labor.
- Conduct admission assessments in a separate admissions area.
- Send women in false or early or latent labor home or keep them in the admissions area.
- Admit women in active labor to the labor and birth unit.

USE APPROPRIATE ASSESSMENT TECHNIQUES TO
- Determine status of the maternal-fetal unit.
- Establish an individualized rationale for initiating labor interventions such as epidural anesthesia, induction or augmentation, amniotomy, cesarean birth.

INITIATE A DOULA PROGRAM THAT
- Provides one-to-one support for women in labor

DEVELOP A PHILOSOPHY OF LABOR MANAGEMENT THAT
- Schedules admission during active labor
- Avoids automatic interventions such as routine induction for spontaneous rupture of membranes at term or postterm pregnancy and cesarean birth for breech presentation, twin gestation, genital herpes, or failure to progress
- Relies on assessment findings reflective of the status of the maternal-fetal unit rather than strict adherence to set ranges for the duration of the stages and phases of labor
- Employs intermittent rather than continuous electronic fetal monitoring of low risk pregnant women
- Focuses on measures that are known to enhance the progress of labor, such as one-to-one support, ambulation, maternal position changes, and nonpharmacologic pain relief
- Establishes criteria for elective cesarean birth and TOL
- Encourages women who have had a previous cesarean birth to participate in TOL to attempt a vaginal birth

TOL, Trial of labor; *VBAC*, vaginal birth after cesarean.

Video: Childbirth (Cesarean)
Spanish Guidelines: Cesarean Birth

as a nurse, nurse-midwife, or doula (Berghella, Baxter, & Chauhan, 2008; Hodnett, Gates, Hofmeyr, & Sakala, 2007).

Indications. Few absolute indications exist for cesarean birth. Today, most of these procedures are performed for conditions that might pose a threat to both mother and fetus if vaginal birth occurred, such as placenta previa or placental abruption (Landon, 2007). Box 22-11 lists common indications for cesarean birth.

Elective cesarean birth. The term *cesarean on request* or *cesarean on demand* refers to a primary cesarean birth without a medical or obstetric indication. One reason given for elective cesarean birth is the belief that the surgery will prevent future problems with pelvic support or sexual dysfunction. However, at this time, evidence is insufficient to recommend elective cesarean birth to prevent urinary or fecal incontinence later in life (Collard et al., 2008/2009; Thorp, 2009). Perinatal mortality is lower with a planned cesarean birth compared with labor and vaginal birth (Landon, 2007). Other reasons women may desire an elective cesarean birth are because of the convenience of planning a date or having control and choice about when to give birth (Williams, 2005).

Currently, only limited data are available comparing cesarean birth on request with planned vaginal birth (ACOG, 2007). In a 2007 Committee Opinion, ACOG lists potential risks of cesarean birth on request that include a longer hospital stay for the woman, an increased risk of respiratory problems for the baby, and greater complications in subsequent pregnancies, including uterine rupture and placental implantation problems. Therefore ACOG recommends that cesarean birth on request not be performed unless a gestational age of 39 weeks has been accurately determined. ACOG does not recommend cesarean birth on request for women who desire additional children because the risks of placenta previa, placenta accreta, and cesarean hysterectomy increase with each cesarean birth (ACOG). The Society of Obstetricians and Gynaecologists of Canada (SOGC) promotes natural childbirth. The organization does not promote elective cesarean birth but believes that the final decision as to the safest route for childbirth rests with the woman and her health care provider (SOGC, 2004).

Forced cesarean birth. A woman's refusal to undergo cesarean birth when indicated for fetal reasons is often described as a *maternal-fetal conflict.* Health care providers are ethically obliged to protect the well-being of both the mother and the fetus; a decision for one affects the other. If a woman refuses a cesarean birth that is recommended because of fetal jeopardy, health care providers must make every effort to find out why she is refusing and provide information that may persuade her to change her mind. If the woman continues to refuse surgery, then health care providers must decide if obtaining a court order for the surgery is ethical. Every effort should be made to avoid this legal step.

Surgical techniques. The skin incision will be either vertical, extending from near the umbilicus to the mons pubis, or transverse (Pfannenstiel incision) in the lower abdomen (Fig. 22-10). The transverse incision, sometimes called the *bikini* incision, is performed more often than the vertical incision. The type of skin incision is generally determined by the urgency of the surgery and the presence of any prior skin incisions (Landon, 2007). The type of skin incision does *not* necessarily indicate the type of uterine incision.

The two main types of uterine incision are the low transverse and the vertical, which may be either low or classic (Fig. 22-11). Ideally the vertical incision is contained

COMMUNITY ACTIVITY

Meet with a midwife in your community physician's office or clinic. Explore the role of a midwife. What information are pregnant women given about measures they can take to enhance the labor process and reduce the possibility of unwanted interventions such as labor augmentation or cesarean birth?

BOX 22-11

Indications for Cesarean Birth

MATERNAL
- Specific cardiac disease (Marfan syndrome, unstable coronary artery disease)
- Specific respiratory disease (Guillain-Barré syndrome)
- Conditions associated with increased intracranial pressure
- Mechanical obstruction of the lower uterine segment (tumors, fibroids)
- Mechanical vulvar obstruction (condylomata)
- History of previous cesarean birth

FETAL
- Nonreassuring fetal status
- Malpresentation (e.g., breech or transverse lie)
- Active maternal herpes lesions
- Maternal human immunodeficiency virus with a viral load >1000 copies/ml
- Congenital anomalies

MATERNAL-FETAL
- Dystocia (cephalopelvic disproportion, "failure to progress" in labor)
- Placental abruption
- Placenta previa
- Elective cesarean birth

Sources: Duff, P., Sweet, R., & Edwards, R. (2009). Maternal and fetal infections.. In R. Creasy, R. Resnik, & J. Iams (Eds.), *Creasy and Resnik's maternal-fetal medicine: Principles and practice* (6th ed.). Philadelphia: Saunders; Landon, M. (2007). Cesarean delivery. In S. Gabbe, J. Niebyl, & J. Simpson (Eds.), *Obstetrics: Normal and problem pregnancies* (5th ed.). Philadelphia: Churchill Livingstone; Thorp, J. (2009). Clinical aspects of normal and abnormal labor. In R. Creasy, R. Resnik, & J. Iams (Eds.), *Creasy and Resnik's maternal-fetal medicine: Principles and practice* (6th ed.). Philadelphia: Saunders.

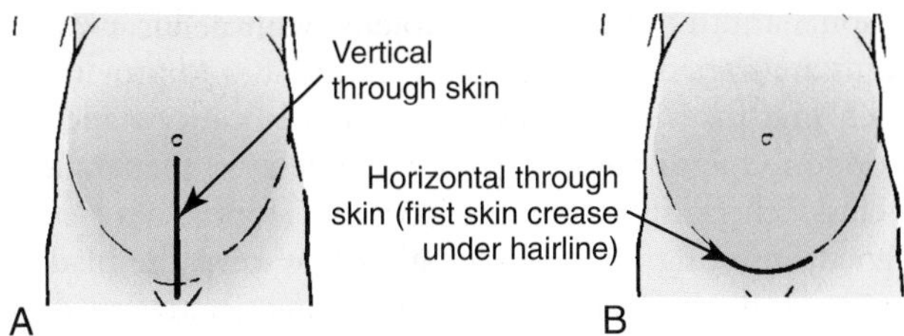

Fig. 22-10 Skin incisions for cesarean birth. **A,** Vertical. **B,** Horizontal (Pfannenstiel).

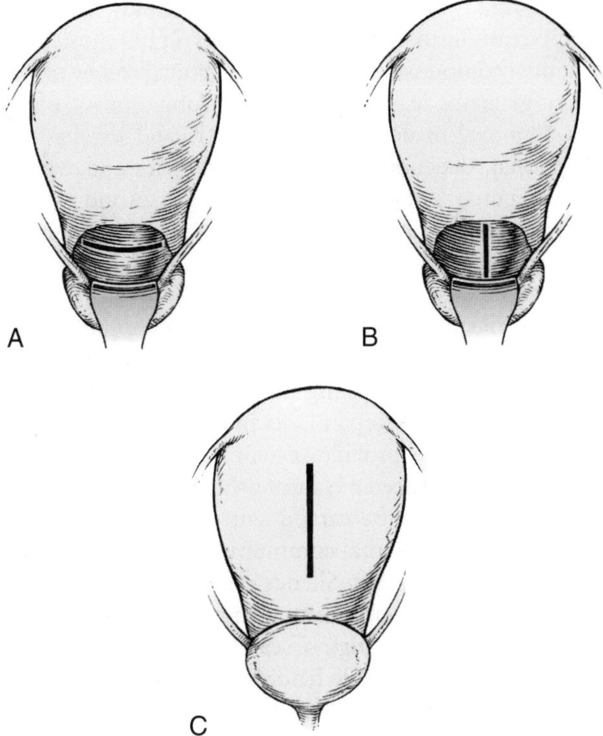

Fig. 22-11 Uterine incisions for cesarean birth. **A,** Low transverse incision. **B,** Low vertical incision. **C,** Classic incision. (From Gabbe, S., Niebyl, J., and Simpson, J. [2007]. *Obstetrics: Normal and problem pregnancies* [5th ed.]. Philadelphia: Churchill Livingstone.)

entirely within the lower uterine segment, but extension into the contractile portion of the uterus (e.g., a classic incision) is common (Fig 22-11, *B* and *C*) (Landon, 2007). Indications for a vertical uterine incision include an underdeveloped lower uterine segment, a transverse lie or preterm breech presentation, certain fetal anomalies such as massive hydrocephalus, and an anterior placenta previa (Landon). Because it is associated with a higher incidence of uterine rupture in subsequent pregnancies than lower-segment cesarean birth, vaginal birth after a classic uterine incision is contraindicated.

The low transverse uterine incision is performed in more than 90% of cesarean births (Fig. 22-11, *A*). Compared with the vertical incision, the transverse incision is preferred because it does not compromise the upper uterine segment, is easier to perform and repair, and is associated with less blood loss; it is also less likely to rupture in subsequent pregnancies (Landon, 2007).

Complications and risks. Possible maternal complications related to cesarean birth include aspiration, hemorrhage, atelectasis, endometritis, abdominal wound dehiscence or infection, urinary tract infection, injuries to the bladder or bowel, and complications related to anesthesia (Thorp, 2009). The fetus may be born prematurely if the gestational age has not been accurately determined. Fetal asphyxia can occur if the uterus and placenta are poorly perfused as a result of maternal hypotension caused by regional anesthesia (epidural or spinal) or maternal positioning. Fetal injuries (scalpel lacerations) can also occur during the surgery (Thorp). In addition to these risks, the woman is at economic risk because the cost of cesarean birth is higher than that of vaginal birth, and a longer recovery period may require additional expenditures.

Anesthesia. Spinal, epidural, and general anesthetics are used for cesarean births. Epidural blocks are popular because women want to be awake for and aware of the birth experience. However, the choice of anesthetic depends on several factors. The mother's medical history or present condition, such as a spinal injury, hemorrhage, or coagulopathy, may rule out the use of regional anesthesia. Time is another factor, especially if an emergency exists and the life of the mother or infant is at stake. In an emergency situation, general anesthesia will most likely be used unless the woman already has an epidural block in effect. The woman herself is a factor. Either she may not know all the options, or she may have fears about having "a needle in her back" or about being awake and feeling pain. She needs to be fully informed about the risks and benefits of the different types of anesthesia so that she can participate in the decision whenever a choice must be made.

Scheduled cesarean birth

Cesarean birth is scheduled or planned if labor and vaginal birth are contraindicated (e.g., complete placenta previa, active genital herpes, positive HIV status with a high viral load), if birth is necessary but labor is not inducible (e.g., hypertensive states that cause a poor intrauterine environment that threatens the fetus), or if this course of action has been chosen by the primary health care provider and the woman (e.g., a repeat cesarean birth).

Women who are scheduled to have a cesarean birth have time to prepare for it psychologically. However, the psychologic responses of these women may differ. Those having a repeat cesarean birth may have disturbing memories of the conditions preceding the initial surgical birth (primary cesarean birth) and of their experiences in the postoperative recovery period. They may be concerned about the added burdens of caring for an infant and perhaps other children while recovering from surgery. Others may feel glad that they have been relieved of the uncertainty about the date and time of the birth and are free of the pain of labor.

Unplanned cesarean birth

The psychosocial outcomes of unplanned or emergency cesarean birth are usually more pronounced and negative when compared with the outcomes associated with a scheduled or planned cesarean birth. Women and their families experience abrupt changes in their expectations for birth, postbirth care, and the care of the new baby at home. This experience may be extremely traumatic for all.

The woman may approach the procedure tired and discouraged after an ineffective and difficult labor. Fear predominates as she worries about her own safety and well-being and that of her fetus. She may be dehydrated, with low glycogen reserves. Because preoperative procedures must be performed rapidly, often little time is available for explaining the procedures and the operation itself. Because maternal and family anxiety levels are high at this time, much of what is said may be forgotten or misunderstood. The woman may experience feelings of anger or guilt in the postpartum period. Fatigue is often noticeable in these women, and they need much supportive care.

Prenatal preparation. A discussion of cesarean birth should be included in all parenthood preparation classes. No woman can be guaranteed a vaginal birth, even if she is in good health and no indication of danger to the fetus exists before the onset of labor. Therefore every woman needs to be aware of and prepared for this possibility.

Childbirth educators stress the importance of emphasizing the similarities and differences between a cesarean and a vaginal birth. In support of the philosophy of family-centered birth, many hospitals have instituted policies that permit fathers and other partners and family members to share in these births as they do in vaginal ones. Women who have undergone cesarean birth agree that the continued presence and support of their partners helped them respond positively to the entire experience.

Preoperative care. Family-centered care is the goal for the woman who is to undergo cesarean birth and for her family. The preparation of the woman for cesarean birth is the same as that made for other elective or emergency surgery. The primary health care provider discusses with the woman and her family the need for the cesarean birth and the prognosis for the mother and infant. A member of the anesthesia care team assesses the woman's cardiopulmonary system and describes the options for anesthesia. Informed consent is obtained for the procedure.

Blood tests are usually ordered a day or two before a planned cesarean birth or on admission to the labor and birth unit. Laboratory tests commonly ordered include a complete blood cell count and blood type and Rh status. Maternal vital signs and FHR continue to be assessed per hospital routine until the operation begins. Intravenous fluids are started to maintain hydration and to provide an open line for the administration of medications and for blood products if needed. Other preoperative preparations include checking to be sure consent forms have been signed, inserting a retention catheter to keep the bladder empty, and administering prescribed preoperative medications. In addition to medications given to prevent aspiration pneumonia, many women receive prophylactic antibiotics to prevent postoperative infection. An abdominal-mons shave or a clipping of pubic hair may be ordered by the primary health care provider. In many instances, thromboembolism deterrent stockings (TED hose) and sequential compression devices (SCD boots) will be placed on the woman's legs to prevent the formation of blood clots. Removal of dentures, nail polish, and jewelry may be optional, depending on hospital policies and type of anesthesia used. If the woman wears eyeglasses and is going to be awake, the nurse should make sure her eyeglasses accompany her to the operating room so she can see her infant.

During the preoperative preparation, the support person is encouraged to remain with the woman as much as possible to provide continuing emotional support (if this action is culturally acceptable to the woman and support person). The nurse provides essential information about the preoperative procedures during this time. Although the nursing actions may be carried out quickly if a cesarean birth is unplanned, verbal communication, particularly an explanation, is important. Silence can be frightening to the woman and her support person. The nurse's use of touch can communicate feelings of care and concern for the woman. If time is available before the birth, the nurse can teach the woman about postoperative expectations and about pain relief, turning, coughing, and deep-breathing measures.

Intraoperative care. Cesarean births occur in operating rooms in the surgical suite or in the labor and birth unit. Staff members from the labor and birth unit may scrub and circulate during the surgery or these functions may be assumed by members of the hospital's surgery staff (Fig. 22-12). If possible, the partner, who is dressed appropriately for the operating room, accompanies the mother to the operating room and remains close to her for continued comfort and support.

The nurse who is circulating may assist with positioning the woman on the birth (surgical) table. The woman is positioned so that her uterus is displaced laterally to prevent compression of the inferior vena cava, which causes decreased placental perfusion. This task is usually accomplished by placing a wedge under the hip or tilting the table to one side. The woman's legs should be strapped to the table to ensure proper positioning during the surgery.

If the partner is not allowed or chooses not to be present, the nurse can stay in communication with him or

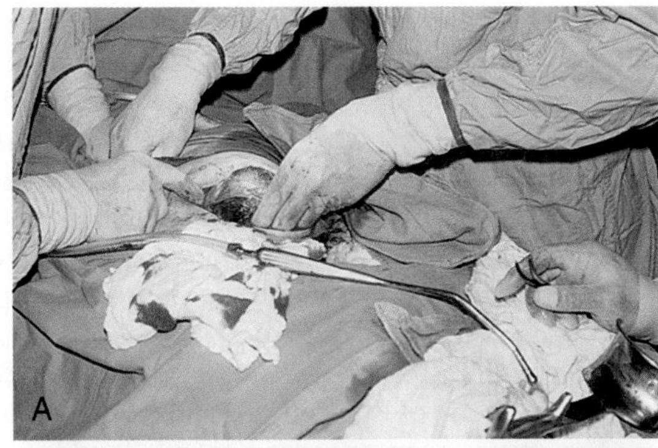
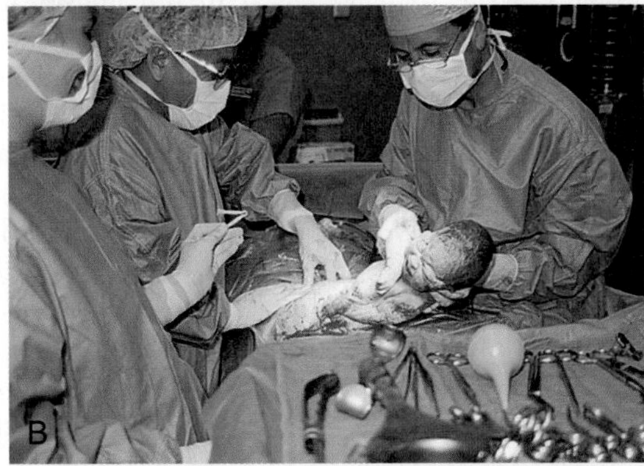
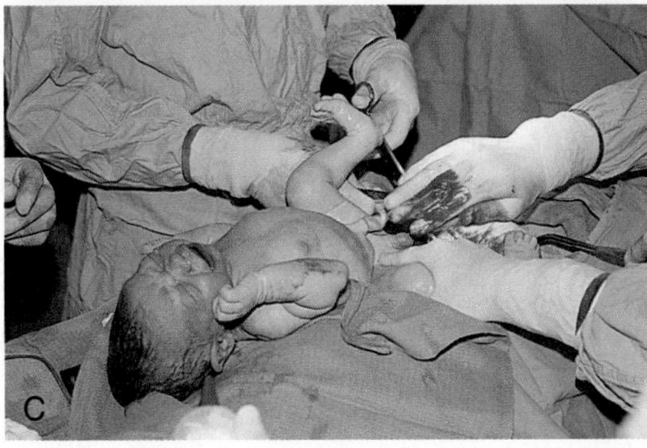

Fig. 22-12 Cesarean birth. **A,** "Bikini" incision has been made, the muscle layer is separated, the abdomen is entered, and the uterus has been exposed and incised; suctioning of amniotic fluid continues as head is brought up through the incision. Note small amount of bleeding. **B,** The neonate's birth through the uterine incision is nearly complete. **C,** A quick assessment is performed; note extreme molding of head resulting from cephalopelvic disproportion. (Courtesy Marjorie Pyle, RNC, Lifecircle, Costa Mesa, CA.)

her and give progress reports whenever possible. If the woman is awake during the birth, the nurse, anesthesia care provider, or both can tell her what is happening and provide support. She may be anxious about the sensations she is experiencing, such as the coldness of solutions used to prepare the abdomen and pressure or pulling during the actual birth of the infant. She may also be apprehensive because of the bright lights or the presence of unfamiliar equipment and masked and gowned personnel in the room. Explanations can help decrease the woman's anxiety.

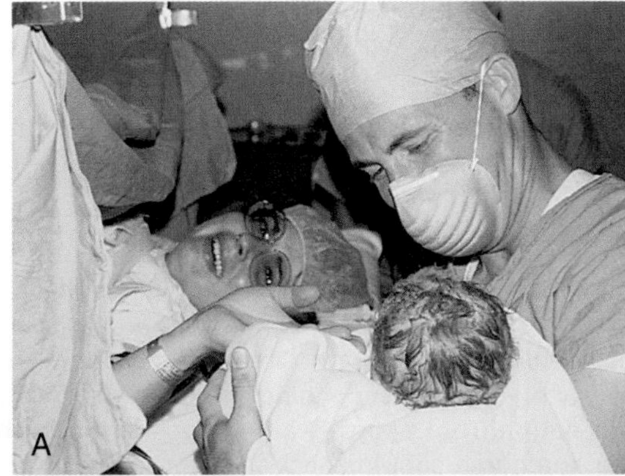
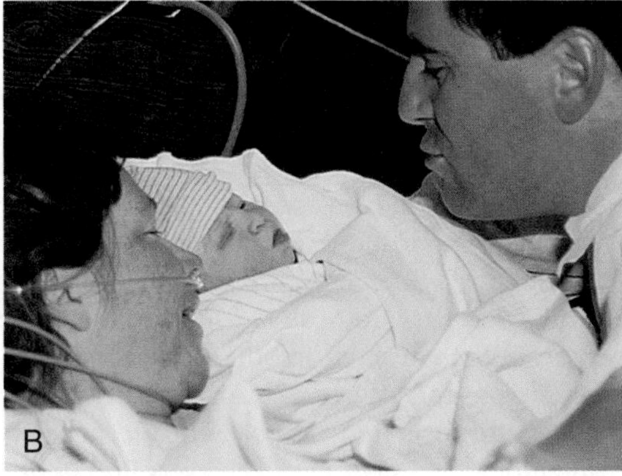

Fig. 22-13 **A,** Parents and their newborn. The physician manually removes the placenta, suctions the remaining amniotic fluid and blood from the uterine cavity, and closes the uterine incision, peritoneum, muscle layer, fatty tissue, and finally the skin, while the new family shares some time together. **B,** Parents become better acquainted with their newborn while mother rests after surgery. (Courtesy Marjorie Pyle, RNC, Lifecircle, Costa Mesa, CA.)

A nurse from the labor and birth unit usually is present to provide care for the infant. In addition, a pediatrician or a nurse team skilled in neonatal resuscitation may also be present for the surgery because these infants are considered to be at risk until evidence of physiologic stability exists after the birth. A crib with resuscitation equipment is readied before surgery. Personnel who are responsible for care are expert not only in resuscitative techniques, but also in their ability to detect normal and abnormal infant responses. After birth, if the infant's condition permits and the mother is awake, the baby may be placed skin-to-skin on the mother or can be given to the woman's partner to hold (Fig. 22-13). The infant whose condition is compromised is transported after initial stabilization to the nursery for observation and the implementation of appropriate interventions. In some institutions the partner may accompany the infant; if not, personnel keep the family informed of the infant's progress, and parent-infant contacts are initiated as soon as possible.

If family members cannot accompany the woman during surgery, they are directed to the surgical or obstetric waiting room. The physician then reports on the condition of the mother and child to the family members after the birth is completed. Family members may be allowed to accompany the infant as he or she is transferred to the nursery, giving them an opportunity to see and admire the new baby.

LEGAL TIP **Disclosure of Patient Information**

Some mothers or fathers want the privilege of informing family and friends of the infant's gender (if it was not known before birth) or other information about the birth. Before responding to requests for such information from people waiting outside the birthing area, the nurse should check to see if the mother has given consent for such information to be released.

Immediate postoperative care. Once surgery is completed the mother is usually transferred to a postanesthesia recovery area. After a cesarean birth, women have both postoperative and postpartum needs that must be addressed. They are surgical patients, as well as new mothers. Nursing assessments in this immediate postbirth period follow agency protocol and include the degree of recovery from the effects of anesthesia, postoperative and postbirth status, and degree of pain. A patent airway is maintained, and the woman is positioned to prevent possible aspiration. Vital signs are taken every 15 minutes for 1 to 2 hours or until stable. The condition of the incisional dressing, the fundus, and the amount of lochia are assessed, as well as the intravenous intake and the urine output through the Foley catheter. The woman is helped to turn and to perform coughing, deep-breathing, and leg exercises. Medications for pain relief should be administered before postoperative pain becomes severe.

If the baby is present, the mother and her partner are given some time alone with him or her to facilitate bonding and attachment. Breastfeeding can be initiated if the mother feels like trying. The woman is ready for discharge from the recovery area once her condition is stable and the effects of anesthesia have worn off (i.e., she is alert, oriented, and able to feel and move extremities).

Postoperative or postpartum care. The attitude of the nurse and other health team members can influence the woman's perception of herself after a cesarean birth. The caregivers should stress that the woman is a new mother first and a surgical patient second. This attitude helps the woman perceive herself as having the same problems and needs as other new mothers while requiring supportive postoperative care. See Care Path: Cesarean Birth without Complications for an overview of the care this woman will require.

The women's physiologic concerns for the first few days may be dominated by pain at the incision site and pain resulting from intestinal gas. For the first 24 hours after surgery, pain relief may be provided by epidural opioids, patient-controlled analgesia, or intravenous or intramuscular injections. After this time, women are generally changed to oral analgesics. Other comfort measures such as position changes, splinting of the incision with pillows, and relaxation and breathing techniques (e.g., those learned in childbirth classes) may be implemented (see Patient Instructions for Self-Management box: Postpartum Pain Relief after Cesarean Birth).

Women are often the best judges of what their bodies need and can tolerate, including the postoperative ingestion of foods and fluids. They are usually kept on nothing-by-mouth status or given "sips and chips" (sips of clear fluids and teaspoons of crushed ice) until bowel sounds return. The diet is then advanced to full liquids. After women are passing flatus, they can resume a regular diet (Gilbert, 2007). Intravenous fluids are usually discontinued as soon as the woman is tolerating liquids orally. Ambulation and rocking in a rocking chair may relieve gas pains. Avoiding gas-forming foods and carbonated beverages and drinking liquids through a straw may help minimize them (see Patient Instructions for Self-Management box: Postpartum Pain Relief after Cesarean Birth).

Daily care includes perineal care, breast care, and routine hygienic care. The woman may shower after the incisional dressing is removed, usually on the first postoperative day (if showering is acceptable according to the women's cultural beliefs and practices). The indwelling urinary catheter is also generally removed on the first postoperative day. The woman is encouraged to be out of bed and ambulating several times each day as soon as the urinary catheter is removed. The nurse assesses the woman's vital signs, incision, fundus, and lochia according to hospital policies, procedures, or protocols. Breath sounds, bowel sounds, circulatory status of the lower extremities, and urinary and bowel elimination also are assessed. In addition, noting maternal emotional status is important.

During the postpartum period the nurse can also provide care that meets the psychologic and teaching needs of mothers who have had cesarean births. The nurse can explain postpartum procedures to help the woman participate in her recovery from surgery. The nurse can also help the woman plan care and visits from family and friends that will allow adequate rest periods. Providing information on and assistance with infant care can facilitate adjustment to her role as a mother. The woman is supported as she breastfeeds her baby by receiving individualized assistance to hold and position the baby comfortably at her breast. Use of the side-lying or football hold positions and supporting the newborn with pillows can enhance comfort and facilitate successful breastfeeding. The partner can be included in infant teaching sessions and in explanations about the woman's recovery. The couple should also be encouraged to express their feelings about the birth experience. Some parents are angry, frustrated, or disappointed that a vaginal birth was not possible. Some women express feelings of low self-esteem or a negative self-image; others express relief and gratitude that the baby is healthy and safely born. Having the nurse who

CARE PATH Cesarean Birth without Complications: Expected Length of Stay—48 to 72 Hours

	IMMEDIATE POSTOPERATIVE CESAREAN	BY FOURTH HOUR AFTER ADMISSION TO PP UNIT	5-24 HOURS	25-48 HOURS	BY DISCHARGE
ASSESSMENTS					
Admission assessments	Recovery room or PACU admission assessment complete	PP admission assessment and care plan completed			
Vital signs	Every 15 min × 1 hr; every 30 min × 1 hr, WNL	Every 4-8 hr, WNL	Every 4-8 hr, WNL	Every 4-8 hr, WNL	Every 8 hr, WNL
Postpartum assessment	Every 15 min × 1 hr; every 30 min × 1 hr, WNL	Every 4-8 hr, WNL	Every 4-8 hr, WNL	Every 8-12 hr, WNL	Every 8-12 hr, WNL
Abdominal incision	Dressing dry and intact	Dressing dry and intact	Dressing dry and intact	Dressing off or changed, incision intact	Incision intact; staples may be removed and Steri-Strips in place, incision WNL
Genitourinary	Retention catheter output >30 ml/hr	Retention catheter output >30 ml/hr	Retention catheter output >30 ml/hr; usually discontinued by 24 hours	Catheter discontinued, output >100 ml/void or 240 ml/8 hr	Urine output >240 ml/8 hr
Gastrointestinal		Absent or hypoactive BS	Hypoactive to active BS	Active BS + flatus	Active BS + flatus; may or may not have BM
Musculoskeletal	Alert or easily aroused, can move legs	Alert and oriented, moving all extremities	Ambulating with help	Ambulating unassisted	Ambulating ad lib
Bonding	Evidence of parent-infant bonding; first breastfeeding if desired		Parent-infant bonding continues	Parent-infant bonding progressing	
Laboratory tests			Intrapartal CBC results on chart or computer; determine Rh status and need for anti-Rh globulin; check for rubella immunity	PP HCT WNL, give anti-Rh globulin if indicated	Give rubella vaccine if indicated
INTERVENTIONS					
IV	IV continues	IV continues	IV continues	IV may be discontinued	
Diet	NPO	Ice chips, sips of clear liquids	Clear liquids, advance as tolerated	Regular diet or as tolerated	Regular diet
Perineal care		Pericare by nurse	Pericare with help	Self-pericare	
Activity	Bed rest	Bed rest	OOB × 3 with help, ADLs assisted, assisted to comfortable position to hold and feed baby	Holds baby comfortably, ambulates without assistance, ADLs unassisted	Activity ad lib

Continued

CARE PATH *Cesarean Birth without Complications: Expected Length of Stay—48 to 72 Hours—cont'd*

	IMMEDIATE POSTOPERATIVE CESAREAN	BY FOURTH HOUR AFTER ADMISSION TO PP UNIT	5-24 HOURS	25-48 HOURS	BY DISCHARGE
Pulmonary care	Patent airway; oxygen discontinued	TCDB every 2 hr with splinting, incentive spirometry every hour if ordered, lungs clear	TCDB every 2 hr, continue incentive spirometry if ordered while awake; lungs clear	TCDB as needed; lungs clear	
Medications	Oxytocin added to IV Pain control: analgesics, IV, or epidural narcotic as ordered	Oxytocin continued Pain control: analgesics—PCA, IM, PO, or epidural narcotic as ordered	Oxytocin may be discontinued Pain control: IM, PO, PCA narcotics or analgesics as needed	Oxytocin discontinued Pain control: PO analgesics, NSAIDs as needed; PCA discontinued; stool softener, PNV as ordered	Rx filled or given to take home
Teaching, discharge plan	Breastfeeding, positioning, leg exercises	Verbalize understanding of unit routines, how to achieve rest, TCDB, involution, pain control	*Self:* comfort measures and care; reinforce TCDB and positioning; introduce teaching videos, lactation promotion or suppression *Infant:* handwashing, infant safety, positioning for feeding and burping; if breastfeeding, then positioning baby, latching on, timing, removing from breast	*Self:* diet; activity and rest; bowel and bladder function; perineal care *Infant:* bonding; parent concerns; feeding; infant bath, cord care; need for car seat; newborn characteristics; circumcision care if procedure performed; answer questions	*Self:* home care, signs of complications (infections, bleeding), normal psychologic adjustments, normal ADLs; resumption of sexual activities; contraception; identification of support system at home; self-concept issues related to cesarean birth. Inform whom to call if problems; review need to keep follow-up appointment; provide information about community resources; provide copy of home care instructions *Infant:* parents to demonstrate infant care; reinforce use of booklets for infant care, whom to call if problems; discuss immunization needs; review need to keep follow-up appointments

ADLs, Activities of daily living; *BM,* bowel movement; *BS,* bowel sounds; *CBC,* complete blood count; *HCT,* hematocrit; *IM,* intramuscularly; *IV,* intravenous; *NPO,* nothing by mouth; *NSAIDs,* nonsteroidal antiinflammatory drugs; *OOB,* out of bed; *PACU,* postanesthesia care unit; *PCA,* patient-controlled analgesia; *PNV,* prenatal vitamins; *PO,* by mouth; *PP,* postpartum; *Rx,* prescription; *TCDB,* turn, cough, deep breathe; *WNL,* within normal limits.

PATIENT INSTRUCTIONS FOR SELF-MANAGEMENT

Postpartum Pain Relief after Cesarean Birth

INCISIONAL

- Splint incision with a pillow when moving or coughing.
- Use relaxation techniques such as music, breathing, and dim lights.

GAS

- Walk as often as you can.
- Do not eat or drink gas-forming foods, carbonated beverages, or whole milk.
- Do not use straws for drinking fluids.
- Take antiflatulence medication if prescribed.
- Lie on your left side to expel gas.
- Rock in a rocking chair.

PATIENT INSTRUCTIONS FOR SELF-MANAGEMENT

Signs of Postoperative Complications After Discharge Following Cesarean Birth

Report the following signs to your health care provider:

- Temperature exceeding 38° C (100.4° F)
- Urination: painful urination, urgency, cloudy urine
- Lochia: heavier than a normal menstrual period, clots, odor
- Cesarean incision: redness, swelling, bruising, foul-smelling discharge or bleeding, wound separation
- Severe, increasing abdominal pain

was present during the birth visit to help fill in "gaps" about the experience may be helpful.

Discharge after cesarean birth usually occurs by the third postoperative day. The time is often determined by criteria established by the woman's insurance carrier or the federal government (e.g., diagnosis-related groups). The Newborn's and Mother's Health Protection Act of 1996 provides for a length of stay of up to 96 hours for cesarean births. These criteria may not coincide with the woman's physical or psychosocial readiness for discharge. Some states have added home care provisions for mothers who meet appropriate criteria for discharge and choose to leave sooner than the allowed length of stay. This policy recognizes that home care is less costly than hospital care and in most cases is more beneficial for recovery.

The nurse provides discharge teaching to prepare women for self-care and newborn care in a limited time while trying to ensure that the woman is comfortable and able to rest. Discharge teaching and planning should include information about nutrition; measures to relieve pain and discomfort; exercise and specific activity restrictions; time management that includes periods of uninterrupted rest and sleep; hygiene, breast, and incision care; timing for resumption of sexual activity and contraception; signs of complications (see Patient Instructions for Self-Management box: Signs of Postoperative Complications); and infant care.

Trial of labor

A **trial of labor (TOL)** is the observance of a woman and her fetus for a reasonable period (e.g., 4-6 hours) of spontaneous active labor to assess the safety of vaginal birth for the mother and infant. By far the most common reason for a TOL is if the woman wishes to have a vaginal birth after a previous cesarean birth. During a TOL the woman is evaluated for the occurrence of active labor, including adequate contractions, engagement and descent of the presenting part, and effacement and dilation of the cervix.

The nurse assesses maternal vital signs, FHR, and contractions and is alert for signs of potential complications. If complications develop, the nurse is responsible for initiating appropriate actions, including notifying the primary health care provider, and for evaluating and documenting the maternal and fetal responses to the interventions. Nurses must recognize that the woman and her partner are often anxious about her health and well-being and that of their baby. Supporting and encouraging the woman and her partner and providing information regarding progress can reduce stress, enhance the labor process, and facilitate a successful outcome.

Vaginal birth after cesarean

Indications for primary cesarean birth, such as dystocia, breech presentation, or fetal distress, are often nonrecurring. Therefore a woman who has had a cesarean birth may subsequently become pregnant, experience no contraindications to labor and vaginal birth during the pregnancy, and choose to attempt a **vaginal birth after cesarean (VBAC).** Box 22-12 lists selection criteria suggested by ACOG for identifying candidates for VBAC. The overall VBAC success rate is approximately 70% to 80% (Landon, 2007). The benefits of VBAC include a shorter maternal hospital stay, less blood loss, fewer infections, and fewer thromboembolic events than with cesarean birth. Risks associated with VBAC include uterine rupture, hysterectomy, operative injury, and neonatal morbidity (ACOG, 2004).

Spontaneous labor is more likely to result in a successful VBAC than labor that has been induced or augmented (ACOG, 2004). Women most likely to have a successful VBAC are those who are younger than 35 years, whose fetus weighs less than 4000 g, and whose previous cesarean was performed for some reason other than failure of descent in second stage labor (Thorp, 2009). Not everyone is enthusiastic about TOL and VBAC. After being fully informed about the risks and benefits, more than 25% of potential candidates choose to have a repeat cesarean birth instead (Thorp).

Critical Thinking/Clinical Decision Making

Trial of Labor for Vaginal Birth after Cesarean (TOL/VBAC)

Heather, a 28-year-old G2 P1 gave birth by cesarean during her last pregnancy. During her routine prenatal visit at 32 weeks of gestation, Heather tells the nurse that she really wants to have a vaginal birth this time. Heather asks, "What do you think? Can I try for a VBAC?"

1. Evidence—Does the nurse have sufficient evidence at this time to advise Heather about the safety and feasibility of a trial of labor (TOL) for vaginal birth after cesarean (VABC)? If not, what data should be collected?
2. Assumptions—What assumptions can be made about the following issues related to TOL and VBAC?
   a. Risks that Heather faces if she chooses a TOL for VBAC
   b. Criteria that must be met for Heather to attempt a TOL for VBAC
   c. Labor management practices that facilitate a successful VBAC
   d. Labor management techniques that should be avoided during a TOL for VBAC
3. What implications and priorities for nursing care can be drawn at this time?
4. Does the evidence objectively support your conclusion?
5. Do alternative perspectives to your conclusion exist?

Case Study: Postdate Pregnancy

BOX 22-12

Selection Criteria for Vaginal Birth After Cesarean

- One or two previous low-transverse cesarean births
- Clinically adequate pelvis
- No other uterine scars or history of previous rupture
- Physicians immediately available throughout active labor capable of monitoring labor and performing an emergency cesarean birth if necessary

Data from American College of Obstetricians and Gynecologists (ACOG): *Vaginal birth after previous cesarean delivery* (ACOG Practice Bulletin No. 115), Washington, DC, 2010, Author.

If a woman chooses TOL, attention should be paid to her psychologic, as well as physical, needs during the TOL. Anxiety increases the release of catecholamines and can inhibit the release of oxytocin, thus delaying the progress of labor and possibly leading to a repeat cesarean birth. To alleviate such anxiety the nurse can encourage the woman to use breathing and relaxation techniques and to change positions to promote labor progress. The woman's partner can be encouraged to provide comfort measures and emotional support. Collaboration among the woman in labor, her partner, the nurse, and other health care providers often results in a successful VBAC. If a TOL does not proceed to vaginal birth, the woman will need support and encouragement to express her feelings about having another cesarean birth. This outcome should *not* be labeled as a failed VBAC.

POSTTERM PREGNANCY, LABOR, AND BIRTH

A **postterm pregnancy** (also sometimes called a *postdate* or *prolonged pregnancy*) is one that extends beyond the end of week 42 of gestation, or 294 days from the first day of the last menstrual period (LMP). The incidence of postterm pregnancy is estimated to be between 4% and 14% (Resnik & Resnik, 2009). Many pregnancies are misdiagnosed as prolonged. The use of first-trimester ultrasound for pregnancy dating in recent years has confirmed that the LMP, traditionally used for pregnancy dating, is much less reliable as a predictor of true gestational age than other methods. Therefore use of the LMP alone for pregnancy dating tends to greatly overestimate the number of postterm gestations (Divon, 2007; Resnik & Resnik).

The exact cause of postterm pregnancy is still unknown. However, clearly the timing of labor is determined by complex interactions among the fetus, the placenta and membranes, the uterine myometrium, and the cervix. For example, congenital primary fetal adrenal hypoplasia and placental sulfatase deficiency cause low estrogen production. Decreased estrogen levels may prevent normal cervical ripening and cause the delayed onset of labor. Although postterm pregnancy is more common in primiparous women than in other women, a woman who experiences one postterm pregnancy is more likely than others to experience it again in subsequent pregnancies (Divon, 2007; Resnik & Resnik, 2009).

Maternal and Fetal Risks

Maternal risks are often related to labor dystocia, such as increased risk for perineal injury related to fetal macrosomia. Interventions such as induction of labor with prostaglandins or oxytocin, forceps- or vacuum-assisted birth, and cesarean birth are more likely to be necessary. Each of these interventions, of course, carries its own set of risks. The woman may also experience fatigue, physical discomfort, and psychologic reactions such as depression, frustration, and feelings of inadequacy as she passes her estimated date of birth. Relationships with close friends and family members may become strained, and the woman's negative feelings about herself may be projected as feelings of resentment toward the fetus (Gilbert, 2007).

Another complication associated with postterm pregnancy is abnormal fetal growth. Although the risk of having a small-for-gestational-age infant is increased, only 10% to 20% of postterm fetuses are undernourished. Macrosomia (birth weight >4000 g) occurs far more often than in a term pregnancy. Macrosomia occurs when the placenta continues to provide adequate nutrients to support fetal growth after 40 weeks of gestation. Macrosomic infants have an increased risk for birth injuries caused by difficult forceps-assisted births and shoulder dystocia (Resnik & Resnik, 2009).

Other fetal risks associated with postterm gestation are related to the intrauterine environment. After 43 to 44 weeks of gestation the placenta begins to age. Enlarging areas of infarction and increased deposition of calcium and fibrin in its tissue decrease the placenta's reserve and may affect its ability to oxygenate the fetus. Decreased amniotic fluid (<400 ml), oligohydramnios, is the complication most frequently associated with postterm pregnancy. Because of the decreased amount of amniotic fluid, a potential likelihood exists for cord compression and resulting fetal hypoxemia (Gilbert, 2007). Other potential complications include meconium-stained amniotic fluid, an increased chance of meconium aspiration, and low Apgar scores. Oligohydramnios magnifies the effect of meconium staining. Having less than the normal amount of amniotic fluid available to dilute it makes the meconium thicker and stickier than it would otherwise be (Resnik & Resnik, 2009).

Dysmaturity syndrome occurs in approximately 20% of neonates born after postterm pregnancies. Dysmaturity syndrome is characterized by dry, cracked, peeling skin; long nails; meconium staining of the skin, nails, and umbilical cord; and perhaps loss of subcutaneous fat and muscle mass. Babies born with dysmaturity syndrome usually regain their weight quickly and exhibit few long-term neurologic problems (Gilbert, 2007).

CARE MANAGEMENT

The management of postterm pregnancy is still controversial. However, because perinatal morbidity and mortality increase greatly after 42 weeks of gestation, pregnancies are not usually allowed to continue after this time. In the United States, most physicians induce labor at 41 weeks of gestation. An alternative approach is to initiate twice-weekly fetal testing at 41 weeks of gestation. The testing generally consists of either a BPP or an NST along with an assessment of amniotic fluid volume. (See Chapter 19 for further discussion of these tests.) Currently, evidence is insufficient to determine which of the two management approaches is better (Resnik & Resnik, 2009).

During the postterm pregnancy period the woman is encouraged to assess fetal activity daily, assess for signs of labor, and keep appointments with her primary health care provider (see Patient Instructions for Self-Management box: Postterm Pregnancy). The woman and her family should be encouraged to express their feelings (e.g., frustration, anger, impatience, fear) about the prolonged pregnancy and should be helped to realize that these feelings are normal. At times the emotional and physical strain of a postterm pregnancy may seem overwhelming. Referral to a support group or another supportive resource may be needed.

> **PATIENT INSTRUCTIONS FOR SELF-MANAGEMENT**
>
> **Postterm Pregnancy**
>
> - Perform daily fetal movement counts.
> - Assess for signs of labor.
> - Call your primary health care provider if your membranes rupture or if you perceive a decrease in or no fetal movement.
> - Keep appointments for fetal assessment tests or cervical checks.
> - Go to the hospital soon after labor begins.

During labor the fetus of a woman with a postterm pregnancy should be continuously monitored electronically for a more accurate assessment of the FHR and pattern. Inadequate fluid volume can lead to compression of the cord, which results in fetal hypoxia that is reflected in variable or prolonged deceleration patterns. If oligohydramnios is present, an amnioinfusion may be performed to restore amniotic fluid volume to maintain a cushioning of the cord. See Chapter 11 for additional information on amnioinfusion.

OBSTETRIC EMERGENCIES

Meconium-Stained Amniotic Fluid

Meconium-stained amniotic fluid indicates that the fetus has passed meconium (first stool) at some time before birth. Meconium-stained amniotic fluid is green in color. The consistency of the meconium fluid is often described as either thin (light) or thick (heavy), depending on the amount of meconium present. Three possible reasons for the passage of meconium are as follows: (1) It is a normal physiologic function that occurs with maturity (meconium passage being infrequent before weeks 23 or 24, with an increased incidence after 38 weeks) or with a breech presentation; (2) it is the result of hypoxia-induced peristalsis and sphincter relaxation; and (3) it may be a sequel to umbilical cord compression–induced vagal stimulation in mature fetuses.

The major risk associated with meconium-stained amniotic fluid is the development of meconium aspiration syndrome (MAS) in the newborn. MAS causes a severe form of aspiration pneumonia that occurs most often in term or postterm infants who have passed meconium in utero. Current thought is that MAS most likely results from a long-standing intrauterine process rather than from aspiration immediately after birth as respirations are initiated (Rosenberg, 2007).

The presence of a team skilled in neonatal resuscitation is required at the birth of any infant with meconium-stained amniotic fluid. When meconium-stained amniotic fluid is present, the American Academy of Pediatrics (AAP) and the American Heart Association (AHA) Neonatal Resuscitation Program no longer recommends routine suctioning of the newborn's mouth and nose on the perineum (after the head is out but before the rest of the baby is born) followed by endotracheal suctioning after birth. Instead, management of a newborn with meconium-stained amniotic fluid is based only on assessment of the baby's condition at birth. No clinical studies warrant basing tracheal suctioning guidelines simply on meconium consistency (AAP & AHA, 2006) (see the Emergency box: Immediate Management of the Newborn with Meconium-Stained Amniotic Fluid for specific interventions).

NURSING ALERT *Every* birth should be attended by at least one person whose only responsibility is the baby and who is capable of initiating resuscitation. Either that person or someone else who is immediately available should have the skills required to perform a complete resuscitation, including endotracheal suctioning to remove meconium, if necessary.

Animation: Shoulder Dystocia

Shoulder Dystocia

Shoulder dystocia is an uncommon obstetric emergency that increases the risk for fetal and maternal morbidity and mortality during the attempt to deliver the fetus vaginally. It is a condition in which the head is born, but the anterior shoulder cannot pass under the pubic arch. Fetopelvic disproportion related to excessive fetal size (>4000 g) or maternal pelvic abnormalities may be a cause of shoulder dystocia, although up to half of all cases of shoulder dystocia occur with fetuses of smaller size (Lanni & Seeds, 2007; Thorp, 2009). Other risk factors for shoulder dystocia include maternal diabetes, a history of shoulder dystocia with a previous birth, and prolonged second-stage labor. In half of all cases of shoulder dystocia, however, no risk factors are identified (Thorp). During second-stage labor the nurse should observe for retraction of the fetal head against the perineum immediately after emergence (turtle sign), an early warning sign of shoulder dystocia (Thorp).

Fetal injuries are usually caused either by asphyxia related to the delay in completing the birth or by trauma from the maneuvers used to accomplish the birth. Complications related to trauma include brachial plexus and phrenic nerve injuries and fracture of the humerus or clavicle. The most serious complication is brachial plexus injury (Erb palsy), which occurs in 10% to 20% of infants born after shoulder dystocia. If brachial plexus injuries are recognized early and treated properly, 80% to 90% heal completely. Therefore permanent neurologic injury is rare (Thorp, 2009). The major maternal complications associated with shoulder dystocia are postpartum hemorrhage and rectal injuries (Thorp).

Management

Many maneuvers such as suprapubic pressure and maternal position changes have been suggested and tried to free the anterior shoulder. Suprapubic pressure can be applied (Fig. 22-14) in an attempt to push the anterior shoulder under the symphysis pubis (Lanni & Seeds, 2007).

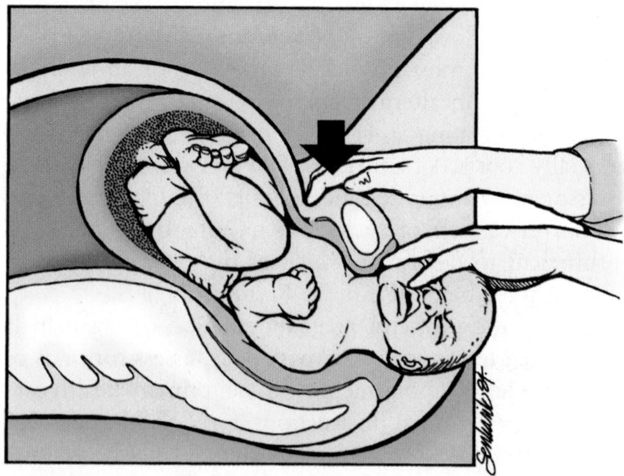

Fig. 22-14 Application of suprapubic pressure. (From Gabbe, S., Niebyl, J., & Simpson, J. [2007]. *Obstetrics: Normal and problem pregnancies* [5th ed.]. Philadelphia: Churchill Livingstone.)

EMERGENCY

Immediate Management of the Newborn with Meconium-Stained Amniotic Fluid

BEFORE BIRTH

- Assess amniotic fluid for the presence of meconium after rupture of membranes.
- If the amniotic fluid is meconium stained, gather equipment and supplies that might be necessary for neonatal resuscitation before the birth.
- Have at least one person capable of performing endotracheal intubation on the baby present at the birth.

IMMEDIATELY AFTER BIRTH

- Assess the baby's respiratory efforts, heart rate, and muscle tone.
- Suction only the baby's mouth and nose, using either a bulb syringe or a 12 or 14 French suction catheter if the baby has:
  - Strong respiratory efforts
  - Good muscle tone
  - Heart rate >100 beats/min
- Suction below the vocal cords using an endotracheal tube to remove any meconium present before many spontaneous respirations have occurred or assisted ventilation has been initiated if the baby has:
  - Depressed respirations
  - Decreased muscle tone
  - Heart rate <100 beats/min

Source: American Academy of Pediatrics (AAP) & American Heart Association (AHA). (2006). *Textbook of Neonatal Resuscitation* (5th ed.). Elk Grove Village, IL: AAP and Dallas, TX: AHA.

In the McRoberts maneuver (Fig. 22-15) the woman's legs are flexed apart, with her knees on her abdomen (Lanni & Seeds, 2007). This maneuver causes the sacrum to straighten, and the symphysis pubis rotates toward the mother's head. The angle of pelvic inclination is decreased, which frees the shoulder. Suprapubic pressure can be applied at this time. The McRoberts maneuver is the preferred method when a woman is receiving epidural anesthesia.

Having the woman move to the hands-and-knees position (the Gaskin maneuver), squatting position, or lateral recumbent position also has been used to resolve cases of shoulder dystocia. However, use of the Gaskin maneuver requires that the woman be mobile, with no significant loss of motor function caused by regional anesthesia. Additionally, a wide and stable surface must be available (Lanni & Seeds, 2007).

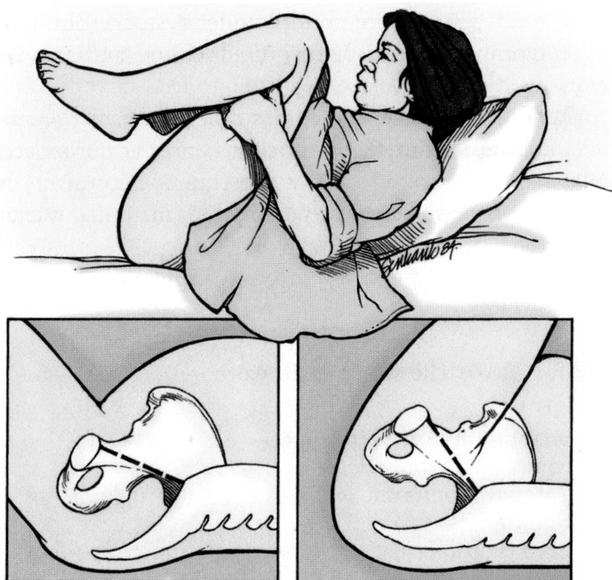

Fig. 22-15 McRoberts maneuver. (From Gabbe, S., Niebyl, J., & Simpson, J. [2007]. *Obstetrics: Normal and problem pregnancies* [5th ed.]. Philadelphia: Churchill Livingstone.)

When shoulder dystocia is diagnosed, the nurse should stay calm and immediately call for additional assistance (i.e., extra nurses, anesthesia care provider, neonatal resuscitation team). The nurse then helps the woman assume the position or positions that may facilitate birth of the shoulders, assists the primary health care provider with these maneuvers and techniques during birth, and documents the maneuvers. The nurse also provides encouragement and support to reduce anxiety and fear.

Newborn assessment should include examination for fracture of the clavicle or humerus, as well as brachial plexus injuries and asphyxia (Thorp, 2009). Maternal assessment should focus on early detection of hemorrhage and trauma to the vagina, perineum, and rectum.

Prolapsed Umbilical Cord

Animation: Cord Prolapse

Prolapse of the umbilical cord occurs when the cord lies below the presenting part of the fetus. Umbilical cord prolapse may be occult (hidden rather than visible) at any time during labor whether or not the membranes are ruptured (Fig. 22-16, *A* and *B*). Most commonly seen is frank (visible) prolapse directly after rupture of membranes, when gravity washes the cord in front of the presenting part (Fig. 22-16, *C* and *D*). Contributing factors include a long cord (longer than 100 cm), malpresentation (breech or transverse lie), or an unengaged presenting part.

If the presenting part does not fit snugly into the lower uterine segment (e.g., as in hydramnios), when the membranes rupture, a sudden gush of amniotic fluid may cause the cord to be displaced downward. Similarly, the cord may prolapse during amniotomy if the presenting part is

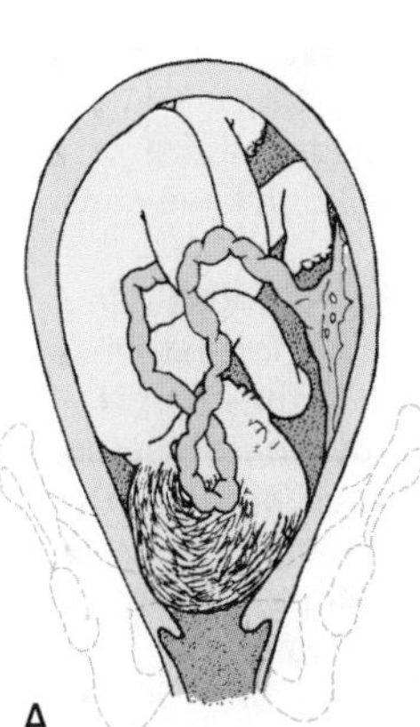

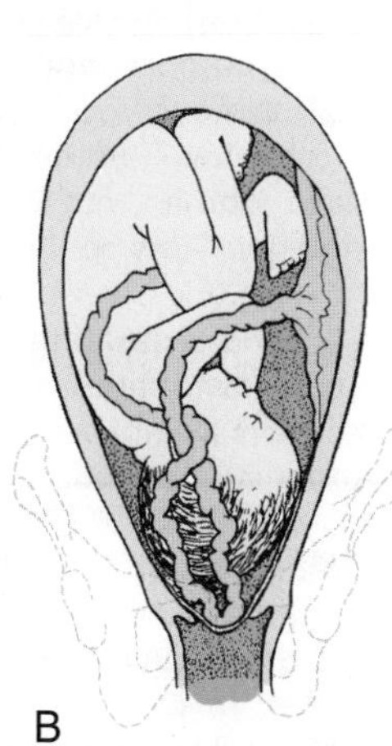

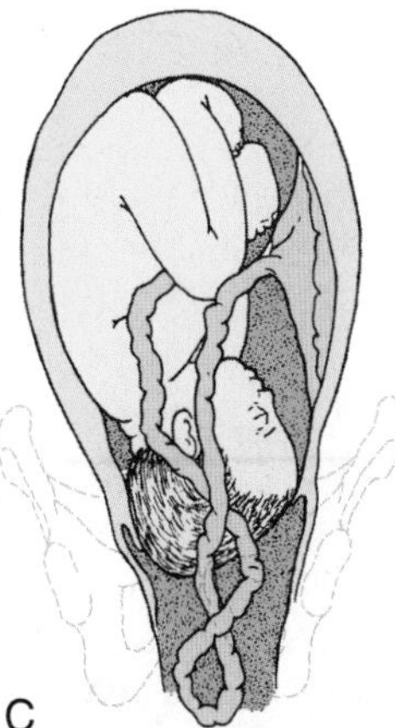

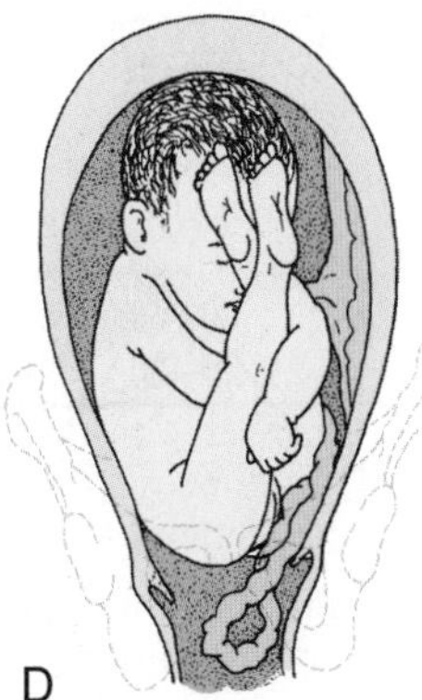

Fig. 22-16 Prolapse of umbilical cord. Note pressure of presenting part on umbilical cord, which endangers fetal circulation. **A,** Occult (hidden) prolapse of cord. **B,** Complete prolapse of cord. Note that membranes are intact. **C,** Cord presenting in front of the fetal head may be seen in vagina. **D,** Frank breech presentation with prolapsed cord.

high. A small fetus may not fit snugly into the lower uterine segment; as a result the likelihood of cord prolapse increases.

Management

Prompt recognition of a prolapsed umbilical cord is important because fetal hypoxia resulting from prolonged cord compression (i.e., occlusion of blood flow to and from the fetus for more than 5 minutes) usually results in central nervous system damage or death of the fetus. Pressure on the cord may be relieved by the examiner putting a sterile gloved hand into the vagina and holding the presenting part off of the umbilical cord (Fig. 22-17, *A* and *B*). The woman may also be assisted into a position such as a modified Sims (Fig. 22-17, *C*), Trendelenburg, or knee-chest (Fig. 22-17, *D*) position in which gravity keeps the pressure of the presenting part off the cord. If the cervix is fully dilated, a forceps- or vacuum-assisted birth can be performed for the fetus in a cephalic presentation; otherwise, a cesarean birth is likely to be performed. Nonreassuring FHR patterns, inadequate uterine relaxation, and bleeding also can occur as a result of a prolapsed umbilical cord. Indications of and immediate interventions for prolapsed cord are presented in the Emergency box: Prolapsed Cord. Ongoing assessment of the woman and her fetus is critical to determine the effectiveness of each action taken. The woman and her family are often aware of the seriousness of the situation; therefore the nurse must provide support by giving explanations for the interventions being implemented and their effect on the status of the fetus.

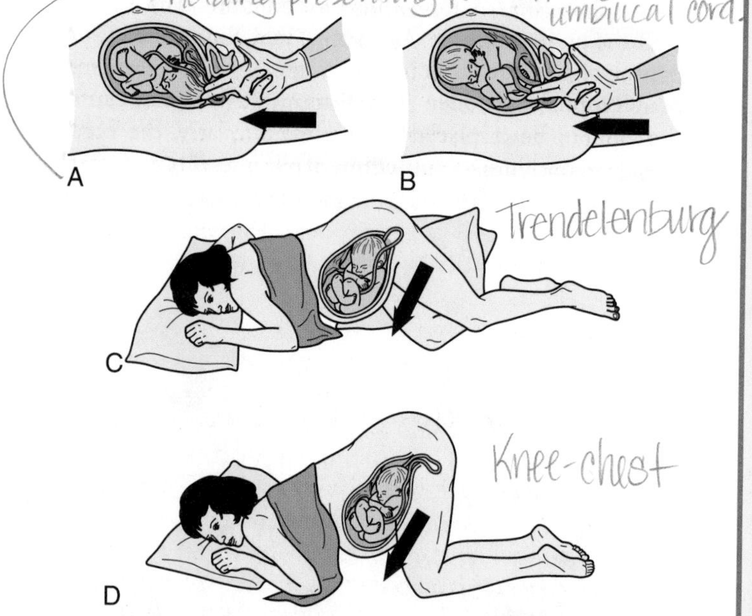

Fig. 22-17 *Arrows* indicate direction of pressure against presenting part to relieve compression of prolapsed umbilical cord. Pressure exerted by examiner's fingers in **A,** vertex presentation, and **B,** breech presentation. **C,** Gravity relieves pressure when woman is in modified Sims position with hips elevated as high as possible with pillows. **D,** Knee-chest position.

Rupture of the Uterus

Rupture of the uterus, in which complete nonsurgical disruption of all uterine layers takes place, is a rare but very serious obstetric injury that occurs in 1 in 2000 births (Francois & Foley, 2007; Landon, 2007). During labor and birth the major risk factor for uterine rupture is a TOL for attempted VBAC. The likelihood of uterine rupture depends on both the type and the location of the previous uterine scar. Uterine rupture occurs most often with a previous classic incision (Landon). Other risk factors include labor induction, multiple prior cesarean births or other types of uterine surgery, multiparity, and trauma (Francois & Foley).

Uterine dehiscence, sometimes called *incomplete uterine rupture,* is separation of a prior scar. It may go unnoticed unless the woman undergoes a subsequent cesarean birth or other uterine surgery. The potential for maternal or fetal

EMERGENCY

Prolapsed Umbilical Cord

SIGNS

- Variable or prolonged deceleration during uterine contraction.
- Woman reports feeling the cord after membranes rupture.
- Cord is seen or felt in or protruding from the vagina.

INTERVENTIONS

- Call for assistance.
- Have someone notify the primary health care provider immediately.
- Glove the examining hand quickly, and insert two fingers into the vagina to the cervix. With one finger on either side of the cord or both fingers to one side, exert upward pressure against the presenting part to relieve compression of the cord (Fig. 22-17, *A* and *B*). Do not move your hand! Another person may place a rolled towel under the woman's right or left hip.
- Place woman into the extreme Trendelenburg or a modified Sims position (Fig. 22-17, *C*) or a knee-chest position (Fig. 22-17, *D*).
- If cord is protruding from vagina, wrap loosely in a sterile towel saturated with warm sterile normal saline solution. Do not attempt to replace cord into cervix.
- Administer oxygen to the woman by nonrebreather facemask at 8-10 L/min until birth is accomplished.
- Start intravenous fluids or increase existing drip rate.
- Continue to monitor fetal heart rate continuously, by internal fetal scalp electrode, if possible.
- Explain to woman and support person what is happening and the way it is being managed.
- Prepare for immediate vaginal birth if cervix is fully dilated or cesarean birth if it is not.

complications as a result of uterine dehiscence is negligible given that separation of a prior scar does not result in hemorrhage (Landon, 2007).

Signs and symptoms vary with the extent of the uterine rupture. The most common finding is a nonreassuring FHR tracing, including variable and late decelerations, bradycardia, and absent or minimal variability. A loss of fetal station may also occur. The woman may experience constant abdominal pain, uterine tenderness, a change in uterine shape, and cessation of contractions (Francois & Foley, 2007). She may also exhibit signs of hypovolemic shock caused by hemorrhage (i.e., hypotension, tachypnea, pallor, and cool, clammy skin). If the placenta separates, the FHR will be absent. Fetal parts may be palpable through the abdomen.

Management

Prevention is the best treatment. Women who have had a previous classic cesarean birth are advised to not labor or attempt vaginal birth in subsequent pregnancies. Those at risk for uterine rupture are assessed closely during labor. Women whose labor is induced with oxytocin or prostaglandins (especially if their previous birth was cesarean) are monitored for signs of uterine tachysystole because contractions that occur too frequently or last too long can precipitate uterine rupture. If tachysystole occurs, the oxytocin infusion is discontinued or decreased, and a tocolytic medication may be given to decrease the intensity of the uterine contractions (see Emergency box: Uterine Tachysystole with Oxytocin p. 702). After giving birth, the woman is assessed for excessive bleeding, especially if the fundus is firm and signs of hemorrhagic shock are present.

If rupture occurs, management depends on the severity. A small rupture may be managed with a laparotomy and birth of the infant, repair of the laceration, and blood transfusions, if needed. Hysterectomy may be necessary if the rupture is large and difficult to close or if the woman is hemodynamically unstable (Francois & Foley, 2007).

The nurse's role in this situation may include starting intravenous fluids, transfusing blood products, administering oxygen, and assisting with the preparation for immediate surgery. Supporting the woman's family and providing information about the treatment is important during this emergency. The associated fetal mortality rate is high (50%-75%), and the maternal mortality rate may be high if the woman is not treated immediately (Cunningham et al., 2005). Providing information about spiritual support services or suggesting that the family contact their own support system may be warranted.

Amniotic Fluid Embolism

Amniotic fluid embolism (AFE), also known as *anaphylactoid syndrome of pregnancy,* is a rare but devastating complication of pregnancy. It is characterized by the sudden, acute onset of hypoxia, hypotension, or cardiac arrest, and coagulopathy. AFE occurs during labor, during birth, or within 30 minutes after birth. This combination of sudden respiratory and cardiovascular collapse, along with coagulopathy, is similar to that observed in patients with anaphylactic or septic shock. In both of these conditions, a foreign substance is introduced into the circulation, resulting in disseminated intravascular coagulation, hypotension, and hypoxia (Martin & Foley, 2009).

In AFE the foreign substance that initiates the condition is presumed to be present in amniotic fluid that is introduced into the maternal circulation. However, the exact factor that initiates AFE has not been identified. In the past, particles of fetal debris (e.g., vernix, hair, skin cells, or meconium) found in amniotic fluid were thought to be responsible for initiating the syndrome. However, fetal debris can be found in the pulmonary circulation of most normal laboring women. Also, fetal debris is identified in only 78% of women who are diagnosed with AFE (Martin & Foley, 2009). Although AFE is rare, the mortality rate is 61% or higher (Martin & Foley). Approximately 50% of the neonates who survive have neurologic impairment (Schoening, 2006).

Maternal factors (including multiparity, tumultuous labor, placental abruption, and oxytocin induction of labor) and fetal problems (including macrosomia, death, and meconium passage) have been associated with an increased risk for the development of AFE (Cunningham et al., 2005).

Management

The immediate interventions for AFE are summarized in the Emergency box: Amniotic Fluid Embolism. Care must be instituted immediately. Cardiopulmonary resuscitation is often necessary. If cardiopulmonary arrest occurs, for optimal fetal survival, a perimortem cesarean birth should be accomplished within 5 minutes (Lu & Curet, 2007). The nurse's immediate responsibility is to assist with the resuscitation efforts. See Chapter 21 for further discussion of cardiopulmonary resuscitation in the pregnant woman.

If the woman survives, she is usually moved to a critical care unit. Additional interventions will likely include replacing blood and clotting factors and maintaining adequate hydration and blood pressure. The woman is usually placed on mechanical ventilation. Invasive cardiac monitoring may also be required (Martin & Foley, 2009).

Support of the woman's partner and family is needed; they will be anxious and distressed. Brief explanations of what is happening are important during the emergency and can be reinforced after the immediate crisis is over. If the woman dies, emotional support and involvement of the perinatal loss support team or other resource for grief counseling is needed. Referral to grief and loss support groups would be appropriate (see Chapter 24). The nursing staff also may need help in coping with feelings and emotions that result from a maternal death.

EMERGENCY

Amniotic Fluid Embolism (Anaphylactoid Syndrome of Pregnancy)

SIGNS

- Respiratory distress:
  - Restlessness
  - Dyspnea
  - Cyanosis
  - Pulmonary edema
  - Respiratory arrest
- Circulatory collapse:
  - Hypotension
  - Tachycardia
  - Shock
  - Cardiac arrest
- Hemorrhage:
  - Coagulation failure: bleeding from incisions, venipuncture sites, trauma (lacerations); petechiae, ecchymoses, purpura
  - Uterine atony

INTERVENTIONS

- Oxygenate:
  - Administer oxygen by nonrebreather facemask at 8-10 L/min or by resuscitation bag delivering 100% oxygen.
  - Prepare for intubation and mechanical ventilation.
  - Initiate or assist with cardiopulmonary resuscitation. Tilt pregnant woman 30 degrees to side to displace uterus.
- Maintain cardiac output and replace fluid losses:
  - Position woman on her side.
  - Administer intravenous fluids.
  - Administer blood products: packed cells, fresh frozen plasma.
  - Insert indwelling catheter, and measure hourly urine output.
- Correct coagulation failure.
- Monitor fetal and maternal status.
- Prepare for emergency birth once woman's condition is stabilized.
- Provide emotional support to woman, her partner, and family.

KEY POINTS

- Preterm labor is uterine contractions with cervical change that occurs between 20 and 37 weeks of pregnancy; preterm birth is any birth that occurs before the completion of 37 weeks of pregnancy.
- The cause of preterm labor is unknown and is assumed to be multifactorial; therefore predicting with certainty which women will experience preterm labor and birth is impossible.
- Because the onset of preterm labor is often insidious and can be mistaken for normal discomforts of pregnancy, nurses should teach all pregnant women how to detect the early symptoms of preterm labor and to call their primary health care provider when symptoms occur.
- Bed rest, a commonly prescribed intervention for preterm labor, has many serious side effects and has never been shown to decrease preterm birth rates.
- The best reasons for tocolytic therapy are to achieve sufficient time to administer glucocorticoids in an effort to accelerate fetal lung maturity and reduce the severity of respiratory complications in infants born preterm and to allow time for transporting the woman before birth to a center equipped to care for preterm infants.
- If fetal or early neonatal death is expected, the parents and members of the health care team need to discuss the situation before the birth and decide on a management plan that is acceptable to everyone.
- Vigilance for signs of infection is a major part of the care for women with preterm PROM.
- Dystocia results from differences in the normal relations among any of the five factors affecting labor and is characterized by differences in the pattern of progress in labor.
- Uterine contractility is increased by the effects of oxytocin and prostaglandin and is decreased by tocolytic agents.
- Cervical ripening using chemical or mechanical measures can increase the success of labor induction.
- Expectant parents benefit from learning about operative obstetrics (e.g., forceps-assisted, vacuum-assisted, or cesarean birth) during the prenatal period.
- The basic purpose of cesarean birth is to preserve the life or health of the mother and her fetus.
- Unless contraindicated, vaginal birth is possible after a previous cesarean birth.
- Labor management that emphasizes one-to-one support of the laboring woman by another woman (e.g., doula, nurse, nurse-midwife) can reduce the rate of cesarean birth.
- A postterm pregnancy poses a risk to both the mother and the fetus.
- Obstetric emergencies (e.g., meconium-stained amniotic fluid, shoulder dystocia, prolapsed cord, rupture of the uterus, AFE) occur rarely but require immediate intervention to preserve the health or life of the mother and fetus or newborn.

Audio Chapter Summaries Access an audio summary of these Key Points on evolve

References

Albers, L. (2007). The evidence for physiologic management of the active phase of the first stage of labor. *Journal of Midwifery & Women's Health, 52*(3), 207-215.

American Academy of Pediatrics (AAP) & American College of Obstetricians and Gynecologists (ACOG). (2007). *Guidelines for perinatal care* (6th ed.). Washington, DC: ACOG.

American Academy of Pediatrics (AAP) & American Heart Association (AHA). (2006). *Textbook of Neonatal Resuscitation* (5th ed.). Elk Grove Village, IL: AAP and Dallas, TX: AHA.

American College of Obstetricians and Gynecologists (ACOG). (1999). Induction of labor. *ACOG Practice Bulletin No. 10.* Washington, DC: ACOG.

American College of Obstetricians and Gynecologists. (ACOG). (2003). Management of preterm labor. *ACOG Practice Bulletin No. 43.* Washington, DC: ACOG.

American College of Obstetricians and Gynecologists (ACOG). (2004). Vaginal birth after a previous cesarean delivery. *ACOG Practice Bulletin No. 54.* Washington, DC: ACOG.

American College of Obstetricians and Gynecologists (ACOG). (2007). Cesarean delivery on maternal request. *ACOG Committee Opinion No. 394.* Washington, DC: ACOG.

American College of Obstetricians and Gynecologists (ACOG). (2009). Intrapartum fetal heart rate monitoring: Nomenclature, interpretation, and general management principles. *ACOG Practice Bulletin No. 106.* Washington, DC. ACOG.

Battista, L. R., & Wing, D.A. (2007). Abnormal labor and induction of labor. In S. Gabbe, J. Niebyl, & J. Simpson (Eds.). *Obstetrics: Normal and problem pregnancies* (5th ed.). Philadelphia: Churchill Livingstone.

Berghella,V., Baxter, J., & Chauhan, S. (2008). Evidence-based labor and delivery management. *American Journal of Obstetrics & Gynecology, 199*(5), 445-454.

Cherouny, P., Federico, F., Haraden, C., Leavitt Gullo, S., & Resar, R. (2005). *Idealized design of perinatal care.* IHI Innovation Series white paper. Cambridge, MA: Institute for Healthcare Improvement. Internet document available at www.ihi.org (accessed June 23, 2009).

Clark, S., Simpson, K., Knox, G., & Garite, T. (2009). Oxytocin: New perspectives on an old drug. *American Journal of Obstetrics and Gynecology 200*(35), e1-35, e6.

Cleary-Goldman, J., Chitkara, U., & Berkowitz, R. (2007). Multiple gestations. In S. Gabbe, J. Niebyl, & J. Simpson (Eds.). *Obstetrics: Normal and problem pregnancies* (5th ed.). Philadelphia: Churchill Livingstone.

Collard, T., Diallo, H., Habinsky, A., Hentschell, C., & Vezeau, T. (2008/2009). Elective cesarean section: Why women choose it and what nurses need to know. *Nursing for Women's Health, 12*(6), 480-488.

Cunningham, F., Leveno, K., Bloom, S., Hauth, J., Gilstrap, L., & Wenstrom, K. (2005). *Williams obstetrics* (22nd ed.). New York: McGraw-Hill.

Divon, M. (2007). Prolonged pregnancy. In S. Gabbe, J. Niebyl, & J. Simpson (Eds.). *Obstetrics: Normal and problem pregnancies* (5th ed.). Philadelphia: Churchill Livingstone.

Francois, K., & Foley, M. (2007). Antepartum and postpartum hemorrhage. In S. Gabbe, J. Niebyl, & J. Simpson (Eds.), *Obstetrics: Normal and problem pregnancies* (5th ed.). Philadelphia: Churchill Livingstone.

Freda, M. (2006). It's time for preconception health! *MCN American Journal of Maternal Child Nursing, 31*(6), 346.

Friedman, E. (1989). Normal and dysfunctional labor. In W. Cohen, D. Ackers, & E. Friedman (Eds.). *Management of Labor* (2nd ed). Rockville, MD: Aspen.

Gennaro, S., Shults, J., & Garry, D. (2008). Stress and preterm labor and birth in black women. *Journal of Obstetric, Gynecologic, and Neonatal Nursing, 37*(5), 538-545.

Gilbert, E., (2007). *Manual of high risk pregnancy and delivery* (4th ed.). St. Louis: Mosby.

Hodnett, E., Gates, S., Hofmeyr G., & Sakala, C. (2007). Continuous support for women during childbirth. In *The Cochrane Database of Systematic Reviews* 2007, Issue 3. Art. No.: CD 003766.

Iams, J. & Romero, R. (2007). Preterm birth. In S. Gabbe, J. Niebyl, & J. Simpson (Eds.), *Obstetrics: Normal and problem pregnancies* (5th ed.). Philadelphia: Churchill Livingstone.

Iams, J., Romero, R., & Creasy, R. (2009). Preterm labor and birth. In R. Creasy, R. Resnik, & J. Iams (Eds.), *Creasy and Resnik's maternal-fetal medicine: Principles and practice* (6th ed.). Philadelphia: Saunders.

Landon, M. (2007). Cesarean delivery. In S. Gabbe, J. Niebyl, & J. Simpson (Eds.), *Obstetrics: Normal and problem pregnancies* (5th ed.). Philadelphia: Churchill Livingstone.

Lanni, S., & Seeds, J. (2007). Malpresentations. In S. Gabbe, J. Niebyl, & J. Simpson (Eds.), *Obstetrics: Normal and problem pregnancies* (5th ed.). Philadelphia: Churchill Livingstone.

Lu, E., & Curet, M.J. (2007). Surgical procedures in pregnancy. In S. Gabbe, J. Niebyl, & J. Simpson (Eds.), *Obstetrics: Normal and problem pregnancies* (5th ed.). Philadelphia: Churchill Livingstone.

Macones, G., Hankins, G., Spong, C., Hauth, J., & Moore, T. (2008). The 2008 National Institute of Child Health and Human Development Workshop Report on Electronic Fetal Monitoring: Update on definitions, interpretation, and research guidelines. *Journal of Obstetric, Gynecologic, and Neonatal Nursing, 37*(5), 510-515.

Mahlmeister, L. (2008). Best practices in perinatal care: Evidence-based management of oxytocin induction and augmentation of labor. *Journal of Perinatal and Neonatal Nursing, 22*(4), 259-263.

Malone, F., & D'Alton, M. (2009). Multiple gestation: Clinical characteristics and management. In R. Creasy, R. Resnik, & J. Iams (Eds.), *Creasy and Resnik's maternal-fetal medicine: Principles and practice* (6th ed.). Philadelphia: Saunders.

Maloni, J., & Park, S. (2005). Postpartum symptoms after antepartum bedrest. *Journal of Obstetric, Gynecologic, and Neonatal Nursing, 34*(2), 163-171.

Martin, J., Hamilton, B., Sutton, P., Ventura, S., Menacker, F., Kirmeyer, S., et al. (2009). Births: Final data for 2006. *National Vital Statistics Reports* (*Vol. 57,* No. 7). Hyattsville, MD: National Center for Health Statistics. Internet document available at http://www.cdc.gov/nchs/data/nvsr/nvsr57/nvsr57_07.pdf (accessed March 17, 2009).

Martin, S., & Foley, M. (2009). Intensive care monitoring of the critically ill pregnant patient. In R. Creasy, R. Resnik, & J. Iams (Eds.), *Creasy and Resnik's maternal-fetal medicine: Principles and practice* (6th ed.). Philadelphia: Saunders.

Meis, P., & Society for Maternal-Fetal Medicine. (2005). 17 hydroxyprogesterone for the prevention of preterm delivery. *Obstetrics & Gynecology, 105* (5 Pt 1), 1128-1135.

Mercer, B. (2007). Premature rupture of the membranes. In S. Gabbe, J. Niebyl, & J. Simpson (Eds.), *Obstetrics: Normal and problem pregnancies* (5th ed.). Philadelphia: Churchill Livingstone.

Mercer, B. (2009a). Assessment and induction of fetal pulmonary maturity. In R. Creasy, R. Resnik, & J. Iams (Eds.), *Creasy and Resnik's maternal-fetal medicine: Princi-*

ples and practice (6th ed.). Philadelphia: Saunders.

Mercer, B. (2009b). Premature rupture of the membranes. In R. Creasy, R. Resnik, & J. Iams (Eds.), *Creasy and Resnik's maternal-fetal medicine: Principles and practice* (6th ed.). Philadelphia: Saunders.

Moleti, C.A. (2009). Trends and controversies in labor induction. *MCN American Journal of Maternal Child Nursing, 34*(1), 40-47.

Nielsen, P., Galan, H., Kilpatrick, S., & Garrison, E. (2007). Operative vaginal delivery. In S. Gabbe, J. Niebyl, & J. Simpson (Eds.), *Obstetrics: Normal and problem pregnancies* (5th ed.). Philadelphia: Churchill Livingstone.

Resnik, J., & Resnik, R. (2009). Post-term pregnancy. In R. Creasy, R. Resnik, & J. Iams (Eds.), *Creasy and Resnik's maternal-fetal medicine: Principles and practice* (6th ed.). Philadelphia: Saunders.

Rideout, S. (2005). Tocolytics of pre-term labor: What nurses need to know. *AWHONN Lifelines, 9*(1), 56-61.

Roberts, J., & Hanson, L. (2007). Best practices in second stage labor care: Maternal bearing down and positioning. *Journal of Midwifery & Women's Health, 52*(3), 238-245.

Romero, R., & Lockwood, C. (2009). Pathogenesis of spontaneous preterm labor. In R. Creasy, R. Resnik, & J. Iams (Eds.), *Creasy and Resnik's maternal-fetal medicine: Principles and practice* (6th ed.). Philadelphia: Saunders.

Rosenberg, A. (2007). The neonate. In S. Gabbe, J. Niebyl, & J. Simpson (Eds.), *Obstetrics: Normal and problem pregnancies* (5th ed.). Philadelphia: Churchill Livingstone.

Schoening, A. (2006). Amniotic fluid embolism: Historical perspectives and new possibilities. *MCN American Journal of Maternal Child Nursing, 31*(2), 78-83.

Simpson, K., & Knox, G. (2009). Oxytocin as a high-alert medication: Implications for perinatal patient safety. *MCN American Journal of Maternal Child Nursing, 34*(1), 8-15.

Society of Obstetricians and Gynaecologists of Canada (SOGC). (2004). News. C-sections on demand–SOGC's position. *Birth, 31*(2), 154.

Stremler, R., Hodnett, E., Petryshen, P., Stevens, B., Weston, J., & Willan, A. (2005). Randomized controlled trial of hands-and-knees positioning for occipito-posterior position in labor. *Birth, 32*(4), 243-251.

Thorp, J. (2009). Clinical aspects of normal and abnormal labor. In R. Creasy, R. Resnik, & J. Iams (Eds.), *Creasy and Resnik's maternal-fetal medicine: Principles and practice* (6th ed.). Philadelphia: Saunders.

Williams, D. (2005). The top 10 reasons elective cesarean section should be on the decline. *AWHONN Lifelines, 9*(1), 23-24.

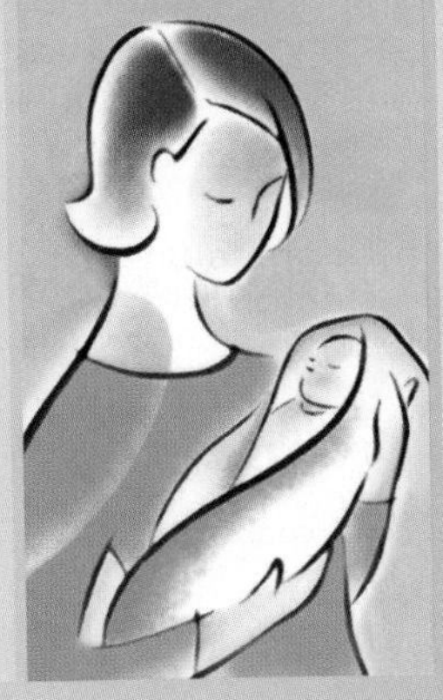

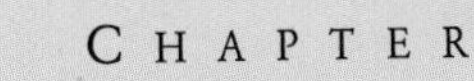

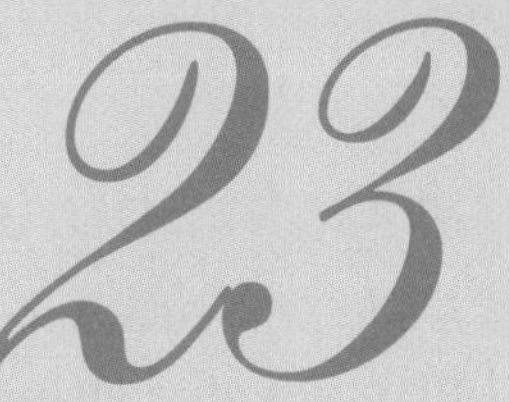

CHAPTER 23 Postpartum Complications

DEITRA LEONARD LOWDERMILK

LEARNING OBJECTIVES

- *Identify the causes, signs and symptoms, possible complications, and medical and nursing management of postpartum hemorrhage.*
- *Differentiate the causes of postpartum infection.*
- *Summarize the assessment and care of women with postpartum infection.*
- *Describe thromboembolic disorders, including incidence, etiologic factors, signs and symptoms, and management.*
- *Describe the sequelae of childbirth trauma.*
- *Discuss postpartum emotional complications, including incidence, risk factors, signs and symptoms, and management.*
- *Summarize the role of the nurse in the home setting in assessing potential problems and managing care of women with postpartum complications.*

KEY TERMS AND DEFINITIONS

endometritis Postpartum uterine infection, often beginning at the site of the placental implantation

hemorrhagic (hypovolemic) shock Clinical condition in which the peripheral blood flow is inadequate to return sufficient blood to the heart for normal function, particularly oxygen transport to the organs or tissue

inversion of the uterus Condition in which the uterus is turned inside out such that the fundus intrudes into the cervix or vagina

mastitis Infection in a breast, usually confined to a milk duct, characterized by influenza-like symptoms and redness and tenderness in the affected breast

mood disorders Disorders that have a disturbance in the prevailing emotional state as the dominant feature; cause is unknown

pelvic relaxation Lengthening and weakening of the fascial supports of pelvic structures

postpartum depression (PPD) Depression occurring within 4 weeks of childbirth, lasting longer than postpartum blues and characterized by a variety of symptoms that interfere with activities of daily living and care of the baby

postpartum hemorrhage (PPH) Excessive bleeding after childbirth; traditionally defined as a loss of 500 ml or more after a vaginal birth and 1000 ml after a cesarean birth

postpartum psychosis Syndrome characterized by depression, delusions, and thoughts by the mother of harming herself or her infant

puerperal infection Infection of the pelvic organs during the postbirth period; also called postpartum infection

subinvolution Failure of a part (e.g., the uterus) to reduce to its normal size and condition after enlargement from functional activity (e.g., pregnancy)

thrombophlebitis inflammation of a vein with secondary clot formation

urinary incontinence (UI) Uncontrollable leakage of urine

uterine atony Relaxation of uterus; leads to postpartum hemorrhage

WEB RESOURCES

Additional related content can be found on the companion website at evolve
http://evolve.elsevier.com/Lowdermilk/Maternity/

- NCLEX Review Questions
- Critical Thinking Exercise: Postpartum Complications
- Critical Thinking Exercise: Postpartum Depression
- Nursing Care Plan: Postpartum Depression
- Nursing Care Plan: Postpartum Hemorrhage

Collaborative efforts of the health care team are needed to provide safe and effective care to the woman and family experiencing postpartum complications. This chapter focuses on hemorrhage, infection, sequelae of childbirth trauma, and psychologic complications.

POSTPARTUM HEMORRHAGE

Definition and Incidence

Postpartum hemorrhage (PPH) continues to be a leading cause of maternal morbidity and mortality in the United States and worldwide (American College of Obstetricians and Gynecologists [ACOG], 2006; Johnson, Gregory, & Niebyl, 2007). It is a life-threatening event that can occur with little warning and is often unrecognized until the mother has profound symptoms. PPH has been traditionally defined as the loss of more than 500 ml of blood after vaginal birth and 1000 ml after cesarean birth. A 10% change in hematocrit between admission for labor and postpartum or the need for erythrocyte transfusion also has been used to define PPH (Francois & Foley, 2007). However, defining PPH is not a clear-cut issue. The diagnosis is often based on subjective observations, with blood loss often being underestimated by as much as 50% (Cunningham, Leveno, Bloom, Hauth, Gilstrap, & Wenstrom, 2005).

Traditionally, PPH has been classified as early or late with respect to the birth. Early, acute, or primary PPH occurs within 24 hours of the birth. Late or secondary PPH occurs after 24 hours and up to 6 to 12 weeks postpartum (ACOG, 2006; Francois & Foley, 2007). Today's health care environment encourages shortened stays after birth, thereby increasing the potential for acute episodes of PPH to occur outside the traditional hospital or birth center setting.

Etiology and Risk Factors

Considering the problem of excessive bleeding with reference to the stages of labor is helpful. From birth of the infant until separation of the placenta the character and quantity of blood passed may suggest excessive bleeding. For example, dark blood is probably of venous origin, perhaps from varices or superficial lacerations of the birth canal. Bright blood is arterial and may indicate deep lacerations of the cervix. Spurts of blood with clots may indicate partial placental separation. Failure of blood to clot or remain clotted indicates a pathologic condition or coagulopathy such as disseminated intravascular coagulation (DIC) (Francois & Foley, 2007).

Excessive bleeding may occur during the period from the separation of the placenta to its expulsion or removal. Commonly, such excessive bleeding is the result of incomplete placental separation, undue manipulation of the fundus, or excessive traction on the cord. After the placenta has been expelled or removed, persistent or excessive blood loss is usually the result of atony of the uterus or inversion of the uterus into the vagina. Late PPH may be the result of subinvolution of the uterus, endometritis, or retained placental fragments (Francois & Foley, 2007). Risk factors for PPH are listed in Box 23-1.

BOX 23-1

Risk Factors for Postpartum Hemorrhage

- Uterine atony
  - Overdistended uterus
    - Large fetus
    - Multiple fetuses
    - Hydramnios
    - Distention with clots
  - Anesthesia and analgesia
    - Conduction anesthesia
  - Previous history of uterine atony
  - High parity
  - Prolonged labor, oxytocin-induced labor
  - Trauma during labor and birth
    - Forceps-assisted birth
    - Vacuum-assisted birth
    - Cesarean birth
- Unrepaired lacerations of the birth canal
- Retained placental fragments
- Ruptured uterus
- Inversion of the uterus
- Placenta accreta, increta, percreta
- Coagulation disorders
- Placental abruption
- Placenta previa
- Manual removal of a retained placenta
- Magnesium sulfate administration during labor or postpartum period
- Chorioamnionitis
- Uterine subinvolution

Uterine Atony

Uterine atony is marked hypotonia of the uterus. Normally, placental separation and expulsion are facilitated by contraction of the uterus, which also prevents hemorrhage from the placental site. The corpus is in essence a basket weave of strong, interlacing smooth-muscle bundles through which many large maternal blood vessels pass (see Fig. 2-3). If the uterus is flaccid after detachment of all or part of the placenta, brisk venous bleeding occurs, and normal coagulation of the open vasculature is impaired and continues until the uterine muscle is contracted.

Uterine atony is the leading cause of PPH, complicating approximately 1 in 20 births (Francois & Foley, 2007). It is associated with high parity, hydramnios, a macrosomic fetus, and multifetal gestation. In such conditions the uterus is "overstretched" and contracts poorly after the birth. Other causes of atony include traumatic birth, use of halogenated anesthesia (e.g., halothane) or magnesium sulfate, rapid or prolonged labor, chorioamnionitis, and use of oxytocin for labor induction or augmentation (Francois & Foley). PPH in a previous pregnancy is a predominant risk factor for recurrent PPH (Kominiarek & Kilpatrick, 2007).

Lacerations of the Genital Tract

Lacerations of the cervix, vagina, and perineum are also causes of PPH. Hemorrhage related to lacerations should be suspected if bleeding continues despite a firm, contracted uterine fundus. This bleeding can be a slow trickle, an oozing, or frank hemorrhage. Factors that influence the causes and incidence of obstetric lacerations of the lower genital tract include operative birth, precipitate birth, congenital abnormalities of the maternal soft parts, and contracted pelvis. Size, abnormal presentation, and position of the fetus; relative size of the presenting part and the birth canal; previous scarring from infection, injury, or operation; and vulvar, perineal, and vaginal varicosities also can cause lacerations.

Extreme vascularity in the labial and periclitoral areas often results in profuse bleeding if laceration occurs. Hematomas also may be present.

Lacerations of the perineum are the most common of all injuries in the lower portion of the genital tract. These lacerations are classified as first, second, third, and fourth degree (see Chapter 12). An episiotomy may extend to become either a third- or fourth-degree laceration.

Prolonged pressure of the fetal head on the vaginal mucosa ultimately interferes with the circulation and may produce ischemic or pressure necrosis. The state of the tissues in combination with the type of birth may result in deep vaginal lacerations, with consequent predisposition to vaginal hematomas.

Pelvic hematomas may be vulvar, vaginal, or retroperitoneal in origin. Vulvar hematomas are the most common. Pain is the most common symptom, and most vulvar hematomas are visible. Vaginal hematomas occur more commonly in association with a forceps-assisted birth, an episiotomy, or primigravidity (Francois & Foley, 2007). During the postpartum period, if the woman reports a persistent perineal or rectal pain or a feeling of pressure in the vagina, a thorough examination is made. However, a retroperitoneal hematoma may cause minimal pain, and the initial symptoms may be signs of shock (Francois & Foley).

Cervical lacerations usually occur at the lateral angles of the external os. Most lacerations are shallow, and bleeding is minimal. More extensive lacerations may extend into the vaginal vault or into the lower uterine segment.

Retained Placenta

Nonadherent retained placenta

Retained placenta may result from partial separation of a normal placenta, entrapment of the partially or completely separated placenta by an hourglass constriction ring of the uterus, mismanagement of the third stage of labor, or abnormal adherence of the entire placenta or a portion of the placenta to the uterine wall. Placental retention because of poor separation is common in very preterm births (20-24 weeks of gestation).

Management of nonadherent retained placenta is by manual separation and removal by the primary health care provider. Supplementary anesthesia is not usually needed for women who have had regional anesthesia for birth. For other women, administration of light nitrous oxide and oxygen inhalation anesthesia or intravenous (IV) thiopental facilitates uterine exploration and placental removal. After this removal the woman is at continued risk for PPH and for infection.

Adherent retained placenta

Abnormal adherence of the placenta occurs for reasons unknown, but it is thought to result from zygotic implantation in an area of defective endometrium such that no zone of separation is present between the placenta and the decidua. Attempts to remove the placenta in the usual manner are unsuccessful, and laceration or perforation of the uterine wall may result, putting the woman at great risk for severe PPH and infection (Cunningham et al., 2005).

Unusual placental adherence may be partial or complete. The following degrees of attachment are recognized:

- *Placenta accreta*–slight penetration of myometrium by placental trophoblast
- *Placenta increta*–deep penetration of myometrium by placenta
- *Placenta percreta*–perforation of uterus by placenta

Bleeding with complete or total placenta accreta may not occur unless separation of the placenta is attempted. With more extensive involvement, bleeding will become profuse when removal of the placenta is attempted. Cesarean hysterectomy is indicated in approximately two thirds of women. If future fertility is desired, uterine conserving techniques may be attempted. Blood component replacement therapy is often necessary (Francois & Foley, 2007).

Inversion of the Uterus

Inversion of the uterus after birth is a potentially life-threatening but rare complication. The incidence of uterine inversion is approximately 1 in 2500 births (Francois & Foley, 2007), and the condition may recur with a subsequent birth. Uterine inversion may be partial or complete. Complete inversion of the uterus is obvious; a large, red, rounded mass (perhaps with the placenta attached) protrudes 20 to 30 cm outside the introitus. Incomplete inversion cannot be seen but must be felt; a smooth mass will be palpated through the dilated cervix. Contributing factors to uterine inversion include uterine malformations, fundal implantation of the placenta, manual extraction of the placenta, short umbilical cord, uterine atony, leiomyomas, and abnormally adherent placental tissue (Francois & Foley). The primary presenting signs of uterine inversion are hemorrhage, shock, and pain in the absence of a palpable fundus abdominally.

Prevention–always the easiest, cheapest, and most effective therapy–is especially appropriate for uterine inversion. The umbilical cord should not be pulled on strongly unless the placenta has definitely separated.

Subinvolution of the Uterus

Late postpartum bleeding may occur as a result of subinvolution of the uterus. Recognized causes of **subinvolution** include retained placental fragments and pelvic infection.

Signs and symptoms include prolonged lochial discharge, irregular or excessive bleeding, and sometimes hemorrhage. A pelvic examination usually reveals a uterus that is larger than normal and that may be boggy.

CARE MANAGEMENT

Medical management

Early recognition and acknowledgment of the diagnosis of PPH are critical to care management. The first step is to evaluate the contractility of the uterus. If the uterus is hypotonic, management is directed toward increasing contractility and minimizing blood loss.

Hypotonic uterus. The initial management of excessive postpartum bleeding is firm massage of the uterine fundus (Hofmeyr, Abdel-Aleem, & Abdel-Aleem, 2008). Expression of any clots in the uterus, elimination of any bladder distention, and continuous IV infusion of 10 to 40 units of oxytocin added to 1000 ml of lactated Ringer's or normal saline solution also are primary interventions. If the uterus fails to respond to oxytocin, a 0.2-mg dose of ergonovine (Ergotrate) or methylergonovine (Methergine) may be given intramuscularly to produce

Critical Thinking/Clinical Decision Making

Postpartum Hemorrhage

You are a member of the interdisciplinary team for the labor and birth unit at your hospital. The team has been asked to develop a protocol for managing postpartum hemorrhage (PPH). Your assignment is to identify the nursing role during the early postpartum period. What will you include in your report?

1. Evidence—Is evidence sufficient to draw conclusions about information to include in the report about the nurse's role in caring for the woman with early PPH?
2. Assumptions—Describe underlying assumptions about each of following issues:
   a. Women at high risk for early PPH
   b. Frequent assessments in the early postpartum period
   c. Use of uterotonic medications for PPH
3. What implications and priorities need to be included in this report?
4. Does the evidence objectively support your conclusion?
5. Do alternative perspectives to your conclusion exist?

sustained uterine contractions. However, administering a 0.25-mg dose of a derivative of prostaglandin $F_{2\alpha}$ (carboprost tromethamine) intramuscularly is more common. It can also be given intramyometrially at cesarean birth or intraabdominally after vaginal birth (Francois & Foley, 2007). Prostaglandin E_2 (Dinoprostone) 20 mg vaginal or rectal suppository and rectal (800 mcg to 1000 mcg) administration of misoprostol also are used (American College of Obstetricians and Gynecologists, 2006). (See Medication Guide for a comparison of drugs used to manage PPH.) In addition to the medications used to contract the uterus, rapid administration of crystalloid solutions or blood or blood products or both will be needed to restore the woman's intravascular volume (Francois & Foley).

NURSING ALERT Use of ergonovine or methylergonovine is contraindicated in the presence of hypertension or cardiovascular disease. Prostaglandin $F_{2\alpha}$ should be used cautiously in women with cardiovascular disease or asthma (Francois & Foley, 2007).

Oxygen can be given by nonrebreather face mask to enhance oxygen delivery to the cells. A urinary catheter is usually inserted to monitor urine output as a measure of intravascular volume. Laboratory studies usually include a complete blood cell count with platelet count, fibrinogen, fibrin-split products, prothrombin time, and partial thromboplastin time. Blood type and antibody screen are initiated if not previously performed (Cunningham et al., 2005).

Medication Guide

Drugs Used to Manage Postpartum Hemorrhage

DRUG	ACTION	SIDE EFFECTS	CONTRAINDICATIONS	DOSAGE AND ROUTE	NURSING CONSIDERATIONS
Oxytocin (Pitocin)	Contraction of uterus; decreases bleeding	Infrequent: water intoxication, nausea and vomiting	None for PPH	10 to 40 units/L diluted in lactated Ringer's solution or normal saline at 125 to 200 milliunits/min IV; or 10 to 20 units IM	Continue to monitor vaginal bleeding and uterine tone
Methylergonovine (Methergine)*	Contraction of uterus	Hypertension, nausea, vomiting, headache	Hypertension, cardiac disease	0.2 mg IM every 2-4 hr up to five doses; may also be given intrauterine or orally	Check blood pressure before giving, and do not give if >140/90 mm Hg; continue monitoring vaginal bleeding and uterine tone
15-Methylprostaglandin $F_{2\alpha}$ (Prostin/15m; Carboprost, Hemabate)	Contraction of uterus	Headache, nausea and vomiting, fever, tachycardia, hypertension, diarrhea	Avoid with asthma or hypertension	0.25 mg IM or intrauterine every 15-90 min up to eight doses	Continue to monitor vaginal bleeding and uterine tone
Dinoprostone (Prostin E_2)	Contraction of uterus	Headache, nausea and vomiting, fever, chills, diarrhea	Avoid with hypotension	20 mg vaginal or rectal suppository every 2 hr	Continue to monitor vaginal bleeding and uterine tone
Misoprostol (Cytotec)	Contraction of uterus	Headache, nausea and vomiting, diarrhea	History of allergy to prostaglandins	800 to 1000 mcg rectally once	Continue to monitor vaginal bleeding and uterine tone

Sources: American College of Obstetricians and Gynecologists (ACOG). (2006). *Postpartum hemorrhage. ACOG Practice Bulletin No.76.* Washington, DC: ACOG; Francois, K., & Foley, M. (2007). Antepartum and postpartum hemorrhage. In S. Gabbe, J. Niebyl, & J. Simpson (Eds.), *Obstetrics: Normal and problem pregnancies* (5th ed.). Philadelphia: Churchill Livingstone.

IM, Intramuscularly; *IV,* intravenously; *PPH,* postpartum hemorrhage.

*Information about methylergonovine may also be used to describe ergonovine (Ergotrate).

If bleeding persists, bimanual compression may be considered by the obstetrician or nurse-midwife. This procedure involves inserting a fist into the vagina and pressing the knuckles against the anterior side of the uterus and then placing the other hand on the abdomen and massaging the posterior uterus with it. If the uterus still does not become firm, manual exploration of the uterine cavity for retained placental fragments is implemented. If the preceding procedures are ineffective, surgical management may be the only alternative. Surgical management options include vessel ligation (uteroovarian, uterine, hypogastric), selective arterial embolization, and hysterectomy (Cunningham et al., 2005; Francois & Foley, 2007).

Bleeding with a contracted uterus. If the uterus is firmly contracted and bleeding continues, the source of bleeding still must be identified and treated. Assessment may include visual or manual inspection of the perineum, vagina, uterus, cervix, or rectum and laboratory studies (e.g., hemoglobin, hematocrit, coagulation studies, platelet count). Treatment depends on the source of the bleeding. Lacerations are usually sutured. Hematomas may be managed with observation, cold therapy, ligation of the bleeding vessel, or evacuation. Fluids and blood replacement may be needed (Francois & Foley, 2007).

Uterine inversion. Uterine inversion is an emergency situation requiring immediate recognition, replacement of the uterus within the pelvic cavity, and correction of associated clinical conditions. Tocolytics (e.g., magnesium sulfate, terbutaline) or halogenated anesthetics may be given to relax the uterus before attempting replacement (Francois & Foley, 2007). Medical management of this condition includes repositioning the uterus, giving oxytocin after the uterus is repositioned, and treating shock (Francois & Foley).

Subinvolution. Treatment of subinvolution depends on the cause. Ergonovine, 0.2 mg every 4 hours for 2 or 3 days, and antibiotic therapy are the most common medications used (Cunningham et al., 2005). Dilation and curettage may be needed to remove retained placental fragments or to debride the placental site.

Herbal remedies

Herbal remedies have been used with some success to control PPH after the initial management and control of bleeding, particularly outside the United States. Some herbs have homeostatic actions, whereas others work as oxytocic agents to contract the uterus (Tiran & Mack, 2000). Box 23-2 lists herbs that have been used and their actions. However, published evidence of the safety and efficacy of herbal therapy is lacking. Evidence from well-controlled studies is needed before recommendation for practice can be made (Born & Barron, 2005).

Nursing interventions

PPH may be sudden and even exsanguinating. The nurse must therefore be alert to the symptoms of hemorrhage and hypovolemic shock and be prepared to act quickly to minimize blood loss (Fig. 23-1 and Box 23-3). Immediate assessments, nursing diagnoses, expected outcomes of care, and interventions are listed in the Nursing Process box: Postartum Hemorrhage.

BOX 23-2

Herbal Remedies for Postpartum Hemorrhage*

HERB	ACTION
Witch hazel	Homeostatic
Lady's mantle	Homeostatic
Blue cohosh	Oxytocic
Cotton root bark	Oxytocic
Motherwort	Promotes uterine contraction; vasoconstrictive
Shepherd's purse	Promotes uterine contraction
Alfalfa leaf	Increases availability of vitamin K; increases hemoglobin; may promote uterine contraction
Nettle	Increases availability of vitamin K; increases hemoglobin; may promote uterine contraction
Raspberry leaf	Homeostatic; promotes uterine contraction
Yarrow	Homeostatic

Sources: Beal, M. (1998). Use of complementary and alternative therapies in reproductive medicine. *Journal of Nurse-Midwifery, 43*(3), 224-233; Born, D., & Barron, M. (2005). Herbal use in pregnancy: What nurses need to know. *MCN The American Journal of Maternal/Child Nursing, 30*(3), 201-208; Skidmore-Roth, L. (2010). *Mosby's handbook of herbs and natural supplements* (4th ed.). St. Louis: Mosby; Tiran, D., & Mack, S. (Eds.). (2000). *Complementary therapies for pregnancy and childbirth* (2nd ed.). Edinburgh: Baillière Tindall.

*Continued research is needed to determine efficacy of these herbal remedies.

BOX 23-3

Noninvasive Assessments of Cardiac Output in Postpartum Patients Who Are Bleeding

- Palpation of pulses (rate, quality, equality)
  - Arterial
  - Blood pressure
- Auscultation
  - Heart sounds and murmurs
  - Breath sounds
- Inspection
  - Skin color, temperature, turgor
  - Level of consciousness
  - Capillary refill
  - Neck veins
  - Mucous membranes
- Observation
  - Presence or absence of anxiety, apprehension, restlessness, disorientation
- Measurement
  - Urinary output
  - Pulse oximetry

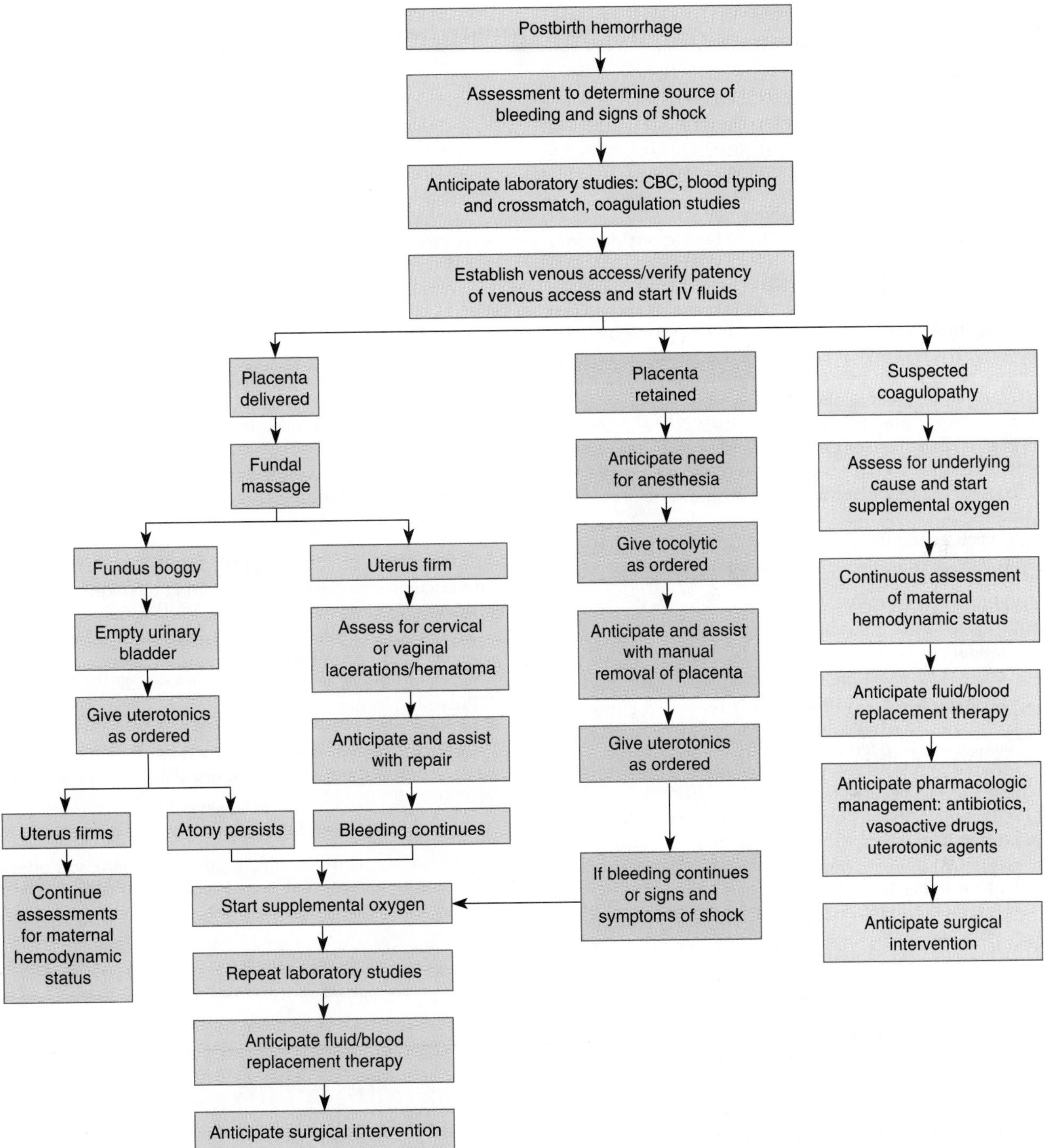

Fig. 23-1 Nursing assessments for postpartum bleeding.
CBC, Complete blood cell count; *IV,* intravenous; *s/s,* signs and symptoms; *uterotonics,* medications to contract the uterus.

After the bleeding has been controlled the care of the woman with lacerations of the perineum is similar to that of women with episiotomies (analgesia as needed for pain and hot or cold applications as necessary). The need for increased roughage in the diet and increased intake of fluids is emphasized. Stool softeners may be used to assist the woman in reestablishing bowel habits without straining and putting stress on the suture lines.

NURSING ALERT To prevent injury to the suture line a woman with third- or fourth-degree lacerations is not given rectal suppositories or enemas or digital rectal examinations.

The care of the woman who has experienced an inversion of the uterus focuses on immediate stabilization of hemodynamic status. This situation requires close observation of her response to treatment to prevent shock or fluid

NURSING PROCESS *Postpartum Hemorrhage*

ASSESSMENT

- Review the woman's history for factors that cause a predisposition to postpartum hemorrhage (PPH) (see Box 23-1).
- Assess the fundus to determine whether it is firmly contracted at or near the level of the umbilicus.
- Assess bleeding for color and amount.
- Inspect the perineum for signs of lacerations or hematomas.
- Assess vital signs every 15 minutes during the first 2 hours after birth to identify trends related to blood loss (e.g., tachycardia, tachypnea, decreasing blood pressure). However, vital signs may not be reliable indicators of shock immediately postpartum because of the physiologic adaptations of this period.
- Assess for bladder distention because a distended bladder can displace the uterus and prevent contraction.
- Assess the skin for warmth and dryness; nail beds should be checked for color and promptness of capillary refill.
- Collect specimens or review reports of laboratory studies, specifically hemoglobin and hematocrit levels.

NURSING DIAGNOSES

Nursing diagnoses for women experiencing PPH include the following:

- *Deficient fluid volume* related to:
  - Excessive blood loss secondary to uterine atony, lacerations, or uterine inversion
- *Risk for imbalanced fluid volume* related to:
  - Blood and fluid volume replacement therapy
- *Risk for infection* related to:
  - Excessive blood loss or exposed placental attachment site
  - Multiple invasive procedures
- *Risk for injury* related to:
  - Attempted manual removal of retained placenta
  - Administration of blood products
  - Operative procedures
- *Fear* or *anxiety* related to:
  - Threat to self
  - Deficient knowledge regarding procedures and operative management
- *Risk for impaired parenting* related to:
  - Separation from infant secondary to treatment regimen
- *Ineffective (peripheral) tissue perfusion* related to:
  - Excessive blood loss and shunting of blood to central circulation

EXPECTED OUTCOMES OF CARE

Expected outcomes of care for the woman experiencing PPH may include that the woman will do the following:

- Maintain normal vital signs and laboratory values.
- Develop no complications related to excessive bleeding.
- Express an understanding of her condition, its management, and discharge instructions.
- Identify and use available support systems.

PLAN OF CARE AND INTERVENTIONS

Immediate nursing care of the woman with PPH includes:

- Assessing vital signs, bleeding, and fundus
- Administering medication per protocol or orders
- Establishing or maintaining venous access
- Notifying the primary health care provider
- Providing explanations about interventions to woman and her family

(Care for specific problems that caused the bleeding as well as discharge instructions, are discussed in the text beginning on p. 726.)

EVALUATION

The nurse can be reasonably assured that care was effective to the extent that the expected outcomes were achieved.

overload. If the uterus has been repositioned manually, care must be taken to avoid aggressive fundal massage.

Discharge instructions for the woman who has had PPH are similar to those for any postpartum woman. In addition, the woman should be told that she will probably feel fatigue, even exhaustion, and will need to limit her physical activities to conserve her strength. She may need instructions in increasing her dietary iron and protein intake and iron supplementation to rebuild lost red blood cell (RBC) volume. She may need assistance with infant care and household activities until she has regained strength. Some women have problems with delayed or insufficient lactation and postpartum depression. Referrals for home care follow-up or to community resources such as support groups may be needed. (See Nursing Care Plan: Postpartum Hemorrhage.)

HEMORRHAGIC (HYPOVOLEMIC) SHOCK

Hemorrhage may result in **hemorrhagic (hypovolemic) shock.** Shock is an emergency situation in which the perfusion of body organs may become severely compromised and death may occur. Physiologic compensatory mechanisms are activated in response to hemorrhage. The adrenal glands release catecholamines, causing arterioles and venules in the skin, lungs, gastrointestinal tract, liver, and kidneys to constrict. The available blood flow is diverted to the brain and heart and away from other organs, including the uterus. If shock is prolonged, the continued reduction in cellular oxygenation results in an accumulation of lactic acid and acidosis (from anaerobic glucose metabolism). Acidosis (reduced serum pH) causes arteriolar vaso-

NURSING CARE PLAN *Postpartum Hemorrhage*

NURSING DIAGNOSIS Deficient fluid volume related to postpartum hemorrhage

Expected Outcome *Woman will demonstrate fluid balance as evidenced by stable vital signs, prompt capillary refill time, and balanced intake and output.*

Nursing Interventions/*Rationales*

- Monitor vital signs, oxygen saturation, urine specific gravity, and capillary refill *to provide baseline data.*
- Measure and record amount and type of bleeding by weighing and counting saturated pads. If woman is at home, teach her to count pads and save any clots or tissue. If woman is admitted to the hospital, save any clots and tissue for further examination *to estimate the type and amount of blood loss for fluid replacement.*
- Provide a quiet environment *to promote rest and decrease metabolic demands.*
- Give an explanation of all procedures *to reduce anxiety.*
- Begin intravenous access with an 18-gauge or larger needle for infusion of isotonic solution as ordered *to provide fluid or blood replacement.*
- Administer medications as ordered, such as oxytocin, methylergonovine, or prostaglandin F_{2a}, *to increase contractility of the uterus.*
- Insert an indwelling urinary catheter *to provide most accurate assessment of renal function and hypovolemia.*
- Prepare for surgical intervention as needed *to stop the source of bleeding.*

NURSING DIAGNOSIS Ineffective tissue perfusion related to hypovolemia

Expected Outcome *Woman will have stable vital signs, oxygen saturation, arterial blood gases, and adequate hematocrit and hemoglobin.*

Nursing Interventions/*Rationales*

- Monitor vital signs, oxygen saturation, arterial blood gases, and hematocrit and hemoglobin *to assess for hypovolemic shock and decreased tissue perfusion.*
- Assess for any changes in level of consciousness *to assess for evidence of hypoxia.*
- Assess capillary refill, mucous membranes, and skin temperature *to note indicators of vasoconstriction.*
- Give supplementary oxygen as ordered *to provide additional oxygenation to tissues.*
- Suction as needed, insert oral airway, *to maintain clear, open airway for oxygenation.*
- Monitor arterial blood gases *to provide information about acidosis or hypoxia.*
- Administer sodium bicarbonate if ordered *to reverse metabolic acidosis.*

NURSING DIAGNOSIS Anxiety related to sudden change in health status

Expected Outcome *Woman will verbalize that anxious feelings are diminished.*

Nursing Interventions/*Rationales*

- Using therapeutic communication, evaluate the woman's understanding of events *to provide clarification of any misconceptions.*
- Provide calm, competent attitude and environment *to aid in decreasing anxiety.*
- Explain all procedures *to decrease anxiety about the unknown.*
- Allow the woman to verbalize feelings *to permit clarification of information and promote trust.*
- Continue to assess vital signs or other clinical indicators of hypovolemic shock *to evaluate if the psychologic response of anxiety intensifies physiologic indicators.*

NURSING DIAGNOSIS Risk for infection related to blood loss and invasive procedures as a result of postpartum hemorrhage

Expected Outcomes *Woman will verbalize understanding of risk factors. Woman will demonstrate no signs of infection.*

Nursing Interventions/*Rationales*

- Maintain Standard Precautions, and use good handwashing technique when providing care *to prevent the introduction or spread of infection.*
- Teach the woman to maintain good handwashing technique (particularly before handling her newborn) and to maintain scrupulous perineal care with frequent change and careful disposal of perineal pads *to prevent the spread of microorganisms.*
- Monitor vital signs *to detect signs of systemic infection.*
- Monitor level of fatigue and lethargy, evidence of chills, loss of appetite, nausea and vomiting, and abdominal pain, *which are indicative of extent of infection and serve as indicators of the status of infection.*
- Monitor lochia for foul smell and profusion *as indicators of the infection state.*
- Assist with collection of intrauterine cultures or other specimens for laboratory analysis *to identify the specific causative organism.*
- Monitor laboratory values (i.e., white blood cell count, cultures) *for indicators of the type and status of infection.*
- Ensure adequate fluid and nutritional intake *to fight infection.*
- Administer and monitor broad-spectrum antibiotics if ordered *to prevent infection.*
- Administer antipyretics as ordered and necessary *to reduce elevated temperature.*

dilation; venule vasoconstriction persists. A circular pattern is established; that is, decreased perfusion, increased tissue anoxia and acidosis, edema formation, and pooling of blood further decrease the perfusion. Cellular death occurs. (See the Emergency box for assessments and interventions for hemorrhagic shock.)

CARE MANAGEMENT

Medical Management

Vigorous treatment is necessary to prevent adverse sequelae. Medical management of hypovolemic shock involves restoring circulating blood volume and treating the cause

EMERGENCY

Hemorrhagic Shock

ASSESSMENTS	CHARACTERISTICS
• Respirations	• Rapid and shallow
• Pulse	• Rapid, weak, irregular
• Blood pressure	• Decreasing (late sign)
• Skin	• Cool, pale, clammy
• Urinary output	• Decreasing
• Level of consciousness	• Lethargy → coma
• Mental status	• Anxiety → coma
• Central venous pressure	• Decreased

INTERVENTIONS

- Summon assistance and equipment.
- Start intravenous infusion per standing orders.
- Ensure patent airway; administer oxygen.
- Continue to monitor status.

of the hemorrhage (e.g., lacerations, uterine atony, or inversion). To restore circulating blood volume a rapid IV infusion of crystalloid solution is given at a rate of 3 ml infused for every 1 ml of estimated blood loss (e.g., 3000 ml infused for 1000 ml of blood loss). Packed RBCs are usually infused if the woman is still actively bleeding and no improvement in her condition is noted after the initial crystalloid infusion. Infusion of fresh-frozen plasma may be needed if clotting factors and platelet counts are below normal values (Cunningham et al., 2005; Francois & Foley, 2007).

Nursing Interventions

Hemorrhagic shock can occur rapidly, but the classic signs of shock may not appear until the postpartum woman has lost 30% to 40% of blood volume. The nurse must continue to reassess the woman's condition, as evidenced by the degree of measurable and anticipated blood loss, and mobilize appropriate resources.

Most interventions are instituted to improve or monitor tissue perfusion. The nurse continues to monitor the woman's pulse and blood pressure. If invasive hemodynamic monitoring is ordered, the nurse may assist with the placement of the central venous pressure (CVP) or pulmonary artery (Swan-Ganz) catheter and monitor CVP, pulmonary artery pressure, or pulmonary artery wedge pressure as ordered (Gilbert, 2007).

Additional assessments to be made include evaluating skin temperature, color, and turgor, as well as assessing the woman's mucous membranes. Breath sounds should be auscultated before fluid volume replacement, if possible, to provide a baseline for future assessment. Inspection for oozing at the sites of incisions or injections and assessment of the presence of petechiae or ecchymosis in areas not associated with surgery or trauma are critical in the evaluation for DIC.

Oxygen is administered, preferably by nonrebreathing facemask, at 10 to 12 L/min to maintain oxygen saturation. Oxygen saturation should be monitored with a pulse oximeter, although measurements may not always be accurate in a woman with hypovolemia or decreased perfusion. Level of consciousness is assessed frequently and provides an additional indication of blood volume and oxygen saturation (Gilbert, 2007). In early stages of decreased blood flow the woman may report "seeing stars" or feeling dizzy or nauseated. She may become restless and orthopneic. As cerebral hypoxia increases, she may become confused and react slowly or not at all to stimuli. Some women complain of headaches (Curran, 2003). An improved sensorium is an indicator of improved perfusion.

Continuous electrocardiographic monitoring may be indicated for the woman who is hypotensive or tachycardic, continues to bleed profusely, or is in shock. A Foley catheter with a urometer is inserted to allow hourly assessment of urinary output. The most objective and least invasive assessment of adequate organ perfusion and oxygenation is urinary output of at least 30 ml/hr (Cunningham et al., 2005). Blood may be drawn and sent to the laboratory for studies that include hemoglobin and hematocrit levels, platelet count, and coagulation profile.

Fluid or Blood Replacement Therapy

Critical to successful management of the woman with a hemorrhagic complication is the establishment of venous access, preferably with a large-bore IV catheter. The establishment of two IV lines facilitates fluid resuscitation. Vigorous fluid resuscitation includes the administration of crystalloids (lactated Ringer's, normal saline solutions), colloids (albumin), blood, and blood components (Francois & Foley, 2007). Fluid resuscitation must be closely monitored because fluid overload may occur. Intravascular fluid overload occurs more frequently with colloid therapy compared with other fluids. Transfusion reactions may follow the administration of blood or blood components, including cryoprecipitates. Even in an emergency, each unit must be checked per hospital protocol. Complications of fluid or blood replacement therapy include hemolytic reactions, febrile reactions, allergic reactions, circulatory overload, and air embolism.

LEGAL TIP **Standard of Care for Bleeding Emergencies**

The standard of care for obstetric emergency situations such as PPH or hypovolemic shock is that provision should be made for the nurse to implement actions independently. Policies, procedures, standing orders or protocols, and clinical guidelines should be established by each health care facility in which births occur and should be agreed on by health care providers involved in the care of obstetric patients.

COAGULOPATHIES

When bleeding is continuous and no identifiable source is found, a coagulopathy may be the cause. The woman's coagulation status must be assessed quickly and continuously. The nurse may draw and send blood to the laboratory for studies. Abnormal results depend on the cause and may include increased prothrombin time, increased partial thromboplastin time, decreased platelets, decreased fibrinogen level, increased fibrin degradation products, and prolonged bleeding time. Causes of coagulopathies may be pregnancy complications such as idiopathic thrombocytopenic purpura (ITP) or von Willebrand disease and DIC (see Chapter 21 for discussion of DIC).

Idiopathic Thrombocytopenic Purpura

ITP is an autoimmune disorder in which antiplatelet antibodies decrease the life span of the platelets. Thrombocytopenia, capillary fragility, and increased bleeding time are diagnostic findings. ITP may cause severe hemorrhage after cesarean birth or from cervical or vaginal lacerations. The incidence of postpartum uterine bleeding and vaginal hematomas is also increased. Neonatal thrombocytopenia can result, but serious bleeding is unusual (Rosenberg, 2007).

Medical management focuses on control of platelet stability. If ITP was diagnosed during pregnancy, the woman likely was treated with corticosteroids or IV immunoglobulin. Platelet transfusions are usually given when bleeding is significant. A splenectomy may be needed if the ITP does not respond to medical management (Samuels, 2007).

von Willebrand Disease

von Willebrand disease (vWD), a type of hemophilia, is probably the most common of all hereditary bleeding disorders (Samuels, 2007). Although von Willebrand disease is rare, it is among the most common congenital clotting defects in U.S. women of childbearing age. It results from a deficiency or defect in a blood clotting protein called von Willebrand factor (vWF). Symptoms include recurrent bleeding episodes such as nose bleeds or after tooth extraction, bruising easily, prolonged bleeding time (the most important test), factor VIII deficiency (mild to moderate), and bleeding from mucous membranes. (Samuels).

The woman may be at risk for bleeding for up to 4 weeks postpartum. The treatment of choice is administration of desmopressin, which promotes the release of vWF and factor VIII. It can be given nasally, intravenously, or orally. Transfusion therapy with plasma products that have been treated for viruses and contain factor VIII and vWF (e.g., Humate-P, Alphanate) may also be used (Lee & Abdul-Kadir, 2005; Samuels, 2007).

THROMBOEMBOLIC DISEASE

Thrombosis results from the formation of a blood clot or clots inside a blood vessel and is caused by inflammation **(thrombophlebitis)** or partial obstruction of the vessel. Three thromboembolic conditions are of concern in the postpartum period:

1. *Superficial venous thrombosis*–involvement of the superficial saphenous venous system
2. *Deep venous thrombosis*–involvement varies but can extend from the foot to the iliofemoral region
3. *Pulmonary embolism*–complication of deep venous thrombosis occurring when part of a blood clot dislodges and is carried to the pulmonary artery, where it occludes the vessel and obstructs blood flow to the lungs

Incidence and Etiology

The incidence of thromboembolic disease in the postpartum period varies from approximately 1 in 1000 to 1 in 2000 women (Pettker & Lockwood, 2007). The incidence has declined in the last 20 years because early ambulation after childbirth has become the standard practice. The major causes of thromboembolic disease are venous stasis and hypercoagulation, both of which are present in pregnancy and continue into the postpartum period. Other risk factors include operative vaginal birth, cesarean birth, history of venous thrombosis or varicosities, obesity, maternal age older than 35 years, multiparity, infection, immobility, and smoking. Women with associated genetic risk factors are also at risk (Pettker & Lockwood).

Clinical Manifestations

Superficial venous thrombosis is the most frequent form of postpartum thrombophlebitis. It is characterized by pain and tenderness in the lower extremity. Physical examination may reveal warmth, redness, and an enlarged, hardened vein over the site of the thrombosis. Deep vein thrombosis is more common during pregnancy than after the birth and is characterized by unilateral leg pain, calf tenderness, and swelling (Fig. 23-2). Physical examination may reveal redness and warmth, but many women may have few if any symptoms (Pettker & Lockwood, 2007). A positive Homans sign may be present, but further evaluation is needed because the calf pain may be attributed to other causes, such as a strained muscle resulting from the birthing position (Pettker & Lockwood). Acute pulmonary embolism is characterized by dyspnea and tachypnea (>20 breaths/min). Other signs and symptoms frequently seen include tachycardia (>100 beats/min), apprehension, cough, hemoptysis, elevated temperature, syncope, and pleuritic chest pain (Cunningham et al., 2005; Pettker & Lockwood).

Physical examination is not a sensitive diagnostic indicator for thrombosis. Venography is the most accurate method for diagnosing deep venous thrombosis; however, it is an invasive procedure that is associated with serious complications. Noninvasive diagnostic methods are commonly used; these methods include real-time and color Doppler ultrasound. Cardiac auscultation may reveal

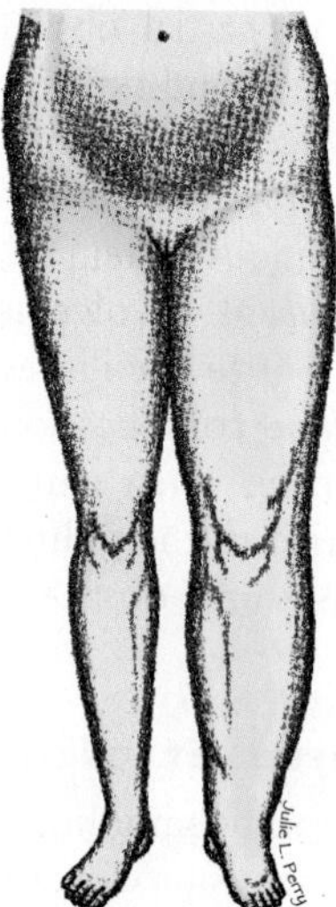

Fig. 23-2 Deep vein thrombophlebitis.

murmurs with pulmonary embolism. Electrocardiograms are usually normal. Arterial oxygen pressure may be lower than normal (Katz, 2007a; Pettker & Lockwood, 2007).

CARE MANAGEMENT

Medical Management

Superficial venous thrombosis is treated with analgesia (nonsteroidal antiinflammatory agents), rest with elevation of the affected leg, and elastic stockings (Cunningham et al., 2005; Katz, 2007a). Local application of heat also may be used. Deep venous thrombosis is initially treated with anticoagulant (usually continuous IV heparin) therapy, bed rest with the affected leg elevated, and analgesia. After the symptoms have decreased, the woman may be fitted with elastic stockings to use when she is allowed to ambulate. IV heparin therapy continues for 3 to 5 days or until symptoms resolve. Oral anticoagulant therapy (warfarin) is started during this time and will be continued for approximately 3 months. Continuous IV heparin therapy is used for pulmonary embolism until symptoms have resolved and is followed by subcutaneous heparin or oral anticoagulant therapy for up to 6 months (Pettker & Lockwood, 2007).

Nursing Interventions

In the hospital setting, nursing care of the woman with a thrombosis consists of continued assessments: inspection and palpation of the affected area; palpation of peripheral pulses; checking Homans sign; measurement and comparison of leg circumferences; inspection for signs of bleeding; monitoring for signs of pulmonary embolism, including chest pain, coughing, dyspnea, and tachypnea; and respiratory status for presence of crackles. Laboratory reports are monitored for prothrombin or partial thromboplastin times. The woman and her family are assessed for their level of understanding about the diagnosis and their ability to cope during the unexpected extended period of recovery.

Critical Thinking Exercise: Postpartum Complications

Interventions include explanations and education about the diagnosis and the treatment. The woman will need assistance with personal care as long as she is on bed rest; the family should be encouraged to participate in the care if that is what she and they wish. While the woman is on bed rest, she should be encouraged to change positions frequently but to avoid placing the knees in a sharply flexed position, which could cause pooling of blood in the lower extremities. She should also be cautioned to avoid rubbing the affected area, given that this action can cause the clot to dislodge. Once the woman is allowed to ambulate, she is taught how to prevent venous congestion by putting on the elastic stockings before getting out of bed.

Heparin and warfarin are administered as ordered, and the physician is notified if clotting times are outside the therapeutic level. If the woman is breastfeeding, she is assured that neither heparin nor warfarin is excreted in significant quantities in breast milk. If the infant has been discharged, the family is encouraged to bring the infant for feedings as permitted by hospital policy; the mother can also express milk to be sent home.

Pain can be managed with a variety of measures. Position changes, elevating the leg, and application of moist warm heat may decrease discomfort. Administration of analgesics and antiinflammatory medications may be needed.

NURSING ALERT Medications containing aspirin are not given to women receiving anticoagulant therapy because aspirin inhibits synthesis of clotting factors and can lead to prolonged clotting time and increased risk of bleeding.

The woman is usually discharged home with oral anticoagulants and will need explanations about the treatment schedule and possible side effects. If subcutaneous injections are to be given, the woman and family are taught how to administer the medication and about site rotation. The woman and her family also should be given information about safe care practices to prevent bleeding and injury while she is receiving anticoagulant therapy, such as using a soft toothbrush and using an electric razor. She also will need information about follow-up with her health care provider to monitor clotting times and to make sure the correct dose of anticoagulant therapy is maintained. The woman also should use a reliable method of contraception if taking warfarin, because this medication is considered teratogenic. Oral contraceptives are contraindicated because of the increased risk for thrombosis (Gilbert, 2007).

POSTPARTUM INFECTIONS

Postpartum infection, or **puerperal infection,** is any clinical infection of the genital canal that occurs within 28 days after miscarriage, induced abortion, or childbirth. The definition used in the United States continues to be the presence of a fever of 38° C or more on 2 successive days of the first 10 postpartum days (not counting the first 24 hours after birth) (Cunningham et al., 2005). Puerperal infection is probably the major cause of maternal morbidity and mortality throughout the world; endometritis is the most common cause. In the United States, it occurs after approximately 2% of vaginal births and 10% to 15% of cesarean births (Katz, 2007b). Other common postpartum infections include wound infections, mastitis, urinary tract infections (UTIs), and respiratory tract infections.

The most common infecting organisms are the numerous streptococcal and anaerobic organisms. *Staphylococcus aureus,* gonococci, coliform bacteria, and clostridia are less common but serious pathogenic organisms that also cause puerperal infection. Postpartum infections are common in women who have concurrent medical or immunosuppressive conditions or who had a cesarean or operative vaginal birth. Intrapartal factors such as prolonged rupture of membranes, prolonged labor, and internal maternal or fetal monitoring also increase the risk of infection (Duff, 2007). Factors that predispose the woman to postpartum infection are listed in Box 23-4.

Endometritis

Endometritis is the most common cause of postpartum infection. It usually begins as a localized infection at the placental site (Fig. 23-3) but can spread to involve the entire endometrium. Incidence is higher after cesarean birth than it is after vaginal birth. Assessment for signs of endometritis may reveal a fever (usually greater than 38° C), increased pulse, chills, anorexia, nausea, fatigue and lethargy, pelvic pain, uterine tenderness, or foul-smelling, profuse lochia (Duff, 2007). Leukocytosis and a markedly increased RBC sedimentation rate are typical laboratory findings of postpartum infections. Anemia also may be present. Blood cultures or intracervical or intrauterine bacterial cultures (aerobic and anaerobic) should reveal the offending pathogens within 36 to 48 hours.

BOX 23-4

Predisposing Factors for Postpartum Infection

PRECONCEPTION OR ANTEPARTAL FACTORS

- History of previous venous thrombosis, urinary tract infection, mastitis, pneumonia
- Diabetes mellitus
- Alcoholism
- Drug abuse
- Immunosuppression
- Anemia
- Malnutrition

INTRAPARTAL FACTORS

- Cesarean birth
- Operative vaginal birth
- Prolonged rupture of membranes
- Chorioamnionitis
- Prolonged labor
- Bladder catheterization
- Internal fetal or uterine pressure monitoring
- Multiple vaginal examinations after rupture of membranes
- Epidural anesthesia
- Retained placental fragments
- Postpartum hemorrhage
- Episiotomy or lacerations
- Hematomas

Wound Infections

Wound infections also are common postpartum infections but often develop after the woman is at home. Sites of infection include the cesarean incision and the episiotomy or repaired laceration site. Predisposing factors are similar to those for endometritis (see Box 23-4). Signs of wound infection include erythema, edema, warmth, tenderness, seropurulent drainage, and wound separation. Fever and pain also may be present.

Urinary Tract Infections

UTIs occur in 2% to 4% of postpartum women. Risk factors include urinary catheterization, frequent pelvic examinations, epidural anesthesia, genital tract injury, history of UTI, and cesarean birth. Signs and symptoms include dysuria, frequency and urgency, low-grade fever, urinary retention, hematuria, and pyuria. Costovertebral angle tenderness or flank pain may indicate upper UTI. Urinalysis results may reveal *Escherichia coli,* although other gram-negative aerobic bacilli also may cause UTIs (see Chapter 21 for further discussion).

Mastitis

Mastitis affects approximately 1% to 10% of women soon after childbirth, most of whom are first-time mothers who are breastfeeding (Newton, 2007). Mastitis is almost always unilateral and develops well after the flow of milk has been established (Fig. 23-4). The infecting organism is generally

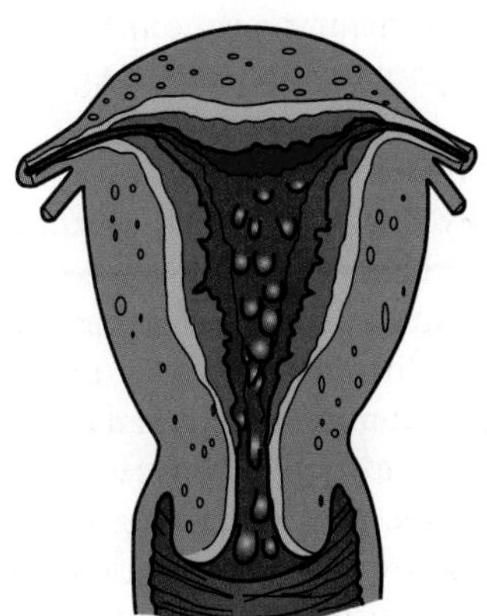

Fig. 23-3 Postpartum infection—endometritis.

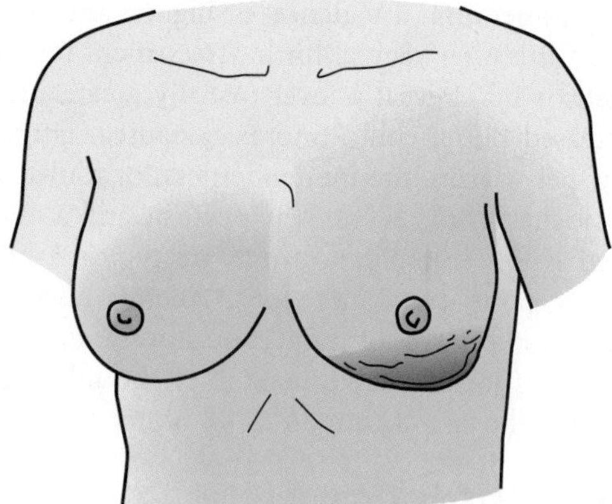

Fig. 23-4 Mastitis.

the hemolytic *S. aureus.* An infected nipple fissure is usually the initial lesion, but the ductal system is involved next. Inflammatory edema and engorgement of the breast soon obstruct the flow of milk in a lobe; regional, then generalized, mastitis follows. If treatment is not prompt, mastitis may progress to a breast abscess.

Symptoms rarely appear before the end of the first postpartum week and are more common in the second to fourth weeks. Chills, fever, malaise, and local breast tenderness are noted first. Localized breast tenderness, pain, swelling, redness, and axillary adenopathy also may occur.

CARE MANAGEMENT

Signs and symptoms associated with postpartum infection were discussed with each infection. Laboratory tests usually performed include a complete blood count, venous blood cultures, and uterine tissue cultures. Nursing diagnoses for women experiencing postpartum infection are listed in Box 23-5.

The most effective and least expensive treatment of postpartum infection is prevention. Good maternal perineal hygiene with thorough handwashing is emphasized. Strict adherence by all health care personnel to aseptic techniques during childbirth and the postpartum period is very important.

Medical management of endometritis consists of IV broad-spectrum antibiotic therapy (e.g., cephalosporins, penicillins, clindamycin, and gentamicin) and supportive care, including hydration, rest, and pain relief. Antibiotic therapy is usually discontinued 24 hours after the woman is asymptomatic (Duff, 2007).

Nursing measures including assessments of lochia, vital signs, and changes in the woman's condition continue during treatment. Comfort measures depend on the symptoms and may include cool compresses, warm blankets, perineal care, and sitz baths. Teaching should include side effects of therapy, prevention of spread of infection, signs and symptoms of worsening condition, and adherence to the treatment plan and the need for follow-up care.

BOX 23-5

Nursing Diagnoses for Women Experiencing Postpartum Infection

- Deficient knowledge related to:
  - Cause, management, course of infection
  - Transmission and prevention of infection
- Impaired tissue integrity related to:
  - Effects of infection process
- Acute pain related to:
  - Mastitis
  - Puerperal infection
  - Urinary tract infection
- Interrupted family processes related to:
  - Unexpected complication to expected postpartum recovery
  - Possible separation from newborn
  - Interruption in process of realigning relationships after the addition of the new family member
- Risk for impaired parenting related to:
  - Fear of spread of infection to newborn

Women may need to be encouraged or assisted to maintain mother-infant interactions and breastfeeding (if allowed during treatment).

Treatment of wound infections may combine antibiotic therapy with wound débridement. Incisions may be opened and drained. Nursing care includes frequent wound and vital sign assessments and wound care (e.g., irrigation and dressing changes). Comfort measures for perineal wounds include sitz baths, warm compresses, and perineal care. Teaching includes good hygiene techniques (e.g., changing perineal pads front to back, handwashing before and after perineal care), self-care measures, and signs of worsening conditions to report to the health care provider. The woman is usually discharged to home for self-care or home nursing care after treatment is initiated in the inpatient setting.

Medical management for UTIs consists of antibiotic therapy, analgesia, and hydration. Postpartum women are usually treated on an outpatient basis; therefore teaching should include instructions on how to monitor temperature, bladder function, and appearance of urine. The woman also should be taught about signs of potential complications and the importance of taking all antibiotics as prescribed. Other suggestions for prevention of UTIs are discussed in Chapter 21.

Because mastitis rarely occurs before the postpartum woman who is breastfeeding is discharged, teaching should include warning signs of mastitis and counseling about the prevention of cracked nipples. Management includes support of breasts, local application of heat (or cold), adequate hydration, analgesics, and antibiotic therapy (e.g., dicloxacillin or flucloxacillin). Lactation can be maintained by emptying the breasts every 2 to 4 hours by breastfeeding, manual expression, or breast pump (Katz, 2007b) (see Chapter 18 for further information).

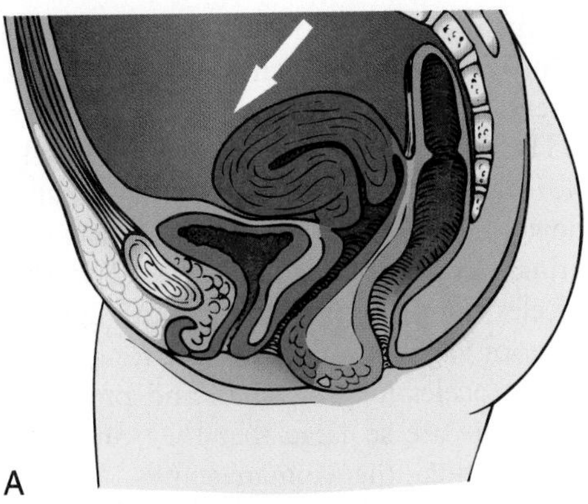

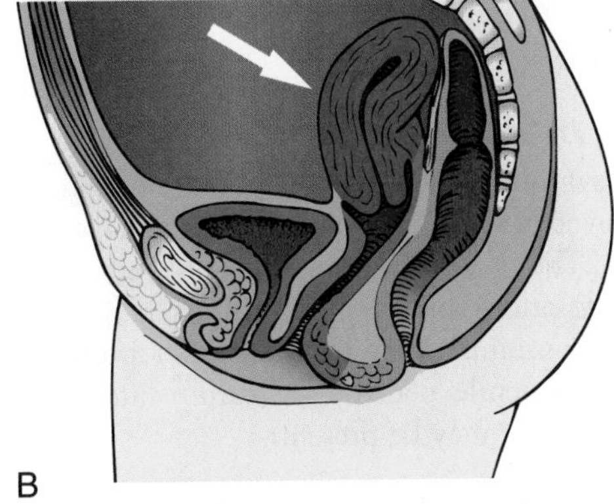

Fig. 23-5 Types of uterine displacement. **A,** Anterior displacement. **B,** Retroversion (backward displacement of uterus).

Postpartum women are usually discharged by 48 hours after birth and signs of infection may not be present until after this time. Nurses in birth centers and hospital settings must be able to identify women at risk for postpartum infection and to provide anticipatory teaching and counseling before discharge. After discharge, telephone follow-up, hot lines, support groups, lactation counselors, home visits by nurses, and teaching materials (videos, written materials) are all interventions that can be implemented to prevent or increase recognition of postpartum infections. Home care nurses must be able to recognize signs and symptoms of postpartum infection and also must be able to provide the appropriate nursing care for women who need follow-up home care.

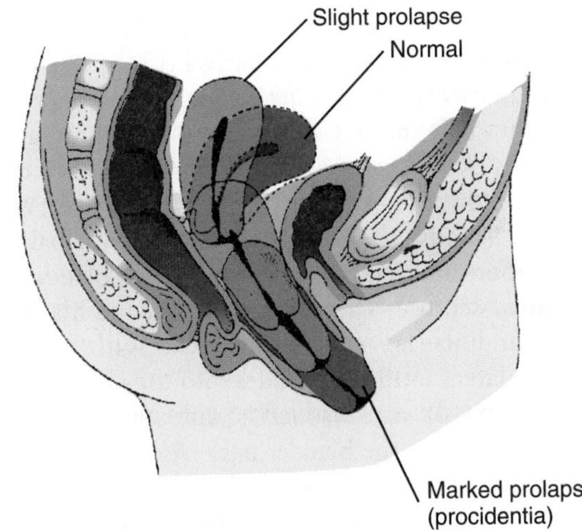

Fig. 23-6 Prolapse of uterus.

SEQUELAE OF CHILDBIRTH TRAUMA

Women are at risk for problems related to the reproductive system from the age of menarche through menopause and the older years. These problems include structural disorders of the uterus and vagina related to pelvic relaxation and urinary incontinence. They can be a delayed result of childbearing. For example, the structures and soft tissues of the vagina and bladder may be injured during a prolonged labor, during a precipitous birth, or when cephalopelvic disproportion occurs. Defects can also occur in women who have never been pregnant.

Uterine Displacement and Prolapse

The round ligaments normally hold the uterus in anteversion, and the uterosacral ligaments pull the cervix backward and upward (see Fig. 4-2). Uterine displacement is a variation of this normal placement. The most common type of displacement is posterior displacement, or retroversion, in which the uterus is tilted posteriorly and the cervix rotates anteriorly. Other variations include retroflexion and anteflexion (Fig. 23-5).

By 2 months postpartum the ligaments should return to normal length, but in approximately one third of women the uterus remains retroverted. This condition is rarely symptomatic, but conception may be difficult because the cervix points toward the anterior vaginal wall and away from the posterior fornix, where seminal fluid pools after coitus. If symptoms occur, they may include pelvic and low back pain, dyspareunia, and exaggeration of premenstrual symptoms.

Uterine prolapse is a more serious type of displacement. The degree of prolapse can vary from mild to complete. In complete prolapse, the cervix and body of the uterus protrude through the vagina and the vagina is inverted (Fig. 23-6).

Uterine displacement and prolapse can be caused by congenital or acquired weakness of the pelvic support structures (often called **pelvic relaxation**). In many cases, problems can be related to a delayed but direct result of childbearing. Although extensive damage may be noted and repaired shortly after birth, symptoms related to pelvic relaxation most often appear during the perimenopausal period, when the effects of ovarian hormones on pelvic tissues are lost and atrophic changes begin. Pelvic trauma, stress and strain, and the aging process are also contributing causes. Other causes of pelvic relaxation include reproductive surgery and pelvic radiation.

Clinical manifestations

Generally, symptoms of pelvic relaxation relate to the structure involved: urethra, bladder, uterus, vagina, cul-de-sac, or rectum. The most common complaints are pulling and dragging sensations, pressure, protrusions, fatigue, and low backache. Symptoms may be worse after prolonged standing or deep penile penetration during intercourse. Urinary incontinence may be present.

Cystocele and Rectocele

Cystocele and rectocele almost always accompany uterine prolapse, causing the uterus to sag even further backward and downward into the vagina. *Cystocele* (Fig. 23-7, *A*) is the protrusion of the bladder downward into the vagina that develops when supporting structures in the vesicovaginal septum are injured. Anterior wall relaxation gradually develops over time as a result of congenital defects of supports, childbearing, obesity, or advanced age. When the woman stands, the weakened anterior vaginal wall cannot support the weight of the urine in the bladder; the vesicovaginal septum is forced downward, the bladder is stretched, and its capacity is increased. With time the cystocele enlarges until it protrudes into the vagina. Complete emptying of the bladder is difficult because the cystocele sags below the bladder neck. *Rectocele* is the herniation of the anterior rectal wall through the relaxed or ruptured vaginal fascia and rectovaginal septum; it appears as a large bulge that may be seen through the relaxed introitus (Fig. 23-7, *B*).

Clinical manifestations

Cystoceles and rectoceles are often asymptomatic. If symptoms of cystocele are present, they may include complaints of a bearing-down sensation or that "something is in my vagina." Other symptoms include urinary frequency, retention, incontinence, and possible recurrent cystitis and UTIs. Pelvic examination will reveal a bulging of the anterior wall of the vagina when the woman is asked to bear down. Unless the bladder neck and urethra are damaged, urinary continence is unaffected. Women with large cystoceles complain of having to push upward on the sagging anterior vaginal wall to be able to void.

Rectoceles may be small and produce few symptoms, but some are so large that they protrude outside of the vagina when the woman stands. Symptoms are absent when the woman is lying down. A rectocele causes a disturbance in bowel function, the sensation of "bearing down," or the sensation that the pelvic organs are falling out. With a very large rectocele, having a bowel movement may be difficult. Each time the woman strains during bowel evacuation the feces are forced against the thinned rectovaginal wall, stretching it more. Some women facilitate evacuation by applying digital pressure vaginally to hold up the rectal pouch.

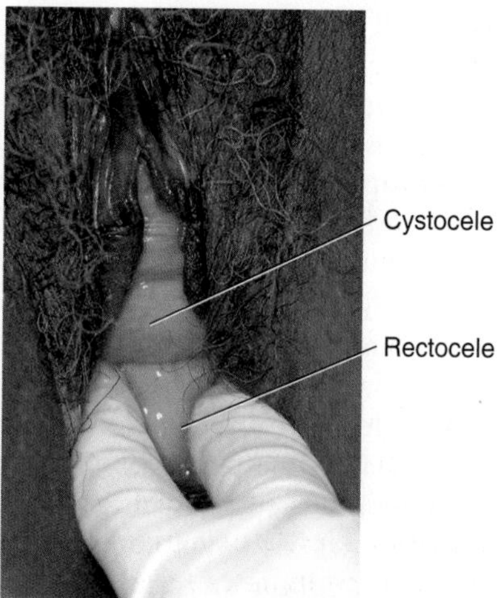

Fig. 23-7 Cystocele and rectocele. (From Seidel, H., Ball, J., Dains, J., & Benedict, G. [2006]. *Mosby's guide to physical examination* [6th ed.]. St. Louis: Mosby.)

Urinary Incontinence

Urinary incontinence (UI) affects young and middle-aged women, with the prevalence increasing as the woman ages (Sampselle, 2003). Although nulliparous women can have UI, the incidence is increased in women who have given birth and also increases with parity (Sampselle). Conditions that disturb urinary control include stress incontinence because of sudden increases in intraabdominal pressure (such as from sneezing or coughing); urge incontinence, caused by disorders of the bladder and urethra, such as urethritis and urethral stricture, trigonitis, and cystitis; neuropathies such as multiple sclerosis, diabetic neuritis, and pathologic conditions of the spinal cord; and congenital and acquired urinary tract abnormalities.

Stress incontinence may follow injury to bladder neck structures. A sphincter mechanism at the bladder neck compresses the upper urethra, pulls it upward behind the symphysis, and forms an acute angle at the junction of the posterior urethral wall and the base of the bladder (urethrovesiculo angle) (Fig. 23-8). To empty the bladder the sphincter complex relaxes, and the trigone contracts to open the internal urethral orifice and pull the contracting bladder wall upward, forcing urine out. The angle between the urethra and the base of the bladder is lost or increased if the supporting pubococcygeus muscle is injured; this change, coupled with urethrocele, causes incontinence. Urine spurts out when the woman is asked to bear down or cough in the lithotomy position.

Clinical manifestations

Involuntary leaking of urine is the main sign. Episodes of leaking are common during coughing, laughing, and exercise.

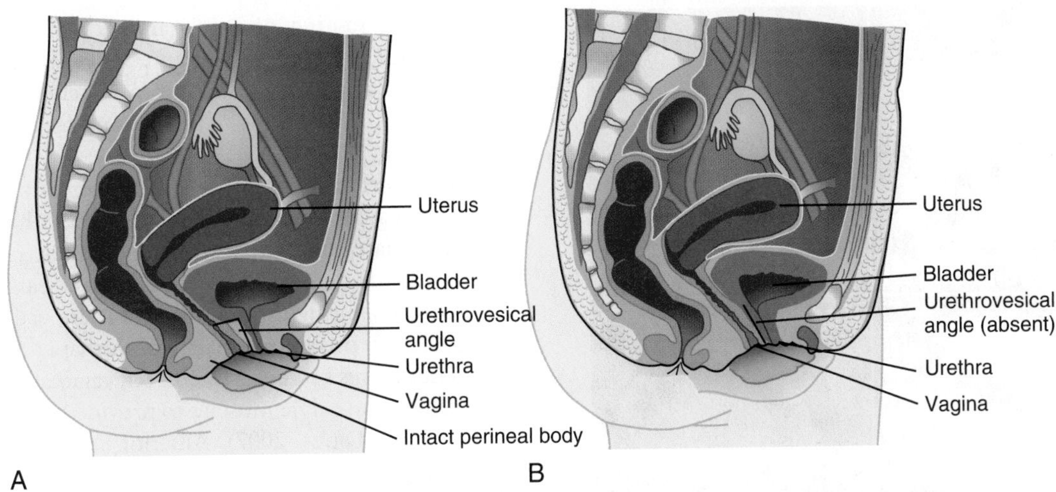

Fig. 23-8 Urethrovesical angle. **A,** Normal angle. **B,** Widening (absence) of angle.

Genital Fistulas

Genital fistulas are perforations between genital tract organs. Most occur between the bladder and the genital tract (e.g., vesicovaginal); between the urethra and the vagina (urethrovaginal); and between the rectum or sigmoid colon and the vagina (rectovaginal) (Fig. 23-9). Genital fistulas may also be a result of a congenital anomaly, gynecologic surgery, obstetric trauma, cancer, radiation therapy, gynecologic trauma, or infection (e.g., in the episiotomy).

Clinical manifestations

Signs and symptoms of vaginal fistulas depend on the site but may include presence of urine, flatus, or feces in the vagina; odors of urine or feces in the vagina; and irritation of vaginal tissues.

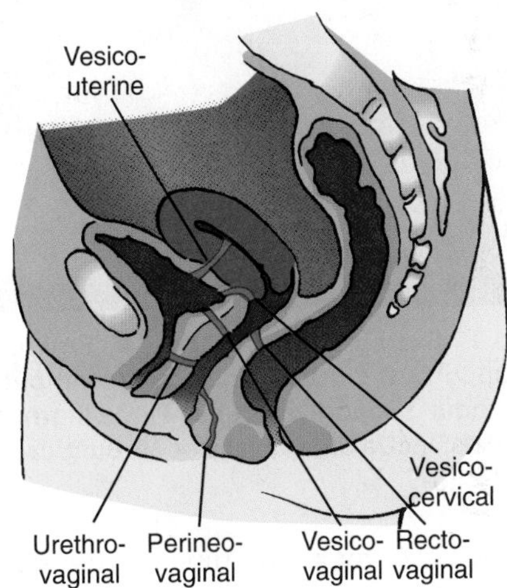

Fig. 23-9 Types of fistulas that may develop in vagina, uterus, and rectum. (From Monahan F., Sands, J. K., Neighbors, M., Marek, J. F., & Green, C. J. (2007). Phipps' medical-surgical nursing: Health and illness perspectives (8th ed.). St. Louis: Mosby.

CARE MANAGEMENT

Assessment for problems related to structural disorders of the uterus and vagina focuses primarily on the genitourinary tract, the reproductive organs, bowel elimination, and psychosocial and sexual factors. A complete health history is obtained, and a physical examination and laboratory tests are performed to support the appropriate medical diagnosis. The nurse needs to assess the woman's knowledge of the disorder, its management, and the possible prognosis.

The health care team works together to treat the disorders related to alterations in pelvic support and to assist the woman in the management of her symptoms. In general, nurses working with these women can provide information and self-care education to prevent problems before they occur, to manage or reduce symptoms and promote comfort and hygiene if symptoms are already present, and to recognize when further intervention is needed. This information can be part of all postpartum discharge teaching or can be provided at postpartum follow-up visits in clinics or physician or nurse-midwife offices or during postpartum home visits.

Interventions for specific problems depend on the problem and the severity of the symptoms. If discomfort related to uterine displacement is a problem, several interventions can be implemented to treat uterine displacement. Kegel exercises (see p. 54) can be performed several times daily to increase muscle strength. A knee-chest position performed for a few minutes several times a day can correct a mildly retroverted uterus. A fitted pessary device may be inserted in the vagina to support the uterus and hold it in the correct position (Fig. 23-10). Usually, a

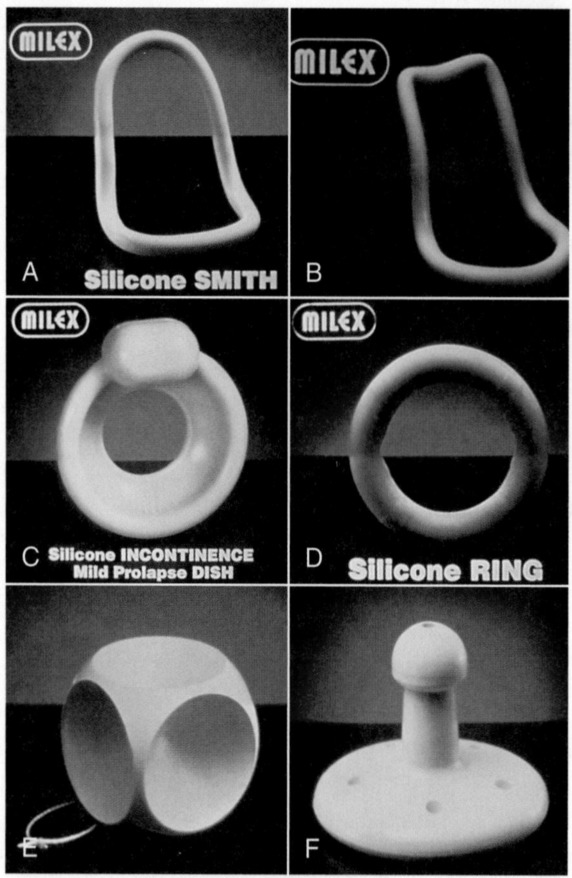

Fig. 23-10 Examples of pessaries. **A,** Smith. **B,** Hodge without support. **C,** Incontinence dish without support. **D,** Ring without support. **E,** Cube. **F,** Gellhorn. (Courtesy Milex Products, Inc., a division of CooperSurgical, Trumbull, CT.)

pessary is used only for a short time because it can lead to pressure necrosis and vaginitis. Good hygiene is important; some women may be taught to remove the pessary at night, cleanse it, and replace it in the morning. If the pessary is always left in place, regular douching with commercially prepared solutions or weak vinegar solutions (1 tablespoon to 1 quart of water) to remove increased secretions and keep the vaginal pH at 4 to 4.5 is suggested. After a period of treatment, most women are free of symptoms and do not require the pessary. Surgical correction is rarely indicated.

Treatment for uterine prolapse depends on the degree of prolapse. Pessaries may be useful in mild prolapse to support the uterus in the correct position. Estrogen therapy also may be used in the older woman to improve tissue tone. If these conservative treatments do not correct the problem, or if the degree of prolapse is significant, abdominal or vaginal hysterectomy is usually recommended (Lentz, 2007).

Treatment for a cystocele includes use of a vaginal pessary or surgical repair. Anterior repair (colporrhaphy) is the usual surgical procedure and is usually performed for large, symptomatic cystoceles. The procedure involves a surgical shortening of pelvic muscles to provide better support for the bladder. An anterior repair is often combined with a vaginal hysterectomy. Kegel exercises may be beneficial for symptoms of urinary and fecal incontinence (Lentz, 2007).

Small rectoceles may not need treatment. The woman with mild symptoms may get relief from a high-fiber diet and adequate fluid intake, stool softeners, or mild laxatives. Vaginal pessaries may be effective. Large rectoceles that are causing significant symptoms are usually repaired surgically. A posterior repair (colporrhaphy) is the usual procedure. This surgery is performed vaginally and involves shortening the pelvic muscles to provide better support for the rectum (Lentz, 2007). Anterior and posterior repairs may be performed at the same time and with a vaginal hysterectomy.

Mild to moderate UI can be significantly decreased or relieved in many women by bladder training and pelvic muscle (Kegel) exercises (Bersuk, 2007; Sampselle, 2003). Other management strategies include pelvic flow support devices (i.e., pessaries), vaginal estrogen therapy, serotonin-norepinephrine reuptake inhibitors, electrical stimulation, insertion of an artificial urethral sphincter, and surgery (e.g., anterior repair) (Dwyer & Kreder, 2005; Kielb, 2005; Lentz, 2007).

Nursing care for women with UI includes assessment for depression that can result from decreased quality of life and functional status (Melville, Delaney, Newton, & Katon, 2005). Women also may need guidance about changes in lifestyle (e.g., losing weight) and education about pelvic muscle exercises.

Nursing care of the woman with a cystocele, rectocele, or fistula requires great sensitivity because the woman's reactions are often intense. She may become withdrawn or hostile because of embarrassment caused by odors and soiling of her clothing that are beyond her control. She may have concerns about engaging in sexual activities because her partner is repelled by these problems. The nurse may tactfully suggest hygiene practices that reduce odor. Commercial deodorizing douches are available, or noncommercial solutions such as chlorine solution (1 teaspoon of chlorine household bleach to 1 quart of water) may be used. The chlorine solution is also useful for external perineal irrigation. Sitz baths and thorough washing of the genitals with unscented, mild soap and warm water help. Sparse dusting with deodorizing powders can be useful. If a rectovaginal fistula is present, enemas given before leaving the house may provide temporary relief from oozing of fecal material until corrective surgery is performed. Irritated skin and tissues may benefit from use of a heat lamp or application of an emollient ointment. Hygienic care is time consuming and may need to be repeated frequently throughout the day; protective pads or pants may need to be worn. All of these activities can be demoralizing to the woman and frustrating to her and her family.

POSTPARTUM PSYCHOLOGIC COMPLICATIONS

Mental health disorders have implications for the mother, the newborn, and the entire family. Such conditions can interfere with attachment to the newborn and family integration, and some may threaten the safety and well-being of the mother, newborn, and other children.

Mood Disorders

Mood disorders are the predominant mental health disorder in the postpartum period, typically occurring within 4 weeks of childbirth (American Psychiatric Association [APA], 2000). Many women experience a mild depression, or "baby blues," after the birth of a child. Others can have more serious depressions that can eventually incapacitate them to the point of being unable to care for themselves or their babies. Nurses are strategically positioned to offer anticipatory guidance, to assess the mental health of new mothers, to offer therapeutic interventions, and to refer when necessary. Failure to do so may result in tragic consequences.

The *Diagnostic and Statistical Manual of Mental Disorders* contains the official guidelines for the assessment and diagnosis of psychiatric illness (APA, 2000). However, specific criteria for **postpartum depression (PPD)** are not listed. Instead, postpartum onset can be specified for any mood disorder either without psychotic features (i.e., PPD) or with psychotic features (i.e., postpartum psychosis) if the onset occurs within 4 weeks of childbirth (APA).

Etiology and risk factors

The cause of PPD may be biologic, psychologic, situational, or multifactorial. It affects 13% of women worldwide. In a comprehensive review of the literature, Bina (2008) found that cultural practices could positively or negatively affect the development of PPD. A personal history or a family history of mood disorder, mood and anxiety symptoms in the antepartal period, as well as postpartum blues also increases the risk for PPD (APA, 2000; Milgrom et al., 2008). Beck (2008a, 2008b) published an integrative review of 141 studies of what nurse researchers internationally have contributed to the state of the science on postpartum depression. One aspect was in identifying risk factors. Beck described at least five instruments that have been developed since 1990 to assess risk factors or symptoms of PPD. The most common risk factors that have been identified are discussed in a later section.

Postpartum depression without psychotic features

PPD is an intense and pervasive sadness with severe and labile mood swings and is more serious and persistent than postpartum blues. Intense fears, anger, anxiety, and despondency that persist past the baby's first few weeks are not a normal part of postpartum blues. Occurring in approximately 10% to 15% of new mothers, these symptoms rarely disappear without outside help. Approximately 50% of these mothers do not seek help from any source (Dennis & Chung-Lee, 2006). The occurrence of PPD among teenage mothers is approximately 50% more than that for older mothers (Driscoll, 2006). Young mothers (younger than 20 years) and those with a high school education or less are less likely to seek help and have higher rates of PPD than other women (Mayberry, Horowitz, & Declercq, 2007).

The symptoms of postpartum major depression do not differ from the symptoms of nonpostpartum mood disorders except that the mother's ruminations of guilt and inadequacy feed her worries about being an incompetent and inadequate parent. In PPD the woman may have odd food cravings (often sweet desserts) and binges with abnormal appetite and weight gain. New mothers report an increased yearning for sleep, sleeping heavily but awakening instantly with any infant noise, and an inability to go back to sleep after infant feedings.

A distinguishing feature of PPD is irritability. These episodes of irritability may flare up with little provocation, and they may sometimes escalate to violent outbursts or dissolve into uncontrollable sobbing. Many of these outbursts are directed against significant others ("He never helps me.") or the baby ("She cries all the time and I feel like hitting her."). Women with postpartum major depressive episodes often have severe anxiety, panic attacks, and spontaneous crying long after the usual duration of baby blues.

Many women feel especially guilty about having depressive feelings at a time when they believe they should be happy. They may be reluctant to discuss their symptoms or their negative feelings toward the infant. A prominent feature of PPD is rejection of the infant, often caused by abnormal jealousy (APA, 2000). The mother may be obsessed by the notion that the offspring may take her place in her partner's affections. Attitudes toward the infant may include disinterest, annoyance with care demands, and blaming because of her lack of maternal feeling. When observed, she may appear awkward in her responses to the baby. Obsessive thoughts about harming the child are very frightening to her. In many instances, she does not share these thoughts because of embarrassment, but when she does, other family members become very frightened.

Critical Thinking Exercise: Postpartum Depression

Medical management. The natural course is one of gradual improvement over the 6 months after birth. Supportive treatment alone is not efficacious for major PPD. Pharmacologic intervention is needed in most instances. Treatment options include antidepressants, anxiolytic agents, and electroconvulsive therapy (ECT). Alternative therapies such as herbs, dietary supplements, massage, aromatherapy, and acupuncture may be helpful (Weier & Beal, 2004). Psychotherapy focuses on the mother's fears and concerns regarding her new respon-

EVIDENCE-BASED PRACTICE

Assessing for Postpartum Depression

Pat Gingrich

ASK THE QUESTION

What is the best way to assess for postpartum depression?

SEARCH FOR EVIDENCE

Search Strategies: Professional organization guidelines, meta-analyses, systematic reviews, randomized controlled trials, nonrandomized prospective studies, and retrospective studies since 2006.

Databases Searched: CINAHL, Cochrane, Medline, National Guideline Clearinghouse, TRIP Database Plus, and the websites for Association of Women's Health, Obstetric, and Neonatal Nurses and Society of Obstetricians and Gynaecologists of Candada.

CRITICALLY ANALYZE THE EVIDENCE

Postpartum depression (PPD) is a serious and insidious disease that can rob a new family of valuable nurturing time. Using data on U.S. women from the Pregnancy Risk Assessment Monitoring System (PRAMS), the Centers for Disease Control and Prevention (CDC) reported a prevalence of PPD in the first year after birth ranging from 11.7% to 20.4% (CDC, 2008). Risk factors for PPD included young age, low socioeconomic status, and use of Medicaid benefits. The CDC recommends incorporating PPD information into existing programs for high risk women, such as intimate partner violence services.

A large prospective study of 40,000 Australian women found risk factors for PPD included previous history of depression, especially current or antenatal anxiety or depression, and low partner support (Milgrom et al., 2008). The authors recommend interventions targeted to women with current depression or anxiety and low social support.

IMPLICATIONS FOR PRACTICE

In an update on the evidence-based guidelines of the Registered Nurses' Association of Ontario, nurses are encouraged to give individualized, flexible care; assess early and often, offering the Edinburgh Postnatal Depression Score (EPDS) as the most well-tested screening tool for patient self-test; intervene swiftly for a score greater than 12 on the EPDS, or if any evidence of self-harm ideation on score item #10 or in clinical judgment; and encourage peer support group participation (McQueen, Montgomery, Lappan-Gracon, Evans, Hunter, 2008).

The Postpartum Social Support Questionnaire shows preliminary promise as a valid and reliable screening tool (Hopkins & Campbell, 2008).

A systematic review of telephone support revealed that proactive telephone support decreases the symptoms of PPD. Other postpartum benefits included preventing smoking relapse and promoting breastfeeding (Dennis, Kingston, 2008).

Nurses can also help by teaching women self-care, especially symptoms and risk factors for PPD, help them to feel safe and empowered in discussing their mental and social health, and facilitate adequate social and partner support. Women and their families should be given written resources in their native language and emergency telephone numbers to call. Last but not least, follow-up is a powerful tool for detection and deterrence of PPD.

References:

Center for Disease Control and Prevention. (2008). Prevalence of self-reported postpartum depression symptoms—17 states, 2004-2005. *MMWR Morbidity and Mortality Weekly Report, 57*(14), 361-366.

Dennis, C., & Kingston, D. (2008). A systematic review of telephone support for women during pregnancy and the early postpartum period. *Journal of Obstetric, Gynecologic & Neonatal Nursing, 37*(3), 301-314.

Hopkins, J., & Campbell, S. (2008). Development and validation of a scale to assess social support in the postpartum period. *Archives of Women's Mental Health, 11*(1), 57-65.

Milgrom, J., Gemmill, A., Bilszta, J., Hayes, B., Barnett, B., Brooks, J., et al. (2008). Antenatal risk factors for postnatal depression: A large prospective study. *Journal of Affective Disorders, 108*(1-2), 147-157.

McQueen, K., Montgomery, P., Lappan-Gracon, S., Evans, M., & Hunter, J. (2008). Evidence-based recommendations for depressive symptoms in postpartum women. *Journal of Obstetric Gynecologic & Neonatal Nursing, 37*(2), 127-136.

sibilities and roles, as well as monitoring for suicidal or homicidal thoughts. For some women, hospitalization is necessary.

Nursing Care Plan: Postpartum Depression

Postpartum depression with psychotic features

Postpartum psychosis is a syndrome most often characterized by depression (as described previously), delusions, and thoughts by the mother of harming either the infant or herself (Kaplan & Sadock, 2005). A postpartum mood disorder with psychotic features occurs in 1 to 2 per 1000 births and may occur more often in primiparas (Kaplan & Sadock). Once a woman has had one postpartum episode with psychotic features, a 30% to 50% likelihood of recurrence exists with each subsequent birth (APA, 2000).

Symptoms often begin within days after the birth, although the mean time to onset is 2 to 3 weeks and almost always within 8 weeks of birth (Kaplan & Sadock, 2005). Characteristically, the woman begins to complain of fatigue, insomnia, and restlessness and may have episodes of tearfulness and emotional lability. Complaints regarding the inability to move, stand, or work are also common. Later, suspiciousness, confusion, incoherence, irrational statements, and obsessive concerns about the baby's health and welfare may be present (Kaplan & Sadock). Delusions may be present in 50% of all women with this disorder and hallucinations in approximately 25%. Auditory hallucinations that command the mother to kill the infant can also occur in severe cases. When delusions are present, they are often related to the infant. The mother may think the infant is possessed by the devil, has special powers, or is destined for a terrible fate (APA, 2000). Grossly disorganized behavior may be exhibited as a disinterest in the infant or an inability to provide care. Some women will insist that something is wrong with the baby or accuse nurses or family members of hurting or poisoning him or her.

NURSING ALERT Nurses are advised to be alert for mothers who are agitated, overactive, confused, complaining, or suspicious.

A specific illness included in depression with psychotic features is bipolar disorder. This mood disorder is preceded or accompanied by manic episodes, characterized by elevated, expansive, or irritable moods. Clinical manifestations of a manic episode include at least three of the following symptoms that have been significantly present for at least 1 week: grandiosity, decreased need for sleep, pressured speech, flight of ideas, distractibility, psychomotor agitation, and excessive involvement in pleasurable activities without regard for negative consequences (APA, 2000). Because these women are hyperactive, they may not take the time to eat or sleep, which leads to inadequate nutrition, dehydration, and sleep deprivation. While in a manic state, mothers will need constant supervision when caring for their infants. Mostly, they will be too preoccupied to provide child care.

Medical management. A favorable outcome is associated with a good premorbid adjustment (before the onset of the disorder) and a supportive family network (Kaplan & Sadock, 2005). Because mood disorders are usually episodic, women may experience another episode of symptoms within a year or two of the birth. Postpartum psychosis is a psychiatric emergency, and the mother will probably need psychiatric hospitalization. Antipsychotics and mood stabilizers such as lithium are the treatments of choice. If the mother is breastfeeding, some sources advise caution while prescribing some agents (ACOG, 2008; Newport & Stowe, 2006.). Antipsychotics and lithium should be avoided in breastfeeding mothers, but other mood stabilizers may be compatible with breastfeeding (see later discussion). Having contact with her baby is usually advantageous for the mother if she so desires, but visits must be closely supervised. Psychotherapy is indicated after the period of acute psychosis is past.

CARE MANAGEMENT

Even though the prevalence of PPD is fairly well established, it often remains undetected because women are hesitant to report symptoms of depression even to their own health care providers (McQueen, Montgomery,

NURSING PROCESS *Postpartum Depression*

ASSESSMENT

- Listen actively and demonstrate a caring attitude because women may not volunteer unsolicited information about their depression.
- Observe for signs of depression.
- Ask appropriate questions to determine moods, appetite, sleep, energy and fatigue levels, and ability to concentrate. An example of how to initiate a conversation is, "Now that you have had your baby, how are things going for you?"
- Use a screening tool to assess whether the depressive symptoms have progressed from postpartum blues to postpartum depression (PPD) (see text).
- If depression is identified, ask if the mother has thought about hurting herself or the baby.

NURSING DIAGNOSES

- *Risk for self-directed (mother) or other-directed (children) violence* related to:
  - PPD
- *Situational low self-esteem in the mother* related to:
  - Stresses associated with role changes
- *Disabled family coping* related to:
  - Increased care needs of mother and infant
- *Risk for impaired parenting* related to:
  - Inability of depressed mother to attach to infant
- *Risk for injury to newborn* related to:
  - Mother's depression (inattention to infant's needs for hygiene, nutrition, safety) and psychotropic medications via breast milk

EXPECTED OUTCOMES OF CARE

Specific measurable criteria can be developed based on the following general outcomes:

- The mother will no longer be depressed.
- The mother's and infant's physical well-being will be maintained.
- The family will cope effectively.
- Family members will demonstrate continued healthy growth and development.
- The infant will be fully integrated into the family.

PLAN OF CARE AND INTERVENTIONS

- Teach signs and symptoms of PPD to woman and family.
- Provide information about community resources for PPD, including mental health therapists and support groups; refer if needed.
- Provide teaching about psychotropic medications if ordered, including risks of breastfeeding (see text discussion).
- Provide information on alternative therapies as needed or requested (see text discussion).

EVALUATION

The nurse can be assured that care has been effective if the physical well-being of the mother and infant is maintained, the mother and family are able to cope effectively, and each family member continues to show a healthy adaptation to the presence of the new member of the family.

Lappan-Gracon, Evans, & Hunter, 2008). The following discussion identifies ways to assess for symptoms of PPD and describes the treatment options (see the Nursing Process box: Postpartum Depression).

Postpartum Depression Screening Tools

Examples of screening tools are the Edinburgh Postnatal Depression Scale (EPDS), the Postpartum Depression Predictors Inventory (PDPI), and the Postpartum Depression Screening Scale (PDSS). The EPDS is a self-report assessment designed specifically to identify women experiencing PPD. It has been used and validated in studies in numerous cultures and is viewed as a valid screening tool for PPD (Lintner & Gray, 2006). The assessment tool asks the woman to respond to 10 statements about the common symptoms of depression. The woman is asked to choose the response that is closest to describing how she has felt for the past week (Cox, Holden, & Sagovsky, 1987).

Through focused research over at least a decade, Beck has developed and continues to refine the PDPI (PDPI-R [Revised]) (Beck, 2001, 2002) and the PDSS (Beck & Gable, 2002). The PDPI-R consists of 13 risk factors related to PPD. The PDSS is a 35-item Likert response scale that assesses for seven dimensions of depression: sleeping or eating disturbances, anxiety or insecurity, emotional lability, mental confusion, loss of self, guilt or shame, and suicidal thoughts (Beck, 2008a). Both published tools are designed to be used by nurses and other health care providers to elicit information from the woman during an interview to assess risk. Areas assessed include the predictors of depression as listed in Box 23-6.

In addition, a simple two-item tool has been developed that nurses can use that has been shown to be effective in identifying women at risk for PPD. Ask, "Are you sad and depressed?" and "Have you had a loss of pleasurable activities?" An affirmative answer to both questions suggests that depression is likely (Jesse & Graham, 2005).

If any initial assessment reveals some question that the woman might be depressed, a formal screening is helpful in determining the urgency of the referral and the type of provider.

BOX 23-6

Risk Factors for Postpartum Depression

- Low self-esteem
- Stress of child care
- Prenatal anxiety
- Life stress
- Lack of social support
- Marital relationship problems
- History of depression
- "Difficult" infant temperament
- Postpartum blues
- Single status
- Low socioeconomic status
- Unplanned or unwanted pregnancy

Sources: Beck, C. (2001). Predictors of postpartum depression: An update. *Nursing Research, 50*(5), 275-282; Beck, C. (2002). Revision of the postpartum depression predictors inventory. *Journal of Obstetric, Gynecologic, and Neonatal Nursing, 31*(4), 394-402.

Nursing Interventions

Nursing care on the postpartum unit

The postpartum nurse must observe the new mother closely for any signs of tearfulness and conduct further assessments as necessary. PPD must be discussed by nurses to prepare new parents for potential problems in the postpartum period (see Patient Instructions for Self-Management box: Coping with Postpartum Blues, p. 427). The family must be able to recognize the symptoms and know where to go for help. Written materials that explain what the woman can do to prevent depression could be used as part of discharge planning.

Mothers are often discharged from the hospital before the blues or depression occurs. If the postpartum nurse is concerned about the mother, a mental health consultation should be requested before the mother leaves the hospital. Routine instructions regarding PPD should be given to the person who comes to take the woman home; for example, "If you notice that your wife (or daughter) is upset or crying a lot, please call the postpartum care provider immediately—don't wait for the routine postpartum appointment."

NURSING ALERT Because the newborn may be scheduled for a checkup before the mother's 6-week checkup, nurses in well-baby clinics or pediatrician offices should be alert for signs of PPD in new mothers and be knowledgeable about community referral resources.

PATIENT INSTRUCTIONS FOR SELF-MANAGEMENT

Activities to Prevent Postpartum Depression

- Share knowledge about postpartum emotional problems with close family and friends.
- Take care of yourself: Eat a balanced diet, exercise on a regular basis, and get enough sleep. Ask someone to take care of the baby so that you can get a full night's sleep.
- Share your feelings with someone close to you; do not isolate yourself at home.
- Do not overcommit yourself or feel as though you need to be a superwoman.
- Do not place unrealistic expectations on yourself.
- Do not be ashamed of having emotional problems after your baby is born—it happens to approximately 15% of women.

Nursing care in the home and community

Postpartum home visits can reduce the incidence of or complications from depression. A brief home visit or telephone call at least once a week until the new mother returns for her postpartum visit may save the life of a mother and her infant; however, these contacts may not be feasible or available. Supervision of the mother with emotional complications may become a prime concern. Because depression can greatly interfere with her mothering functions, family and friends may need to participate in the infant's care. The extended family and friends can use this time to determine what they can do to help, and the nurse can work with them to ensure adequate supervision of the woman and their understanding of the woman's mental illness.

When the woman has PPD, a partner often reacts with confusion, shock, denial, and anger and feels neglected and blamed. Both the woman and her partner need an opportunity to express their needs, fears, thoughts, and feelings in a nonjudgmental environment. The nurse can talk with the woman about how her condition is hard for her partner too and that he is probably very worried about her. Men often withdraw or criticize when they are deeply worried about their significant others. The nurse can provide opportunities for the partner to verbalize feelings and concerns, help the partner identify positive coping strategies, and be a source of encouragement for the partner to continue supporting the woman. Even if the mother is severely depressed, hospitalization can be avoided if adequate resources can be mobilized to ensure safety for both mother and infant. The nurse in home health care will need to make frequent telephone calls or home visits to do assessment and counseling. Community resources that may be helpful are temporary child care or foster care, homemaker service, Meals on Wheels, parenting guidance centers, mother's-day-out programs, and telephone support groups or other support programs.

Referral. Women with moderate to severe PPD should be referred to a mental health therapist, such as an advanced practice psychiatric nurse, for evaluation and therapy to prevent the effects that PPD can have on the woman and on her relationships with her partner, baby, and other children (Lintner & Gray, 2006). Inpatient psychiatric hospitalization may be necessary. This decision is made when the safety needs of the mother or children are threatened.

Providing safety. When depression is suspected, the nurse asks, "Have you thought about hurting yourself?" If delusional thinking about the baby is suspected, the nurse asks, "Have you thought about hurting your baby?" Four criteria can be used to assess the seriousness of a suicidal plan: (1) method, (2) availability, (3) specificity, and (4) lethality. Has the woman specified a method? Is the method of choice available? How specific is the plan? If the method is concrete and detailed, with access to it right at hand, the suicide risk increases. How lethal is the method? The most lethal method is shooting, with hanging a close second. The least lethal is slashing one's wrists. Medication overdose can also be used to cause death.

NURSING ALERT Suicidal thoughts or attempts are one of the most serious symptoms of PPD and require immediate assessment and intervention (Lintner & Gray, 2006).

Psychiatric hospitalization

Women with postpartum psychosis are a psychiatric emergency and must be referred immediately to a psychiatrist who is experienced in working with women with PPD, who can prescribe medication and other forms of therapy, and who can assess the need for hospitalization.

LEGAL TIP **Legal Commitment**

If a woman with PPD is experiencing active suicidal ideation or harmful delusions about the baby and is unwilling to seek treatment, legal intervention may be necessary to commit the woman to a psychiatric inpatient setting for treatment.

If the infant is allowed in the hospital psychiatric setting, the reintroduction of the baby to the mother can occur at the mother's own pace. A schedule is set for increasing the number of hours the mother cares for the baby over several days, culminating in the infant staying overnight in the mother's room. This method allows the mother to experience meeting the infant's needs and giving up sleep for the baby, a difficult situation for new mothers even under ideal conditions. The mother's readiness for discharge and caring for the baby is assessed. Her interactions with her baby are also carefully supervised and guided. A postpartum nurse is often asked to assist the psychiatric nursing staff in assessment of the mother-infant interactions.

Psychotropic medications

PPD is usually treated with antidepressant medications. If the woman with PPD is not breastfeeding, antidepressants can be prescribed without special precautions. The

COMMUNITY ACTIVITY

Analyze research findings on effectiveness of screening tools used by nurses in your community to identify women with postpartum depression (PPD). Evaluate community resources for women with PPD as to accessibility and cost. Develop a plan for improving assessment and care of postpartum patients with PPD.

commonly used antidepressant drugs are often divided into four groups: selective serotonin reuptake inhibitors (SSRIs), heterocyclics (including the tricyclic antidepressants [TCAs]), monoamine oxidase inhibitors (MAOIs), and other antidepressant agents not in the above classifications (ACOG, 2008) (Table 23-1).

The SSRIs are prescribed more frequently today than other groups of antidepressant medications. They are relatively safe and carry fewer side effects than TCAs. The most frequent side effects with the SSRIs are gastrointestinal disturbances (nausea, diarrhea), headache, and insomnia. In approximately one third of patients the SSRIs reduce libido, arousal, or orgasmic function (Keltner, 2007a).

TCAs cause many central nervous system (CNS) and peripheral nervous system (PNS) side effects. A common CNS effect is sedation, which can easily interfere with mothers caring for their babies. A mother could fall asleep while holding the baby and drop him or her, or she could have trouble getting fully awake during the night to care for the baby. Other side effects include weight gain, tremors, grand mal seizures, nightmares, agitation or mania, and extrapyramidal side effects. Anticholinergic side effects include dry mouth, blurred vision (usually temporary), difficulty voiding, constipation, sweating, and orgasm difficulty (Keltner, 2007a).

Hypertensive crisis is the main reason that MAOIs are not prescribed more frequently than other psychotropic medications. The woman should be taught to watch for signs of hypertensive crisis–throbbing, occipital headache, stiff neck, chills, nausea, flushing, retroorbital pain, apprehension, pallor, sweating, chest pain, and palpitations (Keltner, 2007a). This crisis is brought on by the woman eating foods that contain tyramine, a sympathomimetic pressor amine, which is normally broken down by the enzyme monoamine oxidase. The nurse must do extensive teaching about the avoidance of foods that contain tyramine such as aged cheeses, nuts, soy sauce, preserved meats, and tap beers (National Headache Foundation, 2009).

The woman taking mood stabilizers (see Table 23-1) must be taught about the many side effects, and especially, for those on lithium, the need to have serum lithium levels assessed every 6 months. Women with severe psychiatric syndromes such as schizophrenia, bipolar disorder, or psychotic depression will probably require antipsychotic medications (see Table 23-1). Most of these antipsychotic medications can cause sedation and orthostatic hypotension, both of which can interfere with the mother being able to safely care for her baby. They can also cause PNS effects such as constipation, dry mouth, blurred vision, tachycardia, urinary retention, weight gain, and agranulocytosis. CNS effects may include akathisia, dystonias, parkinsonism-like symptoms, tardive dyskinesia (irreversible), and neuroleptic malignant syndrome (potentially fatal) (Keltner, 2007b, 2007c).

Psychotropic medications and lactation. A major clinical dilemma is the psychopharmacologic treatment of women with PPD who want to breastfeed their infants. In the past, women were told to discontinue lactation. Current beliefs are that although most drugs will diffuse into breast milk, instances in which breastfeeding has to be discontinued are very few (Pigarelli, Kraus, & Potter, 2005). Several factors influence the amount of drug an infant will receive through breastfeeding: the amount of milk produced, the composition of the milk (mature milk versus colostrum), the concentration of the medication, and the extent to which the breast was emptied during a previous feeding (Menon, 2008; Pigarelli et al.). Infants also vary in their ability to absorb, metabolize, and excrete ingested medication. Premature infants may not have optimal liver function, and kidney function does not reach maturity until 2 to 4 months of age.

The U.S. Food and Drug Administration (FDA) has not approved any psychotropic medication for use during lactation. However, most of the medications listed in the position statement from the American Academy of Pediatrics (AAP) are compatible with breastfeeding (AAP, 2001) (see Table 23-1 for risk of taking common psychotropic medications during lactation). Almost all of the psychotropic medications are drugs for which the effects on the breastfeeding newborn are "unknown but still may be of concern." The reason for the concern is that although the medications appear to be in low concentrations in breast milk (commonly a milk-to-serum ratio of 0.5 to 1.0), many drugs have a long half-life, and levels may build up in plasma and tissue of nursing infants. Medications that have shorter half-lives tend to accumulate less, and those that are more protein bound do not cross into breast milk as well (Pigarelli et al., 2005). Because all psychotropic medications pass through breast milk to the infant, the risks associated with the use of such medication must be weighed against the benefits associated with breastfeeding for both mother and infant (Menon, 2008).

The elapsed time between maternal dosing and infant feeding has been shown to affect the amount of antidepressant medication to which the breastfed infant is exposed. If the mother is using a once-daily medication, administration at bedtime may be advised to increase the interval to the next feeding (Pigarelli et al., 2005). For medications taken multiple times per day, administration of medication immediately after a breastfeeding session will give the longest interval to allow back diffusion of drug from the breast milk as the mother's serum concentration decreases (Lawrence & Lawrence, 2005).

The long-term neurobehavioral effects of infant exposure to psychotropic medications through breastfeeding are unknown. When selecting psychotropic medications for breastfeeding women, choose those with the greatest documentation of prior use, lowest FDA risk category,

TABLE 23-1

Psychiatric Medications and Lactation Risks

	LACTATION RISK AAP*	CATEGORY HALE†
ANTIDEPRESSANT MEDICATIONS		
Selective serotonin reuptake inhibitors		
Citalopram (Celexa)	NR	L3
Escitalopram (Lexapro)	4	L3 in older infants
Fluoxetine (Prozac)	4	L2 in older infants; L3 in neonates
Fluvoxamine (Luvox)	4	L2
Paroxetine (Paxil)	4	L2
Sertraline (Zoloft)	4	L2
Tricyclics		
Amitriptyline (Elavil)	4	L2
Amoxapine (Asendin)	4	L2
Clomipramine (Anafranil)	4	L2
Desipramine (Norpramin)	4	L2
Doxepin (Sinequan)	4	L5
Imipramine (Tofranil)	4	L2
Nortriptyline (Pamelor)	4	L2
Monoamine oxidase inhibitors		
Phenelzine (Nardil)	NR	Unknown
Tranylcypromine (Parnate)	NR	Unknown
Other antidepressants		
Bupropion (Wellbutrin) IR and SR	4	L3
Maprotiline (Ludiomil)	NR	L3
Mirtazapine (Remeron)	NR	L3
Trazodone (Desyrel)	4	L2
Venlafaxine (Effexor)	NR	L3
ANTIANXIETY MEDICATIONS		
Alprazolam (Xanax)	4	L3
Buspirone (BuSpar)	NR	L3
Chlordiazepoxide (Librium)	NR	L3
Clonazepam (Klonopin)	NR	L3
Clorazepate (Tranxene)	NR	L3
Diazepam (Valium)	4	L3; L4 if used chronically
Flurazepam (Dalmane)	4	L3
Lorazepam (Ativan)	4	L3
Temazepam (Restoril)	4	L3
Triazolam (Halcion)	NR	L3
MOOD STABILIZERS		
Carbamazepine (Tegretol XR)	6	L2
Gabapentin (Neurontin)	NR	L3
Lamotrigine (Lamictal)	4	L3
Lithium carbonate (Eskalith)	5	L4
Topiramate (Topamax)	NR	L3
Valproic acid (Depakene, Depakote, Depakote ER)	6	L2
ANTIPSYCHOTIC MEDICATIONS		
Traditional antipsychotics		
Chlorpromazine (Thorazine)	4	L3
Fluphenazine (Prolixin)	NR	L3
Haloperidol (Haldol)	4	L2
Perphenazine (Trilafon)	4	L3
Thioridazine (Mellaril)	NR	L4
Thiothixene (Navane)	NR	L4
Trifluoperazine (Stelazine)	4	Unknown
Atypical antipsychotics		
Aripiprazole (Abilify)	NR	L3
Clozapine (Clozaril)	4	L3
Loxapine (Loxitane)	NR	L4
Olanzapine (Zyprexa)	NR	L2
Quetiapine (Seroquel)0	4	L4
Risperidone (Risperdal)	NR	L3
Ziprasidone (Geodon)	4	L4

*Source: Hale, T. (2004). *Medications and mother's milk* (11th ed.). Amarillo, TX: Pharmasoft.

†American Academy of Pediatrics (AAP) Committee on Drugs. (2001). The transfer of drugs and other chemicals into human milk. *Pediatrics, 108*(3), 776-789.

ER, XR, Extended release; *IR,* intermediate release; *SR,* sustained release.

Ratings: L2 = drug studied in limited number of breastfeeding women with no adverse effects in infant OR evidence is remote; L3 = no controlled studies OR studies show minimal nonthreatening effects; L4 = possibly hazardous.

NR = not rated; 4 = drug in which the effect on nursing infants is unknown but may be of concern; 5 = drugs associated with significant effects on some breastfed infants, thus caution is advised if used for nursing mothers; 6 = maternal medication usually compatible with breastfeeding.

fewest or no metabolites, and fewest side effects (ACOG, 2008; Newport & Stowe, 2006).

Nursing implications

When breastfeeding women have emotional complications and need psychotropic medications, referral to a mental health care provider who specializes in postpartum disorders is preferred. The woman should be informed of the risks and benefits to her and her infant of the medications to be taken. Depressed women will need the nurse to reinforce the need to take antidepressants as ordered. Because antidepressants do not exert any effect for approximately 2 weeks and usually do not reach full effect for 4 to 6 weeks, many women discontinue taking the medication on their own. Patient and family teaching should reinforce the schedule for taking medications in conjunction with the infant's feeding schedule and to continue taking the medication until therapeutic effects occur.

Other treatments for postpartum depression

Other treatments for PPD include complementary or alternative therapies (e.g., yoga, massage, relaxation techniques), ECT, and psychotherapy. Alternative therapies may be used alone but are often used with other treatments for PPD. Safety and efficacy studies of these alternative therapies are needed to ensure that care and advice is based on evidence (Lintner & Gray, 2006; Weier & Beal, 2004).

NURSING ALERT St. John's wort is often used to treat depression. It has not been proven safe for women who are breastfeeding.

ECT may be used for women with PPD who have not improved with antidepressant therapy. Psychotherapy in the form of group therapy or individual (interpersonal) therapy also has been used with positive results alone and in conjunction with antidepressant therapy; however, more studies are needed to determine what types of professional support are most effective (Dennis & Hodnett, 2007).

Postpartum Onset of Panic Disorder

Approximately 3% to 5% of women develop panic disorder or obsessive-compulsive disorder in the postpartum period. Panic attacks are discrete periods in which the sudden onset of intense apprehension, fearfulness, or terror occurs (APA, 2000). During these attacks, symptoms such as shortness of breath, palpitations, chest pain, choking, smothering sensations, and fear of losing control are present. Women have intrusive thoughts about terrible injury done to the infant, such as stabbing or burns, sometimes by themselves. Rarely do they harm the baby. Nurses need only to listen to hear symptoms of panic disorder. Usually, these women are so distraught that they will share with whomever will listen. In many instances the family has tried to tell them that what they are experiencing is normal, but they know differently.

CARE MANAGEMENT

Medical management

Treatment is usually a combination of medications, education, psychotherapy, and cognitive behavioral interventions, along with an attempt to identify any medical or physiologic contributors. Antidepressants such as SSRIs are the treatment of choice (Kirkwood & Melton, 2005), and most of the SSRIs are approved in the United States for the treatment of panic disorder and obsessive-compulsive disorder.

Nursing Considerations

The following nursing interventions are suggested:

- Education is a crucial nursing intervention. New mothers should be provided with anticipatory guidance concerning the possibility of panic attacks during the postpartum period. Preparing for the attacks may help decrease their unexpected, terrifying nature (Beck, 1998; Driscoll, 2006).
- Women can be reassured that feeling a sense of impending doom and fear of insanity during panic attacks is common. These fears are temporary and disappear once the panic attack is over (Beck, 1998).
- Nurses can help women identify panic triggers that are particular to their own lives. Keeping a journal can help identify the triggers (Peeke, 2008).
- Family and social supports are helpful. The new mother is encouraged to put usual chores on hold and to ask for and accept help.
- Support groups allow these mothers to experience comfort in seeing others in similar circumstances.
- Sensory interventions such as music therapy and aromatherapy are nonintrusive and inexpensive.
- Behavioral interventions such as breathing exercises and progressive muscle relaxation can be helpful (Peeke, 2008).
- Cognitive interventions such as positive self-talk training, reframing and redefining, and reassurance can help a woman learn to change the way she feels or acts even in situations that do not change (National Women's Health Resource Center, 2008).
- Exercise may be helpful for some women, particularly if they have low levels of gamma aminobutyric acid (Peeke, 2008).

KEY POINTS

- PPH is the most common and most serious type of excessive obstetric blood loss.
- Hemorrhagic (hypovolemic) shock is an emergency situation in which the perfusion of body organs may become severely compromised, leading to significant risk of morbidity or death for the mother.
- The potential hazards of the therapeutic interventions may further compromise the woman with a hemorrhagic disorder.
- Clotting disorders are associated with many obstetric complications.
- The first symptom of postpartum infection is usually fever greater than 38° C on 2 consecutive days in the first 10 postpartum days (after the first 24 hours).
- Prevention is the most effective and inexpensive treatment of postpartum infection.
- Structural disorders of the uterus and vagina related to pelvic relaxation and UI may be a delayed result of childbearing.
- Bladder training and pelvic muscle exercises can significantly decrease or relieve mild to moderate UI.
- Mood disorders account for most mental health disorders in the postpartum period.
- Identification of women at greatest risk for postpartum depression can be facilitated by use of various screening tools.
- Suicidal thoughts or attempts are one of the most serious symptoms of postpartum depression.
- Antidepressant medications are the usual treatment for postpartum depression; however, specific precautions are needed for breastfeeding women.

Audio Chapter Summaries Access an audio summary of these Key Points on evolve

References

American Academy of Pediatrics (AAP) Committee on Drugs. (2001). The transfer of drugs and other chemicals into human milk. *Pediatrics, 108*(3), 776-789.

American College of Obstetricians and Gynecologists (ACOG). (2006). *Postpartum hemorrhage. ACOG Practice Bulletin No. 76*. Washington, DC: ACOG.

American College of Obstetricians and Gynecologists (ACOG). (2008). Use of psychiatric medications during pregnancy and lactation. *ACOG Practice Bulletin No. 92*. Washington, DC: ACOG.

American Psychiatric Association (APA). (2000). *Diagnostic and statistical manual of mental disorders* (4th ed., text revision). Washington, DC: American Psychiatric Association Press.

Beck, C. (1998). Postpartum onset of panic disorder. *Journal of Nursing Scholarship, 30*(2), 131-135.

Beck, C. (2001). Predictors of postpartum depression: An update. *Nursing Research, 50*(5), 275-282.

Beck, C. (2002). Revision of the postpartum depression predictors inventory. *Journal of Obstetric, Gynecologic, and Neonatal Nursing, 31*(4), 394-402.

Beck, C. (2008a). State of the science on postpartum depression: What nurse researchers have contributed–part 1. *MCN The American Journal of Maternal/Child Nursing, 33*(2), 122-126.

Beck, C. (2008b). State of the science on postpartum depression: What nurse researchers have contributed–part 2. *MCN The American Journal of Maternal/Child Nursing, 33*(3), 151-156.

Beck, C., & Gable, R. (2002). *Postpartum depression screening scale manual.* Los Angeles: Western Psychological Services.

Bersuk, K. (2007). A strong pelvic floor: How nurses can spread the word. *Nursing for Women's Health, 11*(1), 54-62.

Bina, R. (2008). The impact of cultural factors upon postpartum depression: A literature review. *Health Care for Women International, 29*(6), 568-592.

Born, D., & Barron, M. (2005). Herbal use in pregnancy: What nurses need to know. *MCN The American Journal of Maternal/Child Nursing, 30*(3), 201-208.

Cox, J., Holden, J., & Sagovsky, R. (1987). Detection of postnatal depression. Development of the 10-item Edinburgh Postnatal Depression Scale. *British Journal of Psychiatry, 150*, 782-786.

Cunningham, F. G., Leveno, K., Bloom, S., Hauth, J., Gilstrap, L., & Wenstrom, K. (2005). *Williams obstetrics* (22nd ed.). New York: McGraw-Hill.

Curran, C. (2003). Intrapartum emergencies. *Journal of Obstetric, Gynecologic, and Neonatal Nursing, 32*(6), 802-813.

Dennis, C., & Chung-Lee, L. (2006). Postpartum depression helpseeking barriers and maternal treatment preferences: A qualitative systematic review. *Birth, 33*(4), 323-331.

Dennis C., & Hodnett, E. (2007). Psychosocial and psychological interventions for treating postpartum depression. In *The Cochrane Database of Systematic Reviews*, 2007, Issue 4, CD 006116.

Driscoll, J. (2006). Postpartum depression: How nurses can identify and care for women grappling with this disorder. *AWHONN Lifelines, 10*(5), 400-409.

Duff, P. (2007). Maternal and perinatal infection-bacterial. In S. Gabbe, J. Niebyl, & J. Simpson (Eds.), *Obstetrics: Normal and problem pregnancies* (5th ed.). Philadelphia: Churchill Livingstone.

Dwyer, N., & Kreder, K. (2005). Conservative strategies for the treatment of stress urinary incontinence. *Current Urology Report, 6*(5), 371-375.

Francois, K., & Foley, M. (2007). Antepartum and postpartum hemorrhage. In S. Gabbe, J. Niebyl, & J. Simpson (Eds.), *Obstetrics: Normal and problem pregnancies* (5th ed.). Philadelphia: Churchill Livingstone.

Gilbert, E. (2007). *Manual of high risk pregnancy & delivery* (4th ed.). St. Louis: Mosby.

Hofmeyr, G., Abdel-Aleem, H., & Abdel-Aleem, M. (2008). Uterine massage for preventing postpartum haemorrhage. In *The Cochrane Database of Systematic Reviews*, 2008, Issue 3, CD 006431.

Jesse, D., & Graham, M. (2005). Are you sad and depressed? Brief measures to identify women at risk for depression in pregnancy. *MCN The American Journal of Maternal/Child Nursing, 30*(1), 40-45.

Johnson, T., Gregory, K., & Niebyl, J. (2007). Preconception and prenatal care: Part of the continuum. In S. Gabbe, J. Niebyl, & J. Simpson (Eds.), *Obstetrics: Normal and problem pregnancies* (5th ed.). Philadelphia: Churchill Livingstone.

Kaplan, H., & Sadock, B. (2005). *Kaplan & Sadock's comprehensive textbook of psychiatry*. Philadelphia: Lippincott Williams & Wilkins.

Katz, V. (2007a). Postoperative counseling and management In Katz, V., Lentz, G., Lobo, R., & Gershenson, D. (Eds.), *Comprehensive gynecology* (5th ed.). Philadelphia: Mosby.

Katz, V. (2007b). Postpartum care. In S. Gabbe, J. Niebyl, & J. Simpson (Eds.), *Obstetrics: Normal and problem pregnancies* (5th ed.). Philadelphia: Churchill Livingstone.

Keltner, N. (2007a). Antianxiety drugs. In N. Kelter, L. Schwecke, & C. Bostrum (Eds.), *Psychiatric nursing* (5th ed.). St Louis: Mosby.

Keltner, N. (2007b). Antidepressant drugs. In N. Kelter, L. Schwecke, & C. Bostrum (Eds.), *Psychiatric nursing* (5th ed.). St Louis: Mosby.

Keltner, N. (2007c). Antimanic drugs. In N. Kelter, L. Schwecke, & C. Bostrum (Eds.), *Psychiatric nursing* (5th ed.). St Louis: Mosby.

Kielb, S. (2005). Stress incontinence: Alternatives to surgery. *International Journal of Fertility and Women's Medicine*, *50*(1), 24-29.

Kirkwood, C., & Melton, S. (2005). Anxiety disorders. I: Generalized anxiety, panic, and social anxiety disorders. In J. DiPiro, R. Talbert, G. Yee, G. Matzke, B. Wells, & M. Posey (Eds.), *Pharmacotherapy: A pathophysiologic approach* (6th ed.). New York: McGraw-Hill.

Kominiarek, M., & Kilpatrick, S. (2007). Postpartum hemorrhage: A recurring pregnancy complication. *Seminars in Perinatology*, *31*(3), 159-166.

Lawrence, R., & Lawrence, R. (2005). *Breastfeeding: A guide for the medical profession* (6th ed.). Philadelphia: Mosby.

Lee, C., & Abdul-Kadir, R. (2005). von Willebrand disease and women's health. *Seminars in Hematology*, *42*(1), 42-48.

Lentz, G., (2007). Anatomic defects of the abdominal wall and pelvic floor. In V. Katz, G., Lentz, R. Lobo, & D. Gershenson (Eds.), *Comprehensive gynecology* (5th ed.). Philadelphia: Mosby.

Lintner, N., & Gray, B. (2006). Childbearing and depression: What nurses need to know. *AWHONN Lifelines*, *10*(1), 50-57.

Mayberry, L., Horowitz, J., & Declercq, E. (2007). Depression symptom prevalence and demographic risk factors among U.S. women during the first 2 years postpartum. *Journal of Obstetric, Gynecologic, and Neonatal Nursing*, *36*(6), 542-549.

McQueen, K., Montgomery, P., Lappan-Gracon, S., Evans, E., & Hunter, J. (2008). Evidence-based recommendations for depressive symptoms in postpartum women. *Journal of Obstetric, Gynecologic, and Neonatal Nursing*, *37*(2), 127-136.

Melville, J., Delaney, K., Newton, K., & Katon, W. (2005). Incontinence severity and major depression in incontinent women. *Obstetrics and Gynecology*, *106*(3), 585-592.

Menon, S. (2008). Psychotropic medication during pregnancy and lactation. *Archives of Gynecology and Obstetrics*, *277*(1), 1-13.

Milgrom, J., Gemmill, A., Bilszta, J., Hayes, B., Barnett, B., Brooks, J., et al. (2008). Antenatal risk factors for postnatal depression: A large prospective study. *Journal of Affective Disorders*, *108*(1-2), 147-157.

National Headache Foundation. (2009). *Tyramine*. Internet document available at www.headaches.org (accessed January 7, 2009).

National Women's Health Resource Center. (2008). Women and anxiety disorders. *National Women's Health Report*, *30*(1), 1-7.

Newport, D., & Stowe, Z. (2006). Psychopharmacology during pregnancy and lactation. In A. Schatzberg, & C. Nemeroff (Eds.), *Essentials of clinical psychopharmacology* (2nd ed.). Washington, DC: American Psychiatric Publishing.

Newton, E. (2007). Breastfeeding. In S. Gabbe, J. Niebyl, & J. Simpson (Eds.), *Obstetrics: Normal and problem pregnancies* (5th ed.). Philadelphia: Churchill Livingstone.

Peeke, P. (2008). Anxiety: Things you can do to beat it. *National Women's Health Report*, *30*(1), 8.

Pettker, C., & Lockwood, C. (2007). Thromboembolic disorders. In S. Gabbe, J. Niebyl, & J. Simpson (Eds.), *Obstetrics: Normal and problem pregnancies* (5th ed.). Philadelphia: Churchill Livingstone.

Pigarelli, D., Kraus, C., & Potter, B. (2005). Pregnancy and lactation: Therapeutic considerations. In J. DiPiro, R. Talbert, G. Yee, G. Matzke, B. Wells, & M. Posey (Eds.), *Pharmacotherapy: A pathophysiologic approach* (6th ed.). New York: McGraw-Hill.

Rosenberg, A. (2007). The neonate. In S. Gabbe, J. Niebyl, & J. Simpson (Eds.), *Obstetrics: Normal and problem pregnancies* (5th ed.). Philadelphia: Churchill Livingstone.

Sampselle, C. (2003). Behavior interventions in young and middle-aged women: Simple interventions to combat a complex problem. *American Journal of Nursing*, *103*(Suppl., March 2003), 9-19.

Samuels, P. (2007). Hematologic complications of pregnancy. In S. Gabbe, J. Niebyl, & J. Simpson (Eds.), *Obstetrics: Normal and problem pregnancies* (5th ed.). Philadelphia: Churchill Livingstone.

Tiran, D., & Mack, S. (Eds.). (2000). *Complementary therapies for pregnancy and childbirth* (2nd ed.). Edinburgh: Baillière Tindall.

Weier, K., & Beal, M. (2004). Complementary therapies and adjuncts in the treatment of postpartum depression. *Journal of Midwifery & Women's Health*, *49*(2), 96-104.

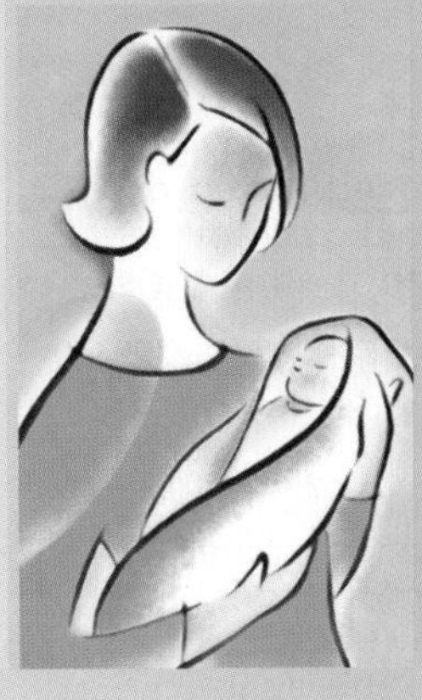

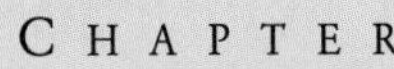

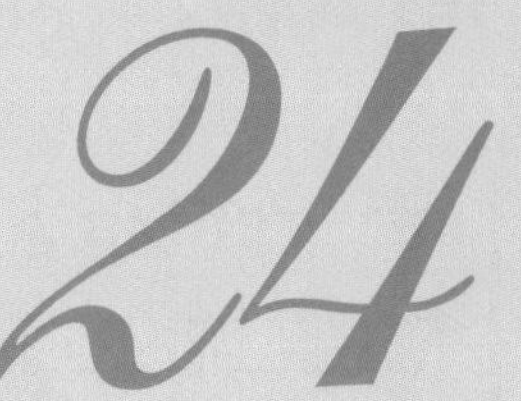

CHAPTER 24

The Newborn at Risk

SHANNON E. PERRY

LEARNING OBJECTIVES

- *Compare and contrast the physical characteristics of preterm, late preterm, term, and postterm neonates.*
- *Discuss respiratory distress syndrome and the approach to treatment.*
- *Compare methods of oxygen therapy for the high risk infant.*
- *Describe nursing interventions for nutritional care of the preterm infant.*
- *Discuss the pathophysiologic mechanism of retinopathy of prematurity and bronchopulmonary dysplasia (chronic lung disease), and identify the predisposing risk factors.*
- *Describe the treatment of the infant with meconium aspiration.*
- *Describe risk factors associated with the birth and transition of an infant of a mother with diabetes.*
- *Summarize the assessment and care of the newborn with soft-tissue, skeletal, and nervous system injuries caused by birth trauma.*
- *Describe methods used to identify clinical signs of infection in the newborn.*
- *Identify the effects of maternal use of alcohol, heroin, methadone, marijuana, methamphetamine, cocaine, and smoking tobacco on the fetus and newborn.*
- *Describe the assessment of a newborn exposed to recreational drugs in utero.*
- *Compare characteristics of neonatal Rh and ABO incompatibility.*
- *Plan developmentally appropriate care for the high risk infant.*
- *Develop a plan to address the unique needs of parents of high risk infants.*
- *Describe emotional, behavioral, cognitive, and physical responses commonly experienced during the grieving process associated with perinatal loss.*
- *Identify specific nursing interventions to meet the special needs of parents and their families related to perinatal loss and grief.*

KEY TERMS AND DEFINITIONS

ABO incompatibility Hemolytic disease that occurs when the mother's blood type is O and the newborn's is A, B, or AB

alcohol-related birth defect (ARBD) Congenital abnormality or anomaly resulting from excessive maternal alcohol intake during pregnancy characterized by typical craniofacial and limb defects, cardiovascular defects, intrauterine growth restriction, and developmental delay; newer terminology for *fetal alcohol syndrome* (FAS)

alcohol-related neurodevelopmental disorder (ARND) Disorder in infants affected by prenatal exposure to alcohol but who do not meet the criteria for FAS; previously termed *fetal alcohol effects* (FAE)

barotrauma Physical injury resulting from changing air pressure, often associated with ventilatory assistance in preterm infants

bereavement The feelings of loss, pain, desolation, and sadness that occur after the death of a loved one

continuous positive airway pressure (CPAP) Means of infusing oxygen or air under a preset pressure via nasal prongs, a facemask, or an endotracheal tube

Coombs test Indirect: determination of Rh-positive antibodies in maternal blood; direct: determination of maternal Rh-positive antibodies in fetal cord blood; positive test result indicates the presence of antibodies or titer

KEY TERMS AND DEFINITIONS—cont'd

corrected age Taking into account the gestational age and the postnatal age of a preterm infant when determining expectations for development

developmental care Care that takes into consideration the gestational age and condition of the infant and promotes the development of the infant

developmental dysplasia of the hip (DDH) Abnormal development of the hip joint, resulting in instability of the hip causing one or both of the femoral heads to be displaced from the acetabulum (hip socket)

erythroblastosis fetalis Hemolytic disease of the newborn usually caused by isoimmunization resulting from Rh incompatibility or ABO incompatibility

exchange transfusion Replacement of 75% to 85% of circulating blood by withdrawal of the recipient's blood and injection of a donor's blood in equal amounts, the purposes of which are to prevent an accumulation of bilirubin in the blood above a dangerous level, to prevent the accumulation of other by-products of hemolysis in hemolytic disease, and to correct anemia and acidosis

extracorporeal membrane oxygenation (ECMO) Oxygenation of blood external to body using cardiopulmonary bypass and a membrane oxygenator, used primarily for newborns with refractory respiratory failure or meconium aspiration syndrome

grief Physical, emotional, social, and cognitive response to a loss such as the death of a loved one

hydrops fetalis Most severe expression of fetal hemolytic disorder with high mortality, a possible sequela to maternal Rh isoimmunization; infants exhibit gross edema (anasarca), cardiac decompensation, and profound pallor from anemia

inborn error of metabolism Group of recessive disorders caused by a metabolic defect that results from the absence of or change in a protein, usually an enzyme, and mediated by the action of a certain gene

kangaroo care Skin-to-skin infant care, especially for preterm infants, that provides warmth to infant; infant is placed naked or diapered against the mother's or the father's bare chest and is covered with the parent's shirt or a warm blanket

late preterm (near term) infant An infant born between 34⅐ and 36⁶⁄₇ weeks of gestation, regardless of birth weight

mechanical ventilation Respiratory support technique used to provide predetermined amount of oxygen; requires intubation

meconium aspiration syndrome (MAS) Function of fetal hypoxia; with hypoxia the anal sphincter relaxes and meconium is released; reflex gasping movements draw meconium and other particulate matter in the amniotic fluid into the infant's bronchial tree, obstructing the airflow after birth

neonatal abstinence syndrome Signs and symptoms associated with drug withdrawal in the neonate

neutral thermal environment (NTE) Environment that enables the neonate to maintain a normal body temperature with minimum use of oxygen and energy

nonnutritive sucking Use of a pacifier by infants; may include thumb or fingers

respiratory distress syndrome (RDS) Condition resulting from decreased pulmonary gas exchange, leading to retention of carbon dioxide (increase in arterial partial pressure of carbon dioxide [pCO_2]); most common neonatal causes are prematurity and perinatal asphyxia, and maternal diabetes mellitus; also called *hyaline membrane disease*

thrush Fungal infection of the mouth or throat characterized by the formation of white patches on a red, moist, inflamed mucous membrane, caused by *Candida albicans*

TORCH Infections caused by organisms that damage the embryo or fetus; acronym for *t*oxoplasmosis, other (e.g., syphilis), *r*ubella, *c*ytomegalovirus, and *h*erpes simplex

trophic feedings Very small feedings given to stimulate maturation of the gut

WEB RESOURCES

Additional information related to the content in Chapter 24 can be found on the companion website at evolve

http://evolve.elsevier.com/Lowdermilk/maternity/

- NCLEX Review Questions
- Critical Thinking Exercise: Patent Ductus Arteriosus
- Critical Thinking Exercise: Fetal Alcohol Syndrome
- Nursing Care Plan: The Drug-Exposed Newborn
- Nursing Care Plan: Fetal Death: 24 Weeks of Gestation
- Nursing Care Plan: The High Risk Preterm Newborn
- Nursing Care Plan: The Infant of a Mother with Diabetes Mellitus
- Spanish Guidelines: Intensive Care Nursery: Parent Teaching on First Visit

Modern technology and expert nursing care have made important contributions to improving the health and overall survival of high risk infants. However, infants who are born considerably before term and survive are particularly susceptible to the development of sequelae related to their preterm birth.

High risk infants are most often classified according to birth weight, gestational age, and predominant pathophysiologic problems (Box 24-1). Intrauterine growth rates may differ among infants; factors such as heredity, placental insufficiency, and maternal disease influence intrauterine growth and birth weight. The classification system in the box encompasses birth weight and gestational age.

Other infants may be born at risk because of conditions or circumstances that are superimposed on the normal course of events associated with birth and the adjustment to extrauterine existence. These situations include birth trauma, congenital anomalies, infection, and maternal substance abuse. Birth trauma includes physical injuries a neonate sustains during labor and birth. Congenital anomalies include such conditions as gastrointestinal (GI) malformations, neural tube defects (NTDs), abdominal wall defects, and cardiac defects.

At times the nurse is able to anticipate problems, such as when a woman is admitted in premature labor or when a congenital anomaly is diagnosed by ultrasound before birth. At other times the birth of a high risk infant is unanticipated. In either case the personnel and equipment necessary for immediate care of the infant must be available.

BOX 24-1

Classification of High Risk Infants

CLASSIFICATION ACCORDING TO SIZE

Low-birth-weight (LBW) infant: an infant whose birth weight is less than 2500 g, regardless of gestational age

Very-low-birth-weight (VLBW) infant: an infant whose birth weight is less than 1500 g

Extremely-low-birth-weight (ELBW) infant: an infant whose birth weight is less than 1000 g

Late preterm (near term) infant: an infant born between 34$\frac{0}{7}$ and 36$\frac{6}{7}$ weeks of gestation, regardless of birth weight*

Appropriate-for-gestational-age (AGA) infant: an infant whose birth weight falls between the 10th and 90th percentiles on intrauterine growth curves

Small-for-date (SFD) or small-for-gestational-age (SGA) infant: an infant whose rate of intrauterine growth was restricted and whose birth weight falls below the 10th percentile on intrauterine growth curves

Large-for-gestational-age (LGA) infant: an infant whose birth weight falls above the 90th percentile on intrauterine growth charts

Intrauterine growth restriction (IUGR): found in infants whose intrauterine growth is restricted (sometimes used as a more descriptive term for the SGA infant)

Symmetric IUGR: growth restriction in which the weight, length, and head circumference are all affected

Asymmetric IUGR: growth restriction in which the head circumference remains within normal parameters while the birth weight falls below the 10th percentile

CLASSIFICATION ACCORDING TO GESTATIONAL AGE

Premature (preterm) infant: an infant born before completion of 37 weeks of gestation, regardless of birth weight

Full-term infant: an infant born between the beginning of 38 weeks and the completion of 42 weeks of gestation, regardless of birth weight

Postmature (postterm) infant: an infant born after 42 weeks of gestational age, regardless of birth weight

CLASSIFICATION ACCORDING TO MORTALITY

Live birth: birth in which the neonate manifests any heartbeat, breathes, or displays voluntary movement, regardless of gestational age

Fetal death: death of the fetus after 20 weeks of gestation and before birth, with absence of any signs of life after birth

Neonatal death: death that occurs in the first 27 days of life; early neonatal death occurs in the first week of life (Late neonatal death occurs at 7 to 27 days.)

Perinatal mortality: total number of fetal and early neonatal deaths per 1000 live births

*NOTE: Definitions on near-term (late preterm) vary among experts, but Engle (2006) suggests the above, which corresponds to 239th day to 259th day from first day of last menstrual period.

PRETERM INFANT

Preterm infants, those born before 37 weeks of gestation, are at risk because their organ systems are immature and they lack adequate physiologic reserves to function in an extrauterine environment. The range of birth weight and physiologic problems varies widely among preterm infants as a result of increased survivability among those who weigh less than 1000 g. However, the lower the weight and the gestational age are, the lower the chances are of survival among infants born preterm. Preterm birth is responsible for almost two thirds of infant deaths. The cause of preterm birth is largely unknown; however, the incidence of preterm birth is highest among low socioeconomic groups, which is likely a result of the lack of comprehensive prenatal health care. Other factors associated with preterm birth include gestational hypertension, maternal infection, multifetal pregnancy, HELLP syndrome (*h*emolysis, *el*evated *l*iver enzymes, and *l*ow *p*latelet count occurring in association with preeclampsia), premature dilation of the cervix, and placental or umbilical cord conditions that affect the fetus' reception of nutrients.

The potential problems and care needs of the preterm infant weighing 2000 g differ from those of the term or postterm infant of equal weight. The presence of physiologic disorders and anomalies affects the infant's response to treatment. These conditions include necrotizing enterocolitis, growth failure, bronchopulmonary dysplasia, intraventricular-periventricular hemorrhage, and retinopathy of prematurity. (See Table 24-2 on pp. 762-763).

Opinions vary about the practical and ethical dimensions of resuscitation of extremely low-birth-weight (ELBW) infants (infants whose birth weight is 1000 g or less). Ethical issues associated with resuscitation of these infants include whether to resuscitate, who should make that decision, whether the cost of resuscitation is justified, and whether the benefits of technology outweigh the burdens on the infant, family, and society in relation to the quality of the infant's life.

Late-Preterm Infant

With the advent of managed care, attempts to cut health care costs were made. Infants who appeared to be "near" term began to be treated much the same as term infants, thus avoiding the excess costs of neonatal intensive care for infants who appeared to be healthy. **Late-preterm infants** (infants born between $34\frac{0}{7}$ and $36\frac{6}{7}$ weeks of gestation) may be able to make an effective transition to extrauterine life; however, such infants, by nature of their limited gestation, remain at risk for problems related to thermoregulation, hypoglycemia, hyperbilirubinemia, sepsis, and respiratory function (Bakewell-Sachs, 2007). Experts now recommend that infants born between 34 and $36\frac{6}{7}$ weeks gestation be called late-preterm infants rather than near-term infants (Engle, 2006; Engle, Tomashek, & Wallman, 2007). Late-preterm infants comprise approximately 70% of the total preterm infant population and the mortality rate for this group is significantly higher than that of term infants (7.9 per 1000 live births versus 2.4 per 1000 live births, respectively) (Tomashek, Shapiro-Mendoza, Davidoff, & Petrini, 2007). Because birthweights of late-preterm infants often range from 2000 to 2500 g and they appear relatively mature in comparison to the smaller less mature infant they may be cared for in the newborn nursery; within this setting, risk factors for late-preterm infants may be overlooked. The Association of Women's Health, Obstetric, and Neonatal Nurses (AWHONN) published a *Late-Preterm Assessment Guide* (Santa-Donato, Medoff-Cooper, Bakewell-Sachs, Frazer Askin, & Rosenberg, 2007) for the education of perinatal nurses regarding the late-preterm infant's risk factors and appropriate care and follow up (Table 24-1) (see also Chapter 18).

Nursing Care Plan: The High Risk Preterm Newborn

CARE MANAGEMENT

For the high risk infant, an accurate assessment of gestational age (see Chapter 17) is critical in helping the nurse identify the potential problems the newborn can experience. The response of preterm, late preterm, and postterm infants to extrauterine life is different from that of term infants. By understanding the physiologic basis of these differences the nurse can assess these infants; determine the response of the preterm, late-preterm, or postterm infant; and anticipate potential problems.

Respiratory function

An effective respiratory pattern is usually quickly established in nonstressed newborns, as evidenced by vigorous activity, adequate tissue perfusion, and pink or acrocyanotic color. However, infants with a potential for respiratory depression at birth because of asphyxia, maternal analgesia or illness, pulmonary immaturity, or congenital malformations may exhibit cyanosis, gasping or ineffective respirations, decreased tissue perfusion, retractions, nasal flaring, tachypnea, decreased muscle tone, or a combination of these problems.

Numerous problems may affect the respiratory system of preterm infants and may include the following:

- Decreased number of functional alveoli
- Deficient surfactant levels
- Smaller airway lumen
- Decreased tracheal cartilage
- Greater obstruction of respiratory passages
- Insufficient calcification of the bony thorax
- Circulating hormones (prostaglandins) that may affect cardiovascular function
- Immature and fragile pulmonary vasculature
- Distance between functional alveoli and capillary bed, especially in ELBW infants

In combination, these deficits severely hinder the infant's respiratory efforts and can produce **respiratory distress** or respiratory failure. Early signs of respiratory distress include tachypnea, nasal flaring, and expiratory grunting. Depending on the severity of the respiratory distress and the cause, retractions can begin as subcostal, intercostal, or suprasternal. Increasing respiratory effort (e.g., paradoxical breathing patterns, retractions, nasal flaring, expiratory grunting, tachypnea, or apnea) indicates increasing distress. As a result of pulmonary immaturity and residual function, very low-birth-weight (VLBW) and ELBW infants may progress rapidly from respiratory distress to complete respiratory failure. Initially a compromised infant's color can be cyanotic centrally or pale. Acrocyanosis is a normal finding in the neonate, but central cyanosis indicates poor oxygenation.

Periodic breathing is a respiratory pattern commonly seen in preterm infants. Such infants exhibit 5- to 10-second respiratory pauses followed by 10 to 15 seconds of compensatory rapid respirations. Such periodic breathing should not be confused with apnea, which is a cessation of respirations of 20 seconds or more. The nurse must be prepared to provide supplemental oxygen and artificial ventilation as necessary when the newborn demonstrates an inability to initiate or maintain adequate respiratory function.

TABLE 24-1

Late-Preterm Infant Assessment and Interventions

RISK FACTORS	ASSESSMENT	INTERVENTIONS*
Respiratory distress (RD)	Assess for cardinal signs of RD (nasal flaring, grunting, tachypnea, central cyanosis, retractions), for presence of apnea especially during feedings, and for hypothermia, hypoglycemia.	Perform gestational age assessment; observe for signs of RD; monitor oxygenation by pulse oximetry; provide supplemental oxygen judiciously.
Thermal instability	Monitor axillary temperature every 30 min immediately postpartum until stable; thereafter every 1-4 hr, depending on gestational age and ability to maintain thermal stability.	Provide skin-to-skin care in immediate postpartum period for stable infant; implement measures to prevent excess heat loss (adjust environmental temperature, avoid drafts); bathe only after thermal stability has been maintained for 1 hr.
Hypoglycemia	Monitor for signs and symptoms of hypoglycemia; assess feeding ability (latch on, nipple feeding); assess thermal stability, signs and symptoms of RD; monitor bedside glucose in infants with additional risk factors (mother with diabetes, prolonged labor, RD, poor feeding).	Initiate early feedings of human milk or formula; avoid dextrose water or water feedings; provide intravenous dextrose as necessary for hypoglycemia.
Jaundice	Observe for jaundice in first 24 hr; evaluate maternal-fetal history for additional risk factors that may cause increased hemolysis and circulating levels of unconjugated bilirubin (Rh, ABO, spherocytosis, bruising); assess feeding method, voiding, stooling patterns.	Monitor transcutaneous bilirubin, and note risk zone on hour-specific nomogram (Fig. 17-8).
Feeding problems	Assess suck-swallow and breathing; assess for RD, hypoglycemia, thermal stability; assess latch-on, maternal comfort with feeding method; weight loss no more than 10% of birth weight.	Initiate early feedings—human milk or formula; ensure maternal knowledge of feeding method and signs of inadequate feeding (sleepiness, lethargy, color changes during feeding, apnea during feeding, decreased or absent urinary output).

Source: Santa-Donato, A., Medoff-Cooper, B., Bakewell-Sachs, S., Frazer Askin, D., & Rosenberg, S. (2007). *Late preterm infant assessment guide.* Washington, DC: Association of Women's Health, Obstetric and Neonatal Nurses.
*This list is not exhaustive of nursing interventions; additional interventions include those discussed under the care of the high risk infant in this chapter.

Cardiovascular function

Evaluation of heart rate and rhythm, color, blood pressure, perfusion, pulses, oxygen saturation, and acid-base status provides information on cardiovascular status. The nurse must intervene if symptoms of hypovolemia, shock, or both are found. These symptoms include prolonged capillary refill (>3 seconds), pale color, poor muscle tone, lethargy, tachycardia initially then bradycardia, and continued respiratory distress despite the provision of adequate oxygen and ventilation. Hypotension may initially be present or can occur in some infants as a late sign of shock.

Blood pressure (BP) is monitored routinely in the sick neonate by either internal or external means. Direct recording with arterial catheters is often used but carries the risks inherent in any procedure in which a catheter is introduced into an artery. An umbilical venous catheter can also be used to monitor the neonate's central venous pressure. Oscillometry (Dinamap) is a noninvasive, effective means for detecting alterations in systemic BP (hypotension or hypertension) and for identifying the need to implement appropriate therapy to maintain cardiovascular function.

Body temperature

Preterm infants are susceptible to temperature instability as a result of numerous factors. Factors that place preterm infants at risk for temperature instability include the following:

- Large surface area in relation to body weight
- Minimal insulating subcutaneous fat
- Limited stores of brown fat (an internal source for the generation of heat present in normal term infants)
- Decreased or absent reflex control of skin capillaries (vasoconstriction)
- Inadequate muscle mass activity
- Poor muscle tone, resulting in more body surface area being exposed to the cooling effects of the environment
- An immature temperature regulation center in the brain
- Increased insensible water loss
- Decreased ability to increase oxygen consumption
- Decreased caloric intake

The goal of thermoregulation is a **neutral thermal environment (NTE)**, which is the environmental temperature at which oxygen consumption and metabolic rate are minimal but adequate to maintain the body temperature (Blackburn, 2007). The NTE range for preterm infants weighing less than 1000 g is very narrow, and the prediction of NTE for each infant is impossible. Extremely immature infants may require environmental temperatures equal to skin and core temperature or possibly higher to achieve thermoneutrality (Blackburn). With knowledge of the four mechanisms of heat transfer (i.e., convection, conduction, radiation, evaporation) the nurse can create an environment for the preterm infant that promotes temperature stability (see Chapter 16). Given that overheating produces an increase in oxygen and calorie consumption, the infant is also jeopardized if he or she becomes hyperthermic (apnea and flushed color may indicate hyperthermia). The preterm infant is not able to sweat and thus dissipate heat.

Central nervous system function

The preterm infant's central nervous system (CNS) is susceptible to injury as a result of the following problems:

- Birth trauma causing damage to immature intracranial structures
- Bleeding from fragile capillaries
- Impaired coagulation process, including prolonged prothrombin time
- Recurrent hypoxic and hyperoxic episodes
- Predisposition to hypoglycemia
- Fluctuating systemic BP with concomitant variation in cerebral blood flow and pressure

In the preterm neonate, neurologic function is dependent on gestational age, associated illness factors, and predisposing factors such as intrauterine asphyxia, which can cause neurologic damage. Clinical signs of neurologic dysfunction can be subtle, nonspecific, or specific. Five categories of clinical manifestations should be thoroughly evaluated in the preterm infant: seizure activity, hyperirritability, CNS depression, elevated intracranial pressure (ICP), and abnormal movements such as decorticate posturing. Primary and tendon reflexes are generally present in preterm infants by 28 weeks of gestation; evaluation of these reflexes should be part of the neurologic examination. Ongoing assessment and documentation of these neurologic signs are needed both for the purposes of discharge teaching and for making follow-up recommendations.

Nutrition status

The initial goal of neonatal nutrition in the preterm infant is to prevent catabolism and excess fluid loss. Once the infant's respiratory and cardiac functions are stabilized, the goal of nutrition is to promote optimal growth and development. The preterm infant's metabolic functions are compromised by a limited store of nutrients, a decreased ability to digest proteins and absorb nutrients, and immature enzyme systems.

The nurse must continuously assess the infant's nutritional status. Preterm infants often require gavage or intravenous (IV) feedings instead of oral feedings, depending on the gestational age, birth weight, and existing illness factors such as respiratory distress.

Renal function

The preterm infant's immature renal system is unable to (1) excrete metabolites and drugs adequately, (2) concentrate urine, or (3) maintain acid-base, fluid, or electrolyte balance. Therefore intake and output, as well as specific gravity, are assessed. Laboratory tests are performed to assess acid-base and electrolyte balance. Medication levels are monitored in preterm infants because metabolism via renal and hepatic routes is often hindered. Because of the great variability in drug metabolism, serum levels are obtained to ensure an adequate therapeutic range for treatment and to prevent toxicity.

Hematologic status

The preterm infant is predisposed to hematologic problems because of the following conditions:

- Increased capillary fragility
- Increased tendency to bleed (prolonged prothrombin time and partial thromboplastin time)
- Decreased production of red blood cells (RBCs) resulting from physiologic rapid decrease in erythropoiesis after birth
- Large amount of fetal hemoglobin (up to 80% of the total volume)
- Loss of blood attributable to frequent blood sampling for laboratory tests
- Decreased RBC survival related to the relatively larger size of the RBC and its increased permeability to sodium and potassium
- Decreased levels of circulating albumin

Infants are assessed for any evidence of bleeding from puncture sites, the GI tract, and pulmonary system. They are also examined for signs of anemia (e.g., decreased hemoglobin and hematocrit levels, pale skin, increased apnea, lethargy, tachycardia, poor weight gain). In high risk infants the amount of blood withdrawn for laboratory testing is monitored.

Infection prevention

Even though protection from infection is an integral part of all newborn care, preterm and sick infants are particularly susceptible to infectious organisms. As with all aspects of care, strict handwashing is the single most important measure to prevent nosocomial infections. Personnel with known infectious disorders are barred from the unit until they are no longer infectious. Standard Precautions are instituted in all nursery areas as a method of infection control to protect infants and staff.

Neonates are highly susceptible to infection as a result of diminished nonspecific (inflammatory) and specific (humoral) immunity, such as impaired phagocytosis, delayed chemotactic response, minimal or absent immunoglobulin A (IGA) and immunoglobulin M (IgM), and decreased complement levels. Because of the infant's poor response to pathogenic agents, in most instances, no local inflammatory reaction is seen at the portal of entry to signal an infection, and the resulting symptoms tend to be vague and nonspecific. Consequently, diagnosis and treatment may be delayed. Preterm and term infants exhibit various nonspecific signs and symptoms of infection (Box 24-2). Early identification and treatment of sepsis is essential.

BOX 24-2

Signs and Symptoms of Neonatal Infection

Many are subtle and nonspecific
- Temperature instability
- Hypothermia—most common
- Hyperthermia—rarely

Central nervous system changes
- Lethargy
- Irritability
- Altered level of consciousness

Changes in color
- Cyanosis, pallor
- Mottling (marbling)
- Jaundice

Cardiovascular instability
- Poor perfusion
- Hypotension
- Bradycardia or tachycardia
- Prolonged capillary refill (>3 seconds)

Respiratory distress
- Tachypnea or bradypnea
- Apnea
- Retractions, nasal flaring, grunting

Gastrointestinal problems
- Feeding intolerance, increased residuals (when gavage fed)
- Vomiting
- Diarrhea
- Bloody stools (frank or occult positive)
- Abdominal distention

Metabolic instability
- Glucose instability
- Metabolic acidosis

Other
- Electrolyte imbalance
- Decreased urinary output

Interventions

The best environment for fetal growth and development is in the uterus of a healthy, well-nourished woman. The goal of care for the preterm infant is to provide an extrauterine environment that approximates a healthy intrauterine environment so as to promote normal growth and development. Medical and nursing personnel, respiratory therapists, occupational and physical therapists, dietitians, social workers, care managers, and pharmacists work as a team to provide the intensive care needed.

The admission of a preterm newborn to the intensive care nursery is usually an emergency situation. When required, resuscitation is started in the birthing unit, and warmth and oxygen are provided during transport to the nursery. A rapid initial assessment is performed to determine the infant's need for lifesaving treatment.

Physical care

The preterm infant's environmental support typically consists of the following equipment and procedures:

- Incubator or radiant warmer to control body temperature (NTE)
- Oxygen administration, depending on infant's pulmonary and circulatory status
- Electronic monitoring of respiratory and cardiac function
- Assistive devices for positioning the infant
- Clustering of care and minimization of stimulation and handling

Various metabolic support measures that may be instituted consist of the following:

- Parenteral fluids to support nutrition, hydration, and fluid and electrolyte balance
- IV access for fluids, parenteral nutrition, and to facilitate medication administration

- Blood work to monitor arterial blood gases (ABGs), blood glucose level, and electrolytes and other diagnostic studies (C-reactive protein, white blood cell [WBC] count with differential, hemoglobin, and hematocrit) as indicated

Maintain body temperature

The preterm infant is susceptible to heat loss and its complications (see Fig. 16-2 on p. 444). In addition, low-birth-weight (LBW) infants may be unable to increase their metabolic rate because of impaired gas exchange, caloric intake restrictions in relation to high expenditure, or poor thermoregulation. Transepidermal water loss is greater than in the term infant because of skin immaturity in ELBW and VLBW infants (i.e., those weighing less than 1000 g and 1500 g, respectively) and can contribute to temperature instability. The preterm infant should be transferred from the birth room in a prewarmed incubator; ELBW infants may be placed in a polyethylene bag to decrease heat and water loss (Fig. 24-1). Skin-to-skin contact (kangaroo care) between the stable preterm infant and parent is a viable option for interaction because of the maintenance of appropriate body temperature by the infant (see p. 767 for further discussion of kangaroo care).

Preterm and other high risk infants are cared for in the NTE created by use of an external heat source. A probe applied to the infant is attached to an external heat source supplied by a radiant warmer or a servo-controlled incubator. Optimal thermoneutrality cannot be predicted for every preterm infant's needs. The American Academy of Pediatrics and the American Heart Association Neonatal Resuscitation Program recommends that the first axillary temperature not be below 36.5° C (Kattwinkel, 2006). Standard guidelines for maintaining NTE in the LBW infant are published (Blake & Murray, 2006). Further research is needed to define an NTE for the ELBW infant.

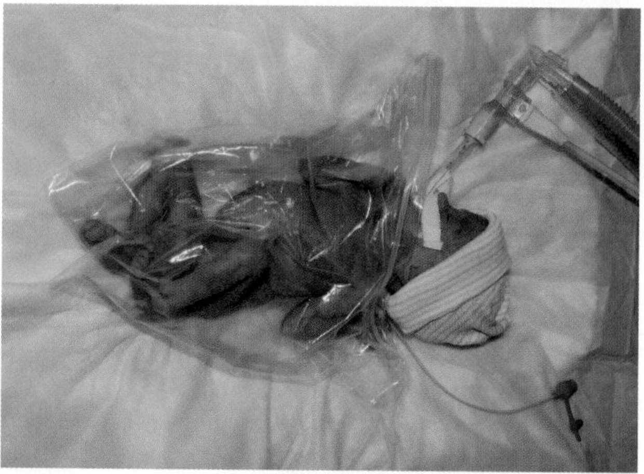

Fig. 24-1 Preterm infant in polyethylene bag to protect against heat loss. (Courtesy Cheryl Briggs, RN, Annapolis, MD.)

Care of the hypothermic infant. Rapid changes in body temperature may cause apnea and acidosis in the neonate. Therefore the warming of a hypothermic infant should occur over a period of hours. Rapid rewarming may cause apnea, and too slow rewarming increases metabolic distress and oxygen consumption. Rewarming must therefore be individualized for each infant according to the illness and the ability to produce heat. To accomplish this task the infant is placed either under a radiant warmer or in an incubator with a servo-control mechanism. Experts suggest that rewarming proceed at a rate of 1° to 2° C per hour. Appropriate guidelines for rewarming the hypothermic infant should be consulted for further information.

Oxygen therapy

The goals of oxygen therapy are to provide adequate oxygen to the tissues, prevent lactic acid accumulation resulting from hypoxia, and at the same time avoid the potentially negative effects of hyperoxia and free radicals. Numerous methods have been devised to improve oxygenation (Fig. 24-2). All of these methods require that the gas be warmed and humidified before entering the respiratory tract. If the infant does not require mechanical ventilation, oxygen can be supplied by plastic hood placed over the infant's head, by nasal cannula, or by nasal continuous positive airway pressure (CPAP) to supply

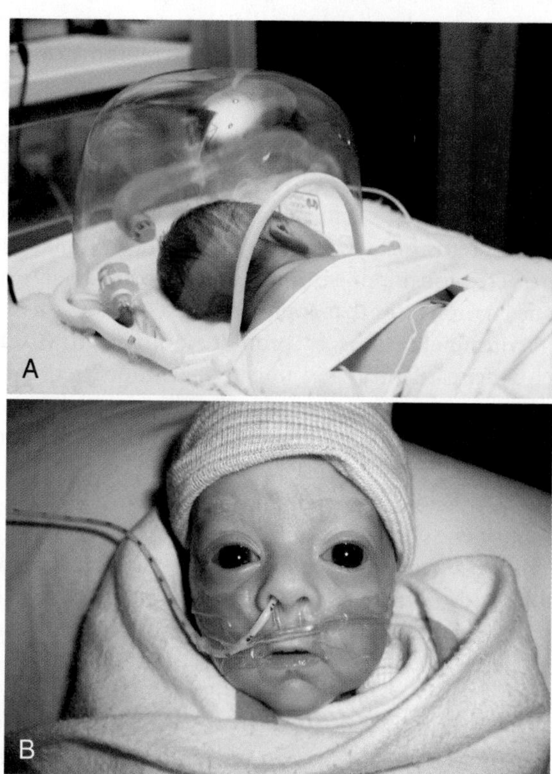

Fig. 24-2 **A,** Infant under hood. **B,** Infant with nasal cannula and indwelling gavage tube. (**A,** Courtesy Leslie Altimier, MSN, RN, TriHealth, Cincinnati, OH; **B,** Courtesy Cheryl Briggs RN, Annapolis, MD.)

variable concentrations of humidified oxygen. Because oxygen therapy is not without inherent hazards, each infant must be closely monitored to prevent hyperoxemia and hypoxemia.

Mechanical ventilation (respiratory support providing predetermined amount of oxygen through endotracheal tube) must be implemented if other methods of therapy cannot correct abnormalities in oxygenation. Ventilator settings are determined by the infant's particular needs. The ventilator is set to provide a predetermined amount of oxygen to the infant during spontaneous respirations and to provide mechanical ventilation in the absence of spontaneous respirations. Newer technologies in ventilation allow oxygen to be delivered at lower pressures and in assist modes, thereby preventing the overriding of the infant's spontaneous breathing and providing distending pressures within a physiologic range, decreasing **barotrauma** and associated complications such as pneumothorax and pulmonary interstitial emphysema.

Neonatal resuscitation

In 2010 the American Heart Association published neonatal resuscitation guidelines (Kattwinkel, Perlman, Aziz, et al., 2010). A rapid assessment of infants can identify those who do not require resuscitation: those born at term gestation, with no evidence of meconium or infection in the amniotic fluid, those who are breathing or crying, and those with good muscle tone. If any of these characteristics is absent, the infant should receive the following actions in sequence: (1) initial steps in stabilization: provide warmth by placing the baby under a radiant warmer, position the head in a position to open the airway, clear the airway with a bulb syringe or suction catheter, dry the baby, stimulate breathing, and reposition the baby; (2) ventilation; (3) chest compressions; and (4) administration of epinephrine or volume expansion or both. The decision to move from one category of action to the next is based on the assessment of respirations, heart rate, and color. Rapid decision making is imperative; 30 seconds are allotted for each step. The condition of the infant is reevaluated and the decision made whether to progress to the next step (Fig. 24-3).

Resuscitation of asphyxiated newborns with 21% oxygen rather than 100% oxygen shows promise. Proponents for room air resuscitation suggest that fewer complications are associated with oxidative stress and hyperoxemia when room air is administered. The 2010 American Heart Association resuscitation standards for neonatal resuscitation stress that resuscitation may begin with no supplemental oxygen (i.e., 21% or room air) but that if the infant's condition does not improve within 90 seconds, supplemental oxygen should be available for use. The stated goal is to minimize oxygen free radicals by preventing hyperoxia using supplemental oxygen at levels less than 100% (Kattwinkel, et al., 2010). A review of several studies indicates that neonatal mortality is reduced by 30% to 40% when room air instead of 100% oxygen is used for neonatal resuscitation (Saugstad, 2007). Fluctuations in oxygen saturation are also deemed harmful. Experts recommend that oxygen saturations for ELBW infants be maintained between 85% and 93% but definitely not exceeding 95% (Saugstad). Rates of retinopathy of prematurity and bronchopulmonary dysplasia are reduced in infants whose arterial oxygen saturation (SaO_2) is kept between 93% and 95%.

Surfactant replacement therapy

Surfactant is a surface-active phospholipid secreted by the alveolar epithelium. Acting much the same as a detergent, this substance reduces the surface tension of fluids that line the alveoli and respiratory passages, resulting in uniform expansion and maintenance of lung expansion at low intraalveolar pressure. Without surfactant, infants are unable to keep their lungs inflated and therefore exert a great deal of effort to reexpand the alveoli with each breath. With increasing exhaustion, infants are able to open fewer and fewer alveoli. This inability to maintain lung expansion produces widespread atelectasis.

Surfactant can be administered as an adjunct to oxygen and ventilation therapy (see Medication Guide: Surfactant Replacement). Generally, infants born before 32 weeks of gestation do not have adequate amounts of pulmonary surfactant to survive extrauterine life. In many centers the use of prophylactic surfactant is reserved for infants younger than 29 weeks who will likely have respiratory distress syndrome (RDS) (see Table 24-2) (Hagedorn, Gardner, Dickey, & Abman, 2006). The American Academy of Pediatrics (AAP) Committee on Fetus and Newborn (Engle & AAP Committee on Fetus and Newborn, 2008) recommends the use of surfactant in infants with RDS as soon as possible after birth, especially ELBW infants and those not exposed to maternal antenatal steroids. The administration of antenatal steroids to the mother and surfactant replacement has decreased the incidence of RDS and concomitant morbidities.

Additional therapies

Inhaled nitric oxide (INO), **extracorporeal membrane oxygenation (ECMO)**, and liquid ventilation are additional therapies used in the treatment of respiratory distress and respiratory failure in neonates. INO is used in term and late preterm infants with conditions such as persistent pulmonary hypertension, meconium aspiration syndrome, pneumonia, sepsis, and congenital diaphragmatic hernia to decrease or reverse pulmonary hypertension, pulmonary vasoconstriction, acidosis, and hypoxemia. Nitric oxide is a colorless, highly diffusible gas that can be administered through the ventilator circuit blended with oxygen. INO therapy may be used in conjunction with surfactant replacement therapy, high-frequency ventilation, or ECMO.

ECMO may be used in the management of term infants with acute severe respiratory failure for the same condi-

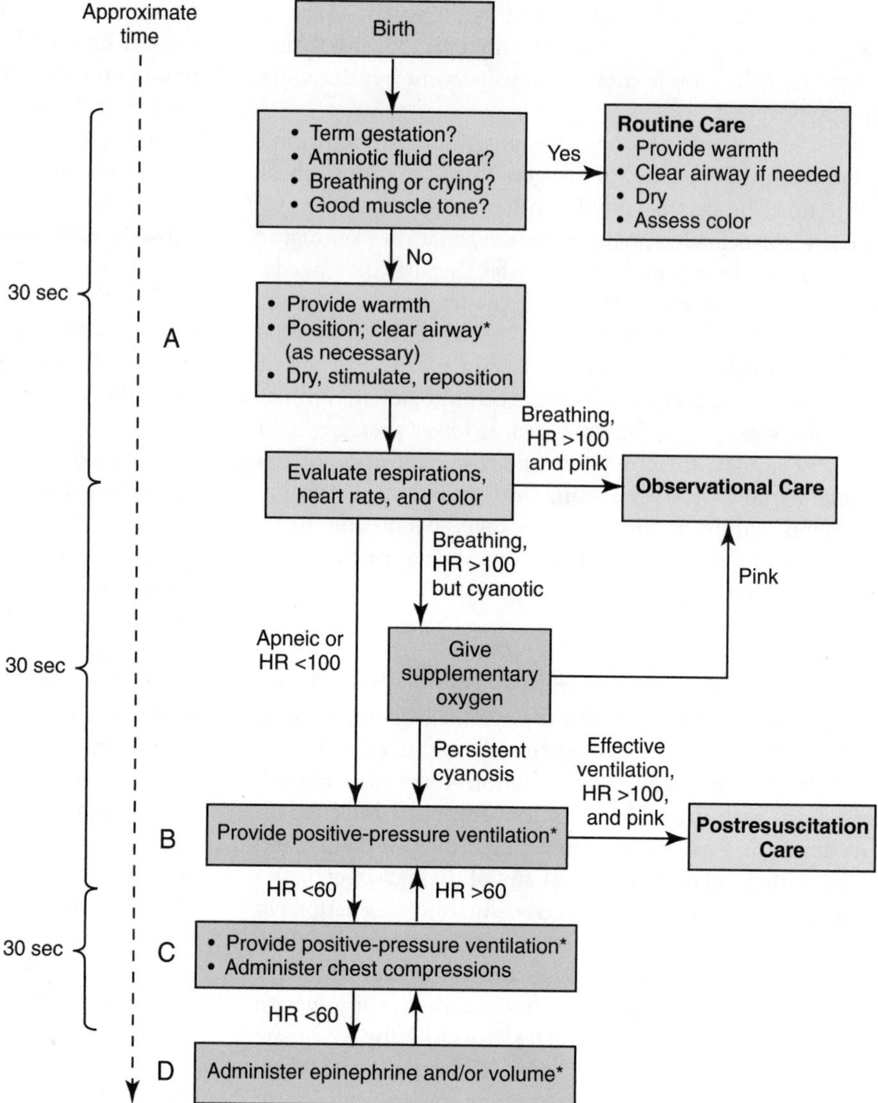

Fig. 24-3 Neonatal resuscitation flow algorithm. (From American Heart Association. [2005]. Neonatal resuscitation guidelines. *Circulation, 112*(24 Suppl) IV-188-IV-195.

tions as those mentioned for INO. This therapy involves a modified heart-lung machine, although in ECMO the heart is not stopped, and blood does not entirely bypass the lungs. Blood is shunted from a catheter in the right atrium or right internal jugular vein by gravity to a servo-regulated roller pump, pumped through a membrane lung where it is oxygenated, through a small heat exchanger where it is warmed, and then returned to the systemic circulation via a major artery such as the carotid artery to the aortic arch. ECMO provides oxygen to the circulation, allowing the lungs to "rest," and decreases pulmonary hypertension and hypoxemia in such conditions as persistent pulmonary hypertension of the newborn, congenital diaphragmatic hernia, sepsis, meconium aspiration, and severe pneumonia. ECMO is not used in preterm infants younger than 34 weeks of gestation because of the anticoagulant therapy required in the pump and circuits, which can increase the potential for intraventricular hemorrhage in such infants. In some centers the success of high-frequency ventilation and INO has greatly decreased the demand for and use of ECMO.

Weaning from respiratory assistance

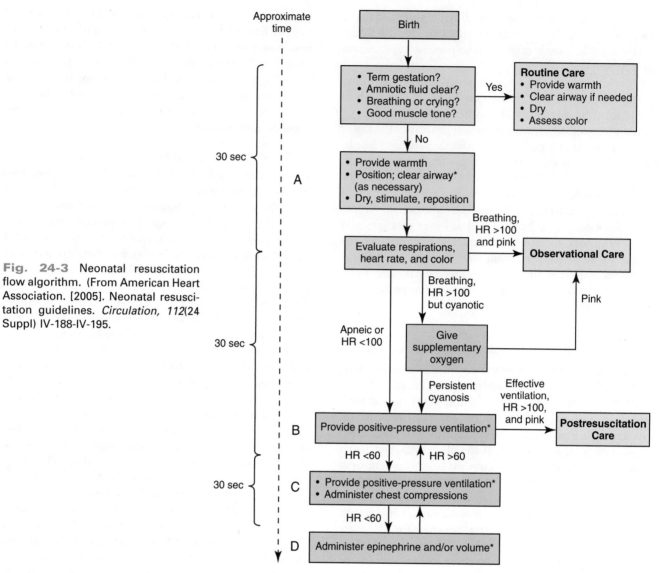

The infant is ready to be weaned from respiratory assistance when the ABG and SaO_2 levels are maintained within normal limits and the infant is able to establish spontaneous ventilation sufficient to maintain acid-base balance. A spontaneous, adequate respiratory effort must be present and the infant must show improved muscle tone during increased activity. Weaning is accomplished in a stepwise and gradual manner, which may consist of the infant being extubated, placed on nasal CPAP, and then weaned to oxygen by means of a hood or nasal cannula. Throughout

Medication Guide

Surfactant Replacement

Bovine lung extract—beractant (Survanta); artificial surfactant—colfosceril palmitate (Exosurf)

ACTION

These medications provide exogenous surfactant to correct deficiency in lung immaturity.

INDICATIONS

Surfactants are used in the prevention and treatment of respiratory distress syndrome in premature infants. For *prevention,* the drug is administered within 15 minutes of birth to infants with clinical manifestations of surfactant deficiency or with a birth weight less than 1250 g. For *treatment,* the drug is administered to infants with a confirmed diagnosis of respiratory distress syndrome, preferably within 8 hours of birth.

DOSAGE AND ROUTE

Dosage depends on the drug used. Administer via endotracheal tube.

ADVERSE EFFECTS

Adverse reactions include respiratory distress immediately after administration and bradycardia and oxygen desaturation.

NURSING CONSIDERATIONS

Observe the infant's condition for changes. Diuresis may occur with improvement. Ventilator settings may need changing as the infant's ability to oxygenate increases.

the weaning process the infant's oxygen levels are monitored by pulse oximetry, transcutaneous partial pressure of oxygen ($tcPO_2$) monitoring, and by assessing blood gas levels.

Frequent skin assessments are essential when the infant is receiving supplemental oxygen with any of the methods described herein but particularly in infants with poor perfusion and in those requiring equipment that comes in continuous contact with the infant's skin (e.g., nasal CPAP, nasal cannula, pulse oximetry probes). A greater-than-normal incidence of skin breakdown is noted in infants and children who require the use of medical devices (e.g., nasal prongs, pulse oximetry probes) (Noonan, Quigley, & Curley, 2006).

Some infants are not able to be weaned from all oxygen support by the time of discharge from the hospital and may require home oxygen therapy for several months. Bronchopulmonary dysplasia or congenital anomalies such as repaired congenital diaphragmatic hernia or tracheal defect or a neurologic insult with resultant dysfunction may preclude weaning.

The parents need to be given consistent information and be reassured about the infant's respiratory progress. Decisions regarding the nature of continued interventions should be included in a multidisciplinary plan of care, and the therapy should be explained frequently to the family.

Nutrition care

Optimal nutrition is critical in the management of LBW and preterm infants, but difficulties exist in providing for their nutritional needs. The various mechanisms for ingestion and digestion of foods are not fully developed; the more immature the infant is, the greater the problem will be. In addition, the nutritional requirements for this group of infants are not known with certainty. All preterm infants are at risk because of poor nutritional stores and several physical and developmental characteristics.

An infant's need for rapid growth and daily maintenance must be met in the presence of several anatomic and physiologic disabilities. Although some sucking and swallowing activities are demonstrated before birth and in premature infants, coordination of these mechanisms does not occur until approximately 32 to 34 weeks of gestation, and they are not fully synchronized until 36 to 37 weeks. Initial sucking is not accompanied by swallowing, and esophageal contractions are uncoordinated. The gag reflex may not be developed until 36 weeks of gestation. Consequently, infants are highly prone to aspiration and its attendant dangers. As infants mature, the suck-swallow pattern develops but is slow and ineffectual, and these reflexes may also become easily exhausted.

The amount and method of feeding are determined by the size and condition of the infant. Nutrition can be provided by either the parenteral or enteral route or by a combination of the two. Infants who are ELBW, VLBW, or critically ill are often initially fed exclusively by the parenteral route because of their inability to digest and absorb enteral nutrition. Illness factors resulting in hypoxia and major organ immaturity further preclude the use of enteral feeding until the infant's condition has stabilized. Necrotizing enterocolitis has previously been associated with enteral feedings in acutely ill or distressed infants (see Necrotizing Enterocolitis, Table 24-2).

Total parenteral nutrition (TPN) support of acutely ill infants can be accomplished quite successfully with commercially available IV solutions specifically designed to meet the infant's nutritional needs, including protein, amino acids, trace minerals, vitamins, carbohydrates (dextrose), and fat (lipid emulsion). Evidence supports early (within hours of birth) introduction of parenteral nutrition, in particular amino acids, lipids, and protein, and the introduction of minimal enteral feedings **(trophic feedings)** within the first 5 days of life. These interventions increase neurodevelopmental outcome and prevent growth failure often witnessed in ELBW infants (Anderson & Gardner, 2006; Ehrenkranz, 2007).

TABLE 24-2

Complications of Prematurity

COMPLICATION	RISK FACTORS	PATHOPHYSIOLOGY	SIGNS	TREATMENT
Respiratory distress syndrome (RDS)	Prematurity, perinatal asphyxia, hypovolemia, male infant, Caucasian race, maternal diabetes, second-born twin, familial predisposition, maternal hypotension, cesarean birth without labor, hydrops fetalis, third-trimester bleeding (Hagedorn et al., 2006)	Deficient surfactant leads to progressive atelectasis, loss of functional residual capacity, and ventilation-perfusion imbalance with an uneven distribution of ventilation Decreased oxygenation, central cyanosis, and metabolic or respiratory acidosis and an increase in pulmonary vascular resistance Right-to-left shunting and a reopening of the ductus arteriosus and foramen ovale (Hagedorn et al., 2006)	Tachypnea; grunting; nasal flaring; intercostal, or subcostal retractions; hypercapnia; respiratory or mixed acidosis; pallor; hypotension and shock; crackles, poor air exchange, and occasionally apnea	RDS is self-limiting—respiratory symptoms usually abate after 72 hours Establish and maintain adequate ventilation and oxygenation to prevent ventilation-perfusion mismatch and atelectasis Administer exogenous surfactant at or shortly after birth Maintain neutral thermal environment (NTE) Monitor arterial blood gas values (Table 24-3) Maintain fluid and nutrition balance Use positive-pressure ventilation, continuous positive airway pressure, and oxygen therapy as needed
Patent ductus arteriosus (PDA)	Ductal closure: term infant—hours or days; preterm infant—may be delayed as a result of decreased oxygenation and circulating hormones (prostaglandins)	Ductus constricts and closes after birth with increase in oxygenation, levels of circulating prostaglandins, and the muscle mass Closure is also influenced by catecholamines, low pH, bradykinin, and acetylcholine Failure of ductus to close after birth = patent ductus arteriosus	Systolic murmur, active precordium, bounding peripheral pulses, tachycardia, tachypnea, crackles, and hepatomegaly Systolic murmur heard best at second or third intercostal space at upper left sternal border Active precordium caused by increased left ventricular stroke volume	Medical management: ventilatory support, fluid restriction, diuretics, and indomethacin Surgical ligation performed when PDA is clinically significant and medical management has failed Supportive nursing care: NTE, adequate oxygenation, meticulous fluid balance, and parental support

Periventricular-intraventricular hemorrhage (PV-IVH)	Capillary bleeding caused by factors such as trauma, asphyxia; prematurity, hypoglycemia, acidosis, rapid volume expansion, blood transfusion	Bleeding into the subependymal germinal matrix; may extend into the lateral ventricles	Usually asymptomatic; some infants experience decreased hematocrit, glucose instability respiratory acidosis, apnea, hypotonia, stupor, ashen color, respiratory distress	Recognize factors that increase risk of PV-IVH, intervene to decrease risk of bleeding, provide supportive care to infants who have bleeding episode Initiate early breast feeding because breast feeding significantly reduces the incidence of this implication
Necrotizing enterocolitis (NES)	Preterm birth; majority of cases occur after feedings have been introduced	Acute inflammatory disease of the gastrointestinal (GI) mucosa, commonly complicated by perforation Intestinal ischemia, colonization by pathogenic bacteria, and substrate (formula feeding) in the intestinal lumen	Signs are nonspecific: decreased activity, hypotonia, pallor, recurrent apnea and bradycardia, decreased oxygen saturation, respiratory distress, metabolic acidosis, oliguria, hypotension, decreased perfusion, cyanosis, temperature instability GI symptoms: abdominal distention, increasing or bile-stained residual gastric aspirates, vomiting (bile or blood), grossly bloody stools, abdominal tenderness, and erythema of the abdominal wall (Roaten, Bensard, & Price, 2006)	Care is supportive and preventive for bowel perforation Oral or tube feedings discontinued to rest GI tract; nasogastric tube inserted and placed to low suction, parenteral therapy (often by total parenteral nutrition); systemic antibiotic therapy; surgical resection and anastomosis if perforation or clinical deterioration occurs
Retinopathy of prematurity (ROP)	Prematurity, supplemental oxygen with oxygen tensions that are too high	Oxygen tensions that are too high for level of retinal maturity initially cause vasoconstriction After oxygen therapy is discontinued, neovascularization occurs in the retina and vitreous, with capillary hemorrhages, fibrotic resolution, and possible retinal detachment Results in scar tissue and visual impairment	No external signs; diagnosed using retinal examination and scleral depression	Prevention and early detection of preterm birth Circumferential cryopexy, laser photocoagulation, vitamin E therapy, and decreasing the intensity of ambient light
Bronchopulmonary dysplasia (BPD) (chronic lung disease)	Prematurity, low birth weight, less than 28 wks of gestation, mechanical ventilation and supplemental oxygen	Lung injury in infants who require mechanical ventilation and supplemental oxygen (Dudell & Stoll, 2007)	Tachypnea, retractions, nasal flaring, increased work of breathing, exercise intolerance (to handling and feeding), and tachycardia (Hagedorn et al., 2006)	Oxygen therapy, nutrition, fluid restriction, and medications (e.g., diuretics, corticosteroids, and bronchodilators)

Type of nourishment. The type, mode, and volume of feedings and the infant's feeding schedule are based on the assessment of the weight of the infant, pattern of weight gain or loss, presence or absence of suck and swallow reflexes, behavioral readiness to take oral feedings, physical condition, residual from previous feeding if being gavage fed, malformations (especially GI defects), and renal function, including urinary output and laboratory values.

Human milk is the best source of nutrition for term and preterm infants. Even small preterm infants (28 to 36 weeks) are able to breastfeed if they have adequate sucking and swallowing reflexes and no other contraindications, such as respiratory complications or concurrent illness, are present. Preterm infants who are breastfed rather than bottle fed demonstrate fewer oxygen desaturations, absence of bradycardia, warmer-than normal skin temperature, and improved coordination of breathing, sucking, and swallowing (Gardner, Snell, & Lawrence, 2006). Mothers who wish to breastfeed their preterm infants are encouraged to pump their breasts until their infants are sufficiently stable to tolerate breastfeeding. Appropriate guidelines for the storage of expressed mother's milk should be used to decrease the risk of milk contamination and destruction of its beneficial properties (Jones & Tully, 2006).

Commercially available preterm formulas are cow's milk–based, whey-predominant, and have a higher concentration of protein, calcium, and phosphorus than term formulas to meet the unique needs of the preterm infant (AAP Committee on Nutrition, 2004). Most preterm formulas are either 22 cal/oz or 24 cal/oz. The preparation of powdered formula for preterm infants should be carefully performed under strict aseptic technique, preferably in a pharmacy, and the formula properly refrigerated to prevent infection (AAP Committee on Nutrition). Human milk with fortifier (protein, phosphorus, and calcium) is recommended for LBW preterm infants because it increases weight gain and improves bone mineralization better than nonfortified human milk (Lawrence & Lawrence, 2005). Supplementation with iron, vitamin D, and multivitamins may be considered in exclusively breastfeed LBW infants.

NURSING ALERT Contamination of powdered infant formula in hospitals by *Enterobacter sakazakii* has been associated with serious neonatal infections, necrotizing enterocolitis, and mortality. When possible, alternatives to powdered formula should be chosen; otherwise, such formula should be carefully mixed in a designated preparation room using aseptic technique. Continuous infusion of powdered formula should not exceed 4 hours.

Hydration. Preterm infants often receive supplemental parenteral fluids to supply additional calories, electrolytes, or water. Adequate hydration is particularly important in preterm infants because their extracellular water content is higher than in term infants (70% in full-term infants and up to 90% in preterm infants), their body surface is relatively larger than in term infants, and the capacity for osmotic diuresis is limited in preterm infants' underdeveloped kidneys. Therefore these infants are highly vulnerable to fluid depletion. Nurses must monitor fluid status by daily (or more frequent) weights and accurate intake and output of all fluids, including medications and blood products.

Alterations in behavior, alertness, or activity level in these infants receiving IV fluids can signal an electrolyte imbalance, hypoglycemia, or hyperglycemia. The nurse is also observant for tremors or seizures in the VLBW or ELBW infant, because these neurologic signs can indicate hyponatremia or hypernatremia. Weight gain from fluid overload in the sick preterm infant can occur as a result of fluid retention (renal failure), inappropriate fluid administration (parenteral), or congestive heart failure. An increased fluid gain can result in the opening of a previously closed patent ductus arteriosus (PDA), thus exacerbating associated illness. Growing preterm infants, especially those with chronic lung disease (bronchopulmonary dysplasia [BPD]), on oral electrolyte supplements should be assessed for rapid weight gain that can result in pulmonary congestion, PDA, and electrolyte imbalance (see Table 24-2).

Elimination patterns. Frequency of urination, as well as the amount, color, pH, and specific gravity of the urine, is assessed. The assessment of bowel movements includes frequency of stooling and character of the stool, as well as the presence of constipation, diarrhea, or loss of fats (steatorrhea). Infants with unexplained abdominal distention are assessed thoroughly to rule out the presence of necrotizing enterocolitis or obstruction of the GI tract.

Oral feeding. Nourishment by the oral route is preferred for the infant who has adequate strength and GI function. Breast milk may be fed by breast, bottle, or gavage. Formula may be fed by bottle or gavage. Preterm infants may be put to breast for practice feeds and nonnutritive suckling as soon as medically stable.

Gavage feeding. Gavage feeding is a method of providing breast milk or formula through a nasogastric or orogastric tube (Fig. 24-4). Gavage feeding can be accomplished either with a tube inserted at each feeding (bolus) or continuously through an indwelling feeding tube. Breast milk or formula can be supplied intermittently using a syringe with gravity-controlled flow, or it can be given continuously using an infusion pump. The type of fluid instilled is recorded with every syringe change. The volume of the continuous feedings is recorded hourly, and the residual gastric aspirate is measured before each feeding. Residuals of less than a quarter of a feeding can be refed to the infant, depending largely on unit protocol. Feeding may be stopped if the residual is greater than 2 to 4 ml/kg or a 1-hour volume and is not resumed until the

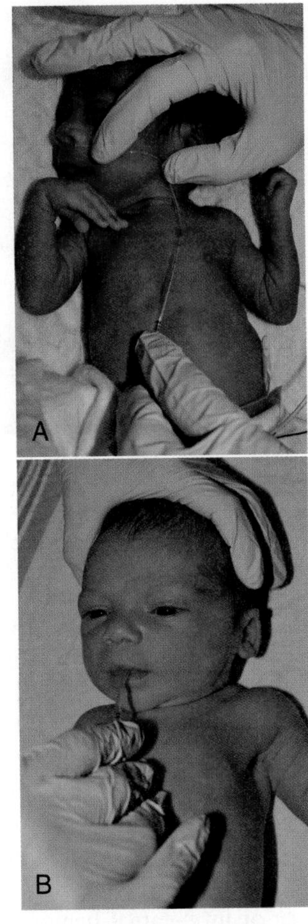

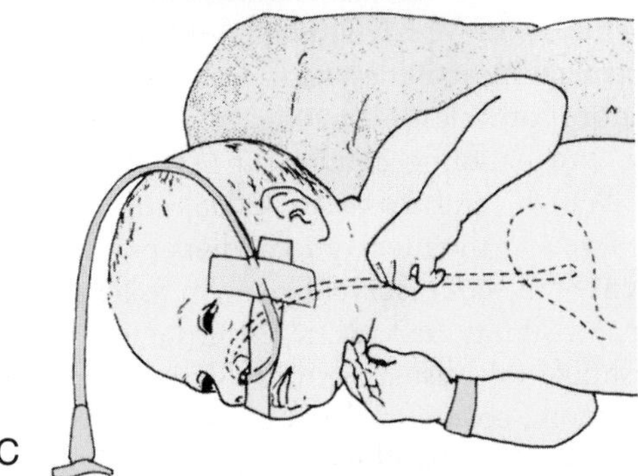

Fig. 24-4 Gavage feeding. **A,** Measurement of gavage feeding tube from tip of nose to earlobe and to midpoint between end of xiphoid process and umbilicus. Baby's nose should face the ceiling when the measurement is done. Tape may be used to mark correct length on tube. **B,** Insertion of gavage tube using orogastric route. **C,** Indwelling gavage tube, nasogastric route. After feeding by orogastric or nasogastric tube, infant is propped on right side or placed prone (preterm infant) for 1 hour to facilitate emptying of stomach into small intestine. Note rolled towel for support. (**A** and **B,** courtesy Cheryl Briggs, RNC, Annapolis, MD.)

Procedure

Inserting a Gavage Feeding Tube

EQUIPMENT

- Infant feeding tube
- For infants less than 1 kg, size 4-Fr tube
- For infants more than 1 kg, size 5-Fr to 6-Fr
- Stethoscope
- Sterile water (lubricant)
- Syringe: 5 to 10 ml
- Tape, optional transparent dressing
- Gloves

1. Measure the length of the gavage tube from the tip of the nose to the earlobe to the midpoint between the xiphoid process and the umbilicus (see Fig. 24-4, *A*). Mark the tube with indelible ink or a piece of tape.
2. Lubricate the tip of the tube with sterile water and insert gently through the nose or mouth (see Fig. 24-4, *B*) until the predetermined mark is reached. Placement of the tube in the trachea will cause the infant to gag, cough, or become cyanotic.
3. Check correct placement of the tube by:
   a. Pulling back on the plunger to aspirate stomach contents. Lack of stomach aspirate or fluid is not necessarily evidence of improper placement. Aspiration of respiratory secretions may be mistaken for stomach contents; however, the pH of the stomach contents is much lower (more acidic) than the pH of respiratory secretions.
   b. Injecting a small amount of air (1-3 ml) into the tube while listening for gurgling by using a stethoscope placed over the stomach. Ensure that the tube is inserted to the mark; air entering the stomach may be heard even if the tube is positioned above the gastroesophageal (cardiac) sphincter.
   c. Abdominal or chest radiography. This is the only definitive way to verify tube placement.
4. Using tape or a transparent dressing, secure the tube in place and tape it to the cheek to prevent accidental dislodgment and incorrect positioning (see Fig. 24-4, *C*).
   a. Assess the infant's skin integrity before taping the tube.
   b. Edematous or very preterm infants should have a pectin barrier placed under the tape to prevent abrasions, or a hydrocolloid adhesive should be used to prevent epidermal stripping.
5. Tube placement *must* be assessed before each feeding.

Source: Anderson, M., Wood, L., Keller, J., & Hay, W. (2011). Enteral nutrition. In S. Gardner, B. Carter, M. Enzman-Hines, & J. Hernandez (Eds.). *Merenstein & Gardner's handbook of neonatal intensive care* (7th ed.). St. Louis: Mosby.

infant can be assessed for a possible feeding intolerance (Anderson & Gardner, 2006).

The orogastric route of gavage feedings may be preferred because most infants are preferential nose breathers. However, some infants do not tolerate oral tube placement. The procedure for inserting a gavage feeding tube is described in the Procedure box.

Gastrostomy feeding. Gastrostomy feeding involves the surgical placement of a tube through the skin of the abdomen into the stomach. With percutaneous gastrostomy insertion, feedings are often started within hours of insertion. Feedings by gravity are performed slowly over 20 to 30 minutes. Special care must be taken to prevent a rapid bolus of the fluid because this event may lead to abdominal distention, GI reflux into the esophagus, diarrhea with malabsorption, or respiratory compromise. Meticulous skin care at the tube insertion site is necessary to prevent skin breakdown or infection. Accurate assessments of intake and output are needed to monitor renal function and the adequacy of fluid and calorie intake.

Advancing infant feedings. Feedings are advanced from passive (parenteral and gavage) to active (nipple and breastfeeding) as warranted by the infant's physical status and ability to tolerate feedings. The infant's sucking patterns and demonstration of a quiet alert state can also be used to determine readiness to nipple feed. Feedings are advanced slowly and cautiously. If feedings are advanced too rapidly, vomiting, diarrhea, abdominal distention, and apneic episodes can result. The parents should be encouraged to interact by talking and making eye contact with the infant during feedings.

Nonnutritive sucking. For the infant who requires gavage or parenteral feedings, **nonnutritive sucking** on a pacifier during the gavage procedure may improve oxygenation and facilitate earlier transition to breastfeeding or nipple feeding. Nonnutritive sucking may lead to decreased energy expenditure with reduced restlessness.

Mothers of preterm infants should be encouraged to let their infant start sucking at the breast during kangaroo care; some infants' suck and swallow reflexes may be coordinated as early as 32 weeks of gestation.

Skin care

The skin of preterm infants is characteristically immature relative to that of full-term infants. Because of its increased sensitivity and fragility, the use of alkaline-based soap that might destroy the acid mantle of the skin is avoided. Vernix caseosa has benefits for the preterm infant's skin. Vernix acts as an epidermal barrier, decreases bacterial contamination of the skin through its antimicrobial peptides and proteins, and decreases transepidermal water loss (Lund, Kuller, Raines, Ecklund, Archambault, & O'Flaherty, 2007). Experts recommend that a validated skin assessment tool such as the Braden Q Scale or the Neonatal Skin Condition Score (NSCS) be used once daily to evaluate the high risk infant's skin condition so as to implement interventions aimed at minimizing skin breakdown (Curley, Razmus, Roberts, & Wypij, 2003; Lund & Osborne, 2004).

Environmental concerns

Infants in neonatal intensive care units (NICUs) are exposed to high levels of auditory input from the various machine alarms, which can have adverse effects (Fig. 24-5). The noise level in an NICU is 20 db higher than in a well-baby nursery. Experts recommend that the overall continuous sound level not exceed 55 db (Haubrich, 2007). The infant's hearing may be damaged if she or he is exposed to a constant decibel level of 90 db or frequent decibel swings higher than 110 db.

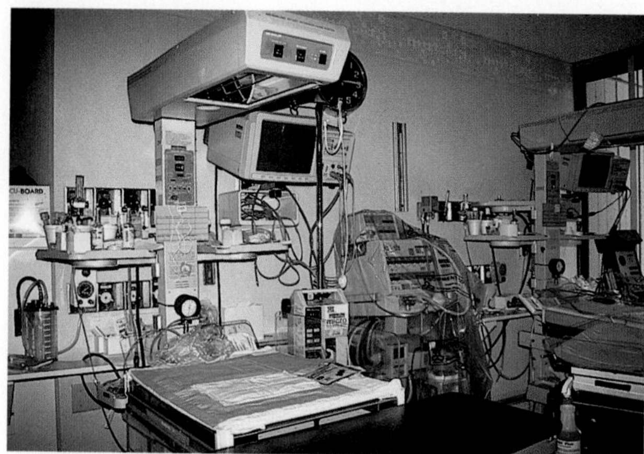

Fig. 24-5 Although necessary, neonatal intensive care unit equipment may contribute to significant environmental stimulation. Note bed, wall oxygen attachments, monitor, ventilator, incubator, and pumps, all of which have alarm systems. (Courtesy Marjorie Pyle, RNC, Lifecircle, Costa Mesa, CA.)

The noise level that results from monitoring equipment, alarms, and general unit activity has been correlated with the incidence of intracranial hemorrhage, especially in the ELBW or VLBW infant. Personnel should reduce noise-generating activities, such as closing doors (including incubator portholes), listening to loud radios, talking loudly, and handling equipment (e.g., trash containers). Byers, Waugh, and Lowman (2006) suggest monitoring sound levels in the nursery to address problem areas.

Twenty-four-hour surveillance of sick infants implies maximal visibility and, in many instance, bright lights. Units should establish a night-day sleep pattern by darkening the room, covering cribs with blankets, or placing eye patches over the infant's eyes at night. Infants need scheduled rest periods during which the lights are dimmed, the incubators are covered with blankets, and the infants are not disturbed for handling of any kind (Holditch-Davis, Blackburn, & VandenBerg, 2007). Sleep periods should be undisturbed for at least 50 minutes to allow complete sleep cycles. Infants' eyes should be shielded from bright procedure lights to prevent potential harm. Many experts suggest that the human face, especially a parent's face, is the best visual stimulus and that visual stimuli be kept to a minimum early in development.

Effects of environmental hazards can be potentiated by some drugs used for infant therapy. Diuretics (especially furosemide [Lasix]), ototoxic antibiotics such as gentamicin and kanamycin, and antimalarial agents can potentiate noise-induced hearing loss. Routine hearing screening should be performed on all infants before discharge (see Fig. 16-15).

Nurses can modify the environment to provide a neurodevelopmentally supportive milieu. In this way the infant's neurobehavioral and physiologic needs can be better met, the infant's developing organization can be supported, and growth and development fostered. Table 24-2 provides a list of complications of prematurity.

Developmental care

Much attention has been focused on the effects of early developmental intervention on both normal and preterm infants. Infants respond to a wide variety of stimuli, and the atmosphere and activities of the NICU are overstimulating. Consequently, infants in the NICU are subjected to *inappropriate* stimulation that can be harmful. Nursing care activities, such as taking vital signs, changing the infant's position, weighing, and changing diapers, are associated with frequent periods of hypoxia, oxygen desaturation, and elevated ICP. The more immature the infant is, the less able he or she is to habituate to a single procedure, such as taking an oscillometric BP, without becoming overstimulated. The caregiver uses the infant's own behavior and physiologic functioning as the basis for planning care and providing interventions. Through caregiver observation, the infant's strengths, thresholds for disorganization, and areas in which the infant is vulnerable can be identified.

Developmental care supports the infant's unique ability to achieve behavioral state organization. It is tailored to the developmental level and tolerance of each infant based on a comprehensive behavioral assessment. Using the developmental model of supportive care, the nurse closely monitors physiologic and behavioral signs to promote organization and well-being of the preterm infant. Infants are handled with slow, restricted movements (some infants are unstable if moved abruptly), and their random movements are controlled with limbs held flexed close to their bodies during turning or other position changes. This *containment* or *facilitated tucking* may also be used before invasive procedures such as heel stick to reduce distress. A nest constructed by placing blanket rolls underneath the bed sheet helps infants maintain an attitude of flexion when prone or side lying.

Although it must be individually adjusted, skin-to-skin contact (kangaroo care) and short periods of gentle massage can help reduce stress in preterm infants (Fig. 24-6). The parent wears a loose-fitting, open-front top that has a modified marsupial-like pocket carrier for the infant. The undressed (except for diaper) infant is placed in a vertical position on the parent's bare chest, which permits direct eye contact, skin-to-skin sensations, and close proximity. Skin-to-skin contact between parent and infant, in addition to being a safe and effective method for VLBW infant-parent acquaintance, can have a positive healing effect for

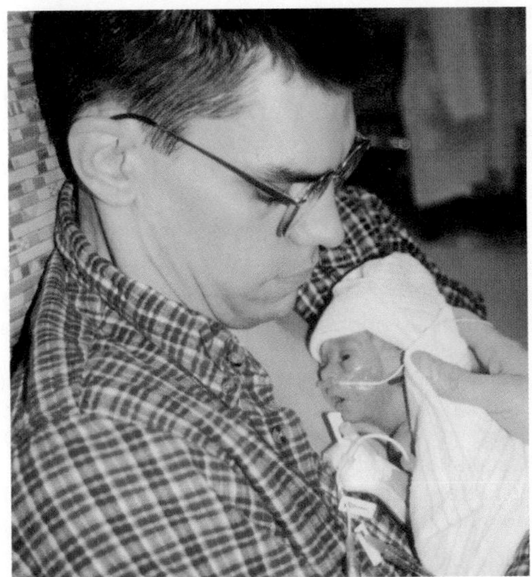

Fig. 24-6 Father providing kangaroo care. (Courtesy Judy Meyr, St. Louis, MO.)

the mother who had a high risk pregnancy. Additional benefits of skin-to-skin care include early contact with mechanically ventilated infants, maintenance of neonatal thermal stability and oxygen saturation, increased feeding vigor, maintenance of organized state, decreased pain perception during painful heel sticks, and minimal untoward effects of being held (Conde-Agudelo & Belizan, 2003; Dodd, 2005). The National Association of Neonatal Nurses developed a clinical practice guideline for the stable healthy preterm infant aged 30 weeks or more of gestation (Ludington-Hoe, Morgan, & Abouelfettoh, 2008) (see Evidence-Based Practice box).

Cobedding of twins (or *multiples*) is another developmental intervention that has been implemented in neonatal intensive care and newborn nurseries to provide an improved environment for neonatal growth and development. Cobedding involves placing twins or other multiples together in the same crib or incubator. Twins who are cobedding have improved thermoregulation, have significantly fewer apnea and bradycardia episodes than infants not cobedded, gain weight more quickly than their single counterparts, and have decreased length of stay. Parental satisfaction is also significantly increased with cobedded newborns. One major concern with cobedding is cross-transmission of infection between the neonates, but increased infection rates have not occurred with cobedding (LaMar & Dowling, 2006).

When infants have reached sufficient developmental organization and stability, interventions are designed and implemented to support their growing abilities. Nurses and parents become adept at learning to read infants' behavioral cues and supplying appropriate interventions. Clues include both approach and avoidance behaviors. *Approach behaviors* that are supported and enhanced include tongue

EVIDENCE-BASED PRACTICE

Skin-to-Skin (Kangaroo) Contact for Term and Preterm Infants

Pat Gingrich

ASK THE QUESTION

What are the benefits of kangaroo care (skin-to-skin contact)?

SEARCH FOR EVIDENCE

Search Strategies: Professional organization guidelines, meta-analyses, systematic reviews, randomized controlled trials, nonrandomized prospective studies, and retrospective studies since 2006.

Databases Searched: CINAHL, Cochrane, Medline, National Guideline Clearinghouse, TRIP Database Plus, and the websites for Academy of Breastfeeding Medicine, Association of Women's Health, Obstetric, and Neonatal Nurses, Centers for Disease Control and Prevention, and Lamaze International.

CRITICALLY ANALYZE THE EVIDENCE

Kangaroo care (skin-to-skin contact) has proved to be so significantly beneficial to the infant and the mother, the father, or both that it is now promoted by most maternal-newborn professional organizations (American Academy of Pediatrics, Academy of Breastfeeding Medicine, Association of Women's Health, Obstetric and Neonatal Nurses, Lamaze, National Institute for Health and Clinical Excellence, and Joanna Briggs Institute). A Cochrane systematic review found that placing the dried newborn on the mother's bare abdomen at birth, covered with a warm towel and early, frequent breastfeeding regulate newborn temperature, decrease stress hormones and crying, promote bonding, and encourage exclusive breastfeeding duration (Moore, Anderson, & Bergman, 2007). As noted in this chapter, a program of skin-to-skin contact and frequent breastfeeding (10-12 times in 24 hours) regulates blood glucose for most term infants within minutes or hours.

For vulnerable preterm infants, these benefits may be even more protective. A randomized controlled trial (RCT) comparing kangaroo care with typical care for preterm infants, 32 to 36 weeks of gestation, showed significant exclusive breastfeeding outcomes out to 6 months (Hake-Brooks & Anderson, 2008). Besides breastfeeding and thermoregulation, another RCT concluded that regular skin-to-skin contact helps preterm infants better organize their sleep-awake states into more mature patterns (Ludington-Hoe et al., 2006).

Painful procedures can add to the stress hormones of the already fragile preterm neonate. A single-blind randomized crossover trial of 61 very preterm infants (gestational ages 28-32 weeks) compared the Premature Infant Pain Profile (PIPP) (heart rate, facial actions, and oxygen saturation) of infants currently being held in skin-to-skin contact during heel stick with those swaddled in incubators. The very preterm infants in kangaroo care had significantly lower PIPP scores than the controls (Johnston et al., 2008).

IMPLICATIONS FOR PRACTICE

Skin-to-skin contact between parents and newborns, even premature infants, is now an accepted way to promote well-being, foster bonding, encourage breastfeeding, and facilitate maturation. The parents feel "needed" and "more comfortable" participating in this highly beneficial intervention (Johnson, 2007). Preterm babies who receive pumped breast milk are not receiving the natural skin-to-skin contact; therefore nurses can advocate for a trial of kangaroo care, as tolerated. Even though very preterm infants cannot tolerate the stimulation, late preterm infants can benefit a great deal from a policy of kangaroo care.

Mother-preterm infant pairs should never be left alone during kangaroo care, especially in the first few hours of life, and will need frequent nursing assessment for signs of instability.

References:

Hake-Brooks, S. J., & Anderson, G. C. (2008). Kangaroo care and breastfeeding of mother-preterm infant dyads 0-18 months: A randomized, controlled trial. *Neonatal Network, 27*(3), 151-159.

Johnson, A. N. (2007). The maternal experience of kangaroo holding. *Journal of Obstetetric, Gynecologic and Neonatal Nursing, 36*(6), 568-573.

Johnston, C. C., Filion, F., Campbell-Yeo, M., Gouley, C., Bell, L., McNaughton, K., et al. (2008). Kangaroo mother care diminishes pain from heel lance in very preterm neonates: A crossover trial. *BMC Pediatrics, 8*, 13. Internet document available at www.biomedcentral.com., 1471-2431-8-13 (accessed Oct. 16, 2009).

Ludington-Hoe, S. M., Johnson, M. W., Morgan, K., Lewis, T., Gutman, J., Wilson, P. D., et al. (2006). Neurophysiological assessment of neonatal sleep organization: Preliminary results of a randomized, controlled trial of skin contact with preterm infants. *Pediatrics, 117*(5), e909-e923. Internet document available at pediatrics.aappublications.org, doi: 10.1542/peds.2004-1422 (accessed July 3, 2008).

Moore, E. R., Anderson, G. C., & Bergman, N. (2007). Early skin-to-skin contact for mothers and their healthy newborn infants. In *The Cochrane Database of Systematic Reviews*, 2007, Issue 3, CD 003519.

TABLE 24-3

Normal Arterial Blood Gas Values for Neonates

VALUE	RANGE
pH	7.35-7.45
Arterial oxygen pressure (PaO_2)	60-80 mm Hg
Carbon dioxide pressure ($PaCO_2$)	35-45 mm Hg
Bicarbonate (HCO_3^-)	18-26 mEq/L
Base excess	(−5) to (+5)
Oxygen saturation	92%-94%

Source: Wood, A. & Jones, D. (2011). Acid-base homeostasis and oxygenation. In S. Gardner, B. Carter, M. Enzman-Hines, & J. Hernandez (Eds.). *Merenstein & Gardner's handbook of neonatal intensive care* (7th ed.). St. Louis: Mosby.

extension, hand clasp, hand-to-mouth movements, sucking, looking, and cooing. Signs of stress or fatigue that signal the infant's need for "time-out" include but are not limited to the following: mottled, flushed, dusky, pale or gray skin; tachypnea, pauses, gasping, sighing; tremors, startles, twitches; hiccups, gagging, choking, spitting up, grunting and straining as if having a bowel movement; coughing, sneezing, yawning; arm or leg extensions, one or both arms outstretched with fingers splayed in salute gesture; and oxygen desaturation.

When the infant is stable and mature enough to begin developmental intervention, activities are individualized according to each infant's cues, temperament, state, behavioral organization, and particular needs. Intervention periods are short (e.g., 2 to 3 minutes of voices, 5 minutes of quiet music). Hearing and vestibular interventions are initiated earlier than visual stimulation. One type of intervention at a time is applied to allow for assessment and evaluation of the infant's tolerance and response. Teaching parents to respond to the infant's individual cues is an important function of the NICU nurse. Parents, siblings, and health care providers are encouraged to adhere to the established developmental care plan to avoid disruption in sleep-wake cycles and minimize inappropriate stimuli.

The NICU Network Neurobehavioral Scale (NNNS), developed by the National Institutes of Health, provides an assessment of neurologic, behavioral, and stress-abstinence function in the neonate. The test combines items from other tests such as the Neonatal Behavioral Assessment Scale (NBAS), stress-abstinence items developed by Finnegan (1985), and a complete neurologic examination, which includes primitive reflexes and active and passive tone (Law, Stroud, LaGasse, Niarua, Liu, & Lester, 2003).

Growth and Development Potential

Although predicting with complete accuracy the growth and development potential of each preterm newborn is impossible, some findings support an anticipated favorable outcome in the absence of ongoing medical sequelae that can affect growth, such as bronchopulmonary dysplasia, necrotizing enterocolitis, and CNS problems. The lower the birth weight is, the greater the likelihood will be of negative sequelae. The growth and development milestones (e.g., motor milestones, vocalization, and body growth) are corrected for gestational age until the child is approximately 3 years of age.

The age of a preterm newborn is calculated by subtracting the number of weeks born before 40 weeks of gestation from the chronological age. For example, a 6-month-old (chronological age) infant born at 32 weeks of gestation would have a **corrected age** of 4 months. The infant's responses are accordingly evaluated against the norm expected for a 4-month-old infant. Therefore, in the infant born preterm, chronological age is not equal to corrected age (AAP Committee on Fetus and Newborn, 2004).

An effective discharge plan should include frequent outpatient follow-up with a primary care practitioner and developmental specialist for monitoring growth and achievement of appropriate developmental milestones.

Parental Adaptation to Preterm Infant

Parents who give birth to a preterm infant have a much different experience than parents who give birth to a full-term infant. Because of this difference, parental attachment and adaptation to the parental role may differ as well.

Parental tasks

Parents must accomplish several psychologic tasks before effective relationships and parenting patterns can evolve. These tasks include the following:

- Experiencing anticipatory grief over the potential loss of the infant. The parent grieves in preparation for the infant's possible death, although the parent clings to the hope that the infant will survive. Anticipatory grieving can begin during labor and often lasts until the infant dies or shows evidence of surviving.
- Acceptance by the mother of her failure to give birth to a healthy, full-term infant. Grief and depression typify this phase, which persists until the infant is out of danger and is expected to survive.
- Resuming the process of relating to the infant. As the infant's condition begins to improve and the infant gains weight, feeds by nipple (breast or bottle), and is weaned from the incubator, the parent can begin the process of developing an attachment to the infant that was interrupted by the infant's critical condition at birth.
- Learning how this infant differs in special needs and growth patterns, caregiving needs, and growth and development expectations.
- Adjusting the home environment to the needs of the new infant. Visitors may be limited to reduce the risk of exposure to pathogens, and the environmental temperature may be altered to optimize conditions for the infant.

Grandparents and siblings also react to the birth of the preterm infant. Parents must deal with the grief of grandparents and the bewilderment and anger of the infant's siblings at the apparent disproportionate amount of parental time spent with the newborn.

Parents progress through stages as they interact with their preterm infants, from maintaining an *en face* position and stroking and touching their infant (Fig. 24-7) to assuming some child care activities such as feeding, bathing, and diapering the infant.

Parental maladaptation

The incidence of physical and emotional abuse is increased in infants who, because of preterm birth or high risk condition, are separated from their parents for a time after birth. Physical abuse includes varying degrees of poor nutrition, poor hygiene, and bodily harm. Emotional abuse ranges from subtle disinterest to outright dislike of the infant. Appropriate resources should be made available to assess the parent's feelings regarding the preterm infant's birth. In addition, proper guidance and counseling are made available, including posthospital discharge, to help families adjust to and care for the preterm infant. The ultimate goal is for the family to accept the infant and incorporate this new member into the existing family structure (see Critical Thinking/Clinical Decision Making box).

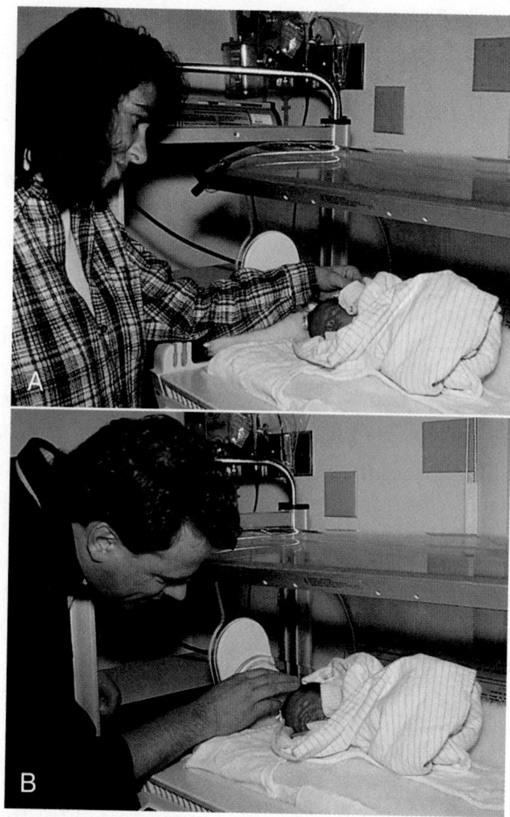

Fig. 24-7 **A,** Mother interacts with her preterm infant by touch. **B,** Father interacts with his newborn by stroking and touching infant with fingertips. (Courtesy Michael S. Clement, MD, Mesa, AZ.)

Critical Thinking/Clinical Decision Making

Late Preterm Infant

A 2013-g (4-lb 7-oz) male infant is born at an estimated gestational age of 35 weeks. The parents are very excited about this birth because they have been trying to become pregnant for 6 years. The baby is placed on the mother's (Lucia's) abdomen after birth for skin-to-skin contact but does not breastfeed. The nurse assessing the baby notes that he has some mild grunting, nasal flaring, and intercostal retractions; he is taken to the transitional nursery for further evaluation and treatment. Jorge, the father, speaks little English but asks when they will be able to hold their son again. Lucia is crying and asks to have her baby brought back to her as soon as his condition is stable because she really wants to breastfeed him.

1. Evidence—Is evidence sufficient to draw conclusions about what to tell Lucia and Jorge about their infant son?
2. Assumptions—What assumptions can be made about the following?
   a. The mother's and the father's reaction to their son's birth
   b. The infant's expected progress
   c. The possibility of Lucia breastfeeding the baby
3. What implications and priorities for nursing care can be drawn at this time?
4. Does the evidence objectively support your conclusion?
5. Do alternative perspectives to your conclusion exist?

Factors surrounding the birth may predispose parents to reject the infant subconsciously or overtly. These factors might include parental anxiety, unmet personal expectations surrounding the birth experience, a heavy financial burden because of the cost of the infant's care, unresolved anticipatory grief, threat to self-esteem, the infant being the product of an unwanted pregnancy, or marital discord. The goal of health professionals is early identification of inadequate coping skills and potentially dysfunctional parenting so that further problems can be prevented and early intervention accessed.

The nursing process in the care of the late preterm and preterm infant is outlined in the Nursing Process box.

POSTMATURE INFANT

Postterm infants are those whose gestation is prolonged beyond 42 weeks, regardless of birth weight; the infant is called *postmature.* These infants may be large-for-gestational-age (LGA) or small-for-gestational-age (SGA) infants, but their weight is most often appropriate for gestational age (AGA). The nurse must be able to assess the infant for signs of postmaturity and must be alert to potential complications. The cause of prolonged pregnancy is unknown. Postmaturity can be associated with placental insufficiency, resulting in a newborn who has a thin, emaciated appearance (dysmature) at birth because of loss of subcutaneous fat and muscle mass. Meconium staining of the fingernails may be noted, the hair and nails may be long, and vernix may be absent. The skin may peel off. Not all postmature infants show signs of dysmaturity; some continue to grow in utero and are large at birth.

Perinatal mortality is significantly increased in the postmature fetus and neonate. During labor and birth, increased oxygen demands of the postmature fetus may not be met. Insufficient gas exchange in the postmature placenta increases the likelihood of intrauterine hypoxia, which may result in the passage of meconium in utero, thereby increasing the risk for meconium aspiration syndrome. Of all the deaths of postmature newborns, one half occur during labor and birth, approximately one third occur before the onset of labor, and one sixth occur in the newborn period.

Meconium Aspiration Syndrome

Meconium staining of the amniotic fluid can be indicative of nonreassuring fetal status, especially in a vertex presentation. It appears in 10% to 15% of all births and occurs primarily in term and postterm births (Dudell & Stoll, 2007). Many infants with meconium staining exhibit no signs of depression at birth; however, the presence of

NURSING PROCESS Late Preterm and Preterm Infant Care

ASSESSMENT

The late preterm or preterm infant must undergo an initial physical assessment for life-threatening problems. The stable infant may undergo a cursory gestational age assessment to identify potential risk factors (see pp. 474 and 487-490).

NURSING DIAGNOSES

After assessment the nursing diagnoses for infants and their parents may include the following:

- *Ineffective breathing pattern* related to:
  - Decreased number of functional alveoli
  - Surfactant deficiency
  - Immature respiratory control
  - Increased pulmonary vascular resistance
- *Ineffective thermoregulation* related to:
  - Immature central nervous system thermoregulatory control
  - Increased heat loss to environment and inability to produce heat
  - Greater body surface exposed to environment
  - Decreased brown fat reserves to produce body heat
- *Risk for infection* related to:
  - Invasive procedures
  - Decreased immune response
  - Ineffective skin barrier
- *Anxiety (parental)* related to:
  - Lack of knowledge about infant's condition
  - Lack of knowledge regarding infant's prognosis (uncertain outcome)
  - Inability to perform expected caregiving activities
  - Neonatal intensive care unit environment noise and high-tech care

EXPECTED OUTCOMES OF CARE

Expected outcomes can apply both to the infant and to the parents. Expected outcomes are presented in patient-centered terms and include that the infant will do the following:

- Maintain adequate physiologic functioning (airway, breathing, circulation)
- Receive adequate nutrition for growth
- Maintain stable body temperature
- Remain free of infection
- Experience appropriate parent-infant interactions

Expected outcomes for the parents include that they will do the following:

- Perceive the infant as a family member
- Provide infant care confidently and competently
- Experience pride and satisfaction in the care of the infant
- Organize their time and energies to meet the love, attention, and care needs of the other members of the family, as well as their own needs

PLAN OF CARE AND INTERVENTIONS

- Maintain neutral thermal environment.
- Maintain nutritional status using oral, gavage, or intravenous feeding as appropriate.
- Monitor amount of blood withdrawn for laboratory tests.
- Maintain Standard Precautions.

Numerous other nursing interventions are discussed in the text (see also Table 24-1).

EVALUATION

The nurse can be reasonably assured that care was effective to the extent that the expected outcomes for care have been achieved.

meconium in the amniotic fluid necessitates close supervision of labor and monitoring of fetal well-being. The presence of a team skilled in neonatal resuscitation is required at the birth of any infant with meconium-stained amniotic fluid (Fig. 24-8). The mouth and nares of the infant are no longer routinely suctioned on the perineum before the infant's first breath. However, for infants with meconium staining who are not vigorous, endotracheal suctioning should be performed immediately (American Heart Association, 2005).

If meconium is not removed from the airway at birth, it can migrate down to the terminal airways, causing mechanical obstruction and leading to **meconium aspiration syndrome (MAS)**. The fetus may have aspirated meconium in utero, which can cause a chemical pneumonitis. These infants may develop persistent pulmonary hypertension of the newborn (PPHN), further complicating their management. Infants with MAS who received surfactant had improved oxygenation, decreased severity of respiratory failure, and reduced need for ECMO and fewer leaks (Engle & AAP Committee on Fetus and Newborn, 2008).

Persistent Pulmonary Hypertension of the Newborn

Persistent pulmonary hypertension of the newborn (PPHN) is a term applied to the combined findings of pulmonary hypertension, right-to-left shunting, and a structurally normal heart. PPHN may occur either as a single entity or as the main component of MAS, congenital diaphragmatic hernia, RDS, hyperviscosity syndrome, or neonatal pneumonia or sepsis. PPHN is also called *persistent fetal circulation* because the syndrome includes reversion to fetal pathways for blood flow (see Fig. 5-12).

After birth, both the foramen ovale and the ductus arteriosus close in response to various biochemical processes, pressure changes within the heart, and dilation of

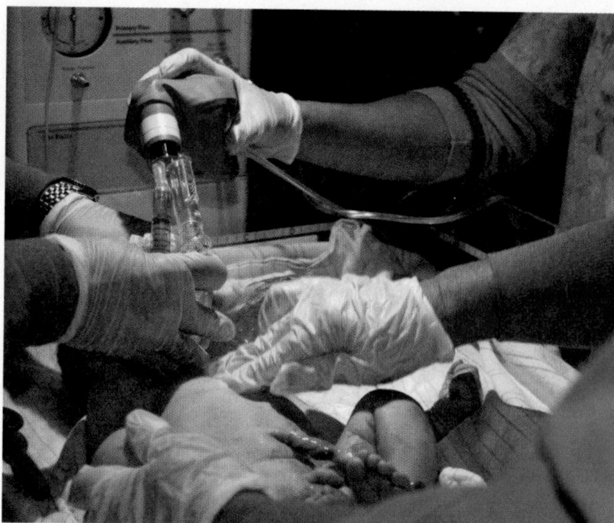

Fig. 24-8 Infant being resuscitated at birth. Meconium was present on the abdomen and umbilical cord. Infant was not breathing, and heart rate was 65 beats/min at birth. Respirations and heart rate were normal at 2 minutes. (Courtesy Shannon Perry, Phoenix, AZ.)

the pulmonary vessels. This dilation allows virtually all of the cardiac output to enter the lungs, become oxygenated, and provide oxygen-rich blood to the tissues for normal metabolism. Any process that interferes with this transition from fetal to neonatal circulation may precipitate PPHN. PPHN characteristically proceeds into a downward spiral of exacerbating hypoxia and pulmonary vasoconstriction. Prompt recognition and aggressive intervention are required to reverse this process.

The infant with PPHN is typically born at term or postterm and exhibits tachycardia and cyanosis. Within minutes or hours the infant's condition progresses to severe respiratory compromise with concomitant acidosis, which further compromises pulmonary perfusion and deteriorating oxygenation. Management depends on the underlying etiologic factors of the persistent pulmonary hypertension. The use of INO, ECMO (see previous discussion), and high-frequency ventilation has improved the chances of survival of these infants.

OTHER PROBLEMS RELATED TO GESTATION

Small-for-Gestational-Age Infants and Intrauterine Growth Restriction

Infants who are SGA (i.e., weight is below the 10th percentile expected at term) or infants who have intrauterine growth restriction (IUGR) (i.e., rate of growth does not meet expected growth pattern) are considered high risk, with the perimortality rate 5 to 20 times greater than that for the healthy term infant (Kliegman, 2006).

Various conditions can affect and impede growth in the developing fetus. Conditions occurring in the first trimester that affect all aspects of fetal growth (e.g., infections, teratogens, chromosomal abnormalities) or extrinsic conditions early in pregnancy result in symmetric IUGR (i.e., head circumference, length, weight are all less than the 10th percentile). Conditions causing symmetric growth restriction result in an SGA infant, usually with a head circumference that is smaller than that of a term infant and reduced brain capacity. Growth restriction in later stages of pregnancy, as a result of maternal or placental factors, results in asymmetric growth restriction (with respect to gestational age, weight will be less than the 10th percentile, whereas length and head circumference will be greater than the 10th percentile). Infants with asymmetric IUGR have the potential for normal growth and development. Abnormal fetal size may indicate an adaptive response, with diminished fetal weight-sparing brain growth.

Care of the SGA infant is based on the clinical problems present and is the same given to preterm infants with similar problems. Gas exchange is supported by maintaining a clear airway and preventing cold stress. Hypoglycemia is treated with oral feedings (e.g., breast, formula) or intravenous dextrose as the infant's condition warrants. An external heat source (radiant warmer or incubator) is used until the infant is able to maintain an adequate body temperature. Nursing support of parents is the same as that given to parents of preterm infants.

Common problems that affect SGA (IUGR) infants are perinatal asphyxia, meconium aspiration (discussed previously), immunodeficiency, hypoglycemia, polycythemia, and temperature instability.

Perinatal asphyxia

Commonly, IUGR infants have been exposed to chronic hypoxia for varying periods before labor and birth. Labor is a stressor to the normal fetus; it is an even greater stressor for the growth-restricted fetus. The chronically hypoxic infant is severely compromised by a normal labor and has difficulty compensating after birth. The alert, wide-eyed appearance of the newborn is attributed to prolonged fetal hypoxia. Appropriate management and resuscitation are essential for the depressed infant.

The birth of the SGA newborn with perinatal asphyxia may be associated with a maternal history of heavy cigarette smoking; gestational hypertension; low socioeconomic status; multifetal gestation; gestational infections such as rubella, cytomegalovirus, and toxoplasmosis; advanced diabetes mellitus; and cardiac problems. Sequelae to perinatal asphyxia include MAS and hypoglycemia.

Hypoglycemia and hyperglycemia

All high risk infants are at risk for the development of hypoglycemia. Infants who experience physiologic stress may experience hypoglycemia as a result of a decreased glycogen supply, inadequate gluconeogenesis, or overutilization of glycogen stored during fetal and postnatal life. Preterm infants may also become hypoglycemic as a result of inadequate intake and increased metabolic demands as a result of illness factors. Evidence to support the concept that the preterm or high risk infant can tolerate lower levels of serum glucose any better than healthy term infants is insufficient (Blackburn, 2007) (see Chapter 17, p. 494, for discussion of hypoglycemia). The SGA infant, not unlike the preterm infant, is at increased risk for hypoglycemia as a result of decreased fetal stores and decreased rate of gluconeogenesis.

Hyperglycemia is defined as a blood glucose level greater than 125 mg/dl (whole blood) or a plasma glucose level of 145 to 150 mg/dl (Blackburn, 2007). This condition is seen primarily in ELBW and VLBW infants receiving parenteral nutrition with dextrose concentrations of 5% or higher. Hyperglycemia can be just as harmful to the preterm infant as hypoglycemia. Increased circulating levels of glucose can lead to osmotic changes, increased urine output, and fluid shifts in the already compromised CNS of the preterm infant. The net result of hyperglycemia can be cellular dehydration and intraventricular hemorrhage. Preterm infants undergoing stress such as surgical intervention can also become hyperglycemic with increased catecholamine release, which inhibits insulin release and glucose utilization (Blackburn). Therefore ELBW and VLBW infants should be monitored closely for both hypoglycemia and hyperglycemia during the acute phase of illness, while receiving parenteral nutrition, and perioperatively.

Heat loss

SGA infants are particularly susceptible to temperature instability as a result of decreased brown fat deposits, decreased adipose tissue, large body surface exposure, and, in many instances, poor flexion, as well as decreased glycogen storage in major organs such as the liver and heart. Therefore close attention must be given to maintain an NTE. Nursing considerations focus on maintenance of thermoneutrality to promote recovery from perinatal asphyxia because cold stress jeopardizes such recovery.

Large-for-Gestational-Age Infants

The LGA infant is defined as an infant weighing 4000 g or more at birth. An infant is considered LGA despite gestation when the weight is above the 90th percentile on growth charts or two standard deviations above the mean weight for gestational age. The LGA infant is at greater risk for morbidity than the SGA and preterm infant; such infants have an increased incidence of birth injuries, asphyxia, and congenital anomalies such as heart defects (Stoll & Adams-Chapman, 2007).

All pregnancies of longer than 42 weeks of gestation must be thoroughly evaluated. All large fetuses are monitored during a trial of labor, and preparation is made for a cesarean birth if nonreassuring fetal status or poor progress of labor occurs. LGA newborns may be preterm, term, or postterm; they may be infants of diabetic mothers; or they may be postmature. Each of these problems carries special concerns. Regardless of coexisting potential problems, the LGA infant is at risk by virtue of size alone.

The nurse assesses the LGA infant for hypoglycemia and trauma resulting from vaginal or cesarean birth. Any specific birth injuries are identified and treated appropriately.

Infants of Diabetic Mothers

Nursing Care Plan: The Infant of a Mother with Diabetes Mellitus

All infants born to mothers with diabetes (IDMs) are at some risk for complications. The degree of risk is influenced by the severity and duration of maternal disease.

Pathophysiology

The mechanisms responsible for the problems seen in IDMs are not fully understood. Congenital anomalies are believed to be caused by fluctuations in blood glucose levels and episodes of ketoacidosis in early pregnancy. Later in pregnancy, when the mother's pancreas cannot release sufficient insulin to meet increased demands, maternal hyperglycemia results. The high levels of glucose cross the placenta and stimulate the fetal pancreas to release additional insulin. The combination of the increased supply of maternal glucose and other nutrients, the inability of maternal insulin to cross the placenta, and increased fetal insulin results in excessive fetal growth called macrosomia (see the discussion that follows).

Hyperinsulinemia accounts for many of the problems the fetus or infant develops. In addition to fluctuating glucose levels, maternal vascular involvement or superimposed maternal infection adversely affects the fetus. Normally, maternal blood has a more alkaline pH than carbon dioxide–rich fetal blood. This phenomenon encourages the exchange of oxygen and carbon dioxide across the placental membrane. When the maternal blood is more acidotic than the fetal blood, such as during ketoacidosis, little carbon dioxide or oxygen exchange occurs at the level of the placenta. The mortality for the unborn infant resulting from an episode of maternal ketoacidosis may be as high as 50% or more (Kalhan & Parimi, 2006).

The single most important factor influencing fetal well-being is the euglycemic status of the mother. Indications are that some neonatal conditions (macrosomia, hypoglycemia, polyhydramnios, preterm birth, and perhaps fetal lung immaturity) may be eliminated, or the incidence decreased, by maintaining tight control of maternal glucose levels within narrow limits. Tight glucose control is defined as the maintenance of maternal blood glucose levels between 100 and 120 mg/dl.

Problems seen in infants of diabetic mothers (IDMs) include the following:

- Congenital anomalies occur in 7% to 10% of IDMs; the incidence is greatest in SGA infants. The most commonly occurring anomalies involve the cardiac, musculoskeletal, and central nervous systems. CNS anomalies include anencephaly, encephalocele, meningomyelocele, and hydrocephalus (see Table 24-10). The musculoskeletal system may be affected by caudal regression syndrome (i.e., sacral agenesis, with weakness or deformities of the lower extremities, malformation and fixation of the hip joints, shortening or deformity of the femurs).
- Macrosomia: At birth the typical LGA infant has a round, cherubic ("tomato" or cushingoid) face, chubby body, and a plethoric or flushed complexion (Fig. 24-9). The infant has enlarged internal organs (i.e., hepatosplenomegaly, splanchnomegaly, cardiomegaly) and increased body fat, especially around the shoulders. The placenta and umbilical cord are larger than average. The brain is the only organ that is not enlarged. IDMs may be LGA but physiologically immature. The macrosomic infant is at risk for RDS, hypoglycemia, hypocalcemia and hypomagnesemia, cardiomyopathy, polycythemia, and hyperbilirubinemia. The excessive shoulder size in these infants often leads to dystocia. Macrosomic infants born vaginally or by cesarean birth after a trial of labor may incur birth trauma.
- Birth injury (resulting from macrosomia or method of birth) and perinatal asphyxia occur in 20% of infants of gestational diabetic mothers and 35% of IDMs. Examples of birth trauma include cephalhematoma; paralysis of the facial nerve (seventh cranial nerve) (Table 24-10); fracture of the clavicle or humerus (see Table 24-10); brachial plexus paralysis, usually Erb-Duchenne (right upper arm) palsy (see Table 24-10); and phrenic nerve paralysis, invariably associated with diaphragmatic paralysis.

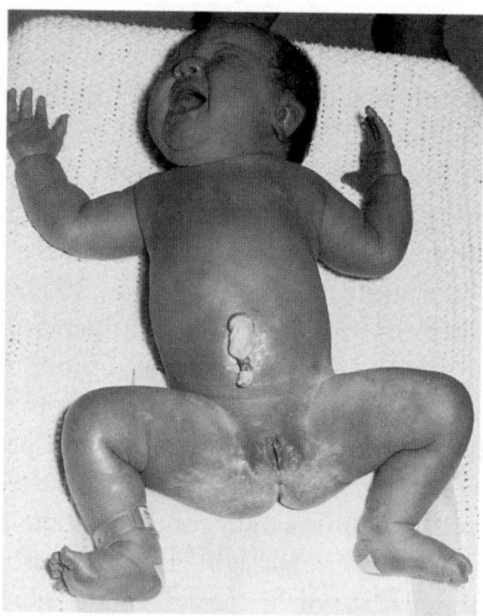

Fig. 24-9 Macrosomic newborn. (From O'Doherty, N. [1986]. *Neonatology: Micro atlas of the newborn.* Nutley, NJ: Hoffmann-La Roche.)

- RDS: IDMs are four to six times more likely than normal infants to develop RDS. In the fetus exposed to high levels of maternal glucose, synthesis of surfactant may be delayed because of the high fetal serum level of insulin. In the IDM the presence of phosphatidylglycerol in the amniotic fluid is the best predictor of normal neonatal respiratory function.
- Hypoglycemia affects many IDMs. After constant exposure to high circulating levels of glucose, hyperplasia of the fetal pancreas occurs, resulting in hyperinsulinemia. With clamping of the umbilical cord, the fetal glucose supply is cut off. The neonate's blood glucose level falls rapidly because of fetal hyperinsulinism.
- Cardiomyopathy: Two types of cardiomyopathy can occur. Hypertrophic cardiomyopathy (HCM) is characterized by a hypercontractile and thickened myocardium. The ventricular walls are thickened, as is the septum, which in severe cases results in outflow tract obstructions. The mitral valve is poorly functioning. In nonhypertrophic cardiomyopathy (non-HCM) the myocardium is poorly contractile and overstretched. The ventricles are increased in size, but outflow is not obstructed. Most infants are asymptomatic, but severe outflow obstruction may cause left ventricular heart failure. HCM may be treated with a beta-adrenergic blocker (e.g., propranolol to decrease contractility and heart rate). A cardiotonic agent is used to treat non-HCM (e.g., digoxin to increase contractility and decrease heart rate). The abnormality usually resolves in 3 to 12 months.
- Hyperbilirubinemia and polycythemia: IDMs are at increased risk of developing hyperbilirubinemia (see Chapter 17). Many IDMs are also polycythemic. Polycythemia increases blood viscosity, thereby impairing circulation. In addition, this increased number of RBCs to be hemolyzed increases the potential bilirubin load that the neonate must clear. Bruising associated with birth of a macrosomic infant will contribute further to high bilirubin levels.

Nursing care

Ideally, planning for the IDM begins during the antenatal period. Pediatric NICU staff members are present at the birth. Implementation of care depends on the neonate's particular problems. If the maternal blood glucose level was well controlled throughout the pregnancy, the infant may require only monitoring. Because euglycemia is not always possible, the nurse must promptly recognize and treat any consequences of maternal diabetes that arise.

ACQUIRED AND CONGENITAL PROBLEMS

A challenge for the nurse is the birth of an infant at risk because of conditions or circumstances that are superimposed on the normal course of events associated with birth and the adjustment to extrauterine existence. The infant may be considered high risk because of birth trauma, maternal substance abuse, infection, or congenital anomalies. Birth trauma includes physical injuries a neonate sustains during labor and birth. Congenital anomalies include such conditions as GI malformations, NTDs, abdominal wall defects, and cardiac defects (see Table 24-10).

The nurse is sometimes able to anticipate problems, such as when a woman is admitted in premature labor, or a congenital anomaly is diagnosed by ultrasound before birth. At other times the birth of a high risk infant is unanticipated. In either case the personnel and equipment necessary for immediate care of the infant must be available (see Table 24-10).

Birth Trauma

Birth trauma (injury) is physical injury sustained by a neonate during labor and birth. It remains an important source of neonatal morbidity.

Most birth injuries are avoidable, especially if a thorough assessment of risk factors and appropriate planning of birth occur. The use of fetal ultrasonography allows antepartum diagnosis of certain fetal conditions that may be treated in utero or shortly after birth. Elective cesarean birth can be chosen for some pregnancies to prevent significant birth injury. A small percentage of serious birth injuries are unavoidable despite skilled and competent obstetric care, such as in especially difficult or prolonged labor or when the infant is in an abnormal fetal presentation. Some injuries cannot be anticipated until the specific circumstances are encountered during childbirth. Emergency cesarean birth may provide a last-minute salvage, but in these circumstances the injury may be truly unavoidable. The same injury might be caused in several ways; for example, a cephalhematoma could result from an obstetric technique such as forceps birth or vacuum extraction or from pressure of the fetal skull against the maternal pelvis.

Many injuries are minor and resolve readily in the neonatal period without treatment. Other trauma requires some degree of intervention; few are serious enough to be fatal. The nurse's contributions to the welfare of the newborn begin with early observation of the newborn's transition. The prompt reporting of signs that indicate deviations from normal permits early initiation of appropriate therapy. Table 24-4 provides an overview of birth injuries. Soft-tissue injuries that commonly occur at birth are discussed in Chapter 17. Caput succedaneum and cephalhematoma are discussed in Chapter 16.

The parents need support in handling these infants because they are often fearful of hurting them. Parents are encouraged to practice handling, changing, and feeding the affected neonate under the guidance of nursery personnel, which increases their confidence and knowledge and facilitates attachment. A plan for follow-up therapy is developed with the parents so that the times and arrangements for therapy are acceptable to them.

NEONATAL INFECTIONS

Sepsis

Sepsis (the presence of microorganisms or their toxins in the blood or other tissues) continues to be one of the most significant causes of neonatal morbidity and mortality. Maternal IgM does not cross the placenta. IgG levels in term infants are equal to maternal levels; however, in preterm infants the amount of IgG is directly proportional to gestational age (Stoll & Adams-Chapman, 2007). IgA and IgM require time to reach optimal levels after birth. Neonatal neutrophils are present in term infants but have decreased functional capabilities; response to infections is sluggish. Phagocytosis is less efficient than it is in older infants. The gut mucosal barrier in the infant is initially immature in both term and preterm infants; this barrier is enhanced by the ingestion of human colostrum, which contains antiinfective properties.

Table 24-5 outlines risk factors for neonatal sepsis. Special precautions for preventing infection, as well as prompt recognition when it occurs, are necessary for optimal newborn care. Neonatal infections may be acquired in utero, at birth or shortly thereafter, and nosocomially.

Early-onset sepsis is acquired in the perinatal period; infection can occur from direct contact with organisms from the maternal gastrointestinal and genitourinary tracts. The most common infecting organism is *Escherichia coli,* whereas group B streptococci (GBS) rates remain low (Stoll et al, 2005). *E. coli,* which may be present in the vagina, accounts for approximately one half of all cases of sepsis caused by gram-negative organisms. GBS is an extremely virulent organism in neonates, with a high (50%) death rate in affected infants. Early-onset sepsis is associated with a history of preterm labor, prolonged rupture of membranes (>18 hours), maternal fever during labor, and chorioamnionitis (Venkatesh, Merenstein, Adams, & Weisman, 2006).

Late-onset sepsis, occurring approximately at 7 to 30 days of age, may include maternally derived infection or nosocomial infection; the offending organisms are usually staphylococci, *Klebsiella* organisms, enterococci, *E. coli,* and *Pseudomonas* or *Candida* species (Stoll & Adams-Chapman, 2007). Coagulase-negative staphylococci are commonly found to be the cause of septicemia in ELBW and VLBW infants. Additional infections of concern include methicillin-resistant *Staphylococcus aureus* (MRSA), vancomycin-resistant enterococci, and multidrug-resistant gram-negative pathogens (Stoll & Adams-Chapman). Bacterial invasion can occur through sites such as the umbilical stump; the skin; mucous membranes of the eye, nose, pharynx, and ear; and internal systems such as the respiratory, nervous, urinary, and gastrointestinal systems.

Viral (perinatally acquired) infections may cause miscarriage, stillbirth, intrauterine infection, congenital malformations, and acute neonatal disease. Other viral infections such as respiratory syncytial virus (RSV), rotavirus, herpes, influenza, and varicella may occur in the NICU. Fungal

TABLE 24-4

Types of Birth Injuries

SITE OF INJURY	TYPE OF INJURY	TREATMENT
Scalp	Caput succedaneum (see Fig. 16-5, *A*)	None necessary
	Cephalhematoma (see Fig. 16-5, *B*)	None necessary
	Subgaleal hemorrhage (see Fig. 16-5, *C*)	Replacement of lost blood and clotting factors
Skull	Linear fracture	None necessary
	Depressed fracture	Possible elevation of depressed area (with breast pump)
Intracranial	Epidural hematoma Subdural hematoma (laceration of falx, tentorium, or superficial veins) Subarachnoid hemorrhage Cerebral contusion Cerebellar contusion Intracerebellar hematoma	Provide supportive care; monitor neurologic signs; establish intravenous access, observe for and manage seizures; prevent increased intracranial pressure.
Spinal cord (cervical)	Vertebral artery injury Intraspinal hemorrhage Spinal cord transection or injury	
Plexus	Erb-Duchenne palsy 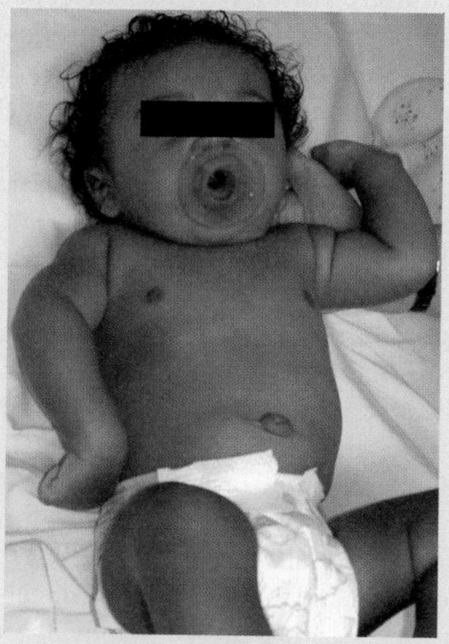 Erb-Duchenne paralysis in newborn infant. Moro reflex is absent in right upper extremity. Recovery was complete. (From Chung, K. C., Yang, L. J.-S., McGillicuddy, J. E. [2012]. *Practical management of pediatric and adult brachial plexus palsies*, Philadelphia: Saunders.)	Abduct arm 90 degrees with external shoulder rotation, forearm supination, and extension at the wrist with the palm facing the infant's face (Adams-Chapman & Stoll, 2007). Initiate passive range-of-motion exercises of the shoulder, wrist, elbow, and fingers in latter part of first week. Splint wrist with padding in the fist.

TABLE 24-4

Types of Birth Injuries—cont'd

SITE OF INJURY	TYPE OF INJURY	TREATMENT
Cranial and peripheral nerve	Facial nerve injury (facial paralysis caused by pressure on facial nerve; often by forceps) 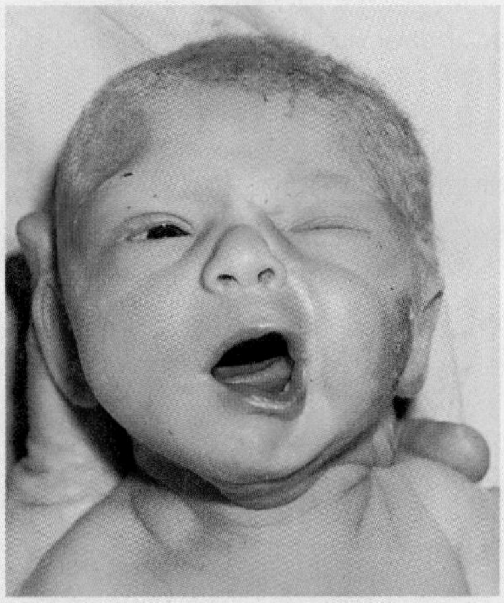 Facial paralysis 15 minutes after forceps birth. Absence of movement on affected side is especially noticeable when infant cries. (From O'Doherty, N. [1986]. *Neonatology: Micro atlas of the newborn.* Nutley, NJ: Hoffmann-La Roche.)	Instill artificial tears daily to prevent drying of conjunctiva, sclera, and cornea. Tape eye closed to prevent accidental injury. Aid infant to suck; help mother with feeding techniques. Surgery if nerve fibers are torn.
Skeletal		
Clavicle 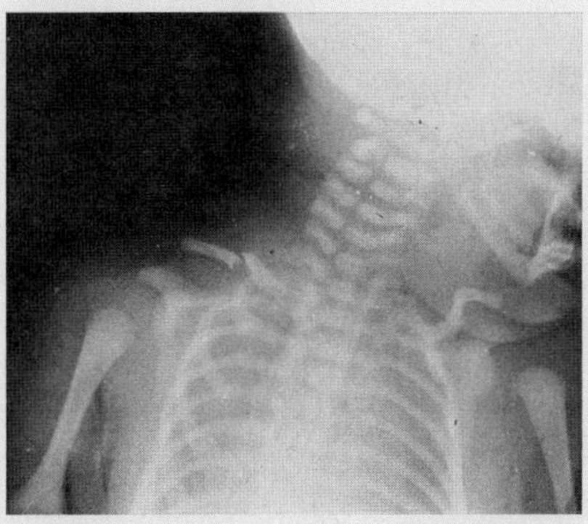 Fractured clavicle after shoulder dystocia. (From O'Doherty, N. [1986]. *Neonatology: Micro atlas of the newborn.* Nutley, NJ: Hoffmann-La Roche.)	Most common fracture during birth; fracture is usually in the middle third of the clavicle.	Careful handling
Humerus	Fracture during difficult birth	Gentle handling; containment of arm against chest
Femur	Fracture during difficult birth	Immobilization with slings, splints, or swaddling

Source: Verklan, M.T. & Lopez, S.M. (2011). Neurologic disorders. In S. Gardner, B. Carter, M. Enzman-Hines, & J. Hernandez (Eds.). *Merenstein & Gardner's handbook of neonatal intensive care* (7th ed.). St. Louis: Mosby.

TABLE 24-5
Risk Factors for Neonatal Sepsis

Maternal	Low socioeconomic status
	Late or no prenatal care
	Poor nutrition
	Substance abuse
	Recently acquired sexually transmitted infection
	Untreated focal infection (urinary tract infection, vaginal, cervical)
	Systemic infection
	Fever
Intrapartum	Premature rupture of fetal membranes
	Maternal fever
	Chorioamnionitis
	Prolonged labor
	Premature labor
	Use of fetal scalp electrode
Neonatal	Multiple gestation
	Male
	Birth asphyxia
	Meconium aspiration
	Congenital anomalies of skin or mucous membranes
	Metabolic disorders (e.g. galactosemia)
	Absence of spleen
	Low birth weight
	Preterm birth
	Malnourishment
	Formula feeding
	Prolonged hospitalization
	Mechanical ventilation
	Umbilical artery catheterization or use of other vascular catheters

Source: Edwards, M. (2006). Postnatal bacterial infections. In R. Martin, A. Fanaroff, & M. Walsh (Eds.), *Fanaroff and Martin's neonatal-perinatal medicine: Diseases of the fetus and infant* (8th ed.). Philadelphia: Mosby.

TABLE 24-6
Signs of Sepsis

SYSTEM	SIGNS
Respiratory	Apnea, bradycardia
	Tachypnea
	Grunting, nasal flaring
	Retractions
	Decreased oxygen saturation
	Acidosis
Cardiovascular	Decreased cardiac output
	Tachycardia
	Hypotension
	Decreased perfusion
Central nervous	Temperature instability
	Lethargy
	Hypotonia
	Irritability, seizures
Gastrointestinal	Feeding intolerance
	Abdominal distention
	Vomiting, diarrhea
Integumentary	Jaundice
	Pallor
	Petechiae
Metabolic	Hypoglycemia
	Hyperglycemia
	Metabolic acidosis
Hematologic	Thrombocytopenia
	Neutropenia

Source: Edwards, M. (2006). Postnatal bacterial infections. In R. Martin, A. Fanaroff, & M. Walsh (Eds.), *Fanaroff and Martin's neonatal-perinatal medicine: Diseases of the fetus and infant* (8th ed.). Philadelphia: Mosby.

infections are of greatest concern in the immunocompromised or preterm infant. Occasionally, fungal infections such as **thrush** are found in otherwise healthy term infants.

Septicemia refers to a generalized infection in the bloodstream. Pneumonia, the most common form of neonatal infection, is one of the leading causes of perinatal death. Bacterial meningitis occurs in approximately 0.2 to 0.4 cases per 1000 live births, with an increased rate in preterm infants. Gastroenteritis is sporadic, depending on epidemic outbreaks. Local infections such as conjunctivitis and omphalitis occur commonly. Infection continues to be a significant factor in fetal and neonatal morbidity and mortality.

CARE MANAGEMENT

The prenatal record is reviewed for risk factors associated with infection and the signs and symptoms suggestive of infection. Maternal vaginal or perineal infection may be transmitted directly to the infant during passage through the birth canal. Psychosocial history and a history of sexually transmitted infections may indicate possible human immunodeficiency virus (HIV), hepatitis B virus, herpes simplex virus, or cytomegalovirus infection.

Perinatal events are also reviewed. Ascending infection may occur after prolonged premature rupture of membranes, prolonged labor, or intrauterine fetal monitoring. A maternal history of fever during labor or the presence of foul-smelling amniotic fluid may also indicate the presence of infection. Antibiotic therapy initiated during labor should be noted. The neonate's gestational age, maturity, birth weight, and sex all affect the incidence of infection. Sepsis occurs approximately twice as often and results in a higher mortality in male than in female infants. The neonate is assessed for respiratory distress, skin abscesses, rashes, and other indications of infection.

The earliest clinical signs of neonatal sepsis are characterized by a lack of specificity. The nonspecific signs include lethargy, poor feeding, poor weight gain, and irritability. The nurse or parent may simply note that the infant is just not doing as well as before. A differential diagnosis may be difficult to determine because signs of sepsis are similar to signs of noninfectious neonatal problems such as hypoglycemia and respiratory distress. Table 24-6 outlines the clinical signs associated with neonatal sepsis.

Laboratory studies are important. Specimens for cultures include blood, cerebrospinal fluid, stool, and urine. A complete blood cell count with differential is obtained to determine the presence of bacterial infection or increased or decreased WBC count (the latter is an ominous sign). The total neutrophil count, immature to total neutrophil ratio, absolute neutrophil count, and C-reactive protein may be used to determine the presence of sepsis. Detection of viral DNA or antibodies by polymerase chain reaction amplification in fluids is also an important diagnostic tool (Frenkel, 2005). Treatment with antibiotics is initiated after blood cultures are obtained in neonates; in high risk infants with significant illness, antiviral or antibiotic treatment may begin once cultures are obtained; and, once the pathogen is identified, antibiotic, antiviral, or antifungal therapy may be modified.

Nursing Interventions

Nursing is directly or indirectly responsible for minimizing or eliminating environmental sources of infectious agents in the nursery. Measures to be taken include effective handwashing, Standard Precautions, thorough cleaning of contaminated equipment, frequent replacement of used equipment (changing intravenous and nasogastric tubing per hospital protocol and cleaning resuscitation and ventilation equipment, intravenous pumps, and incubators), and disposal of contaminated linens and diapers in an appropriate manner. Overcrowding must be avoided in nurseries. Guidelines for space, visitation, and general infection control in areas where newborns receive care have been established and published (American Academy of Pediatrics [AAP] and American College of Obstetricians and Gynecologists [ACOG], 2007).

NURSING ALERT Artificial and long natural fingernails worn by nurses have been associated with serious neonatal infection and morbidity from *Pseudomonas aeruginosa* (Moolenaar et al., 2000) and *Klebsiella* organisms in the NICU (Gupta et al., 2004).

Breastfeeding or feeding the newborn breast milk from the mother is encouraged. Breast milk provides protective mechanisms (see Chapter 18).

Administering medications, taking precautions when performing treatments, and following isolation procedures are also interventions to be considered in the prevention and treatment of neonatal sepsis.

Care must be taken in suctioning secretions from any newborn's oropharynx or trachea. Routine suctioning is not recommended and may further compromise the infant's immune status, as well as cause hypoxia and increase ICP. Isolation procedures are implemented as indicated according to hospital policy. Isolation protocols change rapidly, and the nurse is urged to participate in continuing education and in-service programs to remain up to date.

Perinatally-Acquired Infections

The occurrence of certain maternal infections during early pregnancy is known to be associated with various congenital malformations and disorders. An acronym that is often used in clinical practice is **TORCH**, which stands for *t*oxoplasmosis, *o*ther (gonorrhea, hepatitis B, syphilis, varicella-zoster virus, parvovirus B19, and HIV), *r*ubella, *c*ytomegalovirus, and *h*erpes simplex virus) (Table 24-7). With the advent of newer diagnostic methods, these viral infections can be diagnosed in utero and interventions planned based on the availability of intrauterine treatments.

SUBSTANCE ABUSE

Critical Thinking Exercise: Fetal Alcohol Syndrome

Certain maternal behaviors result in perinatal risk. Maternal habits hazardous to the fetus and neonate include recreational drug abuse, tobacco smoking, and alcohol consumption. All of these substances cross the placenta and enter the breast milk. Other than alcohol and tobacco use, cocaine and marijuana are the most commonly used substances by pregnant women. Physiologic signs of withdrawal have been reported in neonates of mothers who use to excess such drugs as barbiturates, alcohol, opioids, or amphetamines. Prescription opioids such as oxycodone (Percodan, OxyContin) have been identified as increasingly popular drugs of abuse that may cause withdrawal symptoms in neonates (Sander & Hays, 2005). Mothers in substance abuse treatment receiving methadone may give birth to an infant who exhibits withdrawal symptoms requiring treatment. Almost 50% of pregnancies of women addicted to opioids result in LBW infants who are not necessarily preterm. Alcohol is a teratogen that produces CNS effects that may not be evident for years. Maternal ethanol use during gestation can lead to a readily identifiable fetal alcohol syndrome (FAS), an **alcohol-related birth defect (ARBD)**, or a constellation of neurobehavioral and cognitive problems that may be identified only by maternal history and behavioral characteristics, **alcohol-related neurodevelopmental disorder (ARND)**. An important point to note is that newborns exposed to drugs in utero are not addicted in a behavioral sense, yet they may experience mild to strong physiologic signs as a result of the exposure. A more descriptive term for such infants is *drug-exposed newborn,* which implies intrauterine drug exposure.

Nursing Care Plan: The Drug-Exposed Newborn

The adverse effects of exposure of the fetus to drugs are varied; many of these effects may not be identified until the child enters school. Critical determinants of the effect of the drug on the fetus include the specific drug, the dosage, the route of administration, the genotype of the mother or fetus, and the timing of the drug exposure. Fig. 24-10 shows critical periods in human embryogenesis and the teratogenic effects of drugs. Table 24-8 summarizes the effects of commonly abused substances on the fetus and neonate.

Nursing care of affected infants involves the same assessment and observations that are employed for any high-risk infant. Strategies to provide individualized developmental care are aimed at reducing noxious environmental stimuli and helping the infant achieve self-regulation. Special emphasis is placed on monitoring weight gain,

Text continued on p. 786.

TABLE 24-7

Infections Affecting Newborns

	TORCH INFECTIONS			
	INFECTION	CAUSATIVE AGENT	TREATMENT	EFFECTS/COMPLICATIONS
T	Toxoplasmosis	Protozoan, *Toxoplasma gondii* found in feces of cats and raw meat from animals that graze in contaminated fields	Pyrimethamine and oral sulfadiazine; folic acid to prevent anemia	More than 70% of affected infants are free of symptoms. Preterm birth, IUGR, microcephaly, hydrocephaly, microphthalmos, chorioretinitis, CNS calcification, thrombocytopenia, jaundice, fever, petechiae or maculopapular rash, 10%-15% of infants die, 85% have severe psychomotor problems or mental retardation by age 2 to 4 years, and 50% have visual problems by age 1 year.
O	Other: Gonorrhea	*Neisseria gonorrhoeae* Acquired through ascending infection or during birth	Eye prophylaxis (e.g., 0.5% erythromycin ointment) at birth to prevent ophthalmia neonatorum. If mild infection, single dose IM or IV ceftriaxone is administered.	Neonatal conjunctivitis, gonococcal arthritis, septicemia, meningitis, vaginitis, and scalp abscesses Infant may die from overwhelming infection.
	Syphilis 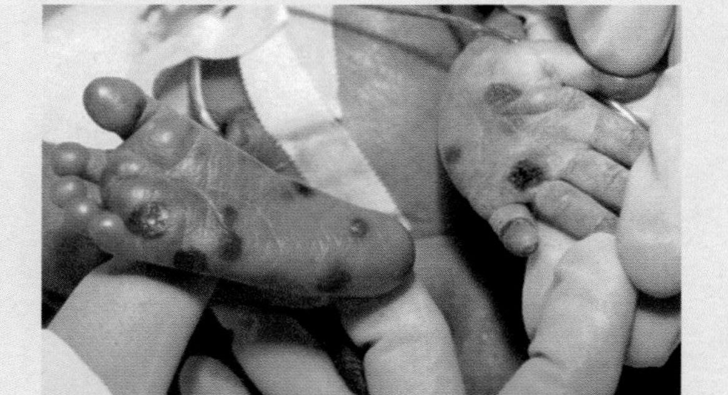 Neonatal syphilis lesions on hands and feet (Courtesy Mahesh Kotwal, MD, Phoenix, AZ.)	Spirochete, *Treponema pallidum:* fetal infestation with the spirochete is blocked by Langhans layer in the chorion until between 16 and 18 wks of gestation.	Aqueous crystalloid penicillin G, 50,000 units/kg/dose IV every 12 hours for the first 7 days of life, then every 8 hours for a total of 10 days, or procaine penicillin, 50,000 units/kg/dose IM in a single daily dose for 10 days. Penicillin G or procaine penicillin G; erythromycin if infant sensitive to penicillin	Preterm labor; neurosyphilis, deafness, Hutchinson teeth (notched incisors), saber shins, joint involvement, saddle nose (depressed bridge), gummas (soft, gummy tumors) over the skin and other organs, and interstitial keratitis (inflammation of the cornea), snuffles (copious, clear, serosanguineous mucus discharge from nose), hydropic, anemia, hepatosplenomegaly, copper colored maculopapular dermal rash on palms of hand, soles of feet, diaper area, around mouth and anus Condylomata around anus; rhagades (circumoral radiating scars)

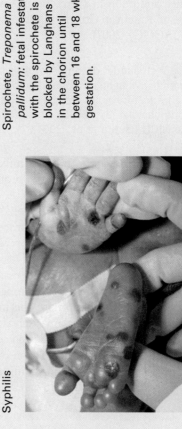

Varicella zoster (chicken pox)	Varicella zoster virus	Varicella-zoster immune globulin (VariZIG) at birth for infants who mothers developed chickenpox between 5 days before birth and 48 hours after birth Acyclovir for infants with generalized involvement and pneumonia (Myers, Seward, & LaRussa, 2007) ***Preterm infants*** exposed to chickenpox should receive either Acyclovir or VariZIG (AAP Committee on Infectious Diseases, 2006).	***First half of pregnancy:*** limb atrophy, neurologic and eye abnormalities, IUGR ***Last few days of pregnancy:*** clinical varicella; neonatal mortality 30% (Sauerbrei & Wutzler, 2007)
Hepatitis B virus (HBV)	HBV	If mother has antibodies for hepatitis B surface antigen (HbsAg) or developed hepatitis during pregnancy or the postpartum period, give infant hepatitis B immunoglobulin (HBIG) in first 12 hours of life and hepatitis B vaccine with additional doses at 1 and 6 months. Infants not exposed to maternal HBV should receive the vaccine before discharge from the birth hospital. Breastfeeding is permitted.	***Preterm birth:*** The transmission rate of HBV to the newborn ranges from 70% to 90% when the mother is seropositive for both HbsAg and HBe antigen (HbeAg) (AAP Committee on Infectious Diseases, 2006); acute hepatitis (mortality 75% in severe cases), chronic hepatitis, cirrhosis of the liver, liver cancer years later.
Human parvovirus B19 (fifth disease or "slapped cheek illness")	Parvovirus B19	Intrauterine transfusion to treat anemia (De Jong, de Haan, Kroes, Beersma, Oepkas, & Walther, 2006).	Miscarriage, fetal hydrops, IUGR Pericardial, pleural, and peritoneal effusions are common and fatal if not treated immediately, with cardiac failure from anemia being the most common cause of death.

Continued

TABLE 24-7

Infections Affecting Newborns—cont'd

	TORCH INFECTIONS			
	INFECTION	CAUSATIVE AGENT	TREATMENT	EFFECTS/COMPLICATIONS
	Human immunodeficiency virus (HIV)	Human immunodeficiency virus; mother-to-fetus transmission transplacentally (13% to 39%) or in breast milk (14%) (AAP Committee on Infectious Diseases, 2006).	Zidovudine antepartum, intrapartum, and neonatally (transmission decreased to 5% to 8%); HAART (transmission decreased to 1% to 2%) (AAP Committee on Infectious Diseases, 2006). Neonatal dose: 2 mg/kg/dose orally every 6 hours or 1.5 mg/kg IV every 6 hours.	Growth failure, parotitis, and recurrent or persistent upper respiratory infections; immunodeficiency which progresses to death. In the first year of life, lymphadenopathy and hepatosplenomegaly are common. Fever, chronic diarrhea, chronic dermatitis, interstitial pneumonitis, persistent thrush, and AIDS-defining opportunistic infections (*Candida* and *pneumocystis carinii* pneumonia), cytomegalovirus (CMV) infection, cryptosporidiosis, herpes simplex or herpes zoster, and disseminated varicella.
R	Rubella (German or 3-day measles)	Rubella virus	Rubella vaccination for nonimmune mothers before pregnancy. Treat affected infant symptomatically.	Abnormalities most severe if mother contracts disease in first trimester. Hearing loss, cataracts or glaucoma, hypogammaglobulinemia, diabetes mellitus type 1, hepatosplenomegaly, lymphedema, IUGR, jaundice, hepatitis, thrombocytopenic purpura with petechiae, and the characteristic blueberry muffin lesions (dermal microphthalmos)

C	CMV infections 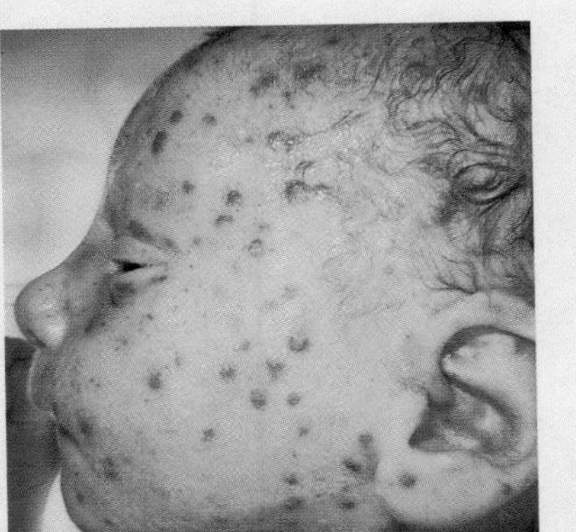 Neonatal cytomegalovirus infection. Typical rash seen in a severely affected infant. (Courtesy David A. Clarke, Philadelphia, PA.)	CMV in utero infection; breast milk	Ganciclovir decreases viral replication and severity of neurologic and auditory damage; drug is toxic to bone marrow; AAP Committee on Infectious Diseases (2006) does not recommend routine use.	Miscarriage, stillbirth, congenital illness. IUGR, microcephaly, rash, jaundice, hepatosplenomegaly, anemia, chorioretinitis, microcephaly, mental retardation, and neuromuscular deficits, thrombocytopenia, hyperbilirubinemia, intracranial, periventricular calcification, inclusion bodies in cells sedimented from freshly voided urine or in liver biopsy specimens. Sensorineural hearing impairment, learning disabilities
H	Herpes simplex virus (HSV) infection 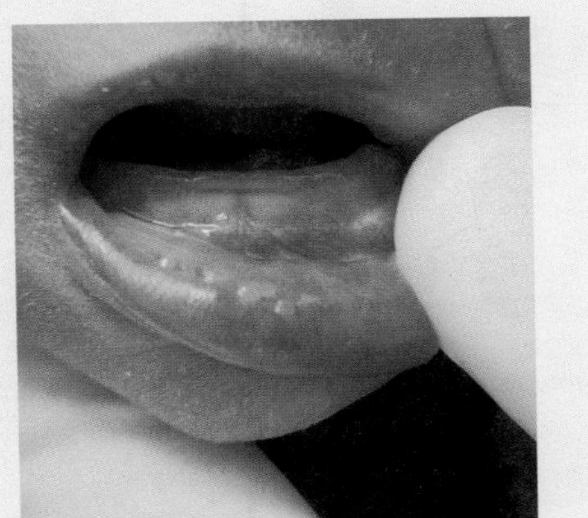 HSV oral lesions. (Courtesy David A. Clarke, Philadelphia, PA.)	Herpes simplex virus; infected transplacentally, ascending infection, directly during passage through birth canal from mother with primary HSV infection, from infected personnel or family	Prophylactic topical eye ointment (vidarabine, iododeoxyuridine, or trifluridine) is administered for 5 days to prevent keratoconjunctivitis; parenteral acyclovir for neonatal herpes.	***Fetus***: IUGR, preterm ***Infant***: severe, often fatal systemic illness, encephalitis, chorioretinitis, severe psychomotor restriction, with intracranial calcifications, microcephaly, hypertonicity, and seizures; eye involvement, including microphthalmos, cataracts, chorioretinitis, blindness, and retinal dysplasia Some infants have oral lesions, patent ductus arteriosus, limb anomalies, and recurrent skin vesicles, with a short life expectancy.

Continued

TABLE 24-7

Infections Affecting Newborns—cont'd

BACTERIAL INFECTIONS			
INFECTION	**CAUSATIVE AGENT**	**TREATMENT**	**EFFECTS/COMPLICATIONS**
Strep	Group B *Streptococcus*	Penicillin and an aminoglycoside (AAP Committee on Infectious Diseases, 2006)	Respiratory illness mimicking severe RDS; neonatal sepsis and meningitis, septic shock; neurologic damage
E. coli	*Escherichia coli*	Aminoglycosides or third-generation cephalosporins (Lott, 2007)	Sepsis, meningitis, infection in other body systems (e.g., urinary tract)
Tuberculosis (TB)	*Mycobacterium tuberculosis*	***Infants at risk of contracting TB:*** vaccinate with Calmette-Guérin bacillus ***Infancy:*** isoniazid, rifampin, pyrazinamide and streptomycin or kanamycin; pyridoxine should always be given with isoniazid or to breast fed infants whose mothers are being treated with isoniazid (Venkatesh, Merenstein, Adams, & Weisman, 2006).	***Congenitally acquired:*** otitis media, pneumonia, hepatosplenomegaly, enlarged lymph glands, or disseminated disease ***Contracted after birth:*** pneumonia, necrosis of lung tissue, death
Chlamydia	*Chlamydia trachomatis*	Oral erythromycin (AAP Committee on Infectious Diseases, 2006) or sulfonamide for 2-3 weeks (risk of infantile hypertrophic pyloric stenosis is increased with erythromycin)	Neonatal conjunctivitis and pneumonia; if untreated trachoma can develop.
FUNGAL INFECTION			
INFECTION	**CAUSATIVE AGENT**	**TREATMENT**	**EFFECTS/COMPLICATIONS**
Candida (formerly moniliasis)	*Candida albicans*	Topical application of 1 ml nystatin (Mycostatin) over surfaces of oral cavity 1 hour before or after feeding 4 times a day; amphotericin B (Fungizone), clotrimazole (Lotrimin, Mycelex), fluconazole (Diflucan), or miconazole (Monistat, Micatin) given intravenously, orally, or topically; topical fungicide at each diaper change for diaper dermatitis. If breastfeeding, mother may need treatment with systemic antifungal medication.	Oral candidiasis (thrush or mycotic stomatitis; white plaques on oral mucosa, gums, and tongue), diaper dermatitis (intensely erythematous, sharply demarcated, scalloped edge) on perianal area, inguinal folds, and lower portion of the abdomen

AIDS, Acquired immunodeficiency syndrome; *CNS,* central nervous system; *HAART,* highly active antiretroviral therapy; *IM,* intramuscular; *IUGR,* intrauterine growth restriction; *IV,* intravenous; *RDS,* respiratory distress syndrome.

TABLE 24-8

Summary of Neonatal Effects of Commonly Abused Substances

SUBSTANCE	NEONATAL EFFECTS
Alcohol 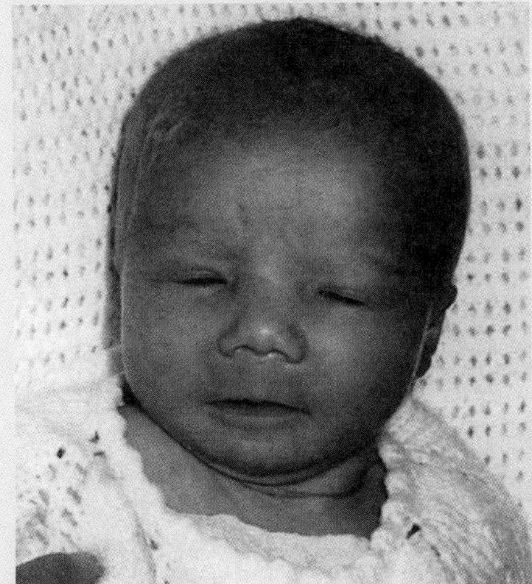 Infant with fetal alcohol syndrome (From Markiewicz, M., & Abrahamson E. [1999]. *Diagnosis in color: Neonatology.* St. Louis: Mosby.)	*Fetal alcohol syndrome* (FAS): craniofacial features vary, may include short eyelid opening, flat midface, flat upper lip groove, thin upper lip; microcephaly; hyperactivity; developmental delays; attention deficits *Alcohol-related neurodevelopmental disorder (ARND):* varying forms of FAS, cognitive, behavioral and psychosocial problems without typical physical features
Cocaine	CNS stimulant and peripheral sympathomimetic. Preterm birth, small for gestational age, microcephaly, poor feeding, irregular sleep patterns, diarrhea, visual attention problems, hyperactivity, difficult to console, hypersensitivity to noise and external stimuli, irritability, developmental delays, congenital anomalies such as prune belly syndrome (i.e., distended, flabby, wrinkled abdomen caused by lack of abdominal muscles)
Heroin	Increased rate of stillbirth, low birth weight, small for gestational age, meconium aspiration, microcephaly, neurobehavioral problems, irritability, tachypnea, feeding difficulties, vomiting, high-pitched cry, seizures, 74-fold increase in SIDS (Minozzi, Amato, Vecci, & Davoli, 2008); physical dependence in the fetus and increased risk of exposure to infections including hepatitis B and C virus and HIV
Marijuana	Possible neonatal tremors, low birth weight, growth restriction, meconium staining
Methadone	Therapy for heroin addiction. Methadone withdrawal more severe and prolonged than withdrawal from heroin. Signs of withdrawal include tremors, irritability, state lability, hypertonicity, hypersensitivity, vomiting, mottling, and nasal stuffiness; disturbed sleep pattern. Incidence of SIDS increased.
Methamphetamine	Effects dose related; small for gestational age, preterm birth, abruptio placenta, perinatal mortality, poor weight gain, lethargy, cleft lip and palate and cardiac defects, emotional disturbances and delays in gross and fine motor coordination, behavioral problems later in childhood
Phencyclidine ("angel dust")	Abnormal motor behavior such as irritability, jitteriness, and hypertonicity
Phenobarbital	Found in high levels in the fetal liver and brain. Because of its slow metabolic rate, withdrawal onset is generally 2 to 14 days after birth and duration is approximately 2 to 4 months. Irritability, crying, hiccups, and sleepiness mark the initial response. During the second stage, the infant is extremely hungry, regurgitates and gags frequently, and demonstrates episodic irritability, sweating, and a disturbed sleep pattern.
Tobacco	Preterm birth; low birth weight; increased risk for sudden infant death syndrome; increased risk for bronchitis, pneumonia, developmental delays
Caffeine	Caffeine consumption more than 150 mg/day associated with IUGR and low birth weight.

CNS, Central nervous system; *HIV,* human immunodeficiency virus; *IUGR,* intrauterine growth restriction; *SIDS,* sudden infant death syndrome.

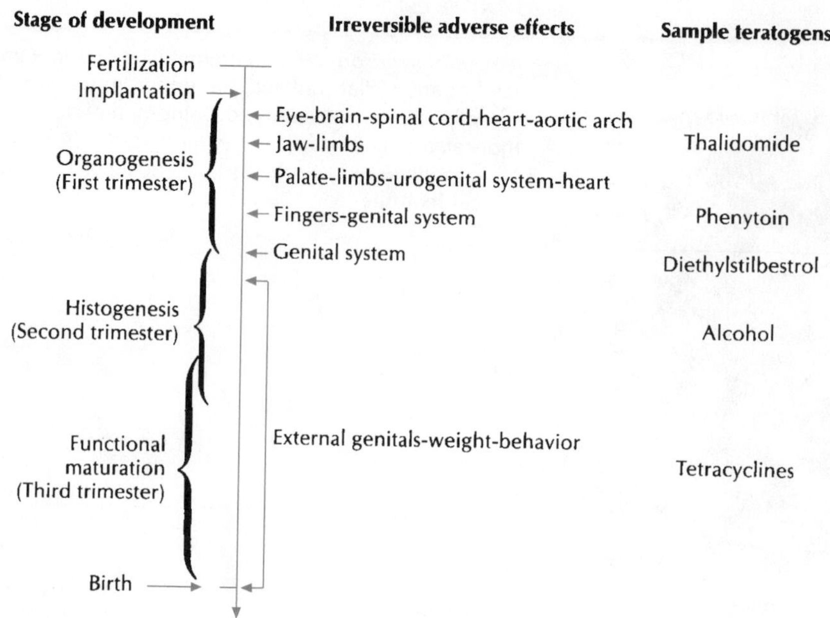

Fig. 24-10 Critical periods in human embryogenesis. (From Reed, M. D., Aranda, J. V., & Hales, B. F. [2006]. Developmental pharmacology. In R. J. Martin, A. A. Fanaroff, & M.C. Walsh [Eds.], *Fanaroff and Martin's neonatal-perinatal medicine: Diseases of the fetus and infant* [8th ed.]. Philadelphia: Saunders.)

TABLE 24-9

Signs of Neonatal Abstinence Syndrome

SYSTEM	SIGNS
Gastrointestinal	Poor feeding, vomiting, regurgitation, diarrhea, excessive sucking
Central nervous	Irritability, tremors, shrill cry, incessant crying, hyperactivity, little sleep, excoriations on face, convulsions
Metabolic, vasomotor, respiratory	Nasal congestion, tachypnea, sweating, frequent yawning, increased respiratory rate >60 breaths/min, fever >37.2° C

analyzing feeding behaviors, and devising strategies to promote nutritional intake.

Neonatal abstinence syndrome (NAS) is the term used to describe the set of behaviors exhibited by the infant exposed to chemical substances in utero (Table 24-9). Fig. 24-11 provides an example of a neonatal abstinence scoring system for assessing withdrawal symptoms. Because many women are multidrug users, the newborn initially may exhibit a variety of withdrawal manifestations.

The NICU Network Neurobehavioral Scale (NNNS), developed by the National Institutes of Health, provides an assessment of neurologic, behavioral, and stress-abstinence function in the neonate. The test combines items from other tests such as the Neonatal Behavioral Assessment Scale (NBAS), stress-abstinence items developed by Finnegan (see Fig. 24-11), and a complete neurologic examination, which includes primitive reflexes and active and passive tone (Law, Stroud, LaGasse, Niaura, Liu, & Lester, 2003; Lester & Tronick, 2004).

Nursing care of the drug-exposed neonate involves supportive therapy for fluid and electrolyte balance, nutrition, infection control, individualized developmental care, and respiratory care. Swaddling, holding, reducing environmental stimuli, and feeding as necessary can be helpful in easing withdrawal. Specific suggestions for providing care to infants experiencing withdrawal are listed in the Teaching Guidelines box.

HEMOLYTIC DISORDERS

Hyperbilirubinemia, physiologic jaundice, pathologic jaundice, and kernicterus are discussed in Chapter 17.

Hemolytic Disease of the Newborn

Hemolytic disease occurs when the blood groups of the mother and newborn are different; the most common of these are RhD factor and ABO incompatibilities. Hemolytic disorders occur when maternal antibodies are present naturally or form in response to an antigen from the fetal blood crossing the placenta and entering the maternal circulation. The maternal antibodies of the IgG class cross the placenta, causing hemolysis of the fetal RBCs, resulting in fetal anemia and often neonatal jaundice and hyperbilirubinemia.

NEONATAL ABSTINENCE SCORING SYSTEM

SYSTEM	SIGNS AND SYMPTOMS	SCORE	AM	PM	COMMENTS
CENTRAL NERVOUS SYSTEM DISTURBANCES	Excessive High Pitched (Or other) Cry Continuous High Pitched (Or other) Cry	2 3			Daily Weight
	Sleeps <1 Hour After Feeding Sleeps <2 Hours After Feeding Sleeps <3 Hours After Feeding	3 2 1			
	Hyperactive Moro Reflex Markedly Hyperactive Moro Reflex	2 3			
	Mild Tremors Disturbed Moderate-Severe Tremors Disturbed	1 2			
	Mild Tremors Undisturbed Moderate-Severe Tremors Undisturbed	3 4			
	Increased Muscle Tone	2			
	Excoriation (Specific Area)	1			
	Myoclonic Jerks	3			
	Generalized Convulsions	5			
METABOLIC/VASOMOTOR/RESPIRATORY DISTURBANCES	Sweating	1			
	Fever <101 (99°-100.8° F/37.2°-38.2° C) Fever >101 (38.4° C and higher)	1 2			
	Frequent Yawning (>3-4 Times/Interval)	1			
	Mottling	1			
	Nasal Stuffiness	1			
	Sneezing (>3-4 Times/Interval)	1			
	Nasal Flaring	2			
	Respiratory Rate >60/min Respiratory Rate >60/min with Retractions	1 2			
GASTROINTESTINAL DISTURBANCES	Excessive Sucking	1			
	Poor Feeding	2			
	Regurgitation Projectile Vomiting	2 3			
	Loose Stools Watery Stools	2 3			
	TOTAL SCORE				
	INITIALS OF SCORER				

Fig. 24-11 Neonatal Abstinence Scoring (NAS) system, developed by L. Finnegan. (From Nelson, N. [1990]. *Current therapy in neonatal-perinatal medicine* [2nd ed.]. St. Louis: Mosby.)

TEACHING GUIDELINES

Care of the Infant Experiencing Withdrawal

- Decrease stimuli: dim lights, decrease noise levels.
- Arrange nursing activities to decrease exogenous stimulation.
- Provide adequate nutrition and hydration; monitor intake and output.
- Put the infant in a sitting position with chin tucked down for feeding.
- Encourage breastfeeding (if mother is negative for human immunodeficiency virus).
- Weigh daily to detect fluid losses or caloric intake.
- Promote positive maternal-infant relationships.
- Place the awake infant in a side-lying position with the spine and legs flexed.
- Position the infant's hands in midline with the arms at the side.
- Carry the infant in a flexed position.
- Protect hyperactive infants from skin abrasions on the knees, toes, and cheeks that are caused by rubbing on bed linens while in a prone position while awake; supine position for sleep is preferred.
- When interacting with the infant, introduce one stimulus at a time when the infant is in a quiet, alert state. Watch for time-out or distress signals (e.g., gaze aversion, yawning, sneezing, hiccups, arching, mottled color).
- When the infant is distressed, swaddle in a flexed position and rock in a slow, rhythmic fashion.
- Monitor and record activity level.
- Pharmacologic treatment to decrease withdrawal side effects includes phenobarbital, morphine, diluted tincture of opium (paregoric), or methadone.

Rh incompatibility

Rh incompatibility occurs when an RhD-negative mother has an RhD-positive fetus that inherits the dominant Rh-positive gene from the father. The Rh blood group consists of several antigens. (Because D is the most prevalent Rh antigen the following discussion focuses on RhD isoimmunization.) If the mother is Rh-negative and the father is Rh-positive and homozygous for the Rh factor, all the offspring will be Rh-positive. If the father is heterozygous for the factor, then a 50% chance exists that each infant born of the union will be Rh-positive and a 50% chance that each will be Rh-negative. An Rh-negative fetus is in no danger because it has the same Rh factor as the mother. An Rh-negative fetus with an Rh-positive mother is also in no danger. Only the Rh-positive offspring of an Rh-negative mother is at risk. From 10% to 15% of all Caucasian couples and approximately 5% of African-American couples have Rh incompatibility. Incompatibility is rare in Asian couples. The incidence of Rh sensitization and resulting hemolytic disease of the newborn has decreased dramatically since the development of Rh_o(D) immune globulin in 1968.

The pathogenesis of Rh incompatibility is as follows: Hematopoiesis in the fetus, or the formation of blood cells, begins as early as the eighth week of gestation; in up to 40% of pregnancies, these cells pass through the placenta into the maternal circulation. When the fetus is Rh-positive and the mother Rh-negative, the mother forms antibodies against the fetal blood cells: first IgM antibodies that are too large to pass through the placenta and then IgG antibodies that can cross the placenta. The process of antibody formation is called *maternal sensitization*. Sensitization may occur during pregnancy, birth, induced abortion or miscarriage, or amniocentesis. Usually, women become sensitized in their first pregnancy with an Rh-positive fetus but do not produce enough antibodies to cause lysis (destruction) of the fetal blood cells. In subsequent pregnancies, antibodies form in response to repeated contact with the antigen from the fetal blood, and lysis results. The overall incidence of isoimmunization in Rh negative mothers who are at risk is less than 10% and only 5% of mothers with isoimmunization have babies with hemolytic disease (Stoll, 2007). Multiple gestations, abruptio placentae, placenta previa, manual removal of the placenta, and cesarean birth increase the incidence of transplacental hemorrhage and the risk of isoimmunization.

Severe Rh incompatibility results in marked fetal hemolytic anemia because the fetal erythrocytes are destroyed by maternal Rh-positive antibodies. Although the placenta usually clears the bilirubin generated by the RBC breakdown, in extreme cases, fetal bilirubin levels increase. The fetus compensates for the anemia by producing large numbers of immature erythrocytes to replace those hemolyzed, thus the name for this condition: **erythroblastosis fetalis**. In **hydrops fetalis**, the most severe form of this disease, the fetus has marked anemia, as well as cardiac decompensation, cardiomegaly, and hepatosplenomegaly. Hypoxia results from the severe anemia. In addition, because of the decreased intravascular oncotic pressure involved, fluid leaks out of the intravascular space, resulting in generalized edema, as well as effusions into the peritoneal (ascites), pericardial, and pleural (hydrothorax) spaces. The placenta is often edematous, which, along with the edematous fetus, can cause the uterus to rupture.

Intrauterine or early neonatal death may occur as a result of hydrops fetalis, although intrauterine transfusions and early delivery of the fetus may avert this. Intrauterine transfusion involves the infusion of Rh-negative, type O blood into the umbilical vein. The frequency of intrauterine transfusions may vary according to institution and fetal hydropic status, but it may be as often as every 3 to 4 weeks until 35 weeks of gestation (Moise, 2007).

ABO incompatibility

ABO incompatibility is more common than Rh incompatibility but causes less severe problems in the affected infant by comparison. It occurs if the fetal blood type is A, B, or AB and the maternal type is O. ABO incompatibility occurs rarely in infants with type B blood born to mothers with type A blood. The incompatibility arises because naturally occurring anti-A and anti-B antibodies are transferred across the placenta to the fetus. Unlike the situation that pertains to Rh incompatibility, first-born infants may be affected because mothers with type O blood already have anti-A and anti-B antibodies in their blood. Such a newborn may have a weakly positive direct **Coombs test** (also termed a direct antiglobulin test [DAT]). The cord bilirubin level usually is less than 4 mg/dl, and any resulting hyperbilirubinemia can usually be treated with phototherapy. Exchange transfusions are required only occasionally. Although ABO incompatibility is a common cause of hyperbilirubinemia, it rarely precipitates significant anemia resulting from the hemolysis of RBCs.

Other

A full discussion of the many potential causes of hemolytic jaundice in childhood is not within the scope of this text. However, in some populations, a high incidence of glucose-6-phosphate dehydrogenase (G6PD) deficiency occurs, which can cause an exaggerated jaundice in a newborn within 24 to 48 hours of birth. G6PD RBCs hemolyze at a greater rate than healthy RBCs, thus overwhelming the immature neonatal liver's ability to conjugate the indirect bilirubin. Some of the triggers that potentiate hemolysis include vitamin K, acetaminophen, aspirin, sepsis, and exposure to certain chemicals (Reiser, 2004). Hereditary spherocytosis can also cause serious neonatal hemolytic anemia as a result of high quantities of fetal hemoglobin; jaundice can develop rapidly and require phototherapy (Luchtman-Jones, Schwartz, & Wilson, 2006). Treatment is the same as for any newborn with rapidly rising serum bilirubin levels. Other metabolic and inherited conditions that increase hemolysis and can cause jaundice in the infant include galactosemia, Crigler-Najjar syndrome, and hypothyroidism.

CARE MANAGEMENT

At the first prenatal visit of an Rh-negative woman with a fetus that may be Rh-positive, an indirect Coombs test should be performed to determine whether she has antibodies to the Rh antigen. In this test the maternal blood serum is mixed with Rh-positive RBCs. If Rh-positive RBCs agglutinate, or clump, maternal antibodies are present or the mother has been sensitized. The dilution of the specimen of blood at which clumping occurs determines the titer, or level, of maternal antibodies. This titer indicates the degree of maternal sensitization. A level of 1 : 8 rarely results in fetal jeopardy. If the titer reaches 1 : 16, amniocentesis is performed to determine the delta optical density (ΔOD) of the amniotic fluid to estimate fetal hemolytic process. Rising bilirubin levels may indicate the need for an intrauterine transfusion. Genetic testing allows early identification of paternal zygosity at the RhD gene locus, thus allowing earlier detection of the potential for isoimmunization and precluding further maternal or fetal testing (Moise, 2007).

The indirect Coombs test is repeated at 24 weeks. If the result remains negative, indicating that sensitization has not occurred, the woman is given an intramuscular injection of Rh_o(D) immune globulin. If the test result is positive, showing that sensitization has occurred, the test is repeated at 4- to 6-week intervals to monitor the maternal antibody titer as just described.

At birth, the neonate's cord blood is sent to the laboratory to determine the infant's blood type and Rh status. A direct Coombs test is performed on cord blood to determine the presence of maternal antibodies in the fetal blood. If antibodies are present, the titer, which indicates the degree of maternal sensitization, is measured. The prevention of or prompt therapy for perinatal asphyxia, acidosis, cold stress, sepsis, and hypoglycemia will decrease the newborn's risk for severe hemolytic disease and his or her susceptibility to kernicterus. Early feeding in the stable newborn is also initiated to stimulate stooling and thus facilitate the removal of bilirubin.

If jaundice is present, the cause is determined and therapeutic management is begun. Phototherapy is used to reduce rapidly increasing serum bilirubin levels. See Chapter 17 for a discussion of phototherapy.

Exchange transfusions are needed infrequently because of the decrease in the incidence of severe hemolytic disease in newborns resulting from isoimmunization. Other factors must always be considered as well, particularly the clinical condition of the infant, because it is a procedure with potential complications. Guidelines for the initiation of exchange transfusion in relation to serum bilirubin levels in infants of 35 weeks or more of gestation may be found in the 2004 AAP Subcommittee on Hyperbilirubinemia: *Clinical Practice Guideline*.

Exchange transfusion is accomplished by alternately removing a small amount of the infant's blood and replacing it with an equal amount of donor blood. If the infant has Rh incompatibility, type O Rh-negative blood is used for transfusion; thus the maternal antibodies still present in the infant do not hemolyze the transfused blood. Depending on the infant's size, maturity, and condition, amounts of 5 to 20 ml of the infant's blood are removed at one time and replaced with warmed donor blood. The total amount of blood exchanged approximates 170 ml/kg of body weight, or 75% to 85% of the infant's total blood volume. Preservatives in donor blood lower the infant's serum calcium level; therefore calcium gluconate is often given during the exchange transfusion. The neonate is monitored closely for signs of a blood transfusion reaction, as well as hypotension, temperature instability, and cardiorespiratory compromise.

CONGENITAL ANOMALIES

Congenital defects are reported to occur in 2% to 3% of all live births (Bay, Steele, & Davis, 2007), but this number increases to approximately 6% by 5 years, when more anomalies are diagnosed. In addition, the incidence of congenital malformations in fetuses that are aborted is higher than that in infants who are born alive, thus also adding to the overall incidence. Major congenital defects are the leading cause of death in infants younger than 1 year of age in the United States and account for 20% of neonatal deaths. Although the incidences of other causes of neonatal mortality have decreased, the death rate associated with most congenital anomalies has essentially remained stable since 1932.

Ways of detecting and preventing some of these anomalies are being improved continually, as are some surgical techniques for the care of the fetus with certain anomalies. Promoting the availability of these services to populations at risk challenges community health care systems. An interdisciplinary team approach is vital for providing holistic care: the surgical treatment, rehabilitation, and education of the child, as well as psychosocial and financial assistance for the parents. Parental disappointment and disillusion add to the complexity of the nursing care needed for these infants. (See Table 24-10 for description of congenital anomalies and their treatment. Consult a pediatric textbook for a more definitive explanation of treatment and nursing care.)

CARE MANAGEMENT

Newborn. A collaborative health team approach that includes specialists and community service representatives is needed in the care of the infant with a congenital anomaly. Surgical intervention in the neonatal period may be necessary for the infant requiring either immediate correction or a palliative procedure to relieve the symptoms of the anomaly until definitive correction can be undertaken. The morbidity and mortality rates in neonates are also higher than in older children or adults undergoing similar procedures. However, despite these problems unique to neonates, advances in surgical techniques, fluid and electrolyte management, anesthesia, pain management, and the nursing care given in intensive care nurseries have together been responsible for decreasing the risk of surgery in neonates.

The health care team must be highly skilled to meet the needs of these infants. These needs are similar to those of other high risk infants. In addition to stabilization of the infant's condition (oxygenation and perfusion of tissues), other preoperative interventions, such as nasogastric tube placement for abdominal decompression, pain management, and the maintenance of fluid and electrolyte balance, are implemented to manage specific problems.

Postoperatively the infant is usually returned to the intensive care nursery, where close monitoring is maintained. The infant's respiratory efforts are supported, which often requires mechanical ventilation. Constant surveillance is necessary to detect any respiratory complications resulting from the anesthesia. A pulse oximeter is attached to measure the oxygen saturation and oxygen is provided as needed. An indwelling gastric catheter can be placed to remove gastric secretions, thereby preventing aspiration and distention of the abdomen. The infant's fluid, electrolyte, and acid-base balances are monitored and adjusted as needed. Urinary output is monitored and should equal 1 to 2 ml/kg/hr. Other nursing interventions are focused on caring for the surgical site, maintaining thermoregulation, pain management, and promoting comfort.

Parents and family. Nurses frequently encounter children with a genetic disorder and families in which a risk exists that a disorder may be transmitted to or occur in an offspring. Being alert to situations in which persons can benefit from a genetic evaluation, counseling to be aware of the local genetic resources, aiding the family in finding services, and offering support and care for children and families affected by genetic conditions are some of the responsibilities of nurses. Local genetic clinics can be located through several sites, such as the GeneTests (www.genetests.org). This publicly funded medical genetics information resource developed for physicians and other health care providers is available at no cost to all interested persons.

While the infant is receiving optimal care, the parents also have needs that must be met as they deal with the crisis of having an infant with an abnormal condition. Their reactions are assessed and are likely to be those typical of a grief response. Facilitating their understanding of the information given them about their infant's condition is a vital nursing intervention. A newly diagnosed disorder often requires the implementation of a therapeutic regimen. For example, the disorder may be an **inborn error of metabolism,** such as phenylketonuria (PKU) which requires consistent and rigid adherence to a diet. The family may need help with securing the prescribed formula and in receiving counseling from a clinical dietitian. The importance of maintaining the diet, keeping an adequate supply of special preparations, and avoiding the use of unauthorized substitutions must be impressed on the family. These conditions often require a drastic change in family lifestyle and functioning; families often depend on others for assistance, and family coping skills and resources can be stretched thin with a diagnosis such as PKU, galactosemia, hypothyroidism, or Down syndrome (see Chapter 5 for a discussion of these conditions).

Referral to appropriate agencies is another essential component of the follow-up management, and the nurse should make the parents aware of all possible sources of aid, including pertinent literature, parent groups, and national organizations. Many organizations and foundations, such as the March of Dimes, provide services and counseling for families of affected children. In addition, numerous parent support groups are available. In these settings, parents can share experiences and derive mutual support in coping with problems similar to those of other group members. Nurses must be familiar with the services available in their community that provide assistance and education to families with these special problems.

Text continued on p. 798.

TABLE 24-10

Congenital Anomalies

ANOMALY	DESCRIPTION	TREATMENT
CENTRAL NERVOUS SYSTEM ANOMALIES		
Encephalocele	Herniation of brain and meninges through a skull defect usually at the base of the neck.	Surgical repair and shunting to relieve hydrocephalus.
Anencephaly	Absence of both cerebral hemispheres and the overlying skull. Incompatible with life.	Comfort measures until infant dies of temperature instability and respiratory failure
Spina bifida	Results from failure of the neural tube to close.	
Spina bifida occulta	Posterior portion of the laminas fails to close but the spinal cord or meninges do not herniated or protrude through the defect. Usually asymptomatic.	Usually no treatment necessary; may not be diagnosed unless there are associated problems.
Spina bifida cystica	Includes meningocele and myelomeningocele.	
Meningocele	External sac that contains meninges and CSF and that protrudes through a defect in the vertebral column.	Prenatal diagnosis makes possible a scheduled cesarean birth. Protect the protruding sac from injury, rupture, and central nervous system infection. Position infant on side or prone. Cover lesion with sterile, moist nonadherent dressing; use sterile technique. Surgical repair within the first 24 to 48 hours. May need surgical shunt to prevent increasing hydrocephalus. Provide support and information for parents.
Myelomeningocele 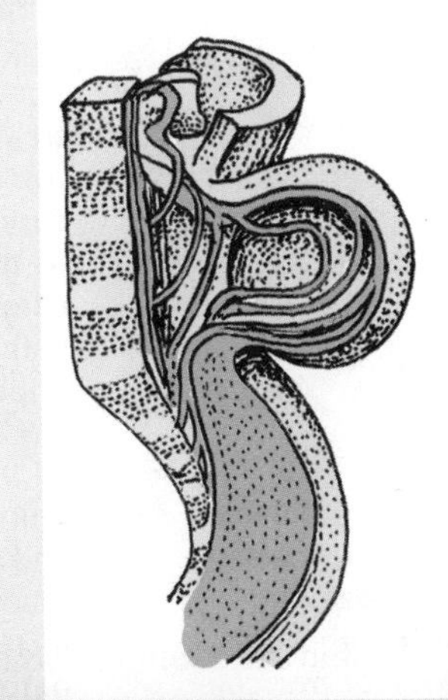 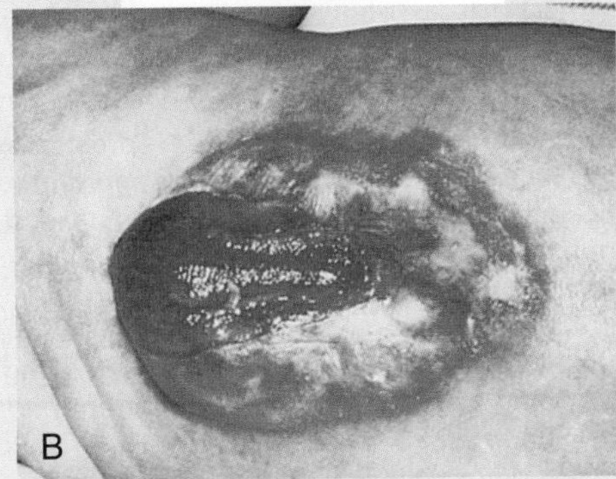 **A,** Myelomeningocele. Note absence of vertebral arches. **B,** Myelomeningocele (ruptured sac exposing defect). (From Zitelli, B. J., & Davis, H. W. [2002]. *Atlas of pediatric physical diagnosis* [4th ed.]. St. Louis: Mosby.)	Similar to meningocele, also contains nerves; infant has motor and sensory deficits below the lesion. Visible at birth, most often in the lumbosacral area. Usually covered with a very fragile, thin membrane that can tear easily, allowing CSF to leak out and providing an entry for infectious agents into the CNS. Hydrocephalus in 90% of children.	

Continued

TABLE 24-10

Congenital Anomalies—cont'd

ANOMALY	DESCRIPTION	TREATMENT
Hydrocephalus 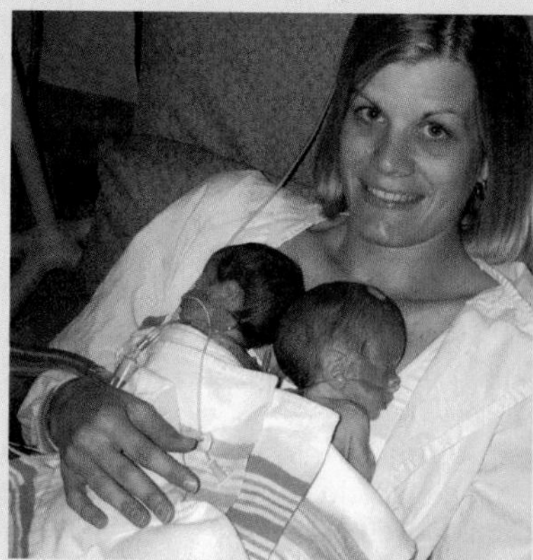 Mother providing kangaroo care to twins; twin on right has hydrocephalus. (Courtesy Cheryl Briggs, RN, Annapolis, MD.)	Ventricles of brain enlarged as a result of an imbalance between the production and absorption of the CSF. Congenital hydrocephalus usually arises as a result of a malformation in the brain or an intrauterine infection. Bulging anterior fontanel and head circumference that increases at abnormal rate.	Surgical shunting soon after birth. Care similar to that of any high risk newborn. Measure head circumference and neurologic assessments frequently. If infant's head is large, place special pressure-sensitive mattress under infant and change position frequently to prevent skin breakdown.
Microcephaly	Head circumference that measures more than three standard deviations below the mean for age and sex. Brain growth is usually restricted and thus mental retardation is common.	Supportive nursing care and medical observation to determine the extent of psychomotor retardation that almost always accompanies this abnormality. No treatment is available. Provide support to parents as they learn to care for a child with cognitive impairment.
CARDIOVASCULAR SYSTEM ANOMALIES (SELECTED)		
Ventricular septal defects 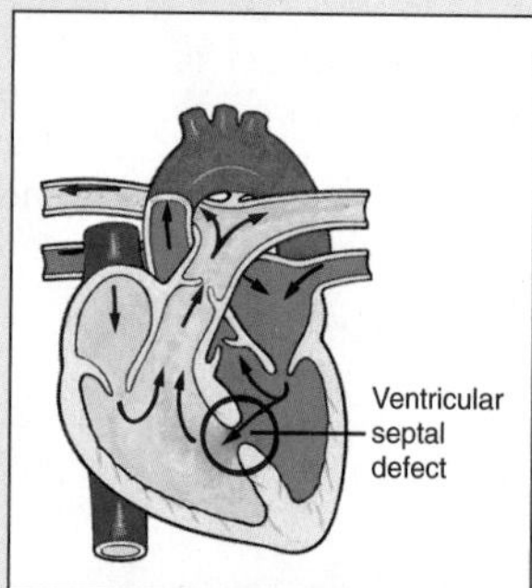 (From Congenital heart abnormalities. Modified from Hockenberry, M., & Wilson, D. [2011]. *Wong's nursing care of infants and children* [9th ed.]. St. Louis: Mosby.)	Abnormal opening between right and left ventricles. VSDs vary in size and may occur in either the membranous or muscular portion of the ventricular septum. Because of higher pressure in the left ventricle, a shunting of blood from the left to the right ventricle occurs during systole. If pulmonary vascular resistance produces pulmonary hypertension, the shunt of blood is then reversed from the right to the left ventricle, with cyanosis resulting.	Administer oxygen and cardiotonic medications to increase cardiac output; medications to prevent closure of the ductus arteriosus (prostaglandin), and diuretic agents as needed for CHF; maintain a thermoneutral environment; and feed using the least strenuous method. Echocardiography and cardiac catheterization to obtain specific information about defect and need for surgical intervention.

TABLE 24-10

Congenital Anomalies—cont'd

ANOMALY	DESCRIPTION	TREATMENT
Tetralogy of Fallot 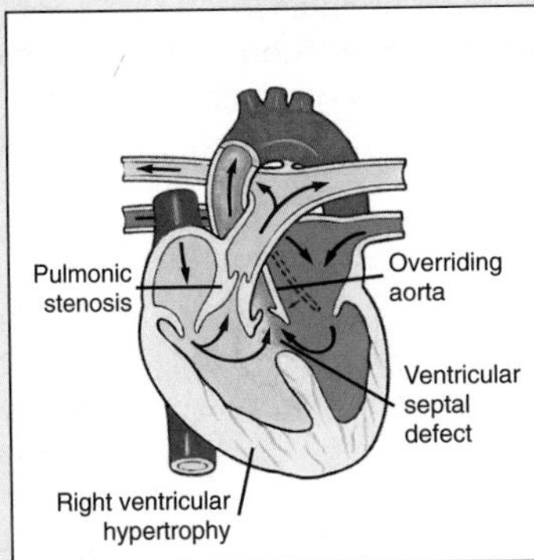 (From Congenital heart abnormalities. Modified from Hockenberry, M., & Wilson, D. [2011]. *Wong's nursing care of infants and children* [9th ed.]. St. Louis: Mosby.)	Four malformations: pulmonary stenosis, overriding aorta, ventricular septal defect, and right ventricular hypertrophy. It is the most common defect, causing cyanosis in children surviving beyond 2 years of age. The severity of symptoms depends on the degree of pulmonary stenosis, the size of the ventricular septal defect, and the degree to which the aorta overrides the septal defect.	
Transposition of the great vessels 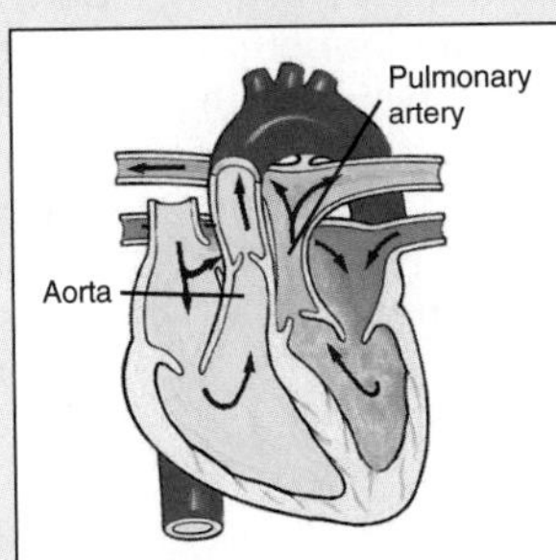 (From Congenital heart abnormalities. Modified from Hockenberry, M., & Wilson, D. [2011]. *Wong's nursing care of infants and children* [9th ed.]. St. Louis: Mosby.)	Pulmonary artery leaves the left ventricle, and the aorta exits from the right ventricle with no communication between the systemic and pulmonary circulation. An abnormal communication between the two circulations must be present to sustain life.	Medical: Administer intravenous prostaglandin E_1 to temporarily increase blood mixing. Surgical: Arterial switch procedure (see pediatric text for details).
Patent ductus arteriosus 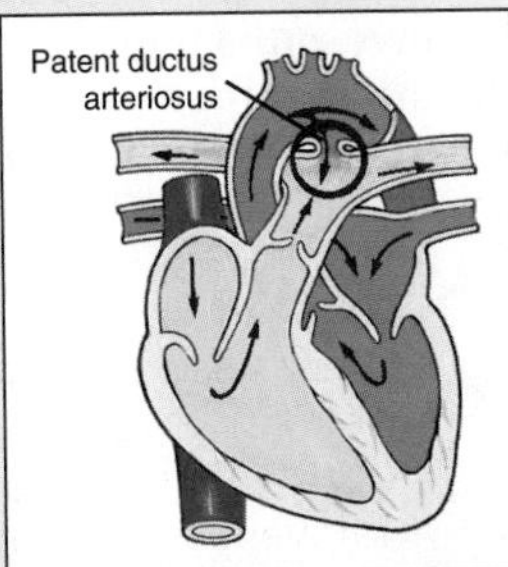 (From Congenital heart abnormalities. Modified from Hockenberry, M., & Wilson, D. [2011]. *Wong's nursing care of infants and children* [9th ed.]. St. Louis: Mosby.)	Vascular connection that, during fetal life, bypasses the pulmonary vascular bed and directs blood from the pulmonary artery to the aorta. Functional closure of the ductus normally occurs soon after birth. If the ductus remains patent after birth, the direction of blood flow in the ductus is reversed by the higher pressure in the aorta (see also p. 762).	Medical: Administer indomethacin. Surgical: division or ligation of the patent vessel.
RESPIRATORY SYSTEM ANOMALIES		
Choanal atresia	Bony or membranous septum located between the nose and the pharynx; may be unilateral or bilateral. Associated with apnea and cyanosis. Diagnosed when unable to insert a nasal catheter.	Supportive care with supplemental oxygen until surgery to correct defect.

Critical Thinking Exercise: Patent Ductus Arteriosus

Continued

TABLE 24-10

Congenital Anomalies—cont'd

ANOMALY	DESCRIPTION	TREATMENT
Congenital diaphragmatic hernia (CDH)	Defect in formation of diaphragm, allowing abdominal organs to be displaced into the thoracic cavity.	Repaired by fetal surgery in some research institutions. High-frequency oscillatory ventilation, conventional mechanical ventilation and extracorporeal membrane oxygenation are used as respiratory support until surgical repair of defect.
GASTROINTESTINAL SYSTEM ANOMALIES		
Cleft lip and palate 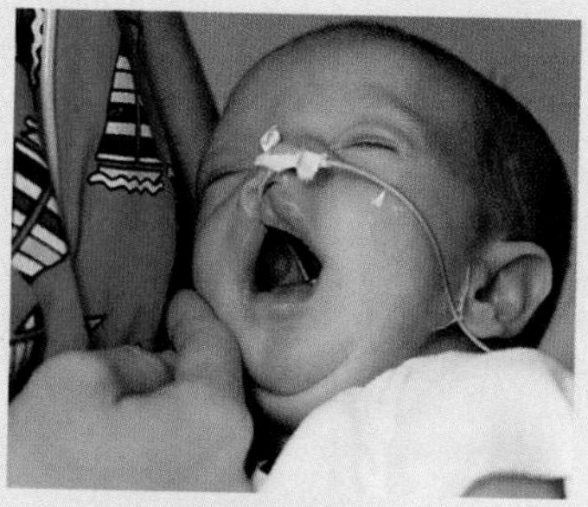 Infant with complete unilateral cleft lip. (From Dickason, E., Silverman, B., & Kaplan, J. [1998]. *Maternal-infant nursing care* [3rd ed.]. St. Louis: Mosby.)	Midline fissure, or opening, in the lip or palate (or both) resulting from failure of the primary palate to fuse.	Surgical repair of cleft lip approximately 3 months of age; hard palate 14-16 months of age, and soft palate by 18 months of age.
Esophageal atresia	Esophagus ends in a blind pouch or narrows into a thin cord, thus failing to form a continuous passageway to the stomach.	Supportive care until surgery is performed. A double-lumen catheter is placed in the proximal esophageal pouch for drainage of swallowed secretions to minimize the possibility of aspiration.
Tracheoesophageal fistula (TEF)	Abnormal connection between the esophagus and trachea.	Maintain thermoregulation, fluid and electrolyte balance, and acid-base balance. Surgical correction consists of ligating the fistula and anastomosing the two segments of the esophagus.

TABLE 24-10

Congenital Anomalies—cont'd

ANOMALY	DESCRIPTION	TREATMENT
Omphalocele 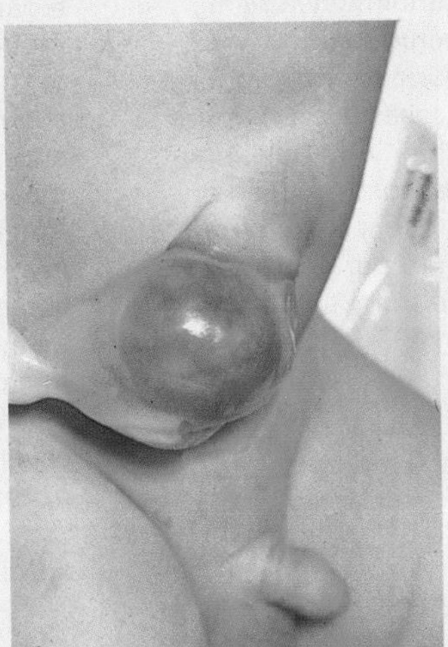 Omphalocele. (From O'Doherty, N. [1986]. *Neonatology: micro atlas of the newborn.* Nutley, NJ: Hoffmann-La Roche.)	Covered defect of umbilical ring into which varying amounts of the abdominal organs may be herniated.	Place infant in an impermeable, clear plastic bowel bag to decrease insensible water losses, maintain thermoregulation, and prevent contamination of the exposed viscera (Roaten, Bensard, & Price, 2006). Antibiotics, fluid and electrolyte replacement, gastric decompression, and thermoregulation are needed. Surgical closure of defect is usually performed soon after birth.
Gastroschisis 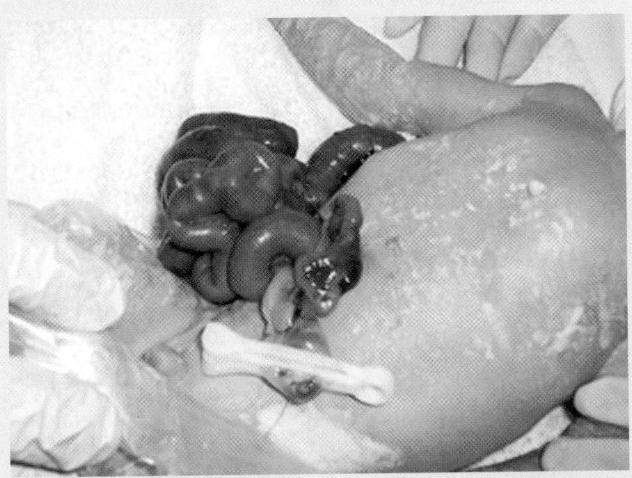 Gastroschisis. (Courtesy Cheryl Briggs, RN, Annapolis, MD.)	Herniation of bowel through defect in the abdominal wall to the right of the umbilical cord. No membrane covers the contents.	Same as for omphalocele; most infants need mechanical ventilation and parenteral nutrition.
Intestinal obstruction	Can occur anywhere in gastrointestinal tract; includes atresia (complete obliteration of the passage); partial obstruction; and malrotation of the intestine.	Supportive until surgical intervention to eliminate obstruction. Oral feedings withheld, nasogastric tube placed for suction, and intravenous therapy provided. Surgery consists of resecting obstructed area of bowel and anastomosing nonaffected bowel.

Continued

TABLE 24-10

Congenital Anomalies—cont'd

ANOMALY	DESCRIPTION	TREATMENT
Anorectal malformation 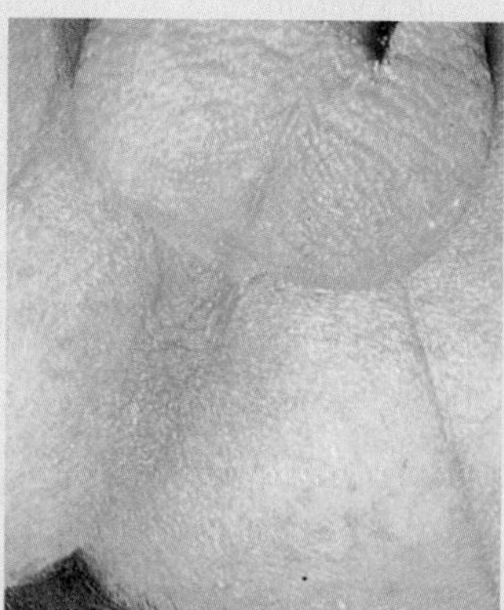 Imperforate anus. (From Chessell, G., Jamieson, M. J., Morton, R., Petrie, J., & Towler, H. [1984]. *Diagnostic picture tests in clinical medicine* [Vol. 2]. St. Louis: Mosby.)	Wide range of congenital disorders involving anus and rectum and genitourinary system in many cases. Occurs more in male than in female infants. Ranges from no anal opening to a fistula from rectum to perineum or genitourinary system.	Extensive surgical repair often required in stages for the more complex types of anorectal malformations. Anomaly may involve stenotic areas, or there may be a thin translucent membrane covering the anal opening.
MUSCULOSKELETAL SYSTEM ANOMALIES		
Developmental dysplasia of the hip (DDH)	Spectrum of disorders related to abnormal development of hip that can develop at any time during fetal life, infancy, or childhood. Characterized by hip joint laxity, subluxation, or dislocation.	Treatment varies with age of child and extent of dysplasia. Maintain hip joint by dynamic splinting with the proximal femur centered in the acetabulum in an attitude of flexion. The Pavlik harness is the most widely used, and with time, motion, and gravity, the hip works into a more abducted, reduced position.
Clubfoot	Complex deformity of ankle and foot that includes forefoot adduction, midfoot supination, hindfoot varus, and ankle equinus. Variations include: ***Talipes varus:*** an inversion or a bending inward ***Talipes valgus:*** an eversion or bending outward ***Talipes equinus:*** plantar flexion in which the toes are lower than the heel ***Talipes calcaneus:*** dorsiflexion, in which the toes are higher than the heels.	Serial casting is begun shortly after birth. Manipulation and casting are repeated frequently (every week) for 8 to 12 weeks. A continuous passive motion (CPM) machine is used to stretch and strengthen muscle groups involved (Faulks & Luther, 2005). A Denis Browne splint can be used to manage feet that correct with casting and manipulation.

TABLE 24-10

Congenital Anomalies—cont'd

ANOMALY	DESCRIPTION	TREATMENT
Polydactyly	Extra digits on hands or feet.	If little or no bone involvement exists, the extra digit is tied with silk suture soon after birth. The finger falls off within a few days, leaving a small scar. When bone involvement exists, surgical repair is indicated.
GENITOURINARY SYSTEM ANOMALIES		
Hypospadias 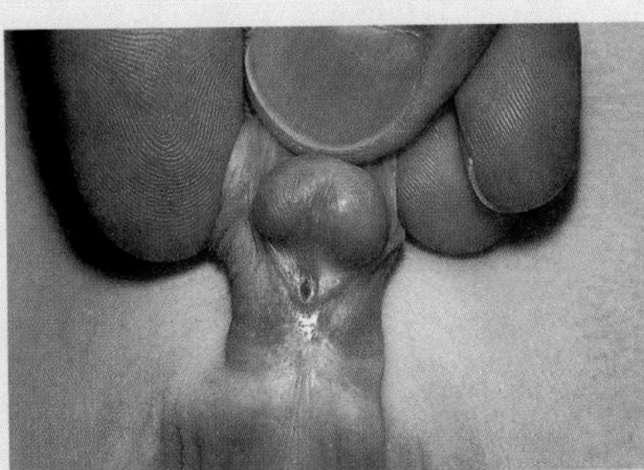 Hypospadias. (Courtesy H. Gil Rushton, MD, Children's National Medical Center, Washington, DC.)	Penile anomalies associated with abnormally located urinary meatus. The meatus can open below the glans penis or anywhere along the ventral surface of the penis, the scrotum, or the perineum.	Mild cases of hypospadias are often repaired for cosmetic reasons and involve a single surgical procedure. Consult urologist before circumcision to see if foreskin is needed for repair.
Epispadias (rare)	Male infants have a widened pubic symphysis and a broad spadelike penis with the urethra opened on its dorsal surface; female infants have a wide urethra and a bifid clitoris.	Surgical correction is necessary, and affected male infants should not be circumcised.
Exstrophy of the bladder 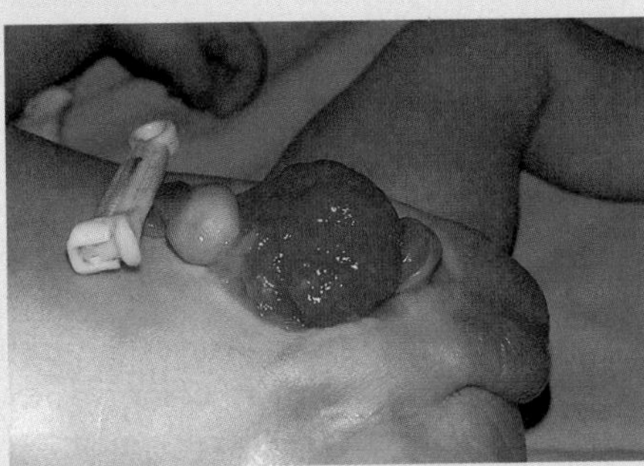 Exstrophy of bladder. (Courtesy H. Gil Rushton, MD, Children's National Medical Center, Washington, DC.)	Bladder anomaly resulting from the abnormal development of the bladder, abdominal wall, and the symphysis pubis that causes the bladder, urethra, and ureteral orifices to all be exposed.	Immediately after birth cover exposed bladder with sterile, nonadherent dressing to protect it until closure can be performed. Preferably close the bladder during the first or second day of life.

Continued

TABLE 24-10

Congenital Anomalies—cont'd

ANOMALY	DESCRIPTION	TREATMENT
Ambiguous genitalia Ambiguous external genitalia (i.e., structure may be enlarged clitoral hood and clitoris or micropenis and bifid scrotum). (Courtesy Edward S. Tank, MD, Division of Urology, Oregon Health Sciences University, Portland, OR.)	Erroneous or abnormal sexual differentiation.	Therapeutic intervention should be started as soon as possible. Assign gender but do not perform irreversible surgery.
Teratoma	Embryonal tumor that can be solid, cystic, or mixed. Composed of at least two and usually three types of embryonal tissue: ectoderm, mesoderm, and endoderm. Teratoma in the newborn may occur in the skull, mediastinum, abdomen, or sacral area; more than one half are located in the sacrococcygeal area.	The treatment of choice is complete surgical resection in the neonatal period.

CHF, Congestive heart failure; *CNS*, central nervous system; *CSF*, cerebral spinal fluid.

ⓔ Spanish Guidelines: Intensive Care Nursery: Parent Teaching on First Visit

A major nursing function is providing emotional support to the family during all aspects of the care of the child born with an anomaly or disorder. The feelings stemming from the real or imagined threat posed by a congenital anomaly are as varied as the people being counseled. Responses can include apathy, denial, anger, hostility, fear, embarrassment, grief, and loss of self-esteem.

Parents can benefit from seeing before-and-after pictures of other babies born with the same defect. Coupled with other verbal and nonverbal supportive care, this visual reassurance can be effective in allaying their concerns.

Families need much information, guidance, and support as they make decisions regarding the care of their infant. Once they have been given the facts and possible consequences and all the assistance they need in problem solving, the final decision regarding a course of action must be their own. Supporting the decision of the family is then incumbent on health care providers.

Support of Parents of a High Risk Neonate

The nurse as support person and teacher shapes the environment and makes caregiving more responsive to the needs of parents and infant. Nurses are instrumental in helping parents learn who their infant is and to recognize behavioral cues in his or her development.

If a high risk birth is anticipated, the family can be given a tour of the NICU or shown a video to prepare them for the sights and activities of the unit. After the birth the parents can be given a booklet, be shown a video, or have someone describe what they will see when they go to the unit to see their infant. As soon as possible the parents should see and touch their infant so that they can begin to acknowledge the reality of the birth and the infant's true appearance and condition (see Fig. 24-1). They will need encouragement to begin to accomplish the psychologic tasks imposed by the preterm birth. A nurse and primary health care provider should be present during the parent's first visit to see the infant for the following reasons:

- To help them "see" the infant rather than focus on equipment (the significance and function of the apparatus that surrounds the infant should be explained.)
- To explain the characteristics normal for an infant of their baby's gestational age (in this way, parents do not compare their infant with a full-term healthy baby.)
- To encourage the parent to express feelings about the pregnancy, labor, and birth and the experience of having a preterm infant
- To assess the parents' perceptions of the infant and determine the appropriate time for them to become actively involved in care

Both parents, but especially the mother, are encouraged to visit the nursery as desired and help with the infant's care. When the family cannot be present physically, staff members devise appropriate methods to keep the family in frequent touch with the newborn, such as daily telephone calls, notes written as if from the infant, video or photographs of the baby (see Community Activity box below).

Support groups for parents of infants in intensive care nurseries are often a source of comfort and encouragement for parents who can feel isolated from peers because of the birth of the preterm infant. These groups encourage parents experiencing anxiety and grief to share their feelings. A parent with NICU experience often makes contact with a new member and provides additional support. These parents provide support for the new NICU parent through hospital visits, telephone contact, and home visits.

Parents of infants in a neonatal intensive care unit have identified the following four central themes for staff to consider when caring for the neonate and family: (1) nurturing the parents, (2) providing accurate and consistent information, (3) clarifying policies for neonatal treatment and family interaction, and (4) helping parents of neonates connect with other parents in the neonatal intensive care unit and graduates of such care (Woodwell, 2002). Ward (2001) developed the 20-item NICU Family Needs Inventory to help identify the particular needs of parents with an infant in the NICU. Perceived needs identified in the initial study included providing information about the infant's condition and treatment plan, answering parents' questions honestly, actively listening to parents' fears and concerns, assisting parents in understanding the infant's responses, and providing assurance.

Some high risk infants can be discharged earlier than expected. Criteria for early discharge require the infant to be physiologically stable, receiving adequate nutrition and gaining weight daily, and to have a stable body temperature in an open bassinet. In addition, screening for hyperbilirubinemia, newborn metabolic and hematologic conditions, and safe transportation (car seat testing), as well as hearing tests, should occur before the preterm infant's discharge; an evaluation of the home environment and resources, as well as appropriate medical follow up, are essential. The parents or other caregivers must exhibit physical, emotional, and educational readiness to assume care of the infant. Ideally the home environment is adequate for meeting the needs of the infant. The parents need to show that they know the way to take the infant's temperature, to recognize the signs and symptoms to report, and to understand the dietary needs of the infant.

COMMUNITY ACTIVITY

A multiparous, single woman has a preterm infant who was born at 28 weeks of gestation and is subsequently transported to a special care nursery in a city 45 miles away from her home town. She is to be discharged tomorrow. The health care team anticipates that the infant will require a stay in the neonatal intensive care unit for at least 6 weeks. What information should the transport team provide the mother? What types of assistance will this mother need now? Identify resources in the community with services that may be beneficial for the woman. Use your community or town as a guide to such resources.

Parent Education

Cardiopulmonary resuscitation

Sudden infant death syndrome (SIDS) is more likely to occur in preterm infants than in term infants; infants discharged from an NICU are approximately twice as likely to die unexpectedly during the first year of life as infants in the general population. Instruction in cardiopulmonary resuscitation (CPR) is essential for parents of all infants but especially for parents of infants at risk for life-threatening events. Risk factors include preterm birth, apnea and bradycardia spells, neurologic immaturity, and the tendency to choke. Before taking the infant home, parents must be able to administer infant CPR. All parents should be encouraged to obtain instruction in CPR at the hospital, local Red Cross, or other community agency. An important point to emphasize is that CPR knowledge does not preclude or substitute for proper positioning of the infant in the crib (i.e., supine) when put to sleep, unless otherwise directed by the primary care physician. In addition, the bed should have a firm mattress and be free of extra blankets, stuffed animals, or toys, which may cause the infant to become entangled and subsequently smothered.

DISCHARGE PLANNING

Discharge planning for the high risk newborn begins early in the hospitalization. Throughout the infant's hospitalization the nurse gathers information from the health care team members and the family. This information is used to determine the infant's and family's readiness for discharge. Discharge teaching for the high risk newborn family is extensive, requires time and planning, and cannot be adequately accomplished on the day of discharge. Information is provided about infant care, especially as it pertains to the particular infant's home care needs (e.g., supplemental oxygen, gastrostomy feedings, follow-up medical visits). Parents should be given the opportunity to spend a night or two in a predischarge room providing care for the infant away from the NICU to become better acquainted with the necessary care and to have a time of transition in which questions may be answered regarding home care. Additional parent teaching should include bathing and skin care; requirements for meeting nutritional needs following discharge; safety in the home, including supine sleep position and prevention of infection (e.g., RSV); and medication administration (see Community Activity box below).

Durable medical equipment and supplies required for the care of the infant in the home should be delivered to the home before the infant is discharged; parents and care providers should have ample opportunity and education in the use of the equipment. Parents of infants being discharged with special needs such as gavage or gastrostomy feedings, nasal cannula oxygen, tracheostomy, or colostomy should receive several days of thoroughly planned education in the procedure before discharge. Preterm infants have a high rate of emergency room visits and readmission to acute care centers; the family absolutely must have a health professional they can contact for questions regarding infant care and behavior once they are home. Parents should obtain an age-appropriate car seat before the discharge of their infant and demonstrate its use with the infant. Car seat safety is an essential aspect of discharge planning, and infants who were born at less than 37 weeks of gestation should have a period of observation in an appropriate car seat to monitor for possible apnea, bradycardia, and decreased SaO_2.

Before discharge, all high risk or preterm infants should receive the appropriate immunizations, metabolic screening, hematologic assessment (bilirubin risk as appropriate), and evaluation of hearing. Successful discharge of high risk infants to their homes requires a multidisciplinary approach. Medical, nursing, social services, and other professionals (physical therapy, occupational therapy, developmental follow-up specialist) are crucial to the smooth transition of these infants and their families to the community and home. If the infant is transported back to the community hospital that referred either the mother before birth or the infant after birth, interfacility communication is essential to continuity of care. Consult a pediatric text for further information on discharge planning.

COMMUNITY ACTIVITY

Contact a local hospital neonatal intensive care unit. Talk with a member of the health care team about discharge teaching for parents who are preparing to take their high risk infant home. Inquire about the following topics: cardiopulmonary resuscitation, oxygen therapy, suctioning, nutrition, and developmental care. Identify resources in the community that assist families to care for high risk infants. Include cost and accessibility of care. What follow-up care is provided for high risk infants after discharge?

TRANSPORT TO AND FROM A REGIONAL CENTER

If a hospital is not equipped to care for a high risk mother and fetus or a high risk infant, transfer to a specialized perinatal or regional tertiary-care center is arranged. Maternal transport ideally occurs with the fetus in utero because of two distinct advantages: (1) neonatal morbidity and mortality are decreased, and (2) the mother and infant are not separated at birth. However, physicians and nurses in all facilities must have the skills and equipment necessary for making an accurate diagnosis and implementing emergency interventions to stabilize the infant's condition until transport can occur (Pettett, Pallotto, & Merenstein, 2006).

Arrangements for transport to an intensive care facility are made as soon as the high risk infant is identified. The infant must be kept warm and adequately oxygenated (including intubation and surfactant replacement as indicated), have vital signs and SaO_2 monitored, and receive an intravenous infusion when indicated. The infant is transported in a specially designed incubator unit containing a complete life-support system and other emergency equipment that can be carried by ambulance, helicopter, or a fixed-wing aircraft. The transport team may consist of physicians, nurse practitioners, nurses, and respiratory therapists. The team must have experience in resuscitation, stabilizations, and provision of critical care during the transport. Teams provide information for the parents about the tertiary center (Box 24-3).

BOX 24-3
Information for Parents about the Tertiary-Care Center

- Exact location of the unit—address, map, waiting area for relatives and friends
- Visiting hours and hospital rules
- Telephone numbers
- Names of individuals likely to be involved with the newborn's care (e.g., primary nurse, neonatologist, clinical manager)
- Information about the special care unit—what it is, what it does
- Location of parking facilities, nearby lodging, and rules regarding visitation by young children (siblings)
- Any particular rules or regulations regarding the special care unit

Source: Rojas, M.A., Shirley, K., & Rush, M.G. (2011). Perinatal transport and levels of care. In S. Gardner, B. Carter, M. Enzman-Hines, & J. Hernandez (Eds.). *Merenstein & Gardner's handbook of neonatal intensive care* (7th ed.). St. Louis: Mosby.

Infants may need to be transferred back (back transport) to the referring facility; however, in most cases the infant is discharged home from the tertiary-care center. Preterm infants who require thermoregulation and gavage feedings may be cared for in community hospitals closer to the parents' home, which allows parents to visit their infant more easily and to work with their personal health care provider on the long-range expected outcomes for the infant. Specialized incubators make these trips possible. However, parents may express mixed feelings about such return transports and may be reluctant to adapt to a different facility and group of caregivers. To minimize some of these concerns, giving the parents very clear information about return transports during the initial discharge planning is important.

GRIEVING THE LOSS OF A NEWBORN

Pregnancy and birth are usually happy events, but they can be associated with loss and grief. For example, the experience of preterm labor and birth or cesarean birth involves loss of the expected pregnancy and birth plans. Parents also may grieve over the sex or appearance of their child. For some parents, loss is associated with the birth of an infant who has a birth defect, genetic disorder, or chronic illness. For other couples, infertility may thwart their plans and desires for parenthood and cause intense feelings of grief.

The death of a twin or baby in a multifetal gestation during pregnancy, labor, birth, or after birth requires parents to parent and grieve at the same time. Parents may feel torn regarding how they should feel. They may have difficulty parenting their surviving child with all the joy and enthusiasm of new parents because their surviving child reminds them of what they have lost. Yet, they may also have difficulty fully grieving their loss because their surviving child demands their attention.

Bereaved parents should be warned that well-meaning family members or friends may say, "Well, at least you have the other baby," implying that there should be no grief because they are lucky to have one at all. Parents need to be able to anticipate insensitivity to their loss and be empowered to say to those people, "That is not how I feel." By simply setting a boundary on what their feelings are, they are able to acknowledge the baby who died and then have an opportunity to share more about their feelings if they so choose.

Nurses have a powerful influence on how parents experience and cope with perinatal loss. Nurses encounter these parents in a variety of settings, including the antepartum, labor and birth, neonatal, postpartum, and gynecologic units of hospitals, and obstetric, gynecologic, and infertility outpatient clinics and general medical offices. Nurses in many inpatient settings have developed protocols that provide clear direction to all staff as to how to help parents through this difficult process. In these settings, nurses have opportunities to provide sensitive and caring interventions to parents. Parents have reported that their nurses were an important resource in helping them cope with their grief (Fig. 24-12).

BOX 24-4

Conceptual Model of Parental Grief

PHASE OF ACUTE DISTRESS

- Shock
- Numbness
- Intense crying
- Depression

PHASE OF INTENSE GRIEF

- Loneliness, emptiness, and yearning
- Guilt
- Anger, resentment, bitterness, irritability
- Fear and anxiety (especially about getting pregnant again)
- Disorganization
- Difficulties with cognitive processing
- Sadness and depression
- Physical symptoms

REORGANIZATION

- Search for meaning
- Reduction of distress
- Reentering normal life activities with more enthusiasm
- Can make future plans, including decision about another pregnancy

Sources: Miles, M. (1980). *The grief of parents … when a child dies.* Oak Brook, IL: Compassionate Friends; Miles, M. (1984). Helping adults mourn the death of a child. In H. Wass & C. Corr (Eds.), *Childhood and death.* New York: Hemisphere.

ⓔ Nursing Care Plan: Fetal Death: 24 Weeks of Gestation

GRIEF RESPONSES

Grief, or **bereavement**, has been described as a cluster of painful responses experienced by individuals coping with the death of someone with whom they had a close relationship, generally a relative or close friend (Lindemann, 1944). Parental grief responses occur in three overlapping phases (Miles, 1984) (Box 24-4). There is an early period of acute distress and shock, followed by a period of intense grief that includes emotional, cognitive, behavioral, and physical responses. The phase of reorganization is reached when parents return to their usual level of functioning in society, although the pain associated with the death remains. The duration of grief varies with the individual, but there is general agreement that grief is a long-term process that can extend for months and years. With a very close relationship such as with one's baby, some aspects of grief never truly end.

FAMILY ASPECTS OF GRIEF

Grandparents and Siblings

It is extremely important for the nurse taking care of these patients to keep in mind that they have an entire family to care for, including especially grandparents and siblings.

Present Thoughts and Feelings About Your Loss

Each of the items is a statement of thoughts and feelings that some people have concerning a loss such as yours. There are no right or wrong responses to these statements. For each item, circle the number that best indicates the extent to which you agree or disagree with the statement at the present time. If you are not certain, use the "neither" category. Please try to use this category only when you truly have no opinion.

		Strongly agree	Agree	Neither agree nor disagree	Disagree	Strongly disagree
1.	I feel depressed.	1	2	3	4	5
2.	I find it hard to get along with certain people.	1	2	3	4	5
3.	I feel empty inside.	1	2	3	4	5
4.	I can't keep up with my normal activities.	1	2	3	4	5
5.	I feel a need to talk about the baby.	1	2	3	4	5
6.	I am grieving for the baby.	1	2	3	4	5
7.	I am frightened.	1	2	3	4	5
8.	I have considered suicide since the loss.	1	2	3	4	5
9.	I take medicine for my nerves.	1	2	3	4	5
10.	I very much miss the baby.	1	2	3	4	5
11.	I feel I have adjusted well to the loss.	1	2	3	4	5
12.	It is painful to recall memories of the baby.	1	2	3	4	5
13.	I get upset when I think about the baby.	1	2	3	4	5
14.	I cry when I think about him/her.	1	2	3	4	5
15.	I feel guilty when I think about the baby.	1	2	3	4	5
16.	I feel physically ill when I think about the baby.	1	2	3	4	5
17.	I feel unprotected in a dangerous world since he/she died.	1	2	3	4	5
18.	I try to laugh, but nothing seems funny anymore.	1	2	3	4	5
19.	Time passes so slowly since the baby died.	1	2	3	4	5
20.	The best part of me died with the baby.	1	2	3	4	5
21.	I have let people down since the baby died.	1	2	3	4	5
22.	I feel worthless since he/she died.	1	2	3	4	5
23.	I blame myself for the baby's death.	1	2	3	4	5
24.	I get cross at my friends and relatives more than I should.	1	2	3	4	5
25.	Sometimes I feel like I need a professional counselor to help me get my life back together again.	1	2	3	4	5
26.	I feel as though I'm just existing and not really living since he/she died.	1	2	3	4	5
27.	I feel so lonely since he/she died.	1	2	3	4	5
28.	I feel somewhat apart and remote, even among friends.	1	2	3	4	5
29.	It's safer not to love.	1	2	3	4	5
30.	I find it difficult to make decisions since the baby died.	1	2	3	4	5
31.	I worry about what my future will be like.	1	2	3	4	5
32.	Being a bereaved parent means being a "second-class citizen."	1	2	3	4	5
33.	It feels great to be alive.	1	2	3	4	5

Scoring Instructions

The total PGS score is arrived at by first reversing all of the items except 11 and 33. By reversing the items, higher scores now reflect more intense grief. Then add the scores together. The result is a total scale consisting of 33 items with a possible range of 33-165.

The three subscales consist of the sum of the scores of 11 items each, with a possible range of 11-55.

Subscale 1 Active Grief	Subscale 2 Difficulty Coping	Subscale 3 Despair
1	2	9
3	4	15
5	8	16
6	11*	17
7	21	18
10	24	20
12	25	22
13	26	23
14	28	29
19	30	31
27	33*	32

*Do not reverse.

Fig. 24-12 The Perinatal Grief Scale (33-item short version). (From Toedter, L., Lasker, J., & Janssen, H. (2001). International comparison of studies using the Perinatal Grief Scale: A decade of research on pregnancy loss. *Death Studies, 25*(3), 205-228.)

The grief of grandparents is often complicated by the fact that they are experiencing intense emotional pain by witnessing and feeling the immense grief of their own child with very few ways to comfort and end their pain. On occasions, some grandparents experience immense "survivor guilt" because they feel the death is out of order as they are alive and their grandchild has died.

The siblings of the expected infant also experience a profound loss. Most children have been prepared for having another child in the family once the pregnancy is confirmed. These children come in all ages and stages of development, and this must be considered in understanding how they view the event and their loss experience. A young child will respond more to the response of the parents, picking up on the fact that they are behaving differently and are extremely sad. This can cause clinging, altered eating and sleeping patterns, or acting out behaviors, yet it is a time when parents have limited patience for responding to and meeting the needs of the child. Older children have a more complete understanding of the loss. School-aged children may be frightened by the entire event, whereas teens may understand fully but feel awkward in responding. Nurses need to help parents recognize and be sensitive to the grief of siblings, include siblings in family grief rituals, and keep the baby alive in the family's memory.

Nurses assist parents in identifying resources needed for support during this difficult time. In addition to family members, the parents may desire the presence of their church minister or hospital chaplain.

CARE MANAGEMENT

Nursing care of mothers and fathers experiencing a perinatal loss begins the first time the parents are faced with the potential loss of their pregnancy or death of their infant. Supportive interventions are important both at the time of the loss and after the parents have returned home (Nursing Process box).

Nursing Interventions

Help actualize the loss

When a loss or death occurs, the nurse should be sure that parents have been honestly told about the situation by their physician or others on the health care team. It is important for their nurse to be with them during this time. With infant death, caregivers should use the words "dead" and "died," rather than "lost" or "gone," to assist the bereaved in accepting this reality. Parents need opportunities to tell their story about the events, experiences, and feelings surrounding the loss. This can help them come to terms with the reality of their loss. Listening to them express their pain and allowing them time to absorb the information are important.

One way of actualizing the loss is to tell the parents the sex of the baby and give them the option of naming the fetus or infant who has died. Choosing a name helps make the baby a member of their family.

NURSING ALERT It is important to be sensitive about naming. This is an individual decision that should never be imposed on parents. Beliefs and needs vary widely among individuals and across cultures and religions. Cultural taboos and rules in some religious faiths prohibit the naming of an infant who has died.

For some mothers and fathers, it is helpful to see the fetus or baby as a way of becoming acquainted and of separating. Many professionals believe that seeing the fetus or baby helps parents face the reality of the loss, reduces painful fantasies, and offers an opportunity for closure. However, encouraging reluctant parents to hold or see their dead child by telling them that not seeing the child could make mourning more difficult is not appropriate. A question such as, "Some parents have found it helpful to see their baby. Would you like time to consider this?" Because the need or willingness to see also may vary between the mother and father, it is extremely important to determine what each parent really wants. This should not be a joint decision made by one person or a decision made for the parents by grandparents or others.

In preparation for the visit with the baby, parents appreciate explanations about what to expect. Descriptions of how the baby looks are important. For example, babies may have red, peeling skin like a bad sunburn, dark discoloration similar to bruises, molding of the head that makes the head look soft and swollen, or birth defects. The nurse should make the baby look as normal as possible, and remember that parents see their baby differently from the way health care professionals do. Bathing the baby, applying lotion to the baby's skin, combing hair, placing identification bracelets on the arm and leg, dressing the baby in a diaper and special outfit, sprinkling powder in the baby's blanket, and wrapping the baby in a pretty blanket conveys to the parents that their baby has been cared for in a special way (Fig. 24-13). If the baby has been in the morgue, he or she can be placed underneath a warmer for 20 to 30 minutes and wrapped in a warm blanket before being brought to the parents. Cold cream rubbed over stiffened joints can help in positioning the baby. The use of powder and lotion stimulates the parent's senses and provides pleasant memories of their baby.

When bringing the baby to the parents, it is important to treat the baby as one would a live baby. Holding the baby close, touching a hand or cheek, using the baby's name, and talking with the parents about the special features of their child conveys that it is acceptable for them to do likewise. If a baby has a congenital anomaly, the nurse can desensitize the family by pointing out aspects of the baby that are normal. Nurses can help parents explore the baby's body as they desire. Parents often seek to identify family resemblance. A good question might be: "Who in your family does Michael resemble?"

NURSING PROCESS *Loss and Grief*

ASSESSMENT

Key areas to address include the following:

- The nature of the parental attachment with the pregnancy or infant, the meaning of the pregnancy and infant to the parent, and the related losses they are experiencing. The meaning of the loss is determined by familial and cultural systems of the parents.
- The circumstances surrounding the loss, including the level of preparation for the loss and the parents' level of understanding about the cause of the loss or death, and any related unresolved issues.
- The immediate response of the mother and father to the loss, whether their responses are complementary or problematic, and how their responses match with their past experiences, personalities, and behavioral and cultural backgrounds.
- The amount and type of support that a couple wants; some prefer to handle the tragedy alone for a time; others want assistance in calling family members, friends, and clergy to be with them and to help them with decisions.

NURSING DIAGNOSES

Nursing diagnoses may include physiologic and psychosocial problems experienced by the individual mother or father, or problems occurring within the couple or family because of the loss and subsequent grief. Examples of nursing diagnoses include the following:

- *Ineffective family coping* related to
  - inability to make decisions as a family
  - difficulties in communication within the family
  - conflicting coping patterns between mother and father
- *Powerlessness* related to
  - high risk pregnancy and birth
  - unexpected cesarean birth
  - inability to prevent the infant's death
- *Interrupted family processes* related to
  - maternal depression leading to changes in role function
  - inadequate communication of feelings between the grieving mother and father
  - lack of expected support from family
  - behavioral and emotional reactions of siblings
  - grief within the family system including grandparents and other relatives
- *Fatigue* and *disturbed sleep pattern* related to
  - inability to fall asleep because of grief
  - waking in the night and thinking about the loss
  - loss of sleep
- *Dysfunctional grieving* related to
  - prolonged denial or avoidance of the loss
  - intense guilt related to the loss
  - continued anger about the loss
  - serious depressive symptoms and despair
  - loss of self-esteem
  - intense grieving patterns that continue for more than a year
  - social isolation due to grief
- *Spiritual distress* related to
  - anger with God
  - confusion about why prayers were not answered

EXPECTED OUTCOMES OF CARE

Expected outcomes are set and priorities assigned in patient-centered terms according to the mutual goals chosen by the patient and the nurse and may include that the woman/family will do the following:

- Actualize the loss.
- Feel supported by the nursing staff throughout their hospital stay and when visiting the clinic.
- Understand the normal grief responses they and others in the family may experience at the time of and after the loss.
- Identify family, spiritual, health care, and community resources for support.

PLAN OF CARE AND INTERVENTIONS

- Interventions and support for parents from the nursing and medical staff after a perinatal loss or infant death are extremely important in their healing. Care must be individualized for each parent and family.
- The cultural and spiritual beliefs and practices of individual parents and families must be considered. The interventions discussed in the text are general ideas about what may be helpful to parents.
- Documentation in the nursing notes of primary concerns, grief responses, health teaching, health care advice, and any referrals of the mother or other family members is essential to ensure continuity and consistency of care.

EVALUATION

The evaluation of nursing care is made more difficult by the shock and numbness of the bereavement process and the varied grief responses of the parents and other family members during hospitalization. The achievement of expected outcomes is assured when positive integration of the perinatal loss is expressed by the family.

Some families may like to have the opportunity to bathe and dress their baby. Although the skin may be fragile, parents can still apply lotion with cotton balls, sprinkle powder, tie ribbons, fasten the diaper, and place amulets, medallions, rosaries, or special toys or mementos in their baby's hands or alongside their baby. Volunteers in communities across the country make special burial clothes to give to parents at this difficult time.

Parents need to be offered time alone with their baby if they wish. They also need to know when the nurse will return and how to call if they should need anything. If at all possible, the family should be placed in a private room and, when possible, the room should have a rocking chair for the parents to sit in when holding their baby. This offers the mother and father special time together with their baby and with other family members (Fig. 24-14). Marking the

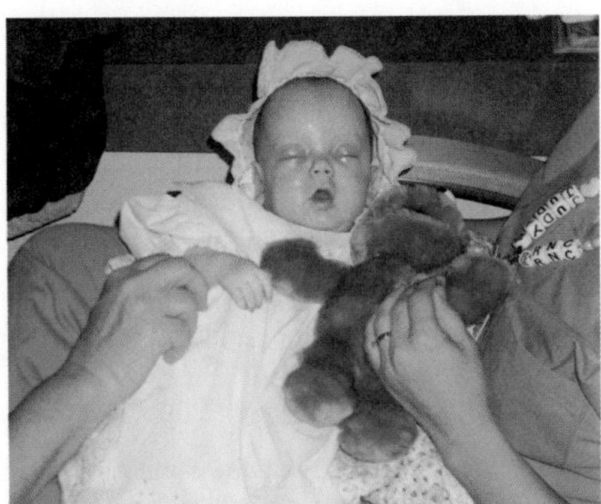

Fig. 24-13 Laura. (Courtesy Amy and Ken Turner, Cary, NC.)

door to the room with a special card can be helpful in reminding the staff that this family has experienced a loss.

It is difficult to predict how long and how often parents will need to spend time with their baby. Some parents need only a few minutes; others need hours. It is extremely painful for some parents to say good-bye to their baby. They will tell the nurse verbally and nonverbally when they are ready. The nurse should watch for cues that the parents have had enough time with their baby, such as when parents are no longer holding their child close to them or have placed the baby back in the crib. Sensitivity to parental needs in actualizing the loss and coping with the reality of the death is essential for their healing. Grandparents should be offered the same opportunities to hold, rock, swaddle, and love their grandchildren so that their grief is started in a healthy way.

Help the parents with decision making

At a time when they are experiencing the great distress of a perinatal loss, and especially if the loss was of an infant, parents have many decisions to make. Mothers, fathers, and extended families look to the medical and nursing staff for guidance in knowing what decisions they must and can make, and in understanding the options related to those decisions (Table 24-11). The hospital chaplain, church minister, or social worker may be helpful to the family in their decision making.

LEGAL TIP **Laws Regarding Live Birth**

Laws in all states govern what constitutes a live birth. In most states a live birth is considered to be any products of conception expelled from a woman that show any signs of life. Signs of life are considered to be any muscle irritability, respiratory effort, or heart rate, regardless of gestational age. All nurses should be knowledgeable about their state laws regarding what constitutes a live birth and what forms must be completed and filed in the case of fetal death, stillbirth, or newborn death.

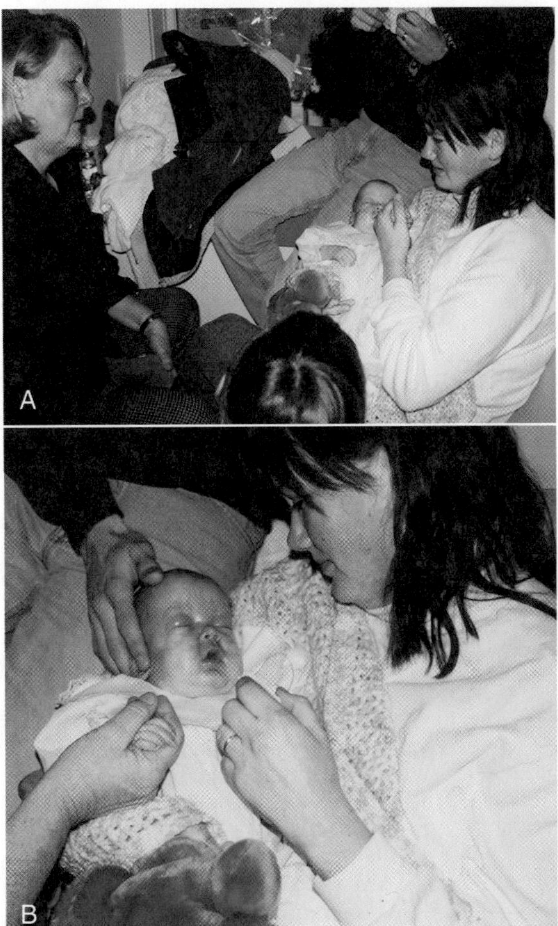

Fig. 24-14 Laura's family members say a special good-bye. (Courtesy Amy and Ken Turner, Cary, NC.)

Final disposition of all identifiable babies, regardless of gestational age, includes burial or cremation. Depending on the cemetery's policies, babies in caskets or the ashes from cremated babies can be buried in a special place designated for babies, at the foot of a deceased relative, in a separate plot, or in a mausoleum. Ashes also may be scattered in a designated area; many states have regulations regarding where ashes can be scattered. A local funeral director or a state's Vital Statistics Bureau should have information about the state's rules, codes, and regulations regarding live births, burial requirements, transportation of the deceased by parents, and cremation.

In making final arrangements for their baby, parents may want a special service. They may choose to have a service in the hospital chapel, visitation at a funeral home or their own home, a funeral service in their own church, or a graveside service. Parents can make any of these services as special, personal, and memorable as they like. They can choose special music, poetry, or prose written by themselves or others.

If the family has decided on a funeral and burial, they still have decisions about what funeral home to call and where to bury the baby. Many couples may be living in

TABLE 24-11

Decisions Parents Must Make

DECISION	PROS	CONS
Autopsy	• May answer question "why" • Helps to process grief and perhaps prevent another loss	• Autopsies are expensive and not covered by insurance • Parents may feel baby has been through enough and prefer not to have further information about cause of death • Some religions prohibit autopsy or limit it
Organ donation (most common is cornea)	• Aid to grief; helps family see something positive associated with their experience	• Prefer to have baby remain intact
Spiritual rituals	• Support of clergy • Baptism when appropriate • Other rituals such as a blessing, a naming ceremony, anointing, ritual of the sick, memorial service, or prayer	• Family chooses to have no religious or spiritual rituals
Disposition of the body	• In most states, if a baby is at least 20 weeks and 1 day of gestational age or is born alive, it is the parents' responsibility to make the final arrangements for their baby • Choices are burial or cremation • A baby younger than 20 weeks of gestation is considered a product of conception, whereas embryos, uterine tubes removed with an ectopic pregnancy, and tissue from a pregnancy obtained during a dilation and curettage are all considered tissue. Many hospitals will make arrangements for free cremation of these infants or tissue.	• Cost of burial or cremation • Responsibility for making arrangements • If hospital arranges for cremation, family will not receive the ashes

an area distant from their family homes, and they may want to bury their child in their hometown or family cemetery. If the family desires cremation, they may want to have the option of obtaining the ashes. It is important to determine whether this will be done by the facility conducting the cremations (e.g., hospitals which cremate the products of conception also dispose of the ashes).

Help the bereaved to acknowledge and express their feelings

One of the most important goals of the nurse is to validate the experience and feelings of the parents by encouraging them to tell their stories and listening with care. At the very least, the nurse should acknowledge the loss with a simple but sincere comment such as "I'm sorry about the baby." Helping the parents to talk about their loss and the meaning it has for their lives and to share their emotional pain is the next step. "Tell me about what happened." Because nurses tend to be very focused on the physical and emotional needs of the mother, it is especially important to ask the father directly about his views of what happened and his feelings of loss.

The nurse should listen patiently during the story of loss or grief, but listening is hard work and can be painful for the helper. The feelings and emotions of expressed grief can overwhelm health care professionals. Being with someone who is terribly sad and crying or sobbing can be extremely difficult. The initial impulse to reduce one's sense of helplessness is to say or do something that you think will reduce their pain. Although such a response may seem supportive at the time, it can stifle the further expression of emotion. Bereaved parents have identified many unhelpful responses given by well-meaning health care professionals, family, and friends. The nurse should resist the temptation to give advice or to use clichés in offering support to the bereaved (Box 24-5).

Bereaved parents have many questions surrounding the event of their loss that can leave them feeling guilty. This is particularly true for mothers. Such questions include "What did I do?" "What caused this to happen?" "What do you think I should have, or could have done differently?" Part of the grief process for bereaved parents is figuring out what happened, their role in the loss, why it happened to them, and why it happened to their baby. The nurse should recognize that the answers to these questions must be answered by the bereaved themselves; it is part of their healing. For example, a bereaved mother might ask, "Do you think that this was caused by painting

BOX 24-5

What to Say and What Not to Say to Bereaved Parents

WHAT TO SAY
- "I'm sad for you."
- "How are you doing with all of this?"
- "This must be hard for you."
- "What can I do for you?"
- "I'm sorry."
- "I'm here, and I want to listen."

WHAT NOT TO SAY
- "God had a purpose for her."
- "Be thankful you have another child."
- "The living must go on."
- "I know how you feel."
- "It's God's will."
- "You have to keep on going for her sake."
- "You're young; you can have others."
- "We'll see you back here next year, and you'll be happier."
- "Now you have an angel in heaven."
- "This happened for the best."
- "Better for this to happen now, before you knew the baby."
- "There was something wrong with the baby anyway."

Used with permission of Bereavement Services. Copyright Lutheran Hospital—La Crosse, Inc., a Gundersen Lutheran Affiliate, La Crosse, WI.

COMMUNITY ACTIVITY

Identify perinatal loss support groups in your community. Attend a support group meeting from an observational perspective. Compare and contrast support modalities. When would you refer a patient? Are referral programs appropriate for all family members? Describe how the nurse can support a family through this difficult time.

the baby's room?" An appropriate response might be, "I understand you need to find an answer for why your baby died, but we really don't know why she died. What are some of the other things you have been thinking about?"

Normalize the grief process and facilitate positive coping

While helping parents share their feelings of pain, it is critical to help them understand their grief responses and feel they are not alone in these painful responses. Most parents are not prepared for the raw feelings that they experience or the fact that these painful, complex feelings and related behavioral reactions continue for many weeks or months. Reassuring them of the normality of their responses and preparing them for the long duration of their grief is important.

The nurse can help parents be prepared for the emptiness, loneliness, and yearning; for the feelings of helplessness that can lead to anger, guilt, and fear; and for the cognitive processing problems, disorganization, difficulty making decisions; and sadness and depression that are part of the grief process. Books and pamphlets about grief, if short and sensitive, can be given to parents to take home. Many parents have reported feelings of fear that they were going crazy because of the many emotions and behavioral responses that leave them feeling totally out of control in the months after the loss.

Nurses can reinforce positive coping efforts and attempt to prevent negative coping (Abboud & Liamputtong, 2005). They can remind the parents of the importance of being patient and being good to themselves during the grief process. Additional suggestions are to encourage attempts to resume normal activities; reinforce and encourage positive ways to hold onto memories of the pregnancy or baby, while letting go; and help the parent to organize a plan for daily activities, if needed. In particular, nurses should discourage overdependence on drugs and alcohol.

Meet the physical needs of the postpartum bereaved mother

The physical needs of a bereaved mother are the same as those of any woman who has given birth. The cruel reality for many bereaved mothers is that their milk may come in with no baby to nurse, their afterpains remind them of their emptiness, and gas pains feel as though a baby is still moving inside. The nurse should ensure that the mother receives appropriate medications to reduce these physical symptoms. Adequate rest, a healthful diet, and sufficient fluids must be offered to replenish her physical strength.

Mothers need postpartum care instructions on discharge. They also need ideas about how to cope with problems with sleep such as decreasing food or fluids that contain caffeine, limiting alcohol and nicotine consumption, exercising regularly, and using strategies for rest such as taking a warm bath or drinking warm milk before bedtime, performing relaxation exercises, listening to restful music, or receiving a massage. Furthermore, the couple needs to be encouraged and supported in maintaining their relationship and keeping open channels of communication. They also need to be prepared for some of the issues related to resuming sexual relations after perinatal loss.

Assist the bereaved in communicating with, supporting, and getting support from the family

Providing sensitive care to bereaved parents means including their families in the grief process. Grandparents and siblings are particularly important when a perinatal loss has occurred. However, it is up to the parents to decide to what extent they want family involved in their grief process. If it is the parents' desire, children, grandparents, extended family members, and friends should be allowed to be involved in the rituals surrounding the death, such as seeing and holding the baby. Such visits afford others the opportunity to become acquainted with the baby, to understand the parents' loss, to offer their support, and to say good-bye (see Fig. 24-14). This experience helps parents explain to their surviving children who their brother or sister was and what death means, offers the children answers to their questions in a concrete manner, and helps the children in expressing their grief (Wilson, 2001). Involving extended family and friends enables the parents to mobilize their social support system of people who will support the family not only at the time of loss but also in the future.

Create memories for parents to take home

Parents may want tangible mementos of their baby to allow them to actualize the loss. Some may want to bring in a previously purchased baby book. Special memory books, cards, and information on grief and mourning are available for purchase by parents or hospitals or clinics through national perinatal bereavement organizations (Box 24-6).

Be concerned about the cultural and spiritual needs of the parents

There are complex differences in the meaning of children and parenthood, the roles of women and men, the beliefs and knowledge about modern medicine, views about death, mourning rituals and traditions, and behavioral expressions of grief among people of differing cultures, ethnicity, and religion (Bennett, Litz, Lee, & Shira, 2005). Thus the nurse must be sensitive to the responses and needs of parents from various cultural backgrounds and religious groups. To do this, nurses need to be aware of their own values and beliefs and acknowledge the importance of understanding and accepting the values and beliefs of others, which may be different or even in conflict (Chichester, 2005). Furthermore, it is critical to understand that the individual and unique responses of a parent to a perinatal loss cannot be entirely predicted by their cultural or spiritual backgrounds. Each mother and father must be approached first as an individual needing support during a profoundly difficult and distressing life experience.

Culture and religious beliefs often affect decision making surrounding stillbirth or death of an infant. Autopsies and/or cremation are not allowed by some religious groups, except under unusual circumstances. Making a decision to end life-sustaining measures may be more difficult for members of some groups. Picture taking may conflict with beliefs of some cultures, such as among some Native Americans, Inuit, Amish, Hindus, and Muslims. In many cultures, decisions do not reside solely in the individual woman or couple but in the extended family. In Muslim families, decisions are made by the father.

Provide sensitive care at and after discharge

Leaving the hospital without a baby in her arms can be a very empty and painful experience for a woman who has experienced a pregnancy loss. It is especially difficult if others are seen leaving with babies; thus the discharge of mothers and fathers who have experienced a perinatal loss should be done with great sensitivity to their feelings. Giving the mother a special flower to carry in her arms can be a thoughtful gesture.

The grief of the mother and her family does not end with discharge; rather it really begins once they return home and start to live their lives without their baby. There are numerous models for providing follow-up care to

BOX 24-6

Creating Memories

- Provide baby's weight, length, and head circumference to the family.
- Footprints and handprints. Sometimes it is difficult to obtain good handprints or footprints. Application of alcohol or acetone on the palms or soles can help the ink adhere to make the prints clearer. When making prints, have a hard surface underneath the paper to be printed. The baby's heel or palm is placed down first, and the foot or hand is rolled forward, keeping the toes or fingers extended. Assistance may be necessary. Tracing around the baby's hands and feet can also be done, although this distorts the actual size. A form of plaster of paris can also be used to make an imprint of the baby's hand or foot.
- Articles that were in contact with or used in caring for the baby including the tape measure used to measure the baby, baby lotions, combs, clothing, hats, blankets, crib cards, and identification bands. Ask parents if they wish to have these articles before giving them to the parents.
- A lock of hair. Parents must be asked for permission before cutting a lock of hair, which can be removed from the nape of the neck where it is not noticeable.
- Pictures are an important memento. Photographs are generally taken whenever there is an identifiable baby and when it is culturally acceptable to the family. It does not matter how tiny the baby is, what the baby looks like, or how long the baby has been dead. Pictures should include close-ups of the baby's face, hands, and feet and photos of the baby clothed and wrapped in a blanket as well as unclothed. If there are any congenital anomalies, close-ups of the anomalies also should be taken. Flowers, blocks, stuffed animals, or toys can be placed in the background to make the picture more special. Parents may want their pictures taken holding the baby. Keeping a camera nearby and taking pictures when parents are spending special time with their baby can provide special memories. Some parents may have their own camera or video camera and would like the nurse to record them as they bathe, dress, hold, or diaper their baby. Other parents may not want a photo at the time of death. The nurse can take photos and place in the medical record for parents if they later decide they want them.

parents after discharge. Programs include hospital-based bereavement teams who provide support during hospitalization and follow-up contacts.

Telephone calls after a loss may be helpful to some parents; however, it must be determined which parents do not want a follow-up call. The calls are made at predictably difficult times such as the first week at home, 1 month to 6 weeks later, 4 to 6 months after the loss, and at the anniversary of the death. Families who experienced a miscarriage, ectopic pregnancy, or death of a preterm baby may appreciate a telephone call on the estimated date of birth. The calls provide an opportunity for parents to ask questions, share their feelings, seek advice, and receive information to help them in processing their grief.

A grief conference can be planned when parents return for an appointment with their doctor, nurses, and other health care providers. At the conference, the loss or death of the infant is discussed in detail, parents are given information about the baby's autopsy report and genetic studies, and they have opportunities to ask the questions that have arisen since their baby's death. Parents appreciate the opportunity to review the events of hospitalization, go over the baby's and/or mother's chart with their primary health care provider, and talk with those who cared for them and their baby during hospitalization. This is an important time to help parents understand the cause of the loss, or to accept the fact that the cause will forever be unknown. This gives health care professionals the opportunity to assess how the family is coping with their loss and provide additional information and education on grief.

Provide postmortem care

Preparation of the baby's body and transport to the morgue depends on the procedures and protocols developed by individual hospitals. The Joint Commission (www.jcaho.org) requires that appropriate care be given to the body after death. Postmortem care can be an emotional and sometimes difficult task for the nurse. However, nurses may find that providing postmortem care helps them find closure in their own grief related to a perinatal loss. This is particularly true for neonatal intensive care nurses who have cared for an infant for several hours, days, or weeks.

KEY POINTS

- Preterm infants are at risk for problems related to the immaturity of their organ systems.
- RDS, retinopathy of prematurity, and chronic lung disease (BPD) are associated with preterm birth.
- High risk infants must be observed for respiratory distress and other early signs of physiologic distress.
- The adaptation of parents to preterm or high risk infants differs from that of parents of full-term infants.
- Parents need special instruction (e.g., CPR, oxygen therapy, suctioning, developmental care) before they take a high risk infant home.
- Infants born to mothers with diabetes (gestational or otherwise) are at risk for congenital anomalies, hypoglycemia, RDS, and birth asphyxia and trauma.
- SGA infants are considered to be at risk because of fetal growth restriction.
- Nonreassuring fetal status among postmature infants is related to the progressive placental insufficiency that can occur in a postterm pregnancy.
- The identification of maternal and fetal risk factors in the antepartum and intrapartum periods is vital for planning adequate care of high risk infants.
- A small percentage of significant birth injuries may occur despite skilled and competent obstetric care.
- Infection in the newborn may be acquired in utero, at birth, in breast milk, or from within the nursery.
- The most common maternal infections during early pregnancy that are associated with various congenital malformations include toxoplasmosis, herpes, cytomegalovirus, rubella, parvovirus B19, and varicella.
- HIV transmission from mother to infant occurs transplacentally at various gestational ages, perinatally by maternal blood and secretions, and by breast milk.
- Maternal-fetal Rh and ABO incompatibility may cause significant hemolysis and jaundice in the neonatal period.
- The injection of Rh_o(D) immune globulin in Rh-negative and Coombs test–negative women minimizes the possibility of isoimmunization.
- The nurse often first observes signs of newborn drug withdrawal (neonatal abstinence syndrome) and acquires information from the maternal history.
- Congenital defects are now the leading cause of death in the first year of life.
- The curative and rehabilitative problems of a child with a congenital disorder are often complex, requiring a multidisciplinary approach to care.
- The supportive care given to the parents of infants with a congenital anomaly or inborn error of metabolism must begin at birth or at the time of diagnosis and continue for years.
- When a baby dies, all members of a family are affected, but no two family members grieve in the same way.
- Therapeutic communication and counseling techniques can help families identify their feelings, feel comfortable in expressing their grief, and understand their bereavement process.
- Follow-up after discharge can be an important component in providing care to families who have experienced a loss.

Audio Chapter Summaries Access an audio summary of these Key Points on evolve

References

Abboud, L., & Liamputtong, P. (2005). When pregnancy fails: Coping strategies, support networks and experiences with health care of ethnic women and their partners. *Journal of Reproductive and Infant Psychology, 23*(1), 3-18.

American Academy of Pediatrics (AAP) and American College of Obstetricians and Gynecologists. (2007). *Guidelines for perinatal care* (6th ed.). Elk Grove Village, IL: AAP.

American Academy of Pediatrics Committee on Infectious Diseases. (2006). *Red book: 2006 report of the committee on infectious diseases* (27th ed.). Elk Grove Village, IL: AAP.

American Academy of Pediatrics Committee on Nutrition. (2004). *Pediatric nutrition handbook* (5th ed.). Elk Grove Village, IL: AAP.

American Academy of Pediatrics Committee on Fetus and Newborn. (2004). Age terminology during the perinatal period. *Pediatrics, 114*(5), 1362-1364.

American Academy of Pediatrics Subcommittee on Hyperbilirubinemia. (2004). Clinical practice guideline: Management of hyperbilirubinemia in the newborn infant 35 or more weeks of gestation. *Pediatrics, 114*(1), 297-316.

Anderson, M. S., & Gardner, S. L. (2006). Enteral nutrition. In G. B. Merenstein. & S. L. Gardner (Eds.), *Handbook of neonatal intensive care* (6th ed.). St. Louis: Mosby.

Bakewell-Sachs, S. (2007). Near-term/late preterm infants. *Newborn & Infant Nursing Reviews, 7*(2), 67-71.

Bay, C. A., Steele, M. W., & Davis, H. (2007). Genetic disorders and dysmorphic conditions. In B. Zitelli, & H. Davis (Eds.), *Atlas of pediatric physical diagnosis* (5th ed.). St. Louis: Mosby.

Bennett, S., Litz, B., Lee, B., & Shira, M. (2005). The scope and impact of perinatal loss: Current status and future directions. *Professional Psychology, Research and Practice 36*(2), 180-187.

Blackburn, S. T. (2007). *Maternal, fetal, and neonatal physiology: A clinical perspective* (3rd ed.). St. Louis: Saunders.

Blake, W. W., & Murray, J. A. (2006). Heat balance. In G. B. Merenstein, & S. L. Gardner (Eds.), *Handbook of neonatal intensive care* (6th ed.). St. Louis: Mosby.

Byers, J. F., Waugh, W. R., & Lowman, L. B. (2006). Sound level exposure of high-risk infants in different environmental conditions. *Neonatal Network, 25*(1), 25-32.

Chichester, M. (2005). Multicultural issues in perinatal loss. *AWHONN Lifelines, 9*(4), 312-320.

Conde-Agudelo, A., & Belizan, J. M. (2003). Kangaroo mother care to reduce morbidity and mortality in low birthweight infants. In *The Cochrane Database of Systematic Reviews,* 2003, Issue 2, CD 002771.

Curley, M. A. Q., Razmus, I. S., Roberts, K. E., & Wypij, D. (2003). Predicting pressure ulcer risk in pediatric patients: The Braden Q scale. *Nursing Research, 52*(1), 22-33.

De Jong, E. P., de Haan, T. R., Kroes, A. C. M., Beersma, M. F. C., Oepkas, D., & Walther, F. J. (2006). Parvovirus B19 infection in pregnancy. *Journal of Clinical Virology, 36*(1), 1-7.

Dodd, V. L (2005). Implications of kangaroo care for growth and development in preterm infants. *Journal of Obstetric, Gynecologic, & Neonatal Nursing, 34*(2), 218-232.

Dudell, G., & Stoll, B. J. (2007). Respiratory tract disorders. In R. M. Kliegman, R. E. Behrman, H.B. Jenson, & B. F. Stanton (Eds.), *Nelson textbook of pediatrics* (18th ed.). Philadelphia: Saunders.

Ehrenkranz, R. A. (2007). Early, aggressive nutritional management for very low birth weight infants: What is the evidence? *Seminars in Perinatology, 31*(2), 48-55.

Ellett, M. L., Croffie, J. M., Cohen, M. D., & Perkins, S. M. (2005). Gastric tube placement in young children. *Clinical Nursing Research, 14*(3), 238-252.

Ellett, M. L., Woodruff, K. A., & Stewart, D. L. (2007). The use of carbon dioxide monitoring to determine orogastric tube placement in premature infants: A pilot study. *Gastroenterology Nursing, 30*(6), 414-417.

Engle, W. A. (2006). A recommendation for the definition of "late preterm" (near-term) and the birth weight–gestational age classification system. *Seminars in Perinatology, 30*(1), 2-7.

Engle, W. A., & American Academy of Pediatrics Committee on Fetus and Newborn. (2008). Surfactant replacement therapy for respiratory distress in the preterm and term neonate. *Pediatrics, 121*(2), 419-432.

Engle, W. A., Tomashek, K. M., & Wallman, C. (2007). Late–preterm infants: A population at risk, *Pediatrics, 120*(6), 1390-1401.

Faulks, S., & Luther, B. (2005). Changing paradigm for the treatment of clubfeet. *Orthopaedic Nursing, 24*(1), 25-30.

Finnegan, L. P. (1985). Neonatal abstinence. In N. Nelson (Ed.), *Current therapy in neonatal perinatal medicine 1985-1986.* Toronto: BC Decker.

Frenkel, L. (2005). Challenges in the diagnosis and management of neonatal herpes simplex virus encephalitis. *Pediatrics, 115*(3), 795-797.

Gardner, S. L., Snell, B. J., & Lawrence, R. A. (2006). Breastfeeding the neonate with special needs. In G. B. Merenstein, & S. L. Gardner (Eds.), *Handbook of neonatal intensive care* (6th ed.). St. Louis: Mosby.

Gupta, A., Della-Latta, P., Todd, B., San Gabriel, P., Haas, J., Wu, F., et al. (2004). Outbreak of extended-spectrum beta-lactamase-producing Klebsiella pneumoniae in a neonatal intensive care unit linked to artificial nails. *Infection Control Hospital Epidemiology, 25*(3), 210-215.

Hagedorn, M. I. E., Gardner, S. L., Dickey, L. A., & Abman, S. H. (2006). Respiratory diseases. In G. B. Merenstein, & S. L. Gardner (Eds.), *Handbook of neonatal intensive care* (6th ed.). St. Louis: Mosby.

Haubrich, K. (2007). Auditory system. In C. Kenner, & J. W. Lott (Eds.), *Comprehensive neonatal nursing care: An interdisciplinary approach* (4th ed.). Philadelphia: Saunders.

Holditch-Davis, D., Blackburn, S. T., & VandenBerg, K. (2007). Newborn and infant neurobehavioral development. In C. Kenner, & J. Lott (Eds.), *Comprehensive neonatal care: An interdisciplinary approach* (4th ed.). St. Louis: Saunders.

Jones, F., & Tully, M.R. (2006). *Best practices for expressing, storing and handling human milk.* Raleigh, N.C.: Human Milk Banking Association of North America.

Kalhan, S. C., & Parimi, P. S. (2006). Disorders of carbohydrate metabolism. In R. J. Martin, A. A. Fanaroff, & M. C. Walsh (Eds.), *Fanaroff and Martin's neonatal-perinatal medicine: Diseases of the fetus and infant* (8th ed.). Philadelphia: Saunders.

Kattwinkel, J. (Ed.). (2006). *Textbook of neonatal resuscitation* (5th ed.). Elk Grove Village, IL: American Academy of Pediatrics and the American Heart Association.

Kattwinkel, J., Perlman, J.M., Aziz, K., et al. (2010). Part 15: Neonatal resuscitation: 2010 American Heart Association guidelines for cardiopulmonary resuscitation and emergency cardiovascular care. *Circulation, 122*(18 Suppl), S909-S919.

Kliegman, R. M. (2006). Intrauterine growth restriction. In R. J. Martin, A. A. Fanaroff, & M. C. Walsh (Eds.), *Fanaroff and Martin's neonatal-perinatal medicine: Diseases of the fetus and infant* (8th ed.). Philadelphia: Saunders.

LaMar, K., & Dowling, D. A. (2006). Incidence of infection for preterm twins cared for in cobedding in the neonatal intensive-care unit. *Journal of Obstetric, Gynecologic, and Neonatal Nursing, 35*(2), 193-198.

Law, K. L., Stroud, L. R., LaGasse, L. L., Niaura, R., Liu, J., & Lester, B. M. (2003). Smoking during pregnancy and newborn neurobehavior. *Pediatrics, 111*(6), 1318-1323.

Lawrence, R. A., & Lawrence, R. M. (2005). *Breastfeeding: A guide for the medical profession* (6th ed.). Philadelphia: Saunders.

Lester, B. M., & Tronick, E. Z. (2004). History and description of the Neonatal Intensive Care Unit Network Neurobehavioral Scale. *Pediatrics, 113*(3), 634-640.

Lindemann, E. (1944). Symptomatology and management of acute grief. *American Journal of Psychiatry, 101*(2), 141-148.

Lott, J. W. (2007). Immune system. In C. Kenner, & J. Lott (Eds.), *Comprehensive neonatal care: An interdisciplinary approach* (4th ed.). St. Louis: Saunders.

Luchtman-Jones, L., Schwartz, A. L., & Wilson, D. B. (2006). The blood and hemopoietic system. In R. J. Martin, A. A. Fanaroff, & M. C. Walsh (Eds.), *Fanaroff and Martin's neonatal-perinatal medicine: Diseases of the fetus and infant* (8th ed.). Philadelphia: Saunders.

Ludington-Hoe, S. M., Morgan, K., & Abouelfettoh, A. (2008). A clinical guideline for implementation of kangaroo care with premature infants of 30 or more weeks' postmenstrual age. *Advances in Neonatal Care, 8*(3 Suppl.), S3-S23.

Lund, C. H., Kuller, J., Raines, D. A., Ecklund, S., Archambault, M. É., & O'Flaherty, P. (2007). *Neonatal Skin Care* (2nd ed.). Washington, D.C.: Association of Women's Health, Obstetric, and Neonatal Nurses.

Lund, C. H., & Osborne, J. W. (2004). Validity and reliability of the Neonatal Skin Condition Score. *Journal of Obstetric, Gynecologic, & Neonatal Nursing, 33*(3), 320-327.

Miles, M. (1984). Helping adults mourn the death of a child. In H. Wass & C. Corr (Eds.), *Childhood and death*, New York: Hemisphere.

Minozzi, S., Amato, L., Vecchi, S., & Davoli, M. (2008). Maintenance agonist treatments for opiate dependent pregnant women. In *The Cochrane Database Systematic Reviews,* 2008, Issue 2, CD 006318.

Moise, K. J. (2007). Red cell alloimmunization. In S. B. Gabbe, J. R. Niebyl, & J. L. Simpson (Eds.). *Obstetrics: Normal and problem pregnancies* (5th ed.). Philadelphia: Churchill Livingstone.

Moolenaar, R. L., Crutcher, J. M., San Joaquin, V. H., Sewell, L. V., Hutwagner, L. C., Carson, L. A., et al. (2000). A prolonged outbreak of *Pseudomonas aeruginosa* in a neonatal intensive care unit: Did staff fingernails play a role in disease transmission? *Infection Control Hospital Epidemiology, 21*(2), 80-85.

Myers, M. G., Seward, J. F., & LaRusso, P. S. (2007). Varicella-zoster virus. In R. M. Kliegman, R. E. Behrman, H. B. Jenson, & B. F. Stanton (Eds.), *Nelson textbook of pediatrics* (18th ed.). Philadelphia: Saunders.

Neal, J. L. (2008). RhD isoimmunization and current management modalities. *Journal of Obstetric, Gynecologic, and Neonatal Nursing, 30*(6), 589-606.

Noonan, C., Quigley, S., & Curley, M. A. Q. (2006). Skin integrity in hospitalized infants and children: A prevalence survey. *Journal of Pediatric Nursing, 21*(6), 445-453.

Pettett, G., Pallotto, E. K., & Merenstein, G. B. (2006). Regionalization and transport in perinatal care. In G. B. Merenstein, & S. L. Gardner (Eds.), *Handbook of neonatal intensive care* (6th ed.). St. Louis: Mosby.

Reiser, D. J. (2004). Neonatal jaundice: Physiologic variation or pathologic process. *Critical Care Nursing Clinics of North America, 16*(2) 257-269.

Roaten, J. B., Bensard, D. D., & Price, F. N. (2006). Neonatal surgery. In G. B. Merenstein & S. L. Gardner (Eds.), *Handbook of neonatal intensive care* (6th ed.). St. Louis: Mosby.

Sander, S. C., & Hays, L. R. (2005). Prescription opioid dependence and treatment with methadone in pregnancy. *Journal of Opioid Management, 1*(2), 91-97.

Santa-Donato, A., Medoff-Cooper, B., Bakewell-Sachs, S., Frazer Askin, D., & Rosenberg, S. (2007). *Late preterm infant assessment guide.* Washington, DC: Association of Women's Health, Obstetric, and Neonatal Nurses.

Sauerbrei, A. & Wutzler, P. (2007). Herpes simplex and varicella-zoster virus infections during pregnancy: Current concepts of prevention, diagnosis and therapy, part 2, Varicella-zoster virus. *Medical Microbiology & Immunology, 196*(2), 95-103.

Saugstad, O. D. (2007). Optimal oxygenation at birth and in the neonatal period. *Neonatology, 91*(4), 319-322.

Stoll, B. J. (2007). Blood disorders. In R. M. Kliegman, R. E. Behrman, H.B. Jenson, & B. F. Stanton (Eds.), *Nelson textbook of pediatrics* (18th ed.). Philadelphia: Saunders.

Stoll, B. J., Hansen, N. I., Higgins, R. D., Fanaroff, A. A., Duara, S., Goldberg, R., Laptook, A., Walsh, M., Oh, W., Hale, E., National Institute of Child Health and Human Development. (2005). Very low birth weight preterm infants with early onset neonatal sepsis: The predominance of gram-negative infections continues in the National Institute of Child Health and Human Development Neonatal Research Network, 2002-2003. *Pediatric Infectious Diseases Journal, 24*(7), 635-639.

Stoll, B. J., & Adams-Chapman, I. (2007). The high-risk infant. In R. M. Kliegman, R. E. Behrman, H. B. Jenson, & B. F. Stanton (Eds.), *Nelson textbook of pediatrics* (18th ed.). Philadelphia: Saunders.

Toedter, L., Lasker, L., & Janssen, H. (2001). International comparison of studies using the Perinatal Grief Scale: A decade of research on pregnancy loss. *Death Studies, 25*(3), 205-228.

Tomashek, K. M., Shapiro-Mendoza, C., Davidoff, M., & Petrini, J. R. (2007). Differences in mortality between late-preterm and term singleton infants in the United States, 1995-2002. *Journal of Pediatrics, 151*(5), 450-456.

Venkatesh, M., Merenstein, G. B., Adams, K., & Weisman, L. E. (2006). Infection in the neonate. In G. B. Merenstein, & S. L. Gardner (Eds.), *Handbook of neonatal intensive care* (6th ed.). St Louis: Mosby.

Ward, K. (2001). Perceived needs of parents of critically ill infants in a neonatal intensive care unit (NICU). *Pediatric Nursing, 27*(3), 281-286.

Wilson, R. (2001). Parents' support of their other children after a miscarriage or perinatal death. *Early Human Development, 61*(2), 55-65.

Woodwell, W. H. (2002). Perspectives on parenting in the NICU. *Advances in Neonatal Care, 2*(3), 161-169.

Appendix
Quality and Safety Competencies

Quality and Safety Education for Nurses (QSEN) is an effort to provide nurses with the competencies to improve the quality and safety of the systems of health care in which they practice (Cronenwett, Sherwood, Barnsteiner, et al., 2007). The competencies for nursing delineated by the Institute of Medicine (IOM) (2003) are patient-centered care, teamwork and collaboration, evidenced-based practice, quality improvement, safety, and informatics. The competencies were adapted by QSEN faculty members and defined by describing essential features of a competent and respected nurse.

CHAPTER 1

- **Patient-Centered Care**
  - Problems with the U.S. Health Care System, p. 4
  - Care during Pregnancy and Childbirth, pp. 7-8
  - Box 1-6 Standards of Care for Women and Newborns, p. 10
  - Ethical Issues in Perinatal Nursing, p. 11
  - The Family in Cultural and Community Context, p. 12
  - Family Nursing, p. 13
  - Cultural Context of the Family, pp. 13-14
  - Childbearing Beliefs and Practices, pp. 15-16
  - Integrating Cultural Competence with the Nursing Care Plan, p. 18
  - Home Care in the Community, pp. 22-23
- **Teamwork and Collaboration**
  - Trends in Nursing Practice, p. 9
  - Community and Home Care, p. 18
  - Community Health Promotion, p. 18
- **Evidence-Based Practice**
  - Problems with the U.S. Health Care System, p. 4
  - Evidence-Based Practice, p. 9
  - Evidence-Based Practice: Searching for and Evaluating the Evidence, p. 9
  - Research in Perinatal Nursing, p. 14
- **Quality Improvement**
  - Involving Consumers and Promoting Self-Management, p. 8
  - Sentinel Events, p. 11
  - Developing Cultural Competence, pp. 17-18
- **Safety**
  - Problems with the U.S. Health Care System, p. 4
  - Risk Management, p. 11
  - Table 1-1 The Joint Commission "Do Not Use" List, p. 11
- **Informatics**
  - High-Technology Care, p. 7
  - Ethical Issues in Perinatal Nursing, p. 11
  - Data Collection and Sources of Community Health Data, pp. 18-20
  - Home Care in the Community, pp. 22-23

CHAPTER 2

- **Patient-Centered Care**
  - Reasons for Entering the Health Care System, p. 36
  - Fertility Control and Infertility, p. 36
  - Cultural Considerations: Female Genital Mutilation, p. 38
  - Gender Issues, p. 38
  - Women with Special Needs, p. 45
  - Pelvic Examination, p. 49
  - Health Protection, p. 56
- **Teamwork and Collaboration**
  - Nutrition, p. 41
- **Evidence-Based Practice**
  - Evidence-Based Practice: Teaching Women Breast Self-Examination: Is it Worthwhile?, p. 32
- **Quality Improvement**
  - Well-Woman Care, p. 36
  - Health Protection, p. 56
- **Safety**
  - Health Risk Prevention, p. 56
  - Health Protection, p. 56

CHAPTER 3

- **Patient-Centered Care**
  - Amenorrhea, p. 61
  - Dysmenorrhea, p. 63
  - Premenstrual Syndrome and Premenstrual Dysphoric Disorder, p. 66
  - Endometriosis, p. 67
  - Nursing Care Plan: Endometriosis, p. 68
  - Sexually Transmitted Infections, pp. 71-72, 75-76
  - Viral Sexually Transmitted Infections, pp. 77-79
  - Benign Problems, pp. 86-87
  - Care Management, p. 91
- **Teamwork and Collaboration**
  - Amenorrhea, pp. 61-62
  - Viral Sexually Transmitted Infections, p. 81
  - Benign Problems, pp. 86-87
- **Evidence-Based Practice**
  - Dysmenorrhea, p. 63
  - Premenstrual Syndrome and Premenstrual Dysphoric Disorder, p. 66

- Evidence-Based Practice: Heavy Menstrual Bleeding: Treatments to Improve Quality of Life, p. 70
- **Safety**
  - Infection Control, p. 84
  - Box 3-4 Standard Precautions, p. 85
- **Informatics**
  - Viral Sexually Transmitted Infections, p. 80

CHAPTER 4

- **Patient-Centered Care**
  - Contraception, p. 97
  - Methods of Contraception, pp. 98, 111
  - Nursing Process: Contraception, p. 98
  - Decision to Have an Abortion, pp. 118-119
  - First-Trimester Abortion, pp. 119-120
  - Second-Trimester Abortion, pp. 120-121
  - Factors Associated with Infertility, p. 122
  - Box 4-5 Religious and Cultural Considerations of Fertility, p. 123
  - Nursing Process: Infertility, p. 124
- **Teamwork and Collaboration**
  - Factors Associated with Infertility, pp. 127, 132
- **Evidence-Based Practice**
  - Evidence-Based Practice: An Ideal Solution: The Intrauterine Device, p. 115

CHAPTER 5

- **Patient-Centered Care**
  - Genetics and Nursing, pp. 137-138
  - Nursing Care Plan: The Family with an Infant Who Has Down Syndrome, p. 146
- **Teamwork and Collaboration**
  - Genetics and Nursing, pp. 137-138
  - Genetic History-Taking and Genetic Counseling Services, p. 138
- **Evidence-Based Practice**
  - Evidence-Based Practice: Genetic Risk Assessment for Breast Cancer, p. 141
- **Quality Improvement**
  - Genetics and Nursing, pp. 137-138

CHAPTER 6

- **Patient-Centered Care**
  - Teaching Guidelines: Home Pregnancy Testing, p. 171
- **Teamwork and Collaboration**
  - General Body System Changes, p. 178

CHAPTER 7

- **Patient-Centered Care**
  - Adaptation to Pregnancy, p. 192
  - Maternal Adaptation, p. 194
  - Paternal Adaptation, p. 196
  - Initial Assessment, pp. 199-201
  - Nursing Process: Prenatal Care, p. 200
  - Collaborative Care, pp. 209-211, 221, 224
  - Patient Instructions for Self-Management: Exercise Tips for Pregnant Women, p. 212
  - Patient Instructions for Self-Management: Posture and Body Mechanics, p. 213
  - Patient Instructions for Self-Management: Safety during Pregnancy, p. 214
  - Nursing Care Plan: Discomforts of Pregnancy and Warning Signs, pp. 222-223
  - Patient Instructions for Self-Management: Sexuality in Pregnancy, p. 225
  - Cultural Influences, p. 226
  - Age Differences, pp. 228-230
  - Nursing Care Plan: Pregnant Adolescent, p. 229
  - Childbirth and Perinatal Education, pp. 231-232
- **Teamwork and Collaboration**
  - Care Management, pp. 198-199
  - Collaborative Care, pp. 207-209, 224
  - Age Differences, p. 230
- **Evidence-Based Practice**
  - Evidence-Based Practice: Exercise and Work in Pregnancy, p. 215
- **Quality Improvement**
  - Care Management, p. 198
- **Informatics**
  - Initial Assessment, p. 199
  - Follow-Up Visits, p. 204

CHAPTER 8

- **Patient-Centered Care**
  - Patient Instructions for Self-Management: Iron Supplementation, p. 247
  - Other Nutritional Issues during Pregnancy, pp. 251-252
  - Diet History, p. 254
  - Adequate Dietary Intake, p. 254
  - Patient Instructions for Self-Management: Nausea and Vomiting, p. 259
  - Cultural Influences, pp. 259-262
  - Nursing Care Plan: Nutrition during Pregnancy, p. 263
- **Evidence-Based Practice**
  - Nutrient Needs During Pregnancy, p. 240
  - Box 8-1 Bariatric Obstetric Care, p. 244
  - Evidence-Based Practice: What Nutritional Supplements, Besides Folic Acid, Promote Optimal Health during Pregnancy? p. 250
  - Other Nutritional Issues during Pregnancy, p. 252

CHAPTER 9

- **Patient-Centered Care**
  - Passageway, p. 271
  - Physiologic Adaptations to Labor, p. 280
- **Evidence-Based Practice**
  - Powers, p. 275

CHAPTER 10

- **Patient-Centered Care**
  - Perception of Pain, p. 285
  - Factors Influencing Pain Response, p. 286
  - Cultural Considerations: Some Cultural Beliefs about Pain, p. 287
  - Nonpharmacologic Management of Discomfort, p. 288

- Nonpharmacologic Interventions, p. 307
- Nursing Process: Management of Discomfort, p. 308
- Nursing Care Plan: Nonpharmacologic Management of Discomfort, p. 309
- Pharmacologic Interventions, pp. 309-312

- **Teamwork and Collaboration**
  - Analgesia and Anesthesia, pp. 300-301
  - Emergency: Maternal Hypotension with Decreased Placental Perfusion, p. 301
  - Pharmacologic Interventions, pp. 309-312
  - Box 10-5 Nursing Interventions for the Woman Receiving Regional Anesthesia or Analgesia, p. 311
- **Evidence-Based Practice**
  - Factors Influencing Pain Response, p. 288
  - Water Therapy, (Hydrotherapy), p. 292
  - Music, p. 292
  - Acupressure and Acupuncture, p. 293
  - Application of Heat and Cold, p. 293
  - Touch and Massage, p. 294
  - Evidence-Based Practice: Regional Pain Relief for Laboring Women, p. 297
- **Safety**
  - Water Therapy (Hydrotherapy), p. 292
  - Analgesia and Anesthesia, pp. 305-306
  - Pharmacologic Interventions, pp. 309-310
- **Informatics**
  - Pharmacologic Interventions, p. 312

CHAPTER 11

- **Patient-Centered Care**
  - Intermittent Auscultation, p. 319
  - Nursing Process: Fetal Heart Rate Monitoring, p. 329
  - Other Methods of Assessment and Intervention, p. 332
  - Box 11-8 Patient and Family Teaching when Electronic Fetal Monitor is Used, p. 333
- **Teamwork and Collaboration**
  - Nursing Management of Abnormal Patterns, p. 330
- **Evidence-Based Practice**
  - Evidence-Based Practice: Fetal Monitoring and the Machine That Goes "Beep," p. 317
  - Fetal Pulse Oximetry, p. 331
  - Amnioinfusion, p. 332
- **Quality Improvement**
  - Intermittent Auscultation, pp. 318-319
  - Electronic Fetal Monitoring, pp. 319-321
  - Fetal Heart Rate Patterns, p. 322
- **Safety**
  - Legal Tip: Fetal Monitoring Standards, pp. 329-330
  - Nursing Management of Abnormal Patterns, p. 330
- **Informatics**
  - Intermittent Auscultation, p. 319
  - Legal Tip: Fetal Monitoring Standards, pp. 329-330
  - Other Methods of Assessment and Intervention, p. 333

CHAPTER 12

- **Patient-Centered Care**
  - Procedure: Tests for Rupture of Membranes, p. 341
  - Assessment, pp. 342-343
  - Cultural Considerations, p. 344
  - Expected Outcomes of Care, p. 352
  - Plan of Care and Interventions, pp. 352, 367, 377, 380-381
  - Nursing Care Plan: Labor and Birth, p. 353
  - Table 12-2 Physical Nursing Care during Labor, pp. 354, 357
  - Box 12-5 Guidelines for Supporting the Father or Significant Other, p. 359
  - Care Management, p. 362
- **Teamwork and Collaboration**
  - Assessment, pp. 337, 376
  - Nursing Alert, p. 349
  - Episiotomy, p. 376
- **Evidence-Based Practice**
  - Evidence-Based Practice: Benefits of Continuous Labor Support, p. 369
  - Plan of Care and Interventions, p. 375
- **Safety**
  - Box 12-3 Standard Precautions during Childbirth, p. 345
  - Legal Tip: Obstetric Triage and EMTALA, p. 338
- **Informatics**
  - Assessment, pp. 337-341, 351, 362
  - Figure 12-2, p. 339
  - Figure 12-4, p. 345
  - Legal Tip: Documentation, p. 370

CHAPTER 13

- **Patient-Centered Care**
  - Neurologic System, p. 390
- **Evidence-Based Practice**
  - Uterus, p. 384

CHAPTER 14

- **Patient-Centered Care**
  - Box 14-3 Teaching Checklist for Postpartum Discharge, p. 395
  - Nursing Process: Physiologic Postpartum Concerns, pp. 396-397
  - Nursing Care Plan: Postpartum Care: Vaginal Birth, p. 398
  - Plan of Care and Interventions, pp. 401-404
  - Care Management: Psychosocial Needs, pp. 407-410
  - Nursing Process: Psychosocial Postpartum Concerns, p. 408
  - Cultural Considerations: Postpartum Period and Family Planning, p. 410
  - Self-Management and Signs of Complications, p. 411
  - Patient Instructions for Self-Management: Resumption of Sexual Intercourse, p. 413
- **Teamwork and Collaboration**
  - Nursing Alert, p. 399
  - Plan of Care and Interventions, p. 402
- **Evidence-Based Practice**
  - Plan of Care and Interventions, pp. 401, 403
  - Evidence-Based Practice: How Soon is Too Soon? Early Discharge after Birth, p. 412
  - Follow-Up after Discharge, p. 414
- **Quality Improvement**
  - Criteria for Discharge, p. 395
- **Safety**
  - Plan of Care and Interventions, p. 399
- **Informatics**
  - Transfer from the Recovery Area, p. 393
  - Plan of Care and Interventions, p. 403

CHAPTER 15

- **Patient-Centered Care**
  - Cultural Considerations: Fostering Bonding in Women of Varying Ethnic and Cultural Groups, p. 419
  - Extended Contact, p. 421
  - Parental Tasks and Responsibilities, p. 424
  - Becoming a Mother, p. 425
  - Nursing Care Plan: Home Care Follow-Up: Transition to Parenthood, p. 426
  - Patient Instructions for Self-Management: Coping with Postpartum Blues, p. 427
  - Becoming a Father, p. 428
  - Adjustment for the Couple, p. 428
  - Age, p. 430
  - Social Support, p. 431
  - Culture, p. 431
  - Nursing Process: Transition to Parenthood, p. 436
- **Teamwork and Collaboration**
  - Parental Attachment, Bonding, and Acquaintance, p. 418
  - Age, p. 430

CHAPTER 16

- **Patient-Centered Care**
  - Table 16-4 Physical Assessment of Newborn, p. 460
- **Teamwork and Collaboration**
  - Skeletal System, p. 451
  - Neurologic Assessment, p. 473
- **Evidence-Based Practice**
  - Cardiovascular System, p. 442

CHAPTER 17

- **Patient-Centered Care**
  - Nursing Process: Care of the Newborn and Family, p. 481
  - Nursing Care Plan: Normal Newborn, p. 483
  - Interventions, pp. 486, 502
  - Collection of Specimens, p. 499
  - Cultural Considerations: Cultural Beliefs and Practices Related to Infant Care, p. 502
  - Intramuscular Injection, p. 504
  - Therapy for Hyperbilirubinemia, p. 506
  - Circumcision, p. 508
  - Assessment of Neonatal Pain, p. 509
  - Teaching Guidelines: Care of the Circumcised Newborn at Home, p. 509
  - Discharge Planning and Teaching, p. 511
  - Teaching Guidelines: Sponge Bathing, pp. 517-518
  - Practical Suggestions for the First Weeks at Home, pp. 519-522
- **Evidence-Based Practice**
  - Evidence-Based Practice: Monitoring for Hypoglycemia, p. 496
- **Safety**
  - Nursing Care Management, p. 479
  - Nursing Care Plan: Normal Newborn, p. 483
  - Interventions, pp. 484, 502
  - Restraining the Infant, p. 501
  - Phototherapy, p. 505
  - Box 17-6 Infant Safety, p. 511
  - Safety: Use of Car Seat, pp. 513-515
  - Teaching Guidelines: Sponge Bathing, pp. 517-518
  - Emergency: Relieving Airway Obstruction, p. 519
  - Emergency: Cardiopulmonary Resuscitation (CPR) for Infants, p. 520
- **Informatics**
  - Nursing Care Plan: Normal Newborn, p. 483

CHAPTER 18

- **Patient-Centered Care**
  - Choosing an Infant Feeding Method, pp. 530-532
  - Cultural Influences on Infant Feeding, p. 532
  - Care Management: The Breastfeeding Mother and Infant, p. 538
  - Nursing Care Plan: Breastfeeding and Infant Nutrition, p. 539
  - Indicators of Effective Breastfeeding, p. 542
  - Patient Instructions for Self-Management: Breast Milk Storage Guidelines for Home Use, p. 548
  - Special Considerations, p. 549
  - Parent Education, p. 555
  - Teaching Guidelines: Formula Preparation and Feeding, p. 557
- **Teamwork and Collaboration**
  - Benefits of Breastfeeding, pp. 529-530
  - Nursing Care Plan: Breastfeeding and Infant Nutrition, p. 539
- **Evidence-Based Practice**
  - Evidence-Based Practice: The Usefulness of Prenatal Breastfeeding Education, p. 531
  - Supplements, Bottles, and Pacifiers, p. 543
  - Special Considerations, p. 553
- **Safety**
  - Nursing Alert, p. 548

CHAPTER 19

- **Patient-Centered Care**
  - Psychologic Considerations Related to High Risk Pregnancy, pp. 561-563
  - Ultrasonography, p. 568
  - Evidence-Based Practice: Having a Baby Later In Life, p. 572
  - Nursing Role in Assessment of the High Risk Pregnancy, p. 578
- **Teamwork and Collaboration**
  - Ultrasonography, p. 566
  - Nursing Role in Assessment of the High Risk Pregnancy, p. 578
- **Evidence-Based Practice**
  - Evidence-Based Practice: Having a Baby Later In Life, p. 572
- **Informatics**
  - Nonstress Test, p. 575
- **Safety**
  - Nursing Alert, p. 571
  - Nursing Alert, p. 572

CHAPTER 20

- **Patient-Centered Care**
  - Antepartum, pp. 586-587, 589, 596
  - Nursing Process: Pregestational Diabetes, p. 588

- Nursing Care Plan: The Pregnant Woman with Pregestational Diabetes, p. 590
- Patient Instructions for Self-Management: Dietary Management of Diabetic Pregnancy, p. 590
- Patient Instructions for Self-Management: Self-Administration of Insulin, p. 592
- Patient Instructions for Self-Management: Self-Testing of Blood Glucose Level, p. 593
- Patient Instructions for Self-Management: Treatment for Hypoglycemia, p. 594
- Patient Instructions for Self-Management: What to Do When Illness Occurs, p. 594
- Thyroid Disorders, p. 600
- Select Cardiovascular Disorders, pp. 603-604
- Nursing Process: Cardiac Disease, p. 606
- Care Management, p. 607
- Nursing Care Plan: The Pregnant Woman with Heart Disease, p. 608
- Patient Instructions for Self-Management: Iron Supplementation, p. 610
- Iron Deficiency Anemia, p. 610
- Neurologic Disorders, p. 615
- Nursing Process: Substance Abuse, p. 619
- Initial Care, pp. 618-620

- **Teamwork and Collaboration**
  - Diabetes Mellitus, p. 581
  - Antepartum, pp. 589, 595
  - Thyroid Disorders, p. 600
  - Cystic Fibrosis, p. 613
  - Initial Care, p. 620
- **Evidence-Based Practice**
  - Evidence-Based Practice: Preconceptional Counseling for Women with Diabetes, p. 585
  - Antepartum, p. 596
  - Substance Abuse, p. 618
- **Safety**
  - Nursing Alert, p. 591
  - Nursing Alert, pp. 599-600
  - Nursing Alert, p. 607
  - Nursing Alert, p. 609
- **Informatics**
  - Legal Tip, pp. 607-608

CHAPTER 21

- **Patient-Centered Care**
  - Mild Gestational Hypertension and Mild Preeclampsia, pp. 631-632
  - Nursing Process: Mild Preeclampsia, p. 632
  - Patient Instructions for Self-Management: Assessing and Reporting Clinical Signs of Preeclampsia, p. 633
  - Patient Instructions for Self-Management: Coping with Activity Restriction, p. 634
  - Patient Instructions for Self-Management: Diet for Severe Preeclampsia, p. 634
  - Severe Gestational Hypertension or Severe Preeclampsia, p. 635
  - Nursing Care Plan: Severe Preeclampsia, pp. 635, 639
  - Box 21-4 Care of the Patient with Preeclampsia Receiving Magnesium Sulfate, p. 637
  - Emergency: Eclampsia, p. 640
  - Hyperemesis Gravidarum, p. 642
  - Patient Instructions for Self-Management: Diet for Hyperemesis, p. 642
  - Early Pregnancy Bleeding, pp. 644, 647
  - Nursing Process: Miscarriage, p. 646
  - Teaching Guidelines: Discharge Teaching for the Woman after Early Miscarriage, p. 647
  - Recurrent Premature Dilation of the Cervix (Incompetent Cervix), p. 648
  - Box 21-5 Nursing Considerations for Women Undergoing Methotrexate Treatment for Ectopic Pregnancy, p. 651
  - Hydatidiform Mole (Molar Pregnancy), p. 652
  - Nursing Process: Placenta Previa, p. 655
  - Late Pregnancy Bleeding, pp. 656, 658
  - Clotting Problems, p. 660
  - Urinary Tract Infections, p. 665
  - Patient Instructions for Self-Management: Prevention of Urinary Tract Infections, p. 666
  - Management, p. 667
  - Box 21-7 Discharge Teaching for Home Care after Surgery, p. 668
- **Teamwork and Collaboration**
  - Severe Gestational Hypertension or Severe Preeclampsia, p. 635
  - Nursing Care Plan: Severe Preeclampsia, p. 635
  - Hemorrhagic Complications, p. 643
  - Nursing Process: Miscarriage, p. 646
  - Early Pregnancy Bleeding, p. 647
  - Tubal Pregnancy Management, p. 650
  - Nursing Process: Placenta Previa, p. 655
  - Management, pp. 667, 670
- **Evidence-Based Practice**
  - Care Management, p. 629
  - Evidence-Based Practice: Preeclampsia Risk Factors and Prevention, p. 630
  - Diet, p. 633
  - Recurrent Premature Dilation of the Cervix (Incompetent Cervix), p. 648
- **Safety**
  - Eclampsia, p. 639
  - Nursing Alert, p. 650
  - Nursing Alert, p. 670
  - Emergency: Cardiopulmonary Resuscitation for the Pregnant Woman, p. 672
- **Informatics**
  - Physical Examination, p. 629

CHAPTER 22

- **Patient-Centered Care**
  - Nursing Process: Preterm Labor, p. 680
  - Nursing Care Plan: Preterm Labor, p. 681
  - Patient Instructions for Self-Management: What to Do if Symptoms of Preterm Labor Occur, p. 682
  - Box 22-6 Nursing Care for Women Receiving Tocolytic Therapy, p. 683
  - Fetal and Early Neonatal Loss, p. 689
  - Management, p. 689
  - Patient Instructions for Self-Management: The Woman with Preterm Premature Rupture of the Membranes, p. 690
  - Dysfunctional Labor, p. 690

- Box 22-7 Back Labor–Occiput Posterior Position Measures to Relieve Back pain and Facilitate Rotation of Fetal Head, p. 692
- Fetal Causes, p. 694
- Nursing Process: Dystocia, p. 696
- Obstetric Procedures, pp. 696, 707-710, 713-714
- Patient Instructions for Self-Management: Postpartum Pain Relief after Cesarean Birth, p. 713
- Patient Instructions for Self-Management: Signs of Postoperative Complications, p. 713
- Shoulder Dystocia, p. 717
- Prolapsed Umbilical Cord, p. 718
- Rupture of the Uterus, p. 719

- **Teamwork and Collaboration**
  - Management of Inevitable Preterm Birth, p. 688
  - Fetal and Early Neonatal Loss, p. 689
  - Fetal Causes, pp. 693-694
  - Care Management, p. 695
  - Obstetric Procedures, pp. 704, 708-709, 714
  - Meconium-Stained Amniotic Fluid, p. 715
  - Anaphylactoid Syndrome of Pregnancy, p. 719
- **Evidence-Based Practice**
  - Predicting Spontaneous Perterm Labor and Birth, pp. 679-680, 682
  - Promotion of Fetal Lung Maturity, p. 684
  - Evidence-Based Practice: Corticosteroids for Lung Maturity in Preterm Labor: One Course or Two? p. 688
  - Position of the Woman, p. 695
  - Cervical Ripening Methods, p. 698
  - Oxytocin, p. 700
  - Augmentation of Labor, p. 702
  - Cesarean Birth, p. 705, 707
- **Safety**
  - Care Management, p. 695
  - Nursing Alert, p. 699
- **Informatics**
  - Legal Tip: Standard of Care–Labor and Birth Complications, p. 695
  - Medication Guide: Oxytocin (Pitocin), p. 701
  - Box 22-9 Assisting with Birth by Vacuum Extraction, p. 704
  - Obstetric Procedures, p. 704

CHAPTER 23

- **Patient-Centered Care**
  - Care Management, pp. 729, 736
  - Nursing Process: Postpartum Hemorrhage, p. 730
  - Nursing Care Plan: Postpartum Hemorrhage, p. 731
  - Nursing Interventions, pp. 734, 744, 748
  - Nursing Process: Postpartum Depression, p. 743
  - Patient Instructions for Self-Management: Activities to Prevent Postpartum Depression, p. 744
  - Nursing Considerations, p. 748
- **Teamwork and Collaboration**
  - Care Management, pp. 728, 739
  - Emergency: Hemorrhagic Shock, p. 732
  - Nursing Interventions, pp. 734, 745
  - Mood Disorders, p. 741
- **Evidence-Based Practice**
  - Care Management, p. 728
  - von Willebrand Disease, p. 733
  - Evidence-Based Practice: Assessing for Postpartum Depression, p. 742
  - Other Treatments for Postpartum Depression, p. 748
- **Safety**
  - Nursing Care Plan: Postpartum Hemorrhage, p. 731
  - Legal Tip: Standard of Care for Bleeding Emergencies, p. 732
  - Providing Safety, p. 745
- **Informatics**
  - Nursing Care Plan: Postpartum Hemorrhage, p. 731

CHAPTER 24

- **Patient-Centered Care**
  - Late-Preterm Infant, p. 756
  - Interventions, pp. 761, 769
  - Parental Adaptation to Preterm Infant, p. 769
  - Nursing Process: Late Preterm and Preterm Infant Care, p. 771
  - Birth Trauma, p. 775
  - Substance Abuse, p. 786
  - Teaching Guidelines: Care of the Infant Experiencing Withdrawal, p. 788
  - Congenital Anomalies, pp. 790, 798
  - Table 24-10 Congenital Anomalies, pp. 791-798
  - Support of Parents of a High Risk Neonate, pp. 798-799
  - Parent Education, p. 799
  - Discharge Planning, pp. 799-800
  - Grieving the Loss of a Newborn, p. 801
  - Nursing Process: Loss and Grief, p. 804
- **Teamwork and Collaboration**
  - Interventions, p. 757
  - Infants of Diabetic Mothers, p. 774
  - Acquired and Congenital Problems, p. 775
  - Congenital Anomalies, p. 790
  - Support of Parents of a High Risk Neonate, p. 799
  - Transport to and from a Regional Center, p. 800
  - Nursing Process: Loss and Grief, p. 804
- **Evidence-Based Practice**
  - Late-Preterm Infant, p. 758
  - Interventions, p. 767
  - Evidence-Based Practice: Skin-to-Skin (Kangaroo) Contact for Term and Preterm Infants, p. 768
- **Safety**
  - Late-Preterm Infant, p. 757
  - Nursing Alert, p. 764
  - Sepsis, pp. 775, 779
- **Informatics**
  - Late-Preterm Infant, p. 756
  - Nursing Process: Loss and Grief, p. 804

References

Cronenwett, L., Sherwood, G., Barnsteiner, J., et al. (2007). Quality and safety education for nurses. *Nursing Outlook*, *55*(3), 122-131.

Institute of Medicine, (2003). *Health professions education: A bridge to quality*. Washington, DC: National Academies Press.

Glossary

ABO incompatibility Hemolytic disease that occurs when the mother's blood is type O and the newborn's blood is type A, B, or AB

abruptio placentae Partial or complete premature separation of a normally implanted placenta

acceleration Increase in fetal heart rate (FHR); usually interpreted as a reassuring sign

acoustic stimulation test Antepartum test to elicit the FHR response to sound; performed by applying a sound source (laryngeal stimulator) to the maternal abdomen over the fetal head

acquaintance Process that parents use to get to know or become familiar with their new infant; an important step in attachment

acrocyanosis Peripheral cyanosis; blue color of hands and feet in most infants at birth that may persist for 7 to 10 days

active phase Phase in the first stage of labor when the cervix dilates from 4 to 7 cm

Adequate Intakes (AIs) Recommended nutrient intakes estimated to meet the needs of almost all healthy persons in the population; are provided for nutrients or age-group categories for which the available information is not sufficient to warrant establishing recommended dietary allowances

afterpains (afterbirth pains) Painful uterine cramps that occur intermittently for approximately 2 or 3 days after birth and that result from contractile efforts of the uterus to return to its normal involuted condition

alcohol-related birth defect (ARBD) Congenital abnormality or anomaly that is the result of excessive maternal alcohol intake during pregnancy; characterized by typical craniofacial and limb defects, cardiovascular defects, intrauterine growth restriction, and developmental delay; newer terminology for fetal alcohol syndrome (FAS)

alcohol-related neurodevelopmental disorder (ARND) Disorder in infants affected by prenatal exposure to alcohol but who do not meet the criteria for FAS; previously termed *fetal alcohol effects (FAE)*

alpha-fetoprotein (AFP) Fetal antigen; elevated levels in amniotic fluid and maternal blood that are associated with neural tube defects

amenorrhea Absence or cessation of menstruation

amniocentesis Procedure in which a needle is inserted through the abdominal and uterine walls to obtain amniotic fluid; used to assess fetal health and maturity

amnioinfusion Infusion of normal saline or lactated Ringer's solution through an intrauterine catheter into the uterine cavity in an attempt to increase the fluid around the umbilical cord and prevent compression during uterine contractions

amniotic fluid index (AFI) Estimation of the amount of amniotic fluid by means of ultrasound to determine excess or decreased levels

amniotomy Artificial rupture of the fetal membranes using a plastic AmniHook or a surgical clamp

analgesia Absence of pain without loss of consciousness

anaphylactoid syndrome of pregnancy Rare complication of pregnancy characterized by the sudden, acute onset of hypoxia, hypotension, or cardiac arrest and coagulopathy that can occur either during labor or during birth or immediately after birth; also known as *amniotic fluid embolism*

anencephaly Congenital deformity characterized by the absence of the cerebrum, cerebellum, and flat bones of the skull

anesthesia Partial or complete absence of sensation with or without loss of consciousness

antenatal glucocorticoids Medications administered to the mother for the purpose of accelerating fetal lung maturity when an increased risk exists for preterm birth between 24 and 34 weeks of gestation

anthropometric measurements Body measurements such as height and weight

Apgar score Numeric expression of the condition of a newborn obtained by rapid assessment at 1 and 5 minutes of age; developed by Virginia Apgar, MD

assisted reproductive therapies (ARTs) Treatments for infertility that include in vitro fertilization procedures, embryo adoption, embryo hosting, and therapeutic insemination

asynclitism Oblique presentation of the fetal head at the superior strait of the pelvis; the pelvic planes and those of the fetal head are not parallel

attachment Specific and enduring affective tie to another person

attitude Relationship of fetal parts to each other in the uterus (e.g., all parts are flexed or all parts are flexed except the neck is extended)

augmentation of labor Stimulation of ineffective uterine contractions after labor has started spontaneously but is not progressing satisfactorily

autoimmune disorders Group of diseases that disrupt the function of the immune system and cause the body to produce antibodies against itself, resulting in tissue damage

autolysis Self destruction of excess hypertrophied tissue

ballottement Diagnostic technique using palpation; a floating fetus, when tapped or pushed, moves away and then returns to touch the examiner's hand

barotrauma Physical injury resulting from changing air pressure; often associated with ventilatory assistance in preterm infants

basal body temperature (BBT) Lowest body temperature of a healthy person taken immediately after awakening and before getting out of bed

baseline fetal heart rate (FHR) Average FHR during a 10-minute period that excludes periodic and episodic changes and periods of significant variability; normal FHR baseline is 110 to 160 beats per minute

becoming a mother Transformation and growth of the mother identity

bereavement Feelings of loss, pain, desolation, and sadness that occur after the death of a loved one

binuclear family Family after divorce in which the child is a member of both the maternal and the paternal nuclear households

biophysical profile (BPP) Noninvasive assessment of the fetus and its environment using ultrasonography and fetal monitoring; includes fetal breathing movements, gross body movements, fetal tone, reactive FHR, and qualitative amniotic fluid volume

biorhythmicity Cyclic changes that occur with established regularity, such as sleeping and eating patterns

biparietal diameter Largest transverse diameter of the fetal head; measured between the parietal bones

birth plan Tool by which parents can explore their childbirth options and choose those that are most important to them

Bishop score Rating system to evaluate inducibility (ripeness) of the cervix; a higher score increases the likelihood of a successful induction of labor

blastocyst Stage in the development of a mammalian embryo, occurring after the morula stage, that consists of an outer layer, or trophoblast, and a hollow sphere of cells enclosing a cavity

bloody show Blood-tinged mucoid vaginal discharge that originates in the cervix and indicates the passage of the mucous plug (operculum) as the cervix ripens before labor and dilates during labor; increases as the cervix dilates during labor

body mass index (BMI) Method of calculating the appropriateness of weight for height (BMI = weight/height^2)

bonding Process by which parents form an emotional relationship with their infant over time

bradycardia Baseline FHR below 110 beats per minute and lasting for 10 minutes or longer

Braxton Hicks contractions or sign Mild, intermittent, painless uterine contractions that occur during pregnancy and become more frequent as pregnancy advances; however, these contractions do not represent true labor and should be distinguished from preterm labor

breast self examination (BSE) Systematic examination of the breasts by the woman

brown fat Source of heat unique to neonates that is capable of greater thermogenic activity than ordinary fat; deposits are found for several weeks after birth around the adrenal glands, kidneys, and neck; between the scapulae; and behind the sternum

caput succedaneum Swelling of the tissue over the presenting part of the fetal head; caused by pressure during labor

cardiac decompensation Condition of heart failure in which the heart is unable to maintain a sufficient cardiac output

carpal tunnel syndrome Syndrome in which edema compresses the median nerve beneath the carpal ligament of the wrist, causing tingling, burning, or numbness in the inner half of one or both hands

cephalhematoma Extravasation of blood from ruptured vessels between a skull bone and its external covering, the periosteum; the swelling is limited by the margins of the affected cranial bone (usually parietals)

cephalopelvic disproportion (CPD) Condition in which the infant's head is of such a shape, size, or position that it cannot pass through the mother's pelvis, or the maternal pelvis is too small, abnormally shaped, or deformed to allow the passage of a fetus of average size

cerclage Use of a nonabsorbable suture to keep a premature dilating cervix closed; usually removed when the pregnancy is at term

cervical funneling Effacement of the internal cervical os

cesarean birth Birth of a fetus by an incision through the abdominal wall and uterus

Chadwick sign Violet color of the vaginal mucous membrane that is visible from approximately the fourth week of pregnancy; caused by increased vascularity

chloasma Increased pigmentation over the bridge of the nose and cheeks of pregnant women and some women who take oral contraceptives; also known as the *mask of pregnancy*

chorioamnionitis Inflammatory reaction in fetal membranes to bacteria or viruses in the amniotic fluid, which then become infiltrated with polymorphonuclear leukocytes

chorionic villi Tiny vascular protrusions on the chorionic surface that project into the maternal blood sinuses of the uterus and help form the placenta and secrete human chorionic gonadotropin (hCG)

chorionic villus sampling (CVS) Removal of fetal tissue from the placenta for genetic diagnostic studies

chromosomes Elements within the cell nucleus that carry genes and are composed of deoxyribonucleic acid (DNA) and proteins

chronic hypertension Systolic pressure of 140 mm Hg or higher or diastolic pressure of 90 mm Hg or higher that is present preconceptionally or occurs before 20 weeks of gestation

chronic lung disease (bronchopulmonary dysplasia) Pulmonary condition affecting preterm infants who have experienced respiratory failure and have been oxygen dependent for more than 28 days

circumcision Excision of the prepuce (foreskin) of the penis, exposing the glans

claiming process Process by which the parents identify their new baby in terms of likeness to other family members, differences, and uniqueness

cleft lip Incomplete closure of the lip (formerly termed *hare lip*)

cleft palate Incomplete closure of the palate or roof of the mouth; a congenital fissure

climacteric Period of a woman's life when she is passing from a reproductive to a nonreproductive state, with regression of ovarian function; cycle during which endocrine, physical, and psychosocial changes occur during the termination of the reproductive years; also called *climacterium*

clonus Spasmodic alternation of muscular contraction and relaxation; counted in beats

Cochrane Pregnancy and Childbirth Database Database of up-to-date systematic reviews and dissemination of reviews of randomized controlled trials of health care

cold stress Excessive loss of heat that results in increased respirations and nonshivering thermogenesis to maintain core body temperature

colostrum Early milk, produced from approximately 16 weeks of pregnancy into the first postpartum days; rich in antibodies, higher in protein and lower in fat than mature milk, with laxative effect to clear meconium and promote excretion of bilirubin.

conception Union of the sperm and ovum, resulting in fertilization; formation of the one-celled zygote

continuous positive airway pressure (CPAP) Means of infusing oxygen or air under a preset pressure via nasal prongs, a facemask, or an endotracheal tube

continuum of care Range of clinical services provided for an individual or group that reflects care given during a single hospitalization or care for multiple conditions over a lifetime

contraception Intentional prevention of pregnancy using a device or practice

contraction stress test (CST) (also called *oxytocin challenge test* [OCT]) Test that stimulates uterine contractions for the purpose of assessing fetal response; a healthy fetus does not react to contractions, whereas a compromised fetus demonstrates late decelerations in the FHR that are indicative of uteroplacental insufficiency

Coombs' test Indirect: determination of Rh-positive antibodies in maternal blood; direct: determination of maternal Rh-positive antibodies in fetal cord blood; positive test result indicates the presence of antibodies or titer

corrected age Taking into account the gestational age and postnatal age of a preterm infant when determining expectations for development

counterpressure Pressure applied to the sacral area of the back during uterine contractions

couplet care One nurse, educated in both maternal and newborn care, functions as the primary nurse for both mother and neonate (also known as *mother-baby care* or *single-room maternity care*)

couvade syndrome Phenomenon of expectant fathers' experiencing pregnancy-like symptoms

Couvelaire uterus Interstitial myometrial hemorrhage after premature separation (abruption) of the placenta; purplish-blue discoloration of the uterus is noted

crowning Phase in the descent of the fetus when the top of the head can be seen at the vaginal orifice as the widest part of the head (biparietal diameter [BPD]) distends the vulva just before birth

cultural competence Awareness, acceptance, and knowledge of cultural differences and adaptation of services to acknowledge and support the culture of the patient

cultural context Setting in which one considers individual and family beliefs and practices (culture)

cultural knowledge Knowledge that includes the beliefs and values about each facet of life; passed from one generation to the next

cultural prescriptions Expected or acceptable practices

cultural proscriptions Forbidden or taboo practices

cultural relativism Learning about and applying the standards of another person's culture to activities within a particular culture

cycle of violence Violence against a woman that usually occurs in a pattern consisting of three phases: a period of increasing tension, an abusive episode, and a period of contrition and kindness

daily fetal movement count (DFMC) Maternal assessment of fetal activity; the number of fetal movements counted within a specified time; also called *kick count*

deceleration Slowing of the FHR attributed to a parasympathetic response and described in relation to uterine contractions. Types of decelerations include:

- **early deceleration** Visually apparent gradual decrease in the FHR before the peak of a contraction and return to baseline as the contraction ends; caused by fetal head compression
- **late deceleration** Visually apparent gradual decrease in FHR, with the lowest point of the deceleration occurring after the peak of the contraction and returning to baseline after the contraction ends; caused by uteroplacental insufficiency
- **prolonged deceleration** Visually apparent decrease (may be either gradual or abrupt) in the FHR of at least 15 beats per minute below the baseline and lasting more than 2 minutes but less than 10 minutes
- **variable deceleration** Visually apparent abrupt decrease in the FHR below the baseline that occurs any time during the uterine contraction phase; caused by the compression of the umbilical cord

decidua basalis Maternal aspect of the placenta that is made up of uterine blood vessels, endometrial stroma, and glands that shed in lochial discharge after birth

demand feeding Feeding in response to feeding cues exhibited by the infant, that indicate the presence of hunger

developmentally appropriate care Care that takes into consideration the gestational age and condition of the infant and promotes the development of the infant

developmental dysplasia of the hip (DDH) Abnormal development of the hip joint, resulting in instability of the hip and causing one or both of the femoral heads to be displaced from the acetabulum (hip socket)

diastasis recti abdominis Separation of the two rectus muscles along the median line of the abdominal wall; often seen in women with repeated childbirths or with a multiple gestation (e.g., triplets)

Dietary Reference Intakes (DRIs) Nutritional recommendations for the United States that consist of the Recommended Dietary Allowances (RDAs), adequate intakes, and tolerable upper intake levels; the upper limit of intake is associated with low risk in almost all members of a population

dilation Stretching of the external cervical os from an opening a few millimeters in size to an opening large enough to allow the passage of the fetus

disseminated intravascular coagulation (DIC) Pathologic form of coagulation in which clotting factors are consumed to such an extent that generalized bleeding can occur; associated with abruptio placentae, eclampsia, intrauterine fetal demise, amniotic fluid embolism, and hemorrhage

Doppler blood flow analysis Use of ultrasound for noninvasive measurement of blood flow in the fetus and placenta

doula Trained assistant who is hired to give the woman support during pregnancy, labor and birth, and postpartum

dysfunctional labor Abnormal uterine contractions that prevent normal progress of cervical dilation, effacement, or descent

dysfunctional uterine bleeding (DUB) Excessive uterine bleeding with no demonstrable organic cause

dysmenorrhea Painful menstruation beginning 2 to 6 months after menarche, related to ovulation or to organic disease such as endometriosis, pelvic inflammatory disease, or uterine neoplasm

dystocia Prolonged, painful, or otherwise difficult labor caused by various conditions associated with the following five factors affecting labor: powers, passage, passenger, maternal position, and maternal emotions

eclampsia Severe complication of pregnancy of unknown cause; occurs more often in primigravida than in multiparous women; characterized by new-onset grand mal seizures in a woman with preeclampsia, occurring during pregnancy or shortly after birth

ectopic pregnancy Implantation of the fertilized ovum outside of the uterine cavity; locations include the uterine tubes, ovaries, and abdomen

effacement Thinning and shortening or obliteration of the cervix that occurs during late pregnancy or labor or both

effleurage Gentle stroking that is used in massage, usually on the abdomen

electronic fetal monitoring (EFM) Electronic surveillance of the FHR by external and internal methods

embryo Conceptus from day 15 of development until approximately the eighth week after conception

en face Face-to-face position in which the parent and infant's faces are approximately 20 cm apart and on the same plane

endometriosis Tissue closely resembling endometrial tissue located outside the uterus

endometritis Postpartum uterine infection that often begins at the site of the placental implantation

engagement In obstetrics, the entrance of the fetal presenting part into the superior pelvic strait and the beginning of the descent through the pelvic canal; the lowest part of the presenting part is usually at or below the level of ischial spines

engorgement Painful swelling of breast tissue that is a result of a rapid increase in milk production and venous congestion causes interstitial tissue edema; impaired milk flow results in the accumulation of milk in the breasts; it most often occurs between the third and fifth postpartum days

engrossment Parent's absorption, preoccupation, and interest in his or her infant; typically used to describe the father's intense involvement with his newborn

entrainment Phenomenon observed in the microanalysis of sound films in which the speaker moves several parts of the body and the listener responds to the sounds by moving in ways that are coordinated with the rhythm of the sounds (infants have been observed moving in time to the rhythms of adult speech but not to random noises or disconnected words or vowels); believed to be an essential factor in the process of maternal-infant bonding

epidural block Type of regional anesthesia that is produced by injection of a local anesthetic alone or in combination with a narcotic analgesic into the epidural (peridural) space

epidural blood patch Patch formed by a few milliliters of the mother's blood occluding a tear in the dura mater around the spinal cord that occurs during the induction of a spinal or an epidural block; its purpose is to relieve headache pain associated with the leakage of spinal fluid

episiotomy Surgical incision of the perineum at the end of the second stage of labor to facilitate birth and to prevent laceration of the perineum

episodic changes Changes from baseline patterns in the FHR that are not associated with uterine contractions

epulis Tumorlike benign lesion of the gingiva that is observed in pregnant women

erythema toxicum Innocuous pink, papular neonatal rash of unknown cause, with superimposed vesicles appearing within 24 to 48 hours after birth and resolving spontaneously within a few days

erythroblastosis fetalis Hemolytic disease of the newborn usually caused by isoimmunization, resulting from Rh incompatibility or ABO incompatibility

ethnocentrism Belief in the rightness of one's own culture's way of doing things

euglycemia Pertaining to a normal blood glucose level; also called *normoglycemia*

evidence-based practice Practice based on knowledge that has been gained through research and clinical trials

exchange transfusion Replacement of 75% to 85% of circulating blood by withdrawal of the recipient's blood and injection of a donor's blood in equal amounts, the purposes of which are to prevent an accumulation of bilirubin in the blood above a dangerous level, to prevent the accumulation of other by-products of hemolysis in hemolytic disease, and to correct anemia and acidosis

extended family Family that includes the nuclear family and other people related by blood

external cephalic version (ECV) Turning of the fetus to a vertex presentation by external exertion of pressure on the fetus through the maternal abdomen

extracorporeal membrane oxygenation (ECMO) Oxygenation of blood external to the body that uses cardiopulmonary bypass and a membrane oxygenator; used primarily for newborns with refractory respiratory failure or meconium aspiration syndrome

family dynamics Interaction and communication among family members

feeding-readiness cues Infant behaviors (e.g., mouthing motions, sucking fist, awakening, crying) that indicate the infant is interested in feeding

Ferguson reflex Reflex contractions (i.e., urge to push) of the uterus after stimulation of the cervix

fern test Appearance of a fernlike pattern found on a microscopic examination of certain fluids such as amniotic fluid

fertility awareness methods (FAMs) Methods of family planning that identify the beginning and end of the fertile period of the menstrual cycle

fertilization Union of an ovum and a sperm

fetal membranes Amnion and chorion surrounding the fetus

fetus Developing human in utero from approximately the ninth week after conception until birth

fibroadenoma Firm, freely movable solitary, solid, benign breast tumor

fibrocystic changes Benign changes in breast tissue

first stage of labor Stage of labor from the onset of regular uterine contractions to full effacement and dilation of the cervix

fontanels Broad areas or soft spots that consist of a strong band of connective tissue, contiguous with cranial bones and located at the junctions of the bones

forceps-assisted birth Vaginal birth in which forceps (i.e., curved-bladed instruments) are used to assist in the birth of the fetal head

fourth stage of labor First 1 to 2 hours after birth

funic soufflé Soft, muffled, blowing sound produced by blood rushing through the umbilical vessels and synchronous with the fetal heart sounds

gamete Mature male or female germ cell; the mature sperm or ovum

gastroschisis Abdominal wall defect at the base of the umbilical stalk

gate-control theory of pain Pain theory used to explain the neurophysiologic mechanism underlying the perception of pain;

the capacity of nerve pathways to transmit pain is reduced or completely blocked by using distraction techniques

genetics Study of a single gene or gene sequences and their effects on the living organism

genogram Pictorial representation of family relationships and health history

genome Complete copy of the genetic material in an organism

genomics Study of the entire DNA structure of all of an organism's genes, including functions and interactions of genes

gestational diabetes mellitus (GDM) Glucose intolerance first recognized during pregnancy

gestational hypertension New onset of hypertension without proteinuria after week 20 of pregnancy

glycosylated hemoglobin A1c Glycohemoglobin, a minor hemoglobin with glucose attached; the glycosylated hemoglobin concentration represents the average blood glucose level over the previous several weeks and is a measurement of glycemic control in diabetic therapy

Goodell sign Softening of the cervix, a probable sign of pregnancy; occurs during the second month

grief Physical, emotional, social, and cognitive response to a loss such as the death of a loved one

growth spurts Times of increased neonatal growth that usually occur at approximately 6 to 10 days, 6 weeks, 3 months, and 6 months; increased caloric needs of the infant prompt more frequent feedings

habituation Psychologic and physiologic phenomenon whereby the response to a constant or repetitive stimulus is decreased

Hegar sign Softening of the lower uterine segment that is classified as a probable sign of pregnancy; may be present during the second and third months of pregnancy and is palpated during the bimanual examination

HELLP syndrome Laboratory diagnosis for a variant of severe preeclampsia that involves hepatic dysfunction, characterized by **h**emolysis, **e**levated **l**iver enzymes, and **l**ow **p**latelet count

hemorrhagic (hypovolemic) shock Clinical condition in which the peripheral blood flow is inadequate to return sufficient blood to the heart for normal function, particularly oxygen transport to the organs or tissue

home birth Planned birth of the child at home; usually performed under the supervision of a midwife

home health care Care that is provided in the home

homosexual (lesbian or gay) family Family that consists of same-sex adults and children who are from previous heterosexual unions, conceived through therapeutic insemination, or adopted

human chorionic gonadotropin (hCG) Hormone that is produced by chorionic villi; the biologic marker in pregnancy tests

hydatidiform mole (molar pregnancy) Gestational trophoblastic neoplasm, usually the result of fertilization of an egg that has no nucleus or an inactivated nucleus

hydramnios (polyhydramnios) Amniotic fluid in excess of 2000 ml

hydrocephalus Accumulation of fluid in the subdural or subarachnoid spaces

hydrops fetalis Most severe expression of fetal hemolytic disorder, a possible sequela to maternal Rh isoimmunization; infants exhibit gross edema (anasarca), cardiac decompensation, and profound pallor from anemia

hyperbilirubinemia Elevated unconjugated serum bilirubin concentrations

hyperemesis gravidarum Abnormal condition of pregnancy characterized by protracted vomiting, weight loss, and fluid and electrolyte imbalance

hyperglycemia Excess glucose in the blood, usually caused by inadequate secretion of insulin by the islet cells of the pancreas or inadequate control of diabetes mellitus

hyperthyroidism Excessive functional activity of the thyroid gland

hypertonic uterine dysfunction Primary dysfunctional labor characterized by uncoordinated, painful, frequent uterine contractions that do not cause cervical dilation and effacement

hypoglycemia Less than a normal level of glucose in the blood; usually caused by the administration of too much insulin, excessive secretion of insulin by the islet cells of the pancreas, or dietary deficiency

hypothermia Body temperature that falls below the normal range (below 35° C); usually caused by exposure to cold

hypothyroidism Deficiency of thyroid gland activity with underproduction of thyroxine

hypotonic uterine dysfunction Weak, ineffective uterine contractions that usually occur in the active phase of labor; often related to cephalopelvic disproportion or malposition of the fetus; secondary uterine inertia

hypoxemia Reduction in arterial oxygen pressure that results in metabolic acidosis by forcing anaerobic glycolysis, pulmonary vasoconstriction, and direct cellular damage

hypoxia Insufficient availability of oxygen to meet the metabolic needs of body tissue

implantation Embedding of the fertilized ovum in the uterine mucosa; nidation

inborn error of metabolism Group of recessive disorders caused by a metabolic defect that results from the absence of or change in a protein, usually an enzyme, and mediated by the action of a certain gene

induced abortion Intentional termination of pregnancy

infertility Impaired fertility, including a prolonged time to conceive or the inability to conceive

integrative health care Complementary and alternative therapies in combination with conventional Western modalities of treatment

intermittent auscultation Listening to fetal heart sounds at periodic intervals using nonelectronic or ultrasound devices placed on the maternal abdomen

intrauterine growth restriction (IUGR) Fetal undergrowth from any cause

inversion of the uterus Condition in which the uterus is turned inside out, resulting in the fundus intruding into the cervix or vagina

inverted nipples Nipples invert rather than evert when stimulated; can interfere with effective latch

involution Return of the uterus to a nonpregnant state after birth

kangaroo care Skin-to-skin infant care, especially for preterm infants, that provides warmth to infant; the infant is placed naked or diapered against the mother or father's bare chest and is covered with the parent's shirt or a warm blanket

karyotype Schematic arrangements of the chromosomes within a cell to demonstrate their numbers and morphologic features

kcal Abbreviation for kilocalorie; unit of heat content or energy equal to 1000 small calories

Kegel exercises Pelvic floor muscle exercises to strengthen the pubococcygeal muscles

kernicterus Pathologic process characterized by the deposition of bilirubin in the brain

ketoacidosis Accumulation of ketone bodies in the blood as a consequence of hyperglycemia; leads to metabolic acidosis

lactation consultant Health care professional who has specialized training and experience working with breastfeeding mothers and infants

lactogenesis Process of breast milk production

lactose intolerance Inherited absence of the enzyme lactase

lanugo Very fine hairs that first appear at 12 weeks; covers the entire body of the fetus by 20 weeks

latch Placement of the infant's mouth over the nipple, areola, and breast, making a seal between the mouth and breast to create adequate suction for milk removal

late preterm birth Birth that occurs between 34 and 36 $^6/_7$ weeks of gestation

late preterm infant Infant born at 34 to 36$^6/_7$ weeks of gestation

latent phase Phase in the first stage of labor when the cervix dilates from 0 to 3 cm

leiomyoma Benign smooth-muscle tumor

Leopold maneuvers Four maneuvers for diagnosing the fetal position by external palpation of the mother's abdomen

letting-go phase Interdependent phase after birth in which the mother and family move forward as a system with interacting members

leukorrhea White or yellowish mucous discharge from the cervical canal or the vagina that may be normal physiologically or caused by pathologic states of the vagina and endocervix

lie Relationship existing between the long axis of the fetus and the long axis of the mother; in a longitudinal lie, the fetus is lying lengthwise or vertically, whereas in a transverse lie, the fetus is lying crosswise or horizontally in the uterus

lightening Sensation of decreased abdominal distention that is produced by uterine descent into the pelvic cavity as the fetal presenting part settles into the pelvis; usually occurs 2 weeks before the onset of labor in nulliparous women

linea nigra Line of darker pigmentation observed in some women during the latter part of pregnancy that appears on the middle of the abdomen and extends from the symphysis pubis toward the umbilicus

lithotomy position Position in which the woman lies on her back with her knees flexed and with abducted thighs drawn up toward her chest; stirrups attached to an examination table can be used to facilitate assuming and maintaining this position

local perineal infiltration anesthesia Process by which a local anesthetic medication is deposited within the tissue to anesthetize a limited region of the body

lochia Vaginal discharge during the puerperium that consists of blood, tissue, and mucus

lochia alba Thin, yellow-to-white, vaginal discharge that follows lochia serosa on approximately the tenth day after birth and may last from 2 to 6 weeks postpartum

lochia rubra Red, distinctly blood-tinged vaginal flow that occurs after birth and lasts 2 to 4 days

lochia serosa Serous, pinkish brown, watery vaginal discharge that occurs after lochia rubra until approximately the tenth day after birth

low-birth-weight (LBW) infants Babies weighing less than 2500 g (5½ lbs) at birth

lumpectomy Removal of a wide margin of normal breast tissue surrounding a breast cancer

macrosomia Large body size as observed in neonates of mothers with pregestational or gestational diabetes

magnetic resonance imaging (MRI) Noninvasive nuclear procedure for imaging tissues with high fat and water content; in obstetrics, uses include the evaluation of fetal structures, placenta, and amniotic fluid volume

mastitis Inflammation of a breast, often associated with infection; usually confined to a milk duct, characterized by influenza-like symptoms, redness, and tenderness in the affected breast

maternal sensitivity Quality of a mother's sensitive behaviors that are based on her awareness, perception, and responsiveness to infant cues and behaviors

mechanical ventilation Respiratory support technique used to provide predetermined amount of oxygen; requires intubation

meconium Greenish black, viscous first stool formed from the amniotic fluid and its constituents during fetal life, intestinal secretions (including bilirubin), and cells (shed from the mucosa)

meconium aspiration syndrome (MAS) Function of fetal hypoxia; with hypoxia the anal sphincter relaxes and meconium is released; reflex gasping movements draw meconium and other particulate matter in the amniotic fluid into the infant's bronchial tree, obstructing the airflow after birth

meiosis Process by which germ cells divide and decrease their chromosomal numbers by one half

menarche Onset, or beginning, of menstrual function

menopause From the Greek words *mensis* (month) and *pausis* (cessation), the actual permanent cessation of menstrual cycles; diagnosed as such after 1 year without menses

menorrhagia Abnormally profuse or excessive menstrual flow

menstrual cycle Complex interplay of events that occur simultaneously in the endometrium, hypothalamus and pituitary glands, and ovaries and results in ovarian and uterine preparation for pregnancy

menstruation Periodic vaginal discharge of bloody fluid from the nonpregnant uterus that occurs from the age of puberty to menopause

metrorrhagia Abnormal bleeding from the uterus, particularly when it occurs at any time other than the menstrual period

microcephaly Abnormally small head size in relation to the rest of the body and underdevelopment of the brain, resulting in some degree of mental retardation

milia Small, white sebaceous glands appearing as tiny, white, pinpoint papules on the forehead, nose, cheeks, and chin of the neonate

milk ejection reflex (MER) Release of milk caused by the contraction of the myoepithelial cells surrounding the milk glands in response to oxytocin; also called the *let-down reflex*

miscarriage Loss of pregnancy that occurs naturally without interference or known cause; also called *spontaneous abortion*

mitosis Process of somatic cell division in which a single cell divides, but both new cells have the same number of chromosomes as the first

modified radical mastectomy Surgery that includes the removal of the breast and fascia over the pectoralis major muscle

molding Overlapping of cranial bones or shaping of the fetal head to accommodate and conform to the bony and soft parts of the mother's birth canal during labor

mongolian spots Bluish gray or dark nonelevated pigmented areas usually found over the lower back and buttocks that are present at birth in some infants, primarily nonwhite, usually fading by school age

monosomy Chromosomal aberration characterized by the absence of one chromosome from the normal diploid complement

Montgomery tubercles Small, nodular prominences (sebaceous glands) on the areolas around the nipples of the breasts that enlarge during pregnancy and lactation

mood disorders Disorders that have a disturbance in the prevailing emotional state as the dominant feature; the cause is unknown

morning sickness Nausea and vomiting that affect some women during the first few months of pregnancy; may occur at any time of day

morula Developmental stage of the fertilized ovum characterized by a solid mass of cells; resembles a mulberry

mosaicism Condition in which some somatic cells are normal, whereas others show chromosomal aberrations

multifetal pregnancy Pregnancy in which more than one fetus is in the uterus at the same time; multiple gestation

mutuality Parent-infant interaction in which the infant's behaviors and characteristics call forth a corresponding set of parental behaviors and characteristics

myelomeningocele External sac containing meninges, spinal fluid, and nerves that protrudes through a defect in vertebral column

Nägele's rule One method for calculating the estimated date of birth or due date

natural family planning (NFP) Contraceptive methods in which a woman abstains from sexual intercourse during the fertile period of her menstrual cycle; no other form of birth control is used during this period

necrotizing enterocolitis Acute inflammatory bowel disorder that occurs primarily in preterm or low-birth-weight neonates; is characterized by ischemic necrosis (death) of the gastrointestinal mucosa, which may lead to perforation and peritonitis; formula-fed infants are at higher risk for this disease

neonatal abstinence syndrome Signs and symptoms that are associated with drug withdrawal in the neonate

neonatal narcosis Central nervous system depression in the newborn caused by an opioid (narcotic); may be signaled by respiratory depression, hypotonia, lethargy, and delay in temperature regulation

neutral thermal environment (NTE) Environment that enables the neonate to maintain a normal body temperature with a minimum use of oxygen and energy

nitrazine test Evaluation of body fluids that uses a test swab to determine the fluid's pH level; urine exhibits an acidic result, and amniotic fluid exhibits an alkaline result

nonnutritive sucking Use of a pacifier by infants; may include thumb or fingers

nonstress test (NST) Evaluation of fetal response (e.g., FHR) to natural contractile uterine activity or to an increase in fetal activity

nuchal cord Encircling of fetal neck by one or more loops of the umbilical cord

nuclear family Family that consists of parents and their dependent children

nutrigenetics Study of the effect of genetic variations on diet and health with implications for susceptible subgroups

nutrigenomics Study of the effect of nutrients on health through the alteration of genome, proteome, and metabolome, noting changes in the physiologic features that result

oligomenorrhea Abnormally light or infrequent menstruation

omphalocele Congenital defect resulting from failure of closure of the abdominal wall or muscles and leading to herniation of abdominal contents through the umbilicus

operculum Plug of mucus that fills the cervical canal during pregnancy

ophthalmia neonatorum Infection in the neonate's eyes; usually the result of gonorrheal, chlamydial, or other infections contracted when the fetus passes through the birth canal (vagina)

opioid (narcotic) agonist analgesics Medications that relieve pain by activating opioid receptors

opioid (narcotic) agonist-antagonist analgesics Medications that combine agonist activity (activates or stimulates a receptor to perform a function) and antagonist activity (blocks a receptor or medication designed to activate a receptor) to relieve pain without causing significant maternal or fetal or newborn respiratory depression

opioid (narcotic) antagonists Medications that reverse the central nervous system depressant effects of an opioid, especially respiratory depression

ovulation Periodic ripening and discharge of the ovum from the ovary, usually 14 days before the onset of menstrual flow

oxytocin Hormone produced by the posterior pituitary gland that stimulates uterine contractions and the release of milk in the mammary glands (let-down reflex); synthetic oxytocin is a medication that mimics the uterine stimulating action of oxytocin

palmar erythema Rash on the surface of the palms sometimes observed in pregnant women

Papanicolaou (Pap) test, smear Microscopic examination using scrapings from the cervix, endocervix, or other mucous membranes that reveal, with a high degree of accuracy, the presence of premalignant or malignant cells

patent ductus arteriosus (PDA) Failure of the fetal ductus arteriosus to close after birth

pelvic inflammatory disease (PID) Infection of internal reproductive structures and adjacent tissues; a disease that is usually secondary to sexually transmitted infections

pelvic relaxation Lengthening and weakening of the fascial supports of the pelvic structures

pelvic tilt (rock) Exercise used to help relieve low back discomfort during menstruation and pregnancy

percutaneous umbilical blood sampling (PUBS) (also called *cordocentesis*) Procedure during which a fetal umbilical vessel is accessed for blood sampling or for transfusions

perimenopause Period of transition of changing ovarian activity before menopause and through the first few years of amenorrhea

periodic changes Changes from baseline of the FHR that occur with uterine contractions

peripartum cardiomyopathy Inability of the heart to maintain an adequate cardiac output; congestive heart failure that occurs during the peripartum

periventricular intraventricular hemorrhage (PV-IVH) Hemorrhage into the ventricles of the brain; a common type of brain injury in preterm infants; prognosis depends on the severity of hemorrhage

pharmacogenetics or pharmacogenomics Study of inherited variations in drug metabolism and response

phototherapy Use of lights to reduce serum bilirubin levels by oxidation of bilirubin into water-soluble compounds that are processed in the liver and excreted in bile and urine

physiologic anemia Relative excess of plasma that leads to a decrease in hemoglobin concentration and hematocrit; a normal adaptation during pregnancy

physiologic jaundice Yellow tinge to the skin and mucous membranes in response to increased serum levels of unconjugated bilirubin; is not usually apparent until after 24 hours; is also called *neonatal jaundice*, physiologic hyperbilirubinemia

pica Unusual oral craving during pregnancy (e.g., for laundry starch, dirt, red clay)

placenta previa Placenta that is abnormally implanted in the thin, lower uterine segment; further classified as complete placenta previa, marginal placenta previa, or low-lying placenta, according to gestational age and placental location in relation to the internal cervical os

plugged milk duct Blockage of milk duct that causes ineffective emptying of the breast

position Relationship of a reference point on the presenting part of the fetus, such as the occiput, sacrum, chin, or scapula, to its location in the front, back, or sides of the maternal pelvis

postpartum blues Let-down feeling, accompanied by irritability and anxiety, which usually begins 2 to 3 days after giving birth and disappears within 1 to 2 weeks; is sometimes called *baby blues*

postpartum depression (PPD) Depression that occurs within 4 weeks of childbirth and lasts longer than postpartum blues; characterized by a variety of symptoms that interfere with activities of daily living and care of the baby

postpartum hemorrhage (PPH) Excessive bleeding after childbirth; traditionally defined as a loss of 500 ml or more after a vaginal birth and 1000 ml after a cesarean birth

postterm pregnancy Pregnancy that extends past 42 weeks of gestation

precipitous labor Rapid or sudden labor lasting less than 3 hours from the onset of uterine contractions to complete birth of the fetus

preconception care Care designed for health maintenance and health promotion for the general and reproductive health of all women of childbearing potential

preeclampsia Vasospastic disease process encountered after 20 weeks of gestation or early in the puerperium that is characterized by hypertension and proteinuria

pregestational diabetes mellitus Diabetes mellitus type 1 or type 2 that exists before pregnancy

premature dilation of the cervix Cervix that is unable to remain closed until a pregnancy reaches term because of a mechanical defect in the cervix; also called *incompetent cervix*

premature rupture of membranes (PROM) Rupture of the amniotic sac and leakage of amniotic fluid before the onset of labor at any gestational age

premenstrual syndrome (PMS) Nervous tension, irritability, weight gain, edema, headache, mastalgia, dysphoria, and lack of coordination that occur during the last few days of the menstrual cycle preceding the onset of menstruation

presentation Part of the fetus that first enters the pelvis and lies over the inlet; may be the head, face, breech, or shoulder

presenting part Part of the fetus that lies closest to the internal os of the cervix

preterm birth Birth that occurs before the completion of 37 weeks of gestation

preterm infant Infant born before 37 weeks of gestation

preterm labor Uterine contractions that cause cervical change and occur between 20 and 37 weeks of gestation

preterm premature rupture of membranes (preterm PROM) PROM that occurs before 37 weeks of gestation

prolapse of the umbilical cord Protrusion of the umbilical cord in advance of the presenting part

prostaglandins (PGs) Substances present in many body tissues that have roles in many reproductive tract functions and are used to induce abortions and for cervical ripening for labor induction

ptyalism Excessive salivation

pudendal nerve block Injection of a local anesthetic at the pudendal nerve root to produce numbness of the genital and perianal regions

puerperal infection Infection of the pelvic organs during the postbirth period; also called *postpartum infection*

puerperium Period between the birth of the newborn and the return of the reproductive organs to their normal nonpregnant state; fourth trimester of pregnancy

pyrosis Burning sensation in the epigastric and sternal region from stomach acid (heartburn)

quickening Maternal perception of fetal movement that usually occurs between weeks 16 and 20 of gestation

radical mastectomy Surgery that includes the total removal of the breast, as well as the underlying pectoralis major and pectoralis minor muscles

reciprocity Type of body movement or behavior that provides the observer with cues, such as the behavioral cues infants provide to parents and parents' responses to cues

Recommended Dietary Allowances (RDAs) Recommended nutrient intakes estimated to meet the needs of almost all (97% to 98%) of the healthy people in the population

reconstituted family Blended, combined, or remarried family; includes stepparents and stepchildren

respiratory distress syndrome (RDS) Condition resulting from decreased pulmonary gas exchange, leading to retention of carbon dioxide (increase in arterial partial pressure of carbon dioxide [PCO_2]); most common neonatal causes are prematurity, perinatal asphyxia, and maternal diabetes mellitus; also called *hyaline membrane disease*

retinopathy of prematurity Complex, multicausal disorder that affects the developing retinal vessels of premature infants, resulting in capillary hemorrhages, fibrotic resolution, and possible retinal detachment; visual impairment may be mild or severe; formerly known as *retrolental fibroplasia*

Ritgen maneuver Technique used to control the birth of the head; upward pressure from the coccygeal region is applied to extend the head during the actual birth

rooting reflex Normal response of the newborn to move toward whatever touches the area around the mouth and to attempt to suck; this reflex usually disappears by 3 to 4 months of age

rupture of membranes (ROM) Integrity of the amniotic membranes is broken either spontaneously (SROM) or artificially (AROM) by amniotomy

second stage of labor Stage of labor from full dilation of the cervix to the birth of the baby

semen analysis Examination of a semen specimen to determine liquefaction, volume, pH, sperm density, and normal morphologic features

sex chromosomes Chromosomes associated with the determination of sex: the X (female) and Y (male) chromosomes; the normal female having two X chromosomes and the normal male having one X and one Y chromosome

sexual response cycle Phases of physical changes that occur in response to sexual stimulation and sexual tension release

shoulder dystocia Condition in which the head is born but the anterior shoulder cannot pass under the pubic arch

sibling rivalry A sibling's jealousy of and resentment toward a new child in the family

simple mastectomy Surgery that includes the removal of the breast without the underlying muscle or fascial tissue

single-parent family Family in which a child lives with one parent because of divorce, separation, death, or desertion; birth to or adoption by a single parent

sleep-wake states Variation in states of newborn consciousness from deep sleep to extreme irritability

spinal anesthesia (block) Regional anesthesia induced by injection of a local anesthetic agent into the subarachnoid space at the level of the third, fourth, or fifth lumbar interspace

squamocolumnar junction Site in the endocervical canal where columnar epithelium and squamous epithelium meet; also called the *transformation zone*

standard of care Level of practice that a reasonable, prudent nurse would provide

station Relationship of the presenting fetal part to an imaginary line drawn between the ischial spines of the pelvis

sterilization Surgical contraceptive procedures intended to be permanent contraception

striae gravidarum Shining reddish lines caused by stretching of the skin, often found on the abdomen, thighs, and breasts during pregnancy; in time, these streaks turn to a fine pinkish white or silver tone in fair-skinned women and brownish in darker-skinned women; also known as *stretch marks*

subinvolution Failure of a part (e.g., the uterus) to reduce to its normal size and condition after enlargement from functional activity (e.g., pregnancy)

suboccipitobregmatic diameter Smallest anterior-posterior diameter of the fetal head; follows a line drawn from the middle of the anterior fontanel to the undersurface of the occipital bone

superimposed preeclampsia New-onset proteinuria in a woman with hypertension before 20 weeks of gestation, a sudden increase in proteinuria if already present in early gestation, a sudden increase in hypertension, or the development of HELLP syndrome

supine hypotension Drop in blood pressure when a woman is lying flat on her back that is caused by impaired venous return when the gravid uterus presses on the ascending vena cava; also known as *vena cava syndrome*

supply-meets-demand system Physiologic basis for milk production; milk volume is produced in response to amount removed from the breast

surfactant Phosphoprotein necessary for normal respiratory function that prevents alveolar collapse (atelectasis)

synchrony Fit between the infant's cues and the parent's response

systemic analgesia Pain relief induced when an analgesic is administered parenterally (subcutaneous [SC], intramuscular [IM], or intravenous [IV] route) and crosses the blood-brain barrier to provide central analgesic effects

tachycardia Baseline FHR above 160 beats per minute and lasting 10 minutes or longer

tachysystole More than five uterine contractions in 10 minutes, averaged over a 30-minute window

taking-hold phase Period after birth characterized by a woman becoming more independent and more interested in learning infant care skills; learning to be a competent mother is an important task

taking-in phase Period after birth characterized by the woman's dependency; maternal needs are dominant, and talking about the birth is an important task

telehealth Use of communication technologies and electronic information to provide or support health care when participants are separated by distance

teratogens Environmental substances or exposures that result in functional or structural disability

therapeutic donor insemination (TDI) Introduction of donor semen by instrument injection into the vagina or uterus for impregnation

therapeutic rest Administration of analgesics and implementation of comfort or relaxation measures to decrease pain and induce rest for management of hypertonic uterine dysfunction

thermogenesis Creation or production of heat, especially in the body

thermoregulation Control of body temperature; the balance between heat loss and heat production

third stage of labor Stage of labor from the birth of the baby to the separation and expulsion of the placenta

thrombophlebitis Inflammation of a vein with secondary clot formation

thrush Fungal infection of the mouth or throat that is characterized by the formation of white patches on a red, moist, inflamed mucous membrane; caused by *Candida albicans*

tocolysis Inhibition of uterine contractions through administration of medications; used as an adjunct to other interventions in the management of fetal compromise related to increased uterine activity

tocolytics Medications used to suppress uterine activity and to relax the uterus in cases of hyperstimulation or preterm labor

TORCH infections Infections caused by organisms that damage the embryo or fetus; is the acronym for **t**oxoplasmosis, **o**ther (e.g., syphilis), **r**ubella, **c**ytomegalovirus, and **h**erpes simplex

transition period Period from birth to 4 to 6 hours later in which the infant passes through a period of reactivity, sleep, and a second period of reactivity

transition phase Phase in the first stage of labor when the cervix dilates from 8 to 10 cm

transition to parenthood Period from the preconception parenthood decision through the first months after birth of the baby during which parents define their parental roles and adjust to parenthood

trial of labor (TOL) Period of observation to determine whether a laboring woman is likely to be successful in progressing to a vaginal birth

trimesters One of three periods of approximately 3 months each into which pregnancy is divided

trophic feedings Very small feedings given to stimulate maturation of the gut

urinary incontinence (UI) Uncontrollable leakage of urine

uterine atony Relaxation of the uterine muscle that may lead to excessive postpartum bleeding and postpartum hemorrhage

uterine contractions Primary powers of labor that act involuntarily to dilate and efface the cervix, expel the fetus, facilitate separation of the placenta, and prevent hemorrhage

uterine resting tone Tension in the uterine muscle between contractions; relaxation of the uterus

uterine souffl é Soft, blowing sound made by the blood in the arteries of the pregnant uterus and synchronous with the maternal pulse

uteroplacental insufficiency (UPI) Decline in placental function (e.g., exchange of gases, nutrients, and wastes) leading to fetal hypoxia and acidosis; evidenced by late decelerations in the FHR in response to uterine contractions

vacuum-assisted birth Birth involving attachment of a vacuum cap to the fetal head (occiput) and application of negative pressure to assist in birth of the fetus

vaginal birth after cesarean (VBAC) Giving birth vaginally after having had a previous cesarean birth

Valsalva maneuver Any forced expiratory effort against a closed airway, such as holding one's breath and tightening the abdominal muscles (e.g., pushing during the second stage of labor)

variability Normal irregularity of fetal cardiac rhythm or fluctuations from the baseline FHR of two cycles or more

vernix caseosa Protective gray-white fatty substance of cheesy consistency covering and protecting the fetal skin

vertex Crown, or top, of the head

vulnerable populations Groups who are at increased risk of developing physical, mental, or social health problems or who are more likely to have worse outcomes from these health problems than the population as a whole

vulvar self-examination (VSE) Systematic examination of the vulva by the woman

walking survey Technique of using one's senses while traveling through a community to obtain information about the sociocultural characteristics and environment, housing, transportation, and local community agencies

warm line Help line, or consultation service, for families to access, most often for support of newborn care and postpartum care after hospital discharge

zygote Cell formed by the union of two reproductive cells or gametes; the fertilized ovum is the result of the union of a sperm and an ovum

Index

Page numbers followed by "f" indicate figures, "t" indicate tables, and "b" indicate boxes.

B

C

E

F

I

J

K

P

Q

R

S

T

U